T0323420

Cornerstones of Attachment Research

Cornerstones of Attachment Research

ROBBIE DUSCHINSKY

Senior University Lecturer, Primary Care Unit, University of Cambridge

Fellow and Director of Studies, Sidney Sussex College

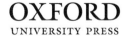

OXFORD
UNIVERSITY PRESS

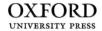

UNIVERSITY PRESS

Great Clarendon Street, Oxford, OX2 6DP,
United Kingdom

Oxford University Press is a department of the University of Oxford.
It furthers the University's objective of excellence in research, scholarship,
and education by publishing worldwide. Oxford is a registered trade mark of
Oxford University Press in the UK and in certain other countries

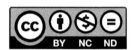
Published in the United States of America by Oxford University Press
198 Madison Avenue, New York, NY 10016, United States of America

British Library Cataloguing in Publication Data
Data available

Library of Congress Control Number: 2020933057

ISBN 978–0–19–884206–4

Printed and bound by
CPI Group (UK) Ltd, Croydon, CR0 4YY

Oxford University Press makes no representation, express or implied, that the
drug dosages in this book are correct. Readers must therefore always check
the product information and clinical procedures with the most up-to-date
published product information and data sheets provided by the manufacturers
and the most recent codes of conduct and safety regulations. The authors and
the publishers do not accept responsibility or legal liability for any errors in the
text or for the misuse or misapplication of material in this work. Except where
otherwise stated, drug dosages and recommendations are for the non-pregnant
adult who is not breast-feeding

Links to third party websites are provided by Oxford in good faith and
for information only. Oxford disclaims any responsibility for the materials
contained in any third party website referenced in this work.

Contents

Introduction

Attachment theory is among the most popular theories of human socioemotional development, with a global research community and widespread interest from clinicians, child welfare professionals, educationalists, and parents. It has been considered 'one of the most generative contemporary ideas' about family life in modern society.[1] It is one of the last of the grand theories of human development that still retains an active research tradition. Indeed, Simpson and Howland have observed that 'perhaps no single theory in the psychological sciences has generated more empirical research during the past 30 years than attachment theory'.[2] Attachment theory and research speak to fundamental questions about human emotions, relationships, and development. They do so in terms that feel experience-near, with a remarkable combination of intuitive ideas and counter-intuitive assessments and conclusions. Over time, attachment theory seems to have become more, rather than less, appealing and popular, in part perhaps due to alignment with current concern with the lifetime implications of early brain development.[3] Emerging reports on the economic costs of insecure attachment may make a further contribution to this appeal over the coming years.[4] In a 2018 survey conducted by the British government of organizations working with children in need of help and protection, attachment theory was, by a large margin, cited as the most frequently used underpinning perspective.[5] Attachment ideas have been used to support

[1] Pittman, J.F. (2012) Attachment orientations: a boon to family theory and research. *Journal of Family Theory & Review*, 4(4), 306–10.

[2] Simpson, J.A. & Howland, M. (2012) Bringing the partner into attachment theory and research. *Journal of Family Theory & Review*, 4(4), 282–9, p.282.

[3] Wastell, D. & White, S. (2017) *Blinded by Science: The Social Implications of Epigenetics and Neuroscience*. Cambridge: Policy Press. Discourses of 'interpersonal neurobiology', and the work of Allan Schore in particular, have been important for the take-up of appeals to attachment within popular and policy discourses emphasising the importance of child development for the brain. See, for example, Schore, A.N. (2001) Effects of a secure attachment relationship on right brain development, affect regulation, and infant mental health. *Infant Mental Health Journal*, 22(1–2), 7–66; and building from Schore's work, Gerhardt, S. (2014) *Why Love Matters: How Affection Shapes a Baby's Brain*, 2nd edn. London: Routledge. Schore's work has been much less influential within the attachment research community. An exception is discussed in Chapter 3.

[4] Bachmann, C.J., Beecham, J., O'Connor, T.G., Scott, A., Briskman, J., & Scott, S. (2019) The cost of love: financial consequences of insecure attachment in antisocial youth. *Journal of Child Psychology & Psychiatry*, 60(12), 1343-50.

[5] In response to the question 'What theories or research do you rely on to inform a plan of how to support a child?' attachment theory was mentioned by 11% of respondents. The next most cited responses were general areas rather than specific theories or research paradigms; and a long way behind, 'mental health' at 5% and 'child development' at 4%. The next most cited specific theory was social learning theory at 1%. Mention of 'attachment disorder' appeared in a further 2.5% of responses. Survey responses to a government inquiry offer little sure knowledge about what these organizations actually do and why. However, the leading position of attachment theory specifically, even compared to 'mental health' and 'child development' as general areas, suggests the position of appeal to attachment as a dominant and apparently authorized discourse within the justification and conceptualization of child welfare practice. Department for Education (2018) Children in need of help and protection: call for evidence. https://www.gov.uk/government/consultations/children-in-need-of-help-and-protection-call-for-evidence. On the contradictions and diversity of uses of attachment discourses in child welfare contexts, see McLean, S., Riggs, D., Kettler, L., & Delfabbro, P. (2013) Challenging behaviour in out-of-home care: use of attachment ideas in practice. *Child & Family Social Work*, 18(3), 243–52; Smith, M., Cameron, C., & Reimer, D. (2017) From attachment to recognition for children in care. *British Journal of Social Work*, 47(6), 1606–23.

recognition of the importance of stable, trusting relationships for children's socioemotional development, with the credibility of links to an established empirical research paradigm.[6] Attachment also provides a framework for interpreting the underlying logic or meaning of the behaviour of children and young people following relational adversities.[7] These qualities have contributed to the popularity of attachment among social workers,[8] clinicians,[9] and health visitors,[10] in training and support provided to foster carers and adoptive parents,[11] in parenting education courses and materials given to parents by health and care professionals,[12] in forensic contexts,[13] and in professional development courses for teachers.[14]

Yet the most well-known account of attachment is in many regards based on certain early claims by John Bowlby and Mary Ainsworth, the originators of attachment theory, at the expense of their own and others' later conclusions and qualifications. Ainsworth herself complained of a tendency to describe psychological theories in terms of early findings and ideas; these enter into circulation, ricochet and rebound among domains of practice, and get repeated and repeated. Later developments, even important ones, become difficult to access

---

[6] The particular utility of attachment ideas for clinicians and child welfare practitioners, increasing the credibility of practice through association with the evidence-base of attachment research, is praised directly in Bennett, C.S. & Nelson, J.K. (2008) Closing thoughts: special issue on attachment. *Clinical Social Work Journal*, 36, 109–11. Concern about many 'attachment-based' therapies as pseudoscience has been raised by Mercer, J. (2019) Conventional and unconventional perspectives on attachment and attachment problems: comparisons and implications, 2006–2016. *Child and Adolescent Social Work Journal*, 36(2), 81–95.

[7] E.g. Haight, W.L., Kagle, J.D., & Black, J.E. (2003) Understanding and supporting parent–child relationships during foster care visits: attachment theory and research. *Social Work*, 48(2), 195–207; Farnfield, S. & Holmes, P. (eds) (2014) *The Routledge Handbook of Attachment: Assessment*. London: Routledge.

[8] An important contribution to the popularity of attachment theory among social workers, especially in the UK, was made by Howe, D., Brandon, M., Hinings, D., & Schofield, G. (1999) *Attachment Theory, Child Maltreatment and Family Support: A Practice and Assessment Model*. London: Palgrave.

[9] For a useful review see Slade, A. & Holmes, J. (2017) *Attachment in Therapeutic Practice*. London: SAGE.

[10] Hogg, S. (2019) *Rare Jewels: Specialised Parent–Infant Relationship Teams in the UK*. London: Parent–Infant Partnership UK. https://www.pipuk.org.uk/sites/default/files/PIPUK%20Rare%20Jewels%20FINAL.pdf. In the UK, National Institute for Health and Care Excellence (NICE) Guidelines for postnatal care state that health visitors should promote the emerging attachment relationship, and that health visitors should assess potential obstacles or problems for this relationship. NICE (2015) Postnatal care up to 8 weeks after birth. London: NICE. https://www.nice.org.uk/guidance/cg37/resources/postnatal-care-up-to-8-weeks-after-birth-pdf-975391596997.

[11] Laybourne, G., Andersen, J., & Sands, J. (2008) Fostering attachments in looked after children: further insight into the group-based programme for foster carers. *Adoption and Fostering*, 32(4), 64–76; Benesh, A.S. & Cui, M. (2017) Foster parent training programmes for foster youth: a content review. *Child & Family Social Work*, 22(1), 548–59.

[12] Wall, G. (2018) 'Love builds brains': representations of attachment and children's brain development in parenting education material. *Sociology of Health & Illness*, 40(3), 395–409. Attachment is a module in the *Ready Steady Baby* book, given to all new parents in Scotland. https://www.nhsinform.scot/ready-steady-baby/pregnancy/relationships-and-wellbeing-in-pregnancy/attachment-and-bonding-during-pregnancy.

[13] Ministry of Justice (2011) *Working with Personality Disordered Offenders: A Practitioner's Guide*. London: HMSO; Baim, C. & Morrison, T. (2011) *Attachment-Based Practice with Adults: Understanding Strategies and Promoting Positive Change*. Hove: Pavilion Publishing; Brown, R. & Ward, H. (2012) *Decision-Making within a Child's Timeframe: An Overview of Current Research Evidence for Family Justice Professionals Concerning Child Development and the Impact of Maltreatment*. London: Childhood Wellbeing Research Centre; Crittenden, P.M., Farnfield, S., Landini, A., & Grey, B. (2013) Assessing attachment for family court decision making. *Journal of Forensic Practice*, 15(4), 237–48.

[14] Geddes, H. (2006) *Attachment in the Classroom: A Practical Guide for Schools*. London: Worth Publishing; Beckh, K. & Becker-Stoll, F. (2016) Formations of attachment relationships towards teachers lead to conclusions for public child care. *International Journal of Developmental Science*, 10(3–4), 103–10; Rose, J., McGuire-Snieckus, R., Gilbert, L., & McInnes, K. (2019) Attachment Aware Schools: the impact of a targeted and collaborative intervention. *Pastoral Care in Education*, 37(2), 162–84. In the UK, NICE has mandated that 'Schools and other education providers should ensure that all staff who may come into contact with children and young people with attachment difficulties receive appropriate training on attachment difficulties' (Recommendations 1.2.1). NICE (2016) Children's attachment: attachment in children and young people who are adopted from care, in care or at high risk of going into care. London: NICE. https://www.ncbi.nlm.nih.gov/pubmed/26741018.

and incorporate, with textbooks and summaries sustaining an outdated caricature.[15] Already in 1968, Ainsworth wrote to Bowlby with concern: 'attachment has become a bandwagon'.[16]

In the helping professions, the idea of attachment theory is well known, and even forms part of the mandatory curriculum for some professions. At the same time, knowledge of developments in attachment theory and research may not be strong. Qualitative research by Furnivall and colleagues found that 'there was a sense that professionals knew the word but not the underlying theory … although there was strong support for the importance of the fundamental concept'.[17] Likewise Morison and colleagues found that staff working in residential childcare generally stated in interview that their practice was informed by attachment theory, but struggled to say exactly how.[18] Bennett and Blome have observed that welfare agencies give lip-service to attachment in providing a support for the credibility of their work, but may provide a protocol-focused organizational culture that ultimately discourages practitioners from gaining expertise regarding attachment research and its implications.[19]

Elizabeth Meins, one of the UK's leading attachment researchers through the 1990s and 2000s, has recently turned her back on the paradigm. She has argued that regardless of the scientific advances made by attachment research, the benefits arising from these have been outstripped by the problems caused by public misunderstandings. Meins' position is unusual. However, it sets out clearly the stakes in the gap between attachment research today and how it is widely understood:

> Somewhere along the line, the idea that early attachment is the best predictor of all aspects of later development has gained credence. We need to get out of our ivory towers and unite in calling out this caricature of our research. I stand by my claim that laying so much emphasis on attachment isn't helpful. Being made to worry about whether you have a secure attachment with your baby won't make you a better parent; healthcare professionals who are provided with oversimplified hype about the predictive power of attachment won't give families good advice; and letting non-experts who think they know the attachment literature loose in the political arena won't result in good policies for children and families.[20]

[15] Ainsworth, M. (1969) CPA oral history of psychology in Canada interview. Unpublished. http://www.feministvoices.com/assets/Women-Past/Ainsworth/Mary-Ainsworth-CPA-Oral-History.pdf: 'I think it was just the way it is so often with textbooks. The things that get into the textbooks are the early publications and they don't ever get around to putting in the later publications, and people write textbooks on the basis of other people's textbooks.' Illustrating the caricature and outright mistakes about attachment research available from textbooks, see Parke, R.D. & Clarke-Stewart, A. (2011) *Social Development*. New York: Wiley.

[16] Ainsworth, M. (1968) *Letter to John Bowlby*, 27 April 1968. PP/Bow/K.4/12: 'Attachment has become a bandwagon. There are so many people now interested in research in this area, and so many approaches, both theoretical and methodological. I am afraid that people will leap in in a half-baked way, that findings will be equivocal or conflicting, and that perhaps interest will move away from "attachment" dismissing it as one more area that did not "pan out".'

[17] Furnivall, J., McKenna, M., McFarlane, S., & Grant, E. (2012) Attachment matters for all: an attachment mapping exercise for children's services in Scotland. Glasgow: Centre for Excellence for Looked after Children in Scotland (CELCIS). www.celcis.org/knowledge-bank/search-bank/attachment-matters-all/.

[18] Morison, A., Taylor, E., & Gervais, M. (2019) How a sample of residential childcare staff conceptualize and use attachment theory in practice. *Child & Youth Services*, DOI: 10.1080/0145935X.2019.1583100.

[19] Bennett, S. & Blome, W.W. (2013) Implementing attachment theory in the child welfare system: clinical implications and organizational considerations. In J.E. Bettmann & D.D. Friedman (eds) *Attachment-Based Clinical Work with Children and Adolescents* (pp.259–83). New York: Springer.

[20] Meins, E. (2017) Reply. *The Psychologist*, 30, 6–9. https://thepsychologist.bps.org.uk/volume-30/march-2017/attachment-public-and-scientific-discourse, p.9.

Meins' remarks suggest the value in taking stock of qualifications, innovations, and amendments made by later researchers in relation to Bowlby's early claims. One important early attempt at such taking stock was *Becoming Attached* by Robert Karen, published in 1994.[21] Karen described the emergence of the attachment paradigm in the work of Bowlby and Ainsworth, and its subsequent elaboration by younger researchers such as Sroufe, Main, and Shaver. Karen interviewed all these researchers, as well as conducting extensive study of their published works until 1992. He documented how attachment theory was introduced by John Bowlby in the 1950s and 1960s. He traced how Bowlby sought to revise psychoanalytic theory in order to create a scientific model that nonetheless retained the strengths of psychoanalysis in relevance to clinical work. The theory was not well received at the time by the psychoanalytic community. However, Karen showed, through the work of Mary Ainsworth, how attachment theory entered into American developmental psychology, where it took firm root, first among Ainsworth's immediate collaborators and then across the subdiscipline. Central to the establishment of attachment theory within developmental psychology, in Karen's account, was Ainsworth's introduction of the Strange Situation procedure, an observational assessment of infant–caregiver attachment relationships using separations and reunions to examine infants' expectations about their caregiver. Ainsworth found that infants' behaviour in the Strange Situation was associated with observations of the care they received at home. Infants who could confidently explore in the Strange Situation and retreat to their caregiver for comfort when distressed were those whose caregiver had been attentive and responsive to their signals over the first year of life. Ainsworth therefore termed this pattern of behaviour 'secure attachment'.

Karen also documented how longitudinal studies by Ainsworth's collaborators and students had shown the value of attachment theory as an approach within developmental psychology, and validated the Strange Situation as a predictive measure. Ainsworth's student Mary Main demonstrated that patterns of behaviour towards each parent in the Strange Situation are largely independent, confirming Ainsworth's interpretation that the behaviours were less individual traits than reflections of infant expectations about particular relationships. Qualities from autobiographical interviews with parents were also found to have predictable associations with their children's behaviour in the Strange Situation. This formed the basis of the introduction of the Adult Attachment Interview. Karen also explored the findings of the Minnesota Longitudinal Study of Risk and Adaptation, led by Alan Sroufe and Byron Egeland. These researchers followed up a large high-risk sample since the 1970s. This longitudinal study has been of particular importance in both supporting and qualifying claims by Bowlby, Ainsworth, and Main about the developmental implications of attachment. Karen also reported another key development: the growth of research on attachment within social psychology, initiated by Phillip Shaver and colleagues, and drawing on self-report assessments of adult attachment.

Karen's book came out at an important moment for attachment research. Bowlby and Ainsworth were no longer available to act as leaders. Main's methodological innovations had been introduced but were still in the process of being validated in other laboratories. Karen

---

[21] Karen, R. (1994) *Becoming Attached.* New York: Warner Books. Karen's book developed an earlier article: Karen, R. (1990) Becoming attached. *The Atlantic*, February. Karen's stock-taking not only was influential for the public reception of attachment theory, but also influenced subsequent attachment research, such as providing a prompt for the development of the 'Circle of Security' intervention: Powell, B., Cooper, G., Hoffman, K., & Marvin, B. (2016) *The Circle of Security Intervention.* New York: Guilford, p.9.

could discuss the Minnesota group's follow-up of their sample from infancy to preschool, but the data from later childhood were still being analysed. And Shaver and colleagues had introduced their early 'love quiz' self-report measure of adult attachment, but the properties of this assessment were subject to significant criticism. The relationship between the developmental psychologists and the social psychologists was relatively hostile, and it was wholly unclear how the ideas and measures of the two traditions would relate to one another. Yet alongside sorrow at the loss of Bowlby and Ainsworth, and tensions over the future direction of attachment research and theory, it was a time of great excitement for the field. The standing of attachment research as a scientific paradigm had been established by the 1980s, and support from research funders had led to a rapid growth in the size of the field by the mid-1990s.[22]

Since Karen's book, there has been substantial academic scholarship exploring the early years of attachment research from a historical perspective. Inge Bretherton, a student and colleague of Ainsworth, and Jeremy Holmes, a clinician and colleague of Bowlby, also published influential celebratory reviews in the early 1990s.[23] Work to document the emergence of Bowlby and Ainsworth's research by academic historians began in the late 1990s, and remains thriving today.[24] There has also been a rich tradition of critical discussion of the relationship between Bowlby's ideas and post-war gender and parenting cultures.[25] However, the important developments in the field of the past 30 years have not been examined by historians, a startling gap in light of the revolutions in theory and method that have taken place in these decades. Peter Fonagy and Chloe Campbell, significant figures in the British attachment research community, have criticised historians of attachment research for focusing too exclusively on Bowlby and Ainsworth, neglecting attention to the ways in which the paradigm has changed over time.[26] These changes are also of great interest for the history of science, illustrating dynamics in the relationship between theory and method in psychological science, debates about the function of categorization, problems in the conceptualization of emotional development, changing appeals to evolutionary theory and ontologies of human nature, and shifts in the relationship between developmental science and its publics. The images of attachment research offered by commentators outside the field are generally outdated, hackneyed, and too often inaccurate.[27] This loses critical psychology access

---

[22] The boom in funding for attachment research in the 1990s is discussed in White, K. & Schwartz, J. (2007) Attachment here and now: an interview with Peter Fonagy. *Attachment: New Directions in Relational Psychoanalysis and Psychotherapy*, 1(1), 57–61.

[23] Bretherton, I. (1992) The origins of attachment theory: John Bowlby and Mary Ainsworth. *Developmental Psychology*, 28(5), 759–75; Holmes, J. (1993) *John Bowlby and Attachment Theory*. London: Routledge.

[24] E.g. Van Dijken, S. (1998) *John Bowlby: His Early Life: A Biographical Journey into the Roots of Attachment Theory*. London: Free Association Books; Mayhew, B. (2006) Between love and aggression: the politics of John Bowlby. *History of the Human Sciences*, 19(4), 19–35; van der Horst, F. (2011) *John Bowlby—From Psychoanalysis to Ethology: Unravelling the Roots of Attachment Theory*. Oxford: Blackwell.

[25] E.g. Birns, B. (1999) I. Attachment theory revisited: challenging conceptual and methodological sacred cows. *Feminism & Psychology*, 9(1), 10–21; Vicedo, M. (2013) *The Nature and Nurture of Love: From Imprinting to Attachment in Cold War America*. Chicago: University of Chicago Press. As Ruck observes, the popularity of the development of attachment theory for historians of science resides at least in part in the fact that 'the theory offers a looking glass into the social foundations and effects of science; the function and logic of scientific controversies and disciplinary hierarchies; and the interrelation of descriptive and prescriptive scientific theories, scientific and popular discourse, and science and ideology all at once' : Ruck, N. (2014) Review: Marga Vicedo. The nature and nurture of love. *Journal of the History of the Behavioral Sciences*, 50(4), 410–11, p.410.

[26] Fonagy, P. & Campbell, C. (2016) Attachment theory and mentalization. In A. Elliott & J. Prager (eds) *The Routledge Handbook of Psychoanalysis in the Social Sciences and Humanities* (pp.115–31). London: Routledge, p.123.

[27] For an example of a work in critical psychology that does little more than repeat stock criticisms with little relevance to contemporary attachment research, see Walsh, R.T.G., Teo, T., & Baydala, A. (2014) *A Critical History and Philosophy of Psychology*. Cambridge: Cambridge University Press.

to an influential and superbly rich case—one relevant to major current concerns such as the history of emotion in the human sciences, debates about psychological categorisation, and ways of imagining human relationships. In turn, attachment research loses effective critical interlocutors.

This book

Cornerstones re-examines the background and current approaches of key laboratories that have contributed to attachment research as it exists today. In this way the book traces the development in a single scientific paradigm through parallel albeit separate lines of inquiry. The laboratories in focus, those examined by Karen, exemplify particular advances and dilemmas the field has faced. *Cornerstones* seeks to use a focus on five research groups as a lens on wider themes and challenges faced by the contemporary field as it has emerged. In doing so, the book uses certain landmarks that suggest some of the fundamental logic, infrastructure, and points of orientation in attachment research as a terrain.

The book in no way aims to be a comprehensive account of attachment research.[28] This scholarship is diverse. It does not form a single totality, but rather a region with points of density and intensity. Both the density and intensity of work within attachment research are structured by research groups, which are shaped by and shape the field. Chapters aim to remain with researchers long enough to offer a sense of their characteristic ways of thinking and tone, to feel them as figures keeping us company—if sometimes quarrelling, sometimes pulling in unison—within the broader history of developments in the field. Readers will note that the book does not contain chapters focusing on the research groups of influential direct students of Ainsworth such as Jude Cassidy, Patricia Crittenden, Roger Kobak, and Bob Marvin, and other research leaders such as Kim Bartholomew, Jay Belsky, Martha Cox, Peter Fonagy, Karlen Lyons-Ruth, Avi Sagi-Schwartz, Sue Spieker, and Marinus van IJzendoorn. A younger cohort of research leaders would also need to be considered in a characterization of contemporary research groups, including—but by no means limited to—Marian Bakermans-Kranenburg, Gurit Birnbaum, Mary Dozier, Robin Edelstein, Pasco Fearon, Chris Fraley, Patrick Luyten, Sheri Madigan, Carlo Schuengel, Jeff Simpson, Gottfried Spangler, and Glenn Roisman. All these figures will feature in the present book, however. And a further book is already underway to examine key research groups that gained prominence only after Karen's *Becoming Attached*. This will include attention to major preoccupations of the 1990s and 2000s, such as studies of attachment and the developing brain.

The concept of a 'generation' can be used pragmatically to characterise members of a cohort who, facilitated by structural factors that suggest commonalities, regard themselves as facing a bundle of common challenges, including delimitation and appraisal of the legacy of an earlier generation.[29] In an important sense, just as Karen was writing at a point of

---

[28] One expression of the sheer scale of the historical background to contemporary attachment research is the six-volume edited work of Slade, A. & Holmes, J. (eds) (2014) *Attachment Theory*. London: Sage. The editors aimed to collect 60 essential papers; however, 119 papers ultimately were judged indispensable. On the diversity of factors involved in canon formation, and above all the importance of subsequent resonance, see Fishelov, D. (2010) *Dialogues with/and Great Books: The Dynamics of Canon Formation*. Eastbourne: Sussex Academic Press.

[29] The idea of generations in attachment research is heuristic rather than intended as a simple statement of fact. Certainly, there are figures who do not fall easily within one generation or the other in terms of age and attitudes; Jude Cassidy, Jay Belsky, Marinus van IJzendoorn, and Gottfried Spangler are all clear examples. And the present book is centrally concerned with changes over time regarding theory, method, and research priorities that do not

transition from the first to the second generation of attachment researchers, this book has been written during a transition from the second to the third generation of attachment researchers. The leaders of the research groups considered in this book have, with the exception of Mikulincer, now retired.[30] Consideration of their work is intended to offer an opportunity to examine the strengths and the limitations, and clarify some of the debates, that have characterized the second generation of attachment researchers and which have formed the context in which a new generation of leaders are inheriting the field of attachment research. In a letter to Mary Main, Bowlby wrote that 'there is no need for the old to learn from the young in order for the population to benefit from youthful innovation. The supersession of an older generation by a younger is sufficient.'[31] Now it is Main's own generation who are putting down their tools, and a new set of research leaders who must take stock of what they have learned, and of what hold this learning has on them.

There are several excellent books that have taken a thematic approach in offering the reader a guide and introduction to contemporary attachment research, most notably the *Handbook of Attachment* edited by Cassidy and Shaver, *Understanding Attachment and Attachment Disorders* by Prior and Glaser, and *Adult Attachment* by Gillath, Karantzas, and Fraley.[32] Thompson, Simpson, and Berlin's *Attachment: The Fundamental Questions* also will offer a systematic stock-taking of the present state of attachment research when it is published next year.[33] However, a thematic approach to synthesis can risk making an area of research appear seamless and without edges. In particular, it can lose track of the social dynamics, debates, and diverging use of the same terminology that organize a field of inquiry and the relationships between research groups. Thompson has argued that this heterogeneity must be captured by any attempt to understand attachment research today, even if it makes for a more intricate story.[34] The chapters of *Cornerstones* draw on a complete analysis of published scholarly and popular works by each research group, as well as unpublished doctoral theses published in English where these were available through inter-library loan.

This signals an important limitation. Much of the imagination, passion, and artistry of research, much of its process and messy creation out of different elements, much of its influence by and influence on social interactions, is hidden in textual records, especially those that go into print.[35] Many of the most vital social dynamics of the field of attachment research do not feature in the textual record. For instance, the available texts offer little vantage on interactions between attachment researchers and clinical and social welfare professionals.

divide by generation. On the concept of 'generations' see Aboim, S. & Vasconcelos, P. (2014) From political to social generations: a critical reappraisal of Mannheim's classical approach. *European Journal of Social Theory*, 17, 165–83.

[30] Ainsworth's first doctoral students at Johns Hopkins graduated in 1972, among them Mary Main; her final doctoral students were Jude Cassidy in 1986 and Carolyn Eichberg in 1987. This means that most of Ainsworth's doctoral students have moved into retirement over the past decade.

[31] Bowlby, J. (1970) *Letter to Mary Main*, 18 November 1970. PP/Bow/J.4/1.

[32] Cassidy, J. & Shaver, P. (eds) (2016) *Handbook of Attachment: Theory, Research, and Clinical Applications*, 3rd edn. New York: Guildford; Prior, V. & Glaser, D. (2006) *Understanding Attachment and Attachment Disorders: Theory, Evidence and Practice*. London: Jessica Kingsley Press; Gillath, O., Karantzas, G.C., & Fraley, R.C. (2016) *Adult Attachment: A Concise Introduction to Theory and Research*. London: Academic Press. See also Holmes, P. & Farnfield, S. (2014) *The Routledge Handbook of Attachment*. London: Routledge.

[33] Thompson, R.A., Simpson, J.A., & Berlin, L. (eds) (2020) *Attachment: The Fundamental Questions*. New York: Guildford.

[34] Thompson, R.A. (2017) Twenty-first century attachment theory. In H. Keller & K. Bard (eds) *The Cultural Nature of Attachment: Contextualizing Relationships and Development* (pp.301–19). Cambridge, MA: MIT Press, p.303.

[35] Schickore, J. (2008) Doing science, writing science. *Philosophy of Science*, 75(3), 323–43.

Some commentators have described attachment theory and research as little more than an ideology for the coercive evaluation, classification, and discipline of families by professionals.[36] In response to such accusations, apologists have countered that attachment theory and research are no different than any other form of knowledge of children and families, and that contemporary attachment research, adequately understood, offers no support for oppression of families.[37] Both claims are likely too flat, masking the diversity within attachment discourses and their changes over time and between contexts. Neither the accusations nor the apologetics are based on empirical research, or on textual evidence. In fact, very little is readily available in the public domain about the circulation of ideas between research and practice.[38] Colleagues and I currently have research on these questions underway, drawing on interviews, focus groups, ethnography, and analysis of a large archive of clinical case records.[39]

Yet even if subject to systematic and important limitations, the written record available for a study of important research groups in the history of attachment is extensive. And I have been grateful to have access to some texts in this area beyond the published record. Chapters draw extensively on materials from the John Bowlby Archive at the Wellcome Collection, the Mary Ainsworth Archive at the Nicholas and Dorothy Cummings Center for the History of Psychology, and the Mary Main and Erik Hesse personal archive (currently being catalogued for the Wellcome Collection).[40] These archives provide access to a treasure trove of unpublished lectures and seminars, correspondence, notes, and speculations, and drafts of published works and coding manuals. For Bowlby, I have been able to access the surviving part of his library at Human Development Scotland (the location of the rest of the Bowlby library is unknown, even to his family!). This has permitted study of relevant marginalia—for instance the annotations on his personal copy of the works of Freud. Mary Main and Erik Hesse have also made available the manuscripts of two major unpublished books from 1986 and 1995, describing the methods and ideas of their Berkeley group. Use of unpublished materials, such as correspondence, has helped this book attend to the lines of continuity and discontinuity over time and between research groups.

For readers less familiar with attachment research, it is hoped that *Cornerstones* can provide a thorough introduction to theories and methods that form the basis for contemporary

---

[36] For example, Smeeton puts this polemically, alleging that 'we watch as the next generation of social workers suffer the consequences of intellectual inbreeding, fumbling through practice with webbed theories and six-fingered methodologies that give up on families unable to reach the optimal state of a "secure pattern" attachment with their child'. Smeeton, J. (2017) From Aristotle to Arendt: a phenomenological exploration of forms of knowledge and practice in the context of child protection social work in the UK. *Qualitative Social Work*, 16(1), 14–28, p.16. See also Garrett, M.P. (2017) Wired: early intervention and the 'neuromolecular gaze'. *British Journal of Social Work*, 48(3), 656–74. Such criticisms are not based on empirical work on how attachment research is conducted, transmitted, or applied.

[37] For example, Ross Thompson's remarks during discussion in Keller, H. & Thompson, R. (2018) Attachment theory: past, present & future, recorded at the 2nd 'Wilhelm Wundt Dialogue', 28 November 2018, Leipzig University, hosted by the Leipzig Research Center for Early Child Development (LFE). https://www.youtube.com/watch?v=_nG5SelEj28.

[38] One of the few studies found that the more training professionals had in attachment theory, the less likely they were to make judgemental comments about parents' caregiving behaviours. McMahon, C., Huber, A., Kohlhoff, J., & Camberis, A.L. (2017) Does training in the Circle of Security framework increase relational understanding in infant/child and family workers? *Infant Mental Health Journal*, 38(5), 658–68.

[39] Some early findings are presented in Reijman, S., Foster, S., & Duschinsky, R. (2018) The infant disorganised attachment classification: 'Patterning within the disturbance of coherence'. *Social Science & Medicine*, 200, 52–58.

[40] Occasional further manuscripts have been made available by other attachment researchers including Chris Fraley, Klaus and Karin Grossmann, and Alan Sroufe.

attachment research. Attention to a number of research groups offers an 'arsenal of exemplars' for how key questions have been approached, as well as clarifying the stakes in debates between researchers and clarifying the meaning of terminology.[41] At the same time, for readers more familiar with attachment research, the book seeks to surprise and defamiliarize. Historical inquiry offers a point of access for considering how an area of scientific practice decides its objects, priorities, and tools, and in doing so can provide a way of refreshing a reader's perspective on the present and its concerns.[42] The interested reader is also advised to review the book's detailed footnotes, many of which explore some of the peculiar catacombs and other structures underneath the more well-known landscapes of attachment research.

Attachment and historical time

Cornerstones is oriented by the perception that, despite their very substantial differences, historical research and attachment research have points of overlap in how they regard time.[43] Several attachment researchers have, in fact, offered substantial—if scattered—commentary on the idea of history, informed by reading in the history and philosophy of science. From early in his career, Bowlby was wholly convinced of the importance of patients' history for making sense of their trajectory through life, including the capacity of the past to shape or influence behaviours without the awareness of the individual themselves. As a clinician, history taking was second nature to him.[44] Beyond this, however, Bowlby was an avid, lifelong reader of social and political history in his spare time. He had a strong belief in the value of slow, in-depth historical research, which reached its culmination in his decision to dedicate his final years to a grand study of the life of Charles Darwin.[45] In Bowlby's time, historians of science tended to shy away from evaluating the ideas of an earlier scientist in light of later developments. This practice was motivated by an effort to truly understand scientific practices in their own context.[46] Bowlby was impatient with this view. Reflecting on his reading of philosophers of science such as Kuhn, Lakatos, and Popper, he had a different image of historical analysis.[47] His book on Darwin treats it as obvious that later scientific developments can help historians understanding what an earlier scientist was attempting to feel out and explore, the constraints they faced, and limitations or tensions within their understanding and terminology.

---

[41] Bowlby, J. (1974) *Marginalia on Kuhn, second thoughts on paradigms*. PP/Bow/H.98: Heavily underlined: 'Acquiring an arsenal of exemplars, just as much as learning symbolic generalisations, is integral to the process by which a student gains access to the cognitive achievements of his disciplinary group' (p.471).

[42] This function of the history of psychology is discussed well in Capshew, J. (2014) History of psychology since 1945: a North American review. In R. Backhouse & P. Fontaine (eds) *A Historiography of the Modern Social Sciences* (pp.144–82). Cambridge: Cambridge University Press.

[43] The links between historical research and attachment research in this regard relate especially to researchers in the developmental tradition. The social psychological tradition of attachment research has offered fewer relevant reflections on the idea of history, reflecting a predominant tendency in the broader discipline of social psychology. However, see Billig, M. (2018) Those who only know of social psychology know not social psychology: a tribute to Gustav Jahoda's historical approach. *Culture & Psychology*, 24(3), 282–93.

[44] Bowlby, J. (c.1932–33) *History taking; methods of examining*. PP/BOW/D.2/13.

[45] Bowlby, J. (1990) *Charles Darwin: A Life*. New York: Norton.

[46] Wilson, A. & Ashplant, T.G. (1988) Whig history and present-centred history. *The Historical Journal*, 31(1), 1–16.

[47] See Bowlby, J. (1982) A case of mistaken identity. *Higher Education Quarterly* 36(4): 328–32; Bowlby, J. (1962) *Notes on Feyerabend*. PP/BOW/H.99; Bowlby, J. (1974) *Marginalia on Kuhn, Second Thoughts on Paradigms*. PP/Bow/H.98.

In the Darwin biography, unpublished materials are treated as different but not necessarily inferior sources of information. Both are asked to play their part in filling out the development of ideas and scientific practices over time. Bowlby felt that history can, and at times should, help 'exhume' the 'archaeological remnant' of ideas that have been lost or thrust into the background over time.[48] He warned that 'so long as our history is hidden from us, so long as we hide our history from ourselves, we are very likely to see the present and future in the terms of the past'.[49] In his view, the history of a research paradigm holds open the possibility of greater critical awareness of its ideas and methods, including a sense of what avenues have been or might be more or less fruitful. This can contribute to greater flexibility and freedom of action in facing contemporary dilemmas. Another potential benefit of historical inquiry, Bowlby held, is that such research can directly contribute to 'the formulation of specific hypotheses and theories', even if this is not its primary purpose.[50]

Bowlby emphasized the 'appalling complexity' of history, whether this is the history of societies, persons, or ideas, since it has to capture 'highly specific interacting events'.[51] Scientific research is partly shaped by the phenomena under investigation. However, Bowlby stated that historians of science, and their emphasis on the social relationships and cultural contexts that underpin research, have had a 'profound influence on my whole conception of what science is and how scientists operate'.[52] In finding a path through this complexity, Bowlby urged that the historian's priority must be on attempting to discern what problems a scientist or a group of scientists were trying to solve.[53] If close attention is paid to the problems that were faced in a particular period, comparison between earlier and later developments need not result in anachronism. Cautions are required when pursuing such a project. We should take care not to collapse the problems faced by different periods and how those problems were understood; we must not assume that words always meant the same thing over time; and we must not assume that later developments were inevitable or necessarily the best path that could have been taken. Nonetheless, Bowlby's book on Darwin strongly evidences a perspective which has gained ground in recent years within the history of science: that earlier and later scientific developments shed light on one another when examined together.[54]

Yet, more than this, Bowlby wondered 'whether something living which has developed historically can ever be restructured without reference to its historical origins as a social institution'.[55] As such, in Bowlby's view, historical awareness may not just be helpful but actually may be a necessary ingredient for the continued vitality of an area of research. This

[48] Bowlby, J. (1976) In Dr Martin Bax. Are Mothers Necessary? Radio 3, October 1976. PP/Bow/F.5/7.

[49] Bowlby, J. (1989) Attachment and Loss: Continuing Education Seminars. Film produced by David Scott May and Marion Solomon. Distributed by Insight Media.

[50] Bowlby, J. & Dahrendorf, R. (1958) Summary of discussions and topics for final session. Seminar delivered to members of the Stanford Conflict Seminar, February 1958. PP/Bow/H.67. See also Chang, H. (2017) Who cares about the history of science? Notes and Records, 71(1), 91–107.

[51] Bowlby, J. (1982) A case of mistaken identity. Higher Education Quarterly, 36(4), 328–32.

[52] Bowlby, J. (1979) The ten books which have most influenced my thought, 24 October 1979. PP/Bow/A.1/8.

[53] Bowlby, J. (1981) Jean Piaget: some reminiscences. The Tavistock Gazette, 5, 3–4, p.4.

[54] Tosh, N. (2003) Anachronism and retrospective explanation: in defense of a present-centred history of science. Studies in History and Philosophy of Science, 34, 647–59; Oreskes, N. (2013) Why I Am a Presentist. Science in Context, 26(4), 595–609; Loison, L. (2016) Forms of presentism in the history of science: rethinking the project of historical epistemology. Studies in History and Philosophy of Science Part A, 60, 29–37.

[55] Bowlby, J. (c.1950) Marginalia on Bronfenbrenner's 'Toward an integrated theory of personality'. PP/Bow/J.9/37.

argument would also be put forward some years later by both historians and developmental psychologists who would describe the use of historical methodology in the critical examination of psychological paradigms as a 'necessary supplement' to the hypothesis-testing tradition of academic psychological research.[56]

Alan Sroufe and the Minnesota group also offered reflections on what it means to know the past, as part of a deep and abiding concern with the nature of continuities and discontinuities in development over time.[57] Like Bowlby, Sroufe was respectful of history and felt that 'it is important to bring forward the lessons of the past and at the same time redraw them with an eye on current problems and current understanding'.[58] For Sroufe, the essential commonality between history and developmental psychology lies in the fact that both acknowledge that early events do not determine later ones. Early events shape what is taken forward from the past in ways that then frame subsequent interactions between individuals, groups, or societies and their wider environments. In this account, the past is not used up but continues to inflect the present, perhaps resourcing and supporting, perhaps depleting or obstructing what is now possible: 'the emerging complexity is not specified by prior features, yet it is founded on them'.[59] Furthermore, in Sroufe's interpretation of the concept of 'development', the present is not the sum of the past. There may well be ways in which earlier forms possessed strengths for particular purposes that have not been passed on to later forms. There remains the potential, in Sroufe's words, for 'lessons from the past'.[60]

Historical entities like attachment research and the structure of a personality can be imagined as a maze of little streets and squares, with houses from various periods nonetheless situated by earlier structures. It is these structures, which continue to both constrain and enable what is built today, that come into view when science or a human personality is considered in historical terms. Both history and developmental science are oriented by an amazing and strange aspect of the human condition: our pasts are both discontinuous with our present and, disconcertingly, still with us. The two disciplines agree that we make our homes on top of and within the standing structures or ruins of our pasts: 'though we may be done with the past, the past is by no means done with us'.[61] This perspective on the past suggests a changed attitude to bereavement, to the extent that aspects of the past remain with

[56] Van IJzendoorn, M. & van der Veer, R. (1984) *Main Currents of Critical Psychology*, p.233, trans. M. Schoen. New York: Irvington Publishers. See also Klempe, S.H. & Smith, R. (eds) (2017) *Centrality of History for Theory Construction in Psychology*. New York: Springer.

[57] The concept of 'development' of course has its own long history. See, for example, Wertheimer, M. (1985) The evolution of the concept of development in the history of psychology. In G. Eckardt, W.G. Bringmann, & L. Sprung (eds) *Contributions to a History of Developmental Psychology* (pp.13–25). Berlin: Mouton; Valsiner, J. (1994) Irreversibility of time and the construction of historical developmental psychology. *Mind, Culture, and Activity*, 1(1–2), 25–42.

[58] Sroufe, L.A. (1996) *Emotional Development*, p.xii. Cambridge: Cambridge University Press.

[59] Sroufe, L.A. (2007) The place of development in developmental psychopathology. In A. Masten (ed.) *Multilevel Dynamics in Developmental Psychopathology: Pathways to the Future: The Minnesota Symposia on Child Psychology*, Vol. 34 (pp.285–99). Mahwah, NJ: Lawrence Erlbaum, p.290.

[60] Sroufe, L.A. (1996) *Emotional Development*, p.xii. Cambridge: Cambridge University Press.

[61] Roisman, G.I., Madsen, S.D., Hennighausen, K.H., Sroufe, L.A., & Collins, A. (2001) The coherence of dyadic behavior across parent–child and romantic relationships as mediated by the internalized representation of experience. *Attachment & Human Development*, 3(2), 156–72, p.169. An example of attachment researchers 'building in the ruins' is the way that the term 'internal working model' has been used by later attachment researchers to show that Bowlby was attentive to change, since these models were 'working', i.e. open to development. However, this was never Bowlby's intention with the term: 'working' just meant that they were applied (Chapter 1). Nonetheless, the word 'working' has made available this subsequent interpretation.

us. Bowlby held that we can even retain the dead as secure attachment figures at a symbolic/representational level, if we can accept the loss whilst taking courage and reassurance from memories and other aspects of the person's legacy.[62]

Both history and developmental science agree that the past shapes what we can build, where, and with what stability. Both disciplines recognize that important aspects of our lives are often best regarded as by-products of the past, rather than immediately functional and well judged in the present. Yet both perceive that this by-product can be used or adapted responsively, that contingency is material and runs deep. In making sense of such contingency, history and developmental science have significant respective commitments that emphasize the social basis of the self, and the effects of this for the knowing subject. As such, Sroufe and colleagues expressed concern that when the legacy of the past is 'unnoticed, disallowed, unacknowledged or forgotten', present-day social practices will likely not be responsive, well judged, or especially resilient to challenges.[63]

In agreement with Bowlby's image of history, *Cornerstones* takes a stance in proactively evaluating aspects of attachment as a research paradigm. Particular attention is paid to aspects of the history of attachment research that have structured or shaped the present, especially those that have become taken-for-granted over time. Ideas are considered for their cogency, terminology for its clarity, and empirical claims are appraised against the available evidence. Appeals by researchers to earlier or contemporary theory or research for authority or support are evaluated both for the accuracy of the commentary and for the function the citation appears designed to serve. This includes analysis of the ways in which interpretations of Bowlby and Ainsworth have served as sites for alignment or struggle between later researchers. Each chapter identifies the strengths and particular insights associated with the work of the research group under discussion, and changes that have occurred over time in methodology and theory, and a section at the close of each chapter considers some potential limitations.

Much of what goes on within a research group occurs behind the scenes. Where the textual record makes this possible, which is not in every case, the biographical contributories to the research priorities of principal investigators are identified in the introduction to each chapter. However, science is a collective work and has a collective legacy. So chapters attempt to consider the perspectives and efforts of the principal investigators within the context of their work with collaborators and as embedded within a wider context. Each chapter seeks to identify the opportunities, debates, and challenges faced by the field of attachment research, and how these were shaped by and shaped the priorities and concerns of particular research groups, leading to the making and remaking of methodology, knowledge, and authority over time. Chapters are intended to be readable as standalones; none necessarily requires knowledge of the others. However, the cumulative work of the book as a whole will permit comparison and evaluation of the positions of different research groups when confronted with related concerns. The book as a whole is also intended to facilitate translation, since differences in method or terminology have often obscured the relationship between the claims of different groups of researchers.

[62] Bowlby, J. (1980) *Loss*. London: Pimlico: 'for many widows and widowers it is precisely because they are willing for their feelings of attachment to the dead spouse to persist that their sense of identity is preserved and they become able to reorganize their lives along lines they find meaningful' (p.98).

[63] Carlson, E.A., Egeland, B., & Sroufe, L.A. (2009) A prospective investigation of the development of borderline personality symptoms. *Development & Psychopathology*, 21(4), 1311–34, p.1315.

One of the primary forms of attachment-based intervention with families is video-feedback. Researchers found that showing caregivers exemplars of 'ideal' parenting on film was counterproductive. It did not serve as a useful model, and instead lowered the feelings of self-worth and self-efficacy of caregivers. However, for a friendly individual to show caregivers a film of their own behaviour with their child, and watch together, noticing interactions in the film and what stemmed from these moments, had a different effect. This technique has been repeatedly found to have a meaningful effect on adults' caregiving behaviour (Chapter 6).[64] *Cornerstones* is written with the analogous hope that looking together at the recent past, with joint attention to how things occurred and what then ensued, may form a basis for clarifying how things stand and whether there might be other ways of acting in the present and future. This will likely not always be comfortable reading for attachment researchers. At the same time, *Cornerstones* is written with affection for the field and its genuine insights into the strange, drunk-dialling human heart.[65]

Both attachment research and its reception have had enough polemics already. Yet achieving measured and sincere evaluation is a complex task. There are structural pressures on historians of science and social historians to take a flatly critical stance towards scientific claims about family life, treating this as an inappropriate incursion of science as ideology. As Latour and Bourdieu have observed, the conditions of academic production, which separate critics in a variety of ways from the practices they are describing, obscure internal differences in the object of study and may contribute to a wish to 'debunk' the scientific work.[66] There has indeed been a tendency in history and sociology to adopt a stance in which psychological knowledge is regarded as a vast smooth power, without artistry or contingency in its formation.[67] Nonetheless, this tendency for the external observer to be somewhat heedless of the demands practice makes on insiders may, in certain regards, be part of what history has to offer. For instance, *Cornerstones* closely examines matters—for instance the items of scales for measuring attachment—that researchers themselves have generally simply taken for granted as workable for practical purposes at a local level. Yet judgements about what is workable by individual researchers can have huge cumulative unintended consequences as the years go by. Part of the specific relevance of historical analysis for research psychology is in the identification and description of such consequences.[68]

Ainsworth highlighted that empirical research always entails compromises. In her view, heterogeneity among research groups can be to the benefit of psychological science as a whole, since the compromises may well be in different places.[69] Similarly, reflecting on the

---

[64] Juffer, F., Bakermans-Kranenburg, M.J., & van IJzendoorn, M.H. (eds) *Promoting Positive Parenting: An Attachment-Based Intervention*. New York: Psychology Press.

[65] Cf. Mykhalovskiy, E., Frohlich, K.L., Poland, B., Di Ruggiero, E., Rock, M.J., & Comer, L. (2018) Critical social science *with* public health: agonism, critique and engagement. *Critical Public Health*, 29(5).

[66] Bourdieu, P. (2000) *Pascalian Meditations*. Stanford: Stanford University Press; Latour, B. (2013) *An Inquiry into Modes of Existence*. Cambridge, MA: Harvard University Press. Illustrative of the 'debunking' narrative is Gaskins, S. (2013) The puzzle of attachment. In N. Quinn & J.M. Mageo (eds) *Attachment Reconsidered: Cultural Perspectives on a Western Theory* (pp.33–66). London: Palgrave.

[67] Sedgwick, E.K. (2003) *Touching Feeling: Affect, Pedagogy, Performativity*. Durham, NC: Duke University Press.

[68] Duschinsky, R. (2019) Attachment and the archive: barriers and facilitators to the use of historical sociology as complementary developmental science. *Science in Context*, 32(3), 309–26.

[69] Ainsworth, M. (1972) Attachment and dependency: a comparison. In J. Gewirtz (ed.) *Attachment and Dependency* (pp.97–137). Washington, DC: Winston: 'In terms of his problem, theoretical orientation, resources, opportunities, and personal style, each investigator chooses his own set of compromises. The interests of science seem likely to be best served in this context by a multiplicity of studies, each with its own compromises, which yet may in aggregate answer the questions' (p.126).

nature of psychological theory, Sroufe has argued that 'embracing a particular model of disturbance is analogous to putting on lenses which may bring some issues or questions into focus while distorting others in ways that may not be obvious to the observer'.[70] As suggested by Ainsworth and Sroufe's reflections, though all contributing to the study of attachment in some sense, the research groups considered in *Cornerstones* have varied strengths and primary concerns. Treating them together, and with attention to their commentary on and elaborations of one another, helps reveal these differences and their wider stakes.[71] It also helps in understanding the priorities, methodological choices, and terminology of each group, which at all times were, in part, structured toward those communicated by or anticipated from other research groups as well as the wider discipline. Essentially, *Cornerstones* aims to acknowledge and understand the point of view of particular researchers and research groups, without assuming that this point of view is the only or best one available in the field, even on their own original ideas and results.[72]

Ordinary and scientific language

One of the recurrent themes of this book is the way in which communication between research groups, and communication with wider publics, has been hindered by confusion about the meaning of concepts. Part of the appeal of attachment research lies in its central reference to experience-near metaphors and terms such as 'attachment', 'mother', 'security', 'sensitivity', 'disorganization', 'coherence', 'anxiety', 'dissociation', and 'trauma'. Yet, equally, part of the difficulty with understanding attachment research is that *not one* of these terms is used by attachment researchers in line with ordinary language, and rarely with the same meaning between research groups.

It is not unusual for terms to take on a life of their own in shaping human perceptions and actions, both in scientific and ordinary language, a life in turn conditioned by the structures and conditions within which the language occurs.[73] The independent life of language has been an especially common issue for psychological discourse, as previous historians have observed.[74] The researchers discussed in this book from Bowlby onwards have themselves been aware of this issue. For instance, Shaver and Brennan have observed that in ordinary language 'depression' can encompass alienation, low self-esteem, helplessness, and dissatisfaction with life. However, psychological researchers may well want to distinguish these states, and investigate their respective contribution to clinical symptoms.[75] Ordinary use of

[70] Sroufe, L.A. (1997) Psychopathology as an outcome of development. *Development & Psychopathology*, 9(2), 251–68, p.251.

[71] Danziger, K. (1994) Does the history of psychology have a future? *Theory & Psychology*, 4(4), 467–84: It is 'when the professional community is divided in some profound way that a critical disciplinary history has a significant contribution to make' (p.478).

[72] Hacking, I. (2002) *Historical Ontology*. Cambridge, MA: Harvard University Press; Collins, H. & Evans, R. (2014) Actor and analyst: a response to Coopmans and Button. *Social Studies of Science*, 44(5), 786–92.

[73] Cavell, S. (1994) *In Quest of the Ordinary: Lines of Skepticism and Romanticism*. Chicago: University of Chicago Press.

[74] E.g. Smith, R. (2013) *Between Mind and Nature: A History of Psychology*. New York: Reaktion Books.

[75] Shaver, P.R. & Brennan, K.B. (1991) Measures of depression and loneliness. In J.P. Robinson, P.R. Shaver, & L.S. Wrightsman (eds) *Measures of Social Psychological Attitudes*, Vol. 1 (pp.195–289). San Diego: Academic Press: 'In addition to being parts of ordinary language, "depression" and "loneliness" are technical terms within psychiatry and clinical psychology .... When ordinary concepts are used technically, definitional confusion may arise ... these emotions are closely related to other states discussed in this book: alienation, low self-esteem, external locus of control (helplessness), and dissatisfaction with life. In ordinary language, this is as it should be; in

the word 'depression' thus diverges from the clinical use of the term—and perhaps both in turn diverge from the term as used in research contexts. Shaver and colleagues have argued that the issue expresses the broader predicament of academic and clinical psychology, which attempt to characterize and support change within the sphere of human everyday life, and therefore begin with the terms and problems of everyday language.[76] And just like everyday life, ordinary language is unruly, multiply invested, and occasionally nutty or treacherous.

However, even if potential confusions with ordinary language is a broader problem for psychology, attachment research has been unusually vulnerable from the start. It is helpful to see that Bowlby was pulled in two directions.[77] On the one hand, he was keen to make use of the advantages of ordinary language. Ordinary language is excellent for doing less precise work, for making evocative claims, and for communicating with diverse audiences in ways that resonate with everyday concerns.[78] It is intrinsically historical and pitted with depth, a reserve of images and connotations. Bowlby wanted to communicate simply and evocatively, making ideas available to a wide public and clinical audiences. He held no tenured academic post, and especially in the 1950s and 1960s, was intent on speaking beyond the academic community to support changes in policy and the lives of children and families. Bowlby also appreciated the flexibility of ordinary language, and the advantages that this could bring to science. He felt that it can be beneficial in the context of working out ideas, to draw on ordinary language without strict definitions 'for, once a definition is laid down, it tends to straitjacket thought and to control what the worker permits himself to observe.'[79]

However, there is also a danger in reliance on ordinary language, which Bowlby came to recognize increasingly over the span of his long career. Use of everyday terms, rich in existing connotations, 'makes it extremely difficult to tie any specialised meaning to any particular word'.[80] Above all, the connotations of a term from ordinary language can inadvertently accompany the word into scientific language. And no amount of scrubbing and qualifying will ever fully hold back these connotations from influencing discussions between scientists, let alone attempts by scientists to communicate with their publics.[81] In a chapter drafted for his final book, Bowlby expressed regret that Darwin's intellectual legacy has been damaged by assuming the ordinary language connotations of terms that he in fact used in a technical sense: 'it has been unfortunate that in his own expositions of his scientific procedures, Darwin uses words and phrases that have misled readers and have resulted in misconceived criticism.' For instance, 'where we would say we built an explanatory model, Darwin refers to

professional social science it is problematic .... Another problem is that the terms "loneliness" and "depression" harbour implicit causal theories' (p.195).

[76] Shaver, P.R., Morgan, H.J., & Wu, S. (1996) Is love a 'basic' emotion? *Personal Relationships*, 3, 81–96, p.83. See also Derksen, M. (1997) Are we not experimenting then? The rhetorical demarcation of psychology and common sense. *Theory & Psychology*, 7(4), 435–56.

[77] Bowlby's predicament can be seen within the wider context of psychoanalysis discourse in the period, which both wanted and repudiated the advantages of ordinary language. This issue is considered well in Abram, J. (2007) *The Language of Winnicott: A Dictionary of Winnicott's Use of Words*. London: Karnac.

[78] Geertz describes common sense as having five experiential properties: it is felt in use as 'natural', 'practical', 'thin'/'simple', 'immethodical', and 'accessible'. Geertz, C. (1983) Common sense as a cultural system. In *Local Knowledge* (pp.73–93). New York: Basic Books.

[79] Bowlby, J. (1980) *Loss*, p.17. London: Pimlico.

[80] Bowlby, J. (1972) Notes towards *Separation*. PP/Bow/K.5./17.

[81] Bowlby, J. (1973) *Separation*, p.118. New York: Basic Books. As a mature scholar, Bowlby regularly warned his students regarding the use of language in their theorizing. E.g. Issroff, J. (2005) *Donald Winnicott and John Bowlby: Personal and Professional Perspectives*. London: Karnac: 'He concentrated on ensuring that language used was not loose, and on keeping speculation to a minimum' (p.26). 'Often he held forth about the importance of language used for conceptualising' (p.27).

himself as 'speculating', giving the false impression that he lacked rigour or reason as he put forward an explanation.[82]

The most basic example of such problems can be seen with the term 'attachment' itself, which Benjafield situates as one of the most characteristic examples of linguistic polysemy in all the history of psychology.[83] There is a gulf between the ordinary connotations of the term and how it is used by attachment researchers. And there is a further gap between narrower and broader uses of the term by Bowlby, and then by subsequent attachment researchers. In ordinary language, the word means to bind something to something else, physically or emotionally. In Bowlby's narrower usage, the word meant a specific set of behaviours and states that facilitate care-seeking. In Bowlby's broader usage, the word meant all and any intimate relationships. Such multiple investments in the term have had a powerful legacy. They have contributed to the intuitive appeal of attachment theory, making it seem user-friendly to diverse publics. And it has contributed to ceaseless miscommunication by and among researchers. 'Attachment' is a fuzzy term, in both the sweet and worst senses. By the 1980s Bowlby admitted ruefully in correspondence that he kept using the word to describe children's care-seeking behaviours 'for purely historical reasons'.[84] This was despite the fact that it necessitated work, time and again, to clarify the distinction between the technical usage and the various connotations of the term, including adjudication between his own earlier multiple uses.

One of the leaders of the second generation of attachment research, Everett Waters, acknowledged that attachment theory is worse than most areas of psychology for muddling ordinary and technical scientific language. In Waters' view, scientists do and likely should use ordinary language regularly, calling on common metaphors and ideas in order to communicate technical notions. This can be a generative process, contributing helpfully to new theoretical and methodological developments, as well as the circulation of forms of knowledge.[85] However, Waters has argued, when scientific and ordinary language are mistaken for one another, the results can be problematic ways that are difficult to notice and redress:

> In psychology, and more so, attachment theory, the words we use to label ideas often get in the way. They misdirect us in what we think we should do next. Many implications that people draw from their knowledge of attachment theory are probably not rigorously derived from the logic of the underlying theory. Take this example: you ask a college class, what kinds of developmental problems might arise from being insecure in your attachment to your mother? They start thinking that insecure sounds like afraid, fearful, anxious, shy, uncomfortable, maybe incompetent, and the reasoning goes on to a conclusion that

---

[82] Bowlby, J. (1987–90) *Darwin's Scientific Achievement*. Cambridge University Library, MS Add. 8884.

[83] Benjafield, J.G. (2016) The digital history of the anglophone vocabulary of psychology: an exploration using Zipfian methods. *History of Psychology*, 19(2), 125–40, p.127.

[84] E.g. Bowlby, J. (1983) *Letter to Helen Block Lewis*, 12 January 1983. PP/Bow/J.9/123: 'As I expect you know, some difficulties have arisen over the best use of the term attachment. For purely historical reasons it seems best now to confine it to protection and comfort-seeking behaviour as seen most obviously in childhood.'

[85] On the costs and gains of metaphor for Bowlby's reception, see Duniec, E. & Raz, M. (2011) Vitamins for the soul: John Bowlby's thesis of maternal deprivation, biomedical metaphors and the deficiency model of disease. *History of Psychiatry*, 22(1), 93–107. The issue is likewise discussed in Fonagy, P. (2003) Some complexities in the relationship of psychoanalytic theory to technique. *The Psychoanalytic Quarterly*, 72(1), 13–47: 'Science regularly employs metaphor in the absence of detailed knowledge of the underlying process. Provided that metaphor is not confused with a full understanding—or, to use Freud's expression, the scaffolding is not mistaken for the building—heuristic considerations might outweigh any disadvantages of such employment' (p.36).

insecure is therefore a bad thing. This is not being deduced from some mechanism that is spelled out in attachment theory. It is merely associative.[86]

Unless we can be sure that others know just what we mean by 'attachment', Waters argued, severe cautions are needed. In fact, 'the less often we use the word "attachment" in this discussion, and the more often we refer specifically to what you are asking about, the better off we'll all be'.[87] However, Waters' warning has gone generally unheeded. Attachment research has had comparatively strong platforms for reporting and synthesizing empirical findings but weak platforms for the critical discussion of concepts and terminology—besides, to an extent, the journal *Attachment & Human Development* and the *Handbook of Attachment*.[88]

Luyten has argued that 'much of the language of … attachment theory may have had its time. There is an unmistakable tendency to reify'.[89] Yet any attempt to replace or bypass unclear terminology related to attachment will be difficult, perhaps even counter-productive, unless the various meanings of concepts within the scientific community are understood. There can be a variety of ways of discerning such meanings, including interviews, focus groups, and Q-sort tasks.[90] However, historical analysis of written material has particular advantages for tracing lines of continuity and discontinuity in the uses of terms. The five research groups considered in this book are cornerstones in the development of the research paradigm as it exists today, and have in many regards set the terms of discussion. They are also, perhaps with the exception of the Minnesota group, the prime originators of the most serious confusions in the use of attachment language. As a result, historical study of the contributions of these research groups and the debates between them offers both an introduction to and a clarification of the central concepts and terminology of attachment research.

Summary of chapters

Chapter 1 focuses on the work of John Bowlby. It describes the lines of agreement and disagreement between Bowlby and the psychoanalytic theory of his day, and the extent of his debt to Robert Hinde and ethology. The chapter clarifies ways in which incompatibilities between psychoanalysis and ethology have contributed to tensions within Bowlby's work and subsequent attachment theory. Access to Bowlby's unpublished correspondence and notes provides the basis for a new interpretation of several of Bowlby's key concepts, including

---

[86] Waters, E. & McIntosh, J. (2011) Are we asking the right questions about attachment? *Family Court Review*, 49(3), 474–82, p.474.

[87] Ibid.

[88] Foucault refers to a 'field of stabilization' for the concepts and methods of a discipline that make recognition of equivalence possible. Attachment research has benefited from allowing many an expansive field of stabilization that allows many phenomena to be recognized as pertaining to ideas relating to attachment. On the concept of 'field of stabilization' see Foucault, M. (1969, 1972) *The Archaeology of Knowledge and the Discourse on Language*, p.103, trans. A.M. Sheridan Smith. New York: Pantheon.

[89] Luyten, P. (2015) Unholy questions about five central tenets of psychoanalysis that need to be empirically verified. *Psychoanalytic Inquiry*, 35(1), 5–23.

[90] For instance, the term 'coherence' has a central place in the conceptualization and coding of the Adult Attachment Interview (Chapter 3). Beijersbergen, Bakermans-Kranenburg, and van IJzendoorn conducted a detailed empirical study in 2006 to see whether attachment researchers used the term 'coherent' in the same way as ordinary language or other academic specialisms. The answer was a resounding 'no'. Beijersbergen, M.D., Bakermans-Kranenburg, M.J., & van IJzendoorn, M.H. (2006) The concept of coherence in attachment interviews: comparing attachment experts, linguists, and non-experts. *Attachment & Human Development*, 8(4), 353–69.

monotropy and aggression. The chapter discusses Bowlby's unpublished book written with Jimmy Robertson in the 1950s and 1960s on the effects of major separations experienced by young children. And the chapter presents previously unavailable ideas from Bowlby's unpublished book on defence mechanisms from the 1960s, which sheds light on his later information processing model. The chapter also pieces together the full story of Bowlby's work with a patient, Mrs Q., the account of which is scattered across a dozen of Bowlby's writings. The chapter closes by discussing some ways in which limitations in Bowlby's work have proven obstacles for later attachment researchers.

Though the terms 'attachment theory' and 'attachment research' are sometimes used interchangeably, attachment as an empirical research paradigm may be regarded as having fully commenced only with Ainsworth's work. Chapter 2 begins by introducing the biographical context of Ainsworth's work, including her early work at Toronto University. Ainsworth's concept of 'security' and her attempt to develop self-report measures of security are reappraised, placing Ainsworth's work in the context of her debt to her teacher Blatz. The chapter then draws on Ainsworth's published and unpublished writings to consider the strengths and limitations of her Uganda ethnography and Baltimore longitudinal study. This helps clarify Ainsworth's goals in her development of a scale to measure sensitivity and in developing the Strange Situation procedure. A central concern of the chapter is close examination of the theoretical commitments contained in Ainsworth's choices in the design of her coding protocols, including the justifications she provided for characterizing individual differences in infant attachment as three categories, and how she handled discrepancies. The chapter also considers the work of Ainsworth's collaborator and student Everett Waters. Waters played a critical role in the validation of Ainsworth's measure, and stimulated an influential debate about the stability of attachment over time. However, he also acknowledged the limitations of the Strange Situation procedure, and developed other measures for assessing attachment in childhood and adulthood based on Ainsworth's ideas. In addition, the chapter addresses other concerns that have been raised regarding Ainsworth's work, including the extent of its cross-cultural validity.

Chapter 3 explores the contributions of Mary Main, Erik Hesse and the Berkeley longitudinal study. The Berkeley group generated the dominant approach to method and theory for the second generation of attachment research, and helped establish the priorities and values of the field over recent decades. Drawing on archival materials, the introduction offers a new interpretation of the development of Main's work. This highlights the fundamental role she gave to attentional processes, and leads to a new account of how Main conceptualized minimizing and maximizing attachment strategies. Recognition of the centrality of attention to Main's theory also helps makes sense of her introduction of the disorganized attachment classification and her development of the Adult Attachment Interview. The chapter draws on two unpublished books by Main to describe her methodological innovations, and how they were achieved, and also to clarify misunderstandings of her goals. This includes discussion of Main and colleagues' use of the concepts of 'disorganization', 'fear', and 'internal working model', and how these related to earlier ideas by Bowlby and Hinde. A particular focus of the chapter is on the six-year systems for assessing attachment developed by Main and colleagues. Relatively little information about these coding systems is in print, and yet close consideration of these methods offers a powerful window into Main's thinking about attachment and development, as well as into her more well-known assessments of infant and adult attachment. The chapter also draws on an examination of the development of the Adult Attachment Interview coding system from the 1980s to the 2000s to offer clarifications regarding Main and Hesse's ideas regarding 'lack of resolution' of loss and trauma. The precise relationship between trauma and dissociation in their thinking—which has often been confused by subsequent attachment researchers—is described, drawing on a major theoretical work by Main and Hesse published only in Italian.

Chapter 4 considers the work of Alan Sroufe, Byron Egeland, and the Minnesota Longitudinal Study of Risk and Adaptation. The Minnesota group has served as a fundamental source of stability and support for the developmental tradition of attachment research. The chapter begins by describing the origins of the Minnesota study in the context of growing policy and academic interest in the consequences of child maltreatment. The chapter presents the first sustained commentary on Sroufe's ideas about emotion, attachment, and development. These ideas were vital to the selection of measures and interpretation of results in the longitudinal study. Headline concepts like 'felt security' were influential for subsequent attachment theory. However, other ideas such as affects as social currency, and intrusive intimacy, are interesting but less well known. The chapter examines the antecedents and sequalae of attachment in the Minnesota study. It then considers the contribution made by the study of attachment at Minnesota to the emergence of developmental psychopathology as a movement within developmental science. This includes consideration of Sroufe, Egeland, and colleagues' distinctive approach to conceptualizing risk and resilience. Two case studies from the Minnesota study are used to illustrate how the multiple, rich assessments conducted over decades offered the research group an encompassing picture of human lives. And the legacy of Sroufe and Egeland is discussed for two former students who have subsequently returned to take leadership roles at Minnesota: Dante Cicchetti and Glenn Roisman. The chapter also discusses ways in which Sroufe and Egeland's theoretical commitment to holism has contributed to both strengths and limitations in their work.

Chapter 5 discusses Phillip Shaver, Mario Mikulincer and the Experiences in Close Relationships scale, the most widely used self-report measure of adult attachment. The chapter begins by revisiting Ainsworth's reasons for abandoning self-report measures of security, and Shaver and Hazan's reason for reigniting this approach. Shaver and Hazen's development of the 'love quiz' and early work on adult attachment is discussed, considering ways in which their ideas converged and diverged from earlier attachment theory. The chapter then explores the creation of the Experiences in Close Relationships scale, which has provided a methodological and theoretical basis for the social psychological tradition of attachment research over subsequent decades. The chapter clarifies Shaver and Mikulincer's approach to conceptualizing and measuring attachment, and secure base use, and minimizing and maximizing strategies. It is anticipated that this will help translation between the social psychological and developmental traditions of attachment research. The chapter also considers original contributions made by Shaver and Mikulincer and colleagues through their inquiries into the relationship of adult attachment styles with sexuality and with religious practices. The chapter closes with examination of the items of the Experiences in Close Relationships scale, and the ways in which the mechanics of the measure have limitations for capturing the implications of both security and trauma for adult attachment.

Acknowledgements

Work on this book has taken five years, during which time I have accumulated an absurd number of debts. A more detailed account of the experience and nature of these accumulated debts can be found in Duschinsky, R. (2019) Attachment and the archive: barriers and facilitators to the use of historical sociology as complementary developmental science. *Science in Context*, 32(3), 309–26.

First off, my apologies are due to my father for failing, as yet, to turn Chapter 3 into a film. I agree that it should be. The reader is welcome to be in touch with advice for casting. More generally, I would be delighted to hear from readers and to learn from their thoughts about attachment research, past and present.

I am grateful to my mother for first encouraging me to read Bowlby as a teenager. Having ideas from attachment theory as a reference point through adolescence and adult development was a true resource. I have also taken courage from witnessing her indomitability in the face of health challenges, as well as her thirst for adventure. Conversations with my wife have likewise contributed directly to this book. *Cornerstones* benefited from her good judgement in appraising forks in the road, her insights as a clinician, her strength in the face of our losses, and from the countless ways in which our relationship makes me happy.

The basis of *Cornerstones* has been access to the John Bowlby, Mary Ainsworth, and Mary Main/Erik Hesse Archives. My first thanks therefore must go to the Wellcome Collection for hosting the Bowlby Archive (reference: PP/Bow/), the Nicholas and Dorothy Cummings Center for hosting the Ainsworth Archive, and to Mary Main, Erik Hesse, and Naomi Gribneau-Bahm at Berkeley for their efforts to make materials available for study (soon to arrive at the Wellcome Collections). These are inexhaustible, miraculous collections, and I feel deeply lucky to have had access to them. This archival research has been enriched by the kindness Mary Main and Erik Hesse have shown me, in the course of years of correspondence and multiple visits. This has been a transformative gift. I have especially appreciated our wider conversations about poetry and family, as well as their patience with my endless questions and criticisms. And—on a personal level—I have appreciated the chance to see, and hopefully learn something from, a marriage so pervaded in every part by affection and security.

Special thanks are due to the Wellcome Trust for making it possible for me to work on this book (Grant WT103343MA), and for encouraging the menagerie of spin-off projects. I have appreciated Dan O'Connor, Tom Bray, Lauren Couch, Jack Harrington, Jenny Haynes, and Ross MacFarlane, among others, for their faith in me. Chapter 3 was enhanced by Mary Sue Moore's generosity in sharing the detailed notes she took during the 1987 Adult Attachment Institute in London.

Among colleagues, I am grateful to Sarah Foster, an ally and friend. Sarah's creativity, meticulousness, and insight have fed this project from the very start, and helped it grow. Thanks are similarly due to Sophie Reijman, who has also been an ally and friend on this journey. It has been a joy and a privilege to work with her. *Cornerstones* is dedicated to Sophie, and to León, her new little one. Marinus van IJzendoorn and Marian Bakermans-Kranenburg have been unstinting in their generosity and care, not least in encouraging Sophie Reijman to come to join me at Cambridge in the first place. I have learnt so much from discussions with them across the themes of this book, and had great fun spending time together.

Affectionate thanks are likewise due to Judith Solomon for having me to stay during her Fulbright Visiting Professorship at Vienna University, a visit that has subsequently formed the basis for many varied and fun conversations. A reader who would like to see 'proceedings' from these conversations might take a look at Duschinsky, R., Greco, M., & Solomon, J. (2015) The politics of attachment: lines of flight with Bowlby, Deleuze and Guattari. *Theory, Culture & Society*, 32(7–8), 173–95; or Solomon, J., Duschinsky, R., Bakkum, L., & Schuengel, C. (2017) Toward an architecture of attachment disorganization: John Bowlby's published and unpublished reflections. *Clinical Child Psychology and Psychiatry*, 22(4), 539–60.

My grateful thanks to Martin Baum, Charlotte Holloway, Janine Fisher, Julie Musk and Lucía Pérez at Oxford University Press for their support for this book.

Chapters of this book have benefited greatly from feedback from Marian Bakermans-Kranenburg, Sasha Ban, Kazuko Behrens, Richard Bowlby, Jean-François Bureau, Betty Carlson, Patricia Crittenden, Tsachi Ein-Dor, Jo Faulkner, Pasco Fearon, Chris Fraley, Lydia Fransham, Pehr Granqvist, Philip Heslop, Erik Hesse, Jeremy Holmes, Juliet Hopkins, Michael Lamb, Mary Main, Karin Maraney, Bob Marvin, Mario Mikulincer, Mary Sue Moore, Mikhael Reuven, Anne Rifkin-Graboi, Glenn Roisman, Avi Sagi-Schwartz, Jessica Saffer, Carlo Schuengel, Judith Solomon, Alan Sroufe, Paul Stenner, Alessandro Talia, Anne Tharner, Ross Thompson, Marinus van IJzendoorn, Marije Verhage, Mary Jo Ward, Everett Waters, and Judy Keiner. I am also grateful to other researchers who have offered encouragement for this work, including but by no means limited to Byron Egeland, Kelly Brennan-Jones, Steve Farnfield, Peter Fonagy, Deborah Jacobvitz, Kasia Kozlowska, Mirjam Oosterman, David Shemmings, Gottfried Spangler, Ruan Spies, Phil Shaver, Miriam and Howard Steele, Frank van der Horst, Sue White, David Wilkins, and Matt Woolgar.

I am grateful to Tommie Forslund and Kate White for all that I have learnt from them in the course of editing the *Attachment Reader* for Wiley and *Trauma and Loss: Key Texts from the John Bowlby Archive* for Routledge. The Bowlby family have been remarkable in their wholehearted support of these endeavours, and their helpful feedback.

At Cambridge, I am grateful to Jonathan Mant and the Primary Care Unit, who provide my academic home and secure base. The last stage of the book's composition has been bewildering and painful on various fronts in terms of losses and family health. Jonathan's kindness has helped make it possible to continue. I have similarly felt fortunate to be part of Sidney Sussex College, which has been a supportive community at every turn. Particular thanks are due to Max Beber, Richard Penty, Brett Gray, and Gary Gerstle for their availability through difficult times. I have benefited from the mentorship of Mary Dixon-Woods, Claire Hughes, and Susan Golombok, who have been role models and ever-thoughtful friends. Finally, I feel deeply fortunate for the intellectual companionship and camaraderie of my immediate research group: Lianne Bakkum, Helen Beckwith, Barry Coughlan, Sarah Foster, Julia Mannes, Sophie Reijman, Sam Reisz, Guy Skinner, and Melody Turner. I am grateful to them for conversations about the ideas contained in this book as they have pursued aligned inquiries with other methodologies. And I am thankful for their unwavering support through the challenges of the last year.

1

John Bowlby and the Tavistock Separation Research Unit

Biographical sketch

John Bowlby reported that his interest in psychological issues was kindled in 1929 whilst working at a school for troubled children, following studies in natural science at Cambridge. There he had 'known an adolescent boy who had been thrown out of a public school for repeated stealing. Although socially conforming, he made no friends and seemed emotionally isolated from adults and peers alike. Those in charge attributed his condition to his having never been cared for during his early years by any one motherly person, a result of his illegitimate birth.'[1] The previous year Bowlby had read Sigmund Freud's *Introductory Lectures on Psychoanalysis*; in light of his experiences at the school, Freud's ideas 'came alive for me', and Bowlby decided to train as a psychoanalyst in London.[2] In 1948 he founded the Separation Research Unit at the Tavistock Clinic and appointed James Robertson as an assistant for a study of the effects on young children of hospitalisation with no or minimal visitation from their parents. In 1950 he expanded the research group, appointing Mary Ainsworth as a clinical postdoctoral researcher (Chapter 2). Reflecting on the observations and ideas of this research group, Bowlby developed his novel theory of the nature of the parent–child relationship, of the role of inhibition as a defence against the expectation of rejection, and the form and nature of grief. This theory found its expression first in a series of articles in the *International Journal of Psychoanalysis,* and then in a trilogy of books: *Attachment, Separation,* and *Loss.* Bowlby's discipline-spanning research made a critical contribution to thinking about human development, offering a model that mitigated important limitations of both behaviourism and psychoanalytic theory. This vital contribution to developmental science, together with his passion for public engagement, has made him one of the most important and influential psychologists of the twentieth century. It has also made him at once one of the most accessible to understand superficially, and one of the most difficult to understand in depth.

Introduction

In an unpublished article from 1969, Bowlby wrote that 'an individual holding an idiosyncratic model of the world or of himself is likely to find himself facing the world alone.'[3] This expectation that individuality and novel ideas will be met with isolation and rejection had a

---

[1] Bowlby, J. (1981) Perspective: a contribution by John Bowlby. *Bulletin of the Royal College of Psychiatrists,* 5(1), 2–4, p.2.

[2] Bowlby, J. (1979) The ten books which have most influenced my thought, 24 October 1979. PP/Bow/A.1/8.

[3] Bowlby, J. (1969) *Anxiety, Stress and Homeostasis.* Unpublished manuscript, April 1969. PP/Bow/H10.

number of sources.[4] Bowlby himself attributed his distrust in others in his professional life in part to the ambush and misunderstanding he received from peers when he first began to present his ideas at the Institute of Psychoanalysis.[5] The expectation of misunderstanding and rejection led to sharp distinctions throughout his life in what Bowlby would reveal to different audiences. The result of this was, in a sense, three John Bowlbys, each with somewhat different motivations, and different tones to their writing, reflecting three anticipated audiences.[6] The human self is, of course, always a multiple thing, even if there is a certain amount of hierarchical organisation. Nonetheless, consideration of three relatively distinct Bowlbys helps make sense of breakdowns of communication between his writings across different forums and eras, and between the audiences of these texts.

The most well known to the public is the Bowlby available in works written for a general audience during the 1950s. These include the famous 1953 *Child Care and the Growth of Love*,[7] but also his articles in popular women's magazines[8] and presentations to professional organisations.[9] Here a tone of sobriety and daring is expressed as authority, even when the evidence was—by his own later admission—'sketchy' or 'inadequate'.[10] In these texts from the 1950s, Bowlby argued that a young child needs their mother 'as an ever-present companion', providing 'the provision of constant attention night and day, seven days a week, and 365 days in the year'.[11] What he hoped to get across, above all, was that young children should have someone they feel confident turning to when alarmed. Bowlby had been clearly informed by his wife, based on her own experience, that 'constant attention' to a child was both an impossible and unhelpful aspiration for mothers.[12] And late in life, he acknowledged that he regretted this statement and the implied demand for ever-present care.[13] In the 1950s, however, the language of total presence had the advantage for Bowlby of appealing to the obviousness and authority of popular British stereotypes about women and children and nature.[14] As has often been remarked, these attitudes were shaped by the context of post-war

---

[4] Van Dijken, S. (1998) *John Bowlby: His Early Life: A Biographical Journey into the Roots of Attachment Theory.* London: Free Association Books; Bowlby, U. (1992) A memoir of John. PP/Bow/P.6/3: John believed that 'his own childhood had been sufficiently unhappy to want him to investigate—but not so unhappy that he had obliterated the subject'.

[5] Bowlby, J. (1984) *Letter to Phyllis Grosskurth, amending discussions of Bowlby in Grosskurth's biography of Klein*, 10 January 1984. PP/Bow/A.5/7.

[6] Bakhtin, M.M. (1981) *The Dialogic Imagination: Four Essays by M.M. Bakhtin.* Austin: University of Texas Press; Showers, C.J. & Zeigler-Hill, V. (2003) Organization of self-knowledge: features, functions, and flexibility. In M.R. Leary & J.P. Tangney (eds) *Handbook of Self and Identity* (pp.47–67). New York: Guilford.

[7] Bowlby, J. (1953) *Child Care and the Growth of Love.* Harmondsworth: Pelican.

[8] See e.g. Bowlby, J. (1954) Should a baby be left to cry? *Parents*, March 1954, pp.32–35; Bowlby, J. (1958) Should mothers of young children work? *Ladies Home Journal* (November) 75, 58–59, 158–61.

[9] E.g. Association for Psychiatric Social Workers (1955) Presentation at the Annual General Meeting 1955: Dr John Bowlby on preventative activities. Modern Records Centre Warwick University. MSS.378/APSW/P/16/6/19-20.

[10] Bowlby, J. (1986) Interview with the BBC. PP/Bow/F.5/8: 'I published this report for the World Health Organisation in 1951, *Maternal Care and Mental Health* … all the evidence was still sketchy, it was inadequate'.

[11] Bowlby, J. (1953) *Child Care and the Growth of Love.* Harmondsworth: Pelican, p.53, 76.

[12] Ross, L.R. (2014) Reading Ursula Bowlby's letters (1939–1940). *Journal of the Motherhood Initiative for Research & Community Involvement*, 5(1), 67–82.

[13] Doyle, C. (1987) A continuing case for keeping children at home. *Daily Telegraph*, 23 June 1987: 'He insists that he has never intended to imply that a continuous relationship should mean every minute of the day, and now adds "intermittent" to "warm and continuous"' as the qualities of care he wished children to receive from their familiar caregivers.

[14] Bowlby less fell into the naturalistic fallacy than emblazoned it on his shield. Bowlby, J. (1990, 2011) John Bowlby: interview by Leonardo Tondo. *Clinical Neuropsychiatry*, 8(2), 159–71: *Tondo*—'Do you agree with the rather simplistic view that the mother may be more important than the father? *Bowlby*— 'That view, I think, is well attested by the information we have … This is the way all societies operate. So my concern is always with human

Britain.[15] Bowlby was knowing and explicit that he was drawing on 'pure prejudice',[16] that in his popular writings he 'exaggerates everything'.[17] Such a strategy helped him get some core ideas heard, even if these were mostly the rind of the views he actually held.

Subsequent attachment researchers have engaged in some whack-a-mole efforts to correct fallacies arising from Bowlby's populist claims about attachment, for instance his overstrong claims about the influence of early experiences or his polemical claims about the responsibilities of mothers. However, this has been at most partially successful in shaping public perceptions of the implications of attachment theory. Some things are irreversible once they are put out into the world. But additionally, even if they could have been reversed, the second generation of attachment researchers generally did little, especially compared to Bowlby, to speak to a wider public.[18] This left Bowlby's early statements in popular works unqualified, contributing to misalignment between the technical positions of attachment theorists and criticisms levelled at popular representations of the paradigm.

Among commentators who have read his work carefully, there has been growing recognition that there is little evidence that Bowlby believed in the positions with which his name became associated in the public imagination.[19] At the same time, it should be recognised that he did little to correct them in his writing for wider publics. In 1954, Donald Winnicott wrote to Bowlby warning of such consequences, and asking Bowlby to issue a public statement

nature, about which I am most confident about Western culture. When I teach my students, I say, "Look, the first thing to remember is that Western society is not a human norm." We behave in a way that human societies have never behaved in the past. If you take human societies over the past hundred thousand years so far as we know and around the world, Western societies are peculiar. We do things in funny ways which may be alright, and it may not. Do not think they are normal. They are not the normal way human beings are meant to behave" … You either go along with human nature or you fight it. If you fight it you get problems. If you don't fight it life is much more comfortable.' (164–5)

[15] E.g. Franzblau, S.H. (1999) Historicizing attachment theory: binding the ties that bind. *Feminism & Psychology*, 9(1), 22–31; Vicedo, M. (2011) The social nature of the mother's tie to her child: John Bowlby's theory of attachment in post-war America. *British Journal for the History of Science*, 44(3), 401–26. Van der Horst has also situated Bowlby's work in the wider context of post-war Europe, especially in the context of his travels in the 1950s. Van der Horst, F.C.P. (2011) *John Bowlby—From Psychoanalysis to Ethology. Unravelling the Roots of Attachment Theory*. Oxford: Blackwell.

[16] Bowlby, J. (1958) Should mothers of young children work? *Ladies Home Journal* (November) 75, 58–59, 158–61, p.158. LeVine has claimed that Bowlby had little awareness of the extent to which he was engaging with contemporary ideologies of family life. Careful examination of the full range of Bowlby's public and private writings indicate that the ideological aspects of Bowlby's popular writings were not simply the result of a lack of self-awareness, but had a decidedly strategic component. LeVine, R.A. (2014) Attachment theory as cultural ideology. In H. Otto & H. Keller (eds) *Different Faces of Attachment: Cultural Variations on a Universal Human Need* (pp.50–65). Cambridge: Cambridge University Press. In sociological perspective, Bowlby's appeal to existing concerns and prejudices of his day may be considered in light of Bourdieu's remark that when attempting to reach a mass market, the 'more directly and completely' must cultural producers direct their goods to 'a pre-existing demand, i.e. to pre-existent interests in established forms'. Bourdieu, P. (1993) *The Field of Cultural Production*. Cambridge: Polity, p.97.

[17] Bowlby, J. (1987) Baby love. *Hampstead and Highgate Express*, 3 April 1987.

[18] For example, Alan Sroufe (Chapter 4) wrote a popular textbook and a handful of newspaper articles primarily focused on the overprescription of ADHD medication. But he did not attempt in a sustained way to speak to wider publics in the manner of Bowlby. In Germany, Klaus and Karin Grossmann were more active in attempting to speak to wider publics and increase public understanding of attachment. See e.g. Grossmann, K. & Grossmann, K. (2011) *Das Geflecht des Lebens*. DVD, Auditorium Netzwerk: Freigegeben ohne Altersbeschränkung. Perhaps the closest to Bowlby in direct engagement with policy-makers and publics has been Peter Fonagy, e.g. Fonagy, P. (2018) Evidence submitted to the Evidence-Based Early-Years Intervention Inquiry. Science and Technology Committee (Commons). http://data.parliament.uk/writtenevidence/committeeevidence.svc/evidencedocument/science-and-technology-committee/evidencebased-early-years-intervention/written/77644.pdf.

[19] E.g. Riley, D. (1983) *War in the Nursery: Theories of the Child and Mother*. London: Virago Press; Thomson, M. (2013) *Lost Freedom: The Landscape of the Child and the British Post-War Settlement*. Oxford: Oxford University Press, p.87.

revealing his belief that there was, in fact, a shortage of nursery care.[20] There is no evidence that Bowlby replied to this letter, and no public statement was issued. Winnicott later reflected on both the advantages and disadvantages of Bowlby's strategy:

> His propaganda for the avoidance of unnecessary breaks in the infant–mother relationship had gone round the world, though I do also feel that the propaganda element necessarily led to a fashion in child care and to the inevitable reactions which follow propaganda.[21]

A good part of the poor relationship between Bowlby and his critics stemmed from this predicament: in the expectation of misunderstanding and rejection, he had simplified and excluded qualifications from his position in writing populist propaganda in the 1950s for the sake of conveying a message that could travel easily between contexts and down through time; as a consequence, he elicited rejection, and was not able to subsequently make full use of feedback in further amending his views. For example, he made harsh and mocking remarks about his feminist critics, unable or unwilling to take on their concerns, for instance regarding his often underspecified claims about the harms of 'separations'.[22]

When asked in 1976 about the discrepancy between statements in his academic writings and those in which he used his position as clinician to speak with authority to the public, Bowlby replied: 'I would defend this; in different roles one is entitled to speak in different voices.'[23] However, at times it was more than a single person speaking in different voices: there seemed to be some cases where communication between the different personae failed or became distorted. For instance, in 1971 he wrote to Michael Rutter 'I think you misrepresent me and mislead the reader' when Rutter attributes to Bowlby the oversimplified positions—such as an undifferentiated use of the concept of 'separation', or a particular focus on the figure of the mother—that are readily evident from Bowlby's early popular writings.[24] Bowlby appeared genuinely baffled as to why he was being misrepresented, apparently having forgotten his earlier statements. For instance, in an article from 1981, Rutter wrote 'Bowlby's argument is that the child's relationship with mother differs from other relationships specifically with respect to its attachment qualities', a passage annotated by Bowlby in his private copy of the article 'Where did he get this idea from?'[25] A thoroughly different man is known to those who read Bowlby's scientific and clinical writings compared to his popular writings.[26] This is surely a good part of why his critics and his successors deal essentially

---

[20] Winnicott, D. (1954, 1987) Letter to Dr J. Bowlby. In F. Robert Rodman (ed.) *The Spontaneous Gesture: Selected Letters of D.W. Winnicott*. London: Karnac, pp.65–66. See also Lewis, J. (2013) The failure to expand childcare provision and to develop a comprehensive childcare policy in Britain during the 1960s and 1970s. *Twentieth Century British History*, 24(2), 249–74.

[21] Winnicott, D. (1953, 1989) John Bowlby. In C. Winnicott, R. Shepherd, & M. Davis (eds) *Psycho-analytic Explorations* (pp.423–32). London: Karnac, p.427.

[22] E.g. Ringold, E.S. (1965) Bringing up baby in Britain. *New York Times*, 13 June 1965: "Dr Bowlby, however, sticks to his guns. Interviewed in his office at the Tavistock clinic he said: "Whenever I hear the issue of maternal deprivation being discussed, I find two groups with a vested interest in shooting down the theory. The Communists are one, for the obvious reason that they need their women at work and thus their children must be cared for by others. The professional women are the second group. They have, in fact, neglected their families. But it's the last thing they want to admit."

[23] Bowlby, J. (1976) Bowlby on latch-key kids: interviews with Dr Nicholas Tucker. *Psychology Today*, Autumn 1976, 37–41, p.38.

[24] Bowlby, J. (1971) *Letter to Michael Rutter*, 6 October 1971. PP/Bow/J.9/161.

[25] Annotations by Bowlby (PP/Bow/J.9/162) on Rutter, M. (1981) Social-emotional consequences of day care for preschool children. *American Journal of Orthopsychiatry*, 51(1), 4–28.

[26] Bowlby's scientific and clinical writings are placed together since the tone and arguments are quite well integrated; there are fewer disparities than with Bowlby's popular writings or his private reflections. Bowlby's routine

with two irreconcilable individuals with the same name, and often seem perplexed by one another. In these scholarly writings, Bowlby presented his 'idiosyncratic model' of the world, laying out its logic. Bowlby's scientific and clinical writings were just as daring as the popular texts, but authority is tempered with sobriety. He was concerned with the particularity of the things he discussed, not the familiar idea of them, even if this demanded dense writing and some loss of ready readability. In general, there is quite a clean division between the lively metaphors and appeal to common sense in Bowlby's popular writings[27] and the somewhat dry prose of his writing for medical audiences and the psychoanalytic community, and in books such as *Personality and Mental Illness* from 1940 and *Attachment, Volume 1* from 1969.[28] True, the division between the populariser and the scholar is not complete. For instance, though mild in comparison with the outright homophobia that can be identified in other psychoanalytic texts in the 1960s, Bowlby leans on metaphors of deficit and futility to characterise gay and lesbian sexualities in explaining his new account of human motivation in passages deep inside *Attachment, Volume 1*.[29] However, the fact that even his most hostile critics have never mentioned these passages evidences the division between his popular and scholarly readers, corresponding to his popular and scholarly texts.[30]

The very content of Bowlby's claims and his use of familiar words was different between his popular works and his scientific and clinical writings—as was the period of their composition: the vast majority of the popular works were published prior to *Attachment, Volume 1* in 1969; the works most read and discussed by subsequent attachment research were published after 1969. In *Attachment, Volume 1*, Bowlby was absolutely explicit that 'almost from the first many children have more than one figure towards whom they direct attachment behaviour; these figures are not treated alike; the role of a child's principal attachment-figure can be filled by others than the natural mother'.[31] In dialogue with academic colleagues, Bowlby stated clearly that, for children, 'provided he sees plenty of his principle figure', whoever this is, 'it is an advantage for him to have others as well'.[32] He specified that he intended the child's primary caregiver when he used the term 'mother', which was standard practice in the psychoanalytic discourse of his day.[33] In his scholarly writings, Bowlby prided himself on a measured and scientific tone largely without feeling, even as he wrote about its causes. He largely avoided polemics, and in his academic writings the characterisation of his London colleagues in the psychoanalytic community was cordial and respectful. Part of Bowlby's discipline-spanning courage came from his deep acknowledgement of the limited status of

---

work as a clinician, and clinical notes, likely represent a further distinct Bowlby. However, there are few available textual traces, except insofar as this work contributed to Bowlby's scholarship or his private reflections. Most of Bowlby's clinical notes are closed still for several decades in the Wellcome Collections.

[27] Duniec, E. & Raz, M. (2011) Vitamins for the soul: John Bowlby's thesis of maternal deprivation, biomedical metaphors and the deficiency model of disease. *History of Psychiatry*, 22(1) 93–107.

[28] Bowlby, J. (1940) *Personality and Mental Illness*. London: Kegan Paul; Bowlby, J. (1957) An ethological approach to research on child development. *British Journal of Medical Psychology*, 30(4), 230–40; Bowlby, J. (1969, 1982) *Attachment, Volume 1*. London: Penguin.

[29] Ibid. pp.130–31.

[30] A partial exception is Vicedo, M. (2011) The social nature of the mother's tie to her child: John Bowlby's theory of attachment in post-war America. *British Journal for the History of Science*, 44(3), pp.401–26, where there is valuable analysis of links between Bowlby's popular and academic writings of the 1950s.

[31] Bowlby, J. (1969, 1982) *Attachment, Volume 1*. London: Penguin, pp.303–4.

[32] Bowlby, J. (1971) *Letter to Michael Rutter*, 6 October 1971. PP/Bow/J.9/161.

[33] Melanie Klein had set a trend in which the word 'mother' (or 'breast') was deployed as a synecdoche for the infant's experience of the caregiving environment in general, rather than referring specifically to the biological mother. See Hinshelwood, R.D. (1989) *A Dictionary of Kleinion Thought*. London: Free Association Books.

theory, as a conjecture to then be appraised against the available evidence.[34] In his notes on the philosopher of science Karl Popper, Bowlby wrote: 'Intelligibility requires the model to be cast in terms mainly of some analogous and better understood set of ideas. Plausibility that it does not affront widely held assumptions.'[35] His daring and genre-busting theoretical works, in this sense, were also set up from the start in expectation of being debated, as part of the scientific process.

Bowlby as populariser treated readers as needing to be coaxed to even the most crude points through appeal to their stereotypes and preconceptions. The scientific and clinical commentator held his audience firmly at bay with a carefully orchestrated remoteness. The Bowlby Archive is also a reflection of another kind of reserve and distrust, evident in the hidden array of wayward, profound thoughts that he did not trust to print. Bowlby's wife described him as 'completely inarticulate' when he tried to talk about feelings.[36] Yet in his private writings and correspondence available in the Archive, Bowlby is visible as a human: with deep feelings, a personal emotional fragility, frequently thoughtful about his personal limitations. (A volume of writings that reflect this 'hidden' Bowlby has recently been published by Duschinsky and White, with the encouragement of the Bowlby family, under the title *Trauma and Loss: Key Texts from the John Bowlby Archive*.)[37] In his notes Bowlby took an interest in monkeys left alone in zoo cages. When angered by visitors, they self-mutilate. Indeed, remarked Bowlby, how like cages are our inhibitions.[38] The Archive reveals the engine-room of Bowlby's thinking behind his inhibitions, in the ordering and transformation of difficult feelings evoked by the world, and by himself, forming the materials for imagination, insight, and propositions. It is this engine that motored his thinking, as he sought sense in the stories he was hearing from veterans from the battlefields of France and the sorrows and symptoms of children.

In the mid-1950s, Bowlby was part of a series of meetings by the 'Psychobiology of the Child' study group, organised by Ronald Hargreaves at the World Health Organisation. The discussants included leading researchers from across the world: Jean Piaget, Erik Erikson, Konrad Lorenz, Margaret Mead, and Ludwig von Bertalanffy. A transcription of the discussions was published. In a strangely unguarded moment, the transcript reveals Bowlby reflecting on his own experiences in considering child development and the predicament of patients seen in his clinical work. 'It seems to me', Bowlby said, 'that the main problem with which we are all faced in the process of growing up is that of making a tolerable and compatible synthesis out of a number of manifestly incompatible components.' Within us are all kinds of positions and elements, including tender feelings and callousness, kindness and cruelty, and 'these things are literally incompatible'. If an individual wishes to benefit from

---

[34] Bowlby, J. (1982) *A Secure Base*. London: Routledge: 'All knowledge is conjectural and ... science progresses through new theories coming to replace older ones when it becomes clear that a new theory is able to make sense of a greater circle of phenomena than are comprehended and explained by an older one and is able to predict new phenomena more accurately.' (84)

[35] Bowlby, J. (*c*.1982) Popper's evolutionary epistemology. PP/Bow/H.98. The passage is heavily underlined in red pen for emphasis.

[36] Ursula Bowlby, cited in Karen, R. (1998) *Becoming Attached: First Relationships and How They Shape Our Capacity to Love*. Oxford: Oxford University Press, p.29.

[37] Duschinsky, R. & White, K. (eds) (2019) *Trauma and Loss: Key Texts from the John Bowlby Archive*. London: Routledge.

[38] Bowlby, J. (1933–36) Research notes for uncompleted PhD. PP/Bow/D.1/2/13: 'Zuckerman describes how monkeys will mutilate themselves if they are alone in their cages and visitors make them angry ... Although not in visitor-cages, humans are often in cages of inhibition.'

these different parts, the first thing is that he must 'own to all these different parts of himself', rather than pretend that they do not exist. And secondly, he must 'gradually relate them in some self-balancing unity'.[39]

There is little unity between Bowlby as populariser, as scholar, and as private thinker through the 1950s and early 1960s. From the late 1960s, the relations between these three personae became more integrated. In this period he came to greater acknowledgement of misunderstandings that had arisen as a result of such divisions, and also to reflect in his theoretical work on the damage that may be done by inhibiting communication between aspects of the self. By the 1970s, with retirement from clinical work, Bowlby further scaled back his activity as a public figure to focus more on his scholarship and his family. He almost exclusively ceased to publish popularizing works after 1969. In discussions with his son, Bowlby explained at the time that he needed to focus on scholarly rather than popular works as he 'could not afford to be taken as a lightweight'.[40] In interview he continued to offer polemical views that played on sexist attitudes towards women.[41] But in the final two decades of Bowlby's life, his central focus was on securing the scholarly standing and clinical relevance of attachment theory—and on pursuing meticulous historical work of the life of Charles Darwin. His desire to influence wider publics was allowed to slide. He made no attempt to update them on developments and qualifications of his position between the 1950s and 1980s, even in late interviews, focusing instead on his classic message of the importance of maternal availability for young children.[42]

The dominance of the three Bowlbys varied over time, with the populariser quiet after 1969 and the academic scholar in much greater ascendance. However, over the span of Bowlby's career, a certain generative interplay can be identified. The private thinker fed the scholar experiences and ideas about intimacy and pain, though these were very thoroughly intellectualised by the time they hit the printed page. The private thinker also fed the populariser his passion and his courage—as well as buffering him from the effects of rejection and misunderstanding, which were anticipated in advance. The scholar permitted the private thinker some order and containment, and gave the populariser credibility. And the populariser provided the private thinker both a spur and an outlet, and provided the scholar a wildly increased audience for key claims. There was, however, a personal price to this self-balancing unity. In the World Health Organisation discussions in the mid-1950s, Margaret Mead responded to Bowlby's remarks by asking a penetrating question: 'What are the conditions of disassociation in which you do or do not own to this part of your personality?' Bowlby's reply

---

[39] Bowlby, cited in Tanner, J.M. & Inhelder, B. (eds) (1958) *Discussions on Child Development: Proceedings of the WTO Study Group of the Psychobiological Development of the Child*, Vol. 3. London: Tavistock, p.207. Use of the first person plural ('the main problem with which we are all faced') is sufficiently unusual to permit a biographical interpretation, especially given the salience of the theme of integration for Bowlby. It should be acknowledged, of course, that this could have simply been a manner of speaking.

[40] Richard Bowlby, personal communication, February 2019. An exception is Bowlby, J. (1974) A guide to the perplexed parent. *New York Times*, 2 March 1974.

[41] E.g. Bowlby, J. (1976) Bowlby on latch-key kids: interviews with Dr Nicholas Tucker. *Psychology Today*, Autumn 1976, 37–41.

[42] E.g. Doyle, C. (1987) A continuing case for keeping children at home. *Daily Telegraph*, 23 June 1987. Careful examination of the interview signals shifts in Bowlby's thinking—even his regret in his use of the term 'continuous' care by mothers in his early writings. Yet the dominant narrative remains remarkably similar to the early popular works, and there is no attempt to explain theoretical developments. Bowlby's lack of explicit attempt to clarify revisions to his picture of child–caregiver relationships was likely supported by a lack of interest in such developments in media forums, where reference to basic stereotypes about mothers and children made for more accessible reading.

is remarkable: 'I think one could refer to the notions of forgivability and unforgivability.'[43] The ultimate question, Bowlby indicates, is whether the parts of oneself can accept one another, can forgive one another, for what may be irreversible.

Bowlby and psychoanalysis

Of special importance for Bowlby's popularizing, scholarly, and private writings was his training and work as a psychoanalytic clinician. His central ideas emerged from within psychoanalytic theory and clinical work. Not least, Bowlby's earliest attention to the term 'attachment' was in annotations from 1942 on *Young Children in War-Time* by Dorothy Burlingham and Anna Freud,[44] where he marked the term wherever it appeared. Bowlby not only underlined but also highlighted and starred the following passages: 'Whenever certain essential needs are not fulfilled, lasting psychological malformations will be the consequence; these essential elements are the need for personal attachment, for emotional stability, and for permanency of educational influence' and 'It is a known fact that children will cling even to mothers who are continually cross and sometimes cruel to them.' That there will be some form of 'attachment of the small child to his mother' seemed to Burlingham and Freud 'to a large degree independent of her personal qualities.'[45] The latter passage was prominently cited 16 years later in Bowlby's foundational article on 'Nature of the child's tie to his mother', published in 1958.[46]

In a late manuscript circulated only to other psychoanalysts,[47] Bowlby explained that, as a young psychoanalyst, he envied colleagues (Donald Winnicott is implied) their clinical intuition and grace. And he saw other peers doing good clinical work in spite of the theories to which they subscribed. However, 'I have not that sort of mind, nor am I strong on intuition. Instead, I tend to apply such theories as I hold in an effort to understand my patient's problems. This works well when the theories are applicable but can be a big handicap when they are not.' Without clinical grace or intuition, Bowlby felt that he had no choice but to develop a new theory. Lay and colleagues succinctly identify that this new theory salvaged five aspects of psychoanalytic theory: '(1) that infants have a complex social and emotional life, (2) that

[43] Tanner, J.M. & Inhelder, B. (eds) (1958) *Discussions on Child Development: Proceedings of the WTO Study Group of the Psychobiological Development of the Child*, Vol. 3. London: Tavistock, p.208. Some legacy of Klein may be felt here, in the idea of forgiveness as psychological integration.

[44] Burlingham, D. & Freud, A. (1942) *Young Children in War-time*. Oxford: Allen & Unwin.

[45] Annotations by Bowlby dated 1942 on Burlingham, D. & Freud, A. (1942) *Young Children in War-time*. Oxford: Allen & Unwin, pp.10, 47. Copy held in the library of Human Development Scotland. Earlier than Burlingham and Freud, Ian Suttie had written that 'instead of an armament of instincts—latent or otherwise—the child is born with a simple attachment-to-mother who is the sole source of food and protection ... the need for a mother is primarily presented to the child mind as a need for company and as a discomfort in isolation'. Suttie I. (1935) *The Origins of Love and Hate.*, London: Free Association Books, p.15. It is possible that the use of the term came to Bowlby via Suttie and/or conversations through the Tavistock or the wider London psychoanalytic scene. In any case, no textual record is available of Bowlby having read Suttie until after Anna Freud. On the link between Bowlby and Suttie see van der Horst, F.C. & van der Veer, R. (2010) The ontogeny of an idea: John Bowlby and contemporaries on mother–child separation. *History of Psychology*, 13(1), 25–45.

[46] Bowlby, J. (1958) Nature of the child's tie to his mother. *International Journal of Psycho-Analysis*, 39, 350–73. Bowlby's first published use of the term 'attachment' would appear in Bowlby, J., Ainsworth, M., Boston, M., & Rosenbluth, D. (1956) The effects of mother–child separation: a follow-up study. *British Journal of Medical Psychology*, 29, 211–47, p.237.

[47] Bowlby, J. (1985, 1991) The role of the psychotherapist's personal resources in the treatment situation. *Bulletin of the British Psychoanalytic Society*, 27(11), 26–30. Published as Chapter 12 in Duschinsky, R. & White, K. (eds) (2019) *Trauma and Loss: Key Texts from the John Bowlby Archive*. London: Routledge.

early experiences can have lifelong implications, (3) that mental representations of early experiences mediate effects on later behavior and development, (4) that defensive processes play a role in affect regulation, and (5) that loss of an attachment figure—at any age—is an emergency and mourning is a process that serves an adaptive affect-regulation function.'[48] Yet despite these continuities, Bowlby perceived three major problems with psychoanalytic theory and method: a weak recognition of actual family experiences in shaping child psychology; a mistaken account of the causes of incompatible elements within the human mind; and a conflation of self-preservative actions and sexuality.

Actual experience

The issue of actual experiences was perhaps the earliest of the three central problems Bowlby found with the psychoanalytic theory of his day. Bowlby's notes from the 1930s and his own retrospective accounts both suggest that Bowlby entered psychoanalytic training in the belief that Freud attributed the emotional problems of his patients to adverse experiences, especially in the context of the family. It was an uncomfortable surprise for him to learn that the psychoanalytic establishment in London, and the work of Melanie Klein in particular, had come to downplay past experience as the basis of symptoms and instead emphasise the role of fantasy.[49] In a record of his dreams from the early 1930s, Bowlby reported a dream in which he was imprisoned by the Nazis. Likely with a certain irony, he interpreted the fantasy material as reflecting his anxiety about how to think about fantasy, the unconscious, and sexuality, and about the status of psychoanalytic knowledge in the society around him.[50] It was not that Bowlby thought that fantasy was unimportant. But he believed that it had come to be badly overemphasised, at the expense of attention to the effects of biographical experiences.

In private conversations or in interview, when Bowlby was asked to explain the origins of attachment theory, he would frequently refer to clinical cases he saw under the supervision of Melanie Klein. These cases encapsulated key problems Bowlby experienced as a young psychoanalyst. From around 1938, he began treatment of a small boy of about three years old, who was hyperactive, anxious, and aggressive. The boy's mother was evidently highly troubled, but Melanie Klein insisted that the mother should just sit outside the room. This made Bowlby uncomfortable. He had previous experience of delivering therapy to families within a Child Guidance Clinic, which had convinced him that 'the problem which as a rule we need to solve is the tension among all the different members of the family.'[51] Three or four months into the treatment of the little boy, the mother was admitted as an inpatient to a mental hospital. Bowlby was appalled that Melanie Klein was not interested in the impact of this on the boy, except insofar as it had the practical effect of interrupting the analysis. World

[48] Lay, K.L., Waters, E., Posada, G., & Ridgeway, D. (1995) Attachment security, affect regulation, and defensive responses to mood induction. *Monographs of the Society for Research in Child Development*, 60(2–3), 179–96, p.179. On continuities between attachment and psychoanalysis see also Eagle, M. (1995) The developmental perspectives of attachment and psychoanalytic theories. In S. Goldberg, R. Muir, & J. Kerr (eds) *Attachment Theory: Social, Developmental & Clinical Perspectives* (pp.123–50). Hillsdale, NJ: Analytic Press.

[49] Bowlby, J. (1933–36) Research notes for MD thesis: 'Anxiety— Essays'. PP/Bow/D.2/46/6; Bowlby, J. (1981) Perspective: a contribution by John Bowlby. *Bulletin of the Royal College of Psychiatrists*, 5(1), 2–4.

[50] Bowlby, J. (c.1933) Dreams. PP/Bow/D.2/45/7.

[51] Bowlby, J. (1949) The study and reduction of group tensions within the family. *Human Relations*, 2, 123–28.

War II halted Bowlby's training as a child analyst: 'When it was over and I was free to resume my training I could not face doing so however: the absurdity of treating young children and neglecting their parents was too much for me.'[52]

In staking out the importance of actual experiences for children, Bowlby developed new terminology. Kleinian theorists had used the term 'internal object' to refer to the image of the parent held by a child. Bowlby was dissatisfied with this term. He felt that it left the 'object' a shimmering abstraction rather than anything concrete. Influenced by the growing interest in cognitive and representational processes of the 1960s,[53] Bowlby offered instead the term 'internal working model'. The term was used by Bowlby to gesture to the cognitive components associated with the attachment behavioural system, as a way to 'broach the large, difficult, and profound questions of how a child gradually builds up his own "internal world"':

> Starting, we may suppose, towards the end of his first year, and probably especially actively during his second and third when he acquires the powerful and extraordinary gift of language, a child is busy constructing working models of how the physical world may be expected to behave, how his mother and other significant persons may be expected to behave, how he himself may be expected to behave, and how each interacts with all the others. Within the framework of these working models he evaluates his situation and makes his plans. And within the framework of the working models of his mother and himself he evaluates special aspects of his situation and makes his attachment plans.[54]

Bowlby's proposal was that early attachment relationships shape cognitive representations that then inform action. This accounts for continuities between children's experiences of early care and their later expectations of their caregivers, and subsequently of other people. The idea of the 'internal working model' was not, as Bretherton has observed, a fully worked out theory. In part it was a metaphor, one that allowed Bowlby above all to highlight in a general and encompassing way that representations, as 'models', should be regarded as tolerably accurate encapsulations of the history of past experiences.[55]

A clear disadvantage was that the 'model' included a huge variety of cognitive content. It is not really clear what the term means, except that it refers to a representation relevant to attachment. At one point or another, most second-generation attachment researchers have stated that Bowlby's gestural use of the term 'internal working models' has made it difficult to generate specific hypotheses using the idea.[56] Indeed, part of the ritualised inheritance

---

[52] Bowlby, J. (1984) *Letter to Phyllis Grosskurth, amending discussions of Bowlby in Grosskurth's biography of Klein*, 10 January 1984. PP/Bow/A.5/7. Bowlby requested that Grosskurth add to her biography of Klein the following passage: 'It was fortunate for Bowlby that the war then intervened. He tells people that it saved him from open conflict with Melanie Klein for which he would not then have been ready.'

[53] See Gardner, H. (1986) *The Mind's New Science: A History of the Cognitive Revolution*. New York: Basic Books.

[54] Bowlby, J. (1969, 1982) *Attachment, Volume 1*. London: Penguin, p.353. Internal working models are 'none other than the internal worlds of traditional psychoanalytic theory seen in a new perspective' (82).

[55] Bowlby, J. (1969, 1982) *Attachment, Volume 1*. London: Penguin, p.82. Bretherton, I. (1998) Internal working models and communication in attachment relationships. In A. Braconnier & J. Sipos (eds) *Le Bébé et les Interactions Précoces* (pp.79–90). Paris: Presses Universitaires de France: 'I would urge, however, that the various metaphors Bowlby … used as tools to think about internal working models are not to be taken too literally.' (79)

[56] See e.g. Crittenden, P.M. (1990) Internal representational models of attachment relationships. *Infant Mental Health Journal*, 11(3), 259–77; Bartholomew, K. (1990) Avoidance of intimacy: an attachment perspective. *Journal of Social and Personal relationships*, 7(2), 147–78; Main, M. (1991) Metacognitive knowledge, metacognitive monitoring, and singular (coherent) vs. multiple (incoherent) models of attachment: some findings and some directions for future research. In P. Marris, J. Stevenson-Hinde, & C. Parkes (eds) *Attachment Across the Life Cycle* (pp.127–59). London: Routledge; Collins, N.L. & Read, S.J. (1994) Cognitive representations of attachment: the structure

of Bowlby's ideas by second-generation attachment researchers was criticism and revision of the concept of the internal working model. It has served as a wide, undefined target onto which each researcher can project his or her own image of what an attachment theory should be. Nonetheless, at the time, there were distinct advantages to the metaphor for Bowlby's purposes. The idea of the 'working model' helped Bowlby to emphasise that expectations about relationships are in constant use, day in and day out, as individuals respond to present demands and forecast future needs.[57] It also helped him emphasise that expectations can lead us to search for confirmatory input. Interpretations by later attachment researchers of the term 'working model' as suggesting 'provisional (in the sense of "working" drafts—changeable plans)'[58] are a *post hoc* reconstruction: Bowlby apparently did not intend this connotation.[59] His most important emphasis in using the term was to contrast the psychoanalytic emphasis on fantasy with his own emphasis on models as tolerably accurate representations of what actually happened in childhood.

As Peter Fonagy and Morris Eagle have noted, Bowlby's opposition between the psychoanalytic theory of his day and his own focus on 'internal working models' that reflected the role of actual childhood experiences was, for polemical reasons, oversimplified.[60] There were analysts like W.R.D. Fairbairn, who held aligned perspectives, as Bowlby himself acknowledged.[61] And Anna Freud chided Bowlby for his depiction of her as a secondary-drive theorist, with a position similar to Klein's; Freud felt that her stance was much closer to Bowlby's in emphasizing the importance of actual experiences of caregiving for understanding anxious and aggressive behaviours by children.[62] Furthermore, it should be highlighted that

and function of working models. In K. Bartholomew & D. Perlman (eds) *Advances in Personal Relationships*, Vol. 5 (pp.53–90). London: Jessica Kingsley; Waters, H.S. & Waters, E. (2006) The attachment working models concept: among other things, we build script-like representations of secure base experiences. *Attachment & Human Development*, 8(3), 185–97.

[57] Bowlby, J. (1988) Developmental psychiatry comes of age. *American Journal of Psychiatry*, 145, 1–10.

[58] Mikulincer, M. & Shaver, P.R. (2003) The attachment behavioral system in adulthood: activation, psychodynamics, and interpersonal processes. In M.P. Zanna (ed.) *Advances in Experimental Social Psychology*, Vol. 35 (pp.53–152). New York: Academic Press, p.60. The idea of working models as changeable, provisional representations is likewise a central theme in many more applied works making appeal to Bowlby, e.g. Johnson, S.M. (2019) *Attachment Theory in Practice*. New York: Guilford.

[59] Alan Sroufe, personal communication, January 2019: 'Bowlby never used "working model" to mean provisional. I asked him explicitly because I kind of liked that idea. He said no, he didn't mean that.'

[60] Fonagy, P. (1999) Points of contact and divergence between psychoanalytic and attachment theories: is psychoanalytic theory truly different. *Psychoanalytic Inquiry*, 19(4), 448–80; Eagle, M. (2013) *Attachment and Psychoanalysis*. New York: Guilford.

[61] Scharff, D.E. & Fairbairn Birtles, E. (1997) From instinct to self: the evolution and implications of W.R.D. Fairbairn's theory of object relations. *International Journal of Psycho-Analysis*, 78, 1085–103: 'Bowlby specifically acknowledged his Fairbairnian orientation in the development of attachment theory and the ethological approach to infant development (personal communication)' (1100). Bowlby's annotations on Fairbairn's writings offer testament to his alignment and agreement with the latter's positions. For instance, he wrote 'crucial points' in the margins when Fairbairn emphasized that even a parent perceived as unkind may still be the person a child will want to turn to for comfort. Annotations by Bowlby on Fairbairn, W.R.D. (1944) Endopsychic structure considered in terms of object-relationships. *International Journal of Psycho-Analysis*, 25, 70–92. Bowlby's copy of this paper is held by Richard and Xenia Bowlby.

[62] Anna Freud urged recognition that the idea of the 'pleasure principle' in psychoanalytic theory was not opposed to the idea of attachment; all it posited was that when impulses or responses were activated for a child, a homeostatic response would be initiated to reduce the feeling of tension or motivation, especially in ways that provide pleasure or comfort. This was therefore aligned with, rather than contrary to, the idea of attachment as a homeostatic system. Freud, A. (1958, 1960, 1969) Discussion of John Bowlby's work on separation, grief and mourning. In A. Freud & D.T. Burlingham (eds) *The Writings of Anna Freud*, Vol. 5 (pp.167–86). New York: International Universities Press. Press. Blum's statement that 'Bowlby's ideas angered just about everyone he knew. Anna Freud dismissed him outright' is a thoroughgoing oversimplification, based on selective reading. Blum, D. (2002) *Love at Goon Park: Harry Harlow and the Science of Affection*. New York: Basic Books, p.59.

Bowlby did not assume that all adult recollection reflected historical experience in any simple way. Unpublished clinical cases from the 1930s to the 1960s and published later reflections show Bowlby's attentiveness in his clinical work to the role of psychological processes that may shape, edit, or distort a patient's account of their actual experiences.[63] In particular, he was interested in the way that early experiences of care could contribute to a tendency to either unrealistically denigrate or idealise attachment figures, and the therapist.[64]

Nonetheless, it is also true that Bowlby's emphasis on actual experience represented a shift in clinical technique and in epistemology. In terms of clinical technique, it oriented his discussions with patients and interpretation of their symptoms towards consideration of past experiences.[65] And in terms of epistemology, Bowlby regarded psychoanalytic knowledge as compatible with other forms of scientific knowledge and measurement. This distinguished Bowlby from even sympathetic members of the London Institute at the time.[66] It was a position that would open the door to both the interdisciplinary synthesis and the focus on concrete observational measures that would lie at the heart of attachment theory. It would also contribute to the backlash of psychoanalysis against attachment theory. In contrast to psychoanalysts who enacted their rebellions more implicitly, the focus on actual experiences at the expense of fantasy has meant that even to this day attachment theory is not formally taught at the British Psychoanalytic Institute.[67] This is highly unfortunate. In a longitudinal follow-up study of children treated at the Anna Freud Centre, Target and Fonagy described several cases in which therapists, having been taught that representations of parents represented fantasy, interpreted children's reports of abuse as such, rather than recognising them as reports of actual events. These children had especially poor long-term outcomes.[68]

There were, then, several important advantages to Bowlby's introduction of the idea of 'internal working models' in negotiating the relationship between his ideas and psychoanalytic perspectives of the day. However, it should be noted that Bowlby's use of the concept incorporated several of the same flaws as the psychoanalytic terms, such as 'object', it was replacing.[69] First, and most significantly, the concept was simply too encompassing, since

[63] Bowlby, J. (undated) Maternal behaviour: humans. PP/Bow/H.136; Bowlby, J. (1979) On knowing what you are not supposed to know and feeling what you are not supposed to feel. *Canadian Journal of Psychiatry*, 24(5), 403–8.

[64] This was the topic of his first published paper: Bowlby, J. (1940) The influence of early environment in the development of neurosis and neurotic character. *International Journal of Psycho-Analysis*, 21, 154–78: 'Every patient who comes to us has a distorted view of his parents . . . Some patients will project all that they feel to be bad in themselves on to their parents and blame and hate their parents. Others will project all the good and idolize their parents' (176). Such reflections on two classes of distortion in adults' perceptions of their parents align with the later position of Mary Main (Chapter 3).

[65] Bowlby, J. (1977, 1979) The making and breaking of affectional bonds. In *The Making and Breaking of Affectional Bonds* (pp.150–88). London: Routledge.

[66] See e.g. Isaacs, S. (1944) *Letter to Major Bowlby*, 20 October 1944. PP/Bow/J.9/111.

[67] Fonagy, P. (2015) Mutual regulation, mentalization, and therapeutic action: a reflection on the contributions of Ed Tronick to developmental and psychotherapeutic thinking. *Psychoanalytic Inquiry*, 35(4), 355–69.

[68] Target, M. & Fonagy, P. (2003) Attachment theory and long-term psychoanalytic outcome: are insecure attachment narratives less accurate? In M. Leuzinger-Bohleber, A.U. Dreher, & J. Canestri (eds) *Pluralism and Unity? Methods of Research in Psychoanalysis* (pp.149–67). London: International Psychoanalytical Association, p.163.

[69] Fonagy attempted to spell out clearly some of the elements Bowlby absorbed within the concept of 'internal working model': 'Four representational systems compose the internal working model (IWM): (1) expectations of interactive attributes of early caregivers created in the first year of life and subsequently elaborated; (2) event representations by which general and specific memories of attachment-related experiences are encoded and retrieved; (3) autobiographical memories by which specific events are conceptually connected because of their relationship to a continuing personal narrative and developing self-understanding; and (4) understanding of the psychological characteristics of other people (inferring and attributing causal motivational mind states, such as desires and emotions, and epistemic mind states, such as intentions and beliefs) and differentiating these states from those of the self.' Fonagy, P. (2001) The human genome and the representational world: the role of early mother–infant

it seemed to refer to any and all cognitive content about how interactions work within relationships between self and others. For instance, the representational model was situated as both a processor of experience and a repository for experiences, with use of the term often bouncing between these two very different meanings. Second, there was a lack of clarity regarding whether the model was specific to a relationship or general across relationships on the model of early experiences.[70] Third, though clearly infants and adults both have expectations about the availability of attachment figures, it is not clear that it makes sense to use the concept of 'model' to refer to both the basic non-representational goal-directed expectancies of infants and the elaborate representations held by adults, given all the differences between them. This was something Bowlby himself acknowledged and mused on in his unpublished notes.[71] In the 1990s, it became general consensus among attachment researchers that preverbal procedural memories of relationship interactions are qualitatively different to the representations informed by memory following verbal development, making an encompassing concept of 'model' wholly misleading.[72] Each of these issues would leave its legacy for future attachment researchers (Chapters 3 and 5).

Causes of psychological conflict

Bowlby made another important challenge to the dominant psychoanalytic discourses of his day. This was in his thinking about the causes of incompatible elements within the human mind. Bowlby praised Freud for drawing 'attention to the fact that human beings are organisms which at times are driven by forces within themselves which they cannot easily control. We fall in love, we lose our tempers, we panic, we are possessed by forces which seem alien to ourselves.'[73] However, it was especially in his account of the nature of these forces that Bowlby departed from Freud. In the psychoanalytic theory of the 1930s and 1940s, ambivalence was a central theoretical concept, considered an inevitable consequence of the incompatibility of human drives. Most critically, psychoanalytic theory suggested that children feel both love and resentment for their parents. The way that this predicament—the Oedipus complex—is resolved was thought to be of the utmost importance for a child's later development. During his analytic training, this was a position that Bowlby initially accepted.[74]

---

interaction in creating an interpersonal interpretive mechanism. *Bulletin of the Menninger Clinic*, 65(3), 427–48, p.436. See also Collins, N.L. & Allard, L.M. (2004) Cognitive representations of attachment: the content and function of working models. In M.B. Brewer & M. Hewstone (eds) *Perspectives on Social Psychology: Social Cognition* (pp. 75–101). Oxford: Blackwell.

[70] Kobak, R., Rosenthal, N., & Serwik, A. (2005) The attachment hierarchy in middle childhood: conceptual and methodological issues. In K.A. Kerns & R.A. Richardson (eds) *Attachment in Middle Childhood* (pp.71–88). New York: Guilford.

[71] E.g. Bowlby, J. (not dated, c. 1955) Thought, conceptualization, language, psycho-analysis. PP/BOW/H.115.

[72] E.g. Bretherton, I. (1985) Attachment theory: retrospect and prospect. *Monographs of the Society for Research in Child Development*, 50, 3–35; Crittenden, P.M. (1990) Internal representational models of attachment relationships. *Infant Mental Health Journal*, 11(3), 259–77; Lyons-Ruth, K. (1999) The two-person unconscious: intersubjective dialogue, enactive relational representation, and the emergence of new forms of relational organization. *Psychoanalytic Inquiry*, 19(4), 576–617.

[73] Bowlby, J., cited in J.M. Tanner & B. Inhelder (eds) (1956) *Discussions on Child Development: Proceedings of the WTO Study Group of the Psychobiological Development of the Child*, Vol 1. London: Tavistock, pp.182–3.

[74] Bowlby, J. (1938, 1950) An examination of the psychological and anthropological evidence. In E.F.M. Durbin & John Bowlby (eds) *Personal Aggressiveness and War* (pp.51–150). New York: Columbia University Press.

By the 1950s, however, Bowlby had become critical of a tendency in Freud and Klein to presume natural individual differences in ambivalence, rather than examining the social and caregiving context that could intensify such a state. For instance, in the Wolf Man case study, Freud wrote of 'the patient's own ambivalence, which he possessed in a high degree of development'.[75] Next to this passage, in marginalia from the mid-1950s in his personal copy of Freud's text, Bowlby wrote: 'How does Freud explain its genesis?'[76] Bowlby's marginalia on the work of Melanie Klein likewise expresses this concern. In *Contributions to Psychoanalysis*, Klein had observed that 'Unpleasant experiences and the lack of enjoyable ones, in the young child, especially lack of happy and close contact with loved people, increase ambivalence, diminish trust and hope and confirm anxieties'.[77] However, elsewhere she had argued against the 'common tendency to over-estimate the importance of unsatisfactory surroundings, in the sense that the internal psychological difficulties, which partly result from the surroundings, are not sufficiently appreciated. It depends, therefore, on the degree of the intrapsychical anxiety, whether or not it will avail much merely to improve the child's environment'.[78] Both passages were underlined and highlighted by Bowlby in his personal copy. In the margins he expressed frustration that according to the second statement, 'because hatred is primal, the vicious cycle is unavoidable'.[79]

Bowlby felt that the role of experiences of care in fanning or calming frustration was only inconsistently acknowledged by Klein, who showed insufficient 'appreciation that hatred itself and therefore intrapsychic conflict can be intensified by bad surroundings'.[80] Bowlby anticipated that if a child receives gentle care that acknowledges their feelings, then conflicts can be relatively easily managed. If a child is led to expect rejection or harshness, or experiences long-term separation from their familiar caregiver, then inner conflicts are intensified.[81] The Oedipal potential for love and hate of primary caregivers was acknowledged by Bowlby as important, since these emotions would stand in necessary conflict within an intense and important relationship. However, Bowlby regarded this potential as the basis for mental ill health only when a child's experiences of the parent had been troubled ones, for instance as a result of neglect, a parent's threats to harm the child, or an inability to keep the child safe.[82]

In conceptualizing the causes of ambivalence, Bowlby strongly appreciated the emphasis Klein placed on the experience of loss, and how consequential this was for development. However, he was frustrated that Klein predominantly thought about loss as a normal developmental stage within a child–parent relationship. For Klein, every parent would sometimes satisfy a child's desires and sometimes disappoint them, contributing to a sense of

---

[75] Freud, S. (1918, 2001) From the history of an infantile neurosis. In *The Standard Edition of the Complete Psychological Works of Sigmund Freud*, Vol. 17 (pp.1–124). London: Vintage, p.116.

[76] Annotations by Bowlby dated 1956 on *The Standard Edition of the Complete Psychological Works of Sigmund Freud*, Vol. 17. Copy held in the library of Human Development Scotland.

[77] Klein, M. (1948) *Contributions to Psychoanalysis*. London: The Hogarth Press and the Institute of Psycho-Analysis, p.314.

[78] Ibid. p.280

[79] Annotations by Bowlby dated 1948 on Klein, M. (1948) *Contributions to Psychoanalysis*. London: The Hogarth Press and the Institute of Psycho-Analysis. Copy held in the library of Human Development Scotland.

[80] Ibid. The debate between Bowlby and Klein on the status of aggression can be situated as one skirmish within a multiparty controversy running over decades on the status of anger within psychoanalytic theory. See Freud, A. (1972) Comments on aggression. *International Journal of Psychoanalysis*, 53, 163–71.

[81] Bowlby, J. (1960) Separation anxiety. *International Journal of Psycho-Analysis*, 41, 89–113.

[82] Bowlby, J. (1953) *The Roots of Parenthood*. London: National Children's Home; Bowlby, J. (1973) *Separation*. London: Pimlico, p.287; Bowlby, J. (1983) *Letter to Dr Marco Bacciagaluppi*, 6 July 1983. PP/Bow/J.9/11.

ambivalence and a sense of loss. Her emblem for this predicament was that of the infant wanting to access the mother's breastmilk, but also feeling envy and destructive feelings towards the breast. Bowlby regarded this account as obscuring the importance of loss as an event that may damage or remove the child–caregiver relationship, rather than solely as taking place inside it. It underplayed the potential causal relationship between experiences of loss and aggression towards caregivers and others.[83]

In 1956, Bowlby wrote to Klein directly, expressing appreciation for her 'insistence on the central importance of the conflict of ambivalence for the loved object starting early in life ... all my own thinking stems from that'. However, he insisted in this letter that Klein was wrong to regard ambivalence about the maternal breast in particular, and relationships with parents in general, as innate.[84] In 1957, he presented 'The nature of the child's tie to his mother' to the British Psychoanalytic Society. A few days prior to the meeting, Bowlby had given a copy of the paper to a colleague. At the meeting, Klein and her followers had clearly received a copy in advance, and were well prepared with an array of hostile remarks. Above all, Bowlby felt that they criticised his emphasis on actual experiences, rather than inherent conflict about feeding, as the origin of feelings of ambivalence within family relationships.[85] Bowlby experienced this ambush as incontrovertible evidence for the rest of his career that his ideas would inevitably be met with rejection. As a by-product, it led to a tendency for Bowlby to throw scorn on any proposal, even coming from Ainsworth, that early feeding experiences could be important for emotional development (Chapter 2).

Self-preservation

A third central problem for Bowlby with the psychoanalytic theory of innate drives was the status of self-preservatory behaviours. Bowlby's first exposure to psychoanalysis was reading the *Introductory Lectures on Psychoanalysis*. In these lectures Freud posited a drive for self-preservation, which would include seeking safety, seeking help, and eating. However, during the period in which Bowlby began training as a psychoanalyst, Freud changed his stance: he posited a sexual drive as primary, which secondarily became altered into a concern with self-preservation through unpleasurable experiences in the world.[86] From his earliest writings, Bowlby was not happy with this shift:

> It must be realised that Freud equates pleasurable and sexual ... Psycho-analytically, the term sexual should be used only to designate pleasurable and should not be used as identical with genital. I think however there is some confusion here. In the act of sucking, Freud distinguishes between the activity of taking nourishment and the pleasure obtained ... On

[83] Bowlby, J. (1960) Separation anxiety. *International Journal of Psychoanalysis*, 41, 89–113, p.108.

[84] Bowlby, J. (1956) *Public letter to Melanie Klein*, 7 February 1956, following presentation of her paper 'A study of envy and gratitude'. PP/Bow/G.1/4.

[85] Bowlby, J. (1984) *Letter to Phyllis Grosskurth, amending discussions of Bowlby in Grosskurth's biography of Klein*, 10 January 1984. PP/Bow/A.5/7.

[86] Young-Bruehl, E. & Bethelard, F. (1999) The hidden history of the ego instincts. *Psychoanalytic Review*, 86(6), 823–51. Bowlby, J. (1933–36) Functional approach to super-ego. PP/Bow/D.2/49: 'Freud uses the term sex to describe all positive sentiments between two people ... These needs clearly are not always sexual—may be nutritive or self-protective e.g. parent–child. The point may be, however, that the sexual impulses are apt to be aroused in such situations.' This early work by Bowlby appears as Chapter 5 in Duschinsky, R. & White, K. (eds) (2019) *Trauma and Loss: Key Texts from the John Bowlby Archive*. London: Routledge.

the other hand he does not make this distinction in describing the reproductive act ... It seems to me that the difficulty has arisen through using the term sexual to equal pleasure in the first instance and then to refer to its reproductive significance in the second.[87]

Bowlby perceived that Freud's 'discovery that symptoms sometimes represented the patient's sexual activity led him into an over-generalisation ... I should like to suggest that symptoms can be excited purely in the interests of avoiding danger-situations.'[88] In this, one influence on Bowlby was likely the concern of evolutionary theory with both survival and reproduction, which had been significant in his undergraduate training in natural sciences at Cambridge. Whereas Freud treated self-preservation as an essentially rational tendency adapted to the perception of experienced reality, in his notes in the 1930s Bowlby set out the position that the self-preservative response has its own intrinsic predispositions and preferences: 'Although the baby neither foresees nor reasons about cold being bad for its health, [this] does not preclude the possibility of its being concerned with an inclination to react to cold with anxiety and to gentle warmth with pleasure. In such a primitive mechanism, I should recognise the gears of the tendency to self-preservation.'[89]

Further reflections on self-preservation were prompted by Bowlby's own experiences of fatherhood. John and Ursula Bowlby's first child, Mary Hamilton, was born in February 1939. Their second, Richard, was born in August 1941; Pia Rose was born in February 1945; finally, Robert was born in April 1948. A traditional upper-class household in this regard, with the additional separations caused by Bowlby's wartime responsibilities, John had no responsibility for feeding the children. Nonetheless, he recalled observing during the 1940s that his young children would seek him out both for affectionate interaction and when alarmed.[90] This ran contrary to the idea, common at the time, that a child's relationship with their parent developed out of the pleasure that came from feeding ('cupboard love'). In this seeking of a familiar caregiver when alarmed, Bowlby saw a tendency to self-preservation, which he distinguished from the 1950s onwards from feeding activity in strict terms (indeed overstrict. See Chapter 2).

This position had a number of major practical consequences. One implication was that affection shown to children would not 'spoil' them and make them anxious about separation, unable to cope without affection. In fact, Bowlby argued, the opposite would be true. Children who feel confident that they are 'cherished' would be less likely to be anxious about separation.[91] Another critical implication was that the signs of depression and grief seen by children in the context of long-term separations from their caregivers should, indeed, be recognised as mourning for this relationship.[92] From the vantage of the present, this seems like an obvious point. However, it ran against psychoanalytic orthodoxy. Even in 1970, major

---

[87] Bowlby, J. (1933–36) Research notes for MD thesis. PP/Bow/D.2/44/3.

[88] Bowlby, J. (1933–36) Mechanisms—symptom-formation. PP/Bow/D.2/44/1.

[89] Bowlby, J. (1933–36) Anxiety: essays. PP/Bow/D.2/46/6.

[90] Bowlby, J. (1986) Attachment theory: new directions. *ACP-Psychiatric UPDATE*, 7(2), panel discussion, Washington 1986. PP/BOW/A.5/1.

[91] Bowlby, J. (1956) The growth of independence in the young child. *Royal Society of Health Journal*, 76, 587–91. The concept of 'cherishing' was an irregular but important one for Bowlby. He refers to the concept in various places, e.g. Bowlby, J. & Robertson, J. (1965) *Protest, Despair and Detachment*. PP/BOW/D.3/38.

[92] Bowlby's attention to the issue of mourning was stimulated by reading Marris, P. (1958) *Widows and their Families*. London: Routledge. Marris's book was unusual for the time in giving consideration to typical as well as atypical mourning processes. The idea that adult and child mourning represents the same process was one Bowlby inherited from Melanie Klein.

psychoanalysts were still claiming that 'mourning as defined by Freud and as observed in the adult is not possible until the detachment from parental figures has taken place in adolescence'.[93]

Bowlby interpreted childhood loss in terms of adult mourning, and adult bereavement in light of children's response to separations: 'Since the evidence makes it clear that at a descriptive level the responses are similar in the two age groups, I believe it to be wiser methodologically to assume that the underlying processes are similar also, and to postulate differences only when there is clear evidence for them'.[94] This transposition between childhood and adulthood proved an influential move for later attachment research. It represented the beginnings of a heuristic, or even a method, within subsequent attachment theory and the development of attachment assessments in which adulthood and childhood are interpreted as on analogy with one another. Above all, adult attachment would be interpreted by the second generation of attachment researchers through analogy and extrapolation from individual differences in infant attachment. In the 1980s, this was Mary Main's approach in developing the Adult Attachment Interview (Chapter 3) and Hazan and Shaver's in the development of the 'love quiz' (Chapter 5). However, more recently, the analogy has been reversed. Researchers such as Fraley and Roisman have deployed ideas about the underlying dimensions of adult attachment as the basis for reimagining individual differences in infant attachment (Chapters 2 and 3).

Following Hinde

Activating and terminating conditions

For Bowlby, the mistaken idea that children cannot mourn their relationships was a consequence of the assumption in psychoanalytic theory that the relationship is secondary, because sexuality is primary. He saw this view as an obstacle to recognition that affectionate bonds are of various kinds and can serve various functions, at an individual level and for humans in general at an evolutionary level. It was in conceptualizing human social responses in the context of research on animal behaviour that Bowlby found strongest support for his thinking about these different kinds and functions of relational behaviour.

In 1951, Bowlby was introduced by Julian Huxley to the work of Lorenz, which revealed an exciting development: that in the study of animal behaviour, careful work was taking place differentiating between behavioural tendencies.[95] Niko Tinbergen, Konrad Lorenz, Karl von Frisch, and colleagues, working under the label of 'ethology', had developed a revolutionary approach to the study of behaviour. This approach took as its central premise the idea that not just biological structures but also sequences of observable behaviour could be the product of evolution through natural selection, contributing in predictable ways to an

---

[93] Nagera, H. (1970) Children's reactions to the death of important objects: A developmental approach. *Psychoanalytic Study of the Child*, 25(1), 360–400.

[94] Bowlby, J. (1963) Pathological mourning and childhood mourning. *Journal of the American Psychoanalytic Association*, 11(3), 500–41, p.521.

[95] Van der Horst, F.C.P. (2011) *John Bowlby—From Psychoanalysis to Ethology. Unravelling the Roots of Attachment Theory*. Oxford: Blackwell.

individual's chances of survival and reproduction.[96] Ethologists asked four questions of behavioural sequences they observed: How did it develop in the individual? What causes it? What is its function? How did it evolve in the species? When these questions are not adequately distinguished, the ethologists warned, researchers will talk past one another about 'adaptiveness', a concept that can refer to any of these levels. They were also worried that the idea of 'adaptiveness' can imply the implicit value judgement that a response is warranted or useful for the individual, when in fact this would need to be demonstrated (Chapter 2).[97] Indeed, the ethologists argued that responses that support survival and reproduction in general may contribute to highly counterproductive behaviours by an individual, depending on circumstances. Similarly, they observed that the current deployment of a behavioural pattern need not be equated with the function for which it evolved. In fact, an action pattern may become active, reach its predictable outcome, and terminate, all without any direct relationship with the function for which it evolved.

Bowlby was primed to take an interest in ethology by his personal passion for birdwatching. Growing up, Bowlby had quite a formal, distant relationship with his mother; however, she was a passionate and knowledgeable naturalist, with a particular delight in birds. Bowlby learnt that he could retain his mother's attention by engaging her about his sightings of birds.[98] Over time, birdwatching became a firm hobby. However, it should also be emphasised that Bowlby was exhilarated by the quality of the research being done in ethology, especially in contrast to the rudimentary observations of human development available in the 1950s: 'They were brilliant, first-rate scientists, brilliant observers, and studying family relationships in other species—relationships which were obviously analogous with that of human beings—and doing it so frightfully well. We were fumbling around in the dark; they were already in brilliant sunshine.'[99]

Critical for Bowlby's engagement with this literature was his friendship with the ethologist Robert Hinde, who he met in 1954. For the next ten years, Hinde read and gave comments on most of Bowlby's scholarly writings, and attended Bowlby's weekly research seminars at the Tavistock.[100] Together, Bowlby and Hinde identified several ways in which debates in ethology could advance psychoanalytic theory. The most important point of intersection and difference was in the theory of motivation. Both Freud and Lorenz tended to think about activity as motivated or inhibited by the availability of a somewhat underdefined notion of 'psychological energy' or 'drive'. Hinde addressed this model in his paper on 'Ethological models and the concept of "drive"', published in 1956.[101] Here Hinde acknowledged that it was possible in general terms for an organism to become exhausted after various forms of energy expenditure. However, from this he argued that it should not be concluded that all forms of behaviour draw from the same psychological energy or drive. The concepts of 'energy' and 'drive', Hinde noted, had become nodes within a taken-for-granted theoretical

[96] Burkhardt Jr, R.W. (2014) Tribute to Tinbergen: putting Niko Tinbergen's 'Four Questions' in historical context. *Ethology*, 120(3), 215–23.

[97] Tinbergen, N. (1963) On aims and methods of ethology. *Zeitschrift Tierpsychology*, 20, 410–33.

[98] See Bowlby's correspondence with his mother, writing from boarding school, 1921–1924. PP/BOW/A.1/17/1.

[99] John Bowlby interview with Robert Keren, 14 and 15 January 1989, cited in Karen, R. (1998) *Becoming Attached: First Relationships and how They Shape Our Capacity to Love*. Oxford: Oxford University Press, p.94.

[100] Bowlby, J. (1977–79) Interview with Alice Smuts and Milton J.E. Senn. PP/BOW/A.5/2. The interview has been published as Chapter 11 in Duschinsky, R. & White, K. (eds) (2019) *Trauma and Loss: Key Texts from the John Bowlby Archive*. London: Routledge.

[101] Hinde, R. (1956) Ethological models and the concept of 'drive'. *British Journal for the Philosophy of Science*, 6(24), 321–31. See also Hinde, R.A. (1959) Unitary drives. *Animal Behaviour*, 7(3), 130–41.

framework; it was time to reappraise the actual behavioural sequences that they were being used to describe and explain. Hinde proposed that, if behaviours are observed closely in comparative perspective across species, different action patterns could be distinguished, along with their activating and terminating conditions. In contrast to the idea of a single reservoir of energy, an advantage of the idea of distinct action patterns was that it was easier to ask the four key ethological questions, considering the development, causation, function, and evolution of behavioural sequences.

Looking back on his career, Bowlby situated Hinde's 1956 paper on drives as one of the most influential works he ever read. It led directly to the account of motivation at the heart of attachment theory.[102] Hinde's approach lent itself, much more than the psychoanalytic notion of drive, to observational and experimental research to identify the activating and terminating conditions of behavioural responses.[103] For instance, Bowlby grudgingly acknowledged, it can happen that babies stop crying when they are exhausted. However, he had no patience with any model of motivation that implied energy or exhaustion. Personally and intellectually, experiences of depletion were generally disavowed by Bowlby, at least until his book on Darwin where they were treated as a symptom of mental illness.[104] He emphasised that babies generally stop crying because the terminating conditions for the crying have been met, for instance when they are picked up.[105] The specific antecedents, processes, and consequences of the crying response and its termination could be studied empirically much more easily than when crying was theorised in terms of psychological energy or drive.

A second reason that the work of the ethologists appealed to Bowlby was that it distinguished between the infants' desire for proximity with familiar caregivers and the desire for nutrition. Lorenz had found that exposure to a familiar moving figure was sufficient to elicit a following response in baby geese, a process he termed 'imprinting'.[106] Lorenz's work was of special interest to Bowlby as it validated his experiences of fatherhood, which suggested that offspring could seek affection and protection from a caregiver based on familiarity, not on the basis of the pleasure of nutrition. The birds studied by Lorenz were not dependent on their parents for food, but could feed themselves by catching insects. Nonetheless, the geese families remained together for at least 12 months.[107] Bowlby discussed these findings with Hinde in 1956, who concluded that they indicated the critical importance of the following

[102] Bowlby, J. (1979) The ten books which have most influenced my thought, 24 October 1979. PP/Bow/A.1/8: 'Robert Hinde (1956) Ethological models and the concept of drive. *British Journal of the Philosophy of Science.* I first met Hinde in 1954 and in the years following read almost all his papers on publication and often before. It was this paper and others of this published around the same time that led me to the concepts of instinctive behaviour presented in *Attachment*.'

[103] Bowlby, J. (1957) An ethological approach to research on child development. *British Journal of Medical Psychology*, 30(4), 230–40.

[104] Bowlby's niece has pointed to Bowlby's disidentification with his disabled younger brother as important in shaping this stance. Hopkins, J. (in press) The need to put things right: a response to Bowlby's chapter 'Hysteria in Children'. *Attachment.* On tiredness as one of the symptoms of Darwin's illness see Bowlby, J. (1990) *Charles Darwin: A Life.* New York: Norton.

[105] A few years later, Ainsworth reported from her Baltimore home observation study that picking a baby up stopped his or her crying 86% of the time: 'this degree of effectiveness is remarkable when one notes that it occurred irrespective of the conditions that activated crying'. Ainsworth, M., Bell, S., & Stayton, D. (1972) Individual differences in the development of some attachment behaviors. *Merrill-Palmer*, 18(2), 123–43, p.132.

[106] Lorenz, K. (1937) The companion in the bird's world. *Auk*, 54, 245–73.

[107] Lorenz, K. (1949, 1952) *King Solomon's Ring.* London: Methuen & Co. Bowlby, J. (1986) Interview with the BBC. PP/Bow/F.5/8: 'First of all you see this following response had nothing to do with food because young geese feed themselves on insects … It's very powerful and these geese families, they stay together for at least 12 months. Very important. So I said well if this is true of some animal species it might be true of humans too.'

response for the safety of offspring, since it emerges even before the sequence of behaviours that would allow a gosling to flee from a threat.[108] This perspective helped Hinde and Bowlby account for findings by animal researchers such as John Paul Scott and Harry Harlow that non-human animals would continue to show a following response, and indeed might intensify their following response, to a caregiver who was unkind or maltreated them.[109]

Whereas Lorenz had depicted 'imprinting' as a mechanism that was either on or off, Hinde's experiments showed that the following response, though initially elicited by a wide range of objects and sounds, was elaborated by practice and subsequently organised around the particular objects that elicited the response. In a passage heavily underlined in Bowlby's personal copy, Hinde made a comparison with the human infant, for whom an incipient following response can often be elicited by even a stranger walking away, a stronger response can be elicited by a sibling, but for whom the full following response will generally occur primarily with a familiar adult caregiver.[110] Though the following response might be primed by the nervous system, it required interaction for its elaboration and specification. For Hinde, this implied that not only behaviour but the motivational response itself was integrated and altered on the basis of experience.

An additional source of discussion between Hinde and Bowlby was the observation by ethologists that behavioural sequences might contain components that are unrelated to the function of the whole. This shed light for the vexed problem of 'infantile sexuality' that had caused significant consternation and confusion for the psychoanalytic community and its publics, especially during the 1930s when Bowlby was training as an analyst.[111] For Bowlby, the work of the ethologists provided an elegant explanation: 'A great tit whilst still a fledgling may, for example, show isolated fragments of reproductive behaviour—snatches of sub-song, nest-building, and copulatory behaviour—but those fragments appear in contexts quite divorced from the context in which they appear in the adult.'[112] Likewise, many of the component sequences of sexual behaviour may well be present in humans already from infancy. And human children can sometimes show these fragments before they become coordinated as the sequences of adult sexual behaviour. However, Bowlby argued, such behaviours do not imply a unitary sexual drive present from birth in all humans.[113]

At a paper read to the Association for the Study of Animal Behaviour in April 1955, Bowlby praised the ethological research community especially for their combination of close observation and evolutionary theory, which led to conceptually precise distinctions between sequences of child to parent safety-seeking responses, parent to child care-providing

[108] Bowlby, J. (1956) Sequence in maturation of drives: notes from discussion with Hinde, August 1956. PP/Bow/H146.

[109] E.g. Harlow, H.F. (1958) The nature of love. *American Psychologist*, 13(12), 673–85; Scott, J.P. (1963) The process of primary socialisation. *Monographs of the Society for Research in Child Development*, 28, 1–47.

[110] Annotations by Bowlby (PP/Bow/H.226) on Hinde, R.A. (1961) The establishment of the parent–offspring relation in birds, with some mammalian analogies. In W.H. Thorpe & O.L. Zangwill (eds) *Current Problems in Animal Behaviour* (pp.175–93). Cambridge: Cambridge University Press.

[111] E.g. Ferenczi, S. (1933, 1980) Confusion of tongues between adults and the child: the language of tenderness and passion. In M. Balint (ed.) *Final Contributions to the Problems and Methods of Psychoanalysis* (pp.156–67). New York: Brunner.

[112] Bowlby, J. (1969, 1982) *Attachment, Volume 1*. London: Penguin, p.157.

[113] This account would, essentially, supplant the psychoanalytic model within the psychoanalytic community over the subsequent decades. Holmes, J. (1998) The changing aims of psychoanalytic psychotherapy: an integrative perspective. *International Journal of Psychoanalysis*, 79, 227–40; Zeuthen, K. & Gammelgaard, J. (2010) Infantile sexuality—the concept, its history and place in contemporary psychoanalysis. *Scandinavian Psychoanalytic Review*, 33(1), 3–12.

responses, and sexuality. Bowlby felt that 'Freud's observations that these are apt to become mixed up with each other, although certainly true, does not necessarily mean that there are not three main responses.'[114] In a later version of this argument, written up for the *British Journal of Medical Psychology* in 1957, Bowlby expressed his exhilaration that ethological researchers were finding common aspects to these behaviour patterns across different species, despite all their vast differences. This raised the prospect that human behaviour, too, could be conceptualised in this way.[115] Behavioural patterns such as child safety-seeking and following responses, care-providing responses, and sexual behaviour might be discerned that, in human evolutionary history, contributed in predictable ways to individual survival or reproductive fitness. This did not mean that the behaviour as seen in any individual member of a species would be serving this function. However, Bowlby felt that this ethological perspective nonetheless offered the potential to shed light on both typical and atypical forms of development in humans.

Discrimination

One quality of following, care provision, and sexual behaviours was that all three seemed to be directed towards preferred targets, even when suitable alternatives were available. In November 1955, Bowlby wrote to the classicist D.C.H. Rieu to ask for help in describing a quality of the following response: 'What I am seeking is a term to denote this tendency to restrict these basic social responses to particular individuals.' He gives the example of the way an infant discerns their mother from among other mothers. Rieu wrote back: 'I think the word you want is "monotropy".'[116] In retrospect there is an important mismatch here. Bowlby was requesting a word to describe the restriction of following behaviour to 'particular individuals'—plural. However, Rieu's term implies the restriction to a single individual—'mono'—of the tendency to 'turn to' the familiar person. It is rather tragic in the fact that Bowlby, whose appeal to ordinary language so often led to misunderstandings of his ideas even as it helped popularise them, unusually sought a new and technical Latinate term on this occasion, but was handed one by Rieu that differed from his request and contributed no less to confusion and polemics.

The term 'monotropy' was first used and defined by Bowlby in a 1958 paper as 'the tendency for instinctual responses to be directed towards a particular individual or group of individuals and not promiscuously towards many'.[117] In a footnote, Bowlby clarifies that the meaning is the same as William James's concept of 'the law of inhibition of instincts by habits', which is the observation that 'when objects of a certain class elicit from an animal a certain sort of reaction, it often happens that the animal becomes partial to the first specimen of the class on which it has reacted'.[118] The idea that 'monotropy' was intended to mean 'restriction on the individuals or groups towards whom a response is directed on the basis of

---

[114] Bowlby, J. (1955) Paper read to the Association for the Study of Animal Behaviour, April 1955. PP/Bow/H.146.

[115] Bowlby, J. (1957) An ethological approach to research on child development. *British Journal of Medical Psychology*, 30(4), 230–40.

[116] Bowlby/Rieu correspondence, November 1955. PP/Bow/H146.

[117] Bowlby, J. (1958) The nature of the child's tie to his mother. *International Journal of Psycho-analysis*, 39(5), 350–73, p.370.

[118] James, W. (1890, 2003) *Psychology: The Briefer Course*. Toronto: Dover Books, p.266.

experience' is also evident in Bowlby's close collaborators, who used the term in this sense.[119] With changes in experience, it is possible for the restriction itself to alter, though this becomes more difficult with time; there is no implication that attachment is limited to one person, or that it is fixed regardless of later experiences.[120] However, this was certainly not the impression of Bowlby's readers. The reasons for this seem clear. In *Attachment, Volume 1* from 1969, the term appears only once: Bowlby referred his reader back to this 1958 discussion for the meaning of this term, but summarised this earlier account of monotropy briefly—and inaccurately—as 'the bias of a child to attach himself especially to one figure'.[121]

It is this latter characterisation that was the public understanding of the term and of Bowlby's position, supported by the literal implication of the word 'monotropy'. This implication became a natural rallying point for Bowlby's critics, as 'monotropy' neatly encapsulated within one word the complicity between Bowlby's dense and scholarly theory and the polemical claims in his popular writings about mothers' natural responsibilities. Later attachment researchers have worked hard to dispel the idea that attachment theory implies monotropy in this sense,[122] but this has been a slow and incomplete process. Some things are, unfortunately, irretrievable. Apparently unaware of his characterisation of the term in *Attachment, Volume 1*, and of the consequences of his appeals to the natural role of mothers in his popular writings of the 1950s, from the 1970s onwards Bowlby expressed dismay that critics insisted on making him a 'straw man', seeking to discredit him through inaccurate characterisation of his discussion of monotropy. He disagreed vehemently with critics who supposed that he introduced the term to imply attachment only to the biological mother, and expressed bafflement in his private notes as to the origin of this view, which he regarded as 'nonsense'.[123]

In fact, 'monotropy' was intended by Bowlby as a technical term for the way that experience leads a response to become oriented towards particular targets. For Bowlby, 'monotropy' was intended to mean a relationship to a particular 'person or place or thing' that is personally significant, based on a felt sense of need, and not superficial or interchangeable with other people, places, or things even if they are somewhat similar.[124] We cherish certain people, places, or things and not others, and this is part of what it is to cherish. This is in contrast to forms of 'liking' where the targets are interchangeable, without hierarchy, but our investment in them is also bloodless. In an unpublished text from 1955 'Notes on child attachment and monotropy', Bowlby wrote: 'Focusing of instinctive responses on individuals. This is the rule—not the exception and allies to all three basic social responses'—presumably

[119] E.g. Hinde (1986) *Ethology*. New York: Fontana, p.230.

[120] See also Hinde, R.A. (1963) The nature of imprinting. In B.M. Foss (ed.) *Determinants of Infant Behaviour*, Vol. 2 (pp.227–30). London: Methuen.

[121] Bowlby, J. (1969, 1982) *Attachment, Volume 1*. London: Penguin, p.249.

[122] See e.g. van IJzendoorn, M.H., Sagi, A., & Lambermon, M.W.E. (1992) The multiple caregiver paradox. Some Dutch and Israeli data. In R.C. Pianta (ed.) *New Directions for Child Development, No. 57. Beyond the Parent: The Role of Other Adults in Children's Lives* (pp.5–25). San Francisco: Jossey-Bass.; Cassidy, J. (1999) The nature of the child's ties. In J. Cassidy & P.R. Shaver (eds) *Handbook of Attachment: Theory, Research, and Clinical Applications* (pp.3–21). New York: Guilford.

[123] Bowlby's correspondence with Peter K. Smith, PP/Bow/J.9/184, discussing Smith, P.K. (1980) Shared care of young children: alternative models to monotropism. *Merrill-Palmer Quarterly of Behavior and Development*, 26(4), 371–89. See also Bowlby's correspondence with Michael Rutter, PP/Bow/J.9.161-2.

[124] Indeed, Bowlby offered the speculative claim that such relationships are the basis for all that constitutes 'deep feeling' within human life. Bowlby, J. (1960) Separation anxiety. *International Journal of Psycho-Analysis*, 41, 89–113: 'It is because of this marked tendency to monotropy that we are capable of deep feelings; for to have a deep attachment to a person (or place or thing) is to have taken them as the terminating object of our instinctual responses.' (101)

child-to-parent following, parent-to-child care, and sexuality—and 'it is in the nature of the instinctive response to focus on an individual, though this may be everything from complete to very partial'.[125] As such, ' "monotropy" is only a special case of discrimination becoming heightened through learning'. The term 'discrimination' captures Bowlby's intention better than monotropy, in fact—and indeed was preferred by Ainsworth.[126]

In the discussions of the 'Psychobiology of the Child' study group at the World Health Organisation in the 1950s, and then later in *Separation* in 1973, Bowlby argued that the discrimination of particular figures occurs in the case of all the basic behavioural responses. The sexual response, for example, is not evoked indiscriminately in adults by any potential stimulus, but has been trained by experience to become restricted to certain kinds of people or situations.[127] There is likewise discrimination in the 'flight' response. We have particular people that make us feel safe, who we turn to when worried or scared.[128] Bowlby made an argument for 'the following response' as another such basic behavioural response, where discrimination occurs regarding its target. Though his focus was on people, Bowlby allowed that objects can also be treated as targets of following and clinging, and sought for 'the intense sense of reassuring comfort' that they can, at least in some regards, provide.[129] Elsewhere Bowlby added that we also have particular institutions, ideas, and places—such as our nation or our place of prayer[130]—that are discriminated by the flight and following responses as signifying safety, which we might seek when alarmed.

Tinbergen called attachments to things or locations in the physical environment 'site attachment', and Bowlby the 'personal environment to which we are attached' in *Separation*.[131] 'Home' as an idea and as a location is a clear example. Bowlby acknowledged that though his focus was generally on 'distress felt and expressed when a person, particularly a child, is separated from his mother figure, distress is felt also on separation from certain familiar objects of other kinds. Attachment to a particular house and environs as home is usual in humans (as it is in animals of other species).'[132] Gruneau Brulin and Granqvist have argued

---

[125] Bowlby, J. (*c*.1955) Notes on child attachment and monotropy. PP/Bow/H146.

[126] E.g. Ainsworth, M. (1964) Patterns of attachment behavior shown by the infant in interaction with his mother. *Merrill-Palmer*, 10(1), 51–58, p.56. More recently, Lyons-Ruth and the Boston Change Process Study Group have suggested describing these discriminated relationships as 'charged'. For them, 'charged' relationships are characterized by some underlying valuation, their priority over other relationships, and sufficient continuity to scaffold trust. Boston Change Process Study Group (2018) Engagement and the emergence of a charged other. *Contemporary Psychoanalysis*, 54(3), 540–59.

[127] Bowlby cited in Tanner, J.M. & Inhelder, B. (1956) *Discussions on Child Development: Proceedings of the WTO Study Group of the Psychobiological Development of the Child*, Vol 1. London: Tavistock, pp.184–5; Bowlby, J. (1973) *Separation*. London: Pimlico. See also Bowlby, J. (1969, 1982) *Attachment, Volume 1*. London: Penguin, pp.137–8.

[128] Bowlby, cited in Tanner, J.M. & Inhelder, B. (1956) *Discussions on Child Development: Proceedings of the WTO Study Group of the Psychobiological Development of the Child*, Vol 1. London: Tavistock, pp.184–5.

[129] Bowlby, J. (1973) *Separation: Anxiety and Anger*. New York: Basic Books: 'Laughlin (1956) has proposed a new term "soteria", as an obverse of phobia, to denote the intense sense of reassuring comfort that a person may get from a "love object", be it a toy ...' (148).

[130] Bowlby, J. (1956) The growth of independence in the young child. *Royal Society of Health Journal*, 76, 587–91, p.589.

[131] Tinbergen, N. (1956) The functions of territory. *Bird Study*, 4(1), 14–27; Bowlby, J. (1973) *Separation: Anxiety and Anger*. New York: Basic Books: 'It is still too little realized, perhaps, that the individuals of a species, so far from roaming at random throughout the whole area of the earth's surface ecologically suitable to them, usually spend the whole of their lives within an extremely restricted segment of it, known as the home range ... each individual has its own relatively small and very distinctive personal environment to which it is attached' (177).

[132] Bowlby, J. (undated) Distress at loss of home: Chapter 3. *c*.1969–1971. PP/Bow/H.55. See also Bowlby, J. (1965) Attachment behaviour: a note after Ciba 1965. Revised Note January 1966. PP/Bow/H.146: 'Further definition of attachment: equilibrium point is proximity to a certain type of object ... Consider also habitat attachment.' It must be acknowledged, however, that Bowlby was inconsistent on this point. Likely in an attempt to hack away at the thicket of wider connotations of the word 'attachment', he came to emphasize that the object of an attachment

that attachment to 'home' is simply a secondary effect of its association with family and attachment figures.[133] This claim seems overstated: the very concepts of a secure base and safe haven (Chapter 2) are metaphors for territorial movement, away from and back to a base in the context of potential threat.[134] Nonetheless, most of Bowlby's published works focus narrowly on attachment relationships with parents, allowing other attachments such as siblings or to home to slide into the background. Such issues would both have to be rediscovered by later researchers, spurred by the primacy of these concerns in fields such as social work and in ecological approaches.[135] Furthermore, Bowlby was unclear regarding what processes exactly led to the discrimination of attachment figures. Main and Fonagy admonished Bowlby for this.[136] In the 1990s, they later argued that discrimination and the basis for selective attachments occur especially when someone, or something, is perceived as contingently responsive to us.

Following and attachment

In historical perspective, without access to comparisons with animal behaviour, and to Robert Hinde in particular, it seems likely that there would have been no attachment theory. This was also Bowlby's own view.[137] Though use of the phrase has dropped away since the mid-1990s, in the 1970s and 1980s researchers used 'ethological attachment theory' as the official name for the paradigm as a way to 'commemorate the influence of ethological theory and research on Bowlby's early thinking'.[138] Key strengths of Bowlby's thinking can be found

relationship had to be human. Stevenson-Hinde, J. (2007) Attachment theory and John Bowlby: some reflections. *Attachment & Human Development*, 9(4), 337–42: 'During the first conference, I recall John emphatically stating, "We cannot allow 'attachment to an umbrella'!" He insisted that "attachment" be used to describe an emotional bond to someone (i.e., a person) usually perceived as older or wiser (e.g., mother or father). While other kinds of bonds undoubtedly exist, they should not be called "attachment," in order to keep some precision in the use of terms' (338). This, exclamation, of course, produces an excluded middle: our feelings for our home are neither the trivial affection we might feel for a favourite umbrella, nor the feelings we have for a parent.

[133] Gruneau Brulin, J. & Granqvist, P. (2018) The place of place within the attachment-religion framework: a commentary on the circle of place spirituality. *Research in the Social Scientific Study of Religion*, 29, 175–85.

[134] The claim that home cannot be a secure base or safe haven would seem to depend on a reification of 'attachment relationship' beyond its constituent elements. Gruneau Brulin and Granqvist claim that home is non-individual, which is implausible. They also claim that it cannot be an object of attachment since it is non-reciprocal. However, reciprocity was never part of either Bowlby or Ainsworth's definition of an attachment relationship.

[135] On attachment to place see e.g. Scannell, L. & Gifford, R. (2013) Comparing the theories of interpersonal and place attachment. In L.C. Manzo & P. Devine-Wright (eds) *Place Attachment. Advances in Theory, Methods and Applications* (pp.23–36). London: Routledge. On attachment to siblings see e.g. Teti, D.M. & Ablard, K.E. (1989) Security of attachment and infant–sibling relationships: a laboratory study. *Child Development*, 1519–28; Farnfield, S. (2009) A modified strange situation procedure for use in assessing sibling relationships and their attachment to carers. *Adoption & Fostering*, 33(1), 4–17.

[136] Fonagy, P., Steele, M., Steele, H., Higgitt, A., & Target, M. (1994) The Emanuel Miller memorial lecture 1992: the theory and practice of resilience. *Journal of Child Psychology and Psychiatry*, 35(2), 231–57; Main, M. (1999) Epilogue. Attachment theory: eighteen points with suggestions for future studies. In J. Cassidy & P. Shaver (eds) *Handbook of Attachment* (pp.845–87). New York: Guilford, p.848.

[137] E.g. Bowlby, J. (1991) Ethological light on psychoanalytic problems. In P. Bateson (ed.) *The Development and Integration of Behaviour: Essays in Honour of Robert Hinde* (pp.301–14). Cambridge: Cambridge University Press: 'The typed drafts of major parts of the first edition of his [Hinde's] *Animal Behaviour* (1966) which he lent me in 1965 when I was starting work on my volume on *Attachment* (1969). Whatever merits my own volume has owed a tremendous debt to his' (303).

[138] Waters, E., Kondo-Ikemura, K., Posada, G., and Richters, J.E. (1991) Learning to love. In M.R. Gunnar & L.A. Sroufe (eds) *Self Processes and Development* (pp.217–55). New York: Psychology Press, p.227. Ainsworth, M. & Bowlby, J. (1991) 1989 APA award recipient addresses: an ethological approach to personality development.

precisely in the revision of psychoanalytic theory on the basis of ethology: the differentiation of behavioural responses; the care in thinking about value of behaviour for the individual and for the species; recognition that the predisposition for certain responses may come pre-programmed but that their expression requires elaboration in the context of experience and learning; the privilege given to observational methodology; and the specification of the following response in birds and mammals, and in comparison with humans.[139] This is a large chunk of attachment theory.

Whereas Bowlby made appeal to the idea of 'love' throughout the 1950s in both his popular and scientific works—most importantly in *Child Care and the Growth of Love*—from 1961 the term was expunged from his vocabulary.[140] Hinde's contribution had made Bowlby acutely aware that the term was too absorptive, that it hid within itself profoundly diverse processes with different causes and consequences. Clinical experience had taught Bowlby time and again that humans can love fiercely even while we fail one another; we can seek comfort even in the absence of love; we can experience affection as claustrophobic and dangerous, as holding us captive.[141] It may appear that 'love' designates an intense and determinate feeling. In fact, however, the term is more a magnet and placeholder for complex and diverse intensities. Even if appeal to 'love' could help Bowlby with intelligibility and plausibility to his readers, Hinde's precise conceptualisation of motivation had shown the necessity of going beyond evocative euphemism. Michael Rutter later situated the replacement of 'love' with 'attachment' as one of the most important landmarks in the history of attachment research.[142]

However, the establishment of attachment theory on the foundation of Hinde's account of the following response also generated problems. Hinde was discussing a specific behavioural pattern: the following, greeting, and clinging response shown by offspring to their parents. And Bowlby and Ainsworth were both insistent that literal following and bodily clinging were essential referents of the term 'attachment'.[143] However, the concept was fused into the metapsychology of psychoanalytic theory, with its focus on the emotional and symbolic

American Psychologist, 46(4), 333–41: 'The distinguishing characteristic of the theory of attachment that we have jointly developed is that it is an ethological approach' (333).

[139] See e.g. Bowlby, J. (1963) Remarks at the MRC Ethology Meeting organised by Bowlby, 23 May 1963. PP/Bow/D.6/5: 'The role of a comparative approach: a) in facilitating observation b) in elucidating the evolution of behaviour c) in taxonomy d) in providing a basis for generalisation e) in leading to an understanding of function' (3).

[140] Bowlby, R. (2017) Growing up with attachment theory—a personal view. *Psychodynamic Psychiatry*, 45(4), 431–9: 'When my father sat down he told us that he was looking for a new term to replace [a] child's "tie." He said the image of a child being tied to mother or mother being tied to a child had become socially unacceptable, and he was thinking of using the child's "attachment" instead. We all groaned and said how boring and why couldn't he use "love" like he had originally? He explained that "love" was not strictly accurate and anyway he had already decided he was going to use attachment from then on' (436).

[141] Bowlby, J. (1985) *Letter to John Byng-Hall*, 12 April 1985. PP/Bow/J.9/45.

[142] Rutter, M., Kreppner, J., & Sonuga-Barke, E. (2009) Emanuel Miller lecture: attachment insecurity, disinhibited attachment, and attachment disorders: where do research findings leave the concepts? *Journal of Child Psychology and Psychiatry*, 50(5), 529–43. In fact, 'love' would always be threatening to return, hammering at the door of attachment research. This was especially the case for the social psychology tradition (Chapter 5), e.g. Hazan, C. & Shaver, P. (1987) Romantic love conceptualized as an attachment process. *Journal of Personality and Social Psychology*, 52(3), 511–24. However, appeal to 'love' is also a feature in some work in the developmental tradition of attachment research. For instance, 'loving' would be one of the scales of the Adult Attachment Interview, and used in the assessment of transcripts as 'earned secure' (Chapter 3).

[143] E.g. Ainsworth, M. (1967) *Infancy in Uganda*. Baltimore: The Johns Hopkins Press: 'Attachment is more than a discrimination between people and implies something far more active—a literal or figurative seeking out, fastening on' (440).

meanings of parent–child relationships.[144] On the one hand, this gave the ethological concept of 'following' a much deeper emotional resonance. On the other hand, it gave a psychoanalytic model greater behavioural specification. The resulting concept, 'attachment', ended up with both narrow and broad meanings (Chapters 2 and 5).[145] Narrowly, attachment could mean the following response and related actions that serve to monitor and maintain access to the caregiver; broadly, the same term could mean an emotionally invested relationship, as a symbolic source of comfort and protection. Bowlby shuttled between these distinct meanings, sometimes intending one, sometimes the other, and sometimes both.

Though this certainly contributed to conceptual muddle, the basis for this movement was in Bowlby's attempts to capture, as best he could, the expression of a cross-species phenomenon in human beings, a species with particular capacities for symbolisation and shared meanings.[146] In Bowlby's unpublished writings and correspondence of the 1950s, his dissatisfaction is visible with this predicament.[147] His basic referent for an expression of the attachment system was of infant proximity-seeking in the context of distress as a means of eliciting care. Part of his positioning against psychoanalytic theory was his emphasis on observable interactions. Yet, for example, he wished to maintain that a widow or widower who experiences security and comfort in remembering their spouse is likewise benefiting from a real and ongoing attachment relationship, even if this is now solely at a symbolic level.[148] Between these two extremes, he knew that most attachment relationships after toddlerhood would have elements of the basic behavioural system and of its symbolic elaboration: 'A child separated from his mother comes to crave both for her love and for its accompanying

---

[144] The centrality of symptom formation through symbolization in psychoanalysis was established in Breuer, J. & Freud, S. (1893–95, 2001) Studies on hysteria. In *The Standard Edition of the Complete Psychological Works of Sigmund Freud*, Vol. 2 (pp.1–305). London: Vintage. Bowlby was especially interested by Rycroft, C. (1956) Symbolism and its relationship to the primary and secondary processes. *International Journal of Psycho-Analysis*, 37, 137–46, and had correspondence with the author (PP/Bow/H.116). Part of the significance of Rycroft's work on symbolization for Bowlby was that it showed that 'the emphasis placed in Kleinian theory on the fact that "psychical reality" and "external reality" are both subjectively real does, I think, tend to obscure the fact that there are none the less essential differences between them, and that psychical reality is itself divisible into one part which is developmentally bound to external reality and another which has been formed by idealization' (141).

[145] For an example of Bowlby taking away implications for relationships in general from a discussion with Hinde of specific aspects of the following response see e.g. Bowlby, J. (1957) Discussion with Hinde, January 1957. PP/ Bow/H.128: 'Attachment behaviour comprises all those responses which subserve the total task of relating to another human being.'

[146] The capacity for symbolization was, in a sense, highlighted by Main and colleagues' 'move to the level of representation' (Chapter 3). However, Main and colleagues did not distinguish the cross-species ethological aspects of attachment from those aspects associated with human symbolic capabilities. Implicit acknowledgement of the issue also appeared in the 1990s in the writings of researchers focused on intersubjectivity and rhythms of parent–infant interaction, e.g. Beebe, B., Lachmann, F., & Jaffe, J. (1997) Mother–infant interaction structures and presymbolic self- and object representations. *Psychoanalytic Dialogues*, 7(2), 133–82; Trevarthen, C. (1998) The concept and foundations of infant intersubjectivity. In S. Braten (ed.) *Intersubjective Communication and Emotion in Early Ontogeny* (pp.15–46). Cambridge: Cambridge University Press. However, concepts of intersubjectivity and rhythm emphasize continuities between presymbolic procedural expectations in relationships and the symbolic capacities that emerge from them. The distinction and potential disjuncture between presymbolic and symbolic senses of the concept of 'attachment' was not drawn out. In the history of attachment research, this distinction appears to have first been made focally and clearly in the application of attachment theory to religious life: Kirkpatrick, L.A. (1999) Attachment and religious representations and behavior. In J. Cassidy & P.R. Shaver (eds) *Handbook of Attachment: Theory, Research, and Clinical Applications* (pp.803–22). New York: Guilford.

[147] E.g. Bowlby, J. (not dated, c.1955) Thought, conceptualization, language, psycho-analysis. PP/BOW/H.115; Bowlby, J. (1955) *Letter to C.F. Rycroft*, 26 April 1955. PP/Bow/H.116.

[148] Bowlby, J. (1980) *Loss*. New York: Basic Books, p.243. The confusion evoked by this stance for later interpretations of Bowlby is detailed in Fraley, C.R. & Shaver, P.R. (2016) Attachment, loss, and grief: Bowlby's views, new developments, and current controversies. In J. Cassidy & P.R. Shaver (eds) *Handbook of Attachment: Theory, Research, and Clinical Applications* (3rd edn, pp.40–62). New York: Guilford.

symbols.'[149] However, the interrelation between cross-species behavioural system and the symbolic elaboration especially characteristic of humans remained a source of theoretical and terminological problems for him, firmly tangled up within his use of the word 'attachment', as well as his difficulties in rooting the mind in the body.[150]

Another conceptual issue made a potent contribution to this confusion. In Bowlby's writings, the *broad* notion of attachment was generally used alongside, specifically, a *narrower* concept of internal working model—to mean the specific symbolic and affective representations made by humans about attachment figures and their availability, and the value of the self to these attachment figures. By contrast, when Bowlby used the concept of attachment *narrowly* to mean the specific ethological following response, it was accompanied by a *broader* concept of internal working model—to mean expectations about the other's likely availability in response to attachment behaviour.[151] This is how infants, puppies, and lambs can have 'internal working models' in *Attachment, Volume 1* even without the capacity for much representational thought: the concept was being used in this second sense, not the first. This is also why more ethologically oriented attachment researchers, such as Kobak, define internal working models very simply as expectations about attachment figures and how interaction with them will go,[152] whereas less ethologically oriented attachment researchers require more elaborate interpretations (Chapter 5).

Already in the 1960s, Hinde was very worried by Bowlby's misleading use of broad and narrow meanings of the concepts of attachment and internal working model. He felt that 'behaviour is diverse: an attempt to squeeze it into a system involving only a few explanatory concepts is liable to lead to one of two results—either facts which do not fit will be ignored, or the concepts will be stretched until they become valueless'.[153] Hinde tried to warn Bowlby, arguing for greater precision in use of the term 'attachment' and what it meant for interpreting observable behaviour. For instance, with early drafts and ideas from *Attachment, Volume 1* in hand, Hinde expressed concern with the way Bowlby was conceptualizing the terminating conditions of attachment behaviour, and the idea of internal working models. He wrote to Bowlby in 1967 directly: 'I think that you sometimes reify the concepts that you are using for explanation as though they were mechanisms.'[154]

[149] Bowlby, J. (1944) Forty-four juvenile thieves: their characters and home-life (II). *International Journal of Psycho-Analysis*, 25, 107–28, p.121.

[150] On this latter point, criticisms of Bowlby are presented by Fonagy, P. & Target, M. (2007) The rooting of the mind in the body: new links between attachment theory and psychoanalytic thought. *Journal of the American Psychoanalytic Association*, 55(2), 411–56. However, Fonagy and Target did not adequately recognize the polysemy of Bowlby's concept of attachment, which hindered their own discussion of attachment and mentalization.

[151] Note Bowlby's wording in his very definition of internal working models as 'starting, we may suppose, towards the end of his first year', in a procedural form, and as developing into but conceptually distinguishable from semantically elaborated internal working models 'during his second and third when [the child] acquires the powerful and extraordinary gift of language'. Bowlby, J. (1969) *Attachment*. London: Penguin, p.353.

[152] Kobak, R. & Esposito, A. (2004) Levels of processing in parent–child relationships: implications for clinical assessment and treatment. In L. Atkinson & S. Goldberg (eds) *Attachment Issues in Psychopathology and Interventions* (pp. 139–66). Mahwah, NJ: Lawrence Erlbaum, p.140.

[153] Hinde, R. (1957) Consequences and goals: some issues raised by Dr Kortland's paper on aspects and prospects of the concept of instinct. *British Journal of Animal Behaviour*, 5, 116–18, p.116.

[154] Hinde, R. (1967) *Letter to John Bowlby*, 28 June 1967. PP/Bow/K.4/11. Hinde would later make the observation in print, looking back on Bowlby's overall contribution to the study of behaviour in Hinde, R. (1991) Relationships, attachment and culture: a tribute to John Bowlby. *Infant Mental Health*, 12(3), 154–63; and Hinde, R. (1991) Commentary. In P. Bateson (ed.) *The Development and Integration of Behaviour: Essays in Honour of Robert Hinde* (pp.411–18). Cambridge: Cambridge University Press.

Seeing insufficient change in Bowlby's stance, in a 1982 chapter Hinde criticised Bowlby on this matter in print. He argued against the implication in Bowlby's writing that evolution had wired human infants to seek proximity as the sole strategy for achieving the set-goal of the attachment behavioural system. This seemed implausible. Natural selection, Hinde felt, would likely 'favour individuals with a range of potential styles from which they select appropriately'.[155] Whilst direct proximity-seeking might be regarded as the desirable response in many circumstances, Hinde emphasised that survival of infants would be more likely if they could adapt to the conditions of care in which they found themselves. They therefore needed alternative strategies for other conditions. Hinde therefore anticipated that evolution would have given humans a repertoire of 'conditional strategies' for responding to caregiving environments where direct proximity-seeking was not possible or effective.[156] The availability of conditional strategies could be anticipated to contribute to survival under such circumstances.

The emphasis on proximity as the goal of the infant attachment behavioural system also had discrepancies with Ainsworth's empirical findings. As Chapter 2 documents, in the 1960s Ainsworth noticed that some infants—those she labelled B1—clearly achieved termination of the attachment behavioural system *without* proximity. Ainsworth also found other infants—who she labelled C—who did not achieve termination of the attachment behavioural system even when they *did* gain proximity, and continued to exhibit behaviours seemingly aiming to retain the attention of their caregiver. Citing Ainsworth's observations as inspiration, across the 1970s and 1980s researchers demonstrated empirically that the caregiver's physical availability facilitated infant exploration in a novel room less effectively than the caregiver's emotional and attentional availability.[157]

Nonetheless, 'proximity' remained enshrined in theory as the terminating condition of the attachment behavioural system; it was only late in his career that Bowlby consistently amended his descriptions of the attachment behavioural system in infancy to specify that it could be terminated by the 'availability', not simply proximity, of the caregiver.[158] However, by this time, a generation of attachment researchers had come of age. For instance

---

[155] Hinde, R.A. (1982) Attachment: some conceptual and biological issues. In C.M. Parkes & J. Stevenson-Hinde (eds) *The Place of Attachment in Human Behavior* (pp.60–76). London: Tavistock, p.71.

[156] Ibid.

[157] Carr, S.J., Dabbs Jr, J.M., & Carr, T.S. (1975) Mother–infant attachment: the importance of the mother's visual field. *Child Development*, 46(2), 331–8; Sorce, J.F. & Emde, R.N. (1981) Mother presence is not enough: effect of emotional availability on infant exploration. *Developmental Psychology*,17(6), 737–45. See also Joffe, L.S., Vaughn, B.E., Barglow, P., & Benveniste, R. (1985) Biobehavioral antecedents in the development of infant–mother attachment. In M. Reite & T. Field (eds) *The Psychobiology of Attachment and Separation* (pp.323–49). Orlando, FL: Academic Press.

[158] A first acknowledgement appears in Bowlby, J. (1973) *Separation: Anxiety and Anger*. New York: Basic Books: 'Accessibility in itself is not enough. Not only must an attachment figure be accessible but he, or she, must be willing to respond in an appropriate way; in regard to someone who is afraid this means willingness to act as comforter and protector. Only when an attachment figure is both accessible and potentially responsive can he, or she, be said to be truly available. In what follows, therefore, the word 'available' is to be understood as implying that an attachment figure is both accessible and responsive' (234). Throughout the 1970s, Bowlby tended still to refer to proximity as the set-goal of the attachment system. His final word, however, is in Bowlby, J. (1991) Ethological light on psychoanalytic problems. In P. Bateson (ed.) *The Development and Integration of Behaviour: Essays in Honour of Robert Hinde* (pp.301–14). Cambridge: Cambridge University Press: 'The goal of attachment behaviour is to maintain certain degrees of proximity to, or of communication with, the discriminated attachment figure(s)' (306). Some of the tensions in Bowlby's account of the set-goal of the attachment system had been discussed already by Bretherton, I. (1980) Young children in stressful situations: the supporting role of attachment figures and unfamiliar caregivers. In G.V. Coelho & P. Ahmed (eds) *Uprooting and Attachment* (pp.179–210). New York: Plenum Press.

'disorganised/disoriented attachment' had already been established by Main and Solomon as behaviour suggesting disruption in an infant's proximity-seeking (Chapter 3).[159] Likewise, severe conceptual difficulties had been experienced as the field attempted to extend Bowlby's model into adulthood (Chapter 5). For instance, in the 1970s Bob Marvin observed patterns of availability-seeking in otherwise secure-seeming three and four year olds in the Strange Situation that did not rely on proximity. This seemed developmentally expectable. Nonetheless, because proximity was not sought by the children in the Strange Situation, in attempting to square his observations with Bowlby's stated theory, he was improbably forced to wonder whether these were even attachment relationships.[160]

As well as his insistence on proximity as the terminating condition for following, a portion of the confusion lay in Bowlby's use of the term 'attachment'. As Rutter later observed, the word 'attachment' was used by Bowlby 'to refer to discrete patterns of behaviour (such as proximity-seeking), to a dyadic relationship, to a postulated inbuilt predisposition to develop specific attachments to individuals, and to the hypothesised internal controlling mechanisms for this predisposition'.[161] 'Attachment' (inbuilt predisposition) means that children show 'attachment' (discrete behaviours) within 'attachments' (dyadic relationships). How does this happen? Attachment! (a hypothesised internal controlling mechanism). Where the different meanings of the term are not clearly held in mind and distinguished, the result is a recipe for clouded and for circular thinking, and a weak basis for identifying theoretical differences and deviations. Bowlby and subsequent attachment researchers only came to acknowledge the contribution of the sprawling connotations of the term 'attachment' to misappropriations of the theoretical tradition in the 1970s. By this time the term, swollen as if infected, had come to define the research paradigm as a whole, and was inextricable.[162]

Ambiguities about the meaning of 'attachment' as the headline concept for Bowlby's theory have had a widespread legacy. Charles and Alexander expressed concern that Bowlby's varied and underspecified uses of the term 'attachment' have permitted many spurious forms of therapy to claim a basis in the subsequent attachment research paradigm.[163] Likewise, where reference to 'attachment' appears within social policy, it is common to find circular and confused reasoning, with the term—and the associated research paradigm—invoked for various

---

[159] Still by 1990 Main was adamant that physical touch with the caregiver was ultimately the set-goal of the attachment system in infancy. Main, M. (1990) Parental aversion to infant-initiated contact is correlated with the parent's own rejection during childhood: the effects of experience on signals of security with respect to attachment. In T.B. Brazelton & K. Barnard (eds) *Touch* (pp.461–95). New York: International Universities Press.

[160] Marvin, R.S. (1977) An ethological–cognitive model for the attenuation of mother–child attachment behavior. In T.M. Alloway, L. Krames, and P. Pliner (eds) *Advances in the Study of Communication and Affect*, Vol. 3 (pp.25–60). New York: Plenum Press, pp.56–7.

[161] Rutter, M. (1995) Clinical implications of attachment concepts: retrospect and prospect. *Journal of Child Psychology and Psychiatry*, 36(4), 549–71, p.551. See also Stern, D. (1985) *The Interpersonal World of the Infant*. New York: Basic Books: 'Attachment is a set of infant behaviours, a motivational system, a relationship between mother and infant, a theoretical construct, and a subjective experience for the infant' (25).

[162] From the 1970s onwards, Bowlby tested out referring to 'care-seeking' rather than 'attachment behaviour', e.g. Bowlby, J. (1986) Attachment, life-span and old age. In J. Munnichs & B. Miesen (eds) *Attachment, Life-Span and Old Age*. Utrecht: Van Loghum, p.11.

[163] Charles, G. & Alexander, C. (2014) Beyond attachment: mattering and the development of meaningful moments. *Relational Child and Youth Care Practice*, 27(3), 26–30: 'Herein lies another problem with "attachment." It is one of those terms which we all think we understand the meaning of but when we actually examine it we find that it has significantly different meanings for different people … Today the term is often a loose metaphor for a relationship-based intervention, and those using the term do not necessarily have an accurate understanding of the concept. The absence of a precise and universally understood definition has led to a wide variety of interpretations of what is a practical "attachment intervention." For example, there are a number of controversial "attachment" treatments based on various forms of "therapeutic holding"' (27).

purposes so long as they can align with the idea of the importance of child–caregiver rela-tionships. So, for instance, in the UK, since the 2010s there have been consistent appeals to Bowlby and the idea of attachment by the political right, who have argued that a policy focus on the early years justifies cuts to other public services, with attachment security presented as an alternative to social security.[164] Much the same goes for 'attachment parenting' dis-courses that, in fact, lack an evidence-base or anything but the most selective and strategic relationship with the tradition of attachment research, and that play off cultural stereotypes about motherhood.[165] Given the common use of the 'attachment' label and the gulf that sep-arates attachment research from these 'attachment parenting' discourses, Ross Thompson observed that 'if you talk to attachment researchers, you will find involuntary wincing—sometimes followed by groaning—when someone brings up attachment parenting'.[166]

Separation

Forty-four thieves

Bowlby's discussions with Hinde and his emerging model of attachment were fed by and in turn contributed to a concern with the role of long-term separations in childhood for subsequent development. Bowlby regarded himself as predisposed to an interest in major separations by his own childhood experiences, such as being sent to boarding school.[167] This interest was then intensified by his early experiences as a clinician. From the late 1930s, Bowlby began work in the London Child Guidance Clinic. Soon after his arrival he saw two cases, one after the other, where the child had been referred for conduct problems.

---

[164] Duschinsky, R., Greco, M., & Solomon, J. (2015) Wait up! Attachment and sovereign power. *International Journal of Politics, Culture, and Society*, 28(3), 223–42. The polyvalence of attachment as a political discourse should be highlighted, however. For uses of attachment theory for a social agenda more aligned with the political left see e.g. Kraemer, S. & Roberts, J. (1996) *The Politics of Attachment: Towards a Secure Society*. London: Free Association Books. There are also a variety of policy texts invoking attachment without a marked political agenda, and instead using the term in a general sense to characterize the value of 'positive' parent–child relationships. See e.g. Scottish Government (2012) *National Parenting Strategy: Making a Positive Difference to Children and Young People through Parenting*. Edinburgh: Scottish Government.

[165] 'Attachment parenting' is one of the most powerful discourses of intensive parenting. It was introduced by Bill and Martha Sears (1993) in *The Baby Book: Everything You Need to Know about your Baby* (Boston: Little and Brown). The Sears already had their ideas in place, but initially called them 'immersion parenting'. Use of the idea of attachment and appeal to Bowlby's authority was post-hoc and strategic, made available by Bowlby's ambiguous and overgeneral statements about the dangers of separation and the need for mothers to spend time with their baby: 'At a talk one time in Pasadena, a grandmother came up to Bill and said she thought the term immersion mothering was a good one, because some moms find themselves "in over their heads." When he told me of this, I realized we needed to change the term to something more positive, so we came up with AP, since the Attachment Theory literature was so well researched and documented, by John Bowlby and others' (http://attachedattheheart. attachmentparenting.org/faq/). On the weak evidence for 'attachment parenting' and its lack of a link with at-tachment research see Chaffin, M. (2006) Report of the APSAC Task Force on Attachment Therapy, Reactive Attachment Disorder, and Attachment Problems. *Child Maltreatment*, 11(1), 76–89; Fairclough, C. (2013) The problem of 'attachment'. In E. Lee, J. Bristow, C. Faircloth, & J. Macvarish (eds) *Parenting Culture Studies* (pp.147–64). London: Palgrave.

[166] Keller, H. & Thompson, R. (2018) Attachment theory: past, present & future. Recorded at the 2nd 'Wilhelm Wundt Dialogue', 28 November 2018, Leipzig University, hosted by the Leipzig Research Center for Early Child Development (LFE). https://www.youtube.com/watch?v=_nG5SelEj28.

[167] Bowlby, J. (1990, 2015) John Bowlby: an interview by Virginia Hunter. *Attachment*, 9, 138–57, p.147. See also Van Dijken, S. (1998) *John Bowlby, his Early Life: A Biographical Journey into the Roots of Attachment Theory*. New York: Free Association Books.

Both had been caught stealing, but more generally were considered rude and disobedient. Bowlby was curious that both of these children had spent nine months in hospital for fever when they were toddlers, during which time they were isolated and separated from their caregivers.

During this period, Bowlby was beginning his training in child psychoanalysis, and reading Klein's works carefully. He was questioning her description of 'loss' only as a normative developmental stage, and her inattention to the possibility of actual separation and loss as consequential experiences for a child. Bowlby found support for his concerns in the fact that, in both of these cases from the Child Guidance Clinic, the parents reported that their children were 'emotionally remote' when they returned home from the hospital. Bowlby found it remarkable that 'these stories were extraordinarily similar. So I generalised from a sample of the two ... I found a lot of other cases and the upshot was that I wrote this monograph', 'Forty-Four Juvenile Thieves'.[168] In this paper, published in 1944, Bowlby examined the records of 44 consecutive cases of children who had been caught stealing, but where the relevant authorities had sent the child to the Child Guidance Clinic rather than to court. Half the referrals had come from schools. These children were compared to unselected control cases from the Clinic with no history of stealing. Fourteen of the 44 thieves he described as 'affectionless' types; of these, 12 had experiences of early separation, compared to 10% of the controls. He proposed a general theory that early separation experiences predispose later conduct problems by disrupting the bases of self-worth and capacity for empathy.[169] A more specific, and speculative, theory linked early separations specifically to delinquency and criminal behaviour.[170]

The importance of separation was, as commentators often note, likely made especially salient by Bowlby's observations of evacuated children during World War II, as part of his work on the Cambridge evacuation survey.[171] In unpublished papers written at the time, Bowlby documented the mental health symptoms shown by these children, which

[168] Bowlby, J. (1986) Interview with the BBC. PP/Bow/F.5/8.

[169] Bowlby, J. (1944) Forty-four juvenile thieves: their characters and home-life (II). *International Journal of Psycho-Analysis*, 25, 107–28. An earlier version of the paper, delivered on 30 November 1937, is available as 'Some unconscious motives in habitual pilfering', PP/BOW/C.3/10/2.

[170] The specific theory linking separations to delinquency has not subsequently been well supported. There are, however, few relevant studies. Ryan and colleagues have reported that group care, as opposed to family or foster care, increases the likelihood of criminal activity: Ryan, J.P., Marshall, J.M., Herz, D., & Hernandez, P.M. (2008) Juvenile delinquency in child welfare: investigating group home effects. *Children and Youth Services Review*, 30(9), 1088–99. In the attachment literature, Allen and colleagues found a concurrent relationship between criminal activity and insecurity with the Adult Attachment Interview: Allen, J. P., Hauser, S.T., & Borman-Spurrell, E. (1996) Attachment theory as a framework for understanding sequelae of severe adolescent psychopathology: an 11-year follow-up study. *Journal of Consulting and Clinical Psychology*, 64(2), 254. By contrast, Brennan and Shaver found no association between self-reported attachment style and criminal activity: Brennan, K.A. & Shaver, P.R. (1998) Attachment styles and personality disorders: their connections to each other and to parental divorce, parental death, and perceptions of parental caregiving. *Journal of Personality*, 66(5), 835–78. For a review see also Schimmenti, A. (2020) The developmental roots of psychopathy: an attachment perspective. In S. Itzkowitz & E.F. Howell (eds) *Psychopathy and Human Evil: Psychoanalytic Explorations*. London: Routledge.

[171] This interpretation of Bowlby was first offered in Chodorow, N. (1978) *The Reproduction of Mothering*. Berkeley: University of California Press, p.75. As well as the clinical cases seen at the Child Guidance Clinic, another experience that may have been relevant to Bowlby's attention to the pathogenic role of separations was his training as a child analyst. Whereas at the Child Guidance Clinic Bowlby generally saw children and their primary caregiver or caregivers together, the technique for child analysis in the 1930s was to meet with the child alone. Bowlby would later recall to his former student Victoria Hamilton that he had been upset by the distress he would cause young children, time and time again, as he would separate the children from their caregiver in the waiting room and take them to the consulting room. Hamilton, V. (2007) The nature of a student's tie to the teacher: reminiscences of training and friendship with John Bowlby. *Attachment*, 1, 334–47.

included 'tempers, sullenness, disobedience, stealing, sleeplessness, bed-wetting, timidity, pains of an undefined sort'.[172] They also seemed disoriented when they saw their parents again, which Bowlby suspected was a bad sign.[173] Bowlby attributed the mental health symptoms of the evacuated children to feelings of being abandoned by their parents. However, he noticed that such symptoms were reduced—though still present—among those children billeted with affectionate foster parents. And he observed that such symptoms were more common when children passed through multiple carers or foster homes with very large carer-to-child ratios.[174] Bowlby noted, too, that these symptoms were shown not just by children who missed kind and affectionate parents but also by those children who had cruel or unkind parents. Ultimately, he reflected, 'it must be remembered that even socially bad homes are nevertheless the child's only harbours in life. Without a home a child feels lost.'[175]

An additional factor, rarely mentioned in commentaries on Bowlby, should also be highlighted as contributing to his attention to long-term separations. Examination of the 'Forty-Four Juvenile Thieves' case study reveals that some form of child maltreatment appears in around half of the case studies, alongside the separations. Maltreatment is not mentioned in Bowlby's discussion, however, which focuses solely on separation as the cause of the children's conduct problems.[176] This was done knowingly. Later, in an interview in 1986, Bowlby acknowledged that working with abusive interactions between parents and their children was 'the run of the mill of what we were doing clinically' in the Child Guidance Clinic.[177] For instance, in an unpublished case history, likely from the early or mid-1960s, Bowlby described the case of Martin, who lived with both parents, but whose experiences of physically abusive punishment from his mother contributed to a tendency to turn to his father for comfort when he was alarmed.[178] However, Bowlby reported in the 1986 interview his perception that abusive caregiving could not be turned into a viable research topic with the tools available in the 1940s: 'My only reason for focusing so exclusively on separation and loss was the fact that one could get comparatively reliable evidence about them whereas during the forties and fifties we had neither manpower nor means of recording less crude variables. As a result of adopting this research strategy, it often appeared that I was unaware of other adverse family events.'[179] In particular, he recalled that one thing that his 'Forty-Four Juvenile Thieves' paper 'misses terribly' was the physical abuse many of the children had also suffered, alongside multiple separations or neglect.[180]

As well as being difficult to measure with the tools of the time, in the 1940s Bowlby felt that a report on the prevalence of abuse among children referred to the Clinic for conduct

[172] Bowlby, J. & Fairbairn, C.N. (c.1939–42) The billeting of unaccompanied school children. PP/Bow/C.5/4/1.

[173] Bowlby, J., Miller, E., & Winnicott, D. (1939) Evacuation of small children. Letter to the Editor of the British Medical Journal, 16 December 1939. In Winnicott, D. (1984) Deprivation and Delinquency (pp.13–14). London: Tavistock.

[174] Bowlby, J. (c.1939–42) Psychological problems of evacuation. PP/Bow/C.5/4/1. This early work by Bowlby appears as Chapter 7 in Duschinsky, R. & White, K. (eds) (2019) Trauma and Loss: Key Texts from the John Bowlby Archive. London: Routledge.

[175] Bowlby, J. & Fairbairn, C.N. (c.1939–42) The billeting of unaccompanied school children. PP/Bow/C.5/4/1.

[176] Follan, M. & Minnis, H. (2010) Forty-four juvenile thieves revisited: from Bowlby to reactive attachment disorder. Child: Care, Health and Development, 36(5), 639–45.

[177] Bowlby, J. (1986) An interview with John Bowlby on the origins and reception of his work. Free Associations, 1, 36–64, p.39.

[178] Bowlby, J. (undated) Untitled case history beginning 'Mrs E. consulted the Clinic about her son Martin', in the file Maternal Behaviour: Humans. PP/Bow/H.136.

[179] Bowlby, J. (1985) Letter to Tirril Harris, 17 September 1985. PP/Bow/J.9/94.

[180] Bowlby, J. (1986) Interview with the BBC. PP/Bow/F.5/8.

problems would raise scandal, and prove unacceptable to public or clinical opinion.[181] The overarching issue of the importance of actual childhood experiences for later development would risk getting lost. The initial priority, Bowlby felt, had to be to support the study of child development as a science.[182] Bowlby castigated his fellow psychoanalysts in 1943 for their hostility towards scientific methodology, indeed any methodology besides clinical observation. He felt that this stance was rendering psychoanalysis increasingly irrelevant to matters of policy or professional practice: 'We find ourselves in a rapidly changing world and yet, as a Society, we have done nothing, I repeat nothing, to meet these changes, to influence them or to adapt to them. That is not the reaction of a living organism but of a moribund one. If our Society died of inertia it would only have met the fate that it has invited.'[183]

To try to be intelligible and credible in context, Bowlby sacrificed reporting the abuse experiences of the children in his clinic in favour of a focus only on documentable separations. This hard decision to focus on loss rather than abuse had to be taken, he believed, so that later researchers, living in a society more frank about family life and with the tools to do more rigorous work, could make child abuse and its prevention the object of scientific measurement. Even with such justifications, it was one of the professional decisions that Bowlby found most difficult to forgive. And in an interview the year he died, Bowlby described that he remained 'appalled' at himself and colleagues: 'Although I was plugging real life events, there were a whole lot of events I didn't give enough attention to. Sexual abuse is one … Physical abuse is another.'[184] In a manuscript circulated only to fellow psychoanalysts late in his career, Bowlby reported that 'I often shudder' when he found himself thinking about the accounts by patients of abuse experiences that he ignored.[185]

The focus on documentable separations was successful in drawing clinical, research, and public attention. However, in certain regards the strategy backfired. In the 1950s Bowlby had something of a tendency to document separations as present or absent, as a crude measure with high reliability. Anyone could check the record and agree that there had been a separation or not. Yet this methodology contributed to a tendency for Bowlby to think and write about separations as merely present or absent, at least until the early 1970s.[186] Kinds of separations were not distinguished. Instead in his early work they were all grouped under the label 'maternal deprivation', and in his later work discussed as 'separation' or 'lack of continuity'. The concept of 'maternal deprivation' had the problem that it implied that the child belonged, specifically, with their mother. Ainsworth repeatedly criticised Bowlby for the fact that at times he used the term 'maternal deprivation' when describing children whose predominant experience had actually been cruelty or abuse from their caregiver, with separation

[181] Bowlby, J. (1984) Violence in the family as a disorder of the attachment and caregiving systems. *American Journal of Psychoanalysis*, 44, 9–27: 'It was, indeed, largely because the adverse behavior of parents toward their children was such a taboo subject in analytic circles when I was starting my professional work that I decided to focus my research on the effects on children of real-life events of another sort, namely separation' (10).

[182] Bowlby, J. (1990, 2011) John Bowlby: interview by Leonardo Tondo. *Clinical Neuropsychiatry*, 8(2), 159–71, p.160.

[183] Bowlby, J. (1943, 1992) Contribution to business meeting. In P. King & R. Steiner (eds) *The Freud–Klein Controversies 1941–45*, 2nd edn. London: Routledge, p.369.

[184] Bowlby, J. (1990, 2015) John Bowlby: an interview by Virginia Hunter. *Attachment*, 9, 138–57, p.156.

[185] Bowlby, J. (1985, 1991) The role of the psychotherapist's personal resources in the treatment situation. *Bulletin of the British Psychoanalytic Society*, 27(11), 26–30, p.29–30. Published as Chapter 12 in Duschinsky, R. & White, K. (eds) (2019) *Trauma and Loss: Key Texts from the John Bowlby Archive*. London: Routledge.

[186] By the 1980s, Bowlby was admonishing colleagues for not being specific enough in their use of the term 'separation', e.g. Bowlby, J. (1985) *Letter to John Byng-Hall*, 12 April 1985. PP/Bow/J.9/45: 'I think one needs to be a little more precise about lengths of separation—words like moderate and prolonged are obscure. I suggest a week or two instead of "moderate", and "longer than that" in place of prolonged.'

only a lesser feature.[187] However, an additional problem was that 'maternal deprivation', 'separation', and 'lack of continuity' were all used in an undifferentiated way, and could connote everything from a child sleeping alone in a room, to use of daycare, to child neglect, to institutionalisation in an orphanage.[188]

In unpublished writings, and in correspondence, Bowlby was quite capable of making these distinctions from the 1940s onwards.[189] Writing to Michael Rutter in 1971, he stated: 'As regards long-term effects of brief experiences, we [Bowlby's research group] have endeavoured to keep an absolutely open mind. The view I have held for some years is rather like Doll's view of smoking. Whilst serious effects are found almost always only by prolonged and heavy smoking, even lighter and less prolonged smoking can have adverse effects *in some people*. Where one draws the line in practice then becomes a matter for private judgement.'[190] This more qualified position in private is unfortunately generally absent in Bowlby's published writings. His tendency to document separation as a binary variable aligned with populist appeal to a stereotyped image, sun-lit and stock, of mother and child as a natural whole. In both his popular and his scholarly writings Bowlby tended to describe separation as a quantitative phenomenon, without qualitative differentiation. In *Separation*, for instance, the qualifications are removed from the comparison previously offered to Rutter, and the claim is made that more separations of any kind are simply wore: 'the effects of separation from mother can be likened to the effects of smoking or of radiation. Although the effects of small doses appear negligible, they are cumulative'.[191] The crude stance on separations in much of Bowlby's published work has been considered mistaken and misleading not only by feminist critics and other researchers, but also by his collaborators, followers, and even Bowlby's own family.[192] It has had, additionally, an abiding impact on perceptions of Bowlby and of attachment theory in general.

[187] E.g. Ainsworth, M. (1962) The effects of maternal deprivation: a review of findings and controversy in the context of research strategy. In *Deprivation of Maternal Care: A Reassessment of its Effects* (pp.87–195). Geneva: WHO, p.99. See also Yarrow, L. (1961) Maternal deprivation: toward an empirical and conceptual re-evaluation. *Psychological Bulletin*, 58, 459–90.

[188] Rutter, M. (1972) *Maternal Deprivation Reassessed*. London: Penguin; Rutter, M. (2002) Maternal deprivation. In M. Bornstein (ed.) *Handbook of Parenting*, 2nd edn (pp.181–202). Mahwah, NJ: Lawrence Erlbaum.

[189] E.g. Bowlby, U. & Bowlby, J. (1940) *Difficult children*. PP/Bow/H7: 'The term—broken home covers a multitude of situations—illustrate. Vague, don't intend to use term but to examine different situations … Broken home does not <u>cause</u> trouble.'

[190] E.g. Bowlby, J. (1971) *Letter to Michael Rutter*, 6 October 1971. PP/Bow/J.9/161.

[191] Bowlby, J. (1973) *Separation: Anxiety and Anger*. New York: Basic Books, p.96. Another contributing factor appears to have been Bowlby's initial difficulties in articulating the distinction between observable attachment behaviour and the invisible attachment behavioural system. Bowlby would often make claims urging parents to always do their best to follow the cues of a child's attachment to ensure their child's wellbeing. To the degree that this refers to the attachment behavioural system, the claim is clearly overstated, and neglects his friend Robert Hinde's criticisms that weaning and other requirements on parents mean that the short-term demands of the attachment system should not always be given priority in facilitating children's long-term security. However, to the degree that Bowlby was implying that parents should follow the dictates of attachment behaviours—such as distress on separation—the result is an even more extreme position. It would imply that any separation is, in itself, potentially harmful. See, for instance, Bowlby, J. (1987) Baby love: an interview. *Hampstead and Highgate Express*, April 1987. PP/Bow/A.5/19: 'The more a child's attachment is respected and responded to, the more he'll feel secure.'

[192] Ainsworth, M. (1962) The effects of maternal deprivation: a review of findings and controversy in the context of research strategy. In *Deprivation of Maternal Care: A Reassessment of its Effects* (pp.87–195). Geneva: WHO, p.101; Bowlby, R. (2005) *Fifty Years of Attachment Theory*. London: Karnac; Vicedo, M. (2011) The social nature of the mother's tie to her child: John Bowlby's theory of attachment in post-war America. *British Journal for the History of Science*, 44(3), 401–26.

Prospective studies of separations

The treatment of any form of caregiver–child separation as equivalent was unwarranted, and to an extent polemical. Bowlby had no evidence on which to base such claims. He did have some limited evidence regarding the consequences of relatively long-term separations in childhood. The 'Forty-Four Juvenile Thieves' paper looked backwards from clinical cases to find potential pathological causes. However, Bowlby was well aware that this research strategy had significant methodological flaws, not least the problem of confirmation bias for pre-existing theoretical ideas.[193] Instead, he advocated a longitudinal methodology, which began by taking children who had experienced a long-term separation and examining its sequelae. Belief in the promise of slow, empirical, longitudinal study of emotional and family life would become a hallmark of attachment research.

In 1946 Bowlby took up a position with clinical and research responsibilities at the Tavistock Clinic in London. There, in 1948, he founded the Separation Research Unit, and hired James Robertson as a research assistant to study children undergoing hospitalisation.[194] Mary Boston and Dina Rosenbluth, child psychotherapy trainees at the Tavistock, also contributed to the research.[195] At the time, it was common policy to keep parents from visiting their children. For infectious diseases this was partly to prevent the spread of infection. However, it was also general policy for non-infectious diseases as well, since children tended to become distressed and difficult for the hospital staff to manage after their parents had visited. Bowlby had long been interested in the predicament of hospitalised children, which he regarded as a natural experiment to test the effects of separation.[196] In the 1930s, he had seen a 15-year-old girl, Joan, in the Child Guidance Clinic:

> Joan was examined because of severe headaches, which had begun when she was ten years old. Since no organic basis could be found and psychical factors were obvious she was treated with psychotherapy. After some weeks she described how she suffered from absent periods which were evidently hysterical dream-states. For periods up to two or three hours her head would feel funny and she would be unable to remember the recent past. Things looked different and seemed unreal. If she went to touch a thing she found it was not there. She herself remarked 'It's as if I'm in a dream'. The episode ended suddenly and other girls at school would tell her she had been staring curiously, 'looking beyond usual things'. . . The episodes began with severe headaches and would come on when she was frightened or anyone was angry. In this case the hysterical headaches and dream-states had begun when she was ten years old after she and her brother had been in hospital with scarlet-fever and diphtheria.[197]

---

[193] Bowlby, J. (1965) Comments on Joffe and Sandler 1965 'Notes on Pain, Depression and Individuation'. PP/Bow/J.9/168-9.

[194] Van der Horst, F.C.P. (2011) *John Bowlby—From Psychoanalysis to Ethology. Unravelling the Roots of Attachment Theory.* Oxford: Blackwell.

[195] Rustin, M. (2007) John Bowlby at the Tavistock. *Attachment & Human Development*, 9(4), 355–9.

[196] Bowlby, J. & Robertson, J. (1965) *Protest, Despair and Detachment.* PP/BOW/D.3/38: 'Separation can be likened to the natural experiments that are exploited by students of nutrition.'

[197] Bowlby, J. (1939) Hysteria in children. In H. Milford (ed.) *A Survey of Child Psychiatry* (pp.80–94). Oxford: Oxford University Press, p.84.

From 1948 Robertson began making direct observations of a sample of children who had been hospitalised. The first outputs from Robertson's research were a film and a 1952 paper entitled 'A two-year-old goes to hospital', which documented the behaviour of a two-and-a-half-year-old girl, Laura, who was hospitalised for eight days.[198] This film helped contribute to recognition of the sorrow major separations can cause children, and to the important movement to change hospital visitation regulations in the 1950s.[199]

Robertson documented that Laura initially showed a great deal of distress and protest. Her affect then turned towards apparent depression, though accompanied by tic-like stress movements. Three months after she returned home, her mother was away in hospital herself, to have a baby. On her mother's return, Laura seemed avoidant and somewhat disoriented on reunion:

> Laura was very excited and keen to return home. Half an hour later she arrived and the mother could hear her banging on the outside door and calling "Mummy, Mummy". But when her mother opened the door, Laura looked at her blankly and said, "But I want my Mummy". For the next two days she did not seem to recognise her mother, and although quite friendly was completely detached. This naturally upset her mother very much. When the father came home an hour or two after Laura's return, Laura was for a few moments mute toward him but then recovered quickly and was friendly and sure of him.[200]

Robertson went on to observe 50 cases, although less than half of these were observed intensively, and the context and kind of hospitalisation was highly diverse.[201] Reviewing these cases, Robertson and Bowlby came to the conclusion that because the children's efforts to regain their familiar caregivers had failed both chronically and painfully, they responded by inhibiting their feelings, and especially their yearning for their family. Bowlby termed this 'detachment'.[202] Ainsworth sought, essentially unsuccessfully, to persuade him that the term was misleading, since Bowlby did not intend to suggest that the child was no longer attached to their caregiver, but that an inhibition was observable that blocked intense feeling and its expression.[203] Robertson and Bowlby proposed that such inhibition was the cause of the depressed affect, the tic-like tension movements, and also the avoidant or disoriented behaviour on reunion.[204] Robertson noted his qualitative impression that children who sustained

[198] Bowlby J., Robertson, J., & Rosenbluth, D. (1952) A two-year-old goes to hospital. *Psychoanalytic Study of the Child*, 7, 82–94. During the war, Robertson had worked with Anna Freud at the Hampstead Nurseries with children, many of whom had been evacuated from London or who had no family to care for them. Freud and colleagues documented avoidant behaviour by young children to caregivers, including following reunions. This likely primed Robertson's interest in the avoidant behaviour shown by Laura and other hospitalized children on reunion. See Burlingham, D. & Freud, A. (1944) *Infants without Families*. London: Allen and Unwin, p.63.

[199] Van der Horst, F.C. & van der Veer, R. (2009) Why we disagree to disagree: a reply to commentaries by Robertson and McGilly, and Lindsay. *Attachment & Human Development*, 11(6), 569–72.

[200] Bowlby J., Robertson, J., & Rosenbluth, D. (1952) A two-year-old goes to hospital. *Psychoanalytic Study of the Child*, 7, 82–94, p.85.

[201] Bowlby, J. & Robertson, J. (1965) *Protest, Despair and Detachment*. PP/BOW/D.3/38.

[202] Bowlby, J. (1960) Separation anxiety. *International Journal of Psycho-Analysis*, 41, 89–113, p.90. See also Southgate, J. (1998) Attachment, intimacy, autonomy. *British Journal of Psychotherapy*, 14, 389–93: 'During my supervision with John … he argued to keep its original meaning on the grounds that once in an attachment space or relational field there is always some form of attachment even if it is disorganized and chaotic' (390).

[203] Ainsworth, M. (1962) *Letter to John Bowlby*, 11 December 1962. Mary Ainsworth papers, Box M3168, Folder 1. For an example of an otherwise careful reader and friend of Bowlby assuming that 'detachment' meant the opposite of attachment see Birtchnell, J. (1987) Attachment—detachment, directiveness—receptiveness: a system for classifying interpersonal attitudes and behaviour. *British Journal of Medical Psychology*, 60(1), 17–27.

[204] Bowlby, J. & Robertson, J. (1965) *Protest, Despair and Detachment*. PP/BOW/D.3/38.

this inhibition of feeling longer, and who received less comfort from staff during the hospitalisation, were those that showed more psychological disturbance once they returned home. These children displayed more anxiety and aggression, and less affection or help-seeking towards their parents; and these affects were also more likely to occur at odd moments, without apparent reason.[205]

Bowlby's confident tone in his academic writing about the impact of the hospitalisations, and crude statements warning about the dangers of separation in his popular writings, led many readers, even sympathetic ones, to assume that he saw a direct relationship between early separations and later behaviour.[206] Hazen and Shaver called this, in their assessment, 'one of the most common misconceptions about attachment theory'.[207] This impression was likely reinforced by a strong tendency in Bowlby's reporting of his own and his analysis or exposition of others' quantitative findings to neglect attention to moderators and interaction effects. One contributing factor may have been Bowlby's lack of expertise in using and interpreting statistical tests for interaction effects in empirical research. In fact Bowlby, in his theoretical writing already from the early 1950, explicitly acknowledged two additional factors that need to be included in any causal model, based on Robertson's observations. The first is that children will have 'differential susceptibility of an inherited kind' to the effects of separation.[208] The other is that the implications of the separation for a child's development will be mediated through the consequences of this event and the child's behaviour for family interactions: 'Most mothers find their children's failure to recognise them and to respond, or their outright rejection of them, on reunion extremely hard to bear, and later, when feelings have thawed, their intense possessiveness and whining mummyishness tries patience to the limit. Events such as these set up vicious circles which undoubtedly play an important part in establishing adverse patterns of behaviour in the personality.'[209] Rather than treating long-term separation itself as solely directly harmful as implied by Bowlby in popular works and papers reporting empirical findings, in theoretical reflections Bowlby emphasised that harms could be expected to be partially mediated through the vicious cycles that could be expected to be established in family relationships.[210]

In fact, to Bowlby's disappointment, the quantitative measures from the Robertson study of the effects of hospitalisation did not supply the evidence he expected of negative

---

[205] Ibid: 'It is our impression, and that of others, that children who have reached a detached state ... "blow up" more easily and more violently event than the ordinary child at home.' An example was Bobby: 'Everyone was punched when necessary—including father—and it was usually possible to detect the immediate reason for it. But his treatment of mother was exceptional in that she was often punched for no apparent reason. At times he would approach her with a bland or smiling face that gave no warning of the severe body blow that was to follow.' See also Robertson, J. & Robertson, J. (1971) Young children in brief separation: a fresh look. *The Psychoanalytic Study of the Child*, 26(1), 264–315.

[206] E.g. Eagle, M. (2013) *Attachment and Psychoanalysis*. New York: Guilford.

[207] Hazan, C. & Shaver, P.R. (1994) Deeper into attachment theory. *Psychological Inquiry*, 5(1), 68–79, p.70.

[208] Bowlby, J. (1953) Some pathological processes set in train by early mother–child separation. *Journal of Mental Science*, 9, 265–72, p.271. The exact meaning of the term 'differential susceptibility' for Bowlby is unclear. It may or may not necessarily imply that genetic factors may be 'for better or for worse', as later for Belsky, van IJzendoorn, and Bakermans-Kranenburg.

[209] Ibid.

[210] Bowlby was pleased with later research findings indicating the mediating role of family relationships on the impact of parental loss in childhood on an individual's later mental health. See PP/BOW/F.4/1:Box 40 and PP/BOW/J.9/19:Box 60 for Bowlby's reflections on and correspondence with Harris, T., Brown, G.W., & Bifulco, A. (1986) Loss of parent in childhood and adult psychiatric disorder: the role of lack of adequate parental care. *Psychological Medicine*, 16(3), 641–59.

consequences of long-term separation.[211] The quality of the data was, by his own admission, unusably poor. Ainsworth later commented that Bowlby had been overconfident in his hypothesis, and so did not take sufficient care in choosing his measures: 'He had expected this to be so conspicuous that he used very crude measures of assessment—teachers' ratings— and centred in on the IQ. Actually there was nothing in the IQ. The IQs of these children were not lower. And the teachers' ratings were not sufficiently sensitive really, to turf up any very conspicuous differences.'[212] These quantitative results were therefore held back from publication. However, the qualitative descriptions made of the children by Robertson during the hospitalisation and on their return home were very rich and suggestive in their detail.[213] Ainsworth later described Robertson's qualitative descriptions as 'entrancing' and 'deeply impressive'.[214] In 1968 she remarked to Bowlby that 'despite all the lapse of time and subsequent research' it is 'still the best' and most revealing descriptions made by early research on attachment.[215] In an oral history conducted in the same period, Ainsworth recalled:

> I was tremendously impressed with this material. Jimmy was a social worker at the time but he has since been qualified as an analyst. His observations were the most sensitive direct observations I had ever encountered. I don't think I have ever encountered anyone who was more perceptive.[216]

One of the most consequential aspects of Robertson's work was the distinction between 'ambivalent' anxiety/preoccupation and 'withdrawn' avoidance. Following separation, these were often—though certainly not always[217]—observed in sequence, with protest at separation followed by flattened affect over time. Robertson also identified related behaviour upon and following reunion. Anxious preoccupation with the parent was often shown by the formerly hospitalised children.[218] And avoidant behaviour was sometimes evident at the moment of reunion with the parents, and could also manifest as withdrawal from the parent in the months after the child returned home.[219] In a paper from 1956 reporting on their follow-up study with the hospitalised children, Bowlby, Ainsworth, and colleagues wrote

[211] Bowlby, J. (1976) Bowlby on latch-key kids: interviews with Dr Nicholas Tucker. *Psychology Today*, Autumn 1976, 37–41: 'I felt that because we had used such very superficial measures we were in no real position to give an adequate account of how these children had developed ... I really don't think the study has much scientific value' (38).

[212] Ainsworth, M. (1969) CPA oral history of psychology in Canada interview. Unpublished. http://www.feminist-voices.com/assets/Women-Past/Ainsworth/Mary-Ainsworth-CPA-Oral-History.pdf.

[213] Though a proportion of the most important data was second-hand. Bowlby, J. & Robertson, J. (1965) *Protest, Despair and Detachment*. PP/BOW/D.3/38: 'As experience accumulated, it came to be realised that the way a child greets his mother on the occasion of his return home is of great interest. This, however, was not realised in our earlier studies and for this reason in all but a few cases our data referring to this event were obtained second-hand.'

[214] Ainsworth, M. (1983, 2013) An autobiographical sketch. *Attachment & Human Development*, 15(5–6), 448–59, p.454.

[215] Ainsworth, M. (1968) *Letter to John Bowlby*, 2 November 1968. Mary Ainsworth papers, Box M3168, Folder 3.

[216] Ainsworth, M. (1969) CPA oral history of psychology in Canada interview. Unpublished. http://www.feminist-voices.com/assets/Women-Past/Ainsworth/Mary-Ainsworth-CPA-Oral-History.pdf.

[217] Van der Horst, F.C. & van der Veer, R. (2009) Separation and divergence: the untold story of James Robertson's and John Bowlby's theoretical dispute on mother–child separation. *Journal of the History of the Behavioral Sciences*, 45(3), 236–52.

[218] That the preoccupied response was a reflection of concern about the availability of the caregiver was confirmed by Bowlby's clinical observations of the possessiveness, anger, and jealousy with which toddlers responded to the birth of a new sibling, especially if the toddler already had a troubled relationship with his or her caregiver. Bowlby, J. (1955) New baby jealousy. *Parents*, December 1955, p.42–4.

[219] Bowlby, J. & Robertson, J. (1965) *Protest, Despair and Detachment*. PP/BOW/D.3/38.

that 'the personality patterns of children who have experienced long separation tend to fall into one or other of these two opposite classes': either (i) 'over-dependent' and 'ambivalent' or (ii) 'mother-rejecting ... having repressed their need for attachment'.[220]

Ainsworth found it thought-provoking that the two major classes of behaviour appeared to be 'opposites'. She expressed her fascination with the 'anxious over-dependence on the one hand, and superficiality and affectionlessness on the other' in the follow-up study, and the way that this seemed to correspond to 'the anxious clinging response following reunion after relatively brief or mild separations on the one hand, and the detachment and failure to re-establish affectional relations after long and severe separations on the other' (Chapter 2).[221] Bowlby, Ainsworth, and colleagues discussed this extensively, and they came increasingly to regard the two classes 'as the prototypes of responses that, when seen in acute and chronic form in older individuals and out of family context, are habitually labelled as psychiatric symptoms. Thus, for example, when the family situation is ignored, it becomes easy to label despair as depression, detachment as psychopathic lack of affect, protest as hysterical.'[222]

However, these observations of hospitalised children were dismissed as circumstantial evidence by Bowlby's critics. For instance, the behaviour of hospitalised children could be rejected as unrepresentative of children who were healthy. Experimental research was needed to support the case, but major separations of human children in experimental research was not morally permissible. Bowlby helped Hinde secure the funds to set up a colony of rhesus monkeys at Madingley, Cambridge.[223] Rhesus monkeys were chosen on the basis of the intimate relationship between infant and mother during early childhood, which made attachment phenomena especially visible. One of many important findings from Hinde's Madingley colony of rhesus monkeys from the 1960s was observation of both the 'classes' of behaviour following separation that had been identified by Bowlby, Ainsworth, and colleagues in their 1956 paper. Spencer-Booth and Hinde studied the effects of separating rhesus monkey infants from their mothers for six days, too long to be treated as an ordinary separation and so able to offer a parallel to hospitalisation. The researchers observed that 'the infants' behaviour during the mothers' absence can only be described as depressed. They sat in the hunched, passive attitude of a subordinate animal.'[224] After reunion, they 'showed exceptionally intense tantrums when rejected by their mothers, and often flung themselves

[220] Bowlby, J., Ainsworth, M., Boston, M., & Rosenbluth, D. (1956) The effects of mother–child separation: a follow-up study. *British Journal of Medical Psychology*, 29, 211–47, p.238. On the two classes as 'opposites' see also Bowlby, J. (1968, 1970) Disruption of affectional bonds and its effects on behavior. *Journal of Contemporary Psychotherapy* 2(2), 75–8: 'In the separated children, two forms of disturbance of affectional behaviour were seen, neither of which were observed in the comparison group of non-separated children. One form is that of emotional detachment; the other, its apparent opposite, i.e., an unrelenting demand to be close to mother' (82). Both responses would be documented again, decades later, by Stovall-McClough and Dozier, observing children one to two years old in the first months after joining a foster-family. Stovall-McClough, K.C. & Dozier, M. (2004) Forming attachments in foster care: infant attachment behaviors during the first 2 months of placement. *Development & Psychopathology*, 16(2), 253–71. Stovall-McClough and Dozier observed that these behaviours may mis-cue the foster-parent about the child's needs. These findings fed into the construction of the Attachment and Biobehavioral Catch-up intervention (Chapter 6).

[221] Ainsworth, M. (1962) The effects of maternal deprivation: a review of findings and controversy in the context of research strategy. In *Deprivation of Maternal Care: A Reassessment of its Effects* (pp.87–195). Geneva: WHO, p.140.

[222] Bowlby, J. (1976) Human personality development in an ethological light. In G. Serban & A. Kling (eds) *Animal Models in Human Psychobiology* (pp.27–36). New York: Plenum Press, p.28.

[223] Bateson, P., Stevenson-Hinde, J., & Clutton-Brock, T. (2018) Robert Aubrey Hinde CBE. 26 October 1923–23 December 2016. *Royal Society Biographical Memoirs*, 65.

[224] Spencer-Booth, Y. & Hinde, R. (1967) The effects of separating rhesus monkey infants from their mothers for six days. *Journal of Child Psychology & Psychiatry*, 7, 179–97, p.187.

violently on to their mothers, or sometimes, when the mother had rejected them, on to aunts':

> A further interesting feature was the way in which the infants could change from being re-laxed to being very upset and clinging without apparent cause. Thus Tim on Days 11 and 12 was recorded as coming off his mother in an apparently calm fashion, then suddenly panicking and going on her geckering. The most dramatic example was that of Linda, who on Day 16 was playing in a very relaxed fashion for about the first 35 min of the watch, then went on the mother and slept. When she awoke she seemed very upset and, terrified, cringed and would hardly leave her mother.[225]

Spencer-Booth and Hinde also documented that 'the deprivation experience accentuated pre-existing individual differences. When the various symptoms were combined to give a distress index, those infants which had been rejected most and/or played the largest role in maintaining proximity before separation were most disturbed after. By contrast, the actual time the infant spent off or at a distance from its mother before separation bore practically no relationship to the disturbance it showed subsequently.'[226] Spencer-Booth and Hinde fur-ther found that all effects were intensified if they separated the infants from their mothers for two six-day periods or for thirteen days.[227] These experimental studies with rhesus monkeys therefore provided further support that depression or detachment could be expected during a major separation from the primary caregiver, and that anxious preoccupation with the caregiver occurred following reunion, especially for those infants who had received the least proactive and nurturing caregiving.

Disorientation

However, the ambivalent and avoidant classes of behaviour were not the only behaviours observed by Robertson that would prove consequential for attachment theory. Robertson identified other anomalous behaviours, especially during separation, but also sometimes on reunion. These were described in detail in an unpublished book of Robertson's observations, written and re-written with Bowlby over the span of about ten years from the mid-1950s to mid-1960s.[228] The central theme that Robertson perceived in these anomalous behaviours was disorientation. Bowlby and Robertson regarded the behaviours as suggesting some dis-ruption of the attachment response. However, what exactly they signified was not clear, and this may have contributed to the decision by Bowlby to hold back the book from publication, alongside Robertson's gradual departure from the Tavistock in the early 1960s. There was also little academic interest during this period in disoriented behaviour as a mental health symptom.[229] Ainsworth regarded the absence of the Robertson and Bowlby book as a major

---

[225] Ibid. p.190.

[226] Hinde, R. & Spencer-Booth, Y. (1970) Individual differences in the responses of rhesus monkeys to a period of separation from their mothers. *Journal of Child Psychology & Psychiatry*, 11, 159–76, p.174.

[227] Hinde, R. & Spencer-Booth, Y. (1971) Effects of brief separation from mothers on rhesus monkeys. *Science* 173(3992), 111–18.

[228] Bowlby, J. & Robertson, J. (1965) *Protest, Despair and Detachment*. PP/BOW/D.3/38.

[229] Ross, C.A. (1996) History, phenomenology, and epidemiology of dissociation. In L.K. Michelson & W.J. Ray (eds) *Handbook of Dissociation: Theoretical, Empirical and Clinical Perspectives* (pp.3–25). New York: Springer;

loss to developmental psychology, and a source of personal sadness given the quality of the observations.[230] The behaviours only came back into central focus in the work of Mary Main, some decades later (Chapter 3).

One sign of disorientation was that behaviour became unmoored from environmental cues for activation and termination. Robertson noted that some children would swing, seemingly without external prompt, between the ambivalent and avoidant classes of behaviour. For instance: 'By about the end of her fifth month at home Jacqueline was frequently seeking "baby cuddles" from her mother not only in the evening but also in the daytime. In these brief moments she would curl up and revel in the mutual indulgence she and mother permitted themselves. But between the extremes of being a helpless sensual "baby" and of being detached and independent there was little behaviour of a moderate and quietly affectionate kind.'[231]

Robertson also documented many signs of disorientation on reunion. He offers a vivid description of Laura's behaviour during a brief visit by her mother to the hospital:

> One of the most striking features about Laura is that, despite being only two years and five months old, she contrived much of the time to control the expression of her grief. Mother announced "I'm going home now". Laura's expression was instantly tense and unhappy. Mother insisted "Don't cry" and pointed an admonitory finger; Laura nodded uncertainly. As her mother left and before she was out of sight Laura turned away with an expression of the deepest misery on her face. The relief of tears, which would have come to most children of that age in that situation, was not available to Laura. As she tried to keep her feelings in check she idly turned the pages of a book, fingered her hair, and both hands fluttered impotently before her face as if she had been momentarily disoriented.[232]

The withdrawn avoidant class of behaviour was, he thought, especially often accompanied by disorientation in relation to the caregiver. Robertson interpreted both disorientation and avoidance as suggesting the 'repression of attachment behaviour'.[233]

A different child showed fear on reunion with her mother. Robertson interpreted this as an effect of disorientation, with the mother misrecognised as a stranger due to repression of the attachment response:

> When they reached home and Mary saw her mother for the first time in six weeks, she screamed and refused to go near her. This rejection continued for several days during which she treated her mother so much as though she was a frightening stranger … Only after a week did Mary begin to show a wish to be near her mother. Then her behaviour moved to the other extreme and she followed mother about continuously as if afraid to let her out of her sight. She became increasingly aggressive towards her sisters, and made several vicious attacks on her new baby brother.[234]

Van der Hart, O. & Dorahy, M.J. (2009) Dissociation: history of a concept. In P.F. Dell & J. O'Neill (eds) *Dissociation and the Dissociative Disorders: DSM-V and Beyond* (pp.3–26). London: Routledge.

[230] Ainsworth, M. (1970) *Letter to John Bowlby*, 28 September 1970. Mary Ainsworth papers, Box M3168, Box 3.
[231] Bowlby, J. & Robertson, J. (1965) *Protest, Despair and Detachment*. PP/BOW/D.3/38. Bowlby's colleagues Heinicke and Westheimer also documented such responses following brief separations. Heinicke, C.M. & Westheimer, I. (1966) *Brief Separations*. Oxford: International Universities Press.
[232] Bowlby, J. & Robertson, J. (1965) *Protest, Despair and Detachment*. PP/BOW/D.3/38.
[233] Ibid.
[234] Ibid.

Another behaviour that Robertson described as having a disoriented quality was freezing when alarmed rather than looking for support from a familiar caregiver. For instance, Vicky showed such behaviour soon after returning from the hospital: 'On the third day her grandmother took her out. Although she had wanted to see the traffic, when she was halfway across a road she suddenly became petrified by fear, and refused to move, while the cars stopped and hooted and people stared.'[235]

Robertson also described forms of disorientation that led to care-seeking behaviours being directed towards strangers rather than familiar caregivers, what might now be referred to as 'disinhibited social engagement'. For example, he described the behaviour of Jacqueline: 'unlike ordinary children of this age, when hurt she did not go to her mother for comfort. Indeed, on an occasion when she bruised a finger quite badly Jacqueline did not turn to her mother but to a visitor who happened to be in the room.'[236] Robertson's impression was that a significant minority of the hospitalised children seemed to show 'a tendency to make shallow relationships with one and all, and thus to be undiscriminating' in their attachment behaviour following their hospitalisation.[237] He described the behaviour of Stephanie: 'Although she had not seen me for 18 months, she was immediately friendly and asked for a ride in my car: she was driven around the avenues without showing anxiety, a response mother commented upon. The parents also expressed a related concern—that she was unable to concentrate on anything for more than a very short time. They linked this, with considerable alarm, to the fact that she had been wandering away from home.'

Behavioural systems

The idea of a behavioural system

In the unpublished Robertson and Bowlby book, the authors described many observations relevant to the disruption of the attachment response: ambivalent behaviour, avoidant behaviour, and various forms of what appeared to be disorientation. However, the interpretation of these observations kept running into trouble, across the various drafts and redrafts of the book. 'Attachment', 'detachment', 'disorientation', 'preoccupation'—all these terms were used at times to refer to observable behaviour and at times to an inferred process at a motivational level. Sometimes they referred to voluntary actions; sometimes to involuntary responses or predispositions. This led the research group in circles at times, as Bowlby became increasingly aware as the 1950s progressed.[238] Bowlby's work on what became attachment theory was driven in part by a desire to develop a conceptual apparatus adequate to the findings of the Separation Research Unit. Indeed, *Attachment, Volume 1* began life as a single theoretical chapter for a book reporting on the empirical work with

---

[235] Bowlby, J. & Robertson, J. (undated, 1950–65?) Cases relating to part II and III. PP/BOW/D.3/11-12.
[236] Bowlby, J. & Robertson, J. (1965) *Protest, Despair and Detachment*. PP/BOW/D.3/38.
[237] Ibid.
[238] Bowlby, J. (1960) Separation anxiety. *International Journal of Psycho-Analysis*, 41, 89–113, p.95.

hospitalised children.[239] The fundamental concept that Bowlby elaborated was that of a 'behavioural system'.

The idea of a behavioural system was developed within ethology.[240] It referred to 'systems postulated as controlling a group of behaviour patterns that together serve to achieve a given biological end'.[241] For Bowlby, the concept was essentially a metaphor, 'conceived on the analogy of a physiological system organised homeostatically to ensure that a certain physiological measure, such as body temperature or blood pressure, is held between appropriate limits'.[242] If these limits are breached, then steps are taken by the individual to alter the environment or itself to regain them, achieving what Bowlby termed the 'set-goal' of the system and re-establishing homeostatic equilibrium.[243] Each behavioural system can recruit various kinds of resources, most visibly behaviours, to respond flexibly to the environment to achieve the set-goal. The concept of a behavioural system therefore presupposes a hierarchy between an overall goal and the means of achieving this goal, which must be assembled and coordinated together.[244]

As such, different behaviours commonly associated with the same system may not correlate, or may even negatively correlate with one another, as they are different paths to the same goal. For instance, crying and smiling directed towards the caregiver may be alternative paths to achieving the availability of an attachment figure; freezing and fleeing alternative paths to avoiding danger for the fear system. The concept of behavioural systems allowed Bowlby to clearly distinguish between the behavioural system (the motivation) and behaviour (the observable actions undertaken in the service of the motivation). Admittedly these terms are sufficiently close, and Bowlby was insufficiently careful in his use of the concepts, that this was and has remained an enduring point of confusion for his readers.[245] However, the distinction between invisible motivation and observable behaviour is sharp enough when Bowlby is being careful, and it was a consequential distinction for subsequent attachment theory and research.

When activated, behavioural systems such as attachment, caregiving, exploration, fear, and aggression initiate a disposition to try to achieve a set-goal. Where past and present information suggest that the environment will be receptive, the motivation finds expression in behaviour. Indeed, in contexts where the environment may demand the intense activation of a behavioural system, but provides only subtle cues, Bowlby observed in *Loss* that normal attentional processes may be sharpened and narrowed, as 'perceptual vigilance'. Such vigilance will lower the threshold at which conditions in the environment stir a slumbering

[239] Ainsworth, M. (1966) *Letter to John Bowlby*, 29 October 1966. Mary Ainsworth papers, Box M3168, Folder 2.

[240] Sevenster, P. (1961) A causal analysis of a displacement activity (Fanning in *Gasterosteus aculeatus* L.). *Behaviour*, 9, 1–170; Baerends, G.P. (1976) The functional organization of behaviour. *Animal Behaviour*, 24, 726–38. The movement of the concept from ethology to attachment theory is discussed further in Grossmann, K. & Grossmann, K. (2012) *Bindungen—das Gefüge psychischer Sicherheit Gebundenes*. Stuttgart: Klett-Cotta.

[241] Hinde, R. (1983) Ethology and child development. In P.H. Mussen (ed.) *Handbook of Child Psychology* (pp.27–93). New York: Wiley, p.57.

[242] Bowlby, J. (1982) Attachment and loss: retrospect and prospect. *American Journal of Orthopsychiatry*, 52(4), 664–78, p.670.

[243] Bowlby, J. (1969, 1982) *Attachment, Volume 1*. London: Penguin, p.69.

[244] Marvin, R.S., Britner, A.A., & Russell, B.A. (2016) Normative development: the ontogeny of attachment in childhood. In J. Cassidy & P.R. Shaver (eds) *Handbook of Attachment: Theory, Research, and Clinical Applications*, 3rd edn (pp.273–90). New York: Guilford.

[245] An important case was that of contemporary social learning theorists, e.g. Gewirtz, J.L. (ed.) (1972) *Attachment and Dependency*. Washington, DC: Winston.

behavioural system to life; it will also increase the intensity of motivation, which will likely be expressed in more elaborate and intense behaviour to achieve the set-goal of the system. This model appeared to Bowlby to account for the clingy behaviour documented by Robertson in children following hospitalisation: the distress of the separation prompted perceptual vigilance regarding proximity to their parents in these children. This led to an intense activation of the attachment system even to minor cues of caregiver unavailability. In turn, the opposite process could explain the 'detached' behaviour of the children who had been hospitalised for some time, and on reunion with their caregiver. Where the environment has come to be perceived as unreceptive and unwelcoming for a behavioural system, the activation and expression of a behavioural system can be inhibited.

Ethologists had used the concept of behavioural systems solely to refer to behaviour.[246] Bowlby expanded the concept, arguing that a behavioural system also recruits *cognitive* aspects, most especially expectations based on repeated past experiences and interactions, and perceptions of the present situations.[247] In *Attachment, Volume 1* he used the term 'internal working models' to characterise these cognitive components of a behavioural system. However, too much has often been made of internal working models as an element in Bowlby's thinking, especially among commentators in the late 1980s and early 1990s who took the internal working model as the ultimate 'content' of qualitative differences in attachment, in part based on an interpretation of Main's work (Chapter 3).[248] In fact, Bowlby used the concept relatively sparingly from the 1970s onwards, though he remained keen to emphasise that behavioural systems have cognitive components.[249]

Furthermore, for Bowlby behavioural systems contain not just behavioural and cognitive components, but also *emotional* aspects. This aspect of behavioural systems is acknowledged but not detailed in *Attachment, Volume 1,* which sought only to secure the argument that affects alter our perception of the point that a behaviour system requires activation or termination.[250] More than in his books, Bowlby's key remarks on the emotional components of behavioural system are generally contained in his publications in psychoanalytic journals— which have generally been little read since the publication of Bowlby's books—as well as in unpublished work. He observed: 'I conceive overt behaviour to be only one component of a motivational system within the organism, and fantasies, thoughts and affects, conscious and unconscious, to be integral to, and other components of, such systems.'[251] Furthermore, some affects, he proposed, accompany the activation of a behavioural system, some to its termination, and others its lack of assuagement. For instance, the sexual system may be accompanied by arousal, its termination by satisfaction and comfort, and its lack of assuagement to yearning and dissatisfaction. The attachment system is accompanied by distress, its termination by comfort, and its lack of assuagement to yearning and dissatisfaction, and eventually despair.[252]

[246] E.g. Baerends, G.P. (1976) The functional organization of behaviour. *Animal Behaviour*, 24, 726–38.

[247] Bowlby, J. (1958) The nature of the child's tie to his mother. *International Journal of Psycho-Analysis*, 39, 350–73, pp.365–6; Bowlby, J. (1980) *Loss*. London: Pimlico, p.348.

[248] E.g. Zeanah, C.H. & Anders, T.F. (1987) Subjectivity in parent–infant relationships: a discussion of internal working models. *Infant of Mental Health Journal*, 8(3), 237–50.

[249] E.g. Bowlby, J. (1982) Outline of attachment theory. PP/Bow/H.260.

[250] Bowlby, J. (1969, 1982) *Attachment, Volume 1.* London: Penguin: 'The process of categorising parts of the environment in terms of fitness to elicit a particular class of behaviour is itself experienced as coloured by the appropriate emotion' (114).

[251] Bowlby, J. (1962) *Defences that Follow Loss: Causation and Function.* PP/Bow/D.3/78.

[252] Bowlby, J. (1960) Separation anxiety. *International Journal of Psycho-Analysis*, 41, 89–113, p.96.

Groundplans of desire

Another important consequence of the concept of behavioural systems was that it allowed Bowlby to circumvent simplistic notions of nature and nurture. Harkness observed that first among the concerns raised by critics of attachment research since the 1970s has been the question 'How can attachment be both biologically based and determined by context?'.[253] The theory of attachment as a behavioural system was Bowlby's answer to this question, though it is not an answer that has been widely or well understood. For Bowlby, humans may be primed to develop behavioural systems along certain lines, but the very assemblage of a system depends upon experience. As Bowlby put it in his notes in the 1960s, discussing the attachment behavioural system: 'What I mean by this is that in an infant's behavioural equipment there is a built-in bias, genetically determined, that in the ordinarily expectable environment leads to the development of object relations. The built-in bias is there from the first: the actual development of object relations takes time.'[254]

Attachment behaviour is neither inevitable nor pre-wired, which is why reference by later researchers to the attachment system as a whole using terms such as 'innate'[255] can be misleading. Behavioural systems are a very specific subset of responses that are neither simply innate nor learnt, and that are not primarily expressions of emotion without environmental responsiveness. On the one hand, behavioural systems are neurologically primed at the level of motivation; they represent behaviour towards particular goals that would increase individual survival or reproductive success, at least in the environment within which humans evolved. However, on the other hand, behavioural systems are assembled out of component behaviours and experiences in a way that is flexibly responsive to the environment, with behaviours used interchangeably to achieve the set-goal. Shaver stated that 'according to Bowlby and Ainsworth, an infant can be viewed as an assembly of behavioural systems'.[256] This is essentially incorrect, or at least suggests a broader use of the concept of 'behavioural system' by Shaver than that of Bowlby and Ainsworth (Chapter 5). For Bowlby and Ainsworth an infant is much more than the sum of behavioural systems: they observed that infants have some almost entirely innate and pre-given responses, and some entirely learnt responses.[257] Additionally, not all behaviours have a set-goal. Some recognisable and patterned responses appeared to Bowlby and Ainsworth to be expressions of overwhelming affect, such as rage and despair, but without being environmentally responsive in a way that recruits component behaviours to achieve a specific end.[258]

For Bowlby, behavioural systems have specific properties, including that they are neither simply innate nor simply learnt, and that they have a set-goal for their termination. In one

[253] Harkness, S. (2015) The strange situation of attachment research: a review of three books. *Reviews in Anthropology*, 44(3), 178–97, p.179.

[254] Bowlby, J. (1965) Comments on Joffe and Sandler 1965 'Notes on Pain, Depression and Individuation'. PP/Bow/J.9/168–9.

[255] E.g. Mikulincer, M. & Shaver, P. (2008) Contributions of attachment theory and research to motivation science. In J.Y. Shah & W.L. Gardner (eds) *Handbook of Motivational Science* (pp.201–16). New York: Guilford, p.204.

[256] Koski, L.R. & Shaver, P.R. (1997) Attachment and relationship satisfaction across the lifespan. In R.J. Sternberg & M. Hojjat (eds) *Satisfaction in Close Relationships* (pp.26–55). New York: Guilford, p.27.

[257] The correspondence between Bowlby and Rene Spitz on smiling addressed just this issue (see PP/Bow/H.169). As an example of a largely pre-given response requiring only sufficient maturation and the absence of a grossly inhibiting environment, Bowlby offered the example of infant sucking. As an example of an essentially learnt response, Bowlby gave the example of throwing a ball.

[258] Bowlby, J. (1973) *Separation*. New York: Basic Books, p.288.

of Bowlby's key metaphors: 'As in the case of a military operation, the master plan gives only main objective and general strategy; each commander down the hierarchy is then expected to make more detailed plans and to issue more detailed instructions for the execution of his part in the master plan.'[259] This phrasing might imply that the activating and terminating points of the attachment system are constant, that only the behaviour is shaped by experience. This was a common misunderstanding of Bowlby's position among his critics, as Ainsworth identified.[260] In fact, Bowlby's claim was more radical: that the very parameters of the motivational system, though predisposed by evolution, are nonetheless also shaped by our encounters with others, such as experiences of expressing behaviour and how this behaviour is received.[261] Not just how, but what and when we desire or do not desire, and what that desire means to us, are inscribed by experience, even if the groundplan of desire may be available from human evolutionary history.

In *Attachment, Volume 1,* Bowlby proposed that, in humans, 'most behavioural systems are to some extent environmentally labile—namely, the form they take in an adult turns in some degree on the kind of environment in which that adult is reared. The advantage of this is that the form ultimately to be taken by the system is in some degree left open so that it can, during development, become adapted to the particular environment in which the individual finds himself.'[262] The complex cognitive capabilities of humans can also permit this flexibility to extend to individual or collective forms of substitution, so that if a desired set-goal is unattainable, some interim, partial, or symbolic form can nonetheless reduce activation of the behavioural system and offer some portion of the emotional rewards of achieving the set-goal.[263]

Nonetheless, experiences cumulatively channel this flexibility. 'Once a human has had experience of reaching a consummatory situation the behaviour that leads to it is likely to become reorganised in terms of a set-goal and a plan hierarchy. That is what appears to occur in sexual behaviour', where early experiences of relationships in general, and in particular of intimacy lit by intensity, serve to channel the later shape and targets of desire.[264] Furthermore, this ontogenetic flexibility is not limitless. A basic quality of behavioural systems is that they require certain kinds of environments for the homeostatic system to operate successfully. A 'feature of control systems that it is important to note is that they can operate effectively only within certain environmental limits. For example, the system responsible for maintaining body temperature is effective only provided the ambient temperature lies within certain limits. Outside those limits it fails.'[265]

[259] Bowlby, J. (1969, 1982) *Attachment, Volume 1,* London: Penguin, p.78.

[260] Ainsworth, M., Blehar, M., Waters, E., & Wall, S. (1978, 2015) *Patterns of Attachment: A Psychological Study of the Strange Situation.* Bristol: Psychology Press, p.11.

[261] In a remarkable statement, Bowlby observed that this gives attachment behaviour a certain developmental and causal priority over the attachment relationship itself: 'Attachment behaviour leads to the development of affectional bonds or attachments, initially between child and parent.' Bowlby, J. (1980) *Loss.* London: Pimlico, p.39.

[262] Bowlby, J. (1969, 1982) *Attachment, Volume 1.* London: Penguin, p.129. Bowlby later reflected that this flexibility is especially potent for humans: 'the longer-lived an individual the more necessary is ontogenetic flexibility to enable it to adapt to changes in the environment'. Bowlby, J. (1982) Evolution theory. PP/Bow/H102.

[263] Bowlby, J. (1957) An ethological approach to research on child development. *British Journal of Medical Psychology,* 30(4), 230–40, p.239.

[264] Bowlby, J. (1969, 1982) *Attachment, Volume 1.* London: Penguin, p.160.

[265] Bowlby, J. (1976) Human personality development in an ethological light. In G. Serban & A. Kling (eds) *Animal Models in Human Psychobiology* (pp.27–36). New York: Plenum Press, p.31. This idea has its origins for Bowlby not only in control systems theory, but also in his reading of Freud. Annotations by Bowlby dated 1960 on the 'Project for a Scientific Psychology' in *Sigmund Freud: The Origins of Psychoanalysis.* Copy held in the library of Human Development Scotland. Bowlby highlighted and starred the passage: 'Every contrivance of a biological

In his popular and early writings, Bowlby tended to imply that the expected environment for an infant was their primary caregiver, generally the mother. However, over time he came to acknowledge that a context with multiple familiar caregivers simply could not lie outside of the bounds of the attachment system's responsiveness. His last published work explicitly stated his mature view that the attachment system 'contributes to the individual's survival by keeping him or her in touch with one or more caregivers',[266] and he told colleagues that 'a baby interacting with and forming trusting (secure) relationships (attachments) with a larger number of significant persons will as a child and later as an adult walk more securely in the world'.[267] For example, in the environment within which humans evolved it would have been quite possible that grandparents would have been on hand when a baby required care.[268] By contrast, he supposed that institutional care, as in orphanages, with a rapid turn-over of paid professional caregivers, was likely outside the limits of what the attachment system had evolved to handle. The attachment system is not pre-given, and requires environmental learning and input, wrapping itself around and elaborating itself on the basis of discriminated relationships. Growing up in an institutional context with continual turnover of professional caregivers, it would be much harder for a child to experience any caregiver as familiar enough to entrain the attachment system and its elaboration.

Five behavioural systems

In his scholarly writings, Bowlby gave particular attention to five behavioural systems: the attachment system; the caregiving system; the exploratory system; the fear system; and aggression. This is not an exclusive list—for instance, Bowlby also described a sexual system; he suggests sleep may have qualities of a behavioural system; and he discussed an affiliative system that organises friendly behaviour towards others. However, attachment, caregiving, exploration, fear, and aggression are the most well-characterised instances in his writings, and will be discussed in turn (Table 1.1).

The attachment behavioural system

In Bowlby's account of behavioural systems, a central place is given to the system's activating and terminating conditions. Activating conditions trigger a motivation and behaviour to achieve the set-goal; achievement of the set-goal deactivates the motivation and its behaviour. Bowlby theorised that the attachment system in infancy is usually comparatively dormant, tasked primarily with monitoring the caregiver's whereabouts and checking in from time to time to ensure that a line of retreat to the caregiver remains open. In this dormant state, the system is also engaged with gaining relevant information about the caregiver and

---

nature has limits to its efficiency, beyond which it fails. Such failures exhibit themselves as phenomena bordering on the pathological' (368).

[266] Bowlby, J. (1991) Ethological light on psychoanalytic problems. In P. Bateson (ed.) *The Development and Integration of Behaviour: Essays in Honour of Robert Hinde* (pp.301–14). Cambridge: Cambridge University Press, p.306.

[267] Bowlby 1984 personal communication, cited in Harwood, I. (2003) Creative use of gender while addressing early attachment, trauma, and cross-cultural issues in a cotherapy group. *Psychoanalytic Inquiry*, 23, 697–712.

[268] Bowlby, J. (1986) Interview with the BBC. PP/Bow/F.5/8.

Table 1.1 Behavioural systems and their parameters in infancy in Bowlby's writing

Behavioural system	Activating condition(s)	Terminating condition	Key component behaviour	Species-level function
Attachment	Alarming stimuli or the potential for separation from familiar caregivers	The perceived availability of a familiar caregiver	Sucking, clinging, crawling, smiling, distress cries	Protection of self from harm (especially predation)
Caregiving	Perceptions of infant need, especially for retrieval	The perceived cessation of infant signals of need	Retrieval, care, encouragement, protection	Protection and support of others
Exploration	Novel and/or complex stimuli	Perceived familiarity	Exploratory manipulation	Learning
Fear	Alarming stimuli or the potential for separation from familiar caregivers	Perceived safety	Startle, wariness, fleeing, hiding, freezing	Escape
Aggression (anger of hope)	Frustration of another behavioural system	Satisfaction of the frustrated behavioural system	Threatening, attack	Coercion

the environment, especially information related to the caregiver's responses to the child's behaviour and to potential cues for danger. When a child is alarmed, the attachment system will prompt attempts to gain proximity with the caregiver.

From the primate researchers Harry Harlow and Robert Zimmermann, Bowlby took the phrase 'haven of safety' to refer to the way that an infant's alarm and motivation to seek their caregiver was terminated once they achieved proximity with the caregiver.[269] However, Bowlby was keen to make clear that the extent of proximity required by the attachment system was flexible, not a biological given. The set-goal of the attachment system may, indeed, abruptly change to specify the degree of proximity more narrowly or more loosely, and this will bring about attachment behaviours of different forms and intensities. Even the same environmental cue, such as a loud and sudden noise, may elicit only a look to the caregiver from an infant when accessibility feels ready and sure, but may elicit swift approach and clinging when the set-goal of the attachment system has been calibrated at full physical contact.

In *Attachment, Volume 1* Bowlby highlighted three conditions as of particular importance to the calibration of the set-goal. A first was past experience: for children who have come to expect that their caregiver might not be accessible when the attachment system is activated, a lower threshold would be set for its activation and a higher threshold for termination. By contrast, for children confident in the accessibility of their caregiver, physical proximity-seeking may only occur at a high threshold, and can be more readily terminated.[270] A second factor that would influence these thresholds, Bowlby suggested, was the extent of current

---

[269] Bowlby, J. (1958) Nature of the child's tie to his mother. *International Journal of Psycho-Analysis*, 39, 350–73; Harlow, H.F. & Zimmermann, R.R. (1958) The development of affectional responses in infant monkeys. *Proceedings of the American Philosophical Society*, 102(5), 501–9.

[270] Bowlby, J. (1973) *Separation: Anxiety and Anger*. New York: Basic Books, p.228–9.

sources of threat. In environments with alarming stimuli, or cues that an unexpected or major separation might occur, the parameters of the attachment system might well be altered.[271] Finally, a third factor that Bowlby thought would especially impact the attachment system's parameters was human cognitive development. With maturation beyond infancy, we have at our disposal more sophisticated strategies for maintaining contact, including verbal communication and mental representation.

As Ainsworth's student Bob Marvin documented in his 1972 doctoral thesis, maturation raises the threshold for the activation of the attachment system, and also the intensity of the attachment behaviours that are likely to be expressed.[272] Infants may cry and seek to cling to their attachment figure following an unexpected separation. By contrast, preschoolers, with greater tools at their disposal for understanding and achieving the caregiver's accessibility, may simply offer a look and smile of greeting. Ultimately the set-goal of the attachment system is not a particular inner state or set of external conditions, Bowlby argued, but a point at their intersection: 'a certain sort of relationship with another specified individual'.[273] Until his final writings, Bowlby generally claimed that this relationship was physical accessibility. Later, taking heed of Ainsworth's observations and arguments, he acknowledged that the 'certain sort of relationship' is, in infancy and across childhood, both the physical and psychological 'availability' of the attachment figure.

Though this was a point generally missed by his critics, and could have been better highlighted, Bowlby regarded few, if any, of the component behavioural sequences of the attachment system as exclusive to it.[274] Behaviours can and often do serve more than one system. The attachment system takes as key early components behavioural sequences such as sucking, clinging, crawling, and smiling.[275] However, sucking is also important for what Bowlby called the 'eating' or 'feeding' behavioural system[276] and what Ainsworth termed the 'food-seeking system' (Chapter 2). The shared components of the following and the food-seeking systems were critical for the conflation of the two in psychoanalytic theory, under the notion of the 'oral stage'.[277] Smiling is not only used for activating caregiver responses, but is more generally critical for the affiliative system, and can be co-opted by the fear system as a form of placation. Developmental maturation also allows behaviours usually characteristic of other systems to be recruited by the attachment system if its usual repertoire for seeking care has not been successful. As discussed below in the section 'The caregiving behavioural

[271] Bowlby, J. (1979) By ethology out of psychoanalysis: an experiment in interbreeding. (The Niko Tinbergen Lecture.) *Animal Behaviour*, 28(3), 649–56, p.651.

[272] Marvin, R.S. (1972) Attachment, exploratory and communicative behavior of two, three and four year old children. Unpublished doctoral dissertation, University of Chicago. Discussed in Bowlby, J. (1973) *Separation: Anxiety and Anger*. New York: Basic Books, p.70.

[273] Bowlby, J. (1969, 1982) *Attachment, Volume 1*. London: Penguin, p.140.

[274] The point would need to be clarified repeatedly by early members of the second generation of attachment researchers. The most important contribution on this score was that of Everett Waters, who also demonstrated the claim empirically (Chapter 2).

[275] Bowlby, J. (1958) The nature of the child's tie to his mother. *International Journal of Psycho-Analysis*, 39, 350–73, p.351.

[276] Bowlby, J. (1980, 1988) Caring for children. In *A Secure Base* (pp.1–21). London: Routledge, p.6; Bowlby, J. (1973) *Letter to Scott Henderson*, 30 July 1973. PP/Bow/J.9/98.

[277] Bowlby, J. (1960) Grief and mourning in infancy and early childhood. *Psychoanalytic Study of the Child*, 15, 9–52: 'I believe that the hypothesis now advanced would have been advocated earlier had it not happened that the phase of attachment to a mother figure was so late in being recognized and had not theory become preoccupied instead on the one hand with primary narcissism and on the other with orality' (14).

system', Bowlby's particular interest was in the recruitment of the caregiving system in the service of the attachment system. However, he also noted how sexuality could be used in the service of the attachment system when other forms of care-seeking have failed, and 'one can regard attempted suicide as an aberrant form of care-eliciting behaviour resorted to by only those who have had very unstable relationships in the past, and who have learned that more normal types of care-eliciting behaviour fail to work. As an aberrant form of attachment behaviour, of course, it is not far removed from total despair.'[278] Behaviours can also serve more than one system at the same time: for instance, Bretherton and Ainsworth argued that coy and submissive behaviour is coordinated by the fear and affiliative systems together.[279] Rough-and-tumble play integrates, stylises, and perhaps ritualises elements from both the exploratory and the anger systems. Close observation of children during such play reveals how aggression and exploration, specifically, can be used in the service of the other.[280] For Bowlby:

> Affect laden behaviour I tend to view in terms of structures built of component bricks. The bricks are relatively stereotyped behaviour patterns, e.g. bird song or sucking, which, according to the species, may be built in or learnt or a combination of both. The larger structure, e.g. courtship or nest building, is less stereotyped and a complex synthesis of these components. Although in principle any component is available for any synthesis, in practice each synthesis tends to select a particular group of components. None the less it is probably usual for certain component items to be utilised in more than one synthesis.[281]

For instance, Bowlby discussed the close relationship between the attachment response and the flight response. These may have many common components, since we often flee to those we turn to with the expectation of protection, though there may be occasions when we do not do so, for instance when we do not perceive such individuals as available to us. Bowlby also expected the attachment and fear behavioural systems to share important cognitive components, such as expectations about the effectiveness of previous attempts to gain safety, and present perceptions of sources of danger.

Another pair of behavioural systems with significant shared components are attachment and sexuality. Ainsworth felt that Bowlby had seriously underplayed the importance and complexity of the sexual system, as part of his attempt to pull away from psychoanalytic theory.[282] This is certainly true of the 1970s and 1980s. However, during the late 1950s, whilst

---

[278] Bowlby, J. (1979) *Letter to Professor K.S. Adam*, 12 February 1979. PP/Bow/J.9.2.

[279] Bretherton, I. & Ainsworth, M.D.S. (1974) Responses of one-year-olds to a stranger in a strange situation. In M. Lewis & L.A. Rosenblum (eds) *The Origin of Fear* (pp.131–64). New York: Wiley. This was also discussed by Tony Ambrose, working within Bowlby's group: Ambrose, T. (1960) The smiling and related responses in early human infancy: an experimental and theoretical study of their course and significance. Unpublished PhD thesis, Birkbeck College, London.

[280] See Attili, G. & Hinde, R.A. (1986) Categories of aggression and their motivational heterogeneity. *Evolution and Human Behavior*, 7(1), 17–27.

[281] Bowlby cited in Tanner, J.M. & Inhelder, B. (1960) *Discussions on Child Development: Proceedings of the WTO Study Group of the Psychobiological Development of the Child*, Vol. 4. London: Tavistock, p.40.

[282] Ainsworth, M. (1997) Peter L. Rudnytsky—the personal origins of attachment theory: an interview with Mary Salter Ainsworth. *Psychoanalytic Study of the Child*, 52, 386–405: 'PLR: Is there any sense in which your view and Bowlby's diverge at all, or is there a complete meeting of the minds? MSA: Well, I think there's more to the oedipal situation than he does. Bowlby just doesn't talk about it' (399); 'In the oedipal situation, there's no question in my mind that in the parents' dynamics there is a lot of sexuality' (402).

Ainsworth was relatively out of contact in Uganda (Chapter 2), comparison of the sexual response and the following response was key to discussions between Bowlby and Hinde. Bowlby discussed the sexual system in some detail during the meetings of the WTO Study Group of the Psychobiological Development of the Child in the late 1950s.[283] In these discussions Bowlby did not consider the activating and terminating conditions of the sexual system. Instead, his focus was on how the sexual response takes component behaviours from attachment relationships: 'certain components in the human sexual response are derived from parent–child response'.[284] Such common components might include affective and cognitive elements such as trust, affection, gentleness, and expectations around what interactions such as acceptance or rebuff will ultimately mean for a relationship. Common aspects might include behavioural components such as gazing, kissing, and coming into close proximity. This account allowed Bowlby to qualify Freud's claim that early relationship patterns are organised as a whole into later sexual desire. For Bowlby, it seemed more cautious and more probable that only some components of earlier patterns are integrated into how adults show affection, enact courtship and sexuality, and provide care to their own offspring.[285] These components are the thin wires connecting early care to later sexuality; there is no inevitable or single line of continuity.

Even if components of the attachment behavioural system ultimately get recruited and repurposed in adulthood, and even if the threshold for activating the system is increased, Bowlby nonetheless claimed that the attachment system remains available throughout life. In an emergency, or when hurt or scared, we are prompted to seek those we know and trust, and feel the more troubled when they are not available.[286] As adults, when alarmed we may seek a spouse, a parent—or, 'more often than might be supposed', adults may look to their own child for reassurance.[287] However, the surplus of meanings assigned to the term

---

[283] Ainsworth does not cite the transcript of these discussions, and she may not have owned a copy.

[284] Tanner, J.M. & Inhelder, B. (1956) *Discussions on Child Development: Proceedings of the WTO Study Group of the Psychobiological Development of the Child*, Vol 1. London: Tavistock, p.184–5. For later considerations of the relationship between the attachment and sexual behavioural systems see e.g. Crittenden, P.M. (1998) Patterns of attachment and sexual behavior: risk of dysfunction versus opportunity for creative integration. In L. Atkinson & K.J. Zucker (eds) *Attachment and Psychopathology* (pp.47–93). New York: Guilford; Diamond, L.M. (2003) What does sexual orientation orient? A biobehavioral model distinguishing romantic love and sexual desire. *Psychological Review*, 110(1), 173–92.

[285] Bowlby cited in Tanner, J.M. & Inhelder, B. (1960) *Discussions on Child Development: Proceedings of the WTO Study Group of the Psychobiological Development of the Child*, Vol 4. London: Tavistock, p.41.

[286] Bowlby, J. (1969) Affectional bonds: their nature and origin. In H. Freeman (ed.) *Progress in Mental Health* (pp.319–27). London: J. & A. Churchill, p.323.

[287] Bowlby, J. (1977, 1979) The making and breaking of affectional bonds. In *The Making and Breaking of Affectional Bonds* (pp.150–88). London: Routledge, p.157. The use of a child as an attachment figure by adults appears to have been deliberately neglected by subsequent attachment research, in part to maintain—against misunderstanding—the characterization of attachment as something a child shows to their adult caregiver. See e.g. Ainsworth, M.D.S. (1991) Attachments and other affectional bonds across the life cycle. In C.M. Parkes, J. Stevenson-Hinde, & P. Marris (eds) *Attachment Across the Life Cycle* (pp. 33–51). London: Routledge: 'We talk of the bond of a mother to her child ... a mother does not normally base her security on her relationship with her child, however eager she may be to give care and nurturance' (40). The primary exception is Doherty, N.A. & Feeney, J.A. (2004) The composition of attachment networks throughout the adult years. *Personal Relationships*, 11(4), 469–88. Forty percent of participants with children reported using their child as a safe haven, as a secure base, and experiencing separation anxiety. However, both the attachment and caregiving systems can prompt separation anxiety and proximity-maintenance. This difficulty disentangling these systems may be a secondary reason why attachment researchers have neglected the phenomenon of use of children as attachment figures by adults.

'attachment' caused Bowlby to swing between two very different positions.[288] On the one hand, 'attachment' was sometimes used broadly to mean early relationships as a whole. With this meaning in mind, Bowlby made strong claims for the influence of attachment on 'a person's whole emotional life', and as the condition of possibility for all later emotional development and mental health.[289] In *Loss*, for instance, he claimed that 'attachments to other human beings are the hub around which a person's life revolves ... From these intimate attachments a person draws his strength and enjoyment of life.'[290] Such claims later contributed to the impression by audiences of attachment theory that individual differences in early attachment are fixed for life (Chapter 2).

On the other hand, when 'attachment' was understood narrowly as a specific behavioural system, Bowlby's stance was rather different. With the narrow ethological meaning in mind, he proposed that influences on this behavioural system in early life could have a pervasive influence on later mental health, but nonetheless tended towards more qualified claims. Human development is very complex, and no single factor is likely to play more than a moderate role. However, for a single behavioural system, Bowlby anticipated that the attachment system would be quite influential and therefore worthy of particular attention. The period of early following and help-seeking has its importance because 'the period when they are most active is also the period when patterns of control and of regulating conflict are being laid down'. It therefore has a particular significance for socio-emotional development.[291] Yet even children who have had 'ghastly experiences' may 'nevertheless develop favourably', with maybe only 20–30% subsequently showing severe problems. Furthermore, those who show severe problems are often those who have experienced combinations of adversities, rather than disruptions of attachment alone.[292] Nonetheless, Bowlby anticipated that individual differences in early attachment experiences would have some implications for later mental health and wellbeing across the spectrum (see also Chapter 4).

In his final years, Bowlby saw the life of Charles Darwin as offering an especially clear case illustrating the importance of the disruption of the attachment system in childhood for later development, and also the emphasis he placed on family interactions for mediating the effects of separation or loss. Especially after seeing visitors or after some other excitement, as an adult Darwin experienced numerous symptoms including gastric pains, vertigo, vomiting,

---

[288] This hinge seems to have been primarily the result of conceptual imprecision. It may at times have served as a 'motte and bailey' rhetorical strategy, with a poorly defendable but expansive outer area and a more defendable but narrower inner position. However, the fact that the term's meaning slides around just as much in Bowlby's private notes suggests that such a strategy was not his intent. On the 'motte and bailey' rhetorical strategy see Shackel, N. (2005) The vacuity of postmodernist methodology. *Metaphilosophy*, 36(3), 295–320.

[289] E.g. Bowlby, J. (1984) Violence in the family as a disorder of the attachment and caregiving systems. *American Journal of Psychoanalysis*, 44, 9–27, p.11.

[290] Bowlby, J. (1980) *Loss*. London: Pimlico, p.442.

[291] Bowlby, J. (1960) Separation anxiety. *International Journal of Psycho-Analysis*, 41, 89–113, p.105; see also Steele, H. & Steele, M. (1998) Response to Cassidy, Lyons-Ruth and Bretherton: a return to exploration. *Social Development*, 7(1), 137–41.

[292] Bowlby, J. (1986) Interview with the BBC. PP/Bow/F.5/8: 'I'm often accused of exaggerating and various people point out that not every child who has had these sorts of experience comes to grief ... First of all, maybe he'll be vulnerable if things go wrong in his life ... Another point is that, supposing it's true that some children having had some pretty ghastly experiences nonetheless develop favourably ... But then the question arises, what percentage of people who contract polio are left with long term paralysis? The answer is less than 1 per cent. The fact is 99 per cent get by. Now in the case of severe maternal deprivation—first of all I think that much more than 1 per cent suffer. I think the percentage is way up in the 20s or 30s. And the other thing is that crippling of personality is much more serious'. See also Bowlby, J. (1971) *Letter to Michael Rutter*, 6 October 1971. PP/Bow/J.9/161: 'The more serious effects of experiences of the type we are discussing are when there are certain special combinations of variables present.'

tremors, cramps, headaches, eczema, anxiety, and a compulsion to wander or search for something without knowing what. There remains much speculation about the cause of these symptoms, and the relative contribution of organic and psychological illness.[293] In *Charles Darwin: A Life*, published in 1990, Bowlby argued that several other symptoms could essentially be explained as panic attacks, caused by the poor integration of behavioural, affective, and cognitive components of the attachment system following the loss of Darwin's mother. The issue was not this disruption of the attachment relationship alone, however. Bowlby instead highlighted that the family insisted that Darwin was not permitted to talk about his mother after she died when he was eight years old. Bowlby speculated that this could have contributed to exciting emotions being misrecognised as threatening ones.[294] In turn, he proposed that this misrecognition may have contributed to Darwin's tendency to hyperventilate, with his body always on the cusp of physiological overarousal.[295] In support of his claims, Bowlby offers evidence that Darwin's symptoms were exacerbated whenever as an adult he felt threatened or experienced a loss.

The caregiving behavioural system

It is sometimes assumed that Bowlby also regarded parental behaviour and feelings as an expression of attachment. This error is more common among Bowlby's critics, who generally privilege his writings of the 1950s and ignore his later qualifications and clarifications.[296] However, such usage can sometime be seen in the work of attachment researchers too, albeit less since the 2000s.[297] It follows some confusing and overextended use of the term 'attachment' by Bowlby in the early 1950s that did include caregiving behaviour. Though he attempted subsequently to distinguish attachment and caregiving, the early work set up a chain reaction that shaped both interpretation of his theory and measurement tools built from it. For instance, the Maternal–Fetal Attachment Scale was introduced by Cranley in 1981 to measure a mother's 'attachment' (feelings of care for) her unborn baby.[298] Such institutionalised uses of 'attachment' to mean caregiving have caused even attachment researchers assiduous about terminology, such as van IJzendoorn and Bakermans-Kranenburg, to

[293] Finsterer, J. & Hayman, J. (2014) Mitochondrial disorder caused Charles Darwin's cyclic vomiting syndrome. *International Journal of General Medicine*, 7, 59–70.

[294] Bowlby, J. (1987–90) Papers on Charles Darwin. Cambridge University Library. MS Add. 8884, marginalia on Liotti, G. (1986) Structural cognitive therapy. In Dryden, W. & Golden, W. (eds) *Cognitive-Behavioural Approaches to Psychotherapy*. Milton Keynes: Open University Press, p.125.

[295] Bowlby, J. (1990) *Charles Darwin: A Life*. New York: Norton, p.6.

[296] Two clear cases are Vicedo, M. (2013) *The Nature and Nurture of Love: From Imprinting to Attachment in Cold War America*. Chicago: University of Chicago Press, and Gottlieb, A. (2014) Is it time to detach from attachment theory? Perspectives from the West African rainforest. In H. Otto & H. Keller (eds) *Different Faces of Attachment: Cultural Variations on a Universal Human Need* (pp.187–214). Cambridge: Cambridge University Press.

[297] Bretherton, I., Biringen, Z., Ridgeway, D., Maslin, C., & Sherman, M. (1989) Attachment: the parental perspective. *Infant Mental Health Journal*, 10(3), 203–21; Waters, E. & Cummings, E.M. (2000) A secure base from which to explore close relationships. *Child Development*, 71(1), 164–72: 'To examine relations between early attachment experience and both secure base use and secure base support skills later in life and to examine them across contexts such as marriage, parenting, caring for adult parents, and requesting care from others. As currently formulated, attachment theory suggests that these are all organized by the same attachment control system' (171).

[298] Cranley, M.S. (1981) Development of a tool for the measurement of maternal attachment during pregnancy. *Nursing Research*, 30(5), 281–4.

refer to 'attachment' when they mean caregiving.[299] Perhaps a source of confusion between caregiving and attachment for Bowlby in his early writings was that there did seem to be common elements. As mentioned earlier, in his mature writings Bowlby identified that some components of the attachment system, like the capacity to communicate about emotion with others, may be recruited when an adult is required to provide care. However, this does not imply that caregiving is a reflection or expression of attachment. The two systems evolved in parallel, and function reciprocally, producing important forms of potential cooperation and friction.[300]

In *Attachment, Volume 1*, Bowlby developed an account of the caregiving behavioural system modelled on his existing ideas regarding the attachment behavioural system. The caregiving system was specifically anchored in the retrieval response, as a reciprocal partner to the infant's following response for maintaining proximity:

> Retrieving can be defined as any behaviour of a parent a predictable outcome of which is that the young are brought either into the nest or close to mother, or both ... The retrieving behaviour of a primate mother gathers the infant into her arms and holds him there. Having a similar outcome to the attachment behaviour of young, it is probably best understood in similar terms—namely, as being mediated by a number of behavioural systems the predictable outcome of which is maintenance of proximity to the infant ... especially when her infant is playing contentedly with other known individuals in the vicinity, a mother may let things be. Yet her tendency to retrieve him is not wholly dormant: she is likely to keep a watchful eye on him.[301]

Yet just as the attachment behavioural system was anchored in the infant's following response, but inserted into a broader image of comfort-seeking and relationship, the caregiving system had a parallel hinge. Like the attachment system, then, Bowlby's notion of the caregiving system sustained an ambiguity between the narrow notion of the retrieval response (and, presumably, related aspects of holding) and a more expansive notion of the provision of 'encouragement, support, help and protection'.[302] In notes from 1978, disliking throughout his career the ambiguity of the word 'empathy', he referred to the key emotional component of the caregiving system as 'concern for the welfare of others'.[303] And in a late interview he emphasised the importance of attentional processes that serve as architecture for the caregiving system.[304] Yet Bowlby's written reflections on the set-goal of the caregiving

[299] Huffmeijer, R., van IJzendoorn, M.H., & Bakermans-Kranenburg, M.J. (2013) Ageing and oxytocin: a call for extending human oxytocin research to ageing populations—a mini-review. *Gerontology*, 59(1), 32–9: 'In (soon-to-be) mothers, increases in plasma oxytocin concentrations over the course of pregnancy have been found to predict greater attachment to the unborn baby' (33).

[300] Bowlby, J. (1986) *Attachment, Life-Span and Old Age*. Eds J. Munnichs & B. Miesen. Utrecht: Van Loghum, p.11. See also Cassidy, J. (2000) The complexity of the caregiving system: a perspective from attachment theory. *Psychological Inquiry*, 11(2), 86–91, p.88.

[301] Bowlby, J. (1969, 1982) *Attachment, Volume 1*. London: Penguin, p.240.

[302] Bowlby, J. (1973) *Letter to Scott Henderson*, 30 July 1973. PP/Bow/J.9/98: the caregiving provided by the caregiving system 'includes rather more' than the bodily contact of the retrieval response and the affects of 'interest, esteem and affection'. In particular, Bowlby urged Henderson to note that caregiving also included 'encouragement, support, help and protection'. On the ambiguity between the 'retrieval' and 'nurturance' models of caregiving in Bowlby see Bell, D.C. & Richard, A.J. (2000) Caregiving: the forgotten element in attachment. *Psychological Inquiry*, 11(2), 69–83.

[303] Bowlby, J. (1978) Caregiving. In 'Emotion and feeling'. PP/Bow/H.5.

[304] Bowlby, J. (1990) Interviewed in *The Nuts and Bolts of Ben Bowlby* (Channel 4). https://licensing.screenocean.com/r/216106.

system are scarce. And the conflation of specific and general set-goals of the caregiving system is a major limitation of his remarks, given their significant differences. Not least, retrieval, following, and attachment are all homeostatic systems at root, whereas the provision of care and nurturance in a wider sense aims to support growth, not a return to equilibrium. Retrieval and encouragement/support also seemed to be modulated and their successful achievement met by potentially quite different affects in the caregiver, including quite different senses of commitment and pleasure.[305] Indeed, subsequent to Bowlby, ethologists have come to distinguish a consoling system from a caregiving system, given their distinctive behavioural repertoires and conditions of activation and termination.[306]

Despite conceptual ambiguity in Bowlby's writings about caregiving, neither the narrow nor the broad notions of the caregiving system implied, as Vicedo has mistakenly claimed, that Bowlby discussed mothers as 'unthinking and natural', acting 'just out of instinct', in behaviour devoid 'of rationality, of choice and of moral value'.[307] Vicedo's description is a reductive characterisation of even Bowlby's populist writings, and as a characterisation of his theoretical texts, it is essentially polemical. Bowlby did not regard parenting behaviours as characteristic only of mothers—though Ainsworth was more critical than Bowlby of the cultural values that assigned responsibility for caregiving to mothers.[308] As mentioned in the section 'The attachment behavioural system', Bowlby regarded all behavioural systems as neurologically primed, but dependent on experience and contextual support for their elicitation, elaboration, and expression. He stated explicitly in relation to caregiving behaviour that his 'view of behavioural development contrasts sharply with both of the older paradigms, one of which, invoking instinct, over-emphasised the preprogrammed component and the other of which, reacting against instinct, overemphasised the learned component. Parenting behaviour in humans is certainly not the product of some unvarying parenting instinct.'[309] In a presentation of his ideas for radio in 1969, Bowlby drew a comparison between parenting behaviour and language. In both cases, humans are predisposed to pay attention to certain cues, and elaborate systems of meaning and practice. However, the nature of these meanings and practices depends on our opportunities for learning, and our induction into

[305] On the important role of the affect 'delight' in the functioning of the caregiving system see e.g. Bernard, K. & Dozier, M. (2011) This is my baby: foster parents' feelings of commitment and displays of delight. *Infant Mental Health Journal*, 32(2), 251–62. Delight and other positive communicated affect may also be a significant relay between the caregiving and attachment behavioural systems. Dozier, M. & Bernard, K. (2019) *Coaching Parents of Vulnerable Infants: The Attachment and Biobehavioral Catch-up Approach*. New York: Guilford: 'In a personal communication (August 2001) Mary Main suggested that parental delight communicates to children how important they are to their parents, a sentiment she indicated Mary Ainsworth shared' (57).

[306] E.g. Burkett, J.P., Andari, E., Johnson, Z.V., Curry, D.C., de Waal, F.B., & Young, L.J. (2016) Oxytocin-dependent consolation behavior in rodents. *Science*, 351(6271), 375–8.

[307] Vicedo, M. (2011) The social nature of the mother's tie to her child: John Bowlby's theory of attachment in post-war America. *British Journal for the History of Science*, 44(3), 401–26, p.423. For an interesting illustration of how the concept of 'maternal instinct' is now treated as a cultural form rather than part of human nature by attachment researchers see Murphy, A., Steele, M., & Steele, H. (2013) From out of sight, out of mind to in sight and in mind: enhancing reflective capacities in a group attachment-based intervention. In J.E. Bettmann & D.D. Friedman (eds) *Attachment-Based Clinical Work with Children and Adolescents* (pp.237–57). New York: Springer. For a plea for a more measured and less polemical discussion of attachment research, and its heterogeneity see Duschinsky, R., van IJzendoorn, M., Foster, S., Reijman, S., & Lionetti, F. (2019) Attachment histories and futures: reply to Vicedo's 'Putting attachment in its place'. *European Journal of Developmental Psychology*, 17(1).

[308] Ainsworth, M.D.S. (1991) Attachments and other affectional bonds across the life cycle. In: C.M. Parkes, J. Stevenson-Hinde, & P. Marris (eds) *Attachment Across the Life Cycle* (pp. 33–51). London: Routledge: 'Nowadays in Western societies these traditional roles are being challenged, and many couples are experimenting with alternative ways of providing adequate care to their infants and young children. The more successful solutions seem to involve the male taking more responsibility for direct caregiving to the children' (42).

[309] Bowlby, J. (1980, 1988) Caring for children. In *A Secure Base* (pp.1–21). London: Routledge, p.5.

cultural systems. For instance, the development of retrieval response/caregiver behaviour is shaped by what opportunities an adult has had to touch children in the past, and the child's own reciprocal signals.[310]

The role of both the motivational and behavioural aspects of the caregiving system, and of the role of learning and culture, can be illustrated by two phenomena that especially concerned Bowlby. A first was the use of threats as part of caregiving, a behaviour that had interested him from his earliest work as a clinician working with families.[311] In *Separation*, threats by caregivers are a central theme. Bowlby acknowledged that threats might well have the ultimate end of retrieval or protection, the two suggested set-goals of the caregiving system depending on whether it was narrowly or broadly construed. For instance, a threat of abandonment by a parent might be used effectively to keep a child nearby or ensure their obedience, where this is considered of special importance.

However, the same behaviour might express the anger behavioural system, or be a compound fed by both the anger and caregiving systems. Bowlby emphasised that threatening as a cultural practice is quite complex for a young child to understand: it is intensely felt and expressed by the parent, but in fact localised and not fully serious. To the degree that the serious-but-not-serious quality of threats can be difficult for children to understand or trust, he worried about the long-term harm verbal threats could have on a child's perception of caregiver availability in times of need.[312] And he argued that verbal threats to hurt or abandon the child by a parent can contribute to conflict between the attachment and fear systems, since threats with a marked aggressive quality by a caregiver would elicit a desire for both approach and avoidance by their child (Chapter 3).[313] In a letter to Henry Hansburg in 1979 he observed that parents may 'insist that no one loves a child who behaves so and so, and that no one will ever love you unless etc. etc. I believe that when a child is exposed to these pressures over many years, the notion of his being unlovable becomes deeply engrained.'[314]

A second phenomenon that especially interested Bowlby was what he termed 'compulsive caregiving' in *The Making and Breaking of Affectional Bonds*, published in 1979.[315] This was the term Bowlby used when caregiving behaviour was shown by an individual as an alternative to seeking care. Children or adults may receive clear signals from their attachment figures that asking for comfort is not permitted or would backfire.[316] However, in providing care themselves, they at least gain some closeness with and availability from their attachment figures. The culturally mandated and practical closeness that caregiving permits allows individuals to achieve the set-goal of the attachment system, even if in a contorted and limited way.[317] The caregiving system is therefore used in the service of the attachment system, a

---

[310] Bowlby, J. (1969) Ape and apex. BBC Radio, recorded 16 October 1969. PP/Bow/F.5/5: 'Our capacity to learn diversity of behaviour is itself genetically determined e.g. speech and language ... Development of maternal behaviour dependent on appropriate experience, cf. Hinde on false dichotomy. Development of mothering greatly helped by 1. Opportunity to touch, examine infant; 2. Smiling of infant.'

[311] Bowlby, J. (1933–36) Anxiety, guilt, etc: old papers. PP/Bow/D.1/2/13

[312] Bowlby, J. (1973) *Separation*. London: Penguin, pp.231–2.

[313] Ibid. p.117. On threatening caregiver behaviour as a predictor of approach/avoidance conflict in infants see Jacobvitz, D., Leon, K., & Hazen, N. (2006) Does expectant mothers' unresolved trauma predict frightened/frightening maternal behavior? Risk and protective factors. *Development & Psychopathology*, 18(2), 363–79.

[314] Bowlby, J. (1979) *Letter to Henry Hansburg*, 21 February 1979. PP/Bow/J.9/90.

[315] Bowlby, J. (1977, 1979) The making and breaking of affectional bonds. In *The Making and Breaking of Affectional Bonds* (pp.150–88). London: Routledge.

[316] Bowlby, J. (1986) *Letter to John Birtchnell*, 14 October 1986. PP/Bow/J.9/22: 'Compulsive caregiving is based mainly on a fear of seeking love for fear of being rejected.'

[317] Bowlby, J. (1980) *Loss*. London: Penguin, p.411.

phenomenon that highlights both that caregiving behaviour in humans is not the product of some unvarying parenting instinct, and that the silent expression of attachment needs may be present even lodged inside child-to-adult caregiving behaviours.

In his book *A Secure Base,* published in 1988, Bowlby gave particular attention to conditions that may reliably elicit caregiving in the place of attachment behaviour, at least from toddlerhood, and the increased cognitive resources for attending to the mind of the caregiver.[318] Child-to-parent caregiving in the place of attachment may be seen when a parent has very severe depression such that the child's attachment signals elicit little or no response except when the child him-/herself helps the parent to cope, for instance through retrieval behaviours shown towards the parent. Child-to-parent caregiving may additionally be elicited if a parent's own attachment system is activated and becomes directed, through circumstances or misdirection as a consequence of conflict, towards the child.[319] Bowlby observed that child-to-parent caregiving responses may also be elicited, and combined with components of the fear system, in placatory behaviour. In such cases, for instance, 'children learn early that it is possible to placate a disturbed and potentially violent mother by constant attention to her wishes. Such apparently placatory behavior has been observed in young abused children, some less than two years old.'[320]

Yet a problem with Bowlby's characterisation of the caregiving system was the ambiguity between its narrow reference, referring primarily to the retrieval response, and its flung spray of wider meanings.[321] Bowlby's inattention to this system and ambiguities in conceptualizing its set-goal contributed to a neglect of the caregiving behavioural system by attachment researchers until the mid-1990s. A re-examination of Bowlby's position by George and Solomon, in the context of a rising cultural concern with 'motherhood as an experience and institution', led to renewed scientific discussion and debate of Bowlby's position.[322] An important point made by George and Solomon was that the mature balance of the caregiving systems with other behavioural systems is critical for the provision of 'good enough' care to a child. They contrasted their account to the image put forward by Bowlby, especially in his

[318] Bowlby, J. (1988) *A Secure Base.* New York: Basic Books.

[319] Personal communication by John Bowlby to Scott Henderson, cited in Henderson, S. (1974) Care-eliciting behavior in man. *Journal of Nervous and Mental Disease,* 159(3), 172–81.

[320] Bowlby, J. (1984) Violence in the family as a disorder of the attachment and caregiving systems. *American Journal of Psychoanalysis,* 44, 9–27, p.18. Crittenden and DiLalla would later distinguish placatory behaviour from caregiving, as different but related behavioural repertoires: Crittenden, P.M. & DiLalla, D.L. (1988) Compulsive compliance: the development of an inhibitory coping strategy in infancy. *Journal of Abnormal Child Psychology,* 16(5), 585–99.

[321] In the 2000s, social psychologists would highlight the significant limitations of Bowlby's image in *Attachment, Volume 1* of retrieval as the central form and symbol of the caregiving system. Mikulincer, M., Shaver, P.R., Gillath, O., & Nitzberg, R.A. (2005) Attachment, caregiving, and altruism: boosting attachment security increases compassion and helping. *Journal of Personality and Social Psychology,* 89(5), 817–39, p.818; Collins, N.L., Guichard, A.C., Ford, M.B., & Feeney, B.C. (2006) Responding to need in intimate relationships: normative processes and individual differences. In M. Mikulincer & G. S. Goodman (eds) *Dynamics of Romantic Love: Attachment, Caregiving, and Sex* (pp.149–89). New York: Guilford.

[322] Solomon, J. & George, C. (1996) Defining the caregiving system: toward a theory of caregiving. *Infant Mental Health,* 17(3), 183–97. See also Stern, D. (1995) *The Motherhood Constellation.* New York: Basic Books; Lieberman, A. (1996) Aggression and sexuality in relation to toddler attachment: implications for the caregiving system. *Infant Mental Health,* 17(3), 276–92; Heard, D. & Lake, B. (1997) *The Challenge of Attachment for Caregiving.* London: Routledge; Feeney, B.C. & Collins, N.L. (2001) Predictors of caregiving in adult intimate relationships: an attachment theoretical perspective. *Journal of Personality and Social Psychology,* 80, 972–94. On changes in public attention to the mother as 'subject' see e.g. Rich, A. (1995) *Of Woman Born: Motherhood as Experience and Institution.* New York: Norton.

early writing, of the caregiving system as the perfect match for the needs of the attachment system and hence the child.[323]

George and Solomon also argued that economic and social supports are important for the effective elaboration and functioning of the caregiving system. This is, in fact, exactly in line with an argument made by Bowlby himself in his book from 1953, *The Roots of Parenthood*, which was not published in America and so was unavailable to George and Solomon. There Bowlby emphasised that caregiving is dependent on the material and social resources available to a parent, which support a caregiver's energy, patience, and courage in the face of the demands of caring for a child. Without support, a caregiver may well 'give up trying', no matter that 'they would like to give their children all that good parents do'.[324] Bowlby condemned government inattention to 'the poverty of mothers with young children' and called on his readers to 'campaign unremittingly until it is remedied'.[325] This was not a campaign that he, however, would pursue over the coming decades. Instead, in his later work this concern with the conditions of the effective functioning of the caregiving system focused on psychological factors. He recognised the role of despair in hindering caregiving. However, after the early 1950s, he did not spell out poverty and isolation as potential contributors to despair. The traumatic loss of Bowlby's close friend, the Labour MP Evan Durbin, in 1948 undoubtedly played a role in this transition in Bowlby's thought.[326]

Besides George and Solomon, another important appraisal of Bowlby's concept of the caregiving system was presented by the anthropologist and primatologist Sarah Hrdy. In her 1999 book *Mother Nature*, Hrdy observed that 'Bowlby's ideas will stand among the greatest contributions made by evolutionary-minded psychologists to human wellbeing.'[327] However, she questioned his assumption in *Attachment, Volume 1* that in the environment within which humans evolved, care would have been provided by a parent alone; the resources required by a human infant are far more than any caregiver could be expected to provide on their own. Hrdy suggested that Bowlby's own biases and popularizing polemics combined with the available ethological and anthropological evidence of the time to paint a false image of mother–infant care, neglecting the necessity of social and economic supports for caregiving. Additionally, Bowlby drew on baboons and rhesus monkeys as his primate models, when in fact contrary evidence was shown from infant-sharing primates like langurs.[328] Whilst infants usually have a relatively small number of primary caregivers, the network of people involved in offering some care to a child may be very wide. Certainly

---

[323] George, C. & Solomon, J. (1999) The development of caregiving: a comparison of attachment theory and psychoanalytic approaches to mothering. *Psychoanalytic Inquiry*, 19(4), 618–46. Seemingly unaware of earlier critiques of Bowlby by Mary Main (Chapter 3) and Solomon and George, anthropologists have developed this point in detail especially over the past decade, e.g. Carlson, V.J. & Harwood, R.L (2014) The precursors of attachment security: behavioral systems and culture. In H. Otto & H. Keller (eds) *Different Faces of Attachment*. Cambridge: Cambridge University Press, 278–303.

[324] Bowlby, J. (1953) *The Roots of Parenthood*. London: National Children's Home, p.16.

[325] Ibid. p.14.

[326] Mayhew, B. (2006) Between love and aggression: the politics of John Bowlby. *History of the Human Sciences*, 19(4), 19–35.

[327] Hrdy, S.B. (1999) *Mother Nature: A History of Mothers, Infants and Natural Selection*. New York: Pantheon, p.xiii.

[328] Hrdy, S.B. (2005) Evolutionary context of human development: the cooperative breeding model. In L.A.C.S. Carter, K.E. Grossmann, S.B. Hrdy, M.E. Lamb, S.W. Porges, & N. Sachser (eds) *Attachment and Bonding: A New Synthesis* (pp. 9–32). Cambridge, MA: MIT Press. More recently, see Myowa, M. & Butler, D.L. (2017) The evolution of primate attachment: beyond Bowlby's rhesus macaques. In H. Keller & K.A. Bard (eds) *The Cultural Nature of Attachment. Contextualizing Relationships and Development* (pp.53–68). Cambridge, MA: MIT Press.

in human evolutionary history, care has not usually been provided by one person alone as Bowlby sometimes implied, especially in his earlier writings.[329]

Hrdy offered no objection to Bowlby's claim that the attachment behavioural system discriminates caregivers, and perhaps even has a hierarchy of attachment figures. However, she proposed that humans have evolved to engage in cooperative care, with mothers, fathers, grandmothers, aunts, siblings, and adult friends all involved, depending on circumstances. And when insufficient economic and social resources and supports are available, caregivers can be expected to divest from their children, reducing their availability as sources of protection.[330] The attachment system evolved in the context of this threat, and it is part of what makes exploration a dangerous activity for an infant who is not sure of the caregiver's availability. Likewise, the potential for an attachment figure to divest from their infant if other demands are pressing is part of what makes a network of attachment figures part of the evolutionary expectable conditions of infant survival.[331] Dragged towards reductionism at times by the narrow version of caregiving as retrieval, Bowlby did not adequately recognise the extent to which the ordinary functioning of the human caregiving behavioural system entails not only direct care, but also bringing additional supports on line for one we care for. And he did not adequately recognise that an integral part of the functioning of the caregiving system entails protecting the one we care about from ourselves, whether this is failures of patience or the wish to abandon the other when we feel overwhelmed. These are important 'anti-goals' of the caregiving behavioural system (Chapter 5).

Hrdy's critique has been well taken at a theoretical level by attachment researchers. In general, attachment researchers emphasise that young children will likely not be significantly harmed, and may even benefit, from high-quality care from several caregivers who develop personal relationships with the child. The primary qualifications that have been offered are that: (i) the child should not be passed around so many people that it proves difficult to develop at least one stable relationship, as is often the case with institutional care; and (ii) insecure attachment is made more likely if an infant is in very extensive daycare (e.g. over 70 hours a week), or (iii) if nights are spent with relative strangers.[332] A primary caregiver by no means needs to be present to the degree that Bowlby claimed in his popular writings of

[329] Hrdy, S.B. (1999) *Mother Nature: A History of Mothers, Infants and Natural Selection*. New York: Pantheon, p.495, discussing Tronick, E.Z., Winn, S., & Morelli, G.A. (1985) Multiple caretaking in the context of human evolution: why don't the Efé know the western prescription for child care? In M. Reite & T. Field (eds) *The Psychobiology of Attachment and Separation* (pp.293–322). Orlando, FL: Academic Press. For a more recent discussion of multiple caregiving see Meehan, C.L. & Hawks, S. (2013) Cooperative breeding and attachment among the Aka foragers. In N. Quinn & J.M. Mageo (eds) *Attachment Reconsidered: Cultural Perspectives on a Western Theory*. London: Palgrave.

[330] Hrdy appears to have been, understandably, unaware of Bowlby who made exactly this point in his 1953 book *The Roots of Parenthood*. The book was not distributed in the USA. Bowlby, J. (1953) *The Roots of Parenthood*. London: National Children's Home.

[331] Hrdy, S.B. (1999) *Mother Nature: A History of Mothers, Infants and Natural Selection*. New York: Pantheon, p.536.

[332] Hazen, N.L., Allen, S.D., Christopher, C.H., Umemura, T., & Jacobvitz, D.B. (2015) Very extensive nonmaternal care predicts mother–infant attachment disorganization: convergent evidence from two samples. *Development & Psychopathology*, 27(3), 649–61; van IJzendoorn, M.H., Bakermans-Kranenburg, M.J., Duschinsky, R., & Skinner, G.C.M. (2019) Legislation in search of 'good-enough' care arrangements for the child: a quest for continuity of care. In J. Dwyer (eds) *Handbook of Children and the Law*. Oxford: Oxford University Press. Belsky and colleagues have, however, found that the extent of non-familial care is associated with a small increase in child conduct problems and impulsivity, with maternal sensitivity as a moderator: e.g. Burchinal, M.R., Lowe Vandell, D., & Belsky, J. (2014) Is the prediction of adolescent outcomes from early child care moderated by later maternal sensitivity? Results from the NICHD study of early child care and youth development. *Developmental Psychology*, 50(2), 542–53.

the 1950s. And Bowlby's use of the term 'mother' to mean a primary caregiver—following common practice in psychoanalytic discourse of his day—should not be taken to imply that a primary caregiver needs to be a mother.

It is false to say of the contemporary field of empirical attachment research, as do Keller and Chaudhary, that it 'aims at demonstrating the uniqueness of the mother–child bond'.[333] If this were the aim, then, paradoxically, greater attention would have been paid to a variety of caregivers in order to comparatively demonstrate the particular qualities of maternal care. Other care providers have sometimes been studied by attachment researchers, for instance daycarers and foster parents.[334] However, these have hardly been comparisons to demonstrate the uniqueness of maternal care, as Keller and Chaudhary allege. Yet Keller and Chaudhary are undoubtedly correct in their criticism that, in practice, attachment research after Bowlby in the developmental tradition has predominantly focused on practice on mother–infant relationships. Comparatively few researchers have been able to access or prioritise the resources for studies of the contributions of wider caregiving networks using the labour-intensive measures of developmental attachment research,[335] though certainly some research has been done on caregiving networks by developmental researchers.[336]

Nonetheless, it is striking, for instance, that not a single study to date has examined infant–grandparent attachment using the Strange Situation, given the widely acknowledged importance of grandparents as alloparents in both human evolutionary history and contemporary societies.[337] The foremost reason why attachment researchers have focused research attention on mothers is that mothers have had primary care responsibilities for infants in America and in Europe, where the majority of attachment researchers are based. However, there are certainly enough infants living with their grandparents for this to have been a viable topic for study at some point since the 1970s. A focus on maternal care may have been partly self-perpetuating for attachment researchers after Bowlby in the developmental tradition, as it made this population the standard for comparability and study of the effects of specific variables on care.[338] A positive recent development, however, are plans over the coming years by Or Dagan and Avi Sagi-Schwartz to pool the raw data from all studies of attachment

[333] Keller, H. & Chaudhary, N. (2017) Is the mother essential for attachment? Models of care in different cultures. In H. Keller & K.A. Bard (eds) *The Cultural Nature of Attachment* (pp.109–37). Cambridge, MA: MIT Press, p.112. This claim rests on a characteristic rhetorical strategy among many critics, in which early statements by Bowlby are used to characterize all subsequent empirical attachment research (Chapter 2).

[334] E.g. Sagi, A., van IJzendoorn, M.H., Aviezer, O., Donnell, F., Koren-Karie, N., Joels, T., & Harl, Y. (1995) Attachments in a multiple-caregiver and multiple-infant environment: the case of the Israeli kibbutzim. *Monographs of the Society for Research in Child Development*, 60(2–3), 71–91.

[335] Keller, H. & Chaudhary, N. (2017) Is the mother essential for attachment? Models of care in different cultures. In H. Keller & K.A. Bard (eds) *The Cultural Nature of Attachment* (pp.109–37). Cambridge, MA: MIT Press.

[336] E.g. van IJzendoorn, M.H. (2005) Attachment in social networks: toward an evolutionary social network model. *Human Development*, 48(1–2), 85–8; De Schipper, J.C., Stolk, J., & Schuengel, C. (2006) Professional caretakers as attachment figures in day care centers for children with intellectual disability and behavior problems. *Research in Developmental Disabilities*, 27, 203–16. There has been a somewhat greater focus on wider networks among attachment researchers in the social psychological tradition, but not with respect to caregiving. Gillath, O., Karantzas, G.C., & Lee, J. (2019) Attachment and social networks. *Current Opinion in Psychology*, 25, 21–5.

[337] Gibson, M.A. & Mace, R. (2005) Helpful grandmothers in rural Ethiopia: a study of the effect of kin on child survival and growth. *Evolution and Human Behavior*, 26(6), 469–82.

[338] However, there has been a growing literature on fathers and on co-parenting (Chapter 4). An important development has been the inclusion of fathers within research on attachment-based interventions: e.g. Iles, J. E., Rosan, C., Wilkinson, E., & Ramchandani, P.G. (2017) Adapting and developing a video-feedback intervention for co-parents of infants at risk of externalising behaviour problems (VIPP-Co): a feasibility study. *Clinical Child Psychology and Psychiatry*, 22(3), 483–99.

to multiple caregivers using standardised measures, to permit statistical analyses with good depth and breadth, and to reconcile questions of comparability.

The exploratory behavioural system

The exploratory behavioural system was first detailed in *Attachment, Volume 1*, though the discussion remained relatively cursory.[339] Following Hinde's earlier discussions, Bowlby argued that the activating conditions of the exploratory behavioural system are 'stimuli that are novel and/or complex'.[340] An additional criterion implicit in Bowlby's account of the exploratory system, but left unstated, is that the stimuli need to have some potential relevance to the individual. In infancy, Bowlby argued that the exploratory system has three elements that often form a sequence: orienting towards the stimulus to gain information and prime responsiveness; approach to the stimulus to examine it; and manipulation or experimentation with the stimulus in order to understand what it can do.[341] The characteristic affect that supports and calibrates the expression of the exploratory system is 'curiosity'.[342] Like attachment, exploration was conceptualised as a homeostatic system, since once relevant novelty and complexity had been examined and understood, the system was expected to terminate. Bowlby situated the exploratory system as equivalent to Winnicott's concept of 'play', highlighting its importance as a system through which a child learns that meanings are partly self-created and partly supported by what the world makes available.[343] The experience of joy requires a world that can still surprise us with things we cherish, especially when we have attachment figures with whom to share discoveries. So Bowlby regarded the exploratory system as implicated in the pleasures that can come from connecting and reconnecting the

[339] The limited acknowledgement of the exploratory system in Bowlby's work might be linked to the scholarly context of the 1960s. Social learning was a pivotal discourse on child development, and one with which Bowlby had some sympathies. Both Bowlby and social learning theorists were concerned with the consistency and responsiveness of caregiving. However, he was keen to distinguish attachment behaviour from the effect of behaviourist conditioning, which was the dominant frame at the time for conceptualizing social learning. A more detailed elaboration of the exploratory system would have confronted Bowlby with the need to tackle social learning theory head-on, which would have been a demanding task, as demonstrated when it eventually fell to Ainsworth to clarify the differences between the attachment and social learning paradigms. See Bowlby, J. (1961) Comment on paper by Dr Gewirtz. In B.M. Foss (ed.) *Determinants of Infant Behaviour* (pp.301–304). London: Methuen; Ainsworth, M. (1972) Attachment and dependency: a comparison. In J. Gewirtz (ed.) *Attachment and Dependency* (pp. 97–137). Washington, DC: Winston. An additional contemporary dynamic was that creativity and play research were just getting off the ground. Attention to the exploratory system may well have been fed by this source, as shown by Bowlby's appeal to Winnicott's concept of creative play. However, theories of creativity and play were still weak when Bowlby was working on *Attachment, Volume 1*.

[340] Bowlby, J. (1969, 1982) *Attachment, Volume 1*. London: Penguin, p.238, discussing Hinde, R.A. (1954) Factors governing the changes in strength of a partially inborn response. 1. The nature of the response, and an examination of its course. *Proceedings of the Royal Society B*, 142, 306–31. Other important sources for Bowlby were Berlyne, D.E. (1950) Novelty and curiosity as determinants of exploratory behaviour. *British Journal of Psychology*, 41, 68–80; Rheingold, H.L. (1963) Controlling the infant's exploratory behavior. In B.M. Foss (ed.) *Determinants of Infant Behaviour*, Vol. 2 (pp.171–217). London: Methuen.

[341] Bowlby, J. (1969, 1982) *Attachment, Volume 1*. London: Penguin, pp.237–38.

[342] Ibid. p.197. See also Marvin, R.S., Britner, A.A., & Russell, B.A. (2016) Normative development: the ontogeny of attachment in childhood. In J. Cassidy & P.R. Shaver (eds) *Handbook of Attachment: Theory, Research, and Clinical Applications* 3rd edn (pp. 273–90). New York: Guilford.

[343] Bowlby, J. (1977, 1979) The making and breaking of affectional bonds. In *The Making and Breaking of Affectional Bonds* (pp.150–88). London: Routledge, p.183–4; cf. Winnicott, D.W. (1967) The location of cultural experience. *International Journal of Psychoanalysis*, 48, 368–72.

self and world, in sustaining their dialogue.[344] As the game 'peek-a-boo' demonstrates, even the absence of the caregiver may offer the pleasure of manipulation and experimentation if it occurs under the aegis of the exploratory behavioural system, and is brief enough not to threaten the dominance of this system.

Ainsworth qualified Bowlby's account through her attention to half-hearted forms of exploration. She identified this kind of play in infants showing avoidant behaviour in the Strange Situation Procedure (Chapter 2). She suggested that these infants were using play to distract themselves from attachment-relevant internal and external cues, thereby suppressing the expression of the attachment system.[345] Likewise, Main later observed that frame-by-frame video analysis of the reunion episodes of avoidant dyads 'reveals that the inanimate object generally has far from the infant's full attention. The infant may, for example, rather frantically turn toward a tale leg and finger it (but with eyes fixed blankly on the wall ahead). Or, in a clumsily decisive move, it may suddenly drop a toy into a box but then close the box on its hand. The general impression is, again, that the infant could not succeed in maintaining its avoidance of the parent without the aid of the object seized.'[346] Here exploration is used as somewhere else to go, a projection of attention away from felt concerns and into the environment.

The contrast between the lacklustre and distracted infant exploration seen in avoidant dyads and true play burnished by lively curiosity led Ainsworth to criticise Bowlby for his account of the exploratory system, which only infrequently drew distinctions between these two forms.[347] Ainsworth suggested that Bowlby had given a place to exploration, but did not take it seriously enough as a behavioural system. His characterisation had focused too much on its behavioural components, at the expense of affective and cognitive components that lead a child to engage in 'actively seeking' information within a social and cultural context.[348] She offered the example of an infant encountering a novel and potentially alarming situation. Before the sequence described by Bowlby of orienting, approaching, and experimenting, Ainsworth asserted that a first stage of the exploratory system in infancy will be social referencing of attachment figures. The caregiver helps offer shape and definition to the infant's world and will often be actively sought to serve as 'referee' for the meaning of the stimulus, especially when there is a question whether its novelty should stimulate exploration and

---

[344] Some of Bowlby's examples are quite culturally specific, e.g. on novelty and pleasure in family holidays, Bowlby, J. (1969, 1982) *Attachment, Volume 1*. London: Penguin, p.41. Whether exploration of complex/novel stimuli can be interpreted as equivalent to Winnicott's concept of 'play' depends on what is understood by the latter term, an understanding shaped in important ways by culture. Lancy, D.F. (2007) Accounting for variability in mother–child play. *American Anthropologist*, 109(2), 273–84.

[345] Ainsworth, M. (1984) Attachment. In N.S. Endler & J. McVicker Hunt (eds) *Personality and the Behavioral Disorders*. New York: Wiley, 559–602, p.565. See also Grossmann, K., Grossmann, K.E., Kindler, H., & Zimmermann, P. (2008) A wider view of attachment and exploration: the influence of mothers and fathers on the development of psychological security from infancy to young adulthood. In J. Cassidy & P.R. Shaver (eds) *Handbook of Attachment: Theory, Research, and Clinical Applications*, 2nd edn (pp.857–79). New York: Guilford.

[346] Main, M. (1981) Avoidance in the service of proximity: a working paper. In K. Immelmann, G.W. Barlow, L. Petrinovich, M. Biggar Main (eds) *Behavioral Development: The Bielefeld Interdisciplinary Project* (pp.651–93). Cambridge: Cambridge University Press, p.554–5.

[347] E.g. Bowlby, J., Robertson, J., & Rosenbluth, D. (1952) A two-year-old goes to hospital. *Psychoanalytic Study of the Child* 7, 82–94, p.83. He also discussed the use of distraction activities in adults: Bowlby, J. (1980) *Loss*. London: Pimlico: 'One or more behavioural systems within a person may be deactivated, partially or completely. When that occurs one or more other activities may come to monopolize the person's time and attention, acting apparently as diversions' (64).

[348] Ainsworth, M. (1992) A consideration of social referencing in the context of attachment theory and research. In S. Feinman (ed.) *Social Referencing and the Construction of Reality in Infancy* (pp.349–67). New York: Plenum Press, p.361.

affiliation or wariness. For Ainsworth, exploration took part of its significance from the long infancy of human beings, and the dense, multifaceted urgency of the human society that infants must learn to navigate. A behavioural system that makes matters that are novel and/or complex attractive for exploration is therefore a great asset, since, alongside staying safe moment-to-moment, the other great task of children is to encounter and learn from the world around them (Chapter 2).[349]

The fear behavioural system

In Bowlby's account, when a stimulus is judged as alarming, two systems may be activated: the attachment system and the fear system. The first third of his book *Separation* was essentially a theory of the fear behavioural system.[350] Bowlby urged recognition that attachment and fear are 'distinct behavioural systems that (a) have the same function, (b) may be elicited by many of the same conditions, (c) are frequently compatible with each other, but (d) can easily be in conflict'.[351] The compatibility of the attachment system and the fear system is that both are oriented towards increasing proximity to safety in contexts of perceived threat. The difference, for Bowlby, is that the attachment system disposes attempts to achieve the availability of attachment figures, whereas the fear system prompts attempts both to escape the threat and to find people or places that have proven safe in the past. Bowlby suggested that the term 'alarm' should be used for concern about a threatening stimulus, and 'anxiety' should be used for concern about the availability of safety, whether due to the presence of danger or questions about the availability of attachment figures.[352] In distinguishing the attachment and fear systems, however, Bowlby left unaddressed whether or how feelings of safety and of security might inflect one another, and how the set-goal of the attachment behavioural system might be conditioned by experiences of the fear behavioural system and its resolution.

---

[349] Ainsworth, M. & Bell, S. (1970) Attachment, exploration, and separation: illustrated by the behavior of one-year-olds in a strange situation. *Child Development*, 41(1), 49–67, p.51. The underdevelopment of the idea of the exploratory system in Bowlby's work is widely acknowledged, e.g. Gullestad, S.E. (2001) Attachment theory and psychoanalysis: controversial issues. *Scandinavian Psychoanalytic Review*, 24, 3–16. Subsequent to Ainsworth, the major sustained interest in the relationship between exploration and attachment has been among clinically-focused commentators, who have been concerned with what attachment research can suggest about moderators of our capacity to explore the minds of others and learn from experience e.g. Fonagy, P., Luyten, P., Allison, E., & Campbell, C. (2017) What we have changed our minds about: part 2. Borderline personality disorder, epistemic trust and the developmental significance of social communication. *Borderline Personality Disorder and Emotion Dysregulation*, 4, 9; Golding, K. & Hughes, D. (2012) *Creating Loving Attachments: Parenting with PACE to Nurture Confidence and Security in the Troubled Child*. London: Jessica Kingsley; Powell, B., Cooper, G., Hoffman, K., & Marvin, B. (2016) *The Circle of Security Intervention*. New York: Guilford.

[350] Bowlby had also been very interested in human fear behaviour since his work as an army psychiatrist. However, the proximal cause of Bowlby's attention to the topic in the early 1970s appears to have been the proposal of fear as a distinct behavioural system by the American developmentalist Gordon Bronson. Bronson, G.W. (1968) The development of fear in man and other animals. *Child Development*, 39(2), 409–31. Bronson observed that the threshold for activation of the fear behavioural system seemed to be lower for institutionally reared human children and monkeys, and that fear of strangers seemed to develop at around the same time as discrimination of attachment figures. However, Bowlby felt that Bronson's distinctions were not adequately sharp between fear, wariness, and anxiety. In a wider context, cultural discourses appealing to and distinguishing 'fear' and 'anxiety' were gaining ground from the late 1960s, and may have contributed to the salience of the topic for Bronson and Bowlby. See Jenkins, P. (2006) *Decade of Nightmares: The End of the Sixties and the Making of Eighties America*. Oxford: Oxford University Press; Bourke, J. (2006) *Fear: A Cultural History*. Emeryville, CA: Shoemaker & Hoard.

[351] Bowlby, J. (1973) *Separation*. London: Penguin, p.117.

[352] Ibid. Appendix III.

Component behaviours of the fear system identified by Bowlby in his notes included the startle response, withdrawal, fleeing, and hiding.[353] Later, on the suggestion of Hinde, he added freezing as another behavioural component of the fear system.[354] This led him to discuss 'three distinct kinds of predictable outcome' of the fear behavioural system '(a) immobility, (b) increased distance from one type of object, and (c) increased proximity to another type of object'.[355] These responses, he proposed, are highly responsive to context: 'When a chimpanzee is startled by a sudden noise or movement nearby, its immediate response is to duck its head and to fling one or both arms across its face; alternatively, it may throw both hands in the air. Occasionally these startle reactions are followed by a hitting-away movement with the back of the hand towards the object, at other times by flight. When the alarming object is another and more dominant chimpanzee, flight is accompanied by loud screaming; when it is anything else, flight is quite silent.'[356] In an unpublished paper from 1973 entitled 'Wariness', Bowlby discussed a continuum of fear responses. At one end was flight and expressions of terror. At the other end was various forms of wary behaviour.[357]

In *Separation*, Bowlby proposed that the activating conditions for the fear system are partly learnt on the basis of experience, but are also partly neurologically primed by human evolutionary history. Children are certainly more likely to fear the dark if they have been told that darkness is dangerous, they have seen others respond with caution to darkness, or if they associate darkness with unhappy experiences. However, Bowlby argued that humans are predisposed to have a lower bar for treating certain cues, such as darkness, as threatening. Other such cues potentiated to have lower bars for activation include being cold and loud sudden noises. Perhaps the most important such cue for danger, Bowlby observed, is the feeling of being alone, or of blocked access to attachment figures.[358] Furthermore, he argued that the bar for activation of the fear behavioural system would fall dramatically where two or more such cues were present at once, and especially when one of these was feeling alone. Where multiple cues to danger occur at once, most adult humans respond with an activation of the fear system.[359]

However, especially in childhood, we may not know how to interpret the cause of such an activation: 'Often, in fact, when we feel impelled to act in a certain way that is readily explicable in terms of biological function, we concoct "reasons" for doing so that bear little or no relation to the causes of our behaviour. For example, a child or adult, who in order to reduce risk is biologically disposed to respond to strange sounds in the dark by seeking his attachment figure, gives as his reason that he is afraid of ghosts.'[360] Bowlby contended that children's actual experiences in situations with such primed cues for danger are likely to be especially important for the later development of mental health problems. For instance, the origins of

---

[353] Bowlby, J. (1968) Types of fear response. PP/Bow/H.209.

[354] Bowlby, J. (1973) *Separation: Anxiety and Anger*. New York: Basic Books: 'Hinde (1970) reports a finding by Hogan that, in chicks, withdrawal occurs from stimuli at high intensity (and some others) whereas freezing is elicited by stimuli that are strange, novel, or surprising' (154).

[355] Ibid. p.114.

[356] Ibid. p.157.

[357] Bowlby, J. (1973) *Wariness*. Unpublished manuscript, June 1973. PP/BOW/J.9/39. The same distinction was used by Bretherton, I. & Ainsworth, M.D.S. (1974) Responses of one-year-olds to a stranger in a strange situation. In M. Lewis & L.A. Rosenblum (eds) *The Origin of Fear* (pp.131–64). New York: Wiley.

[358] Bowlby, J. (1973) *Separation: Anxiety and Anger*. New York: Basic Books, p.119.

[359] Bowlby, J. (1970, 1979) Self-reliance and some conditions that promote it. In *The Making and Breaking of Affectional Bonds* (pp.124–49). London: Routledge, p.147.

[360] Bowlby, J. (1981) Psychoanalysis as a natural science. *International Review of Psycho-Analysis*, 8, 243–56, p.248.

many phobias and paranoid symptoms can be understood as 'intelligible, albeit distorted' re-sponses to historical experiences in contexts with multiple such cues, where a caregiver was not available to help soothe the child and interpret the meaning of their response.[361]

On the basis of analysis of their activating and terminating conditions, Bowlby was clear that the attachment and fear systems were distinct. With Robertson, he had considered the pre-dicament of hospitalised children, who experienced fear but without being able to turn to their caregivers. Part of Bowlby's focus on long-term separations stemmed from his sense that the clinical community and public were not able to acknowledge child abuse by parents. Yet in the early 1970s, the tide was turning on the acknowledgement of child physical abuse within Britain, and within the medical community in particular.[362] The manuscript history of *Separation* sees Bowlby edging slowly towards the claim that the attachment and fear behavioural systems could conflict as a result of directly frightening or abusive actions by the attachment figure. In an early draft of material for *Separation* Bowlby reported having seen a lamb attempting to cross directly into the path of a car, having been startled by the sound of the car and seeing its mother on the other side of the road.[363] In correspondence with Ainsworth, and then in the typescript, Bowlby added consideration of the case of an infant who is confronted with a threatening stimulus, such as a 'barking dog', that lies in the path towards the attachment figure.[364] Reflecting further, in a pencil annotation on the typescript and then in the published version, Bowlby added that 'a special but not unusual situation in which there is conflict between attachment behaviour and withdrawal is when the attachment figure is also the one who elicits fear, perhaps by threats or violence. In such conditions young creatures, whether human or non-human, are likely to cling to the threatening or hostile figure rather than run away from him or her.'[365] A threatening or violent caregiver, Bowlby observed, could be expected to activate the fear and attachment sys-tems, producing conflict between the two behavioural systems (Chapter 3).

The aggression behavioural system

With one exception in *Attachment, Volume 1,* Bowlby did not generally describe aggression as a behavioural system.[366] Yet consideration of the case of the aggression system in closing this section on behavioural systems may help shed light on the boundaries of this concept for Bowlby. He gave aggression only passing and faltering attention.[367] Despite the fact that the subtitle of his book *Separation* is 'Anxiety and Anger', in fact Part I focuses on anxiety, Part

---

[361] Bowlby, J. (1973) *Separation: Anxiety and Anger.* New York: Basic Books, p.210.

[362] Parton, N. (1985) *The Politics of Child Abuse.* Basingstoke: Macmillan; Hacking, I. (1991) The making and molding of child abuse. *Critical Inquiry,* 17(2), 253–88; Ferguson, H. (2004) *Protecting Children in Time: Child Abuse, Child Protection and the Consequences of Modernity.* London: Palgrave.

[363] Bowlby, J. (1973) Draft material towards *Separation.* PP/Bow/K.5./17.

[364] Bowlby, J. (1973) *Letter to Ainsworth,* 29 October, 1973. PP/Bow/J.1/33; Bowlby, J. (1973) *Separation: Anxiety and Anger.* New York: Basic Books: 'Conflict can easily occur, for example, whenever a stimulus situation that elicits both escape and attachment behaviour in an individual happens to be situated between that individual and his attachment figure; a familiar instance is when a barking dog comes between a child and his mother' (116). The typescript is available at PP/Bow/K.5./17.

[365] Bowlby, J. (1973) *Separation: Anxiety and Anger.* New York: Basic Books, p.117. The typescript is available at PP/Bow/K.5./17.

[366] Bowlby, J. (1969, 1982) *Attachment, Volume 1.* London: Penguin: 'In Tom, it can be said, there is a tendency to appraise certain situations in such a way that a behavioural system is activated that results in his attacking his little sister and biting her' (118).

[367] Bowlby's most sustained attention to aggression appears in Durbin, E.F.M. & Bowlby, J. (1939) *Personal Aggressiveness and War.* London: Kegan Paul. Little from this book fed through into his later reflections on

II focuses on fear, and Part III returns essentially to a consideration of anxiety, with the exception of a dozen pages in Chapter 17 (entitled 'Anger, Anxiety, and Attachment').[368] Mary Main later observed that Bowlby's exclusion of aggression as a behavioural system 'has puzzled many clinicians', and emphasises the disparity this has left between theory and empirical research on aggression.[369] Shaver and Mikulincer expressed disappointment with Bowlby for his poor attention to aggression, since it has left attachment theory without a specified place for anger (Chapter 5).[370] And van IJzendoorn and Bakermans-Kranenburg and colleagues felt forced to bypass Bowlby in their development of an intervention with caregivers struggling with aggressive child behaviour.[371]

It may be speculated that aggression was refused the status of a behavioural system because Bowlby wanted to avoid even the slightest implication of acceptance of Melanie Klein's position. Whereas Klein regarded aggression as an innate human drive, Bowlby claimed that most aggression is a response to the frustration of other behavioural system.[372] Certainly this is a point that he reiterates time and again when aggression is under discussion. Yet, as Ainsworth observed, frustration could still then be a behavioural system: it is neurologically primed as a result of human evolutionary history, but requires frustrating experiences for its elaboration, and works to achieve its goals through various behavioural means.[373]

An additional factor may have contributed to Bowlby's wariness in describing aggression as a behavioural system. Bowlby's younger colleagues at the Tavistock recall that he used to think aloud in seminars and conversations about whether the idea of 'aggression' was too much of a catch-all. He was far from certain that it was a single thing.[374] In *Separation*, he described two forms of aggression, only one of which resembled a behavioural system.

aggression in *Separation*. Those who knew Bowlby personally have often remarked that he did not seem at all comfortable with aggression, which may have contributed to a theoretical antipathy.

[368] This emphasis has been echoed by later attachment researchers: for instance, Cassidy's influential introduction to the *Handbook of Attachment* discusses the attachment, caregiving, exploratory, sociable, and fear systems, but does not discuss anger as a behavioural system. Cassidy, J. (1999) The nature of the child's ties. In J. Cassidy & P.R. Shaver (eds) *Handbook of Attachment: Theory, Research, and Clinical Applications* (pp.3–21). New York: Guilford. This selection of behavioural systems was maintained by Cassidy in the second (2008) and third (2016) editions.

[369] Main, M. (1993) Les bébés et leurs colères. In M.C. Busnel (eds) *Le Langage des Bébés, Savons-nous Entendre?* (pp.17–91). Paris: Grancher; Main, M. (1995) Recent studies in attachment: overview, with selected implications for clinical work. In S. Goldberg, R. Muir, & J. Kerr (eds) *Attachment Theory: Social, Developmental and Clinical Perspectives* (pp.407–70). Hillsdale, NJ: Analytic Press, p.460. In work with Jude Cassidy, Main describes the role of aggressive behaviour within displays of dominance from children towards their attachment figures (Chapter 3), but without ever referring this back to Bowlby's discussion of aggression. An important disjuncture lay in the fact that Bowlby's accounts of aggression characterized primarily frustration and protest in the service of attachment, whereas what Cassidy and Main were seeing was more like use of aggression in the service of dominance in the service of attachment.

[370] Shaver, P.R., Segev, M., & Mikulincer, M. (2011) A behavioral systems perspective on power and aggression. In P.R. Shaver & M. Mikulincer (eds) *Human Aggression and Violence: Causes, Manifestations, and Consequences* (pp.71–87). Washington, DC: American Psychological Association, p.71.

[371] Van Zeijl, J., Mesman, J., van IJzendoorn, M.H., et al. (2006) Attachment-based intervention for enhancing sensitive discipline in mothers of 1- to 3-year-old children at risk for externalizing behavior problems: a randomized controlled trial. *Journal of Consulting and Clinical Psychology*, 74(6), 994–1005.

[372] Bowlby, J. (1973) *Separation: Anxiety and Anger*. New York: Basic Books, p.319.

[373] Ainsworth, M. (1997) Peter L. Rudnytsky—the personal origins of attachment theory: an interview with Mary Salter Ainsworth. *Psychoanalytic Study of the Child*, 52, 386–405, p.403.

[374] E.g. Issroff, J. (2005) *Donald Winnicott and John Bowlby: Personal and Professional Perspectives*. London: Karnac: 'Bowlby disliked what he called sometimes "portmanteau" and sometimes "umbrella" or "omnibus" words like "aggression", which covered too many different broad possibilities and created confusion in the way they were used' (56).

The first form was what he termed 'the anger of despair'.[375] In this form of aggression the behaviour occurs primarily as the expression of emotion, spinning within its own loops of intensity, without the environmental responsiveness that would help behaviour to achieve a specific set-goal. The anger of despair, Bowlby argued, 'occurs whenever a person, child or adult, becomes so intensely and/or persistently angry with his partner that the bond between them is weakened, instead of strengthened, and the partner is alienated. Anger with a partner becomes dysfunctional also whenever aggressive thoughts or acts cross the narrow boundary between being deterrent and being revengeful'.[376] The anger of despair is a mood that disbelieves hope; it is premised on the assumption that aggression cannot change the environment.

He contrasted the anger of despair with 'the anger of hope'.[377] This form of anger is elicited by frustration of another behavioural system. It may seek removal of the obstacle. More often, though, it acts upon people or the environment in such a way as might coerce them to yield, permitting the satisfaction of the other system. For instance, Robertson documented a great increase in aggressive behaviour in children following their hospital separations. Bowlby felt that this might be conceptualised as a kind of punishment of the caregivers for the separation by the child, signalling that the experience should not be repeated: 'In its functional form anger is expressed as reproachful and punishing behaviour that has as its set-goals assisting a reunion and discouraging further separation. Therefore, although expressed towards the partner, such anger acts to promote, and not to disrupt, the bond'.[378] The anger of hope is a mood that disbelieves despair; it is premised on the wish that aggression may change the environment.

The anger of hope is a dangerous strategy, and may readily backfire by provoking retaliatory aggression or rejection from the partner or caregiver. As Waters and Sroufe later observed, aggression risks (further) disrupting the trust and patience on which any secure attachment relationship must rest.[379] However, this risk may be better, or be felt to be better, than alternatives, such as being unnoticed or despairing of achieving co-regulation within a relationship.[380] The anger of hope has a good claim to be a behavioural system, especially in light of its clear set-goal. However, perhaps a mark against even the anger of hope as a behavioural system is that it remains the servant of other behavioural systems, and when it achieves independence from them it is as the dysregulated anger of despair. The anger of hope may have seemed to Bowlby as a component behaviour of other behavioural systems, rather than having the status of a behavioural system in itself. However, as Waters and colleagues have argued, such a stance ascribes too little independence to aggressive behaviours, not least since they may be fed by more than one source of frustration.[381] Moreover, several second-generation attachment researchers including Shaver and Fonagy later criticised

[375] Bowlby, J. (1973) *Separation: Anxiety and Anger*. New York: Basic Books, p.285.

[376] Ibid. p.288.

[377] Ibid. p.285.

[378] Ibid. p.287.

[379] Waters, E. & Sroufe, L.A. (1983) A road careened into the woods: comments on Dr Morrison's commentary. *Developmental Review*, 3(1), 108–14, p.223.

[380] Knox, J. (2005) Sex, shame and the transcendent function: the function of fantasy in self development. *Journal of Analytical Psychology*, 50, 617–39: 'I was fortunate enough to hear John Bowlby lecture on one occasion and one comment he made, almost in passing, remains imprinted on my mind—it was that children can survive the experience that their hate may drive a parent away but to have one's love rejected is intolerable' (625).

[381] Waters, E., Posada, G., Crowell, J., & Lay, K.L. (1993) Is attachment theory ready to contribute to our understanding of disruptive behavior problems? *Development & Psychopathology*, 5(1–2), 215–24, p.220.

Bowlby on the grounds that aggression can be evoked in the absence of the frustration of a behavioural system.[382]

The meaning and structures of symptoms

Defence

A central motivation—perhaps the central motivation—for Bowlby's development of a theory of behavioural systems was to account for the development of mental health symptoms in humans. His new model allowed him to consider symptoms that might arise from the interplay or conflict of different systems, from poor alignment between behavioural systems and their social context, or from aspects of the functioning or misfiring of individual systems themselves. Reflecting on his clinical experiences with adults, Bowlby was impressed by the psychoanalytic insight that even an inhibited response not only continues to exist but can develop, 'putting out derivatives and establishing connections' even if these may be contorted by the inhibition.[383] For instance, inhibited behavioural systems, even if they do not influence our behaviour, may nonetheless exert a powerful influence on our judgement and mood, as well as the activation of memories and forms of imagination or daydream.[384] Such processes may influence individuals' experiences even of their own motivations. In *Attachment, Volume 1,* Bowlby wrote that 'reports are usually trustworthy, but psychoanalysts know well that that is not always so. A subject may in fact mis-identify the set-goal of a behavioural system currently active—and such mis-identification may itself be the result of interference by an active system that has a set-goal which is incompatible with the first. This leads to the concept of unconscious wish.'[385]

However, in discussions of such phenomena, Bowlby felt that the concept in common use in the psychoanalytic community, 'defence', was often confusing. The term absorbed a variety of psychological and behavioural activities that aimed to reduce or eliminate experiences that might threaten the integrity or stability of the individual. Bowlby felt that this usage was lazy, and left nameless and soundless many critical psychological processes.[386] He addressed

---

[382] Shaver, P., Schwartz, J., Kirson, D., & O'Connor, C. (1987) Emotion knowledge: further exploration of a prototype approach. *Journal of Personality and Social Psychology,* 52(6), 1061–86, p.1078; Fonagy, P. (2003) The violence in our schools: what can a psychoanalytically informed approach contribute? *Journal of Applied Psychoanalytic Studies,* 5(2), 223–38, p.230.

[383] Annotations by Bowlby dated 1958 on Freud's essay 'Repression' in *The Standard Edition of the Complete Psychological Works of Sigmund Freud,* Vol. 14. Copy held in the library of Human Development Scotland. Highlighted and underlined: 'Repression does not hinder the instinctual representative from continuing to exist in the unconscious, from organising itself further, putting out derivatives and establishing connections' (p.149). Bowlby marginalia: 'Very much my position.'

[384] Bowlby, J. (1980) *Loss.* London: Pimlico: Information about experience 'can be retained long enough outside consciousness in a temporary buffer store for it to influence judgement, autonomic responses and, I believe, mood' (49).

[385] Bowlby, J. (1969, 1982) *Attachment, Volume 1.* London: Penguin, p.138.

[386] Bowlby's concerns resembled closely those of Laplanche and Pontalis: 'When operations as diverse as, say, rationalisation, which brings complex intellectual mechanisms into play, and turning against the self, which is a "vicissitude" of the instinctual aim, are attributed to a single function, and when the same term "defence" connotes such a truly compulsive operation as "undoing what has been done" as well as the search for a form of "working-off" after the fashion of certain kinds of sublimation, then it may well be asked whether the concept in question is a really operational one.' Laplanche, J. & Pontalis, J.B. (1973) *The Language of Psycho-Analysis,* trans. D. Nicholson-Smith. London: Karnac, p.109.

these concerns in a short unpublished book from 1962 entitled *Defences that Follow Loss: Causation and Function*. ('Defences that Follow Loss' recently appeared in *Trauma and Loss: Key Texts from the John Bowlby Archive*, edited by Duschinsky and White.)[387] In this work, Bowlby disparaged the concept of 'defence' as a confused mix of description and explanation. He felt that it also served to mask the important distinction between the inhibition of a motivation and the inhibition of behaviour, and the distinction between the immediate cause and the ultimate function of inhibition. All too often, Bowlby felt, psychoanalysts discussed 'defences' as if they were initiated in order to avoid some foreseeable consequence.[388] For instance, psychoanalytic discussions of obsessive-compulsive symptoms at the time tended to situate them as a defence against Oedipal conflicts. Klein argued that 'obsessional neurosis is an attempt to cure the psychotic conditions which underlie it', which arise from a predicament of experiencing both love and hate for the mother.[389] Bowlby felt that such claims failed to clarify the initiating conditions of obsessional symptoms, the contexts that led them to become enduring, and the evolutionary function obsessive-compulsive behaviours may have served.

In failing to draw such distinctions Bowlby argued that Klein and other contemporary psychoanalysts were unable to distinguish effectively between defensive strategies and strategies for coping.[390] Some forms of defence are evidently under our conscious control; others indicate that conscious control is breaking down. Some forms of defence are helpful for individuals in responding to their environment; others are highly destructive. Yet psychoanalysts were making these distinctions remarkably rarely (with a few, inconsistent exceptions like Donald Fairbairn and Joseph Sandler).[391] In general, Bowlby felt that in psychoanalytic theory 'the relation of defence to healthy control, or to coping processes, has never been clarified. Like Melanie Klein, most analysts hold the view that there are no great differences between them.'[392] The primary current of psychoanalytic thought directed attention away from the question of which defences were able to contribute to individual coping, for instance through offering short-term adaptation to an adverse environment for an individual.

To address this issue Bowlby appealed to the four questions of ethology: (i) the contribution a behaviour may have for species survival or reproduction; (ii) how the behaviour came about in the course of natural selection; (iii) the behaviour's mechanism or how it works; and (iv) how it develops in the individual. To Bowlby, the processes and behaviours subsumed under the term 'defence' likely have very different answers to these questions. However, what they likely have in common, he argued, is that whilst at a species or population level they may

[387] Duschinsky, R. & White, K. (eds) (2019) *Trauma and Loss: Key Texts from the John Bowlby Archive*. London: Routledge.

[388] Bowlby, J. (1962) *Defences that Follow Loss: Causation and Function*. PP/Bow/D.3/78.

[389] Klein, M. (1932) *The Psychoanalysis of Children*. London: Hogarth, p.226.

[390] The concept of coping strategies was just entering the academic literature in the early 1960s. E.g. Murphy, L.B. (1960) Coping devices and defense mechanisms in relation to autonomous ego functions. *Bulletin of the Menninger Clinic*, 24(3), 144–53. The concept would gain ground in academic psychology, until it detonated into widespread use with Lazarus. R.S. & Folkman, S. (1984) Coping and adaptation. In W.D. Gentry (ed.) *The Handbook of Behavioral Medicine* (pp.282–325). New York: Guilford.

[391] Fairbairn, W.R.D. (1929, 1994) Dissociation and repression. In E. Fairbain & D.E. Scharff (eds) *From Instinct to Self: Selected Papers of W.R.D. Fairbairn* (Vol. II). New York: Aronson Publishing; Sandler, J., Joffe, W.G., Baker, S., & Burgner, M. (1965) Notes on obsessional manifestations in children. *The Psychoanalytic Study of the Child*, 20(1), 425–38. Bowlby's annotations on and correspondence with Sandler are of special interested in this regard. Bowlby was intrigued by the fact that Sandler was not always able to hold on to the distinction between cause and function even despite his best efforts. See Bowlby, J. (1965) Comments on Joffe and Sandler 1965 'Notes on Pain, Depression and Individuation'. PP/Bow/J.9/168-9.

[392] Bowlby, J. (1962) *Defences that Follow Loss: Causation and Function*. PP/Bow/D.3/78.

help at times to contribute to survival or reproduction, for a given individual they may be baffling and sometimes counterproductive: 'defensive processes come into action in certain conditions and that they do so without the individual having any more idea of their biological function than the ordinary man has of the function served by his temperature rising when he contracts an infection'.[393] Later, in *Loss*, Bowlby urged that 'the effects of defensive activity must be judged on a number of distinct scales. For example we can ask: what are its effects, beneficial or otherwise, on the personality concerned? what are its effects, beneficial or otherwise, on the members of the person's family? what are its effects, beneficial or otherwise, on the community at large?'[394] However, Bowlby felt that the concepts available for even asking these questions were overloaded and confused in psychoanalytic discourse. This prompted his decision to introduce the concept of segregated systems.

Segregation

Another problem that Bowlby had with the concept of defence as used by the psychoanalytic community of his day was that it seemed to him oriented by the basic image of withdrawal from an aversive source of excitation. However, whereas in some ways the concept of defence was too absorptive, in this regard Bowlby found it too restrictive. Picking apart the concept, Bowlby narrowed in on the idea of the inhibition of behavioural systems.[395] In *Defences that Follow Loss: Causation and Function* in 1962, he introduced for the first time the concept of 'segregated systems'. This concept would be pulling the strings as the governing concept of Bowlby's later thought, but in fact was only introduced in print 18 years later in *Loss*, in a discussion so brief that subsequent researchers have generally not found it clear or usable.[396] *Defences that Follow Loss*, by contrast, engaged in an extended and elaborate discussion of the concept. In this book Bowlby argued that behavioural systems are 'segregated' if there is reduced, distorted, or blocked communication with perception, memory, and/or other behavioural systems. Though there was, intentionally, some overlap between Bowlby's term 'segregation' and Freud's concept of 'repression', Bowlby preferred the former term since he felt that 'repression' had accrued too much baggage, such as implying processes that keep something unconscious. By contrast, segregation could occur between two conscious systems, or between a conscious system and memory or perception.[397] And whereas for Freud,

---

[393] Ibid.

[394] Bowlby, J. (1980) *Loss*. London: Pimlico, p.67.

[395] Bowlby, J. (1961) *Letter to Dr Robert Hinde*, 24 January 1961. PP/Bow/H224: 'The whole psychoanalytic notion of defence is confused and I want to explore the notion that at the time of onset of what is later called repression one motivational system is blocked of expression and another, incompatible with it, evoked: both continue active but out of communication with each other. In the human, one of them is likely to be more accessible to consciousness than the other ... Supposing this is a correct picture of events, the problem now becomes to define the conditions that give rise to this state of affairs and their mode of operation.'

[396] Among the few attachment researchers to have applied the concept are Bretherton, and Solomon and George. It is revealing about the underdeveloped status of the concept in Bowlby's published writings that their treatments differ vastly from one another, and that Bretherton expressed hesitancy as to whether she fully grasped Bowlby's meaning. See Bretherton, I. (2005) In pursuit of the internal working model construct and its relevance to attachment relationships. In K.E. Grossmann, K. Grossmann, & E. Waters (eds) *Attachment from Infancy to Adulthood: The Major Longitudinal Studies* (pp.13–47). New York: Guilford; Solomon, J. & George, C. (2011) Disorganization of maternal caregiving across two generations. In J. Solomon & C. George (eds) *Disorganized Attachment & Caregiving* (pp. 25–51). New York: Guilford.

[397] Bowlby, J. (1962) *Defences that Follow Loss: Causation and Function*. PP/Bow/D.3/78; cf. Bowlby, J. (1956) Annotations on Charles Brenner 'The nature and development of the concept of repression in Freud's writings'. PP/BOW/J.9/33.

repression worked against the dynamic unconscious as a 'cauldron full of seething excitations',[398] for Bowlby segregation was an abstraction used to describe any process that resulted in a blockage or inhibition of communication within or between behavioural systems.

It might be thought that segregation would be regarded by Bowlby as a bad thing. And this has been the impression of Bowlby's readers who have access to only his published discussions of segregation: an apparent denigration of segregation has been part of Bowlby's legacy to later researchers and clinicians, among the very few who have engaged with the concept.[399] Bailey and colleagues, for instance, seem to presume that all segregation must be an effect of trauma.[400] However, such denigration ignores the potential for helpful segregation, through processes that buffer or segment and creatively recompose what is taken in from outside. In fact, in *Defences that Follow Loss,* Bowlby argued in some detail that long-term mental health would be supported by effective communication between mental systems on the basis of relative and flexible forms of segregation, rather than those that were strictly held. He was attentive to the role of segregation within typical development as well as atypical development, and its contribution to mental health, as well as mental ill health.[401] He was specifically interested in 'the functions that in health the segregation processes serve' and gave careful consideration to the idea that segregation should be regarded 'in the same light that Claude Bernard taught us to view physiological illness, namely as the outcome of processes that are beneficial in kind but faulty in amount'.[402]

Bowlby used the term 'selective exclusion' to refer to strategies of behavioural and attentional aversion or withdrawal that enact a flexible and relatively minimal segregation. 'Selective exclusion' may contribute to the mutual enrichment of behavioural systems. Bowlby gives the example of engrossment: selective exclusion of other thoughts, distractions, and daydreams may insulate and protect the effective operation of the exploratory system. Other cases are easy to imagine. For instance, selective exclusion can help preserve sources of private and sustaining joy, warped and wonderful against the flattening bustle of the world. Or to take another example, selective exclusion may be helpfully deployed to keep worries away during relaxation or sleep. The direction and quality of attention would need to be flexible enough to change once work began again. Where this can be achieved, communication between systems ensures that benefits of physical and attentional rest are transferred in the form of feeling genuinely refreshed.

Segregation essentially means that a system is not accepting information from another source, or potentially from any source. Sometimes, as in the case of selective exclusion, this

---

[398] Freud, S. (1933, 2001) New introductory lectures on psychoanalysis. In *The Standard Edition of the Complete Psychological Works of Sigmund Freud*, Vol. 22 (pp.1–182). London: Vintage, p.73. In *Loss*, Bowlby acknowledged some parallels between his concept of segregation and Freud's concept of 'splitting', though he felt that the latter term had accrued too much baggage to offer much clarity. 'Splitting' would later feature within Crittenden's reinterpretation of Bowlby's information processing model: Crittenden, P.M. (2016) *Raising Parents: Attachment, Representation, and Treatment* (2nd edn). London: Routledge.

[399] See e.g. Lemma, A., Target, M., & Fonagy, P. (2011) *Brief Dynamic Interpersonal Therapy: A Clinician's Guide.* Oxford: Oxford University Press: 'Although there is never a direct correspondence between external and internal, as what is internal reflects the operation of defensive processes that distort what is taken in from the outside' (95).

[400] Bailey, H.N., Redden, E., Pederson, D.R., & Moran, G. (2016) Parental disavowal of relationship difficulties fosters the development of insecure attachment. *Revue Canadienne des Sciences du Comportement*, 48(1), 49–59, p.50.

[401] In this regard, *Defences that Follow Loss* is a forerunner of the priorities and concerns of developmental psychopathology (Chapter 4).

[402] Bowlby, J. (1962) *Defences that Follow Loss: Causation and Function.* PP/Bow/D.3/78. On Bernard see Gross, C.G. (1998) Claude Bernard and the constancy of the internal environment. *The Neuroscientist*, 4(5), 380–85.

is a generally beneficial filtering process. However, segregation can also occur because otherwise useful information is experienced as difficult to accept or incompatible with currently held values.[403] This is likely the meaning of Bowlby's claim, cited earlier in the 'Introduction', that the conditions of lack of integration between aspects of the self rest on conditions of forgivability or unforgivability: the critical question for the segregation or desegregation of systems is whether they are willing to accept information from one another, from memory and from the world, recognizing it as content available for inclusion within the system. If the information is regarded as unacceptable or dangerous, it may not be reconciled, causing segregation of the behavioural system.

Defensive exclusion

Bowlby was not concerned about segregation and the incompatibility of behavioural systems so long as 'when they conflict, as habitually they do, regulation is tolerably smooth and efficient'.[404] Some segregation is an inevitable part of being human, and localised and controlled incompatibility can provide a foundation of imagination, creativity, and work–life balance. By contrast, Bowlby felt that rigid and intense segregation can lead to very significant problems.[405] One fundamental consequence of rigid and/or intense segregation is that the system then does not have access to new perceptions, or to reciprocal development with other behavioural systems. Not only does the cognitive component of a segregated behavioural system not receive the benefits of the learning provided by the exploratory system, or conscious reflection, but also the opportunities for feedback and revision are blocked that would usually occur when a behavioural system is expressed.[406] Without such feedback, behavioural systems cannot fully benefit from the opportunities and lessons of the environment. When the behavioural system does get expressed, the result may be too strong or extreme, or clumsily formulated or ineffective.[407]

Furthermore, in Bowlby's account, behavioural systems become active only when their activating conditions are met. As a consequence, to the degree that a behavioural system is segregated from information about these conditions, the system will only be partially activated or not activated at all. When strategies of behavioural and attentional aversion or withdrawal are used to inhibit memories that would otherwise activate a

---

[403] Main would later criticize Bowlby on this point, suggesting that he placed too much emphasis on information that was difficult to accept because integration would be painful, and not enough emphasis on information that was difficult to accept simply as a result of human cognitive biases and developmental processes, such as the difficulties of a three year old in holding in mind contradictory qualities of a single person. Main, M. (1991) Metacognitive knowledge, metacognitive monitoring, and singular (coherent) vs. multiple (incoherent) models of attachment: some findings and some directions for future research. In P. Marris, J. Stevenson-Hinde, & C. Parkes (eds) *Attachment Across the Life Cycle* (pp.127–59). New York: Routledge, p.138–9.

[404] Bowlby, J. (1962) *Defences that Follow Loss: Causation and Function*. PP/Bow/D.3/78.

[405] Indeed, the strength of his emphasis on segregation as a problem in his book on *Loss* would begin a divergence between two rather different trends in subsequent attachment theory: one that focused on whether internal working models were positive, and one that focused on whether behavioural systems were flexibly used and open to revision. The first to call attention to this ambiguity was van IJzendoorn, M.H., Tavecchio, L.W.C., Goossens, F.A., & Vergeer, M.M. (1982) *Opvoeden in geborgenheid: Een kritische analyse van Bowlby's attachmenttheorie*. Amsterdam: Van Loghum Slaterus, pp.61–2.

[406] Bowlby, J. (1964) Segregation of psychic systems. PP/Bow/H10. See also Reisz, S., Duschinsky, R., & Siegel, D.J. (2018) Disorganized attachment and defense: exploring John Bowlby's unpublished reflections. *Attachment & Human Development*, 20(2), 107–34.

[407] Bowlby, J. (1980) *Loss*. London: Pimlico, p.348.

Table 1.2 Selective exclusion of motivation and levels of motivation

Motivation	Exclusion
Level 1: Low	Slight, e.g. daydreaming, free-association
Level 2: Moderate	Moderate. Some degree of concentration but still possible to attend to other Input
Level 3: High	Considerable. Strong concentration and resulting in exclusion of all other input
Level 4: Very high (or persistence of high)	Erratic. Whilst exclusion continues on a considerable scale, there is also a tendency for responses to a wider class of objects than in other conditions of motivation (cf Hinde)

Source: Theory of Defence, JB notes, 1960–63, PP/Bow/H10.

behavioural system, Bowlby referred to 'cognitive disconnection'.[408] The main effect, he proposed, was that strong emotions would seem to appear out of nowhere or be associated with inappropriate objects, since they have been disconnected from their original, provoking source. If cognitive disconnection is the segregation of *memory*, Bowlby offered the term 'defensive exclusion' to refer to the segregation of external *perception*. Cognitive disconnection keeps memory, reflection, and other cognitive processes from causing the activation of a behavioural system. Defensive exclusion keeps new experiences from achieving this same consequence. Both are dynamic properties that block relevant information from having implications for a behavioural system or systems. In turn, 'segregation' is the structure that such processes create or hold in place, a state in which information or its meaning is blocked, thinned, or distorted in such a way as to shape the activating or terminating conditions of a behavioural system. As Crittenden and Bretherton both observed, the exact nature of what is being blocked, thinned, or distorted, and by what agency, is not clear in Bowlby's account of segregated systems.[409] It would seem that segregation can be maintained by various processes. Among these, however, Bowlby gave defensive exclusion special importance. External perception offers the potential to gain from the opportunities and lessons of the environment. Without this, segregation becomes rigid, a situation with particular implications for mental health.

In unpublished notes from the time of *Defences that Follow Loss: Causation and Function*, Bowlby created a table to distinguish between four levels of exclusion (Table 1.2).[410]

Level 1 is exclusion with only the barest drop of defence. It may, for instance, be little more than engrossment in something novel and/or complex, where the alternative would be rumination. Or it might be thinking about food or work when we might otherwise find

---

[408] Ibid. p.66.

[409] Crittenden, P.M. (1997) Truth, error, omission, distortion, and deception: the application of attachment theory to the assessment and treatment of psychological disorder. In S.M. Clancy Dollinger & L.F. DiLalla (eds) *Assessment and Intervention Issues Across the Lifespan* (pp.35–76). London: Lawrence Erlbaum; Bretherton, I. (2005) In pursuit of the internal working model construct and its relevance to attachment relationships. In K.E. Grossmann, K. Grossmann, & E. Waters (eds) *Attachment from Infancy to Adulthood: The Major Longitudinal Studies* (pp.13–47). New York: Guilford.

[410] Bowlby, J. (1960) Theory of Defence. JB notes, 1960-63. PP/Bow/H10.

ourselves getting upset, bringing one behavioural system partly online in order to exclude another a little. Or exclusion with a drop of defence might be identified in the absorption facilitative of endurance during exercise or sport. What Bowlby termed 'the ordinary everyday things of life',[411] its familiar, conventionalised rhythms and language, can also be characterised as Level 1 defensive exclusion. They keep us connected to others but without demanding vulnerability or deeper availability to others—or to ourselves. 'How are you?' 'Fine thanks, how are you?' Such are the 'outer rings' of social stabilisation, Bowlby argued, that keep individual behavioural systems, such as the attachment system, from needing to be activated.[412]

Level 2 is described by Bowlby as 'moderate' exclusion. It is 'still possible to attend to other input'. There is still some allowance, at least, for untidy, troubling experiences. Laugh-or-you'll-cry humour might be offered as an illustration of this level of defensive exclusion, since the distress is walled off yet, if incipiently, personally and socially acknowledged. In Level 3 there is 'exclusion of all other input'. The information permitted through the filter is rigorously and rigidly policed. Finally, at Level 4, 'whilst exclusion continues on a considerable scale, there is also a tendency for responses [to be made] to a wider class of objects than in other conditions of motivation'. The exclusion becomes extended beyond its original objects, for instance excluding not just perception but whole related classes of emotions as well. An example of this exclusion of a 'wider class of objects' is provided by a patient described by Bowlby in the chapter entitled 'Psychoanalysis as Art and Science', who until she was ten years old had 'been terrified of another separation; but then she had "switched off" her anxiety "like a tap", as she put it, and with the anxiety had disappeared most of her emotional life as well.'[413]

In *Defences that Follow Loss: Causation and Function*, Bowlby theorised that defensive exclusion and cognitive disconnection enact a weakening of the integration between or within behavioural systems. Defensive exclusion and cognitive disconnection may, then, contribute to coping when the alternative might otherwise be a greater or more enduring disruption to the system, or to the psychological apparatus that underpins and orchestrates behavioural responses more generally. This is why children especially vulnerable to using segregative processes, because their psychological apparatus is still immature and less resilient to disruption. Defensive exclusion and cognitive disconnection, then, permit a certain kind of resilience in the face of disintegrative threats precisely by accepting some determinate and limited degree of segregation.

On this basis, Bowlby distinguished avoidance and dissociation as different intensities and kinds of defensive exclusion. Some kinds of avoidant response may involve little segregation, just perhaps a turning of attention away from a person, situation, or thing that might otherwise activate a behavioural system.[414] There is some loss of information from reality, but not

---

[411] Bowlby, J. (1940) The influence of early environment in the development of neurosis and neurotic character. *International Journal of Psycho-Analysis*, 21, 154–78, p.173.

[412] Bowlby, J. (1973) *Separation: Anxiety and Anger*. New York: Basic Books: 'the regulatory systems that maintain a steady relationship between an individual and his familiar environment can be regarded as an "outer ring" of life-maintaining systems complementary to the "inner ring" of systems that maintain physiological homeostasis' (180).

[413] Bowlby, J. (1978, 1988) Psychoanalysis as art and science. In *A Secure Base* (pp.43–64). London: Routledge, p.58.

[414] Bowlby, J. (1960) Theory of Defence. JB notes, 1960-63. PP/Bow/H10: 'Hypothetical function of narrowing of attention. Narrowing of attention is achieved by reducing input, but sensory and cognitive. The advantages are: a) to cut-out irrelevant and confusing input; b) to cut-out input that in fact evokes other motivational systems because such system would distract the organism from the task in hand by reducing relevant input; c) to cut-out input that might require abandonment of current organisation of a motivational system, and consequently reorganisation with its attendant layer of inability to act—disorganisation.' Some commentators have assumed

a loss of contact with reality. For instance, we may tune out small occurrences that might otherwise generate impatience or irritation, to keep the aggression system from coming on-line and disrupting our overall plans. This would be Level 1 in Bowlby's taxonomy. It is also possible to have more thorough-going segregation with avoidance, as for instance when access to anger is muted—the threshold for activating the aggression system is raised—for an individual who was made to feel endangered when they displayed anger as a child. Muted access to anger would be Level 2; if anger is essentially unreachable, this would be Level 3.[415]

In the 1950s Robertson observed that withdrawn and avoidant behaviours shown by hospitalised children were often accompanied by disorientated behaviours. However, Bowlby treated dissociation as, in contrast to avoidance, a more extreme form of segregation—more of an emergency break.[416] At a population level, forms of defensive exclusion such as dissociation may have evolved as a way to shut off and thereby protect behavioural systems or other psychological processes from extreme perceptions or memories that might otherwise risk a greater disruption. Instead of segregating certain information from a behavioural system, perception in general is segregated from other mental processes. He speculated that it would specifically be episodic information about occurrences within time and place that would be lost to dissociative processes; general attitudes might well remain unaffected.[417] Bowlby proposed that such a process will produce responses that, unlike avoidance, are not responsive to the environment. This produces the phenomenon of 'coming to' following dissociation.[418] The generalisation of segregation to all sense perceptions for a time suggests that dissociation would be considered by Bowlby as one kind of Level 4 defensive exclusion.

Displays of conflict

Yet defensive exclusion is not always successful. Bowlby found parallels between psychoanalytic theory and the work of ethologists, who had observed odd behaviour by animals experiencing a conflict of motivations, for instance when cued both to approach and to flee.[419]

---

that all 'detached' behaviours observed by Robertson represented dissociative phenomena, e.g. Barach, P. (1991) Multiple personality disorder as an attachment disorder. *Dissociation*, 4, 117–23. Whilst avoidance may perhaps have relevant prospective links with dissociation (Chapter 4), Bowlby's thinking about different kinds of defensive exclusion acknowledges their differences.

[415] A remark by Ursula Bowlby offers an illustration. She described her husband as, for biographical reasons, incapable of feeling the emotion of fear. She considered this an aspect of Bowlby's general inhibition of negative feelings, and a contributing factor to his indomitable courage as a public intellectual and theoretician. Again, this would be Level 3 defensive exclusion. Ursula Bowlby interview with Robert Keren, cited in Karen, R. (1998) *Becoming Attached: First Relationships and how they Shape our Capacity to Love*. Oxford: Oxford University Press, p.469.

[416] Bowlby, J. (1962) *Defences that Follow Loss: Causation and Function*. PP/Bow/D.3/78: 'I am introducing the generic term "to segregate" and "segregated process"; they denote any process that creates barriers to communication and interaction between one psychic system and another ... Other additional terms are required for the many other particular sorts of segregating process.' Handwritten marginal note: 'dissociation'. See also Bowlby, J. (1961) Processes of mourning. *International Journal of Psycho-Analysis*, 42, 317–40, p.336.

[417] Bowlby, J. (1982) Outline of attachment theory. PP/Bow/H.260.

[418] E.g. Bowlby J., Robertson, J., & Rosenbluth, D. (1952) A two-year-old goes to hospital. *Psychoanalytic Study of the Child* 7, 82–94: 'During the hospital experience these splits were relatively brief; after a few minutes of blankness she "came to" and responded to her real mother ... This, perhaps, helps us to understand how during longer experiences of separation this split can develop to a point where integration on reunion with the mother is no longer automatic and the child is unable to link his need for a good mother and his hatred of a frustrating one to an individual woman' (86).

[419] Bowlby, J. (1976) Human personality development in an ethological light. In G. Serban & A. Kling (eds) *Animal Models in Human Psychobiology* (pp.27–36). New York: Plenum Press: Ethology and psychoanalysis fit

Bowlby was fascinated that Hinde had discerned in his study of chaffinches that 'paradoxically, strangeness evokes both escape and curiosity, and that there is a complex balance between the two competing response systems'.[420] Likewise, Hinde observed that the following response show by young birds towards their parents may be disrupted or discoordinated where this competes with another response system, for instance if the parent is also in some way a cue for danger, not uncommon given 'the broad range of stimuli eliciting both following and fleeing at this age'.[421] In such situations, animals show 'conflict behaviours' such as the rapid transition between one tendency and the other, poorly coordinated combinations, freezing in place, misdirected movements, or signs of confusion or tension.[422] Bowlby also considered that anger might be evoked by conflict between two behavioural tendencies, presumably since conflict can obstruct the achievement of one or both tendencies, contributing to frustration.[423]

Bowlby's interest in conflict behaviour was likely primed by having observed several kinds of conflict response in his clinical work. For instance, as an army psychiatrist in World War II, working with veterans on their return from the front, he observed amnesias, loss of bodily control, misdirected and undirected behaviours, out of context anger or anxiety, signs of confusion, and tic-like behaviours or other signs of tension. Bowlby interpreted these behaviours as reflecting veterans' experiences of psychological conflict between feelings of duty and lingering fear from their time at the front.[424] Robertson also reported many of the same behaviours in his description of children during hospitalisation and on their return home. There were also discussions of conflict behaviour in the psychanalytic community. For instance, in 1956, Anna Freud described the case of a 13-month-old infant whose behaviour towards her mother was disrupted by screaming and states of withdrawal. Since these behaviours were only shown in the relationship with the mother, Freud anticipated that they suggested 'some traumatic event' in the history of this relationship, a hypothesis that was later confirmed.[425]

Bowlby came to believe that his concept of segregated systems could account for some forms of conflict behaviour, including when displayed towards attachment figures. On the one hand, conflict could occur between a behavioural system and its defensive exclusion, especially when information from perception or memory for the activation of a behavioural

so well together because 'both were interested in the effect of early experience on later development' and 'in conflict arising from social situations' (28). As well as Robert Hinde, another important influence on Bowlby's reflections on conflict behaviour was von Holst, E. & von Saint Paul, V. (1963) On the functional organisation of drives. *Animal Behaviour*, 11, 1–20. They detail seven kinds of response to the conflict of behavioural responses: display of one toned by the other; averaging of the responses; alternation between the two; each cancelling the other out; the production of a third rather different kind of response (e.g. pecking and feeing becomes threat screeching); the dominance of one which masks weak expressions of the other; display of only one or the other.

[420] Bowlby, J. (1960) Separation anxiety. *International Journal of Psycho-Analysis*, 41, 89–113, p.97.

[421] Hinde, R.A. (1961) The establishment of the parent–offspring relation in birds, with some mammalian analogies. In W.H. Thorpe & O.L. Zangwill (eds) *Current Problems in Animal Behaviour* (pp.175–93). Cambridge: Cambridge University Press, p.185. Passage underlined as of particular note in Bowlby's personal copy of the text. PP/Bow/H.226.

[422] Hinde, R. (1970) *Animal Behavior*, 2nd edn. New York: McGraw-Hill.

[423] Bowlby, J. (1965) Motivation. PP/Bow/H.128.

[424] Bowlby, J. & Soddy, K. (1940) War neurosis memorandum. PP/Bow/C.5/1; Bowlby, J. (1942) Selection and diagnosis in Army: notes for a talk. PP/BOW/C.5/2/3.

[425] Freud, A. (1956, 1969) The assessment of borderline cases. In *The Writings of Anna Freud*, Vol. 5 (pp.301–14). New York: International Universities Press, p.310.

system is particularly salient. For instance, a child who is hurt may seek to exclude distressing information that might otherwise trigger the attachment system, if they have learnt that their caregiver will likely punish them for being upset or displaying a desire for comfort. They may ignore their injury, pretend it does not cause them distress, or keep their attention away from information about their caregiver's whereabouts to avoid the desire to seek the caregiver. However, this exclusion will become increasingly precarious to the degree that the child's injury is especially painful, is experienced as upsetting, or the caregiver is on hand. The result will be conflict between the attachment system and its inhibition, an approach–avoidance conflict, which may be visible in the child's behaviour.

On the other hand, Bowlby was also interested in the forms of conflict that could arise when two behavioural systems were active at the same time. Often, of course, different behavioural systems are easily compatible. This is why, as Ainsworth repeatedly argued, it is a mistake to study behavioural systems in isolation: 'In any situation, the extent to which attachment behaviour occurs depends not only on the strength to which it is activated, but also on the strength of activation of other competing or compatible behavioural systems.'[426] A favourite example for both Bowlby and Ainsworth was that the fear system and the attachment system are often easily reconciled and integrated, in directing an infant away from a perceived threat and towards a haven of safety.[427] Sometimes behavioural systems, whilst somewhat different in their demands, can be combined: for instance where courtship systems and wariness combine to produce flirting behaviour, or the anger and caregiving systems combine to produce harsh forms of discipline.

In other cases, however, Bowlby argued that behavioural systems may come into significant conflict, especially if there has been segregation of one or both, hindering communication and effective compromise.[428] For example, conflicts may arise between the attachment and caregiving systems. The injured child discussed above may have caring responsibilities for a sick parent. This may be one of the reasons why the child feels that their attachment system should be inhibited where possible, since they have learnt that their parent is most responsive when they seem happy and available to meet the parent's wishes.[429] In such a case, however, pain or distress associated with the injury would come into conflict with the child's caregiving system. The child may attempt to achieve the ends of both systems at once. The two systems do have some compatible behaviour, like physical approach to the caregiver. If the child attempts to maintain his caregiving role, this may be undermined or interrupted by distress from the injury. If the child lets the parent know about his injury and conveys his

[426] Ainsworth, M.D.S. (1977) Attachment theory and its utility in cross-cultural research. In: P.H. Leiderman, S.R. Tulkin, & A. Rosenfeld (eds) *Culture and Infancy: Variations in the Human Experience* (pp. 49–67). New York: Academic Press, p.59.

[427] Bretherton, I. & Ainsworth, M.D.S. (1974) Responses of one-year-olds to a stranger in a strange situation. In M. Lewis & L.A. Rosenblum (eds) *The Origin of Fear* (pp. 131–64). New York: Wiley.

[428] This is discussed in the section 'Incompatible behavioural systems: results of simultaneous activation' of Bowlby, J. (1969, 1982) *Attachment, Volume 1*. London: Penguin, pp.97–101.

[429] Bowlby, J. (1986) Transcript of interview by Lange. Wellcome Trust Library Archive. PP/BOW/A.5/16: 'Anxiously avoidant children who have a parent who tends towards rejection ... They are really caught in a classic approach–avoidance conflict. On the one hand they really would love to have affection and support and comfort. They would love to have that sort of relationship. But their attempts to develop such a relationship were met with so many painful rejections in the past that they dare not attempt it again. And they pretend, sometimes convince themselves and convince everyone else, that they get along very well, thank you, without any of that sentimental nonsense ... They are incredibly out of touch with their feelings and out of touch with the situations which evoke their feelings.'

feelings of distress, this may nonetheless be inflected, even distorted, by the child's habitual caregiving response and relative exclusion of the attachment system.

As a general principle, Bowlby suggested that 'whenever a system that has been deactivated becomes in some degree active, such behaviour as is then shown is likely to be ill-organised and dysfunctional'.[430] The smooth resolution of conflicts depends upon systems being able to communicate and compromise. When one behavioural system is active at the expense of a conflicting one that has been segregated, trapdoors are to be found inside our intentions and actions:

> Not only are information and motor response relevant to any one goal narrowly restricted but information and motor responses relevant to some other and perhaps incompatible goal may be allowed through. It is as though an enquiry clerk, when asked about trains to Cornwall, gave information endlessly about the night express to Plymouth, with occasional intrusions about a plane to Rome.[431]

Psychoanalytic theory proposed that conflict between incompatible psychological demands is part of being human. However, the strength of these demands, the extent of their incompatibility, and other challenges may turn such conflict into a source of symptoms, in which one or both of these demands gets expressed in a distorted form. For instance, in a passage highlighted by Bowlby in his personal copy, Karl Abraham suggested that a conflict between the sexual response and its suppression could find outlet in the intensification of hunger: 'The great frequency of hunger attacks in frigid women is very striking … Strong libidinal impulses, against the undisguised appearance of which consciousness protects itself, can be unusually well masked by a feeling of hunger. For hunger is a sensation that can be admitted to oneself and to others.'[432]

Bowlby proposed that conflict behaviours would become stabilised as symptoms of mental ill health to the extent that the situation that evoked the conflict was stable, and especially when it related to a close and enduring relationship. Signs of 'tension, anxiety and depression' may be especially expected to the degree that contradictory responses (or conflict between a response and its defensive exclusion) are felt towards an attachment figure.[433] When access to attachment figures is uncertain, as may occur in conflict situations, this may evoke tension and anxiety. Conflict situations, when they are sustained, also block the satisfaction of at least one behavioural system (and perhaps more). This predicament can contribute to the onset and/or maintenance of depression by provoking a sense that the achievement of the set-goal is impossible, no matter what strategy is deployed.[434]

---

[430] Bowlby, J. (1980) *Loss*. London: Pimlico, p.346.

[431] Bowlby, J. (1962) *Defences that Follow Loss: Causation and Function*. PP/Bow/D.3/78.

[432] Annotations by Bowlby on Abraham, K. (1927) *Selected Papers*. London: Hogarth Press, p.263; not dated but handwriting and reference on p.74 suggest annotations are from 1933. Copy held in the library of Human Development Scotland.

[433] Bowlby cited in Tanner, J.M. & Inhelder, B. (1956) *Discussions on Child Development: Proceedings of the WTO Study Group of the Psychobiological Development of the Child, Vol. 1*. London: Tavistock, p.186.

[434] Bowlby, J. (1974) Psychological processes evoked by a major psychosocial transition. Presented to Tavistock Research Workshop, March 1974. PP/Bow/F.3/90; Bowlby, J. (1989) Foreword to *Emmy Gut's Productive and Unproductive Depression* (pp.xiii–xv), London: Routledge.

Bowlby anticipated that encounters with attachment figures that evoke conflict are powerful sources of anxiety and depression. He identified several reasons for this. Part of the importance of the attachment system in this regard is that it has implications for the individual's basic sense of being intrinsically worthy, acceptable, and capable of being cherished. It therefore has a developmental role in informing the components of other behavioural systems. Another reason for the important role of conflict in relation to attachment figures in prompting anxiety and depression is that our attachment figures are often socially difficult to avoid, not only but especially in childhood. In the chapter 'The making and breaking of affectional bonds', Bowlby speculated that the intensity of emotion in close relationships may serve especially to activate early behavioural, cognitive, and affective components of behavioural systems, so that forgotten wishes and disappointments from childhood become incorporated into present-day behaviour and expectations.[435] This was one aspect of what Bowlby termed the 'risks of intimacy'.[436] It is in good part in response to these risks that closeness gets so thoroughly modulated and ritualised in everyday family life. This reduces occasions that might risk disturbing the others' composure by activating early and raw components of a behavioural system rather than the more mature and well-conditioned components.

Bowlby's interest in the contribution of psychological conflict to depression and anxiety made him enthusiastic about the work of Aaron Beck, and the emergent paradigm of cognitive behavioural therapy. In Bowlby's terms, to the degree that thoughts such as hopelessness in relationships, personal responsibility, and the unacceptability of the self become segregated from feedback, they would in turn reinforce depression and anxiety.[437] In print, Bowlby stated that his model of depression and anxiety was 'cast in the same mould' as that of Beck, and that 'his theory is compatible with mine'.[438] He was especially impressed by the fact that Beck appeared to distinguish between two forms of depression—one anxious and needy, the other avoidant and with reduced affect—that corresponded to the two classes of response to separation that he and Robertson had identified.[439] However, Bowlby felt that, more than Beck, attachment theory highlighted the importance of early experiences in contributing to psychological conflicts. In particular, the theory highlighted the relationship expectations and forms of defensive exclusion that could perpetuate conflicts even after the original situation evoking conflict had ceased.[440]

[435] Bowlby, J. (1977, 1979) The making and breaking of affectional bonds. In The Making and Breaking of Affectional Bonds (pp.150–88). London: Routledge: 'The stronger the emotions aroused in a relationship the more likely are the earlier and less conscious models to become dominant' (168).

[436] Bowlby, J. (1985) Letter to John Byng-Hall, 12 April 1985. PP/Bow/J.9/45: 'You need to clarify what the risks of intimacy are. One risk, which may motivate either child or mother, is fear of rejection; another risk, which may also motivate either partner, is fear of being held captive by the intense attachment behaviour of the other.'

[437] This point is elaborated with case studies in Bowlby, J. (1980) The place of defensive exclusion in depressive disorders. PP/Bow/K.7/94; see also Bowlby, J. (1987) Notes on depression, towards correspondence with Emmy Gut. PP/Bow/B.3/15.

[438] Bowlby, J. (1980) Loss. London: Pimlico, p.249–50. For a recent discussion see Bosmans, G. (2016) Cognitive behaviour therapy for children and adolescents: can attachment theory contribute to its efficacy? Clinical Child and Family Psychology Review, 19(4), 310–28.

[439] Bowlby, J. (1981) Letter to Aaron Beck, 8 October 1981. PP/Bow/J.9/16. See Beck, A. (1983) Cognitive therapy of depression: new perspectives. In P.J. Clayton & J.E. Barrett (eds) Treatment of Depression: Old Controversies and New Approaches (pp.265–90). New York: Raven.

[440] Bowlby, J. (1990, 2011) John Bowlby: interview by Leonardo Tondo. Clinical Neuropsychiatry, 8(2), 159–71, p.167.

In the clinic

Mrs Q

In his last article, written with Mary Ainsworth, Bowlby highlighted especially his work as a clinician with children and families, and additionally the decades in which he ran a mother's group in a wellbaby clinic, 'learning much from his informal observations of mother–child interaction there.'[441] Bowlby was mindful that his theory addressed general tendencies at the level of populations, and had only a probabilistic relationship with any individual, whereas his clinical practice addressed the concrete dynamics of individual lives, each with their particular vitality and equilibrium.[442] In a sense, Bowlby observed in private notes, the clinician experiences the complex human being in front of his as like a work of art: 'The criteria of a work of art are a) sensory and formal vitality (tension, life); and 2) order (balance, equilibrium, and symmetry) ... What is true of a work of art is also true of a human personality.'[443] Bowlby emphasised the need to distinguish between a clinical understanding of tension and order in the lives of individuals and the generalisations of diagnostic or research frameworks, and to establish a productive relationship between the two:

> In the past there has been a deplorable tendency for the experimentalist to despise the clinician's lack of precision and the clinician to reciprocate with contempt for the experimentalist's lack of insight into human nature. Each has stoutly maintained that his own method was the one true way to knowledge. These claims are absurd: each method is indispensable. It is the clinician who usually has the earliest insights, defines the problem, and formulates the first hypotheses. But [through] the detailed minute study of the feelings and motivations of his patients, and the complicated intellectual and emotional repercussions to which they give rise, the clinical worker provides information regarding the relations of psychic and environmental forces which can be obtained in no other way.[444]

During Bowlby's lifetime, there was already a good deal of discussion of the clinical implications of attachment theory.[445] Since then, commentators have described an 'explosion' of texts offering exposition of Bowlby's ideas for practitioner audiences.[446] These works for

---

[441] Ainsworth, M. & Bowlby, J. (1991) 1989 APA award recipient addresses: an ethological approach to personality development. *American Psychologist*, 46(4), 333–41, p.336. The Bowlby Archive contains a wonderful description of the clinic, entitled 'Mothers Discussion Group' from 1967 (PP/Bow/C.6/3). In justifying the benefits of the group Bowlby wrote: 'It is from other mothers that a beginner can learn most. Professional people can add information about different sorts of behaviour and the range of ages at which different developments are likely to occur—but how to cope best is learned from others who are actually confronted with the job.'

[442] Bowlby, J. (1981) Psychoanalysis as a natural science. *International Review of Psycho-Analysis*, 8, 243–56, p.253.

[443] Bowlby, J. (1957–59) Untitled notes responding to the work of John Alford. PP/Bow/B.3/19.

[444] Bowlby, J. (1951) *Maternal Care and Mental Health*. Geneva: World Health Organisation, p.61.

[445] E.g. Belsky, J. & Nezworski, T. (eds) (1988) *Clinical Implications of Attachment*. Hillsdale, NJ: Lawrence Erlbaum; West, M., Sheldon, A., & Reiffer, L. (1989) Attachment theory and brief psychotherapy: applying current research to clinical interventions. *Canadian Journal of Psychiatry*, 34, 369–75; Byng-Hall, J. (1990) Attachment theory and family therapy: a clinical view. *Infant Mental Health Journal*, 11, 228–37.

[446] An important recent contribution to and review of this literature is Slade, A. & Holmes, J. (2017) *Attachment in Therapeutic Practice*. London: SAGE. For a thematic review, calling for a shift in emphasis from theory- to research-based guidance for attachment-inspired therapies see Berry, K. & Danquah, A. (2016) Attachment-informed

practitioner audiences offer both exposition and revision of Bowlby's ideas.[447] However, close readings of Bowlby's clinical remarks have been rare. One contributing factor may have been that the reader of Bowlby's works is presented with his general reflections on his clinical experience, interspersed only occasionally with a paragraph describing a clinical case. These cases generally describe the childhood factors that predisposed a patient to mental health problems, and the precipitating adult context that led them to enter therapy. Bowlby's own efforts, approaches, successes, and failures with patients are almost never reported. The reason appears to be, alongside Bowlby's characteristic reserve, that unlike many psychoanalysts of his day he did not want to give details about his patients in publications without their permission.[448] In the Bowlby Archive in the Wellcome Collection, Bowlby's case files are embargoed until a century after the clinical work took place; as a result, for the most part, his earliest clinical cases will become available in around 2035.[449]

A marked exception, however, is the case of 'Mrs Q', which is discussed repeatedly by Bowlby in six different published treatments, and several unpublished manuscripts, over the span of decades, beginning from *Defences that Follow Loss*. Given its clear exceptionality, Bowlby presumably sought approval from the patient to discuss the case. In both *Separation* and *Loss* the case receives attention on multiple occasions. In lectures on the clinical implications of attachment research, across different countries, he positioned this case as paradigmatic.[450] Putting together the jigsaw puzzle of Bowlby's remarks on the case across his different writings offers an unusual opportunity to see his clinical work with a patient over time.[451]

Bowlby described his introduction to Mrs Q as follows:

Some years ago the doctor at a maternity and child welfare clinic asked me to see a little boy of 18 months who was not eating and was losing weight. His mother was intensely anxious and depressed and had been so since the boy's birth. On enquiry I found that she was terrified lest her son die and was therefore pestering him to eat. She also told me that she had

therapy for adults: towards a unifying perspective on practice. *Psychology and Psychotherapy: Theory, Research and Practice*, 89(1), 15–32. For descriptions of the boom in therapeutic approaches claiming genesis in attachment theory as an 'explosion' see Magnavita, J.J. & Anchin, J.C. (2013) *Unifying Psychotherapy: Principles, Methods, and Evidence from Clinical Science*. New York: Springer, p.67; Johnson, S.M. (2019) *Attachment Theory in Practice*. New York: Guilford, p.22.

[447] E.g. McCluskey, U. (2005) *To Be Met as a Person: The Dynamics of Attachment in Professional Encounters*. London: Karnac Books; Lyons-Ruth, K. (2007) The interface between attachment and intersubjectivity: perspective from the longitudinal study of disorganized attachment. *Psychoanalytic Inquiry*, 26(4), 595–616; Crittenden, P.M., Dallos, R., Landini, A., & Kozlowska, K. (2014) *Attachment and Systemic Family Therapy*. London: McGraw-Hill.

[448] For instance, Bowlby's request of Emmy Gut to use anonymized material from her case, discussed and appraised in Ross, L.R. (2006) Talking theory, talking therapy: Emmy Gut and John Bowlby. *Issues in Mental Health Nursing*, 27(5), 475–97.

[449] There is one early case which is, however, available: Bowlby's clinical notes of a case from 1938 to 1939 (PP/Bow/C.4/23). The reason why these are available appears to be the lack of identifying details in these notes. There are also a series of undated short case histories under the title 'Maternal Behaviour: Humans' (PP/Bow/H.136) in the Bowlby Archive. However, these contain few details about Bowlby's therapeutic practice, and remained unpublished. The case histories were likely written in the early 1960s, and describe cases seen by Bowlby at the Child Guidance Clinic.

[450] Bowlby, J. (1981) Clinical applications: material for lectures. PP/Bow/F.3/103.

[451] The first discussion of 'Mrs Q' is in a 1962 manuscript. The first published mention is 1963, discussing an analysis that has lasted three years. This suggests that the patient is the 'Mrs K' with whom Bowlby conducted detailed clinical interviews between 1960 and 1964, keeping these interviews for reference. These are the only clinical notes Bowlby kept in this way. The 'reports of interviews with Mrs K (mother) (Mother and Child Welfare Clinic)' (PP/BOW/C.6/6-8) are embargoed until the 2060s.

sometimes had impulses to throw the baby out of the window and to commit suicide. Only some months later did she tell me that on occasion she became hysterical, smashed the dishes and battered the baby's pram.[452]

Bowlby characterised Mrs Q as 'one of the most anxious patients I have ever treated'.[453] Mrs Q described her commitment to giving her son a happy childhood, in contrast to her own. In many respects, Bowlby felt, she succeeded very well. However, Mrs Q was dismayed and confused by her own outbursts of violence, which seemed to coincide especially with occasions when her mother came over to visit.[454] Over the first three years of analysis, Bowlby worked with Mrs Q to trace how her experiences as a child had been an important contributory factor to her adult anxiety and aggression. Her parents had been physically violent and threatened to kill one another. Her mother would also, at times, seek to coerce her husband and children by threatening to leave the family unless they did as she said.

Mrs Q experienced feelings of irrational distrust of Bowlby, which puzzled her. In the clinical work, Bowlby used these feelings as a basis for exploring Mrs Q's experiences of attachment relationships. He gave particular attention to Mrs Q's experiences of her mother's threats of suicide: 'Mrs Q. described how on two occasions she had returned from school to find her mother with her head in the gas oven and how at other times her mother would pretend to have deserted by disappearing for half a day. Naturally, Mrs Q. grew up terrified that if she did anything wrong her mother would go.'[455] Additionally, Bowlby explored with Mrs Q how she had become scared of her own capacity for anger, which she had learnt to redirect 'either towards herself or towards something which, or someone who, could not retaliate. When a child, Mrs Q. recalled, she retreated to her room and bit herself severely or attacked her dolls.'[456]

The clinical work was slow. Mrs Q 'claimed for a long while not only that her feelings for her mother were of love, which was true since her mother had many good qualities, but that that must exclude hatred'.[457] However, an important point in the therapy came when she acknowledged that, when she became angry with Stephen, 'she said the most dreadful things, the very same things, in fact, that her mother had said to her when she was a girl':

> Once the facts were known it was possible to arrange some joint sessions with mother and son during which mother, with real regret, acknowledged making the threats and Stephen explained how terrified they made him. Mother assured Stephen that she would never do it really. All was not well thereafter, but recognition that Stephen's fears were well based and an opening of communication between mother and son eased the situation.[458]

---

[452] Bowlby, J. (1979) By ethology out of psychoanalysis: an experiment in interbreeding. (The Niko Tinbergen Lecture.) *Animal Behaviour*, 28(3), 649–56, p.653.

[453] Bowlby, J. (1969) Psychopathology of anxiety: the role of affectional bonds. *British Journal of Psychiatry*, 3, 80–86, p.85.

[454] Bowlby, J. (1984) Violence in the family as a disorder of the attachment and caregiving systems. *American Journal of Psychoanalysis*, 44, 9–27, p.17.

[455] Bowlby, J. (1979) By ethology out of psychoanalysis: an experiment in interbreeding. (The Niko Tinbergen Lecture.) *Animal Behaviour*, 28(3), 649–56, p.653–4.

[456] Ibid.

[457] Bowlby, J. (1973) *Separation: Anxiety and Anger*. New York: Basic Books, p.269.

[458] Ibid. p.270.

Over three years of therapeutic work, Bowlby helped Mrs Q come to acknowledge the anger she felt towards her mother. As this became less segregated, the violent outbursts towards Stephen reduced. Mrs Q came to understand that, as a child, there had been good reason for segregating her anger. Expressions of anger could otherwise provoke her mother to threaten suicide or to abandon her. Additionally, Mrs Q was strictly told not to let anyone else know about her parents' behaviour, which contributed to the segregation by blocking opportunities for feedback and affirmation of her experiences.

Towards the end of the third year of therapeutic work Mrs Q's father died unexpectedly, following an elective operation for cataracts. In the first years of therapy, Mrs Q's account of her father had been 'overtly negative', hiding the positive feelings that she also felt towards him.[459] Following her loss, Mrs Q became intensely depressed, had thoughts of suicide, and also described dissociative symptoms. Among these were anomalous beliefs about her father's death and its cause:

> During the weeks following her father's death, she now told me, she had lived in the half-held conviction that the hospital had made a mistake in identity and that any day they would phone to say he was alive and ready to return home. Furthermore, she had felt specially angry with me because of a belief that, had I been available, I would have been able to exert an influence on the hospital and so enabled her to recover him.[460]

She experienced the sense that her father's home had to be kept exactly as it was because he was very much alive and would be displeased to find anything changed when he returned.[461] Bowlby was struck that Mrs Q appeared to have two distinct sets of thoughts and feelings in operation: one that led her to act as if her father was dead, and another that led her to act as if her father was alive.[462] Yet neither organisation was strictly unconscious: Mrs Q could discuss her experience of holding both views. In *Defences that Follow Loss*, Bowlby observed that Mrs Q's symptoms could not be explained using the conventional psychoanalytic concept of repression, which suggests a division between conscious and unconscious material. 'Mrs Q. is, however, little different,' he mused. Like with repression, 'there is evidence of a psychic system with its accompanying affects and fantasies that is alien to the one with which we as analysts are in communication'. However, in contrast to repression, this system was not unconscious, but nonetheless blocked from communicating with other conscious systems. It is from this set of reflections on the case of Mrs Q that Bowlby, in fact, went on in the manuscript to use the concept of 'segregated systems' for the first time.[463]

Bowlby as therapist

Three key principles can be gleaned from the treatment of Mrs Q and more generally from Bowlby's late writings about his approach to clinical practice. A first was the importance for Bowlby of the clinical transference: the behaviours, affects, and cognitions displayed by

---

[459] Bowlby, J. (1963) Pathological mourning and childhood mourning. *Journal of the American Psychoanalytic Association*, 11(3), 500–41, p.517.

[460] Ibid. p.517.

[461] Bowlby, J. (1980) *Loss*. London: Pimlico, p.151.

[462] Ibid. pp.348–9.

[463] Bowlby, J. (1962) *Defences that Follow Loss: Causation and Function*. PP/Bow/D.3/78.

the patient towards the therapist, which may find their origin in the plans developed on the basis of earlier experiences of family and intimate relationships. In the 1960s, Bowlby had assumed that relationships with attachment components would be formed by children solely on the basis of familiarity with the caregiver. By contrast, in his late writings on therapeutic technique, he situated the successful longer-term therapeutic relationship for adult patients as one with attachment components, in the provision of a secure base.[464] In this, he seems to acknowledge that attachment components could and should form in the relationship with the therapist, not merely due to familiarity, but due to other factors as well. Bowlby appeared to see something about the intimacy of communication within a therapeutic relationship contributing to its status as a relationship with attachment components. This activated the patient's expectations about close relationships, and at the same time provided an opportunity to reflect on them.[465]

In the case of Bowlby's clinical work with Mrs Q, the transference relationship was used to help the patient notice her difficulties around trust. It was on the basis of this recognition about her relationship with Bowlby as therapist that Mrs Q could then be supported to see that trusting a parental figure was a justifiable fear, given her early experiences. Bowlby stated that 'my therapeutic approach is far from original,'[466] and indeed a special attention to transference phenomena was common to the psychoanalysis of his day, especially for Klein and her followers. However, a significant point of contrast was a second principle of his therapeutic technique. Bowlby believed that the therapist's task, where possible, is to address stable patterns of interaction within close relationships, rather than solely problems 'inside' particular individuals.[467] Even though Bowlby tended to treat behavioural systems as properties of individuals, recovery from symptoms of mental ill health is rarely achieved without considering the resourcing of relevant systems, and the contexts and interpersonal meanings that calibrate their circumstances of activation and termination. The case of Mrs Q began with her son, who was not eating. Bowlby sought the origins and eliciting conditions of these symptoms in the meaning of the boy for his mother, Mrs Q, and in her behaviour towards him—and, in turn, the meaning of Mrs Q's behaviours in her biographical and

---

[464] Whether provision of a relationship with attachment components should be the goal of shorter-term work by helping professionals has been debated, e.g. Charles, G. & Alexander, C. (2014) Beyond attachment: mattering and the development of meaningful moments. *Relational Child and Youth Care Practice*, 27(3), 26–30.

[465] Bowlby's copy of *The Standard Edition of the Writings of Sigmund Freud* still retains his bookmark, in Volume 11, marking the following underlined passage: the patient's 'symptoms, to take an analogy from chemistry, are precipitates of earlier experiences in the sphere of love (in the widest sense of the word), and it is only in the raised temperature of his experience of the transference that they can be resolved and reduced to other psychical products.' Freud, S. (1910) Five lectures on psycho-analysis. In *The Standard Edition of the Complete Psychological Works of Sigmund Freud*, Vol. 11 (pp.1–56). London: Hogarth, p.51; Bowlby's copy is held in the library of Human Development Scotland.

[466] Bowlby, J. (1979, 1988) On knowing what you are not supposed to know and feeling what you are not supposed to feel. In *A Secure Base*. London: Routledge, pp.111–33, p.132.

[467] Bowlby, J. (1949) The study and reduction of group tensions within the family. *Human Relations* 2, 123–8, p.123; Bowlby, J. (1969, 1982) *Attachment, Volume 1*. London: Penguin: 'Nothing in child psychiatry has been more significant in recent years than the increasing recognition that the problems its practitioners are called upon to treat are not often problems confined to individuals but are usually problems arising from stable interactional patterns that have developed between two, and more often several, members of a family' (349). Potential links between attachment theory and systemic family therapy have been widely discussed. See e.g. Cowan, P.A. (1997) Beyond meta-analysis: a plea for a family systems view of attachment. *Child Development*, 68(4), 601–603; Akister, J. & Reibstein, J. (2004) Links between attachment theory and systemic practice: some proposals. *Journal of Family Therapy*, 26(1), 2–16; Crittenden, P.M., Dallos, R., Landini, A., & Kozlowska, K. (2014) *Attachment and Systemic Family Therapy*. London: McGraw-Hill; Vetere, A. (2016) Systemic theory and narratives of attachment: integration, formulation and development over time. In M. Borcsa & P. Stratton (eds) *Origins and Originality in Family Therapy and Systemic Practice* (pp.129–39). New York: Springer.

relational context. From the 1950s until the end of his life, Bowlby referred to himself as a 'family psychiatrist', since he put emphasis on seeing and helping the whole family, rather than only the member of the family showing the symptoms of a mental health problem.[468]

In his attention to the familial context, Bowlby felt that his approach was truly one that avoided blaming parents, but instead considered their actions, thoughts, and feelings in turn in a wider context of predisposing, triggering, and sustaining factors. In 'The making and breaking of affectional bonds', Bowlby argued that when connected to the history or situation that has predisposed or elicited it, much parental behaviour that might otherwise seem simply inexplicable comes in fact to make sense—either as a response to a truly distressing situation or as an attempt to avoid reacting to this situation.[469] In a letter to Joan Stevenson-Hinde, he expressed his strong disagreement with the idea common in family therapy circles that 'patterns of interaction has some particular purpose e.g. that of keeping the family together'. Of course, actions to keep a family together may be a conscious intention of individuals. But Bowlby was hostile to interpretations by therapists that symptoms shown by patients could be understood in terms only of their present function. He felt that such accounts were often generated when the therapist did not yet understand enough about the history of the family, its members, and interactions.[470]

A third principle in Bowlby's late writings on technique was that no advice or guidance should be offered until it is clear that the patient or family is able to understand this as an attempt to be supportive rather than critical. Early in his career, Bowlby regarded himself as more non-directive as a therapist than his peers. However, in his late writings on clinical technique, he made more of a space for challenging and guiding patients and families. Such directive interventions were only recommended, though, on the condition that the patient understands that the therapist's 'concern is to help the patient review his own life, to look at his problems in his own way'.[471] Bowlby was worried that unless therapy leads with support, the encounter may in fact harm the patient or family by reinforcing feelings of guilt and despair. Additionally, where the therapist is perceived as showing disregard for the world as the patient sees it, the potential for trust is eroded. The therapist should not be quick to cast their role as the 'representative of reality', contradicting patients' own perspectives.[472] As well as potentially harmful, Bowlby felt such approaches were ineffective at helping change to occur.

---

[468] Bowlby, J. (1986) 'Attachment Theory: New Directions'. ACP-Psychiatric UPDATE 7(2), panel discussion, Washington. PP/BOW/A.5/1. On Bowlby's position in relation to the history of family therapy and systems approaches to family relations see Byng-Hall, J. (1991) An appreciation of John Bowlby: his significance for family therapy. *Journal of Family Therapy*, 13(1), 5–16. For a discussion of societal factors contributing to 'the family' as the unit of concern and intervention see Weinstein, D. (2013) *The Pathological Family: Postwar America and the Rise of Family Therapy*. Ithaca, NY: Cornell University Press.

[469] Bowlby, J. (1977, 1979) The making and breaking of affectional bonds. In *The Making and Breaking of Affectional Bonds* (pp.150–88). London: Routledge, p.170.

[470] Bowlby, J. (1990) *Letter to Joan Stevenson-Hinde*, 26 March 1990. PP/Bow/J.9/186.

[471] Bowlby, J. (1990, 2011) John Bowlby: interview by Leonardo Tondo. *Clinical Neuropsychiatry*, 8(2), 159–71, p.169. Bowlby was reacting to the emphasis in the Kleinian tradition on transference interpretations. He gave particular emphasis to the importance of support, and helping the patient or family get to a point where they can make sense and use of interpretations—much like the concept of 'developmental help' within the Anna Freudian tradition. See Edgcumbe, R. (1995) The history of Anna Freud's thinking on developmental disturbances. *Bulletin of the Anna Freud Centre*, 18(1), 21–34. Bowlby's emphasis, however, led some second-generation attachment researchers to assume that he was arguing only for support, without challenge, in therapy. See e.g. Bretherton, I. (1991) Pouring new wine into old bottles: the social self as internal working model. In M.R. Gunnar and L.A. Sroufe (eds) *Self-Processes and Development: The Minnesota Symposia on Child Development*, Vol. 23 (pp.1–41). Hillsdale, NJ: Lawrence Erlbaum, p.32.

[472] E.g. Bowlby, J. & Parkes, C.M. (1970, 1979) Separation and loss within the family. In *The Making and Breaking of Affectional Bonds* (pp.99–123). London: Routledge, p.114.

In 'Constructions in Analysis', Freud wrote that 'no damage is done if, for once in a way, we make a mistake and offer the patient a wrong construction as the probably historical truth'. Bowlby, in his marginalia, described Freud's stance as 'complacent'.[473]

Given the importance of laying the ground through support, Bowlby divided therapy into two 'phases'.[474] In the first, the therapist should primarily seek to offer companionable support, combined with open-ended exploratory questions. The focus in this first phase should be on present-day experiences and the wider social context, seeking to identify the kinds of situation that repeatedly tend to be difficult or cause problems for the patient or family. These are likely to be those that led to the initiation of therapy, though the patient may or may not be aware of the pattern. For instance, in cases where a behavioural system has been chronically suppressed (Level 3 defensive exclusion), the first task is for the patient to recover a sense of what it might mean for this system to be activated. Where the attachment system of a patient has been subject to full defensive exclusion, the therapist might explore current experiences outside of therapy and within the transference where this system would otherwise be activated, and the thoughts, feelings, and behaviours that occur instead.[475] This entails slow, careful work to support patients to articulate the ecology of their ordinary lives, and the circumstances that prompt the activation or deactivation of behavioural systems and their associated affects.

Both the attachment system and the exploratory system may need to be coaxed online by this combination of support and attention to present-day experiences: the attachment system bringing fruitful material for the transference, and the exploratory system engaging and integrating this material. Past experiences will have already been at least implicit in the first phase, since both the present and our perceptions of it always hold the past within them. Yet, only once the patient or family feel supported to engage the exploratory system to address present-day experiences should the therapist, in the second phase, seek to explore the nature of these feelings in depth, and then consider past experiences that may have contributed to these difficulties. This should include helping the patient or family sort through their feelings about the past and present, to reduce the extent to which these contaminate one another and become confused when decisions are made in the present.[476] In the case of Mrs Q, Bowlby described patiently supporting her towards recognition of the anger she felt towards her mother. The aspect of the therapeutic task which ultimately 'can best wait is consideration of the past since its only relevance lies in the light it throws on the present':

> The sequence may often be for the therapist and patient, working together, first to recognise that the patient tends habitually to respond to a particular type of interpersonal situation in a certain self-defeating way, next to examine what kinds of feeling and expectation such situations commonly arouse in him, and only after that to consider whether he may

---

[473] Annotations by Bowlby dated 1964 on *The Standard Edition of the Complete Psychological Works of Sigmund Freud*, Vol. 23, p.261. Copy held in the library of Human Development Scotland.

[474] Bowlby, J. (1973) *Separation: Anger and Anxiety*. New York: Basic Books, p.354.

[475] Bowlby, J. (1981) Psychoanalysis as a natural science. *International Review of Psycho-Analysis*, 8, 243–56, p.251.

[476] See the three unpublished case histories in 'Maternal behaviour: humans' (PP/Bow/H.136), where this is the common central feature of his therapeutic approach. See also Bowlby, J. (1971) *Letter to Graham Davies*, 15 April 1971. PP/Bow/H.5: 'I see psychoanalytic therapy as an attempt to help a patient explore his own motives, his own model of the world and himself in it, and also to reconsider the validity of that model. Often I believe it is more valuable to raise questions for a patient than to attempt to inform him by means of interpretations ... In helping a patient make these reappraisals, I believe it useful for us to have some knowledge of the conditions that commonly lead an individual to grow up in ignorance of his motives and with more or less distorted models of his world and himself.'

have had experiences, recent or long past, which have contributed to his responding with those feelings and expectations.[477]

Bowlby offered a metaphor: 'If a ball has gone down a dark passage, a child may be frightened to go there and get the ball, but if I say "Look, I will come with you", he may be quite happy. In psychotherapy we act as a companion to a patient who is too frightened to look at what has happened to him in the past. So we accompany him in the exploration.'[478] Bowlby believed that this companion and social point of reference is important because it gives patients the confidence to unlatch their personal hopes and fears from matters of fact, through close scrutiny of both. Bowlby clearly saw the discovery of historical truth in therapy as making some contribution to the reduction in symptoms, since it permitted more effective information-processing in the present.[479] However, just as important was his emphasis on therapy as supporting curiosity and courage within and beyond the therapeutic setting.

Attachment disorders

Also relevant to his work as a clinician, Bowlby made a number of important remarks on the meaning and function of diagnosis. His overall position was that diagnosis is a relevant and valuable clinical tool for medical professionals, but that it should not be mistaken for explanation. From early in his career, he emphasised that development was multiply determined, and would therefore often exceed static characterisations that depicted particular symptoms as manifestations of specific disturbances.[480] In an undated text, archived with material from around 1939 to 1940, Bowlby reflected carefully on the purposes of psychiatric classification in an attempt to develop diagnostic groupings for children under five:

> Classification and diagnosis in child psychiatry is at present in a state of anarchy. Very few of the children seen correspond to any of the classical psychoneuroses or psychoses—the fact unjustly being simply "character-problems". For these character cases there is as yet no good classification for adults, let alone for children … Even in adults it is sometimes difficult to distinguish clearly between the habitual personality and the particular syndrome of symptoms from which the patient is suffering. This difficulty is increased in childhood. Consequently the classification used here is only provisional.[481]

---

[477] Bowlby, J. (1977, 1979) The making and breaking of affectional bonds. In *The Making and Breaking of Affectional Bonds* (pp.150–88). London: Routledge, p.173.

[478] Bowlby, J. (1990, 2011) John Bowlby: interview by Leonardo Tondo. *Clinical Neuropsychiatry*, 8(2), 159–71, p.163.

[479] Fonagy has regularly criticized strands of psychoanalytic theory for treating the discovery of historical truth as the mechanism and target of therapeutic action, e.g. Fonagy, P. & Tallandini-Shallice, M. (1993) On some problems of psychoanalytic research in practice. *Bulletin of the Anna Freud Centre*, 16, 5–22. Bowlby's emphasis on the contribution of defensive exclusion to mental illness, and the curative powers of the reintegration of reality within information processing, do at times veer in this direction. However, suggesting that this may be a structural issue faced by psychotherapy as an activity, in his more recent work on therapeutic technique Fonagy has himself at times become tangled in the same problem, e.g. Fonagy, P. (2016) The role of attachment, epistemic trust and resilience in personality disorder: a trans-theoretical reformulation. *DMM News*, 22 September 2016. http://www.iasa-dmm. org/images/uploads/DMM%20%2322%20Sept%2016%20English.pdf. 'Feeling recognized opens the epistemic path necessary to update the neural nets which in turn enable accurate (resilient) interpretation of reality' (6).

[480] Bowlby, J. (1954) The diagnosis and treatment of psychological disorders in childhood. *Health Education Journal*, 12(2), 59–68, p.62.

[481] Bowlby, J. (undated, *c*.1939) *Diagnostic Groupings for Children Over 5 Years*. PP/Bow/C3/9.

In his early book *Personality and Mental Illness* from 1940, Bowlby acknowledged that 'few people remain the same throughout their lives', and he explored this lack of continuity in the case of mental health symptoms. He pointed out that only rarely do individuals exactly fit the criteria of psychiatric classification, and generally only those with relatively less severe symptoms. Among patients with more severe problems, 'many show at successive periods an unstable personality, symptoms of psycho-neurosis and of psychosis'. Bowlby therefore called it 'absurd' to regard such a patient 'in terms of any one condition. He must be thought of as an individual of certain potentialities, a unity of which the particular traits and symptoms shown at any one moment are but fleeting expression.'[482] Symptoms are not, in such an account, the manifest effect of an underlying and discrete disorder. For instance, low mood, sleeplessness, and a lack of energy are not the expressions of a disorder of 'depression', as distinct from other mental health problems. Rather, Bowlby's account was transdiagnostic. He suggested that the individual represents a unity of potentialities, in this case towards mental health or ill health. Particular symptoms, or even clusters of symptoms that can be grouped as mental disorders, are best considered as consequences of this set of potentialities. He argued that, where early childhood experiences have been positive, this set of potentialities will predispose mental health. By contrast, early adverse experiences will support the intensification and expression of potentialities towards mental ill health across the lifespan.

In his mature thought, Bowlby developed these reflections further. In 'Developmental psychiatry comes of age', published 1988, he insisted that 'a sharp distinction must be drawn between current functioning, measured in terms of presence or absence of psychiatric disorder and personality structure, measured in terms of greater or less vulnerability to adverse life events and situations'.[483] Furthermore, 'the features of personality to which we draw attention are different to those that most clinical instruments are designed to measure and not necessarily correlated with them'.[484] Bowlby considered factors that might contribute to such transdiagnostic, developmental vulnerability. He was especially concerned with the way that the defensive exclusion of attachment-related motivations may deplete possibilities for experiencing life as 'emotionally rich and varied', and contribute variously to distress, aggression, and depression.[485] Bowlby's position implied that attachment processes can readily impact other areas of functioning, but this did not mean that the resulting behaviours are therefore to be considered as attachment.[486] Though he was particularly concerned with attachment, Bowlby was clear that defensive exclusion of other behavioural systems could contribute to a vulnerability to mental illness. Defensive exclusion of the exploratory system could make it difficult for an individual to learn from experience, or from therapy.[487] And loss of access to the prompts of the fear system could lead an individual to enter cruel and painful relationships. Without itself constituting a form of mental illness, Bowlby anticipated that such processes would contribute to the initiation or the maintenance of various mental health symptoms.

From *Separation* onwards, Bowlby emphasised that clinicians and researchers should note the importance of 'developmental pathways', self-reinforcing patterns in children's trajectories

---

[482] Bowlby, J. (1940) *Personality and Mental Illness*. London: Kegan Paul, p.187.

[483] Bowlby, J. (1988) Developmental psychiatry comes of age. *American Journal of Psychiatry*, 145, 1–10, p.6.

[484] Bowlby, J. (1980) *Loss*. London: Pimlico, p.202–203.

[485] Bowlby, J. (1988) Developmental psychiatry comes of age. *American Journal of Psychiatry*, 145, 1–10, p.6.

[486] For a later statement well aligned with this position see Waters, E., Posada, G., Crowell, J., & Lay, K.L. (1993) Is attachment theory ready to contribute to our understanding of disruptive behavior problems? *Development & Psychopathology*, 5, 215–24.

[487] See also Fonagy, P. & Allison, E. (2014) The role of mentalizing and epistemic trust in the therapeutic relationship. *Psychotherapy*, 51(3), 372–80.

towards or away from mental health. Bowlby was inspired by Waddington's description of how cells can initially develop in a variety of different ways, but that once they do begin to develop, they become canalised such that a change from the established pathway requires greater and greater intervention.[488] Bowlby reflected that, with human development conceptualised in terms of pathways, we can expect 'adverse childhood experiences[489] [to] have effects of at least two kinds. First they make the individual more vulnerable to later adverse experiences. Secondly they make it more likely that he or she will meet with further such experiences.'[490] This pathways metaphor suggested a nuanced model of continuities over time:

> All pathways are thought to start close together so that, initially, an individual has access to a large range of pathways along any one of which he might travel. The one chosen, it is held, turns at each and every stage of the journey on an interaction between the organism as it has developed up to that moment and the environment in which it then finds itself. Thus at conception development turns on interaction between the newly formed genome and the intrauterine environment; at birth it turns on interaction between the physiological constitution, including germinal mental structure, of the neonate and the family, or non-family, into which he is born; and at each age successively it turns on the personality structure then present and the family and, later, the wider social environments then current … As development proceeds and structures progressively differentiate, the number of pathways that remain open diminishes.[491]

This model implied for Bowlby that neither knowledge of general patterns nor knowledge of the specific case should be abandoned. Today, this might be discussed in terms of the distinction between 'diagnosis' and 'formulation'.[492] On an individual level, diagnostic

---

[488] Waddington, C.H. (1957) *The Strategy of Genes*. London: Allen & Unwin.

[489] This term would later become the label for an influential self-report measure of adversity and trauma. Felitti, V.J., Anda, R.F., Nordenberg, D., et al. (1998) Relationship of childhood abuse and household dysfunction to many of the leading causes of death in adults: the Adverse Childhood Experiences (ACE) Study. *American Journal of Preventive Medicine*, 14(4), 245–58. If there is a debt to Bowlby's earlier use, it is not acknowledged by Felitti and colleagues. This is discussed by Partridge, S. (2019) Review of 'The Deepest Well: Healing the Long-term Effects of Childhood Adversity' by Nadine Burke Harris. *Attachment*, 13(1).

[490] Bowlby, J. (1981, 1988) The origins of attachment theory. In *A Secure Base* (pp.22–42). London: Routledge.

[491] Bowlby, J. (1973) *Separation*. London: Pimlico, p.412. The importance of the concept of developmental pathways for Bowlby's late thought cannot be overestimated. See for instance the prominent place it receives in his plan for the unpublished book, representing his final position (on the model of Freud's 'Outline of Psychoanalysis'), Bowlby, J. (1982) Outline of attachment theory. PP/Bow/H.260:

> Chapter 1. Historical. A way of conceptualising family influence.
> Chapter 2. Main features: developmental pathways; description of attachment, caregiving, exploration; abuse
> Chapter 3. Cognitive models
> Part II: Pathways of development
> Chapter 4. Pathways to health, including healthy parenting
> Chapter 5. Pathways to anxious attachment & phobia
> Chapter 6. Pathways to depressive disorders. Suicide?
> Chapter 7. Pathways to false self, masked depression
> Chapter 8. Pathways to delinquency & psychosis
> Chapter 9.
> Part III: Applications
> Chapter 10. Prevention and crisis intervention
> Chapter 11. Treatment
> Part IV: Problems of theory
> Chapter 12. Evolutionary theory, control systems, activation, termination function
> Chapter 13. More re cognitive models and defence. Consciousness and unconsciousness
> Chapter 14. Attachment and science'

[492] Johnstone, L. & Dallos, R. (2013) *Formulation in Psychology and Psychotherapy: Making Sense of People's Problems*. London: Routledge.

classifications tell clinicians about what one child may have in common with other children with similar symptoms. They can help clinicians to develop an integrative account of the child's difficulties, encourage more consistent care-planning, and encourage professionals to consider the treatments that may help. Formulation, on the other hand, is an individual approach that considers the ways in which the child is unique from others. Within formulation, assessment of the attachment system and its functioning serves as one part of nuanced thinking about a child's behavioural profile, potential risk factors, and the role of the child's external environment.

In 1980, the 'Infancy, Childhood and Adolescent Disorders' committee of the American Psychiatric Association Diagnostic and Statistical Manual of Mental Disorders (III) (DSM-III) introduced the category of 'reactive attachment disorder in infancy' as a recognised diagnosis. This diagnosis was an attempt to bring within medical assessment practice observations that had been made of specific forms of behaviour shown by institutionalised and former institutionalised children, influenced by Bowlby's 1951 report to the World Health Organisation, as well as other reports.[493] The disorder was, as it was initially proposed, to be diagnosed on the basis of weak infant physical growth, poor social responsiveness, and emotional apathy, as a consequence of grossly inadequate experiences of caregiving. In 1987, the diagnosis was revised to remove the physical growth criterion and adjust the age criterion, and has since seen other changes.[494] It is notable that in the ten years between 1980 and his death in 1990, Bowlby made no public statement discussing this new official diagnosis ostensibly drawing inspiration from his work and using his headline concept of 'attachment'. Some have treated this as implying that the diagnosis was simply a natural expression of Bowlby's position and that he generally approved.[495] However, Bowlby's silence on the advent of 'attachment disorders' more likely reflected discomfort.

The introduction of the attachment disorder diagnosis as a problem of 'attachment' appears to have been based solely on Bowlby's earliest writings on institutionalisation and his diffuse claims about its socioemotional implications, essentially prior to the development of attachment theory from the late 1950s. Justin Call, the primary member of the 'Infancy, Childhood and Adolescent Disorders' committee to discuss Bowlby's work in print, justified the new diagnostic category in 1982 by arguing that 'attachment disorders of infancy are characterised by the absence, disruption, or distortion of normally occurring developmental sequences of attachment behaviors'.[496] Yet he gave no reference to Bowlby's work after 1958.

---

[493] Bakwin, H. (1949) Emotional deprivation in infants. *Journal of Pediatrics* 35, 512–21; Provence, S. & Lipton, R. (1962) *Infants in Institutions*. New York: International Universities Press; Tizard, R. & Rees, J. (1975) The effect of early institutional rearing on the behaviour problems and affectional relationships of four year old children. *Journal of Child Psychology and Psychiatry*, 16, 61–73.

[494] There has been a growing body of research on attachment disorders since 1998, and especially since the increased prominence and detail of the diagnosis in DSM-IV in 1994 and DSM-5 in 2013. These developments in diagnostic practice have been influenced by the pivotal series of studies of children adopted from Eastern European orphanages. See Zeanah, C.H., Smyke, A.T., & Settles, L.D. (2006) Orphanages as a developmental context for early childhood. In K. McCartney & D. Phillips (eds) *Blackwell Handbook of Early Childhood Development* (pp.424–54). Hoboken, NJ: Wiley-Blackwell; Zeanah, C.H., Chesher, T., Boris, N.W., & American Academy of Child & Adolescent Psychiatry (2016) Practice parameter for the assessment and treatment of children and adolescents with reactive attachment disorder and disinhibited social engagement disorder. *Journal of the American Academy of Child & Adolescent Psychiatry*, 55, 990–1003.

[495] E.g. Kanieski, M.A. (2010) Securing attachment: the shifting medicalisation of attachment and attachment disorders. *Health, Risk & Society*, 12(4), 335–44.

[496] Call, J. (1982) Attachment disorders of infancy. In H.I. Kaplan, A.M. Freedman, & Z.B.J. Sadock (eds) *Comprehensive Textbook of Psychiatry*, Vol. 3 (pp.230–68). Baltimore: Williams and Wilkins, p.2587. Repeated in Call, J.D. (1984) Child abuse and neglect in infancy: sources of hostility within the parent–infant dyad and disorders of attachment in infancy. *Child Abuse & Neglect*, 8(2), 185–202, p.190.

This would account for the fact that Call and the DSM interpret the 'disruption' or 'distortion' of attachment to mean primarily extreme deprivation. Call's lack of familiarity with Bowlby's work would also explain why the DSM-III initially limited attachment disorders to infants under eight months—when, in *Attachment, Volume 1,* Bowlby had argued that the attachment system is not likely formed until at least nine months. The DSM criteria displayed no concern to assess disruption to the attachment system, for instance in distinguishing between behaviour in contexts where the attachment system would be activated and behaviour in other contexts. The criteria also situated 'attachment disorder' as a property of the individual child, in contrast to Bowlby's emphasis on the dyadic status of the attachment system in infancy.[497]

The DSM-III was a major event and sent shock-waves through the psychiatric establishment. Even if particulars were regarded as arguable, it appeared to offer the basis for a valid and reliable category-based diagnosis system, in which all symptoms find their logic and cause in an underlying disorder.[498] However, the 'attachment disorder' diagnosis was not a part of this general upsurge of interest and support for diagnostic categorisation. No empirical studies used the category within research until after Bowlby's death.[499] If the idea of an 'attachment disorder' diagnosis without consideration of Bowlby's writings on attachment theory had been put forward in another document, it seems probable that it would have been ignored. Certainly, Call's chapter 'Attachment Disorders in Infancy' in the 1982 *Comprehensive Textbook of Psychiatry,* written to accompany the new DSM diagnosis, has rarely been cited.[500] And in the next edition Call's chapter was replaced by one that largely assimilated the new attachment disorder category into the frame of infant failure to thrive and psychosocial dwarfism.[501]

However, the diagnosis of 'attachment disorder' was hooked inside one of the single most influential medical documents of the twentieth century. The DSM-III contributed to a transformation in mental health assessment to give prominence to diagnosis and diagnostic pathways.[502] Diagnostic categories have been made central to the delivery and administration of clinical services, to clinical resource allocation, and to clinical training. Throughout his career Bowlby was concerned with clean distinctions, where possible, between diagnostic activity and reflection on developmental processes. Furthermore, it is evident that his overall impulse was towards attention to developmental pathways in understanding children's symptoms, and the use of diagnosis only for specific, limited purposes. Bowlby addressed these matters further in a paper presented to the British Psychological Society three years after the publication of the DSM-III (included as Chapter 4 in *Trauma and Loss: Key Texts*

---

[497] Additionally, the Robertson and Bowlby book discussing observations in the 1950s of anomalous and apparently dissociated behaviours of institutionalized children remained unpublished, so Call and colleagues on the 'Infancy, Childhood and Adolescent Disorders' committee did not have access to this subterranean current of attachment theory, which would find full recognition only in the 1980s in the work of Mary Main and Judith Solomon on the 'disorganized/disoriented' attachment classification (Chapter 3).

[498] Mayes, R. & Horwitz, A.V. (2005) DSM-III and the revolution in the classification of mental illness. *Journal of the History of the Behavioral Sciences,* 41(3), 249–67.

[499] Richters, M. & Volkmar, F. (1994) Reactive attachment disorder of infancy or early childhood. *Journal of the American Academy of Child and Adolescent Psychiatry,* 33, 328–32.

[500] Call, J. (1982) Attachment disorders of infancy. In H.I. Kaplan, A.M. Freedman, & Z.B.J. Sadock (eds) *Comprehensive Textbook of Psychiatry,* Vol. 3 (pp.230–68). Baltimore: Williams and Wilkins.

[501] Green, W. (1985) Attachment disorders of infancy and early childhood. In H.I. Kaplan & Z.B.J. Sadock (eds) *Comprehensive Textbook of Psychiatry,* Vol. 4 (pp.1722–31). Baltimore: Williams and Wilkins.

[502] Greco, M. (2016) What is the DSM? Diagnostic manual, cultural icon, political battleground: an overview with suggestions for a critical research agenda. *Psychology & Sexuality,* 7(1), 6–22.

from the John Bowlby Archive). Bowlby denounced the focus of the psychological establishment on category-centric practice:

> The categorists are still searching for diagnostic criteria that distinguish the mentally ill from the normal, though today their search is more likely to be for genetically determined biochemical anomalies than for any behavioural criterion. [On the other hand, there are] those others who, like myself, believe continuity to be a more fruitful perspective.[503]

Bowlby's remarks to the British Psychological Society suggest that he would have endorsed Sroufe's view that 'the circumscribing of attachment problems to specific disorders reveals a failure to grasp the developmental significance of attachment history and the potential power of a developmental approach to psychopathology in general' (Chapter 4).[504] As we saw in the section 'Disorientation', Robertson documented behaviours that resembled the 'attachment disorders' in the children he observed during and following long-term hospitalisation. However, Bowlby decided not to publish his book with Robertson containing these observations, and did not integrate them into his subsequent theorizing. He also kept silent when the attachment disorder diagnosis was introduced into the DSM. These choices, in retrospect, appear to have helped initiate a split between widely circulating clinical discourses of attachment disorder and the bulk of empirical and theoretical work on attachment.

In the context of diagnosis-focused clinical practice, and continued observations of behaviours such as disinhibited social engagement by clinicians—particularly among those in adoption and fostering contexts—later psychiatrists interested in infant mental health, such as Charles Zeanah, acted as if that they had to work with and elaborate the diagnosis that was 'on the books'.[505] Likewise, the World Health Organisation's International Classification of Diseases largely took on the disorder as characterised in the DSM. The Zero to Three manual introduced in 1994 for the assessment of the mental health and development of young children is an exception, with uses of attachment ideas in the manual informed by Bowlby's later work and subsequent attachment research.[506] The Zero to Three manual, however, is grossly subordinate to the DSM in status. It is rarely possible for American clinicians to seek recompense from insurance companies for their work using Zero to Three. The standard remains the DSM diagnoses.

The primary use of the DSM classification in the 1990s was to describe children reared in institutional care, where two profiles could sometimes be seen: withdrawal from all caregivers, and indiscriminate attachment behaviours shown towards caregivers and

[503] Bowlby, J. (1983) Darwin: Psychiatry and Developmental Psychology. Contribution to a Symposium on Darwin and Psychology held at the conference of the British Psychological Society, London, December 1983. PP/BOW/F.3/132.

[504] Sroufe, L.A. (1997) Psychopathology as an outcome of development. *Development & Psychopathology*, 9(2), 251–68, p.263. Bowlby's position would perhaps align with developments in the UK, where clinical guidelines now advise professionals to consider a broader range of problems described as 'attachment difficulties' for children who are adopted or are at risk of going into care, outside of the constraints of the 'attachment disorder' diagnoses. National Institute for Health & Care Excellence (2015) Children's attachment: attachment in children and young people who are adopted from care, in care or at high risk of going into care. NICE Guideline (NG26). https://www.nice.org.uk/guidance/ng26.

[505] E.g. Zeanah, C.H., Mammen, O., & Lieberman, A. (1993) Disorders of attachment. In C.H. Zeanah (ed.) *Handbook of Infant Mental Health* (pp.332–49). New York, Guilford.

[506] Zero to Three/National Center for Clinical Infant Programs (1994) *Diagnostic Classification of Mental Health and Developmental Disorders of Infancy and Early Childhood* (Diagnostic Classification: 0-3). Washington, DC: Zero to Three; Lyons-Ruth, K., Zeanah, C.H., & Benoit, D. (1996) Disorder and risk for disorder during infancy and toddlerhood. In E.J. Mash & R.A. Barkley (eds) *Child Psychopathology* (pp.457–91). New York: Guilford.

non-caregivers. Over subsequent years, the latter has been redescribed as disinhibited social engagement. In general, the relationship between the DSM disorder and the broader field of attachment theory and research has remained unclear, except the repeated observation that attachment disorder may be more likely when children have not had an opportunity to form a selective attachment or attachments.[507] Some clinicians have argued for the narrowing of the attachment disorder to exclude disinhibited social engagement, since its relationship with the attachment system is unclear.[508] Other clinicians have argued for a broader applicability for the concept of attachment disorder.[509] However, mostly the established generation of attachment researchers, with a few exceptions such as Zeanah, Lyons-Ruth, and Spangler,[510] have largely ignored the clinical diagnosis. Several attachment researchers, for instance Sroufe, van IJzendoorn, and Bakermans-Kranenburg, have expressed exasperation with the attachment disorder diagnosis, given its ill-fit with Bowlby's attachment theory or the predominant categories used in mainstream attachment research.[511] There is a sense in these writings that attachment researchers feel powerless to alter the diagnosis, now that it exists. Yet it is also not clear that they would want a diagnostic entity that better reflected attachment theory. In commentaries on the attachment disorder diagnosis by attachment researchers, attachment is frequently depicted as a dyadic phenomenon, incommensurate with individual-focused diagnostic systems like the DSM.[512]

The poor integration between clinical discourses of attachment disorder and the predominant focus of researchers on patterns of attachment has had several consequences. One has been the still relatively weak research base on disinhibited social engagement, and especially the correlates and implications of these behaviours when shown by home-reared

[507] Atkinson, L. (2019) Reactive attachment disorder and attachment theory from infancy to adolescence: review, integration, and expansion. *Attachment & Human Development*, 21, 205–17.

[508] Lyons-Ruth, K., Zeanah, C.H., & Gleason, M.M. (2015) Commentary: should we move away from an attachment framework for understanding disinhibited social engagement disorder (DSED)? A commentary on Zeanah and Gleason (2015) *Journal of Child Psychology and Psychiatry*, 56(3), 223–7.

[509] Minnis, H., Marwick, H., Arthur, J., & McLaughlin, A. (2006) Reactive attachment disorder—a theoretical model beyond attachment. *European Child & Adolescent Psychiatry*, 15(6), 336–42.

[510] E.g. Zeanah, C.H., Smyke, A.T., Koga, S.F., Carlson, E., & Bucharest Early Intervention Project Core Group (2005) Attachment in institutionalized and community children in Romania. *Child Development*, 76(5), 1015–28; Lyons-Ruth, K., Zeanah, C.H., & Gleason, M.M. (2015) Commentary: should we move away from an attachment framework for understanding disinhibited social engagement disorder (DSED)? A commentary on Zeanah and Gleason (2015) *Journal of Child Psychology and Psychiatry*, 56(3), 223–7; Lyons-Ruth, K., Riley, C., Patrick, M.P., & Hobson, R.P. (2019) Disinhibited attachment behavior among infants of mothers with borderline personality disorder, depression, and no diagnosis. *Personality Disorders*, 10(2), 163–72; Spangler, G., Bovenschen, I., Jorjadze, N., et al. (2019) Inhibited symptoms of attachment disorder in children from institutional and foster care samples. *Attachment & Human Development*, 21(2), 132–51. Spangler, like van IJzendoorn and Cassidy, is perhaps best considered an intermediate case for the heuristic contrast between second- and third-generation attachment researchers.

[511] E.g. Sroufe, L.A., Duggal, S., Weinfield, N., & Carlson, E. (2000) Relationships, development, and psychopathology. In A.J. Sameroff, M. Lewis, & S.M. Miller (eds) *Handbook of Developmental Psychopathology* (pp. 75–91). New York: Kluwer Academic/Plenum Press, p.83; van IJzendoorn, M.H. & Bakermans-Kranenburg, M.J. (2003) Attachment disorders and disorganized attachment: similar and different. *Attachment & Human Development*, 5(3), 313–20. See also Allen, B. (2016) A RADical idea: a call to eliminate attachment disorder and attachment therapy from the clinical lexicon. *Evidence-based Practice in Child and Adolescent Mental Health*, 1, 60–71; Lyons-Ruth, K., Bureau, J.F., Riley, C.D., & Atlas-Corbett, A.F. (2009) Socially indiscriminate attachment behavior in the Strange Situation: convergent and discriminant validity in relation to caregiving risk, later behavior problems, and attachment insecurity. *Development & Psychopathology*, 21(2), 355–72; Granqvist, P., Sroufe, L.A., Dozier, M., et al. (2017) Disorganized attachment in infancy: a review of the phenomenon and its implications for clinicians and policy-makers. *Attachment & Human Development*, 19(6), 534–58.

[512] In this, researchers commenting on the attachment disorder diagnosis rather neglect the question of whether, by late childhood and adolescence, expectations about the availability of attachment figures become a partial property of individuals in much the same way as mental health symptoms.

children.[513] A second consequence has been that, in the gap left between the clinical and re-search communities, the development of treatments for 'attachment disorder' have taken on a life of their own, very largely unmoored to research.[514] Clinicians wishing to identify insecurity and attachment-related needs within a diagnosis-focused clinical culture have also been drawn to use of the 'attachment disorder' label.[515] Such clinical uses align with, and may have been sup-ported by, occasional use of the term 'disordered attachments' by researchers to mean simply problems in attachment relationships.[516] Third, the disjointed relationship between clinical sys-tems of diagnosis and the non-diagnostic categories of attachment has hindered the informed integration of attachment research with diagnosis-focused clinical services and clinical training. It can be especially hard for generalist clinicians to know what meaning attachment should have for their work, given that it figures as both a rare clinical diagnosis and a transdiagnostic de-velopmental perspective.[517] Commentators have warned, however, that slippage between the broad and circumscribed uses of the term 'attachment infant disorder' has contributed in some quar-ters to an overdiagnosis of attachment disorders, misuse of appeal to attachment disorder in psychological assessments for family courts, and neglect of children's potential other psycho-logical needs.[518] The gap between clinical discourses and the research paradigm has also been filled at times by inappropriate uses of the disorganised attachment classification, forced to play the role of a quasi-diagnostic category in child welfare practice (Chapter 3).[519]

Some remaining questions

Continuity

Three limitations of Bowlby's theorizing can be identified as of special significance for sub-sequent attachment theory. A first limitation is Bowlby's assumption that early adverse

---

[513] Though see Scheper, F.Y., Groot, C.R., de Vries, A.L., Doreleijers, T.A., Jansen, L.M., & Schuengel, C. (2019) Course of disinhibited social engagement behavior in clinically referred home-reared preschool children. *Journal of Child Psychology and Psychiatry*, 60(5), 555–65.

[514] Chaffin, M., Hanson, R., Saunders, B.E., et al. (2006) Report of the APSAC task force on attachment therapy, reactive attachment disorder, and attachment problems. *Child Maltreatment*, 11(1), 76–89. Allen and Mercer have criticized attachment disorder and interventions to resolve it as, at present, more pseudoscience than sci-ence: Allen, B. (2018) Misperceptions of reactive attachment disorders persist: poor methods and unsupported conclusions. *Research in Developmental Disabilities*, 77, 24–9; Mercer, J. (2019) Conventional and unconventional perspectives on attachment and attachment problems: comparisons and implications, 2006–2016. *Child and Adolescent Social Work Journal*, 36(2), 81–95. Nonetheless, perhaps it can be said that 'attachment disorder' has been integrated into attachment theory as a characterization of children who have had little chance to form attach-ments due to neglect or institutionalization.

[515] Barnes, G.L., Woolgar, M., Beckwith, H., & Duschinsky, R. (2018) John Bowlby and contemporary issues of clinical diagnosis. *Attachment*, 12(1), 35–47.

[516] E.g. Fonagy, P., Target, M., Steele, M., et al. (1997) Morality, disruptive behavior, borderline personality dis-order, crime, and their relationships to security of attachment. In L. Atkinson & K.J. Zucker (eds) *Attachment and Psychopathology* (pp. 223–74). New York: Guilford, p.224.

[517] Turner, M., Beckwith, H., Duschinsky, R., et al. (2019) Attachment difficulties and disorders. *InnovAiT*, 12(4), 173–9.

[518] Woolgar, M. & Baldock, E. (2015) Attachment disorders versus more common problems in looked after and adopted children: comparing community and expert assessments. *Child and Adolescent Mental Health*, 20(1), 34–40; White, S., Gibson, M., Wastell, D., & Walsh, P. (2019) *Reassessing Attachment Theory in Child Welfare*. Bristol: Psychology Press.

[519] Reijman, S., Foster, S., & Duschinsky, R. (2018) The infant disorganised attachment classification: 'Patterning within the disturbance of coherence'. *Social Science & Medicine*, 200, 52–8.

experiences would have strong continuities with later mental health, not only in the extent of symptoms but also in the kinds of symptoms shown. This reflected Bowlby's residual but strong commitment to a psychoanalytic concept of 'identification' in which the parent is set up as a model for the child, together with influence from Bandura's Social Learning Theory and clinical experiences: 'I strongly suspect that the particular form of atypical care-eliciting behaviour selected by a patient is greatly influenced by modelling, the term introduced by Bandura, and roughly equivalent to identification, to describe adopting the same behaviour that one has observed engaged in by others ... More and more in work with parents I have been struck by the extent to which they have adopted the same disciplinary procedures towards their children as they themselves were subjected to—often despite their wish to behave quite otherwise.'[520]

Bowlby felt that there are many factors that keep developmental pathways stable, or even intensify them, once they have begun to develop. Some of these are individual: Bowlby was especially interested in the way that children's expectations, once shaped, guide their subsequent behaviour. He was confident that, shaped by past experiences, 'present cognitive and behavioural structures determine what is perceived and what [is] ignored, how a new situation is construed, and what plan of action is likely to be constructed to deal with it.'[521] Bowlby highlighted the role of social factors in strengthening and steadying developmental pathways: he had theorised that the effects of early long-term separations on later mental health occur at least in part as a result of the fact that the clingy and difficult behaviour children show following such separations may elicit rejecting or hostile responses from caregivers. Yet, beyond their independent influence, Bowlby felt that the reciprocal reinforcement of psychological and social processes was especially critical to the stability of developmental pathways: 'Whatever family pressures led the development of a child to take the pathway he is now on are likely to persist and so to maintain development on that same pathway',[522] and 'whatever expectations are developed during those years tend to persist relatively unchanged throughout the rest of life.'[523]

Throughout his career, Bowlby was attentive to factors that might mediate, buffer, or break continuity between early experiences and later mental health. Sroufe and colleagues are right that 'Bowlby is not deterministic but, rather probabilistic' in his claims.[524] Nonetheless, Bowlby's characterisation of how the attachment system changes in the context of maturation or changes in social environment remained underdeveloped, with the amorphous concept of 'internal working models' picking up the slack, but often not doing so effectively.[525] He profoundly underspecified the relationship between attachment and personality traits: it

---

[520] Bowlby, J. (1973) *Letter to Scott Henderson*, 30 July 1973. PP/Bow/J.9/98. See also Bowlby's undated notes on the concept of identification, PP/BOW/H.117-121. For instance, the note 'Identification—Klein', in which Bowlby writes 'Mrs K. assumes that the copying follows and is a manifestation of introjection. It seems more likely that the identification is in fact the resultant of copying' PP/Bow/H.118 (parentheses suppressed). For Bandura and the concept of modelling see Bandura A. & Menlove F.L. (1968) Factors determining vicarious extinction of avoidance behavior through symbolic modeling. *Journal of Personality & Social Psychology*, 8, 99–108.

[521] Bowlby, J. (1973) *Separation: Anger and Anxiety*. New York: Basic Books, p.417.

[522] Ibid.

[523] Ibid. p.235; see also Bowlby, J. (1984) No such thing as a baby, March 1984. PP/Bow/F.3/136: 'How to explain persistence: a) Parents commonly continue in the way they started; b) virtuous or vicious circles pattern perpetuates itself.'

[524] Sroufe, L.A., Duggal, S., Weinfield, N.S., & Carlson, E. (2000) Relationships, development, and psychopathology. In M. Lewis & A. Sameroff (eds) *Handbook of Developmental Psychopathology*, 2nd edn (pp.75–92). New York: Kluwer Academic/Plenum Press, p.87.

[525] Gilmore, K. (1990) A secure base. Parent–child attachment and healthy human development: by John Bowlby. *Psychoanalytic Quarterly*, 59, 494–8; Crittenden, P.M. (1997) Truth, error, omission, distortion, and

is not clear whether attachment sets early personality, whether it forms the first point in a loose and interruptible chain of social experiences, whether it moderates the relationship between innate qualities and behaviour, or all three (Chapter 5).[526] Implicitly contrasting her position to that of Bowlby, in 1988 Ainsworth reported that 'increasingly, we are concerning ourselves with increasing our understanding of change, and with defining the conditions under which it takes place'.[527] Later attachment researchers would find only partial support for the strength of Bowlby's emphasis on continuity, and would, as Ainsworth hoped, have much to say about change (Chapter 4).

Furthermore, Bowlby's overstrict opposition between 'actual experiences' and 'fantasy' led him to assume that experiences would be mirrored in symptoms, with adults 'continuing to respond in social situations with the very same patterns of behavior that they had developed during early childhood'.[528] So, for instance, in his 1944 'Forty four juvenile thieves' paper he claimed that children who do not receive affection develop an incapacity for affection, which in turn contributes to their delinquency.[529] And in 'Violence in the family', from 1984, he proposed that children who experience one kind of abuse will then show this same kind of abuse to their spouse and children [530] It is true that later research would support the idea that early experiences of neglect, violence, and highly unstable caregiving arrangements will shape developmental pathways and contribute towards the probability that an individual will develop mental health symptoms. However, Bowlby's claim for a specific mirror between early experiences and later symptoms has not been supported. His claims in the 1940s linking early separations and stealing have not been supported. And later research has found that early experiences of abuse make later abusive behaviour more likely, but not necessarily the same form of abuse (Chapter 4).

Emotion

A second consequential limitation of Bowlby's work also stemmed from his overstrict distinction between 'actual experience' and 'fantasy': his underelaboration of the emotional

---

deception: the application of attachment theory to the assessment and treatment of psychological disorder. In S.M. Clancy Dollinger & L.F. DiLalla (eds) *Assessment and Intervention Issues Across the Lifespan* (pp.35–76). London: Erlbaum; Bretherton, I. (2005) In pursuit of the internal working model construct and its relevance to attachment relationships. In K.E. Grossmann, K. Grossmann, & E. Waters (eds) *Attachment from Infancy to Adulthood: The Major Longitudinal Studies* (pp.13–47). New York: Guilford.

[526] This concern has also been discussed by Weinfield, N.S., Whaley, G. & Egeland, B. (2004) Continuity, discontinuity, and coherence in attachment from infancy to late adolescence: sequelae of organization and disorganization. *Attachment & Human Development*, 6(1), 73–97; Fraley, R.C. & Shaver, P.R. (2008) Attachment theory and its place in contemporary personality research. In O. John & R.W. Robins (eds) *Handbook of Personality: Theory and Research*, 3rd edn (pp. 518–41). New York: Guilford. The problem stems in part from the fact that much of Bowlby's early thinking in the 1940s had taken 'personality' as its object; and this thinking was then transferred to 'attachment', without full elaboration of the relationship between the two constructs. On the concept of personality in Bowlby's early work see Bowlby, J. (1940) *Personality and Mental Illness*. London: Kegan Paul.

[527] Ainsworth, M.D.S. (1988) Security. Unpublished discussion paper prepared for the Foundations of Attachment Theory Workshop, convened for the New York Attachment Consortium by G. Cox-Steiner & E. Waters, Port Jefferson, NY. http://www.psychology.sunysb.edu/attachment/online/mda_security.pdf.

[528] Bowlby, J. (1984) Violence in the family as a disorder of the attachment and caregiving systems. *American Journal of Psychoanalysis*, 44, 9–27, p.21. An early critic of Bowlby on this point was Rutter, M. (1972) *Maternal Deprivation Reassessed*. London: Penguin.

[529] Bowlby, J. (1944) Forty-four juvenile thieves: their characters and home-life (II). *International Journal of Psycho-Analysis*, 25, 107–28.

[530] Bowlby, J. (1984) Violence in the family as a disorder of the attachment and caregiving systems. *American Journal of Psychoanalysis*, 44, 9–27, p.21.

components of behavioural systems. In his writings, Bowlby was clear that affects are important components of behavioural systems, and attention to feelings do emerge from time to time in his scholarly writings. He would often repeat the claim that 'A person's whole emotional life—the underlying tone of how he or she feels—is determined by the state of these long-term, committed relationships. As long as they are running smoothly the person is content; when they are threatened, he or she is anxious and perhaps angry; when the person has endangered them by his or her own actions the person feels guilty; when they are broken, the person feels sad; and when they are resumed he or she is joyful.'[531] Such passages have sometimes been cited, especially by those seeking a model for therapeutic practice in attachment theory, to situate Bowlby as the quintessential theorist of human emotional life. However, such accounts depend upon anachronism. Johnson, for example, describes attachment for Bowlby as oriented by a striving for 'felt security' and 'emotion regulation', when in fact these represent the ideas of the later attachment researchers such as Sroufe, Waters, and Cassidy (Chapter 2, 3, and 4).[532] In fact, Bowlby gives the causal role of emotions little space compared to the behavioural and cognitive aspects of his theory, and as a consequence his account is often oversimple. It is never quite clear what relationship Bowlby perceived between emotion and motivation, perhaps because he was often extrapolating across species from ethological models.[533] Compared to Sroufe (Chapter 4), Bowlby generally offered little acknowledgement that moods and other felt states, such as confidence and fatigue, may arise or be held in place by multiple factors.[534] The caregiving system is a clear example: it is sometimes hard to recognise the actual dynamics of caregiving in Bowlby's characterisation of the caregiving behavioural system, for instance in how he neglects to give attention to both the worries and relief of being needed.

Bowlby highlighted the role of emotion only: (i) in modulating the activation and termination of behavioural systems; and (ii) as a consequence of the satisfaction or non-satisfaction of set-goals. Implicit in this is recognition that moods can offer us partially incompatible visions of the world, including of the viability and meaning of other emotions. Yet Bowlby rarely recognised, at least explicitly, the extent to which the fundamental shape and deployment of behavioural systems, including the calibration of their set-goal, can be conditioned by emotions. In his later writings especially, he came to consider the effects of depression and hopelessness. However, the emotional components of behavioural systems make them more varied and fragile than Bowlby generally acknowledged. This fragility can be seen with horrible clarity if we consider how a behavioural system looks when it becomes invested by shame or boredom, two emotions left aside by Bowlby (and, following him, by

---

[531] Ibid. p.11.

[532] Johnson, S.M. (2019) *Attachment Theory in Practice*. New York: Guilford, Chapter 2. See for instance the anachronistic attribution of a focus on 'felt sense' of emotions such as security to Bowlby, rather than Sroufe and Waters, on p.34.

[533] Bell, D.C. & Richard, A.J. (2000) Caregiving: the forgotten element in attachment. *Psychological Inquiry*, 11(2), 69–83, p.73. It is interesting to watch Bowlby ponder the relationship between motivation and emotion in his notes on 'Emotion and feeling', PP/Bow/H.5. These include reflections from the 1970s on emotion theorists such as Tomkins and Izard. His most determinate statement on the relationship between motivation and emotion in these notes seems to be the claim that the two are distinct, and that feelings contribute to the rise of motivations: 'The feeling of being oriented & drawn toward some end gives rise to the sensation of desiring or wanting to achieve that end.' However, he criticized Izard for insufficient attention to 'causal factors', seemingly besides feelings, 'that activate an actual sequence of behaviour'.

[534] One of Bowlby's most sustained considerations of mood is actually in his notes on history-taking from the mid-1930s: see 'History taking; methods of examining', PP/BOW/D.2/13. However, there he was interested in the role of moods as indices of personality, rather than in their cause or effects.

later empirical attachment research).[535] Indeed, except in relation to outright conflict between behavioural systems, in general Bowlby was consistently poor in acknowledging and characterizing states in which motivation becomes half-hearted, bendy, or sleepy, states of velleity rather than concrete intention or outright inhibited action. He also did not consider the way that some affects simultaneously undermine or sustain different behavioural systems. For instance, excitement can facilitate the exploratory system, but qualifies fear. Even during his lifetime, albeit writing in German, Mary Main criticised Bowlby's account of emotions for treating them as 'precipitates': an invisible part of a liquid that becomes a visible solid only after a chemical reaction. The metaphor suggests the role of emotion as a necessary part of behavioural systems, and actually integral to shaping their form—but as only visible, at least to Bowlby, at the end of the reaction as a 'consequence' of behavioural systems.[536]

In undated notes, likely from around 1955, Bowlby asked himself why he continually underplayed fantasy and emotion in his writing. He concluded that the 'reason is partly because we think psychobiological reactions have been neglected by psychoanalysis & partly because research method has led this way. This is not to say that phantasy is unimportant— obviously it comes in & tends to complicate things still further. Roots of phantasy are in the psychobiological responses.'[537] Bowlby evidently had a strong aversion to appeals to the idea of 'fantasy'. Speaking in an interview in 1986, he observed that 'nowadays, the word fantasy has become used in the analytic world to mean any cognitive process. It means conscious wish, it means a daydream, it means expectation.'[538] He regarded this loose use of the concept as obscuring phenomena that he regarded as both important and distinct. He also did not like the way that the term 'fantasy' collapsed distinctions between different ways of relating to the future, such as expectation, wishing, and planning. Such distinctions, he felt, were important for acknowledging the accounts of patients, and maintaining a 'neutral and empathetic position' in relation to what they said about their experiences.[539] In conversations with junior clinicians at the Tavistock, Bowlby used to ask that conversations of fantasy were 'parked', to see how or whether the matter in question could be addressed with greater precision in other ways.[540]

Bowlby's opposition between 'actual experience' and 'fantasy' was criticised by Ainsworth in their correspondence.[541] Ainsworth felt that Bowlby neglecting the emotional aspects of

---

[535] By contrast, shame has been a central theme in clinical elaborations of Bowlby's ideas by Allan and Judy Schore and by Dan Hughes and colleagues: Schore, A.N. (1991) Early superego development: the emergence of shame and narcissistic affect regulation in the practicing period. *Psychoanalysis and Contemporary Thought*, 14(2), 187–250; Hughes, D., Golding, K.S., & Hudson, J. (2015) Dyadic developmental psychotherapy (DDP): the development of the theory, practice and research base. *Adoption & Fostering*, 39(4), 356–65.

[536] Main, M. (1977) Sicherheit und wissen. In K.E. Grossmann (ed.) *Entwicklung der Lernfähigheit in der sozialen Umwelt* (pp.47–95). Munich: Kindler.

[537] Bowlby, J. (undated) Unpublished notes from his filing cabinets. *c.* 1955. PP/Bow/H115.

[538] Bowlby, J. (1986) An interview with John Bowlby on the origins and reception of his work. *Free Associations*, 1, 36–64, p.42.

[539] Bowlby, J. & Parkes, C.M. (1970, 1979) Separation and loss within the family. In *The Making and Breaking of Affectional Bonds* (pp.99–123). London: Routledge, p.123.

[540] This is described amusingly in Issroff, J. (2005) *Donald Winnicott and John Bowlby: Personal and Professional Perspectives*. London: Karnac: 'Bowlby … "parked" the term "fantasy" in what I always imagine to be a quite capacious parking lot in his mind' (56).

[541] Ainsworth, M. (1971) *Comments on the manuscript of* Attachment Volume 2. *Letter to Bowlby*, 16 August 1971. PP/BOW/K.5/62: 'You yourself, naturally, push your own view. And yet I really am convinced (and I am sure that you basically agree) that in many cases both kinds of "dynamics" are at work … It would take only a few alterations of turns of phrase to leave the classical Freudians and Kleinians a little more opportunity to feel that you are asking them to extend their view rather than to abandon it.'

behavioural systems, 'quite deliberately', in order to avoid ceding ground to those trends in psychoanalytic thought that privileged fantasy over past experiences.[542] In the 1980s, this motivation likely aligned with wider trends in cognitive science, in which thought and feeling were opposed, downplaying their interrelation.[543] To give an example, in 'Developmental psychiatry comes of age' in 1988 Bowlby stated that 'to Sigmund Freud is due the credit for having emphasised the influence on how people think, feel, and behave that is exerted by their internal world—namely, by the way they perceive, construe, and structure the events and situations they encounter'.[544] However, Bowlby was well aware that how people 'think, feel and behave' is not equivalent to how people 'perceive, construe and structure'. He equated them deliberately and strategically, to ensure that the cognitive aspect of behavioural systems, and the role of these in shaping emotions, would not be missed. The price, which appeared to be knowingly accepted by Bowlby, was that the role of emotion within behavioural systems, and the relationship between emotion and motivation, would remain hazy. This would leave problems for later attachment theory, for instance in how exactly to conceptualise affects at odds with expressed attachment behaviour (Chapter 3).

Predation and evolution

Bowlby's familiarity with ethology and developments in evolutionary biology, by his own admission, dropped away sharply after the publication of *Attachment, Volume 1*. A consequence was that aspects of his theory remained partially trapped in amber, and especially his knowledge of developments in evolutionary biology.[545] His account of attachment behaviour as a repertoire developed in human evolutionary history to sustain survival was a powerful cross-disciplinary integration of forms of knowledge, and an important plank in the emergence of developmental psychology as a subdiscipline informed by evolutionary theory. Yet Bowlby tended to rigidly emphasise that the evolutionary purpose of the attachment system was to save young children from predation by ensuring proximity to at least one adult. Downplayed in such an account, however, were the other evolutionary advantages of being physically close to a caregiver—advantages that Bowlby apparently knew. One such advantage is that closeness with the caregiver helps support psychobiological regulation. Bowlby stated this himself in 'The nature of the child's tie to his mother' in 1958, citing with approval a discussion by Winnicott.[546] The notion is also implied in Bowlby's use of a thermostat as the central model or metaphor for the attachment system. Another evolutionary advantage of the attachment system is that proximity with a caregiver offers opportunities for nurturance

---

[542] Ainsworth, M. (1997) Peter L. Rudnytsky—the personal origins of attachment theory: an interview with Mary Salter Ainsworth. *Psychoanalytic Study of the Child*, 52, 386–405, p.398.

[543] Waters, E., Corcoran, D., & Anafarta, M. (2005) Attachment, other relationships, and the theory that all good things go together. *Human Development*, 48(1–2), 80–84: 'Bowlby's attachment theory remains a work in progress ... his notion of attachment working models was limited to what could be done with the cognitive psychology of the day' (82).

[544] Bowlby, J. (1988) Developmental psychiatry comes of age. *American Journal of Psychiatry*, 145, 1–10, p.1.

[545] Bowlby, J. (1990, 2011) John Bowlby: interview by Leonardo Tondo. *Clinical Neuropsychiatry*, 8(2), 159–71: 'The main thing about the monkey work has been that, with fairly rigorous experimental designs and methods, they have demonstrated the ill effects of separation and its obvious consequences (Hinde 1966). It is a huge literary reserve which I was fairly familiar with in the 1960s because it was very dramatic but I haven't kept up' (166).

[546] Bowlby, J. (1958) Nature of the child's tie to his mother. *International Journal of Psycho-Analysis*, 39, 350–73, p.356, citing Winnicott, D.W. (1948) Pediatrics and psychiatry. *British Journal of Medical Psychology* 21, 229–40.

and learning. In 1965, Ainsworth wrote to Bowlby arguing against the exclusive focus on predation as the evolutionary function of attachment, and giving the examples of nurturance and learning.[547] These points were not taken up by Bowlby, except tacitly in his characterisation of attachment behaviour as directed towards someone 'stronger and/or wiser'. However, it would appear from correspondence that he regarded 'wiser' to be less a description of the actual properties of an attachment figure, and more a cognitive bias in the perception of the attachment figure when the attachment system is activated.[548]

In 1970, whilst still a doctoral student with Ainsworth, Mary Main nonetheless took Bowlby's side and argued that a desire for learning could not account for the clinging response as part of the attachment system. Opportunities for learning might be 'correlates that "ride on"' the evolutionary function of proximity for protection.[549] However, Main's support for Bowlby's position still offers no argument against physiological regulation and nurturance as possible evolutionary advantages of the attachment system. From the 1980s, physiological regulation and nurturance would be discussed by Myron Hofer as two 'hidden regulators' missed by Bowlby's exclusive focus on the attachment system as protection against predation.[550] Hofer claimed that Bowlby had ignored the 'chronic' advantages that physiological regulation and nurturance offer. The repetitive sequences of physiological regulation and nurturance may even play a role in constituting attachment as a coherently organised system, and infant separation anxiety may reflect a withdrawal response to these sources of regulation as much as a desire for protection. Furthermore, Hofer's perspective implied that attachments are not formed solely on the basis of familiarity, as Bowlby generally suggested, but with familiar sources of biosocial homeostasis. Even an abusive caregiver can be an attachment figure, if they are familiar and provide sufficient physiological regulation and nurturance to be felt as a source of regulation.

Bowlby entirely accepted Hofer's claims. In a warm letter to Hofer in 1983 he agreed on all points. Furthermore, he offered the notable claim that in humans as well as animals, 'internal representations are usually a poor second best' within the operation of behavioural systems,

[547] Ainsworth, M. (1965) *Letter to John Bowlby*, 7 October 1965. Mary Ainsworth papers, Box M3168, Folder 2: 'I was very pleased with your chapter on Instinct Theory … There was one point at which I was jerked out of my "yes" attitude. On page 60 you state that the main function of attachment behaviour is to ensure safety of the young—safety from predators. Of course, you will develop this point fully in your revision of the "Child's Tie" paper. I did not say "no" to your statement, but I did think about functions of maternal behaviour other than protection from predators—specifically nurturance of the young, but also training.' Several of Ainsworth's students have followed her lead on this matter rather than Bowlby's position. See e.g. Waters, E. (2008) Live long and prosper: a note on attachment and evolution. http://www.psychology.sunysb.edu/attachment/gallery/live_long/live_long.html.

[548] Bowlby, J. (1988) *A Secure Base*. London: Routledge p.121. Bowlby, J. (1985) *Letter to Malcom West*, 13 November 1985. PP/Bow/J.9/201: 'I suspect that, in the specific situations in which A's attachment behaviour is activated, A always *regards* the partner B as definitely the more competent to deal with them. And also that, in other situations, the roles of the partners are reversed. Thus, whilst overall each may regard the other as no more competence, etc. than the self, whenever attachment behaviour is activated the roles become complementary rather than reciprocal.'

[549] Main, M. (1970) Infant play and maternal sensitivity in primate evolution. PP/Bow/J.4/1: 'Alternate biological functions have been proposed, chief among them that mother and infant will come together in order that the infant may learn from the mother the behaviours which will promote its survival. The conditions which activate and terminate attachment behaviour and caretaking behaviour, such as alarming events in the environment and the actual attainment of contact or proximity, indicate that Bowlby's explanation is preferable.'

[550] Hofer, M.A. (1983) On the relation between attachment and separation processes in infancy. In R. Plutnik (ed.) *Emotion: Theory, Research and Experience*, Vol. 2 (pp.199–219). New York: Academic Press; Hofer, M.A. (1984) Relationships as regulators: a psychobiologic perspective on bereavement. *Psychosomatic Medicine*, 46(3), 183–97. For a review of the literature on hidden regulators and attachment see Polan, H.J. & Hofer, M. (2016) Psychobiological origins of infant attachment and its role in development. In J. Cassidy & P.R. Shaver (eds) *Handbook of Attachment*, 3rd edn (pp.117–32). New York: Guilford.

which likely much more 'rely on sensorimotor pathways'.[551] However, Bowlby did not integrate such insights into his subsequent published writings on the evolutionary function of the attachment behavioural system. A hint of a somewhat qualified position on the function of the attachment system can be seen only in Bowlby's last publication, and even this is quite limited: 'It contributes to the individual's survival by keeping him or her in touch with one or more caregivers, thereby reducing the risk of harm, for example from cold, hunger or drowning and, in the human's environment of evolutionary adaptedness, especially from predators.'[552]

Bowlby's almost exclusive emphasis on proximity and predation would be criticised in turn by nearly all of the second generation of attachment researchers as part of marking their own emerging voices in the field. Despite this, in the decades following Bowlby's death in 1990, it took a long while for the theory to receive even partial update in light of developments in evolutionary biology.[553] It has not helped that ethology, the original alloparent of the attachment paradigm, has gone into decline since the 1990s, as interest shifted from behavioural sequences to other levels of analysis such as sociobiology and, more recently, gene–environment coevolution.[554] However, the failure of further engagement with changing paradigms in biology has been fed by an internal dynamic within the field of attachment research: since Bowlby, authority about the biological function of behaviour has been part of leadership of the developmental tradition of attachment research, since in part it defines the nature of attachment as a research object and therefore the questions to be asked. With biological theory mixed up with authority and power, this dynamic has helped insulate attachment theory against a continued update of its models, in Bowlby's era and subsequently. Bowlby's ossified account of the relationship between attachment and evolutionary theory contained in the predation model would eventually lead to disagreements between Bowlby and Main, with lasting consequences for attachment as a research programme (Chapter 3). It would later also be significant ammunition for Peter Fonagy and Chloe Campbell's call for a new paradigm to replace attachment research whilst absorbing its strengths (Chapter 6).

Conclusion

See Table 1.3 in the Appendix to this chapter for consideration of key concepts discussed here.

---

[551] Bowlby, J. (1983) *Letter to Myron Hofer*, 29 July 1983. PP/Bow/J.9/102. This correspondence supports the claim of Cassidy and colleagues that Bowlby downplayed non-representational affective and physiological processes as part of his focus on cognitive processes: Cassidy, J., Ehrlich, K.B., & Sherman, L.J. (2013) Child–parent attachment and response to threat: a move from the level of representation. In M. Mikulincer & P.R. Shaver (eds) *Nature and Development of Social Connections: From Brain to Group* (pp.125–44). Washington, DC: American Psychological Association.

[552] Bowlby, J. (1991) Ethological light on psychoanalytic problems. In P. Bateson (ed.) *The Development and Integration of Behaviour: Essays in Honour of Robert Hinde* (pp.301–14). Cambridge: Cambridge University Press, p.306.

[553] An update in light of evolutionary biology would partially take place from the late 1990s especially through the work of Jay Belsky. Belsky, J. (1999) Modern evolutionary theory and patterns of attachment. In J. Cassidy & P.R. Shaver (eds) *Handbook of Attachment* (pp.141–61). New York: Guilford.

[554] Griffiths, P.E. (2008) Ethology, sociobiology, and evolutionary psychology. In S. Sarkar & A. Plutynski (eds) *A Companion to the Philosophy of Biology* (pp.393–414). Oxford: Blackwell. There remain some ethologists who have continued to conduct empirical studies with a focus on sequences of behaviour in the manner of Lorenz and Tinbergen. See e.g. Suomi, S. (2016) Attachment in rhesus monkeys. In J. Cassidy & P.R. Shaver (eds) *Handbook of Attachment* (pp.133–54), 3rd edn. New York: Guilford; Polanco, A., Díez-León, M., & Mason, G. (2018) Stereotypic behaviours are heterogeneous in their triggers and treatments in the American mink, *Neovison vison*, a model carnivore. *Animal Behaviour*, 141, 105–14.

Sroufe argued that 'as is always characteristic of development, whether in an individual or in a scientific field, Bowlby's work both integrates and transforms what went before creating an alternative way of viewing the world without leaving behind critical insights contained in previous viewpoints'.[555] Bowlby described himself as speaking a 'hybrid, bastard language', bringing together concepts from ethology and psychoanalysis, as well as terms from ordinary language.[556] In creating this hybrid combination of discourses, Bowlby's theory could benefit from the precision of Hinde's conceptualisation of behavioural responses, their conditions and their conflicts; the emotional punch and drama of Kleinian theory of intense emotions and defences invested with his own personal and clinical experiences; and the explosive obviousness of the ordinary language connotations of 'attachment', 'separation', 'loss', 'mother', 'love', and others.[557] Attachment theory was able to make an iconic assemblage of the precision, emotional power, and intuitiveness of these elements in ways that quickened the potential of each.[558] Yet, in making an identity, it also retained qualities of these constituent differences. Various faces of this assemblage offered the theoretical basis for an empirical research paradigm, an approach to clinical work with children and adults, and a popular discourse regarding child development and family life.

If Bowlby had remained a theorist only attentive to the precisely defined 'following response', and had not plugged these ethological observations of behavioural sequences into the evocative world of psychoanalytic concerns, the theory would have been much less rich. Hinde himself would later concede this in reflections many years after Bowlby's death.[559] And if Bowlby had achieved his synthesis of ethology and psychoanalysis, but had communicated only in the language of these two disciplines, his ideas would have had a very limited audience. Bowlby's appeals to ordinary language and cultural stereotypes in writing for popular forums helped set his theory alight; it glowed to widespread visibility, even as its qualifications and technical subtlety burned away as fuel. The manner of Bowlby's popular writings helped create what Bourdieu termed 'allodoxia', a 'light', commodified version of a more complex cultural form, appealing to a wider base of constituents without the tools or means to access the original.[560] This is in contrast to forms of popularisation that attempt to convey the intricacy and technical quality of the form, generally by unpacking terms and explaining in longhand or prioritizing the most essential elements, using an accessible style and stories to keep the audience engaged.[561] Certainly not all works of popular science are allodoxia. What characterises allodoxia in psychology is the circulation of a simplified account of the human mind as if it had the same meaning as the technical account of empirical researchers.

---

[555] Sroufe, L.A. (1986) Bowlby's contribution to psychoanalytic theory and developmental psychopathology. *Journal of Child Psychology and Psychiatry*, 27, 841–9, p.841.

[556] Bowlby, J. cited in J.M. Tanner & B. Inhelder (eds) (1956) *Discussions on Child Development: Proceedings of the WTO Study Group of the Psychobiological Development of the Child*, Vol. 1. London: Tavistock, p.184.

[557] Bowlby's passionate focus on what an assemblage can *do*, and not of the price of its formation or use, can be seen clearly in a late interview: Bowlby, J. (1986) An interview with John Bowlby on the origins and reception of his work. *Free Associations*, 1, 36–64: 'What's important about a person's work is what they have contributed. I don't care two pins about their mistakes or their shortcomings or their omissions—what have they contributed?' (63).

[558] Cf. Bartmanski, D. (2012) How to become an iconic social thinker: the intellectual pursuits of Malinowski and Foucault. *European Journal of Social Theory*, 15(4), 427–53.

[559] Hinde, R. (2005) Ethology and attachment theory. In K. Grossman, E. Waters, & K. Grossman (eds) *Attachment from Infancy to Adulthood: The Major Longitudinal Studies* (pp.1–12). New York: Guilford, p.9. See also Petters, D.D. (2019) The attachment control system and computational modeling: origins and prospects. *Developmental Psychology*, 55(2), 227–39.

[560] Bourdieu, P. (1979, 1984) *Distinction*, trans. R. Nice. Cambridge, MA: Harvard University Press.

[561] Bucchi, M. (2013) Style in science communication. *Public Understanding of Science*, 22(8), 904–15.

All science has a 'price for full entry' in terms of theoretical and technical competence and commitment.[562] This price may be paid by specialists through their training as part of formal qualifications or accreditation. Some or all access may also be gained by non-specialists, for instance through reading, depending on the structural barriers to entry and how much socialisation in tacit skills is required.[563] In both cases there remains some recognition of the distinction between technical and non-technical use of concepts. By contrast, the accessibility of elements of Bowlby's popularizing discourses from the 1950s and 1960s offered cut-price tickets to attachment theory, even though these only granted access to a fairly antiquated portion of the fairground, and—the source of much later trouble—looked much the same as full entry tickets. The cut-price popular discourse of attachment was evocative and underdetermined, as well as having the appearance of scientific credibility. This gave it flexibility, urgency, and reach for these diverse constituents concerned with speaking about the nature of family relationships and child development.[564] The language of attachment theory can be experienced as running towards us, calling our name. This was deliberate. Both the circulation of half-truths about attachment and their rhetorical insistence can be regarded, in part, as a by-product of Bowlby's marketing strategy for his scholarly thinking.[565]

In one of his final papers, Bowlby argued that science has two stages, drawing ideas from the philosopher of science Karl Popper. In the first stage, the task is to frame hypotheses. Where possible, this process benefits from 'detailed and first-hand knowledge of the problem ... together with a dose of intuition and imagination'.[566] Raw materials such as ordinary language and clinical anecdote can be relevant elements for this stage of work, alongside all the other resources of the humanities. Bowlby, in fact, chided behaviourism for failing to see such resources as relevant, making the paradigm rather arid and, at times, 'barren' despite its rigour.[567] Nonetheless, even the thin theory of behaviourism, he felt, was better than atheoretical research in psychology, since theory is necessary for the effective planning and interpretation of empirical research as a cumulative endeavour, as well as the design of interventions and public health policies.[568] Looking back over his long career, Bowlby offered the self-criticism that his work had displayed an 'absence of a follow-through', remaining in the first stage of hypothesis-generation.[569] It would only be with the work of Bowlby's colleague Mary Ainsworth that attachment theory would become the basis for attachment research as an empirical research paradigm. Ainsworth's contribution remained exploratory. It was also work in the context of hypothesis-generation, though it was sometimes misrecognised as hypothesis-testing research. However, Ainsworth's development of procedures for measuring individual differences in attachment and related constructs would prove the bedrock of a hypothesis-testing tradition of attachment research within developmental science.

---

[562] Bourdieu, P. (2004) *The Science of Science and Reflexivity*, trans. R. Nice. Chicago: University of Chicago Press, pp.53–4.

[563] Collins, H. & Evans, R. (2018) A sociological/philosophical perspective on expertise: the acquisition of expertise through socialization. In K. Anders Ericsson, R.R. Hoffman, A. Kozbelt, & A.M. Williams (eds) *The Cambridge Handbook of Expertise and Expert Performance* (pp.21–32). Cambridge: Cambridge University Press.

[564] On the practical logic of underdetermined discourses: de Certeau, M. (1984) *The Practice of Everyday Life*, trans. S.F. Rendall. Berkeley: University of California Press; Bourdieu, P. (2000) *Pascalian Meditations*. Stanford: Stanford University Press; Mercer, J. (2015) Revisiting an article about dyadic developmental psychotherapy: the life cycle of a Woozle. *Child and Adolescent Social Work Journal*, 32(5), 397–404; Alexander, J.C. (2016) Dramatic intellectuals. *International Journal of Politics, Culture, and Society*, 29(4), 341–58; Pettit, M. & Young, J.L. (2017) Psychology and its publics. *History of the Human Sciences*, 30(4), 3–10.

[565] See also Duniec, E. & Raz, M. (2011) Vitamins for the soul: John Bowlby's thesis of maternal deprivation, biomedical metaphors and the deficiency model of disease. *History of Psychiatry*, 22(1), 93–107.

[566] Bowlby, J. (1988) Where science and humanism meet. *Group Analysis*, 21, 81–8, p.81.

[567] Ibid.

[568] Bowlby, J. (1982) Attachment and loss: retrospect and prospect. *American Journal of Orthopsychiatry*, 52(4), 664–78, p.676.

[569] Bowlby, J. (1988) Where science and humanism meet. *Group Analysis*, 21, 81–8, p.81.

Appendix

Table 1.3 Some key concepts in Bowlby's writings

Concept	Mistaken for	Technical meaning
Attachment system	The instinctive relationship with a familiar caregiver	The 'attachment system' is a way of describing a form of motivation. The motivation is activated when a person is alarmed. When the person feels that a particular, familiar person—or familiar people—is available and responsive to their concerns, the motivation is reduced. Where the system is strongly activated, some form of contact is generally sought (though this contact may still be verbal rather than touch). This motivation has some basis in evolution, and for this reason is especially easy for humans to develop. However, a great deal about this motivation, including exactly the conditions that prompt and terminate it, are shaped deeply by experiences in relationships. This is why it is misleading to think of attachment as an 'instinct'.
		The attachment system has some characteristic behaviours, but in principle any behaviour can be recruited that helps achieve the goal of attachment figure availability.
		Attachment researchers have debated the conditions that lead to the satisfaction of the attachment system and a reduction in display of attachment behaviour. The physical and attentional availability of a familiar caregiver has been emphasised as terminating conditions in infancy; other attachment researchers, since Sroufe and Waters, have emphasised the infant's 'felt security' as the terminating conditions for the system.
		In general it is agreed that experience, circumstance, and culture can all shape the conditions under which the attachment system is activated, the forms of behaviour recruited by the attachment system, and how these are expressed.
Attachment behaviour	Pre-set behaviours that express attachment as an instinct	Anything in principle can be an attachment behaviour. All that is required is that the behaviour should be clearly directed towards gaining the availability and responsiveness of a familiar person or familiar people. It is not an 'instinctual' pre-set pattern of behaviour.
		Attachment behaviours are observable, whereas the motivation they are presumed to express is inferred.
		The term 'attachment behaviour' was used in two different ways by Bowlby. His most common use of the term was to refer to proximity-seeking and contact-maintaining behaviours, such as smiling, crawling towards the caregiver, clinging, and directed cries to attract the caregiver's attention. These behaviours were understood as direct expressions of the attachment behavioural system.

Table 1.3 Continued

Concept	Mistaken for	Technical meaning
		Sometimes, however, Bowlby also used the term 'attachment behaviour' to refer to any behaviour that occurs in the context of the activation of the attachment system. This could even include withdrawal from the caregiver and attempts at self-reliance by a child who had found that seeking proximity with their caregiver when alarmed or distressed would be counterproductive.
		Often these two meanings are aligned. However, some behaviours, such as when a child shows caregiving behaviour towards a parent, are attachment behaviours in the second sense, but not the first sense. At times this has caused a lack of clarity in discussing such behaviour, its eliciting conditions, and its relationship with the attachment behavioural system.
Attachment bond	Parent–child bonding	Bowlby characterised relationships and their qualities as diverse. Attachment dynamics characterised only some relationships and not others. He therefore distinguished the broad class of affectional bonds, in which members are special to one another and seek to remain in contact. Within this broad class are relationships with attachment dynamics. These are characterised by the fact that the other person is taken to be the object of the attachment behavioural system: there is a disposition to seek this person under conditions of alarm, and a sense of security when this person is reliably available and responsive to concerns.
		The attachment bond is distinct from 'parent–child bonding', the process by which parents develop an affectionate bond with their child and take the child as the familiar target of the caregiving behavioural system.
Attachment relationship	An absolute state characteristic of a child's relationship with their mother	Being an attachment figure is not a yes/no situation. Bowlby proposed that an attachment relationship is present to the extent that an individual is disposed to seek the availability of a familiar other when alarmed. This disposition may exist even if the other is rejecting or abusive.
		Bowlby felt that an individual could have a variety of attachment relationships—including wider kin (e.g. grandparents), divine beings, and also a person's relationship with their physical home. However, he believed that evolution had primed humans to develop these dynamics especially with our familiar caregivers from childhood. Other relationships would be more contingent in the degree to which these dynamics would be expected.

(continued)

Table 1.3 Continued

Concept	Mistaken for	Technical meaning
Major separation	Occasions when the child and parent are not together	Attachment researchers sometimes discuss children experiencing 'major separations'. This is a technical term, which can easily be confusing. What makes a separation 'major' is that the child is alarmed by the absence of their attachment figure, and this alarm continues for long enough that the attachment behavioural system then becomes chronically unresponsive for a long period. In effect, the child appears to give up searching for, calling, or expecting the parent to return. The result is that even when the caregiver is available, the child is not able to use them—at least for a time—to regulate distress. Or, in Bowlby's terms, the behavioural system becomes chronically unresponsive for a period to cues for its activation and/or termination.
		The classic case of a major separation was the long-term hospitalisations observed by James Robertson in the 1950s, in which there were no or few visits to young children over several months.
		Attachment researchers do not regard some use of daycare as a 'major separation' in the technical sense.
Monotropy	The exclusivity and priority of child–*mother* attachment	Bowlby introduced the term 'monotropy' in 1958 with the intention that it would refer to particular, special relationships, shaped by time and habit. Unfortunately, the literal meaning of the term is 'mono' (one) + tropy (turning to). This gave the mistaken impression he meant the exclusive importance of one caregiver for children.
		Bowlby later mostly abandoned the term, given the extent of misapprehension of his meaning.
Caregiving system	The natural capacity of parents, especially mothers, to care for their children	The 'caregiving system' is a way of describing a kind of motivation. A motivation to help is activated when a child or other person in our care is alarmed, and terminated when we have identified and responded to what we understand to be their concerns.
		In his initial description of caregiving as a behavioural system, Bowlby focused on the caregiver's motivation to retrieve infants who are alarmed or in trouble. However, later in his career he described caregiving as more broadly concerned with encouragement, support, help, and protection.
Effects of early experience	The notion that early social experience can be expected at an individual level to strongly determine later emotional and social experience	In his early writings, Bowlby sometimes made claims that implied that every child who receives poor care or who experiences major separations will develop social and emotional problems. From the 1970s onwards, he was more careful, claiming that—on average—poor care or major separations are likely to increase the chances of later social and emotional problems.
		Later attachment researchers have synthesised findings from many studies through meta-analysis, indeed finding that early care does have effects on later socioemotional development, but that early experience does not determine later outcome, and that there are important mediators and moderators.

Table 1.3 Continued

Concept	Mistaken for	Technical meaning
Internal working model	Representations of caregivers, which become generalised to all relationships with development	This is perhaps the single most confusing concept used by attachment researchers. Bowlby used the term in two different ways.
		Firstly, he intended it only to mean that the way the attachment system works depends on expectations based on previous experiences of interaction with caregivers in childhood—and with partners and friends in adulthood. So a synonym for the internal working model, in this sense, in ordinary language is simply 'expectations'. Bowlby's point was that expectations about early relationships can play a role in shaping our assumptions about later social relationships and interactions.
		Both humans and non-humans will have expectations about our caregivers or partners and their availability. However, humans also develop elaborated cognitive and cultural representations about ourselves and our attachment figures. These include narratives and images about the availability of attachment figures, and how we think they feel about us. A second use of the term 'internal working model' by Bowlby was therefore to refer to the specific symbolic and affective representations made by humans about attachment figures and their availability, and the efficacy of attempts to seek them when alarmed.
		When Mary Main and colleagues introduced the Adult Attachment Interview (AAI) in the 1980s, they documented individual differences in the coherence of autobiographical accounts by participants of their childhood. Initially she referred to these differences in speakers' narratives as reflecting differences in 'internal working models' about attachment. By the 1990s, she had abandoned and criticised the use of the term 'internal working model' to refer to these differences. Given the two different meanings above, she felt that the term was confusing and misleading for describing what the AAI was measuring. Main preferred to characterise individual differences in the AAI as reflecting 'states of mind regarding attachment'. However, many attachment researchers still refer to the AAI as measuring internal working models.
Segregation	The inhibition of information; essentially the same as dissociation	In Bowlby's later writings the term 'segregation' is used to refer to a coping strategy in which some information is filtered out of experience. This can be minor and remain flexible: the filter can be raised or dropped as needed. Or the flow of information to or from whole behavioural systems can be blocked over a long period, regardless of the circumstances.
		Bowlby distinguished two forms of segregation. A first was 'defensive exclusion'. Here the filter is placed on perception. So, certain things in the world may not be noticed. Or if noticed, they may not prompt a response. The paradigmatic form of defensive exclusion is the infant in an avoidant attachment relationship, who directs attention away from their caregiver on reunion. In doing so, they filter out information about their situation that might otherwise prompt the activation of the attachment system.

(continued)

Table 1.3 Continued

Concept	Mistaken for	Technical meaning
		A second form of segregation was 'cognitive disconnection'. Here the filter is placed on memory. So, certain memories may not be available. Or if available, they may not be tagged with well-defined and accurate meanings.
		The segregation of information about attachment figures was anticipated by Bowlby to contribute to an individual holding multiple incompatible perceptions and expectations of these figures.
		Bowlby's primary book on segregation, defensive exclusion, and cognitive disconnection remained unpublished. The terms appear only briefly in his published works. As a result, these terms are only used rarely now by attachment researchers.
Multiple attachments	Bowlby felt that a child should always be cared for by their mother	In his early writings Bowlby sometimes made claims that suggested a child should always be cared for by their mother. However, he subsequently regretted these claims. In his mature writing Bowlby saw value in a child having access to multiple secure bases and safe havens, and did not think that one attachment would be at the expense of another.
		Bowlby's final statement was that the attachment system 'contributes to the individual's survival by keeping him or her in touch with one or more caregivers'. The idea of attachment relationships as a network was developed by subsequent researchers such as Avi Sagi-Schwartz and Marinus van IJzendoorn.

Illustrative statement: 'Bowlby argued that early experiences of care within monotropic attachment relationships, such as potential separations, contribute to the later integration or segregation of mental processes, and to the child's own caregiving behaviours when they reach adulthood.'

Mistaken for: Bowlby argued that the quality of the mothers' care, including separations such as maternal employment, will determine children's later mental health and how they parent their own children.

Technical meaning: Bowlby argued that a child's experiences in specific relationships with familiar caregivers will shape and calibrate the operation of the attachment behavioural system. This process may be disrupted, however, by major separations such as being hospitalised without visitation. Disruptions to the attachment system may influence the formation and operation of later mental processes, including coping strategies. Where disruptions lead to fixed or extreme distortions or blockages of attachment-relevant information, a predisposition to mental health problems may be anticipated—though this will be seen at a population level rather than in any given individual. Behaviours, affects, and cognitions that form components of the attachment behavioural system may influence the caregiving system when it develops, since elements may be inherited by or inform the latter system (e.g. expectations about what intimacy entails).

2

Mary Ainsworth and the Strange Situation Procedure

Biographical sketch

Mary Salter took her undergraduate and graduate degrees in psychology in the 1930s at the University of Toronto. Her mentor was the director of the Institute of Child Study, William Emet Blatz. Salter completed her doctorate in 1940, based on Blatz's ideas. Following time in the Canadian Women's Army Corps during World War II, she rejoined the University of Toronto as assistant professor in psychology, and worked with Blatz in developing self-report measures of security and insecurity. During World War II, she worked in personnel for the Canadian Women's Army Corps, attaining the rank of Major. She married Leonard Ainsworth in 1950, and then followed him to London, which is where she met John Bowlby (Chapter 1). In early 1954, Leonard Ainsworth accepted a position in Uganda. Whilst in Uganda with her husband, Mary Ainsworth conducted an observational study of 26 mothers and their infants living in six villages near Kampala. Mary and Leonard Ainsworth left Uganda for Baltimore in late 1955. Mary Ainsworth gained a permanent academic position at Johns Hopkins University in 1958. With funds from the William T. Grant Foundation, she began a study in 1963 of Baltimore infants and their mothers, who were visited regularly until the children were a year old. As a supplement to home observations, Ainsworth invited the mothers and infants for a laboratory-based observational procedure, which she called the Strange Situation. Ainsworth's findings from this study were reported in numerous articles. Drawing on additional results from her students, she co-authored *Patterns of Attachment* in 1978, which presented a thorough report on the Strange Situation as a research methodology.[1] She was unable to secure funds to replicate or extend her results, despite growing recognition of her work and election to Presidency of the Society for Research in Child Development from 1977 to 1979. Yet her pioneering and profound work established attachment as a paradigm within developmental science, offering a way beyond the opposition between frequency counts of behaviours and subjective judgement about relationships. She also mentored an astonishing cohort of developmental psychologists and clinical researchers, first at Johns Hopkins University and then at the University of Virginia.

Introduction

In a letter to Everett Waters in 1985, Bowlby wrote of his intense pride at having had the opportunity to work with Mary Ainsworth. He described Ainsworth and himself as horses in

---

[1] Ainsworth, M., Blehar, M., Waters, E., & Wall, S. (1978, 2015) *Patterns of Attachment: A Psychological Study of the Strange Situation*. Bristol: Psychology Press.

'double harness', pulling the cart along.[2] This beautiful image of a sturdy, effortful partnership glosses over the fact that, at times, Bowlby and Ainsworth pulled in different directions. As Chapter 1 described, Ainsworth identified limitations in Bowlby's ideas on several fronts. She felt that Bowlby oversimplified matters when he claimed proximity as the set-goal of the attachment behavioural system, and protection from predation as its evolutionary function. She disliked his imprecision in discussions of separation, and particularly the way that the term 'maternal deprivation' could absorb anything from occasional use of professional childcare through to abuse and neglect. She was frustrated that her contributions to research on hospitalised children in London in the 1950s resulted in few publications because Bowlby's lack of empirical expertise had led to poor choice of measures. Ainsworth also had concerns about aspects of Bowlby's account of behavioural systems, feeling that he had underplayed the sexual, exploratory, and aggression behavioural systems, and neglected adequate attention to the emotional components of behavioural systems in humans. And yet the image of two horses pulling the cart along is exactly appropriate. Ainsworth's criticisms came from her overall sense of common purpose with Bowlby, bringing her independent intellectual perspective to shared problems, as well as her own interests.[3] In a co-authored article composed largely in the months before Bowlby died and then finished by Ainsworth, the two researchers wrote that 'their contributions to attachment theory and research interdigitated in a partnership that endured for 40 years across time and distance'.[4] The word 'interdigitated' is a characteristically stiff one; Bowlby, especially, was a person with significant capacities for reserve. But the phrase 'enduring across time and distance' was actually a technical one for these two researchers: it defines one of the qualities of an attachment relationship.[5] It comes from the kind of deep happiness in another person that does not require a smile or other marks of informality.

As discussed in Chapter 1, Ainsworth had worked for Bowlby as a clinical postdoctoral researcher within the Separation Research Unit from 1950 to 1953. During this time, they had been colleagues, but Bowlby's group was run according to a strict hierarchy, with Ainsworth conducting empirical work but with little say on research design or theory development. In an interview with Robert Karen, Ainsworth recalled her experiences of Bowlby during this period: 'He made no bones about the fact that he was single-handedly fighting the analytic establishment, that it pained him some, but that he was convinced he was on the right track. It was a long time before I felt any sense of getting close to him or being a friend. But I had no difficulty whatsoever making him into a surrogate father figure—even though he's not much older than I.'[6] They remained in touch after this, including through Ainsworth's period in Uganda, but the correspondence had little impetus. This changed from 1960. In this year, Ainsworth and her husband divorced.[7] She became quite depressed, feeling that

---

[2] Bowlby, J. (1985) *Letter to Everett Waters*, 30 October 1985. PP/Bow/B.3/40.

[3] A definition of genuine partnership was provided by Bowlby as 'when two more or less autonomous beings share a common plan'. A sure sense of common plan is evident between Bowlby and Ainsworth from the 1960s onwards. The definition appears in Bowlby, J. (1969) *Letter to Robert Marvin*, 10 December 1969. PP/Bow/J.9/132.

[4] Ainsworth, M. & Bowlby, J. (1991) 1989 APA award recipient addresses: an ethological approach to personality development. *American Psychologist*, 46(4), 333–41, p.333.

[5] Bowlby J. (1951) *Maternal Care and Mental Health*. Geneva: WHO, p.53; Ainsworth, M.D. (1985) Attachments across the life span. *Bulletin of the New York Academy of Medicine*, 61(9), 792–812.

[6] Interview with Mary Ainsworth by Robert Karen cited in Karen, R. (1998) *Becoming Attached: First Relationships and How They Shape Our Capacity to Love*. Oxford: Oxford University Press, p.133.

[7] All seven men in the cohort of doctoral students who graduated with Ainsworth were married, stayed married, and raised children; in contrast, only one of the six female academics had an enduring marriage, and it was only

her life had become empty.[8] Gradually, she began to work out new plans, and these brought her into a much closer engagement with Bowlby. Ainsworth had read Bowlby's 'The nature of the child's tie to his mother' paper in 1958. The account of attachment behaviours helped her make sense of her observations of Ganda infant–caregiver dyads, in terms of both the maturational processes associated with the following response and the role of caregiving in shaping individual differences.[9]

In 1960 Bowlby came to visit Ainsworth in Baltimore, following his year at the Stanford Institute for Advanced Study. Bowlby discovered Ainsworth's enthusiasm for his recent theoretical work, and the relationship was rekindled on changed terms. Bowlby remained the senior colleague. However, compared to their years working together in London, the relationship gained greater equality and affection, both of which continued to grow over subsequent years. Where Bowlby had found in ethology the heuristic frame that integrated his otherwise diverse observations, Ainsworth found this in Bowlby's work, supporting her thinking about infant behaviour and infant–caregiver interaction.[10] Yet Ainsworth also found in Bowlby's ideas from 1958 onwards a deep and persuasive account of the human condition, offering a unifying perspective on relatedness, development, and how we respond when our needs are not met. She saw in attachment theory qualities that resembled existentialist philosophy in its careful reflection on relationships, the uncomfortable feelings that stem from them, and what these suggest about the nature of a human life.[11]

Following her divorce, Ainsworth also entered into what would be eight years of therapy, which she later described as perhaps 'the most important positive influence on my career'.[12] It is hardly possible to understand Ainsworth's intellectual orientation, and therefore her contribution to developmental science from the 1960s onwards, without attention to this 'most important positive influence'. For this reason, Ainsworth was herself candid about her therapy in autobiographical writings as well as in interview. At the start, therapy initially provided 'some core of stability in what would otherwise be a confused and confusing period'.[13] Over the years, however, Ainsworth felt that she gained a greatly deepened understanding of psychological processes, especially emotional life, its conflicts, and forms of defence or inhibition.[14] In a late interview, Ainsworth recalled the exploration and learning of her time in therapy. She came to acknowledge and understand 'the feelings of warmth, love and security' she received from her relationship with her father. Her mother was jealous of this closeness between father and daughter, and banned her from seeking physical proximity

---

after the breakdown of the marriages that their careers took off. Isaacson, K.L. (2006) Mary Ainsworth and John Bowlby: the development of attachment theory. Unpublished doctoral dissertation, University of California, Davis.

[8] Ainsworth, M. (1983) Mary D. Salter Ainsworth. In N. Felipe Russo & A.N. O'Connell (eds) *Models of Achievement: Reflections of Eminent Women in Psychology* (pp.200–18). New York: Columbia University Press.

[9] Ainsworth, M. (1969) CPA oral history of psychology in Canada interview. Unpublished. http://www.feministvoices.com/assets/Women-Past/Ainsworth/Mary-Ainsworth-CPA-Oral-History.pdf.

[10] Ainsworth, M. (1995) On the shaping of attachment theory and research: an interview with Mary D.S. Ainsworth. *Monographs of the Society for Research in Child Development*, 60(2–3), 2–21: 'Mainly, however, findings obtained with other species have made me feel that I have been on the right track rather than helping me understand the specifics of human babies' behaviour.' (9)

[11] Ainsworth, M. (1965) *Letter to John Bowlby*, 2 February 1965. Mary Ainsworth papers, Box M3168, Folder 2.

[12] Ainsworth, M. (1983, 2013) An autobiographical sketch. *Attachment & Human Development*, 15(5–6), 448–59, p.456.

[13] Ainsworth, M. (1960) *Letter to John Bowlby*, 18 October 1960. Mary Ainsworth papers, Box M3168, Folder 1.

[14] Ainsworth, M. (1983) Mary D. Salter Ainsworth. In N. Felipe Russo & A.N. O'Connell (eds) *Models of Achievement: Reflections of Eminent Women in Psychology* (pp.200–18). New York: Columbia University Press, p.212.

with her father.[15] Though her mother made Ainsworth feel rejected, anger in response to this rejection was unacceptable, to the point that Ainsworth lost access to that emotion: 'I got to the point of not ever being able to feel angry. I would just feel hurt.'[16]

Therapy also helped Ainsworth think through the rubble and emotional fallout that followed her divorce, and especially her grief that she had been unable to have a child.[17] Her one pregnancy had ended in a miscarriage. She would later reflect to Bowlby that she felt that her grief and preoccupied longing for a child ultimately became transfigured into perceptiveness.[18] This entailed an unusual ability to see things from the baby's point of view, through both an awareness of infants' signals and communications and acuity in interpreting them. In a sense, all subsequent attachment researchers after Ainsworth would, one by one, unknowingly light their own work with the spill from this transfigured loss.

As her therapy was coming to an end, Ainsworth composed an important article, 'Object relations, dependency and attachment', published in 1969, comparing Bowlby's ideas with the mainstream psychoanalytic ideas of the day, and highlighting the strengths of both. In particular, she argued that it was in considering the qualities of individual differences that 'psychoanalysts have made a valuable contribution':

> They have not been concerned so much with the quantitative dimension of object rela-
> tions—stronger or weaker love or attachment—as with the qualitative variations among
> different object relations. How ambivalent is the relationship, what admixture of love and
> hate, and how well is the ambivalence resolved? How anxious is the relationship? How is it
> affected by the person's defenses against anxiety?[19]

Ainsworth's stable academic position at Johns Hopkins, her experiences of ethnographic observation in Uganda, and her subsequent thinking about attachment all fed into plans to develop a longitudinal study of infant development, based on detailed observations of Baltimore infants and mothers at home. This plan was difficult to implement. Ainsworth had great trouble finding funds for such a study. Reviewers did not appreciate her desire for in-depth work with a small sample, or her intention to examine many aspects of interaction. And they regarded as unscientific her wish to develop scales after having conducted qualitative analysis to explore emergent findings.[20]

[15] Main, M. (1999) Mary D. Salter Ainsworth: tribute and portrait. *Psychoanalytic Inquiry*, 19(5), 682–736, p.704.

[16] Ainsworth, M. (1997) Peter L. Rudnytsky—the personal origins of attachment theory: an interview with Mary Salter Ainsworth. *Psychoanalytic Study of the Child*, 52, 386–405, p.401.

[17] This sadness remains powerful, however, in Ainsworth's reference to her 'vain longing' for children in Ainsworth, M. (1983, 2013) An autobiographical sketch. *Attachment & Human Development*, 15(5–6), 448–59, p.459.

[18] Ainsworth, M. (1984) *Letter to John Bowlby*, 11 April 1984. PP/BOW/B.3/8: 'Longing gave me some kind of perceptive in terms of which I could understand mother–infant interaction.' See also Maurer, D. (1998) Interview with Mary Ainsworth: never miss an opportunity to hold a baby, 12 May 1998. *Daily Progress*. http://www.psych-ology.sunysb.edu/attachment/gallery/never_miss/nevermiss.htm:'Quite a lot of my wanting my own child played into my life work.' Among the most distinctive characteristics of Ainsworth's written voice is the dignity she gives to young children's gestures and concerns, grounded in meticulous attentiveness to their behaviour, affect, and interaction. Countless illustrations could be offered from works such as Ainsworth, M. (1967) *Infancy in Uganda*. Baltimore: The Johns Hopkins Press. However, even in discussing adult autobiographical discourse, an imaginative concern with the child this adult might once have been is palpable: Ainsworth, M.D.S. & Eichberg, C.G. (1991) Effects on infant–mother attachment of mother's experience related to loss of an attachment figure. In: C.M. Parkes, J. Stevenson-Hinde, & P. Marris (eds) *Attachment Across the Life Cycle* (pp.160–83). New York: Routledge.

[19] Ainsworth, M. (1969) Object relations, dependency and attachment. *Child Development*, 40, 969–1025, p.1002.

[20] Ainsworth, M. (1962) *Letter to John Bowlby*, 3 January 1962. Mary Ainsworth papers, Box M3168, Folder 1.

She eventually received a fraction of the money that she requested from the William T. Grant Foundation, and was able to begin a study in 1963. The multifaceted nature of this longitudinal study allowed Ainsworth to use many of the skills and insights she had previously developed, including attention to feelings of security and insecurity (from Blatz); close observational study (from work with Robertson in London, and then from her Uganda ethnography); and a personal interest in affection, anger, anxiety, the wish for physical contact, and the inhibition of these feelings (from her therapy). Together, these skills and insights combined to give Ainsworth the desire and ability to take on the challenge of empirically examining Bowlby's hypothesis that early relationships with attachment figures would shape the expression of the attachment behavioural system. This was a radical project. Until Ainsworth, hypotheses about defence mechanisms in young children had been mostly regarded as untestable; the skill of even young children in regulating and redirecting affect, familiar to every clinician working with children, had been regarded as outside the domain of science.

Security and independence

Ainsworth's concern with feelings of security originated in the lectures she attended with Blatz. Blatz hypothesised a number of distinct needs including food, sex, rest, and novelty.[21] According to Blatz, feelings of security are generated if an individual feels their actions will not harm access to the meeting of these needs, whether by the individual themselves or by someone else. Security means that it is possible for an individual to try things out, even to fail or retract a commitment, without this having relevance to whether their needs will be met. By contrast, Blatz proposed that feelings of insecurity are caused by concern that needs might be left unmet. Such concerns prompt anxiety and/or the use of defences.[22] Blatz argued that when an individual feels secure this allows them to turn their attention to other matters. As such, in early life, parents who are able to give children confidence in their availability to meet their needs in general will offer what Blatz referred to as a 'secure base' from which to explore the world, headlong and fully, without the need for excessive caution or control.

Ainsworth took from Blatz the idea that against this 'generally secure background, the infant or young child becomes able to tolerate some degree of insecurity'.[23] Security allows the child to accept the uncertainties inherent in human relationships without defensiveness, and to seek support within relationships as needed. Ainsworth followed Blatz in the suggestion that security also forms a feature of a broader experience of life: 'the person feels that he belongs, not only in his more or less intimate relationships, but in the world at large, and that the contribution he has to make is somehow significant in the larger scheme of things. This is in contrast to the feeling of insignificance, helplessness, and isolation that characterises insecurity.'[24] On Ainsworth's interpretation, Blatz's work highlighted that, in a deep

---

[21] Blatz, W.E. (1934) *Human Needs and How They Are Satisfied*. Des Moines: State University of Iowa.

[22] Blatz, W.E. (1940) *Hostages to Peace: Parents and the Children of Democracy*. New York: William Morrow, p.182; see Ainsworth, M.D.S. (1988) Security. Unpublished discussion paper prepared for the Foundations of Attachment Theory Workshop, convened for the New York Attachment Consortium by G. Cox-Steiner & E. Waters, Port Jefferson, NY. http://www.psychology.sunysb.edu/attachment/online/mda_security.pdf.

[23] Ainsworth, M. & Ainsworth, L. (1958) *Measuring Security in Personal Adjustment*. Toronto: University of Toronto Press, p.4.

[24] Ibid. p.46.

sense, the people we need are ultimately independent of us. Others' independence can be regarded as a source of worry or as a source of reassurance, depending on what this freedom has implied in the past. If the independence of others can be the basis of security and reduce anxiety, it can nonetheless also be an irreducible threat, and may even expand the scope of potential anxiety: 'no matter how secure a person may be in his everyday life, his security will be shaken when he first encounters catastrophe, serious illness, injury, or the possibility of death, whether the threat is directed towards himself or towards other people on whom his security depends'.[25]

Blatz's security theory had a powerful appeal for Ainsworth, especially as compared with other theories available at the time. It offered a model of thinking about development in terms of both individual needs and environmental experiences, in which each had a role in shaping the other. Furthermore, the model acknowledged the potential role of different sources of security for one another, so that even if security in family relationships had a particular primacy since it related to a wide variety of needs, this sense of security in family relationships was in turn influenced by various other sources of security or insecurity for a person in childhood and over the lifespan[26]—not least economic insecurity, and the political security of civil rights.[27] For Ainsworth, following Blatz, a feeling that emergencies can or cannot be confidently handled in social relationships, in athletic or cultural activities for instance, can in turn influence the security of family relationships. In this, Blatz's account differed in important ways from the emphasis of the day in psychoanalytic theory on innate drives and the singular primacy of the family, and the emphasis in behaviourist approaches on learned responses.

Indeed, in one of her final publications, Ainsworth would take a Blatzian approach to offer a criticism of attachment research: 'By focusing so closely on intimacies some attachment researchers have come to conceive of them as the only source of security—which is a pity'.[28] The ethological concept of security in the use of the caregiver as a secure base and safe haven was, for Ainsworth, a particular form of a broader concept of security. Other sources of security are not detailed in theoretical terms by Ainsworth, but might include reliable experiences of successful exploration, and reliable experiences of safety when the fear system is activated. Such a broader cross-domain concept of 'security' seems to have been inherited only by Ainsworth's direct students and immediate collaborators, presumably as a result of oral transmission.[29] Shaver and colleagues also later adopted a broader conceptualisation of security, though seemingly without awareness of Ainsworth's stance (Chapter 5).

[25] Ainsworth, M. & Ainsworth, L. (1958) *Measuring Security in Personal Adjustment*. Toronto: University of Toronto Press, p.44.

[26] Ainsworth, M. (1990, 2010) Security and attachment. In R. Volpe (eds) *The Secure Child: Timeless Lessons in Parenting and Childhood Education* (pp.43–53). Charlotte, NC: Information Age Publishing.

[27] Ainsworth, M.D.S. (1980) Attachment and child abuse. In: G. Gerbner, C.J. Ross, & E. Zigler (eds) *Child Abuse: An Agenda for Action* (pp.35–47). Oxford: Oxford University Press; Ainsworth, M. (1965) *Letter to John Bowlby*, 2 February 1965. Mary Ainsworth papers, Box M3168, Folder 2.

[28] Ainsworth, M. (1990, 2010) Security and attachment. In R. Volpe (ed.) *The Secure Child: Timeless Lessons in Parenting and Childhood Education* (pp.43–53). Charlotte, NC: Information Age Publishing, p.49.

[29] E.g. Main, M. (1977) Sicherheit und wissen. In K.E. Grossmann (ed.) *Entwicklung der Lernfahigheit in der sozialen Umwel* (pp.47–95). Munich: Kindler; Sroufe, L.A. (1996) *Emotional Development*. Cambridge: Cambridge University Press; Waters, E. & Cummings, E.M. (2000) A secure base from which to explore close relationships. *Child Development*, 71(1), 164–72; Davies, P.T., Harold, G.T., Goeke-Morey, M.C., & Cummings, E.M. (2002) Child emotional security and interparental conflict. *Monographs of the Society for Research in Child Development*, 67, 1–115.

Both psychoanalytic and behaviourist theories of the 1940s and 1950s presumed that infants would be more clingy and dependent the more their needs were satisfied. They assumed continuities in the form of behaviour with development. Blatz's model led to the exact opposite conclusion. Blatz's perspective suggested that confidence and an appropriate level of self-reliance would grow out of experiences of being able to rely and rest our weight upon others, and of their availability to help us as needed. Though this was not a point made clear by Blatz himself, Ainsworth drew the implication that mutual reliance within family relationships and an independent and confident attitude in other areas of life could be compatible. In fact, Ainsworth concluded, forming close relationships is itself a human need. As a result, insecurity will result if these are not available, and security will provide a springboard for confident and flexible action in other areas such as in school and work.[30]

Harry Harlow and Robert Zimmermann had used the phrase 'haven of safety' to refer to the way that an infant's alarm and motivation to seek their caregiver would be terminated once they achieved proximity with the caregiver.[31] Ainsworth cultivated the concept of 'secure base' to refer to the way that an infant—or, indeed, humans in general—can feel free to explore the world with confidence, as he or she knows that protection and care is available if needed.[32] A secure base permits negative experiences in the world, even pain, to feel more bearable and less overwhelming.[33] Harlow and Zimmerman's 'haven of safety' was about termination of the attachment behavioural system and its associated distress. By contrast, the concept of 'secure base' was not, for Ainsworth, primarily about the achievement of independent self-reliance, as has sometimes been presumed by anthropologist critics.[34] Instead, seen in the context of Ainsworth's debt to Blatz, the secure base concept was more about the role that a person can play in helping another to live a larger life than the latter would be able to on their own, with the freedom to chase and tumble after the world without worry.[35] This

---

[30] Ainsworth, M. & Ainsworth, L. (1958) *Measuring Security in Personal Adjustment*. Toronto: University of Toronto Press, p.32.

[31] Harlow, H.F. & Zimmermann, R.R. (1958). The development of affectional responses in infant monkeys. *Proceedings of the American Philosophical Society*, 102(5), 501–509.

[32] Ainsworth, M. (1964) Patterns of attachment behavior shown by the infant in interaction with his mother. *Merrill-Palmer*, 10(1), 51–8, p.54. The distinction would be further established within attachment theory through becoming the central theme of the Circle of Security intervention: Marvin, R., Cooper, G., Hoffman, K., & Powell, B. (2002) The Circle of Security project: attachment-based intervention with caregiver–pre-school child dyads. *Attachment & Human Development*, 4(1), 107–24.

[33] Ainsworth, M. (1976) *Attachment and Separation in Paediatric Settings*. Unpublished manuscript. PP/Bow/J.1/40: 'Painful procedures may still be painful, but the pain is easier to endure with mother present to give comfort, and more easily recovered from when it is over. On the other hand, all the potential sources of fear and distress may become overwhelming if the child must face them without the security given by the presence of an attachment figure.'

[34] E.g. Harwood, R.L., Miller, J.G., & Irizarry, N.L. (1995) *Culture and Attachment: Perceptions of the Child in Context*. New York: Guilford; Rothbaum, F., Weisz, J., Pott, M., Miyake, K., & Morelli, G. (2000) Attachment and culture: security in the United States and Japan. *American Psychologist*, 55(10), 1093–104; LeVine, R.A. (2004) Challenging expert knowledge: findings from an African study of infant care and development. In U.P. Gielen & J.L. Roopnarine (eds) *Childhood and Adolescence: Cross-Cultural Perspectives and Applications* (pp.149–65). Westport, CT: Praeger.

[35] Waters, E. & McIntosh, J. (2011) Are we asking the right questions about attachment? *Family Court Review*, 49(3), 474–82, p.475. Bowlby would later observe that 'the values of western culture' lead the benefits of a secure base to be 'overlooked, or even denigrated'. Both he and Ainsworth were angered that in the society around them, autonomy and independence were mistakenly supposed to just be default states, unless there was a specific problem. This had led to a neglect of the quiet enormity of the secure base role and an overvaluation of liberal self-reliance. Bowlby, J. (1970, 1979) Self-reliance and some conditions that promote it. In *The Making and Breaking of Affectional Bonds* (pp.124–49). London: Routledge, p.125. Nonetheless, a focus on the haven of safety at the expense of the secure base has occurred within attachment theory and especially in its public representation. See Wall, G. (2018) 'Love builds brains': representations of attachment and children's brain development in parenting education material. *Sociology of Health & Illness*, 40(3), 395–409.

may have been hidden somewhat by the overridingly spatial and territorial image of a secure base,[36] resulting from Ainsworth's insertion of Blatz's concept into the Hinde–Bowlby ethological account of proximity-maintenance.

Ainsworth was the first to attempt to develop empirical measures based on Blatz's idea of security.[37] In her 1958 book *Measuring Security in Personal Adjustment*, Ainsworth reported findings from her use of self-report measures of security, drawing on the skills in measure design and administration from her time as an Army Examiner (personnel selection) during World War II.[38] However, the self-report scales did not generate results that particularly interested her. This work also led her to conclude that individuals with a chronic experience of insecurity, especially from childhood, may develop anxiety and/or defences to such a degree that self-report measures lose validity.[39] Such a person may be 'so handicapped in his communication with others and in insight into his own needs and feelings that pencil-and-paper tests cannot reflect the nature and extent of his maladjustment'.[40] Ainsworth would later conduct a study, which remained unpublished, utilizing the scales to assess patients in a psychiatric hospital. She found that her scales 'did indeed highlight depression. Those emerging with highly insecure scores felt insecure and unhappy and readily said so.' However, her items failed to differentiate patients with anxiety disorders, paranoid and psychotic symptoms, and those with personality disorders.[41] Ainsworth came increasingly to question whether security was, as Blatz had assumed, solely a conscious attitude, measurable in a valid way using self-report methodology.

Caregiving

Uganda

In 1953, Leonard Ainsworth took up a job at the East Africa Institute of Social Research in Kampala, Uganda. Ainsworth joined him for their two-year stay.[42] This was a period of

---

[36] The spatial and territorial underpinnings of the 'secure base' metaphor were materialized by the squares physically marked by Ainsworth on the floor in the original Strange Situation procedure, to help coders—in the absence of videotape—identify infant movement away from and back towards the caregiver.

[37] Salter, M. (1939) The concept of security as a basis for the evaluation of adjustment. Unpublished doctoral thesis, University of Toronto. Cf. Prichard, E. & Ojemann, R.H. (1941) An approach to the measurement of insecurity. *Journal of Experimental Education*, 10(2), 114–18.

[38] Ainsworth, M. & Ainsworth, L. (1958) *Measuring Security in Personal Adjustment*. Toronto: University of Toronto Press.

[39] Ainsworth, M.D.S. (1988) Security. Unpublished discussion paper prepared for the Foundations of Attachment Theory Workshop, convened for the New York Attachment Consortium by G. Cox-Steiner & E. Waters, Port Jefferson, NY. http://www.psychology.sunysb.edu/attachment/online/mda_security.pdf: 'I felt dissatisfied with the validity of my scales because of their inadequate coping with the whole matter of defensive maneuvers.'

[40] Ainsworth, M. & Ainsworth, L. (1958) *Measuring Security in Personal Adjustment*. Toronto: University of Toronto Press, p.17.

[41] Ainsworth, M.D.S. (1988) Security. Unpublished discussion paper prepared for the Foundations of Attachment Theory Workshop, convened for the New York Attachment Consortium by G. Cox-Steiner & E. Waters, Port Jefferson, NY. http://www.psychology.sunysb.edu/attachment/online/mda_security.pdf

[42] On the travel required by women psychologists such as Ainsworth to support their husband's careers, see Johnston, E. & Johnson, A. (2008) Searching for the second generation of American women psychologists. *History of Psychology*, 11(1), 40–72. On the East African Institute of Social Research see Mills, D. (2006) How not to be a 'Government House Pet:' Audrey Richards and the East African Institute for Social Research. In M. Ntarangwi, D. Mills, and M. Babiker (eds) *African Anthropologies* (pp.76–98). London: Zed Books.

growing demands for political independence. The colonial British government seemed to be seeking to encourage Ugandan independence whilst fearing what it might bring.[43] Social scientists were being encouraged by the colonial government to pursue ethnographic and social scientific studies in Uganda, in an attempt to understand and respond to these tensions.[44] Together with her husband, Ainsworth pursued some research explicitly studying political attitudes in Uganda and sociological factors that might contribute to insurrection against the colonial government.[45] This was, in a sense, the 'day job'.

However, Ainsworth's primary concern was to continue the study of early infant–caregiver relationships, which had been the focus of Bowlby's research group. She received funding for this from the anthropologist Audrey Richards, the director of the East Africa Institute of Social Research.[46] The condition of the funding was that Ainsworth pursue research with a significant qualitative, ethnographic component. With Robertson's detailed notes on hospitalised children as a model, Ainsworth embarked on an ethnographic study of 26 mother–infant dyads from villages near to Kampala, visiting families for two hours, twice a month, over a nine-month period. Seeking to offer recompense that would disturb as little as possible the opportunity for naturalistic observation, Ainsworth paid for the healthcare of her participants. The political context of Uganda is notable in its absence from Ainsworth's *Infancy in Uganda*, published in 1967. She seems to have separated her research with the mother–infant dyads from her attitudinal research with her by-then-former husband. The attitudinal research may have had associations with her painful divorce, though it also clearly interested her less. Throughout *Infancy in Uganda*, however, she displayed great attentiveness to the effects of poverty on the care that families could offer their children, as well as other observable aspects of the families' social context.

One early discovery from Ainsworth's observations was the variety of forms of attachment behaviour. Whereas Bowlby had built from Hinde's work in modelling the attachment behavioural system on the following response and approach through locomotion, Ainsworth documented that the attachment behavioural system could be terminated by various other behavioural sequences that predictably led to the caregiver's availability. These included crying, smiling, or vocalisation directed towards the caregiver; scrambling on the mother's body or nestling into her lap; raising arms or clapping in greeting; and crying when she left the house.[47] She found that the infants used these different behavioural sequences flexibly, depending on present context, but that they seemed to have preferred forms of attachment behaviour built up through routine interaction and experience.

Ainsworth suspected that human evolution had led many of these behaviours to be especially easy for children to learn.[48] However, she also emphasised the role of childcare

[43] See Cohen, A. (1957) Uganda's progress and problems. *African Affairs*, 56(223), 111–22.

[44] On the relationship between ethnographic method and colonialism in the period see Asad, T. (1979) Anthropology and the colonial encounter. In G. Huizer &B. Manheim (eds) *Politics of Anthropology: From Colonialism and Sexism Toward a View from Below* (pp.85–96). The Hague: Mouton.

[45] Ainsworth, L.H. & Ainsworth, M.D. (1962) Acculturation in East Africa. I. Political awareness and attitudes toward authority. *Journal of Social Psychology*, 57(2), 391–9; Ainsworth, M.D. & Ainsworth, L.H. (1962) Acculturation in East Africa. II. Frustration and aggression. *Journal of Social Psychology*, 57(2), 401–407.

[46] Ainsworth, M.D. (1983, 2013) An autobiographical sketch. *Attachment & Human Development*, 15(5–6), 448–59: 'I welcomed Dr Richards' directive that there be an anthropological component to the study, for this ensured that I would view current mother–infant interaction and maternal care practices in their cultural context, and I valued the opportunities presented by the institute again to interact with a multidisciplinary team' (455).

[47] Ainsworth, M. (1964) Patterns of attachment behavior shown by the infant in interaction with his mother. *Merrill-Palmer*, 10(1), 51–8.

[48] Ainsworth, M. (1967) *Infancy in Uganda*. Baltimore: The Johns Hopkins Press, p.438.

culture in shaping their possibility, frequency, and intensity of expression. The clearest example was clapping hands in greeting on reunion: Ainsworth saw this frequently among the Ugandan infants, who were enculturated to treat this as a way to express greeting. By contrast, Ainsworth never saw this form of greeting behaviour towards attachment figures among American infants.[49] Ainsworth was also attentive to relationship-level differences that could prompt differences in the display of attachment behaviours. Some children, for example, seemed more or less inclined to physically follow their caregivers. A large part of such preferences seemed to Ainsworth to be shaped by how the caregivers responded when the infant followed them. Another influence seemed to be the position of the relationship within the broader life of the infant: the same child might show different configurations of attachment behaviour towards different caregivers, and at different times. One infant, for instance, tended to preferentially follow her older sister when she was home, even above her mother, but did not necessarily seek to be held. However, when the infant was ill, she showed a strong preference for her mother, and wanted to be held all the time.[50]

One important line of difference among the Ganda infants was that 'there were some babies, who seemed clearly attached to their mothers, who did not dependably cry, follow or cling when their mothers showed signs of leaving'.[51] Some of these infants appeared relatively unruffled by signs of impending separation, seeming confident in the availability of another caregiver, or in the expectation that the separation would be brief and unthreatening. Another set seemed to have had insufficient interaction with their caregiver, for instance if they were often away for long periods; Ainsworth would wonder whether they had, in fact, developed an attachment relationship yet.[52] A further group of infants, however, were clearly attached and seemed concerned about their caregiver's availability, yet did not show attachment behaviours on separation. These infants tended to be those whose caregivers were less responsive to their signals when the child was distressed. However, Ainsworth also noticed that some infants who seemed less confident in their caregiver's availability displaced insistent and frequent attachment behaviours. It appeared to Ainsworth that a child's lack of confidence in their caregiver's responsiveness could be expressed in a variety of ways.

Ainsworth anticipated that an ordinary attachment relationship makes use of proximity-seeking only occasionally, or under circumstances of alarm. Most of the time, interactions to affirm caregiver availability are achieved through expression, movement, gesture, and vocalisation at a distance. It was, on Ainsworth's observation, only 'the anxious infant who requires close physical contact with his mother, and who is not content to maintain interaction through a middle distance at least part of the time'.[53] For instance, one mother had to work very long hours in a desperate effort to establish a new garden in order to ensure

---

[49] Ibid. p.340.

[50] Ibid. p.307.

[51] Ainsworth, M. (1964) Patterns of attachment behavior shown by the infant in interaction with his mother. *Merrill-Palmer*, 10(1), 51–8, p.52.

[52] Ainsworth, M. & Bowlby, J. (1991) 1989 APA award recipient addresses: an ethological approach to personality development. *American Psychologist*, 46(4), 333–41: In Uganda, Ainsworth 'divided the babies into three groups: securely attached, insecurely attached, and non-attached … Nonattached babies were left alone for long periods by unresponsive mothers but, because they were the youngest in the sample, Ainsworth now believes that they may merely have been delayed in developing attachment' (337).

[53] Ainsworth, M. (1964) Patterns of attachment behavior shown by the infant in interaction with his mother. *Merrill-Palmer*, 10(1), 51–8, p.58.

food for the family, and left the baby with a neighbour during this time. Even when mother and baby were together, the mother was too tired to respond with patience to her child. Ainsworth described 'a vicious spiral' in some of the dyads in her sample in which 'the baby's fussy demands exasperated the mother, who then overtly or covertly rejected the baby, who in turn responded to the rejection by anxiety and by increasing his demands'.[54] Reflecting on these behavioural observations, Ainsworth identified that diverse forms of attachment behaviour could generally have the predictable outcome of increasing proximity with the caregiver, but that some repetoires seemed to risk alienating the caregiver. However, at the time of writing *Infancy in Uganda*, Bowlby's control system model of the attachment behavioural system was not yet available to Ainsworth for interpreting her observations.

Ainsworth's study utilised qualitative observation and also the construction of quantitative scales. As she analysed her quantitative data, an unexpected finding emerged. Two variables stood out as predictors of infants who appeared to be able to effectively use their caregiver as a secure base and safe haven.[55] One was the quantitative amount of care provided by the mother. This supported Bowlby's emphasis on the importance of hours of care by a primary caregiver (Chapter 1). Ainsworth, however, distrusted the finding. Though she felt she lacked firm data, her general impression was that it was not the amount of care, but—at least above a minimum threshold—how the care was provided that most contributed to security. She interpreted the finding as indicating that whilst quality of care is most important for security, the caregiver's understanding of her child's signals can be hindered if there is insufficient opportunity to learn about them. The qualities and the quantitative extent of care were both, she suspected, also shaped by the attitude of the caregivers towards their infants.[56]

A second variable that stood out as a good predictor of use of the caregiver as a secure base and safe haven in Ainsworth's Uganda data was the extent to which the mothers could give a lively account when interviewed about their infant. This was not so much details of the child's schedule as 'idiosyncracies and sensitive little things that testify to a mother's interested perception'.[57] This was unexpected: it was not obvious why a mother's capacity to talk freely and fully with Ainsworth should be associated with her infant's behaviour towards her when worried or on separation. Ainsworth concluded again that both the mother's capacity to offer an effective interview about her caregiving and her infant's attachment behaviour reflected the depth and fluency of her engagement in the caregiving role.[58] The relationship between maternal coherence in interview and infant attachment behaviours would recur as a central theme in the work of Ainsworth's student Mary Main (Chapter 3).[59]

[54] Ainsworth, M. (1967) *Infancy in Uganda*. Baltimore: The Johns Hopkins Press, p.392.

[55] A third predictor was the mother's enjoyment of breastfeeding.

[56] Ainsworth, M. (1959) *Letter to John Bowlby*, 18 September 1959. Mary Ainsworth papers, Box M3168, Folder 1.

[57] Ainsworth's 'Excellence as Informant' scale, unpublished, cited by Bretherton, I. (2013) Revisiting Mary Ainsworth's conceptualization and assessments of maternal sensitivity–insensitivity. *Attachment & Human Development*, 15(5–6), 460–84, p.467.

[58] Ainsworth, M. (1959) *Letter to John Bowlby*, 18 September 1959. Mary Ainsworth papers, Box M3168, Folder 1; Ainsworth, M. (1967) *Infancy in Uganda*. Baltimore: The Johns Hopkins Press, p.398.

[59] See also Bailey, H.N., Redden, E., Pederson, D.R., & Moran, G. (2016) Parental disavowal of relationship difficulties fosters the development of insecure attachment. *Revue Canadienne des Sciences du Comportement*, 48(1), 49–59.

The Baltimore study

Her observations in Uganda confirmed for Ainsworth the value of exploratory observational research with mother–infant dyads in the home. As discussed in the 'Introduction', after joining Johns Hopkins University in 1958, she was successful in obtaining a grant to begin a short-term longitudinal study from 1963. The study was undertaken to examine the role of caregiving factors in shaping the development of infant attachment relationships and attachment behaviour. Fifteen families were observed from 1963 to 1964 by Ainsworth and her assistant Barbara Wittig; eleven families were observed from 1966 to 1967 by Ainsworth's assistants Bob Marvin and George Allyn, thanks to additional funding from the National Institute of Child Health and Human Development (NICHD). Baltimore during this period was in the process of losing its industrial base, and the net population of the city was in decline. However, this demographic shift comprised two trends: a rapid decline in the white middle-class population of the city, and a less rapid but still substantial increase in the African-American population, living in poverty and facing substantial discrimination.[60] Ainsworth wanted to understand infant–caregiver interaction under favourable socio-economic conditions in order to reduce confounds and complexity for her exploration of the role of caregiver–infant interaction on attachment. As a result, she sought a sample of white and middle-class families, recruiting through paediatricians. Visits were made approximately every three weeks from three weeks after the child's birth to 54 weeks . They generally took place during office hours, with the consequence that the mother was home with the baby and the father was out at work. Ainsworth reported that visits, at least in the first wave of work, lasted around four hours, resulting in 72 hours of home observation for each dyad.[61] 'It is a very onerous and time-consuming research', Ainsworth wrote, 'but it has captured me heart and soul'.[62]

Looking back a few years later, Ainsworth reported that she felt that her study had aligned with a growing interest from the scientific community and the public in the naturalistic development of children and in family relationships.[63] Ainsworth's observers were responsive to overtures by the mother, baby, or others in the house, since to do otherwise would have been rude and disruptive. However, they otherwise kept from interfering with ongoing activities, and above all avoided any implied judgement of the mother's behaviour. The observers wrote what they saw, and after the visit narrated an account onto tape. These records used 'common English usage in describing behaviour, with all of its advantages and disadvantages. The advantages were that the descriptions were vivid; the disadvantages were that the same verbal labels might be used to describe different behaviours, with only the qualifying words and the context serving to differentiate them, whereas different verbal labels might be used with reference to behaviours that were essentially similar.'[64] Observers made

[60] Levine, M.V. (2000) A third-world city in the first world: social exclusion, racial inequality, and sustainable development in Baltimore, Maryland. In R. Stren & M. Polese (eds) *The Social Sustainability of Cities: Diversity and the Management of Change* (pp.123–56). Toronto: University of Toronto Press.

[61] Ainsworth, M. & Bowlby, J. (1991) 1989 APA award recipient addresses: an ethological approach to personality development. *American Psychologist*, 46(4), 333–41, p.337.

[62] Ainsworth, M. (1966) *Letter to Bruno Klopfer*, 22 September 1966. Mary Ainsworth papers, Box M3168, Folder 8.

[63] Ainsworth, M. (1967) *Letter to Martin James*, 23 February 1967. Mary Ainsworth papers, M3170, Folder 1.

[64] Blehar, M. & Ainsworth, M. (1978) *Close Bodily Contact*. Unpublished manuscript. PP/Bow/J.1/49.

home visits individually and took written notes; observer reliability was not assessed, except on a few occasions when Ainsworth accompanied one of her students on a visit.

Whilst the Baltimore sample was generally reported in print by Ainsworth as a randomly selected community sample, albeit all middle-class, in fact in a late interview she acknowledged that 'the pediatricians who recruited potential participants for us tended to select women who interested them—"this one is a charmer, that one puzzles me, I wonder how motherhood will work out for this one"—and that this led to our getting a particularly diverse group'.[65] This approach to recruitment may have somewhat increased potential lines of difference between participants, making contrasts sharper. At a statistical level, it made it more likely that Ainsworth's data would appear to be categorically rather than dimensionally distributed, compared to the population from which the sample is drawn. This effect would likely have been intensified by the fact that Barbara Wittig only wrote up half of her observations many months after her home visits, contributing to sharper contrasts through potential recollection biases.[66] As Ainsworth and her group began to analyse the data, they began to notice such a distribution. In a letter to Bowlby from 1967, Ainsworth wrote:

> One of my impressions of my current sample is so bizarre that I hesitate to mention it. I can dichotomise my mother–infant pairs. On one side are the good mothers with the normally-attached infants and on the other side are the non-good mothers with infants who are not normally attached. The not-good mothers are diverse and so are their infants. But, and this is the bizarre part, there seems to be no truly middle or average group. Our ratings reflect this. Usually rating scales tend to lump most cases in the middle ... I find our ratings tend towards the extremes with the middle of the scales scarcely represented in the sample. At first I scolded my team for halo effect, and urged them to judge the variables separately and to feel free to use the scale-points intermediate between the extremes—but when we went into it more deeply, and really tried to get rid of the halo effect it looks as though there is another genuine effect which truly does dichotomise the sample.[67]

The sharpening of certain contrasts in the data may have helped Ainsworth and colleagues find order within the astonishing detail of the information they had collected. Yet it may also have overstrengthened certain signals, such as perhaps the centrality of caregiver sensitivity for secure attachment, discussed below.[68]

---

[65] Ainsworth, M. (1995) On the shaping of attachment theory and research: an interview with Mary D.S. Ainsworth. *Monographs of the Society for Research in Child Development*, 60(2–3), 2–21, p.11–12.

[66] Ainsworth, M. (1965) *Letter to John Bowlby*, 22 June 1965. Mary Ainsworth papers, Box M3168, Folder 2: 'For two years, I set myself to believing that I had found a good assistant, and to ignoring the obvious deficiencies in her performance. Suddenly, there was a moment of truth. I found that she had written up fewer than half of the visits that she had made to the babies in our sample. She has been catching up ever since, and will probably not finish catching up until the end of September.'

[67] Ainsworth, M. (1967) *Letter to John Bowlby*, 9 April 1967. Mary Ainsworth papers, Box M3168, Folder 2.

[68] Another example, consequential for the next chapter, was that two-thirds of the infants classified as part of avoidant dyads in the Ainsworth sample showed extensive conflict behaviours according to the home observation data. These avoidant dyads were more troubled than, in retrospect, might be expected from a representative community sample. This may have contributed to Main's initial assumption that avoidant attachment and conflict behaviour would go together, until she and colleagues came to the conclusion that conflict behaviour could cut across the Ainsworth classifications (Chapter 3). Main, M. (1981) Avoidance in the service of proximity: a working paper. In K. Immelmann, G.W. Barlow, L. Petrinovich, & M. Biggar Main (eds) *Behavioral Development: The Bielefeld Interdisciplinary Project* (pp.651–93). Cambridge: Cambridge University Press, p.664.

Sensitivity

Perhaps the most important contribution made by the Ainsworth's home observation study was her development of a construct, 'sensitivity', which sought to capture this quality of care-giving.[69] This construct would have as much influence on the direction of subsequent attachment research as Bowlby's headline term 'attachment', though not on reception of the theory by the public, practitioners, and researchers in other fields. The term 'sensitivity' was used by Ainsworth from the late 1960s in a wholly technical sense, described in her unpublished manuscript 'Sensitivity vs. Insensitivity to the Baby's Signals Scale'. This manuscript would eventually appear in print only in the 2015 reissue of *Patterns of Attachment* by Waters.[70] In Ainsworth's usage, the term 'sensitivity' referred to the ability of the caregiver to 'perceive and to interpret accurately the signals and communications implicit in her infant's behavior, and given this understanding, to respond to them appropriately and promptly'.[71] Conversely, insensitive caregiving had the same four components in reverse: less awareness of the child's signals; inaccuracies in interpreting them; inappropriate responses to the signals; and a lack of timeliness in these responses. Until that point, researchers in developmental psychology had tended to regard relationships as incalculable aspects of human life: too 'squidgy' and amorphous to measure in themselves.

The first component of sensitivity was 'awareness'. Ainsworth conceptualised awareness in terms of the 'threshold' at which a caregiver would become responsive to infant cues: at a higher threshold, only the baby's most blatant and obvious communications prompt a response, whereas caregivers with 'the highest thresholds seem often oblivious, and are, in effect, highly inaccessible'.[72] A high threshold for awareness of infant cues also contributes, Ainsworth suggested, to poor accuracy in interpreting them, since when these signals do break through to the caregiver's awareness, they do so without contextual information such as what prompted them. This means that interactions are often less satisfying, and can be poorly coordinated, incomplete, or even somewhat fragmentary. However, even caregivers with a low threshold for awareness may have poor accuracy for interpreting infant signals if 'perception is distorted by projection, denial, or other marked defensive operations'.[73] When caregivers are able to perceive and to interpret signals accurately, the child's whole behavioural repertoire takes on signal value, as having relevance for understanding the infant's experience and the implications that stem from this.[74]

---

[69] Ainsworth's first use of the term 'sensitivity' was in *Infancy in Uganda*, but it was used there essentially as a descriptor, without a technical meaning yet. Ainsworth, M. (1967) *Infancy in Uganda*. Baltimore: The Johns Hopkins Press, p.397.

[70] Ainsworth, M., Blehar, M., Waters, E., & Wall, S. (1978, 2015) *Patterns of Attachment: A Psychological Study of the Strange Situation*. Bristol: Psychology Press.

[71] Ainsworth, M. (1969) Sensitivity vs. insensitivity to the baby's signals scale. http://www.psychology.sunysb.edu/attachment/measures/content/ainsworth_scales.html. Some but not all aspects of the sensitivity scale and construct were described in Stayton, D.J., Hogan, R., & Ainsworth, M. (1971) Infant obedience and maternal behavior: the origins of socialization reconsidered. *Child Development* 42(4), 1057–69, p.1060–61.

[72] Ainsworth, M. (1969) Sensitivity vs. insensitivity to the baby's signals scale. http://www.psychology.sunysb.edu/attachment/measures/content/ainsworth_scales.html.

[73] Ibid.

[74] Ainsworth, M.D.S. (1977) Social development in the first year of life: maternal influences on infant–mother attachment. In: J.M. Tanner (ed.) *Developments in Psychiatric Research* (pp.1–20). London: Hodder & Stoughton, p.6.

As Waters and colleagues observed, a problem with the term 'sensitivity' is that it comes with familiar, ordinary language connotations: 'Sensitivity suggests warmth, tenderness, and attention to detail.'[75] If this were what Ainsworth's scale measured, these would be qualities that, in theory, could be assessed with a checklist. They would also be overtly ethnocentric as a cultural ideal of parenting.[76] It is unsurprising that these ordinary language connotations were what Ainsworth's critics presumed that she meant, since the scale itself remained unpublished! In fact, however, what Ainsworth operationalised with her scale was—mostly—something quite different to what her critics presumed. It is true that at times she slid towards the everyday language connotations of sensitivity in using 'warm' as a characterisation of the sensitive caregiver; this led many later attachment researchers to include warmth in their assessments of sensitivity or extrapolation of assessments of sensitivity of caregiving provided to older children.[77] However—contrary to Bowlby's expectations[78]—Ainsworth herself found that maternal warmth was not associated with infant attachment security in her Uganda data.[79]

In fact, Main recalled that Ainsworth's work on the sensitivity scale was actually prompted by the finding that there was no association between maternal warmth and infant behaviour in the Strange Situation.[80] Later researchers, including Egeland and colleagues (Chapter 4), confirmed that many caregivers can be warm and display tenderness without being sensitive in Ainsworth's technical sense.[81] Ainsworth's construct of 'sensitivity' primarily captured the extent to which caregivers detect and successfully interpret behaviours that may convey their child's experience, and offer a relevant response in a timely manner. This was an assessment more of the form than the content of interactions, allowing for a huge variety of ways in which these formal features may be met within caregiving practices, whilst also anchoring these features in concrete examples.[82]

[75] Waters, E., Petters, D., & Facompre, C. (2013) Epilogue: reflections on a Special Issue of Attachment & Human Development in Mary Ainsworth's 100th year. *Attachment & Human Development*, 15(5–6), 673–81, p.676.

[76] LeVine, R.A. & Norman, K. (2001) The infant's acquisition of culture: early attachment reexamined in anthropological perspective. In C.C. Moore & H.F. Mathews (eds) *The Psychology of Cultural Experience* (pp.83–104). Cambridge: Cambridge University Press; Mageo, J.M. (2013) Toward a cultural psychodynamics of attachment: Samoa and US comparison. In N. Quinn & J. Mageo (eds) *Attachment Reconsidered: Cultural Perspectives on a Western Theory* (pp.191–214). New York: Palgrave.

[77] Ainsworth, M. (1969) Sensitivity vs. insensitivity to the baby's signals scale. http://www.psychology.sunysb. edu/attachment/measures/content/ainsworth_scales.html; Mesman, J. & Emmen, R.A. (2013) Mary Ainsworth's legacy: a systematic review of observational instruments measuring parental sensitivity. *Attachment & Human Development*, 15(5–6), 485–506; Bohr, Y., Putnick, D.L., Lee, Y., & Bornstein, M.H. (2018) Evaluating caregiver sensitivity to infants: measures matter. *Infancy*, 23(5), 730–47. Among the studies to have included warmth in indexing sensitivity, the most important is the NICHD study: NICHD Early Child Care Research Network (1999) Child care and mother–child interaction in the first three years of life. *Developmental Psychology*, 35, 1399–413.

[78] For Bowlby's emphasis on maternal 'warmth' see e.g. Bowlby, J. (1953) *Child Care and the Growth of Love*. Harmondsworth: Pelican, p.77.

[79] Ainsworth, M.D.S. (1988) Security. Unpublished discussion paper prepared for the Foundations of Attachment Theory Workshop, convened for the New York Attachment Consortium by G. Cox-Steiner & E. Waters, Port Jefferson, NY. http://www.psychology.sunysb.edu/attachment/online/mda_security.pdf.

[80] Main, M. (1999) Mary D. Salter Ainsworth: Tribute and portrait, *Psychoanalytic Inquiry*, 19(5) 682–736.

[81] See e.g. Egeland, B., & Farber, E. A. (1984). Infant-mother attachment: Factors related to its development and changes over time. *Child Development*, 753–71; Bailey, H.N., Bernier, A., Bouvette-Turcot, A.A., Tarabulsy, G.M., Pederson, D.R., & Becker-Stoll, F. (2017). Deconstructing maternal sensitivity: Predictive relations to mother-child attachment in home and laboratory settings. *Social Development*, 26(4), 679–93.

[82] Grossmann, K. & Grossmann, K. (2012) *Bindungen—das Gefüge psychischer Sicherheit Gebundenes*. Stuttgart: Klett-Cotta; Mesman, J., van IJzendoorn, M., Behrens, K., et al. (2016) Is the ideal mother a sensitive mother? Beliefs about early childhood parenting in mothers across the globe. *International Journal of Behavioral Development*, 40(5), 385–97. Dozier and Bernard conclude that sensitivity in Ainsworth's technical sense is a universal good, which can be achieved in various culturally specific ways; they therefore take a principled stance in adapting the delivery but not the basic tenants of their Attachment and Biobehavioral Catch-up intervention

Ainsworth's concept of attending to the infant's signals has been interpreted by some critics as ethnocentric. They construe Ainsworth as ascribing a kind of liberal autonomy to the infant, and valuing autonomy and individual will over connectedness and joint needs.[83] Certainly there is evidence that Ainsworth personally valued acknowledgement of infant autonomy: another of her scales—'Interference with baby's ongoing behavior'—characterised the 'highly interfering mother' as one with 'no respect for her baby as a separate, active, and autonomous person.'[84] However, it is not clear that criticism of Ainsworth's liberal values applies to the sensitivity scale, and may have been influenced by the connotation of the word 'sensitivity' as non-conflictual interaction; the criticism does not appear to be grounded in observation of how coders actually use the scale in practice.

Various critics have interpreted Ainsworth's notion of sensitivity as mandating that 'the normative imperative is to take the infant's cue',[85] an oppressive demand on mothers. Again, this interpretation seems shaped by the lack of availability of Ainsworth's sensitivity scale, showing actually what it measured. For a caregiver to respond to signals does not necessarily mean obedience to a child's dictates. The sensitive caregiver, Ainsworth proposed, 'acknowledges the baby's wishes even though she does not unconditionally accede to them', since much of what is 'for the baby's own good is done contrary to his wishes'.[86] The caregiver is supporting the infant to achieve a sense that there is contingency between the infant's activity and the activity of the world, even when this contingency and acknowledgement of agency comes together with a response that is contrary to the baby's wishes. There is some ambiguity in Ainsworth's account on this matter, however. Despite having acknowledged that much of what is done for the baby's own good is contrary to his wishes, the highest point on the sensitivity scale identifies a caregiver who 'nearly always gives B what he indicates that he wants, although perhaps not invariably so'. The difference between acknowledgement of infancy signals and following of infant signals is a somewhat unstable distinction for Ainsworth, in part because she underspecified what actually is being signalled.

The signals Ainsworth anticipated that a sensitive caregiver will attend to include the baby's 'tempo, state and communications'.[87] However, tempo, state, and communications are quite different phenomena, and responding to them has quite different challenges and consequences. Not least, an important aspect of sensitivity is the active support of helping a child interpret their state—for instance, whether they feel hurt after falling over—rather than the

when applying it in different cultures. Dozier, M. & Bernard, K. (2019) *Coaching Parents of Vulnerable Infants: The Attachment and Biobehavioral Catch-up Approach.* New York: Guilford, p.231.

[83] LeVine, R.A. (2004) Challenging expert knowledge: findings from an African study of infant care and development. In U.P. Gielen & J.L. Roopnarine (eds) *Childhood and Adolescence: Cross-Cultural Perspectives and Applications* (pp.149–65). Westport, CT: Greenwood Publishing. Keller, H. (2018) Parenting and socioemotional development in infancy and early childhood. *Developmental Review*, 50, 31–41.

[84] Ainsworth, M. (1969) Cooperation vs. interference with baby's ongoing behavior. http://www.psychology. sunysb.edu/attachment/measures/content/ainsworth_scales.html. Rothbaum and Morelli mistakenly attribute this quote to Ainsworth's sensitivity scale in their accusation that the latter is ethnocentric. Rothbaum, F. & Morelli, G. (2005) Attachment and culture: bridging relativism and universalism. In W. Friedlmeier, P. Chakkarath, & B. Schwarz (eds) *Culture and Human Development: The Importance of Cross-Cultural Research to the Social Sciences.* Lisse: Swets & Zeitlinger, p.103.

[85] White, S., Gibson, M., Wastell, D., & Walsh, P. (2019) *Reassessing Attachment Theory in Child Welfare.* Bristol: Psychology Press. See also Vicedo, M. (2013) *The Nature and Nurture of Love: From Imprinting to Attachment in Cold War America.* Chicago: University of Chicago Press, Chapter 7.

[86] Ainsworth, M. (1969) Sensitivity vs. insensitivity to the baby's signals scale. http://www.psychology.sunysb. edu/attachment/measures/content/ainsworth_scales.html.

[87] Ibid.

passive receipt of pre-formed signals from an 'autonomous' infant.[88] Admittedly, even advocates of Ainsworth's coding system acknowledged that it is relatively poor at explicitly
indexing caregiver behaviour that pre-empts infant signals, so that these are not shown.[89]
Ainsworth's overarching point, however, was that detection and response to tempo, state,
and communications are all part of sensitivity, as are responses that attend to the baby's experience as a whole, rather than necessarily either following their wishes or waiting for their
signals. Some forms of insensitivity can come from lack of awareness or inaccurate interpretation of tempo, state, and communications. But Ainsworth believed that significant insensitivity is most likely when caregivers are geared largely by their own experience, rather
than taking that of the infant into account. This did not imply ascription of full autonomy or
personhood to the baby or the assumption that a baby, like a liberal citizen, can be assumed
to know his or her own wishes.[90] It did, however, imply some attribution to the baby of a capacity for experience relevant to the caregiver's actions, revealed to some extent in the baby's
mood and behaviour.[91]

Ainsworth identified that her measure of sensitivity had a high degree of stability over
time in her Baltimore sample, a finding replicated by later researchers working with samples of caregiver–infant dyads drawn from the community.[92] Later researchers also found
that, remarkably, even if Ainsworth's sensitivity scale was built for observations of infant–
caregiver interactions, the principles could readily be extrapolated to different ages without
needing to be recast. The construct of sensitivity as the perception and accurate interpretation of signals, together with a prompt and appropriate response, has as much relevance
for setting boundaries with a toddler as it does in identifying the needs of an infant.[93] Yet,
already in infancy there are varied important aspects of caregiving that are not reducible to

[88] Ainsworth, M. (1992) A consideration of social referencing in the context of attachment theory and
research. In S.Feinman (ed.) *Social Referencing and the Construction of Reality in Infancy* (pp.349–67).
New York: Plenum Press.

[89] Kondo-Ikemura, K. (2001) Insufficient evidence. *American Psychologist*, 56(10), 825. On the issue of forms
of pre-emptive sensitivity see also Keller, H. & Otto, H. (2009) The cultural socialization of emotion regulation
during infancy. *Journal of Cross-Cultural Psychology*, 40(6), 996–1011; Shai, D. & Belsky, J. (2017) Parental embodied mentalizing: how the nonverbal dance between parents and infants predicts children's socio-emotional
functioning. *Attachment & Human Development*, 19(2), 191–219.

[90] For a comparison of attachment theory and liberal political theory see Duschinsky, R., Greco, M., & Solomon,
J. (2015) Wait up! Attachment and sovereign power. *International Journal of Politics, Culture, and Society*, 28(3),
223–42. On the history of concepts of agency see Smith, R. (2015) Agency: a historical perspective. *Annals of
Theoretical Psychology*, 12, 3–29.

[91] Keller has argued that Ainsworth's sensitivity scale is ethnocentric, since there are societies in which 'caregivers do not take the infant's point of view because infants have not (yet) attained personhood status, and it makes
no sense to take the perspective of someone who is not yet a person'. Keller, H. (2018) Parenting and socioemotional development in infancy and early childhood. *Developmental Review*, 50, 31–41, p.38. However, the ascription of personhood is by no means necessarily the same as taking the experience of another into account, which
was Ainsworth's concern.

[92] E.g. Lindhiem, O., Bernard, K., & Dozier, M. (2011) Maternal sensitivity: within-person variability and
the utility of multiple assessments. *Child Maltreatment*, 16(1), 41–50; Joosen, K.J., Mesman, J., Bakermans-
Kranenburg, M.J., & van IJzendoorn, M.H. (2012) Maternal sensitivity to infants in various settings predicts harsh
discipline in toddlerhood. *Attachment & Human Development*, 14(2), 101–17.

[93] Britner, P.A., Marvin, R.S., & Pianta, R.C. (2005) Development and preliminary validation of the caregiving
behavior system: association with child attachment classification in the preschool Strange Situation. *Attachment
& Human Development*, 7(1), 83–102; Mesman, J. & Emmen, R.A. (2013) Mary Ainsworth's legacy: a systematic
review of observational instruments measuring parental sensitivity. *Attachment & Human Development*, 15(5–6),
485–506; Hallers-Haalboom, E.T., Groeneveld, M.G., Endendijk, J.J., Linting, M., Bakermans-Kranenburg, M.J.,
& Mesman, J. (2017) Mothers' and fathers' sensitivity with their two children: a longitudinal study from infancy to
early childhood. *Developmental Psychology*, 53(5), 860–72.

awareness and accurate interpretation of the child's signals.[94] Some of these may be valuable in particular ecological and cultural contexts.[95] Others may have some claim to more general relevance.[96] For instance, an important later addition to Ainsworth's concern with sensitivity has come with growing attention amongst attachment researchers to the caregiving provided by traumatised or abusive parents (Chapter 3).

Ainsworth found that caregiver sensitivity predicted children's cooperativeness, distress, and aggression on brief everyday separations within the home, and other positive aspects of their home behaviour.[97] Later researchers confirmed these findings, and contributed other associations of sensitivity with psychological, linguistic, neurological, and even immuno-logical correlates.[98] For example, Manning, Davies, and Cicchetti documented that caregiver sensitivity fully buffered the association between toddlers' exposure to partner violence and their later behavioural problems and prosocial behaviour. As Manning and colleagues ob-served, this finding was theoretically expectable since sensitivity signals the capacity of the parent to provide a safe base and secure haven, a capacity that can be anticipated to help regulate the difficult feelings evoked for children in violent family contexts.[99] Such associ-ations have provided evidence of predictive validity by confirming Ainsworth's interpret-ation of sensitivity as relevant to a child's later development.

Yet, as well as supporting Ainsworth's concern with sensitivity, later researchers altered some aspects of Ainsworth's approach to measuring it. Caregiver sensitivity has often sub-sequently been assessed in the context of play; this was a significant part of the activity ob-served by the naturalistic observation of Ainsworth and her students.[100] But it is not clear that play is a good environment for understanding attachment processes specifically, especially given that subsequent attachment researchers observed dyads for much briefer periods than Ainsworth's study.[101] It is possible that some infant signals are more attachment-relevant

---

[94] Van IJzendoorn, M.H. & Bakermans-Kranenburg, M.J. (2019) Bridges across the intergenerational trans-mission of attachment gap. *Current Opinion in Psychology*, 25, 31–6.

[95] Yovsi, R.D., Kärtner, J., Keller, H., & Lohaus, A. (2009) Maternal interactional quality in two cultural en-vironments: German middle class and Cameroonian rural mothers. *Journal of Cross-Cultural Psychology*, 40(4), 701–707.

[96] E.g. Whipple, N., Bernier, A., & Mageau, G.A. (2011) Broadening the study of infant security of attach-ment: maternal autonomy-support in the context of infant exploration. *Social Development*, 20(1), 17–32. The question of whether support for child exploration is a universal or a culturally specific contributor to infant attach-ment security is one that has been debated in the cross-cultural research literature, though on the basis of ethno-graphic observation rather than research findings using the standardized attachment measures. See e.g. LeVine, R.A. (2004) Challenging expert knowledge: findings from an African study of infant care and development. In U.P. Gielen & J.L. Roopnarine (eds) *Childhood and Adolescence: Cross-Cultural Perspectives and Applications*, 149–65. Westport, CT: Praeger.

[97] For a summary of all correlates of sensitivity in the Ainsworth Baltimore study see Bretherton, I. (2013) Revisiting Mary Ainsworth's conceptualization and assessments of maternal sensitivity-insensitivity. *Attachment & Human Development*, 15(5–6), 460–84, Table 4.

[98] E.g. Tamis-LeMonda, C.S., Briggs, R.D., McClowry, S.G., & Snow, D.L. (2009) Maternal control and sen-sitivity, child gender, and maternal education in relation to children's behavioral outcomes in African American families. *Journal of Applied Developmental Psychology*, 30(3), 321–31; Vermeer, H.J., van IJzendoorn, M.H., Groeneveld, M.G., & Granger, D.A. (2012) Downregulation of the immune system in low-quality child care: the case of secretory immunoglobulin A (SIgA) in toddlers. *Physiology & Behavior*, 105(2), 161–7; Bernier, A., Dégeilh, F., Leblanc, É., Daneault, V., Bailey, H.N., & Beauchamp, M.H. (2019) Mother–infant interaction and child brain morphology: a multidimensional approach to maternal sensitivity. *Infancy*, 24(2), 120–38.

[99] Manning, L.G., Davies, P.T., & Cicchetti, D. (2014) Interparental violence and childhood adjustment: how and why maternal sensitivity is a protective factor. *Child Development*, 85(6), 2263–78.

[100] Mesman, J. & Emmen, R.A.G. (2013) Mary Ainsworth's legacy: a systematic review of observational instru-ments measuring parental sensitivity. *Attachment & Human Development*, 15(5–6), 485–506.

[101] It may also not be the best context for making cross-cultural comparisons: Lancy, D.F. (2007) Accounting for variability in mother–child play. *American Anthropologist*, 109(2), 273–84. It should be noted that samples with longer observations, for instance the Minnesota Longitudinal Study of Risk and Adaptation (Chapter 4),

than others, though this will be a matter of degree. Leerkes and colleagues drew a distinction between sensitivity to signals suggesting infant distress and sensitivity to non-distress signals. They found that only the former predicted later child attachment, conduct problems, and social competence, as Ainsworth expected. The effect was particularly strong for children who appeared temperamentally inclined to be easily distressed. By contrast, caregiver sensitivity to non-distress signals did not have this effect, at least in the shorter observations used in studies after Ainsworth.[102] Though a qualification of Ainsworth's operationalisation of sensitivity, this finding is exactly in line with her theory, since signals suggesting infant distress would have particular relevance to the attachment behavioural system, and to the provision of a safe haven in particular.

Bowlby vs Ainsworth on feeding

Ainsworth's inquiries in Uganda and in Baltimore sought to examine the caregiving behaviours associated with the development of attachment behaviour and an infant's confidence in his or her caregiver. One form of caregiving behaviour of particular salience at the time was infant feeding, given the emphasis psychoanalysis had placed on the pleasure of feeding in shaping the infant–caregiver relationship. Chapter 1 described how the rejection of Bowlby's 'Child's tie' paper by Klein and her followers in 1957 was a defining moment in his career and contributed in a profound way to his expectation that his ideas would be rejected. In particular, the Kleinians made repeated attacks on Bowlby for underplaying the importance of feeding in the origins of ambivalence within family relationships. As a consequence, only in the most passing references did Bowlby acknowledge that feeding deserved the status of a behavioural system.[103] For the rest of his career, Bowlby heaped scorn on anyone who assigned importance to feeding interactions for later psychological development: 'It seemed to me the feeding variable was totally irrelevant, or almost totally irrelevant.'[104]

However, this put Bowlby at odds with Ainsworth. In Uganda, Ainsworth observed that reductions in breastfeeding, such as weaning, would lead to an increase in attachment behaviour by infants. Her Baltimore home observations led her to the conviction that social interactions around feeding were relevant to the development of the child–parent attachment relationship. In January 1967, she wrote to Bowlby to say that she was 'astonished and—yes—horrified at the tension and anxiety which attended feeding in the majority of infant–mother pairs'. The feeding interaction was clearly one that both caregiver and infant regarded as important, complex, and troubling.[105] Ainsworth did not agree with the Kleinian perspective, or regard feeding as offering insight into an infant's motivational underpinnings. However, she saw the way that infant feeding served as a close interactive behaviour that required skill,

have tended to find an association between sensitivity and attachment even in contexts such as bathing, where attachment-specific signals are less frequent.

[102] Leerkes, E.M. & Zhou, N. (2018) Maternal sensitivity to distress and attachment outcomes: interactions with sensitivity to nondistress and infant temperament. *Journal of Family Psychology*, 32(6), 753–61.

[103] E.g. Bowlby, J. (1980, 1988) Caring for children. In *A Secure Base* (pp.1–21). London: Routledge: 'I regard it as useful to look upon parenting behaviour as one example of a limited class of biologically rooted types of behaviour of which attachment behaviour is another example, sexual behaviour another, and exploratory behaviour and eating behaviour yet others' (6).

[104] Bowlby, J. (1977–79) Interview with Alice Smuts and Milton J.E. Senn. Wellcome Trust Library Archive. PP/BOW/A.5/2.

[105] Ainsworth, M. (1967) *Letter to John Bowlby*, 16 January 1967. Mary Ainsworth papers, Box M3168, Folder 2.

prompted complex emotions in caregivers, and afforded opportunities to observe a higher rate of interaction than during many other activities.

In April, having received an early draft of *Attachment, Volume 1*, Ainsworth was full of enthusiasm for the book. However, she was critical of Bowlby's perception that in order to show the importance of attachment, he must downplay feeding interactions:

> While agreeing with all that you say in the chapters you sent to me, I feel that there is still something to be said about feeding and especially about mother–infant interaction in the feeding situation. I hope that there may be room in your Chapter 10 to restore the balance. I think you have pushed feeding behaviour very much out of the picture ... Far too many people confuse what happens in the so-called 'oral phase' with orality. There is obviously much that goes on in the first year of life that is not linked in any way with hunger, feeding behaviour, nurturance, dependence and the link. Nevertheless in my American sample such a large proportion of the interaction between infant and mother during the first three months of life took place in the feeding situation or relevant to it.[106]

In Ainsworth's home observation data, infant signals related to feeding were a powerful predictor of later attachment.[107] She agreed with Bowlby that this was not because the child's tie to his or her mother occurs because of a need for food. However, Ainsworth's impression from her data was that when infants were hungry, attachment behaviour, not just food-seeking behaviour, became activated.[108] Furthermore, in her observations of infant care practices in Uganda, breastfeeding served as both the major source of infant nutrition and a primary means of soothing infant distress. She wrote to Bowlby that early feeding interactions were emotionally charged, and the extent to which this was handled with sensitivity had ramifications for other forms of interaction in the first year: 'I do think that feeding can become entangled with the development of attachment, and something more is needed here.'[109]

In the final version of *Attachment, Volume 1*, Bowlby discussed the development of the feeding response in infants, and conflict behaviour shown by animals when alarmed by a threat whilst feeding. However, he ignored Ainsworth's concerns. The power imbalance that had characterised their early relationships remained at least partly in place here, as Ainsworth publicly accepted Bowlby's position even though her empirical data on this matter ran contrary. At least in part as a consequence, later attachment researchers generally followed Bowlby's lead, and did not discuss the specific qualities of feeding interactions even when they were used instrumentally to measure sensitivity or infant secure base behaviour.[110]

---

[106] Ainsworth, M. (1967) *Letter to John Bowlby*, 9 April 1967. Mary Ainsworth papers, Box M3168, Folder 2. Though specifically influenced by her Uganda ethnography and Baltimore study, Ainsworth's emphasis on the feeding interaction can be placed in the broader context of American parenting discourses in the 1960s, in which the challenges of infant feeding and its value were being emphasized. See Foss, K.A. (2010) Perpetuating 'scientific motherhood': infant feeding discourse in *Parents* magazine, 1930–2007. *Women & Health*, 50(3), 297–311.

[107] Ainsworth, M.D.S. & Bell, S.M. (1969) Some contemporary patterns of mother–infant interaction in the feeding situation. In A. Ambrose (ed.) *Stimulation in Early Infancy* (pp.133–70). London: Academic Press.

[108] Ainsworth, M. (1984) Attachment. In N.S. Endler & J. McVicker Hunt (eds) *Personality and the Behavioral Disorders* (pp.559–602). New York: Wiley, p.566.

[109] Ainsworth, M. (1967) *Letter to John Bowlby*, 9 April 1967. Mary Ainsworth papers, Box M3168, Folder 2.

[110] An early exception is Egeland, B. & Brunnquell, D. (1979) An at-risk approach to the study of child abuse: some preliminary findings. *Journal of the American Academy of Child Psychiatry*, 18(2), 219–35. However, even in this article, the importance of feeding interactions in predicting child abuse appears clearly in the results but is downplayed in the discussion. Additional more recent exceptions include Britton, J.R., Britton, H.L., & Gronwaldt, V. (2006) Breastfeeding, sensitivity, and attachment. *Pediatrics*, 118(5), 1436–43; Woolley, H.,

Ainsworth would later write that Bowlby's neglect of the topic had ultimately won out: 'the feeding situation has been neglected as a context for mother–infant interaction'.[111] And the direct role of food as a safe haven for many adults, or its role in family life as a symbol of caregiving, has been ignored by researchers.[112] Yet even if the particular issue of feeding interactions was lost, Ainsworth's deeper point was that certain kinds of interaction, like feeding, offer an especially valuable window into the attachment relationship. Another such form of interaction, as we shall see, was brief separations.

The Strange Situation

Origins of the procedure

The Strange Situation procedure was not planned when Ainsworth's project was originally proposed. However, Ainsworth decided to supplement her naturalistic observations with a structured observation more intelligible to the academic psychology journals of the time. She began privately to use the term 'critical situations' as the generic characterisation for any predicament that activated the attachment behavioural system, thereby allowing 'both occurrence and nonoccurrence of expected behaviors' to be observed: 'A baby does not spend his day consistently manifesting a certain degree of attachment to this, that and the other person. The quality and strength of his attachment is likely to be seen only in certain critical situations.'[113] Ainsworth and colleagues had seen feeding operate as just such a critical situation: the interplay of feeding and attachment was intense, complex, and often challenging, and it was this interactional demand on the dyad that made it predictive of later attachment behaviour by the child. Her home observations also led Ainsworth and colleagues to regard the departure of a person from the room as another 'critical situation', and therefore a useful vantage for relevant observation.[114] Furthermore, Bowlby's work strongly emphasised that

Hertzmann, L., & Stein, A. (2008) Video-feedback intervention with mothers with postnatal eating disorders and their infants. In F. Juffer, M.J. Bakermans-Kranenburg, & M.H. van IJzendoorn (eds) *Promoting Positive Parenting: An Attachment-Based Intervention* (pp.111–38). New York: Psychology Press; Tharner, A., Luijk, M.P., Raat, H., et al. (2012) Breastfeeding and its relation to maternal sensitivity and infant attachment. *Journal of Developmental & Behavioral Pediatrics*, 33(5), 396–404; Messina, S., Reisz, S., Hazen, N., & Jacobvitz, D. (2019) Not just about food: attachments representations and maternal feeding practices in infancy. *Attachment & Human Hevelopment*, 23 April, 1–20. Illustrative of the underelaborated position of eating: the relevance of meal-times is acknowledged by Poslawsky and colleagues in the choice of this potentially fraught setting for measuring sensitivity among parents with children with autism. However, the researchers offer no reflection on the relationship between attachment and meal-time practices. Poslawsky, I.E., Naber, F.B., Bakermans-Kranenburg, M.J., van Daalen, E., van Engeland, H., & van IJzendoorn, M.H. (2015) Video-feedback intervention to promote positive parenting adapted to autism (VIPP-AUTI): a randomized controlled trial. *Autism*, 19(5), 588–603.

[111] Ainsworth, M. (1979) Infant–mother attachment. *American Psychologist*, 34(10), 932–7, p.934.

[112] An exception is McCormack, M. (2012) Investigating the association between attachment and binge eating. Unpublished doctoral dissertation, Deakin University, Victoria.

[113] Ainsworth, M. (1963) *Letter to John Bowlby*, 18 July 1963. Mary Ainsworth papers, Box M3168, Folder 1; Ainsworth, M., Bell, S., & Stayton, D. (1972) Individual differences in the development of some attachment behaviors. *Merrill-Palmer*, 18(2), 123–43: 'In the case of attachment behaviors other than crying the coding did not begin with the behavior itself, but rather with a "critical" situation that seemed likely to activate the behavior, so that both occurrence and nonoccurrence of expected behaviors could be counted. Among such critical situations was the departure of a person from the room in which an infant was situated' (126).

[114] Ainsworth, M., Bell, S., & Stayton, D. (1972) Individual differences in the development of some attachment behaviors. *Merrill-Palmer*, 18(2), 123–43.

evolution made children disposed to experience unanticipated separations, even brief, as a potential source of threat—what he would later term a 'natural cue for danger' (Chapter 1). This stress was anticipated to increase the frequency and thus predictability and reliability with which observers could directly examine attachment behaviour. Ainsworth decided to bring her sample into the laboratory to participate in a study entailing brief separations of a few minutes.

Ainsworth was impressed with the work of Bettye Caldwell's Syracuse group, who had combined interviews with mothers and observation of infant behaviour under standardised laboratory settings.[115] However, she felt that Caldwell and colleagues had conducted their study in such a way that it was difficult to cleanly distinguish the role of different behavioural systems in the interpretation of behaviour:

> One of their projects—a study of visual following in the first year of life—is so neatly controlled that its equivocal results give one little chance of sorting out the variables. (The problem is that visual fixation, searching and following may indicate a) attachment; b) keeping the secure base in view; c) curiosity and exploration of a new stimulus; and d) keeping a wary eye on the stranger who is a threat.) In ordinary free observation with the context clearly in mind, it is no real problem to differentiate between these four possibilities. But it is in an experiment in which the four possibilities were not clearly envisaged to begin with.[116]

In 1964, when the first wave of her sample of infants were 11 months old, Ainsworth attempted a study to cleanly distinguish prompts for behavioural systems.[117] Van Rosmalen and colleagues documented that the term 'strange situation' was already in circulation before Ainsworth, to describe a procedure in which the responses of young children to an unfamiliar environment were observed, and compared with other information known about the child's life.[118] 'Strange' here referred to the novelty of the environment for the infant. Ainsworth's Strange Situation was especially indebted to the 'strange situation' of Jean Arsenian, who had examined infant behaviour in response to the novel environment of the laboratory, and in the presence and absence of their mother.[119] Arsenian's sample was drawn from mothers

[115] Caldwell, B.M., Hersher, L., Lipton, E.L., et al. (1963) Mother–infant interaction in monomatric and polymatric families. *American Journal of Orthopsychiatry*, 33(4), 653; Caldwell, B.M. & Hersher, L. (1964) Mother–infant interaction during the first year of life. *Merrill-Palmer*, 10(2), 119–28.

[116] Ainsworth, M. (1963) *Letter to John Bowlby*, 27 June 1963. Mary Ainsworth papers, Box M3168, Folder 1.

[117] Ainsworth, M. (1995) On the shaping of attachment theory and research: an interview with Mary D.S. Ainsworth. *Monographs of the Society for Research in Child Development*, 60(2/3), 2–21: 'I had seen a lot of separations and reunions in the homes, a lot of exploration, a lot of proximity seeking, and a lot of differences in how the baby and the mother behaved in these situations. So constructing the episodes of the Strange Situation wasn't hard at all; as I recall, it took just about half an hour of talking with Barbara Wittig to decide on the episodes and their sequence—it just came naturally' (12).

[118] Van Rosmalen, L., Van der Veer, R., & Van der Horst, F. (2015) Ainsworth's strange situation procedure: the origin of an instrument. *Journal of the History of the Behavioral Sciences*, 51(3), 261–84. See Shirley, M.M. (1942) Children's adjustments to a strange situation. *Journal of Abnormal and Social Psychology*, 37, 201–17. Shirley's work is not cited by Ainsworth in any of her publications but is cited by Arsenian, and by Bowlby, J. (1969, 1982) *Attachment, Volume 1*. London: Penguin, p.247. Michael Lamb (personal communication) recalls that Ainsworth recommended that he read Shirley's paper in 1973. The procedure seems to have also been independently developed by Harlow, who applied the approach to study the exploratory and care-seeking behaviour of baby rhesus monkeys in an unfamiliar environment: Harlow, H.F. (1958) The nature of love. *American Psychologist*, 13, 673–85.

[119] Arsenian, J.M. (1943) Young children in an insecure situation. *Journal of Abnormal and Social Psychology*, 38, 225–49.

and children in a reformatory, and the mothers were permitted only limited access to their children. Arsenian sought to confirm Blatz's idea that, with the caregiver available, children feel more secure and respond to the environment with more exploration and less distress. The availability of security from the caregiver counteracted the 'fear of the strange' prompted by the unfamiliar environment, as did more time in the setting. As well as demonstrating the importance of the caregiver for providing the confidence for exploration, Arsenian also showed that caregiver availability reduced the incidence of crying, and of stereotypic and other anomalous behaviours without 'goal-directedness', and which primarily 'appeared to be determined by a condition of excess tension'.[120]

Following Arsenian, the presence of the caregiver as secure base was expected by Ainsworth to serve as adequate reassurance for most infants. After the novelty of the environment itself, a second prompt was the availability of toys, a little distance away from the caregiver's chair. This was a cue for the exploratory system. Infants were given around three minutes to acclimatise to the room and, should they wish, explore the toys, before a stranger enters. In Uganda, Ainsworth saw that her own entrance, as a relative stranger (and as a white Canadian), provided the most reliable prompt for the display of attachment behaviour by infants.[121] In the Ainworth Strange Situation the stranger begins by sitting quietly and observing the dyad; the stranger then speaks with the caregiver, which conveys to the infant that the caregiver does not regard the stranger as a threat; finally, the stranger attempts interaction with the infant. This was expected to activate the attachment behavioural system another increment. The caregiver then takes leave of and returns to the infant twice. These separations, in turn, ratchet up the activation of the attachment behavioural system further.

The Strange Situation used the combination of separations and the unfamiliar environment to achieve a functional equivalent of instances of availability or unavailability embedded in the wider life of the child.[122] With the behaviour of the caregiver partially standardised, and the attachment behavioural system activated by careful increments, Ainsworth aimed to mobilise the infant's expectations based on what happened when he or she has felt anxiety in the past about the availability of the attachment figure, and allow a viewer to interpret these expectations from observed behaviour. As the episodes of the procedure modulate the infant's anxiety, Ainsworth anticipated that the infant's movement between behavioural systems would be displayed: the interplay of exploration of novelty and attachment behaviour, in the presence and in the absence of a parent.[123]

[120] Ibid. p.227. Arsenian's findings were replicated by Rheingold, H.L. (1969) The effect of a strange environment on the behavior of infants. In B.M. Foss (ed.) Determinants of Infant Behavior, Vol. 4 (pp.137–66). London: Methuen. Ainsworth, M. (1998) Harold Stevenson—SRCD oral history interview. http://srcd.org/sites/default/files/documents/ainsworth_mary_interview.pdf: 'One day, Harriet [Rheingold] and I met at a meeting and I said, "Oh, Harriet, you'd be interested in something I'm currently doing, um, the strange situation …" (Laugh) "You are too? I'm just starting mine".'

[121] Ainsworth, M. (1964) Patterns of attachment behavior shown by the infant in interaction with his mother. Merrill-Palmer, 10(1), 51–8, p.54.

[122] Ainsworth, M., Blehar, M., Waters, E., & Wall, S. (1978, 2015) Patterns of Attachment: A Psychological Study of the Strange Situation. Bristol: Psychology Press: 'Tight control of maternal behaviour is impossible and indeed undesirable. The compromise represented in our procedures turned out to have effected a reasonable degree of standardisation of the situation, while allowing most mothers to behave naturally and fairly comfortably' (41). Cf. Brown, S. (2012) Abstract experimentalism. In N. Wakeford & C. Lury (eds) Inventive Methods (pp.61–75). London: Routledge.

[123] Ainsworth, M. & Bell, S. (1970) Attachment, exploration, and separation: illustrated by the behavior of one-year-olds in a strange situation. Child Development, 41(1), 49–67, pp.50–53.

The Ainsworth Strange Situation was, then, a means for coaxing to visibility infants' expectations about the availability of their caregiver as a secure base and safe haven, and arraying these expectations and their associated affects within physical space and over episodes to make them available for analysis. In this way, the Strange Situation was intended to dramatise a predicament faced in an ordinary, low-level way by the infant–caregiver dyad in everyday life: the question of the extent to which the infants' experiences led them to believe that the caregiver was available when needed. The highly contrived situation was intended to intensify and display specific aspects of real life experience, to be interpreted in the context of home observations of these dyads.[124]

Ainsworth anticipated that, with the attachment behavioural system activated through 'cumulative stresses', infants would be increasingly disposed to seek their caregiver as a safe haven:[125]

> The results are very much in accordance with expectation. Nearly all children explore vigorously when mother is there and not when she is absent; nearly all protest and attempt to follow when she leaves; stranger anxiety is variable, but mother is used as a secure base and/or a haven of safety when a stranger is there.[126]

In general terms, Bowlby's description of the expectable behavioural expression of the attachment system was confirmed. Ainsworth was therefore all the more intrigued, however, by the fact that some of the Baltimore infants made no approach to their caregiver after the first reunion. However, the second separation seemed to activate the attachment behavioural system to an intensity that they abandoned this task, and instead sought their caregiver:

> Two little girls faced the strange situation with remarkable poise, to the extent of interacting with the stranger and offering her toys—only to disintegrate when mother returned for the second time, to cry and cling and carry on, as though they had borne as much as they could, and now could give delayed expression of their distress.[127]

Yet several infants did not display distress even after the second separation, and Ainsworth also noted the display of tension behaviours during reunion, suggesting the strain of holding back the expression of the attachment behavioural system. She wrote to Bowlby:

> A couple of babies who are clearly attached to their mothers showed relatively little stranger anxiety and separation-disturbance, although showing subtle differences in behaviour in the various phases of the strange situation, but they manifested the strain that had been placed upon them by disturbance when the mother returned.[128]

---

[124] Writing under Ainsworth's influence, see Waters, E. & Sroufe, L.A. (1983) Social competence as a developmental construct. *Developmental Review*, 3, 79–97: 'Any single sample of naturalistic behavior, especially if brief, could be unrepresentative and, paradoxically, less revealing of the child's competence in the "real world" than a strategically designed laboratory assessment, in which a child must cope with a problem that regularly (though rarely) occurs in the natural environment' (85). In fact, the similarity of the Strange Situation to ordinary expectable brief infant–caregiver separations has regularly been used by attachment researchers in research ethics applications over the decades.

[125] Ainsworth, M. (1984) Attachment. In N.S. Endler & J. McVicker Hunt (eds) *Personality and the Behavioral Disorders* (pp.559–602). New York: Wiley, p.572.

[126] Ainsworth, M. (1965) *Letter to John Bowlby*, 2 February 1965. PP/Bow/D3/69.

[127] Ibid.

[128] Ibid.

The apparent lack of distress on separation was reminiscent of some of the infants Ainsworth had observed in Uganda, who showed few attachment behaviours in response to separations and reunions with their caregivers. These had often been infants with relatively less-sensitive caregivers, by Ainsworth's ethnographic assessment. The unruffled behaviour of these infants also resembled the avoidant or 'detached' behaviour of some of the long-term hospitalised children seen by Robertson when observed in reunions with their caregivers. Ainsworth quickly concluded that these individual differences in infant behaviour reflected differences in the history of the caregiver–infant relationship.

Forming categories

Within Bowlby's research group at the Tavistock in the early 1960s, Rudolph Schaffer studied 60 infants, who were observed at four-weekly intervals until they were one year of age.[129] Ainsworth acknowledged the importance of this study in documenting the development of attachment behaviour towards the infant's primary caregivers through the first year of life. However, Ainsworth's grounding in Blatz's ideas made her troubled by Schaffer's approach. Schaffer assumed that more attachment behaviour directed towards a figure would indicate more attachment—except in situations like foster-care where an attachment bond may still be in formation.[130] Ainsworth wrote that such a quantitative approach missed important qualitative differences resulting from security, anxiety, and defences.[131] On the one hand, her basis in Blatz's work led her to anticipate that a secure attachment would be associated with less clinging, crying, and following, except when the child needed comfort. When using the caregiver as a secure base for exploration, Ainsworth anticipated that babies would show little attachment behaviour towards the caregiver, except to periodically check in with them and confirm their availability.[132] On the other hand, Ainsworth worried that counting attachment behaviours would be a treacherous research strategy, since a child unsure about the availability of their attachment figure may intensify attachment behaviours, and a child who has learnt that attachment behaviours will be ignored or punished by an attachment figure may show fewer.[133]

[129] Schaffer, H.R. & Emerson, P.E. (1964) The development of social attachments in infancy. *Monographs of the Society for Research in Child Development*, 29(3), 1–77.

[130] See e.g. Ainsworth, M., Blehar, M., Waters, E., & Wall, S. (1978, 2015) *Patterns of Attachment: A Psychological Study of the Strange Situation*. Bristol: Psychology Press. Ainsworth and colleagues propose that the Strange Situation can be used in custody and forensic decision-making: 'A practical situation in which the issue is whether or not to remove a child from his natural parents and place him in a foster or adoptive home, it might be of moment to ascertain whether he has become strongly enough attached to his parent(s) that it would be more traumatic to him to be separated from them or to remain with them' (291). However, Ainsworth's measures did not allow for assessment of strength of attachment. A scale for assessing the strength of attachment in the Strange Situation would later be developed by Betty Carlson, though it has seen little use outside of research contexts. See Zeanah, C.H., Smyke, A.T., Koga, S.F., Carlson, E., & Bucharest Early Intervention Project Core Group (2005) Attachment in institutionalized and community children in Romania. *Child Development*, 76(5), 1015–28.

[131] Ainsworth, M. & Wittig, B. (1969) Attachment and exploratory behaviour of one-year-olds in a Strange Situation. In B.M. Foss (ed.) *Determinants of Infant Behaviour*, Vol. 4 (pp.111–36). London: Metheun, p.112–13.

[132] Ainsworth, M. (1973) *A Secure Base*. Unpublished manuscript. PP/Bow/J.1/33. This claim was soon after supported by Carr, S., Dabbs, J., & Carr, T. (1975) Mother–infant attachment: the importance of the mother's visual field. *Child Development*, 46, 331–8.

[133] Ainsworth, M D.S. (1985) Attachments across the life span. *Bulletin of the New York Academy of Medicine*, 61, 792–812, p.805.

Ainsworth therefore stressed that researchers should not count behaviours in order to assess the 'strength' of an attachment, but take note of qualitative differences in attachment relationships under conditions where the attachment system was anticipated to be activated. When the second wave of her sample reached 11 months, Ainsworth and her team conducted the Strange Situation again with these infant–caregiver dyads. In total, 23 of the 26 dyads in her sample were seen in the Strange Situation. On the basis of these further observations, Ainsworth distinguished three groups. Initially she termed them 'prematurely independent' (6 dyads), 'secure' (13 dyads), and 'disturbed' (4 dyads). However, Bowlby urged that these terms were 'shot through with value judgements & hidden predictions'.[134] He suggested that the labels 'A', 'B', and 'C' should be used instead to avoid prejudging what the individual differences would mean.[135] This was a strategy used by Ainsworth, Robertson, and Bowlby from their earliest work together, analysing Robertson's notes to distinguish different groups of children based on their response to reunion after hospitalisation.[136]

In a letter to Bowlby from 1967, Ainsworth described Group B as 'normally attached'. The attachment behavioural system was activated and expressed in infant behaviour according to the expected increments, and could be deactivated again by the presence of the caregiver. The attachment behaviours shown were various. Infants could crawl or waddle to their caregiver on reunion, lift their arms to be picked up, signal with a directed cry, or clamber up onto the caregiver. Group A initially comprised those dyads with infants who did not show separation anxiety as expected; Ainsworth observed that these infants had a variety of different histories of care. But—at least by the standards of her low-risk sample—her home observations suggested 'a deprivingly disturbed relationship with their mothers'.[137] In 1969 Ainsworth changed the distinction, so that Group A was no longer defined by the lack of separation anxiety but rather classified those infants who did not show more attachment behaviour as the situation contributed greater anxiety, and instead directed their attention and their movements away from their caregiver.[138] Ainsworth found no infants who avoided both the mother and the stranger, contrary the idea that 'avoidance' might simply be regarded as a trait of the individual infant. The groups were not ultimately defined by countable behaviours, but by whether the attachment behavioural system was inferred to have found expression in behaviour (see Table 2.1 for Ainsworth's Strange Situations classifications).

In Patterns of Attachment, reporting results from Ainsworth's original samples plus doctoral projects by her first students, 66% of the total of 106 infants were classified as

---

[134] Bowlby, J. (1967) Letter to Mary Ainsworth, 19 April 1967. Mary Ainsworth papers, Box M3168, Folder 2: 'Terminology. All your terms—securely attached, prematurely independent & disturbed—are shot through with value judgements & hidden predictions.'

[135] Ainsworth, M. (1967) Letter to John Bowlby, 6 August 1967. Mary Ainsworth papers, Box M3168, Folder 2.

[136] Ainsworth, M., Robertson, J., & Bowlby, J. (1953) 'Reunion after prolonged separation', chapters drafted for an unpublished book. PP/BOW/D.3/21; see also Van Rosmalen, L., Van der Veer, R., & Van der Horst, F. (2015) Ainsworth's strange situation procedure: the origin of an instrument. Journal of the History of the Behavioral Sciences, 51(3), 261–84.

[137] Ainsworth, M. (1967) Letter to John Bowlby, 6 August 1967. Mary Ainsworth papers, Box M3168, Folder 2. For Ainsworth's reflections having seen a greater diversity of samples, including higher risk samples and cases of serious child neglect, see Ainsworth, M.D.S. (1980) Attachment and child abuse. In: G. Gerbner, C.J. Ross, & E. Zigler (eds) Child Abuse: An Agenda for Action (pp.35–47). Oxford: Oxford University Press; Crittenden, P.M. & Ainsworth, M.D.S. (1989) Child maltreatment and attachment theory. In D. Cicchetti & V. Carlson (eds) Child Maltreatment: Theory and Research on the Causes and Consequences of Child Abuse and Neglect (pp.432–63). Cambridge: Cambridge University Press.

[138] Ainsworth, M. & Wittig, B. (1969) Attachment and exploratory behaviour of one-year-olds in a Strange Situation. In B.M. Foss (ed.) Determinants of Infant Behaviour, Vol. 4 (pp.111–36). London: Metheun, p.126.

Table 2.1 The Ainsworth Strange Situation Classifications, as outlined in *Patterns of Attachment* (1978)

Attachment classification		Strange Situation Behaviour
A		*Lower proximity-seeking and contact-maintaining on reunion than B or C, together with some proximity-avoiding behaviours. The infant's behaviour, attention and affect are integrated in a coherent way to downplay the communication of distress and keep focus away from the caregiver, e.g. by attention to the toys.*
	A1	Lowest proximity-seeking and contact-maintaining on reunion than B or C; strongest proximity-avoiding behaviours.
	A2	Low to moderate proximity-seeking on reunion. Marked proximity-avoiding behaviours.
B		*Strong proximity-seeking and contact-maintaining on reunion compared to A. Low contact-resisting compared to C. The infant's behaviour, attention and affect integrate in a coherent way which allows distress to be communicated to the caregiver and assuaged, allowing the child to then return calmly to play.*
	B1	Weak proximity-seeking and contact-maintaining. Weaker proximity-avoiding behaviours than A1. Strong communication and affective sharing with their caregiver from a distance. Conceptualised as intermediate between the A and B infants.
	B2	Low to moderate proximity-seeking and marked proximity-avoiding on first reunion. But then strong proximity-seeking and contact-maintaining on second reunion.
	B3	Strong proximity-seeking and contact-maintaining on reunion. No contact-resisting or proximity-avoiding.
	B4	Some proximity-seeking and contact-maintaining prior to separation from the caregiver. Strong proximity-seeking and contact-maintaining prior to separation from the caregiver on reunion. Some contact-resisting.
C		*Marked contact-resisting behaviour. The infant's behaviour, attention and affect integrate in a coherent way which strongly communicates their distress and frustration to the caregiver.*
	C1	Strong proximity-seeking and contact-maintaining on reunion. Strong contact-resisting behaviour punctuates the contact-maintaining, as the child switches between communicating distress and a desire for contact, anger, and a desire to be put down.
	C2	Weak proximity-seeking but moderate to strong contact-maintaining, particularly on second reunion. Moderate contact-resisting.

Group B.[139] The largest proportion of dyads showed a smooth balance between attachment and exploration: with increasing prompts for the attachment behavioural system, attachment behaviour increased; when the caregiver was present, the child was comforted and could return to play. Ainsworth labelled dyads where this pattern of behaviour was shown

---

[139] Ainsworth, M., Blehar, M., Waters, E., & Wall, S. (1978, 2015) *Patterns of Attachment: A Psychological Study of the Strange Situation*. Bristol: Psychology Press, p.230.

as B3. Out of 106 infants, 42% were classified B3, compared to 23% other kinds of B.[140] One kind of Group B response that differed from the prototypical B3 was evident in the difference between infant behaviour on first and second reunion. From the very first, Ainsworth had been interested in the fact that some children showed avoidance on the first reunion, and then attachment behaviours on the second reunion. Their behaviour conveyed a sense that with the increasing activation of the attachment behavioural system, these infants felt that they were no longer able to manage their distress on their own, and that their caregiver would be receptive under such circumstances. Their avoidance thawed as their desire for comfort increased. These dyads were labelled B2.[141]

Another group of infants did not display much separation anxiety or proximity-seeking on reunion, but were unmistakably happy to see their caregiver again on reunion. And the attachment system seemed to be able to be terminated through distance interaction. Ainsworth termed dyads with such infants B1.[142] This ran counter to Bowlby's assumption that proximity would be the set-goal of the attachment behavioural system in infancy, and ultimately led to his qualification in his final writings that the set-goal is caregiver availability (Chapter 1). Nonetheless, Ainsworth and colleagues described B3 as the short and most direct expression of the attachment behavioural system, whereas B1 and B2 were regarded as 'complicated' expressions of the behavioural system.[143] The Ainsworth laboratory considered B1 and B2 as, ultimately, intermediate between Group A and Group B in their Strange Situation behaviour.[144] In work using the Strange Situation by Ainsworth's student Sylvia Bell, an additional subgroup was added for infants who displayed more distress and resistance than the infants of B3 dyads, but who ultimately were able to be comforted by the presence of their caregiver and return to exploration within the Strange Situation.[145]

Ainsworth and her group also distinguished subtypes of Group A. These subtype groupings evolved over time, but had stabilised by the mid-1970s. A1 dyads were characterised by the infant's rigidly held avoidance; A2 dyads were characterised by a partial approach by the infant, succeeded by avoidance. In both cases, the infants ultimately

---

[140] Ibid.

[141] Throughout the 1970s and early 1980s, Ainsworth repeatedly considered splitting the B2 group up, especially after seeing more 18-month Strange Situations. One group of B2 dyads would contain children who were confident in their capacity to self-regulate following the first reunion, but who knew they could approach their caregiver as needed when their anxiety and distress became greater on the second reunion. Another group of B2 dyads contained children who seemed anxious and unhappy, and so avoided on the first reunion, but who could not sustain their avoidance into the second reunion. See e.g. Ainsworth, M. (1981) *Letter to Michael Lamb*. Mary Ainsworth Archive, Box M3173, Folder 4. It is quite possible that where an avoidant strategy seems bent or snapped rather than relaxed into proximity-seeking, this would now generally get coded as D/A, since it would come with other markers of tension. Certainly Ainsworth's concern about the insecure B2s was no longer mentioned after the introduction of the D classification, though this may also have been because the coding system by that point was too well established.

[142] Ainsworth, M., Blehar, M., Waters, E., & Wall, S. (1978, 2015) *Patterns of Attachment: A Psychological Study of the Strange Situation*. Bristol: Psychology Press, p.239.

[143] Ainsworth, M. & Bell, S. (1970) Attachment, exploration, and separation: illustrated by the behavior of one-year-olds in a strange situation. *Child Development*, 41(1), 49–67, p.52.

[144] Blehar, M., Lieberman, A., & Ainsworth, M. (1977) Early face-to-face interaction and its relation to later infant–mother attachment. *Child Development*, 48(1), 182–94, p.186. Ainsworth would later conceptualize the B1 classification as a kind of reserve, observable in other forms with later maturation—personal communication cited in Cassidy, J., Marvin, R., with the Attachment Working Group of the John D. and Catherine T. MacArthur Network on the Transition from Infancy to Early Childhood (1992) Attachment organisation in preschool children: procedures and coding manual. Unpublished manual.

[145] Ainsworth, M.D.S., Bell, S.M., & Stayton, D.J. (1971) Individual differences in strange-situation behavior of one-year-olds. In H.R. Schaffer (ed.) *The Origins of Human Social Relations* (pp.17–58). New York: Academic Press.

did not engage in affective communication with their caregiver, even as the attachment behavioural system was presumed to be incrementally activated by the episodes of the Strange Situation. Instead, a characteristic of the group was that they would often engage with the toys or point out toys to the caregiver precisely when another child showed distress and attachment behaviour. Despite individual differences within the groups, at base the predicaments faced by the Group C and Group A dyads differed from one another. Ainsworth and colleagues offered the dictum that 'the C baby fears that he will not get enough of what he wants; the A baby fears what he wants'.[146] In other words, C babies are not confident in the availability of the caregiver in the Strange Situation to offer the comfort and protection they desire; A babies are concerned that expression of desire for the caregiver will not be effective or, indeed, will backfire by eliciting rebuff or punishment. In *Patterns of Attachment*, 21% of the total of 106 infants were classified as Group A.[147]

Ainsworth put dyads in Group C if the infants did not show the A or B responses.[148] It is curious to see that even in *Patterns of Attachment* as late as 1978, Ainsworth was still using Group C in part as a residual category for generally 'maladaptive' behaviours.[149] However, this was in part a holdover, and was not how she discussed the category with her students and collaborators. Though it began as a residual category, through the late 1960s Ainsworth's comparison of the Strange Situation and home observations led her to identify a common theme in the behaviour of most of the Group C infants: 'They are diverse, but they have in common the trait of low frustration tolerance, and the experience that their own actions have no consistent consequences, because so much that happens to them is the result of the mother's timing, not theirs'.[150]

In the 1960s, Ainsworth and her group came to distinguish two subtypes of Group C behaviour from within the 'mixed bag'.[151] The overall group became characterised as 'babies who were markedly distressed in both separation episodes, and whose behaviour throughout the strange situation showed disturbance of a passive–aggressive nature'.[152] The C1 classification was used for infants whose behaviour towards their caregiver clearly suggested frustration or anger, most notably in resisting being held by the caregiver and less active in maintaining contact. The C2 classification was used when infant behaviour was conspicuously 'passive', though also had more of a tone of anger in their interactions with their caregivers than the Group A or B infants.[153] C1 infants would approach the caregiver on reunion or reach for a pick-up, showing a mixture of attachment behaviours and signs of frustration. By contrast, C2 infants would wail helplessly and gaze beseechingly at the caregiver, without

---

[146] Ainsworth, M., Blehar, M., Waters, E., & Wall, S. (1978, 2015) *Patterns of Attachment: A Psychological Study of the Strange Situation*. Bristol: Psychology Press, p.128.

[147] Ibid. p.230.

[148] Ainsworth, M. (1967) *Letter to John Bowlby*, 6 August 1967. Mary Ainsworth papers, Box M3168, Folder 2.

[149] Ainsworth, M., Blehar, M., Waters, E., & Wall, S. (1978, 2015) *Patterns of Attachment: A Psychological Study of the Strange Situation*. Bristol: Psychology Press, p.62. This role of Group C as a catch-all for anomalous behaviours would finally be officially eliminated by Ainsworth in the mid-1980s, following the introduction of the D classification by Main (Chapter 3).

[150] Ainsworth, M. & Wittig, B. (1969) Attachment and exploratory behaviour of one-year-olds in a Strange Situation. In B.M. Foss (ed.) *Determinants of Infant Behaviour*, Vol. 4 (pp.111–36). London: Metheun, p.134.

[151] Ainsworth, M. (1967) *Letter to John Bowlby*, 16 January 1967. Mary Ainsworth papers, Box M3168, Folder 2: 'I am sure that Group C will become at least two groups rather than the mixed bag it presently is.'

[152] Ainsworth, M. (1967) *Letter to John Bowlby*, 17 October 1967. PP/Bow/K.4/12.

[153] Ainsworth, M. & Wittig, B. (1969) Attachment and exploratory behaviour of one-year-olds in a Strange Situation. In B.M. Foss (ed.) *Determinants of Infant Behaviour*, Vol. 4 (pp.111–36). London: Metheun, p.132.

taking much determinate action to achieve their evident desire for closeness, and without being fully comforted when that closeness was achieved. All of Ainsworth's C2 infants also displayed stereotypic behaviours, such as rocking to themselves;[154] and Ainsworth later wondered whether what she was seeing were infant 'attempts to cope with a threat of psychotic fragmentation' by quite mentally ill mothers.[155]

C1 and C2 infants had in common that the attachment behavioural system had a low threshold for activation and termination: Group C infants were more wary of the stranger than the other children seen in the Strange Situation, and might stop play and show a degree of attachment behaviour even before the first separation. Additionally, following the reunions, they were not comforted or able to return to play. Whereas Group A infants seemed unwilling to permit tension or drama, Group C infants seemed not to permit their resolution. Ainsworth termed Group C 'ambivalent/resistant'. Bowlby regarded this as an unhelpful label since both Group A and Group C infants were ambivalent about contact and comfort from their caregiver: Group A because they felt that they were not permitted to seek their caregiver; Group C because they were not satisfied by the contact and comfort they received.[156] Ainsworth, on the other hand, did not use the term 'ambivalent' to refer to the inner experience of conflict inferred to be common to Group A and Group C infants. Instead, she used the term to refer to the child's observable mingling of contact-seeking and contact-resisting behaviour.[157] In *Patterns of Attachment*, Ainsworth and colleagues reported on the proportions of infants in different groups, drawing on the original Baltimore study and further Strange Situations from studies by Silvia Bell and Mary Main (Chapter 3). Thirteen percent of the 106 infants were classified as C.[158]

Strange Situation scales

Reflecting on the subtypes, Ainsworth came to the conclusion that infants could be distinguished by four kinds of behaviour. She developed scales that took account of '1) the degree of activity and initiative of the behaviour; 2) promptness of the behaviour; 3) frequency of the behaviour; and 4) duration of the behaviour'.[159] These scales have only recently been published as an appendix to the 2015 Psychology Press edition of *Patterns of Attachment*. In the decades before that, they circulated as an unpublished manuscript, passed to individuals attending a training institute. The Ainsworth scales are, in practice, partly a written and partly an oral tradition. Richters, Waters, and Vaughn found that without training in

---

[154] Ainsworth, M.D.S., Bell, S.M., & Stayton, D.J. (1971) Individual differences in strange-situation behavior of one-year-olds. In H.R. Schaffer (ed.) *The Origins of Human Social Relations* (pp.17–58). New York: Academic Press, p.39.

[155] Ainsworth, M. (1980) Infant attachment and maternal care: some implications for psychoanalytic concepts of development. PP/Bow/J.1/53.

[156] Bowlby, J. (1990) *Letter to Sonia Monteiro de Barros*, 6 August 1990. PP/Bow/B.3/40: 'You are quite right to link the two patterns of attachment you refer to, namely "anxious resistant" and "anxious ambivalent". In fact, Mary Ainsworth herself sometimes used "anxious ambivalent" as synonymous with "anxious resistant". I thought that was a mistake since all the insecure patterns of attachment are characterised by ambivalence, sometimes overt and obvious, at others (e.g. avoidant & compulsive caregiving) only covert and potential.'

[157] Ainsworth, M. (1969) *Letter to John Bowlby*, 23 February 1971. Mary Ainsworth Archive, Box M3168, Folder3.

[158] Ainsworth, M., Blehar, M., Waters, E., & Wall, S. (1978, 2015) *Patterns of Attachment: A Psychological Study of the Strange Situation*. Bristol: Psychology Press, p.230.

[159] Ibid. p.51.

using these scales, inter-rater reliability is no better than chance.[160] When the written text is combined with training, three of the scales have incredible clarity and usability, a kind of deftness of touch. These are the proximity-seeking, contact-maintenance, and avoidance scales. Based on examples from a very small sample, Ainsworth managed to characterise infant behaviour in terms of (i) initiative, (ii) promptness, (iii) frequency, and (iv) duration within single dimensions. And this measure has captured the behaviour of the large majority of infants in all subsequent samples with a surprising degree of effectiveness. There is certainly some shoehorning that takes place as coders work with samples with very different caregiving cultures; but, as Behrens observed, what is curious is that there is much less than might be expected.[161]

In the case of proximity-seeking, higher scores have to do with the efforts the infant puts into getting proximity. In the highest score on the scale, 'the baby purposively approaches the adult, creeping, crawling, or walking. He goes the whole way and actually achieves the contact through his own efforts, by clambering up on or grasping hold of the adult.'[162] A lower score is assigned when the initiative, promptness, frequency, or duration is lower. So, for instance, if the baby makes three full approaches to the caregiver, but without completing contact, this scores 4 out of 7. In the case of contact-maintenance, higher scores reflect the initiative of the baby and the duration of contact. As such, even a baby who is held for a long time can receive the lowest possible score—1 out of 7—on contact-maintenance, if when picked up 'he neither clings nor holds on, and when he is put down he makes no protest; if he is not put down he may still be coded (1) if he seems indifferent to being held.'[163] By contrast, a lower score is assigned when desire to maintain contact is less visible, or relatively less effort is engaged to achieve it. For instance, a score of 4 out of 7 is assigned when 'the baby has been held, perhaps clinging a little, perhaps having diminished his crying when picked up; when put down he decisively protests, giving more than a brief cry' or when 'The baby, having been held, is released; he resists release briefly, by attempting to hold on or by clinging briefly, but when this is ineffective he accepts the release without protest and without further effort to maintain contact.'

The avoidance scale emphasises especially promptness, frequency, and duration of attempts to direct attention or behaviour away from the caregiver. However, the initiative taken by the child is also emphasised. The highest score on the scale can only be achieved by an infant who ignores a caregiver attempting to directly attract his or her attention: 'The baby does not greet the mother upon her return in a reunion episode neither with a smile nor with a protest. He pays little or no attention to her for an extended period despite the mother's efforts to attract his attention. He ignores her, and may turn his back on her. If his mother nevertheless picks him up he remains unresponsive to her while she holds him, looking around, interested in other things.'[164] A lower score is assigned if avoidance is persistent but low-keyed or only occasional. A score of 4 out of 7 is assigned, for instance, if 'the baby fails

[160] Richters, J.E., Waters, E., & Vaughn, B.E. (1988) Empirical classification of infant–mother relationships from interactive behavior and crying during reunion. *Child Development*, 59(2), 512–22, p.520.

[161] Behrens, K.Y. (2016) Reconsidering attachment in context of culture: review of attachment studies in Japan. *Online Readings in Psychology and Culture*, 6(1), 7.

[162] Ainsworth, M., Blehar, M., Waters, E., & Wall, S. (1978, 2015) Appendix: Coding of infants' interactive behaviour in the Strange Situation. In *Patterns of Attachment: A Psychological Study of the Strange Situation*. Bristol: Psychology Press.

[163] Ibid.

[164] Ibid.

to greet his mother and ignores her for a time and then takes the initiative in making contact or undertaking interaction, even though the mother has not sought his attention.[165]

Ainsworth also developed a resistance scale, which measures the intensity, frequency, and duration of frustration or aggression directed towards the caregiver, including frustrated resistance to being held. This scale is somewhat less polished and well characterised, likely because incidence of aggression towards the caregiver was less frequent in the Ainsworth sample than proximity-seeking, contact-maintenance, and avoidance. However, the resistance scale has appeared to have equivalent inter-rater reliability to the others. The relevant behaviours are: 'pushing away, throwing away, dropping [toys passed to the infant by the caregiver], batting away, hitting, kicking, squirming to be put down, jerking away, stepping angrily, resistance to being picked up or moved or restrained. More diffuse manifestations are angry screaming, throwing self about, throwing self down, kicking the floor, pouting, cranky fussing, or petulance.'[166] The highest score can be assigned, for instance, if the coder sees the infant enter into 'a full-blown temper tantrum, with angry screaming—the baby either being rigid and stiff or throwing himself about, kicking the floor, batting his hands up and down, and the like'. A lower score is assigned if displays of anger are persistent but low-key or only occasional, for instance if the infant engages in 'persistent low-intensity pouting or cranky fussing' or 'one strong but isolated behavior, accompanied by a cry'.

Why categories?

Infants in dyads classified as Group B were characterised especially by strong proximity-seeking and contact-maintenance following reunion, and relatively low levels of avoidant and resistant behaviour. Infants in dyads classified as Group A were distinguished by low levels of proximity-seeking and contact-maintenance, and high levels of avoidant behaviour. Infants in dyads classified as C1 were distinguished by high levels of infant resistant or frustrated behaviour. C2 dyads were poorly characterised by the four scales, and no independent 'passivity' scale was developed by Ainsworth. Over time, they have subsequently become a rare subclassification—though they are more common in samples drawn from some countries, such as Israel and Japan.[167] Some samples with a significant proportion of neglecting parents also had several C2 infants. One instance is the Minnesota Longitudinal Study of Risk and Adaptation (Chapter 4). In *Patterns of Attachment*, Ainsworth and colleagues reported a discriminant function analysis, drawing on Everett Waters' expertise with this procedure. They found that a two-function model performed extremely well.[168] The first function essentially comprised scores on the avoidance scale for the first and second

---

[165] Ibid.

[166] Ibid.

[167] Crittenden, P.M. (2001) Organization, alternative organizations, and disorganization: competing perspectives on the development of endangered children. *Contemporary Psychology*, 46, 593–6: 'I am reminded of a personal conversation that I had with Ainsworth around the time that samples for training on infant attachment classification were being gathered. Ainsworth lamented a general lack of competence in discerning Type C, fearing that the pattern was being lost, especially the passive C2 subpattern' (595).

[168] Ainsworth, M., Blehar, M., Waters, E., & Wall, S. (1978, 2015) *Patterns of Attachment: A Psychological Study of the Strange Situation*. Bristol: Psychology Press, Chapter 6. The identification of a two-function model was later replicated by other researchers: Richters, J.E., Waters, E., & Vaughn, B.E. (1988) Empirical classification of infant–mother relationships from interactive behavior and crying during reunion. *Child Development*, 59(2), 512–22; Lamb, M., Thompson, R.A., Gardner, W., & Charnov, E.L. (1985) *Infant–Mother Attachment: The Origins and Developmental Significance of Individual Differences in the Strange Situation*. Hillsdale, NJ: Lawrence Erlbaum.

reunions. This distinguished the A from the B and C dyads. Avoidance in the second reunion made a large additional contribution to variance, over and above the first reunion. There was also a negative relationship with the proximity-seeking and contact-maintaining, especially in the second reunion.

The second function was mainly constituted by scores on the resistance scale on first and second reunion, and with crying through the two reunion episodes. This function distinguished the C from the A and B dyads. Contrary to the coding protocols, which give particular weight to the second reunion, in fact the discriminant function analysis revealed that both episodes made the same contribution to variance in classification. Though rare, the best predictor of a C classification was displays of distress before any separation in the Strange Situation, indicating little ability to use the caregiver as a safe base to deal with the novel setting. However, overall, the second function was not as effective as the first. The two-factor model could almost always predict whether a case would be A or B, but misclassified 30% of C dyads. Whereas A/not-A was defined cleanly by the avoidance scale, the C/not-C distinction appeared to include distress and anger, and appeared to also include other elements. For example, Ainsworth developed no scale for passivity, and was not surprised when the C2 infants were poorly characterised by the discriminant function analysis.

Despite limitations in characterizing the C dyads, Ainsworth and colleagues regarded the two-function model as having performed very well. This relative translatability between categories and scales might imply that either can be used by researchers in analysing their data. In *Patterns of Attachment*, Ainsworth and colleagues stated clearly and explicitly that in adopting a categorical approach to their data they did not assume a 'rigid typological concept of the way in which human behaviour is organised, with implications of discontinuity in the various quantitative dimensions'.[169] They held that 'it is inconceivable that any system based on a relatively small sample could comfortably accommodate all patterns'.[170] Nonetheless, they argued in favour of group categorisations in running analyses and reporting data, whilst keeping an eye out for anomalies that suggest the need for revision.

As mentioned above, there was a marked bimodal distribution in Ainsworth's initial data, with few children occupying middle positions on scales of proximity-seeking, contact-maintenance, avoidance, and resistance. This would have made the use of categories rather than dimensions especially intuitive, since both ends of the spectrum were sharpened. The data reported in *Patterns of Attachment* may also have retained a bimodal distribution. For instance, it would seem unimaginable today to recruit a sample which, like Ainsworth's, had 42% B3s. By way of comparison, in the milti-site NICHD sample collected in the 1990s as part of a study of the effects of daycare, there were 224 B3 dyads out of the 1281 seen in the Strange Situation (17.5%). And even this is a substantially higher proportion than most samples that have reported subtype classifications.[171] Against claims by colleagues and contemporaries that attachment phenomena were likely best measured

[169] Ainsworth, M., Blehar, M., Waters, E., & Wall, S. (1978, 2015) *Patterns of Attachment: A Psychological Study of the Strange Situation*. Bristol: Psychology Press, p.55.

[170] Ibid. p.229.

[171] Umemura, T. & Jacobvitz, D.B. (2014) Nonmaternal care hours and temperament predict infants' proximity-seeking behavior and attachment subgroups. *Infant Behavior and Development*, 37(3), 352–65; on the lower rates of B3 in other samples see for instance 12% B3 reported in Van IJzendoorn, M.H., Goossens, F.A., Tavecchio, L.W.C., Vergeer, M.M., & Hubbard, F.O.A. (1983) Attachment to soft objects: its relationship with attachment to the mother and with thumbsucking. *Child Psychiatry & Human Development*, 14(2), 97–105.

dimensionally using scales,[172] in print Ainsworth defended her advocacy of categories with four arguments:

1. A first argument was that categorical measures are appropriate when equivalence is assumed between behaviours with a common goal.[173] This is an effective argument against approaches to the Strange Situation that merely counted the frequency of particular behaviours, a popular approach in the early 1970s.[174] Ainsworth appeared not to have noticed that this argument is not an effective one against the use of her own scales for coding the Strange Situation. The scales already captured the fact that there were a diversity of ways that infants could seek proximity, retain contact with their caregiver, avoid expression of the attachment behavioural system, or display aggression. The fact that Ainsworth's protocols mandated that coders should first score the scales, and then use them in informing a categorical judgement, meant that over time the field accumulated a vast amount of largely unpublished data on scale scores both for Ainsworth's Strange Situation coding system and for all coding measures based on it. As a by-product, an archive of data on scale scores was produced that would, in the 2000s, be a fundamental resource in the revolt of several younger attachment researchers against the Ainsworth categories (Chapter 3).

2. Ainsworth proposed that categories are useful in helping to identify the relevant dimensions.[175] Indeed, Ainsworth's identification of proximity-seeking, contact-maintenance, avoidance, and resistance came out of her initial distinction between Group A and Group B, and then her subsequent attempt to find order within Group C. However, if this was the only function of categories, then it would seem that they would be superseded by the scales. No further dimensional scales have been developed for the Ainsworth Strange Situation (with the exception of the D scale; Chapter 3), so this argument would appear to no longer hold.

3. A third advantage of a category-based system, according to Ainsworth, was that categories sharpen attention to potential causal factors.[176] This was, she believed, in contrast to scales, which flatten different causes of behaviour. So, for instance, both B1 and Group A infants do not show separation anxiety on separation or proximity-seeking on reunion. However, Ainsworth believed that the reason for this is different. B1 infants are able to terminate their attachment behavioural system through distance interaction, whereas Group A infants inhibit signals of their wish to approach their caregiver. However, later attachment researchers would identify that many decisions on the A/B boundary are arbitrary, reducing inter-rater reliability, as the distinction seems dimensional in certain regards. It also remains an open question whether a category-based system has indeed contributed to a better identification of causes. Some second-generation attachment researchers have remained firm defenders of

---

[172] For a review of early arguments in favour of dimensionality see Lamb, M., Thompson, R.A., Gardner, W., & Charnov, E.L. (1985) *Infant–Mother Attachment: The Origins and Developmental Significance of Individual Differences in the Strange Situation.* Hillsdale, NJ: Lawrence Erlbaum, p.281.

[173] Ainsworth, M., Blehar, M., Waters, E., & Wall, S. (1978, 2015) *Patterns of Attachment: A Psychological Study of the Strange Situation.* Bristol: Psychology Press, p.xliv.

[174] E.g. Feldman, S. & Ingham, M. (1975) Attachment behavior: a validation study in two age groups. *Child Development,* 46, 319–30.

[175] Ainsworth, M., Blehar, M., Waters, E., & Wall, S. (1978, 2015) *Patterns of Attachment: A Psychological Study of the Strange Situation.* Bristol: Psychology Press, p.56.

[176] Ibid.

Ainsworth's distinction between avoidant and ambivalent/resistant patterns. But Fonagy has argued that Ainsworth's advocacy of categories precisely directed attention away from the causal mechanisms underlying the behavioural clusters, and away from important psychometric questions about the phenomena.[177] And recently it was remarkable to see Alan Sroufe, one of the primary defenders of a category-based approach to the Strange Situation, writing to acknowledge that 'there also are very few data regarding experiences that lead to resistant versus avoidant attachment. There is a modicum of data suggesting that avoidance results from rejection precisely when the infant signals a tender need (e.g., Ainsworth et al., 1978; Isabella, 1993),[178] but the origins of these two patterns—if indeed they are coherent and distinctive—is not really established.'[179]

4. A fourth advantage proposed by Ainsworth was that categories capture salient information in a 'picture', some of which ends up lost in quantitative scales.[180] A category-based coding system appeared to offer a kind of restricting lighting to focus, highlight, and burnish the scene of observation, keeping contrasts in view even if sometimes they were oversharpened. For instance, a B2 infant shows avoidance and then proximity-seeking. The average of the two proximity-seeking scores may be little higher than a Group A infant, who engages in some proximity-seeking on first reunion, but inhibits attachment behaviour more firmly on second reunion in response to stronger activation of the attachment behavioural system. The Strange Situation prompts activation and deactivation of the attachment behavioural system carefully across episodes, and a purely quantitative approach, at least an unweighted one, would miss this process and its implications.[181] How much difference this would make to prediction was unclear, and the question soon fell away as the Ainsworth coding protocols became taken for granted within developmental science.[182]

---

[177] Fonagy, P. (1999) Points of contact and divergence between psychoanalytic and attachment theories: is psychoanalytic theory truly different? *Psychoanalytic Inquiry*, 19(4), 448–80, p.469.

[178] Ainsworth, M., Blehar, M., Waters, E., & Wall, S. (1978, 2015) *Patterns of Attachment: A Psychological Study of the Strange Situation*. Bristol: Psychology Press; Isabella, R.A. (1993) Origins of attachment: maternal interactive behavior across the first year. *Child Development*, 64(2), 605–621.

[179] Sroufe, L.A. (2016) The place of attachment in development. In J. Cassidy & P.R. Shaver (eds) *Handbook of Attachment: Theory, Research, and Clinical Applications*, 3rd edn (pp.997–1011). New York: Guilford, p.1008.

[180] Ainsworth, M., Blehar, M., Waters, E., & Wall, S. (1978, 2015) *Patterns of Attachment: A Psychological Study of the Strange Situation*. Bristol: Psychology Press, p.57. See also Ainsworth, M. (1981) *Letter to Michael Lamb*, 8 November 1981. Mary Ainsworth Archive, Box M3173, Folder 4: 'I do not think that all of the relevant basis for classification judgment has as yet been captured by the variables we have so far identified and scored.'

[181] In fact, curiously, the only study to investigate this matter empirically and in detail found that the second reunion conveyed only 10% more information than the first reunion. The advantage of the two reunions is that it strengthens the signal received by researchers about the functioning of the attachment behavioural system. Kroonenberg, P.M., Dam, M.V., IJzendoorn, M.H., & Mooijaart, A. (1997) Dynamics of behaviour in the strange situation: a structural equation approach. *British Journal of Psychology*, 88(2), 311–32: 'The second sequence does not add qualitatively new information to what is observed in the first sequence but merely intensifies the behavioural pattern. The replicated nature of the Strange Situation procedure may be one of the reasons for its robustness and its validity despite its relatively short duration' (327–8).

[182] An illustration of this transition can be seen in discussions of the B4 category. In the early 1980s, van IJzendoorn was highly concerned about B4, and urged the need for larger samples to investigate Ainsworth's subtypes, e.g. van IJzendoorn, M.H., Goossens, F.A., Kroonenberg, P.M., & Tavecchio, L.W.C. (1985) Dependent attachment: B-4 children in the strange situation. *Psychological Reports*, 57(2), 439–51. However, by the 2000s when he had data available from many more and much larger samples, van IJzendoorn appears not to have even run the analyses he himself called for two decades earlier. This shift in van IJzendoorn's position offers an especially clear illustration, perhaps even a microcosm, of the broader direction of travel of developmental science in the period. See Roisman, G.I. & van IJzendoorn, M.H. (2018) Meta-analysis and individual participant data synthesis in child development: introduction to the special section. *Child Development*, 89(6), 1939–42. A commitment

In the 1980s, as researchers in the developmental tradition of attachment research were inheriting Ainsworth's measure, they frequently commented that the category-based system captured additional information about the operation of the attachment behavioural system that was not available through the scales alone. Kroonenberg and van IJzendoorn, discussing this argument, expressed concern, however, that no one seemed to know exactly what information exactly was being added, making it a matter of faith.[183] Equally, they worried that no one seemed to know exactly what additional information might be being captured by the scales, compared to categories, other than the fact that continuous measures tend to deal better with individual variation. Both approaches might have pragmatic advantages, but without explicit discussion and testing, it would not always be clear why.[184]

Furthermore, even if categories offer a 'picture', capturing more information than scales, additional information is not always a blessing. In psychology, when overarching and encompassing categories are reified, it is then difficult to separate out the relevant elements from all the other information. The clarity with which relationships with other variables can be picked out is therefore weakened. An important case would be the Group C classification, which is coded on the basis of information about anger, inconsolability, and/or passivity. Yet only inconsolability—understood as anxiety about the availability of the attachment figure—was directly taken up by the social psychology tradition of attachment research. This contribution to differences between the measures of adult attachment has been an under-recognised source of confusion and miscommunication between the social psychology and developmental traditions (Chapter 5).

Considered as a whole, it must be acknowledged that Ainsworth's own writings were ambivalent as to whether categories were pragmatic tools to be taken up or put down as needed, or whether they should be regarded as reflecting truths cut into the nature of individual differences in attachment and a requisite of orthodox attachment research.[185] On the one hand, in *Patterns of Attachment*, Ainsworth and colleagues stated that advocacy of a category-based system was not meant to imply a rigid typological concept of the way in which human behaviour is organised, with implications of discontinuity in the various quantitative dimensions. Yet at other times Ainsworth seemed to imply that the attachment patterns represent distinct kinds of relationship. When questioned by Michael Lamb in correspondence, Ainsworth described herself as 'stubborn' in her conviction that scales will never 'be able to capture everything that should be taken into account when assigning an individual infant to a classification'.[186] Many of Ainsworth's students, including Main (Chapter 3), came to the

to subclassifications was retained in the work of Ainsworth's student Patricia Crittenden, prompting recent debate with van IJzendoorn and colleagues who argued that the fine-grained information captured by subclassifications put at risk scientific credibility, which must be based on aggregation. See Crittenden, P.M. & Spieker, S.J. (2018) DMM vs. ABC+D assessments of attachment in child protection and treatment: reply to van IJzendoorn, Bakermans, Steele, & Granqvist. *Infant Mental Health Journal*, 39(6), 647–51.

[183] Kroonenberg, P.M. & van IJzendoorn, M.H. (1987) Exploring children's behavior in the Strange Situation. In L.W.C. Tavecchio & M.H. van IJzendoorn (eds) *Attachment in Social Networks. Contributions to the Bowlby–Ainsworth Attachment Theory* (pp.379–426). New York: Elsevier, pp.380, 409.

[184] Van IJzendoorn, M.H. & Bakermans-Kranenburg, M.J. (2014) Confined quest for continuity: the categorical versus continuous nature of attachment. *Monographs of the Society for Research in Child Development*, 79(3), 157–67.

[185] Fraley, R.C. & Waller, N.G. (1998) Adult attachment patterns: a test of the typological model. In J.A. Simpson & W.S. Rholes (eds) *Attachment Theory and Close Relationships*. New York: Guilford: 'Ainsworth et al. (1978) are somewhat ambiguous regarding the ontological status of the classificatory groups' (108).

[186] Ainsworth, M. (1981) *Letter to Michael Lamb*, 8 November 1981. Mary Ainsworth Archive, Box M3173, Folder 4.

conclusion that she had discovered 'natural kinds', representing qualitatively different forms of relationships and patterns of child socioemotional development.[187] They acknowledged that scientific constructs are always approximations and simplifications of reality. However, discourses that situated attachment as by nature divided into categories influenced and infiltrated activities such as research design and coding.[188]

The Ainsworth categories were initially important in the 1970s and 1980s in countering social learning theorists, who argued that secure attachment behaviour was caused simply by the mother having reinforced approach when her infant cried. Yet Ainsworth could counter by showing that neither distressed approach nor the absence of distressed approach defined Group B, but rather the use of the caregiver as a secure base and safe haven. Yet, subsequently, the category-based system helped contribute to both the popularity and reifications of attachment theory. A tale about 'three kinds of infants' is one that can carry a tune, and it fitted well with the ascendence of diagnosis-based thinking about psychological processes in the wake of DSM-III (Chapter 1). Even if it was not Ainsworth's intention, then, a significant part of what has rippled out from the coding system for the Strange Situation was an impression of ultimate certainty.[189] The Ainsworth categories were taken as part of, or at least close to, the inner core of the attachment paradigm as a cumulative research endeavour, perhaps with some role as a symbol of the field of attachment research as a differentiated entity. And when the categories were questioned, attachment researchers tended to circle the wagons.

An illustrative case was Chris Fraley and Sue Spieker's 2003 paper 'Are infant attachment patterns continuously or categorically distributed?'[190] From the late 1990s, there had been growing concern across psychological science to replace categories with dimensions in the interests of psychometric precision and statistical power.[191] Influenced by these discussions, Fraley and Spieker held that individual differences in infant attachment were likely influenced by a variety of factors. It would therefore be expectable for these differences to occur by degrees, depending on how much one factor or another was in play. This implied quantitative, not simply qualitative, variability. Fraley, especially, was concerned that a category-based system would not only neglect this variability, but also misdirect discussions of the meaning of attachment: 'Even professional scholars have often misunderstood the theory as implying a strong continuity between early experiences and adult romantic relationships

---

[187] For other interpretations of Ainsworth that treated her categories as reflecting or like natural kinds, see e.g. Bretherton, I. (1990) Communication patterns, internal working models and the intergenerational transmission of attachment relationships. *Infant Mental Health Journal*, 11, 237–51; Crittenden, P.M. (2000) A dynamic–maturational model of the function, development, and organization of human relationships. In R.S.L. Mills & S. Duck (eds) *Developmental Psychology of Personal Relationships* (pp.199–218). New York: Wiley.

[188] See Beauchaine, T.P. & Waters, E. (2003) Pseudotaxonicity in MAMBAC and MAXCOV analyses of rating-scale data: turning continua into classes by manipulating observer's expectations. *Psychological Methods*, 8(1), 3–15.

[189] In the hands of some critics the Strange Situation was treated as some kind of marine mammal, with jaws wide as it moved through the water, ingesting individual differences like krill and exhaling pre-established categories of infants. See e.g. Knudson-Martin, C. (2012) Attachment in adult relationships. *Journal of Family Theory & Review*, 4(4), 299–305; Gaskins, S. (2013) The puzzle of attachment. In N. Quinn & J.M. Mageo (eds) *Attachment Reconsidered* (pp.33–66). London: Palgrave.

[190] Fraley, R.C. & Spieker, S.J. (2003) Are infant attachment patterns continuously or categorically distributed? A taxometric analysis of strange situation behavior. *Developmental Psychology*, 39(3), 387–404.

[191] E.g. Waller, N.G. & Meehl, P.E. (1998) *Multivariate Taxometric Procedures: Distinguishing Types from Continua*. Newbury Park, CA: Sage. For a review of this development see Kendler, K.S., Zachar, P., & Craver, C. (2011) What kinds of things are psychiatric disorders? *Psychological Medicine*, 41(6), 1143–50. This perspective has influenced the design of subsequent attachment measures, for instance Steele, H., Steele, M., & Kriss, A. (2009) *The Friends and Family Interview (FFI) Coding Guidelines*. Unpublished manuscript.

styles. We think that the typological approach ... may help promote the widespread belief that there is a single etiology.'[192]

To support their claims, Fraley and Spieker used taxometric analysis to show that Ainsworth's three patterns of attachment were better modelled as two dimensions: a dimension between avoidance and security, crossed by a dimension between resistance and security. Part of the attractiveness of this proposal was that dimensional scales might well contribute to greater statistical power; differences between dyads in the middle-range would be captured, rather than forcing cases artificially into categories. Another part of the attractiveness of the proposal was that these scales had been coded by researchers as part of making judgements about the categories. So the field could use the already-existing data on the scales from decades of work. Proximity-seeking and the absence of resistance and avoidance could offer an approximation of a dimensional characterisation of security, even if this was imperfect. A disadvantage was that scales are not coded independently, and likely influence the scoring of one another. At least, however, there would be no need to start from scratch.[193]

The Fraley and Spieker paper was initially rejected flat out by *Child Development* as too heretical. Eventually published in *Developmental Psychology*, the paper was met by hostile peer-reviews, and accompanied in print by discouraging replies from other attachment researchers.[194] This may have been prompted by the fact that the initially submitted draft of the Fraley and Spieker paper did, by the authors' own admission, at points adopt quite a strident evaluative tone.[195] Yet, as Fraley set out in his letter to the editor responding to the peer-review feedback, he regarded his position as a defence rather than attack on attachment theory. He was primarily concerned that 'if variation in attachment organisation is continuously distributed—and if it plays a strong role in shaping developmental outcomes—then attachment organisation will appear to have weak effects on other outcomes when studied categorically ... It would be an unsatisfactory state of affairs if the larger field of developmental psychology eventually became disenchanted with the study of attachment for reasons, such as measurement imprecision, that have little to do with the validity of the theory per se.'[196]

[192] Fraley, R.C. & Waller, N.G. (1998) Adult attachment patterns: a test of the typological model. In J.A. Simpson & W.S. Rholes (eds) *Attachment Theory and Close Relationships*. New York: Guilford, p.101.

[193] In fact, until the 2000s, many laboratories destroyed their data regarding the Ainsworth scales, since the focus for publications was on categories alone. This was noted by Lamb, M., Thompson, R.A., Gardner, W., & Charnov, E.L. (1985) *Infant–Mother Attachment: The Origins and Developmental Significance of Individual Differences in the Strange Situation*. Hillsdale, NJ: Lawrence Erlbaum, p.138.

[194] Cummings, E.M. (2003) Toward assessing attachment on an emotional security continuum: comment on Fraley and Spieker (2003). *Developmental Psychology*, 39, 405–408; Cassidy, J. (2003) Continuity and change in the measurement of infant attachment: comment on Fraley and Spieker (2003). *Developmental Psychology*, 39(3), 409–12.

[195] Fraley, C. (2002) *Response to Reviewers, Letter to Douglas M. Teti, Associate Editor of Developmental Psychology*, 30 January 2002. Unpublished text shared by the author: 'The reviewer seems to be supposing hostile and destructive ambitions for our paper that are simply not true' ... "Unfortunately, in the previous draft we did phrase things in a way that might lead a reader to conclude that attachment research based on the categorical model is faulty. As reviewer D noted, for example, we stated that "the typological model is invalid" on page 30 of the previous draft. In that context, we were arguing that the categorical assumption (i.e., that attachment "categories" exist) is not supported by the data. That does not imply, however, that the kinds of factors that are captured by the categorical system are invalid. As reviewer D notes, it is probably the case that the categories have been successful because they capture the relevant dimensions underlying the patterning of attachment behavior. We have revised the manuscript in order to make it clear that we are not challenging or calling into question the significance of attachment theory and research. It is precisely because we believe that this area of inquiry is important and valuable that we have posed the questions that we have in this paper.'

[196] Ibid.

There is often discussion today about opposition between a 'category' and a 'dimension' camp to Strange Situation data. However, in fact, this is something of an artefact. Both sides seem to agree that there are underlying dimensions. The question is whether a dimensional approach to the data would offer better prediction. Author of one of the critical replies to Fraley and Spieker, Alan Sroufe stated in 2000 that 'traditionally, the measurements of security of attachment have been categorical, although it would seem conceptually that there are underlying dimensions'.[197]. In fact, from the late 1980s Sroufe's close colleague Byron Egeland even used group exercises to encourage parents in their STEEP intervention (Chapter 4) to think about aspects of care and parenting as dimensions, as a dimensional perspective was regarded as likely to improve attachment security in the caregiver–infant dyads by contributing to a more 'informed, realistic understanding'.[198]

It is curious that so many years after Fraley and Spieker's paper, the field is yet to see a published comparison of the relative merits of dimensions versus categories in predicting later correlates of interest, such as externalizing behaviours. A first comparison of their relative merits for understanding antecedents of attachment was published only recently, and reported better prediction for the analysis in terms of two latent dimensions.[199] The reasons for the delay in pursuing comparative analysis are not clear, given that such inquiry could have been pursued already on the data available to Fraley and Spieker. One reason may have been that large datasets are needed to adequately address the question.[200] Nonetheless, it can be anticipated that the issue of individual differences in attachment as dimensionally or categorically distributed is likely to be one of the major objects of attention for the third generation of attachment researchers over the coming years, given their greater concern for the psychometric standing of attachment methods and coding systems, and the recent availability of pooled datasets (Chapter 6).

Interpretation of the Strange Situation

The identification of distinct attachment classifications raised the question of their defining characteristics and antecedents. In interpreting the behaviour shown by infants in the

[197] Rutter, M. & Sroufe, L.A. (2000) Developmental psychopathology: concepts and challenges. *Development & Psychopathology*, 12(03), 265–96. A few years earlier, in work with Gail Fury and Elizabeth Carlson, Sroufe had criticised Main and Kaplan's category-based system for coding family drawings at age 6 (Chapter 3) and replaced it with a series of dimensional scales. Fury, G., Carlson, E.A., & Sroufe, A. (1997) Children's representations of attachment relationships in family drawings. *Child Development*, 68(6), 1154–64. Another illustration is offered by Hesse and van IJzendoorn, generally regarded as key defenders of the category-based approach, who—with category-based data available—nonetheless reported their findings in terms of a 9-point scale 'LapseTr', comprising the highest score obtained on either the loss or abuse scale of the Adult Attachment Interview. Hesse, E. & van IJzendoorn, M. (1999) Propensities towards absorption are related to lapses in the monitoring of reasoning or discourse during the Adult Attachment Interview: a preliminary investigation. *Attachment & Human Development*, 1, 67–91.

[198] Egeland, B., Weinfield, N., Bosquet, M., & Cheng, V. (2000) Remembering, repeating, and working through: lessons from attachment-based interventions. In J. Osofsky (ed.) *WHIMH Handbook of Infant Mental Health*, Vol. 4 (pp.35–89). New York: Wiley, p.64–5.

[199] Groh, A.M., Propper, C., Mills-Koonce, R., Moore, G.A., Calkins, S., & Cox, M. (2019) Mothers' physiological and affective responding to infant distress: unique antecedents of avoidant and resistant attachments. *Child Development*, 90(2), 489–505.

[200] Another contributing factor may have been that Main and Solomon decided to code disorganization using a single encompassing scale rather than developing subscales for forms of disorganization, as Main and Hesse later did for frightening/frightened behaviour (Chapter 3). This has made it more difficult to appraise the taxonicity of disorganization.

Strange Situation, Ainsworth and colleagues drew on observations of the dyads at home and particularly caregiving behaviour by the mother. The strong relationship between the two sources of information gave Ainsworth's team confidence that the Strange Situation tapped patterns of attachment, since results were congruent with the history of infant–mother interaction.[201] In publications, Ainsworth felt obliged by the genre of academic writing in developmental psychology in the 1970s and 1980s to present her research as setting out to test hypotheses and, on this basis, discovering correlations. This gave many readers the impression that Ainsworth had more confidence in her findings than she did, and that she was emphasizing the importance of infant–mother interaction over all other factors. In fact, Ainsworth regarded her work as exploratory, seeking to identify previously unnoticed associations between infant attachment behaviour and the infant's history of receiving care, by wading around, up to the knees in her hundreds of hours of observational data.[202] In a letter from 1969 she wrote to Bowlby:

> To discover the interrelationships implicit in these data is my chief talent and all-absorbing aim. I realised that when my own intuitive feel for the data is blocked by our elaborate reliability machinery and do not hesitate to go beyond it. Thus with our attachment–exploration balance classification. I was more concerned to find the "right" basis of classification than to stop with the semi-satisfactory basis that was subject to our reliability-checks. Research is always a compromise—and presumably the most important things are to know what one's own compromise has been and not to attempt to convince either oneself or others that one has done the impossible.[203]

In a letter from 1970, she added: 'Our horrible hypothesis-testing traditional leads us (me and especially my co-authors) to lead the reader to the conclusion that we are claiming successful hypothesis testing, whereas in fact we are presenting a new viewpoint together with one small but "telling" body of evidence that seems congruent with it and hence to offer some support.'[204] Main later recalled that Ainsworth repeatedly applied over subsequent years for funding to conduct a replication of her Baltimore study without success:

> Worrying about the possibility of contaminations among variables which were only identified during the course of the study—she had intended it as a pilot investigation. In her second, planned replication study, she would make no changes, develop no new infant or maternal variables, re-conduct the strange situation procedure with no revisions in her sub-groupings, and hence properly and completely re-test her initial results. However, her applications to granting agencies to conduct this new Baltimore study were repeatedly turned down.[205]

[201] Ainsworth. M.D.S. (1983) Patterns of infant–mother attachment as related to maternal care: their early history and their contribution to continuity. In D. Magnusson & V.L. Allen (eds) *Human Development: An Interactional Perspective* (pp.35–55). New York: Academic Press, p.52.
[202] The ethos of Ainsworth's approach is revealed with remarkable clarity in her letters to Silvia Bell, especially those sent during Ainsworth's sabbatical at Stanford: Ainsworth, M. (1968) *Letter to Silvia Bell*, 2 January 1968. Mary Ainsworth Archive, Box M3169, Folder 6: 'Part of the luck has been capitalisang on differences within the sample. I work back and forth from "cause" to "effect" in the same sample. Under these circumstances it is relatively easy to get everything fitting into place.'
[203] Ainsworth, M. (1970) *Letter to John Bowlby*, 7 August 1969. PP/Bow/K.4/12.
[204] Ainsworth, M. (1970) *Letter to John Bowlby*, 1 September 1970. PP/Bow/K.4/12.
[205] Main M. (1999) Mary D. Salter Ainsworth: tribute and portrait. *Psychoanalytic Inquiry*, 19, 682–776, p.722.

It is important to highlight that in pursuing an interpretation of the Strange Situation in light of infant–mother interaction, Ainsworth was not ruling out the role of fathers on theoretical grounds, though neither did she encourage it. In part this was a distal reflection of the cultural values of the time, which emphasised the importance of maternal care. However, proximally, inattention to fathers was a by-product of Ainsworth's research design: she did not have data on infant–father interaction, since she had conducted her study during office hours in a sample where the fathers all worked away from home. She was also not ruling out that infant temperament could play a role in their behaviour during the Strange Situation procedure. 'Everybody knows that … there is something innate that each child brings', Ainsworth observed.[206] However, she anticipated that these qualities would interact with the caregiving the child received in important ways, and that it would be caregiving that would ultimately make the more important contribution to the Strange Situation classification. Ainsworth was sympathetic, for example, to the idea that some children might be predisposed to resistant behaviour in the Strange Situation as a result of a difficult or fussy temperament.[207] Some colleagues also held that it is probable that 'ambivalent babies differ from others from the beginning of life'.[208] However, Ainsworth and her group felt that the history of caregiving in the dyad was also an important contributing factor to ambivalent/resistant attachment, and that it was of overwhelming importance for secure and avoidant attachment.

Later empirical research supported Ainsworth's general position. Attachment research was an early adopter of a meta-analyses, a technique for the quantification of the combined effect of a set of study outcomes. An especially important contribution to attachment research were the conclusions regarding the role of infant temperament, in the context of raging debates about nature vs nurture in child development. Combining the effect sizes of studies to date, in a paper from 1997 van IJzendoorn and De Wolff reported a correlation of $r = .17$ between infant–mother and infant–father attachment across 14 independent samples, indicating less than 3% overlap in variance.[209] This supported Ainsworth's assumption that only a small proportion of Strange Situation behaviour could be explained by child temperament, unmodified by the particular attachment relationships infants had experienced. Indeed, a later meta-analysis of 69 independent samples by Groh, van IJzendoorn, and colleagues found that infant temperament did have an association with resistant attachment ($r = .15$). However, as expected, it had a very weak association with security ($r = .04$), and no association was found for the avoidant attachment classification.[210] The researchers flagged, however, that assessments of infant temperament are often conducted with the parent present. One of the defining characteristics of the resistant attachment classification is that the attachment behavioural system has a low threshold for activation, and is accompanied

[206] Ainsworth, M. (1997) Peter L. Rudnytsky—the personal origins of attachment theory: an interview with Mary Salter Ainsworth. *Psychoanalytic Study of the Child*, 52, 386–405, p.405.

[207] Ainsworth, M., Blehar, M., Waters, E., & Wall, S. (1978, 2015) *Patterns of Attachment: A Psychological Study of the Strange Situation*. Bristol: Psychology Press, p.182.

[208] Main, M. (1980) Avoidance of attachment figures: index of disturbance. PP/Bow/J.4/1, discussing Waters, E., Vaughn, B.E., & Egeland, B.R. (1980) Individual differences in infant–mother attachment relationships at age one: antecedents in neonatal behavior in an urban, economically disadvantaged sample. *Child Development*, 51(1), 208–16.

[209] Van IJzendoorn, M.H. & Wolff, M.S. (1997) In search of the absent father—meta-analyses of infant–father attachment: a rejoinder to our discussants. *Child Development*, 68(4), 604–609.

[210] Groh, A.M., Narayan, A.J., Bakermans-Kranenburg, M.J., et al. (2017) Attachment and temperament in the early life course: a meta-analytic review. *Child Development*, 88(3), 770–95.

by fussing and distress already when the stranger seeks to engage the child in the Strange Situation before the separations. As such, the temperament assessment *itself* may serve to elicit the resistant attachment pattern, confounding the assessment of temperament with attachment. In line with this supposition, resistance was found to be more strongly associated in the meta-analysis with greater levels of fearful distress, rather than lower levels of the expression of positive emotions.

Secure attachment

Rather than infant temperament, Ainsworth argued that the antecedents of individual differences in attachment lay primarily in experiences of caregiving. This argument was based on close comparison of elements of infant behaviour in the Strange Situation with the infant and the mother's behaviour at home. This comparison revealed that Group B infants cried less than non-B infants, especially in response to the ordinary brief separations of everyday life. They responded more positively to being picked up, and less negatively to being put down. And they were more cooperative to their mother's requests.[211] Ainsworth and colleagues also found an astonishingly strong association between the Group B classification and caregiver sensitivity: $r(21) = .78$. The association was even stronger for the prototypical B3 subtype. This was in contrast, in the data Ainsworth had available, to the non-significant association between child behaviours in the first few months of life and the Group B classification at 11 months.[212] The strong correlation with caregiver sensitivity implied that Group B represented infants who anticipated that their signals would be heeded by their caregiver. Ainsworth therefore reinstated the label 'secure' as the name for Group B, which she had initially left aside on Bowlby's urging as too value-laden.

In retrospect, this was an unfortunate decision in some ways, as the term 'security' has its own connotations that differ from Ainsworth's intended meaning of the term. Or at least, Ainsworth failed to clarify that she intended the term in a technical sense, one that departed from ordinary language. Admittedly there is no ready alternative single word in English that conveys a sense of confidence in the other's availability and responsiveness. Nonetheless, other choices could have been made by Ainsworth, such as to retain the label 'Group B', or to discuss 'care-confident' or 'availability-trusting' infants, though both are ungainly constructions. Yet the term 'secure' was already value-laden in Ainsworth's time, and furthermore has subsequently been infiltrated by a whole range of connotations.[213] Not least, the rapid rise of

[211] Ainsworth, M. (1984) Attachment. In N.S. Endler & J. McVicker Hunt (eds) *Personality and the Behavioral Disorders* (pp.559–602). New York: Wiley, p.574.

[212] Ibid. The exact tests conducted by Ainsworth are not described, so what child behaviours she examined remains unclear. And other researchers, in fact, found associations between early child orienting behaviours and later attachment, even with caregiving included in the model. The earliest such finding was Grossmann, K., Grossmann, K.E., Spangler, G., Suess, G., & Unzner, L. (1985) Maternal sensitivity and newborns' orientation responses as related to quality of attachment in northern Germany. *Monographs of the Society for Research in Child Development*, 50(1–2), 233–56.For a more recent discussion see Spangler, G. (2013) Individual dispositions as precursors of differences in attachment quality: why maternal sensitivity is nevertheless important. *Attachment & Human Development*, 15(5–6), 657–72.

[213] Harwood, R.L., Miller, J.G., & Irizarry, N.L. (1995) *Culture and Attachment: Perceptions of the Child in Context*. New York: Guilford: 'The concept of "security", although technically similar to a sense of psychological safety, has become laden with an array of values and ideals peculiar to mainstream U.S. discourse: the "secure" person is self-confident, independent, and able to utilise his or her talents and abilities to the fullest, but also has the capacity to be empathetic and to relate to others. In short, the "secure" individual is one who embodied U.S. ideals of optimal socioemotional development—ideals that may or may not translate well into the meaning

morally laden discourses about security in contemporary 'risk society' has helped failures of security connote danger and destruction.[214] A semantic mapping exercise conducted by Waters with psychology students found that they used the connotations of the word to make spurious assumptions. For instance, it was assumed that 'security' for Ainsworth meant confident, and therefore someone socially dominant.[215] Sociologists have observed that the connotations of Ainsworth's terms have helped support both the popularisation and popular misconceptions of attachment ideas, including moralizing narratives in which insecure babies have been broken by their caregivers.[216] Ainsworth's students, especially those with clinical training, have made much the same point. The eminent clinician Alicia Lieberman, a graduate student of Ainsworth's, offered a rare criticism of her teacher for failing to adequately clarify that the meaning of 'security' differed from ordinary language. Lieberman alleged that attachment researchers since Ainsworth have slid about unsteadily between various connotations of the term 'secure attachment'.[217] Other attachment researchers also trained as clinicians, for instance Pasco Fearon, have made the same point.[218]

Though warned about the unhelpful connotations of the term 'secure' by Bowlby, Ainsworth felt that this Blatzian concept captured the infant confidence in the caregiver's availability, a confidence that seemed to be reflected in behaviour and that was at least somewhat stable over time. Use of a term from everyday language also perhaps appealed to help signal that there would be multiple contributories to a sense of confidence in the availability of others, not just early care. Furthermore, use of a term with strong and evocative meanings in ordinary language, even if they were rather misleading, may have been attractive for supporting interest in the nascent area of attachment research, though there is no evidence to suggest that this was intentional on Ainsworth's part. Ultimately, Ainsworth felt that she could rest on the etymological meaning of 'security' as being without concern or worry.[219] Not only were Group B infants able to use their caregiver effectively as a secure base and safe

systems of other cultural groups' (143–4); Weisner, T.S. (2005) Attachment as a cultural and ecological problem with pluralistic solutions. *Human Development*, 48(1–2), 89–94: 'Using the word "secure" assumes that there is, in cultures everywhere, a positive valence for development associated with that behavior profile' (91). Bowlby did not help matters in his characterization of the diverse perceived virtues of the Apollo 13 astronauts in terms of their attachment security. Bowlby, J. (1970, 1979) Self-reliance and some conditions that promote it. In *The Making and Breaking of Affectional Bonds* (pp.124–49). London: Routledge, p.129. See Laubender, C. (2019) From the bomb to Apollo 13: Bowlby and the Cold War. *The Psychologist*, 32, 76–9.

[214] E.g. Huysmans, J. (1998) Security! What do you mean? From concept to thick signifier. *European Journal of International Relations*, 4(2), 226–55; Harrington, C. & Shearing, C. (2017) *Security in the Anthropocene: Reflections on Safety and Care*. New York: Columbia University Press.

[215] Everett Waters, personal communication, July 2019.

[216] Thornton, D.J. (2011) Neuroscience, affect, and the entrepreneurialization of motherhood. *Communication and Critical/Cultural Studies*, 8(4), 399–424; Wall, G. (2018) 'Love builds brains': representations of attachment and children's brain development in parenting education material. *Sociology of Health & Illness*, 40(3), 395–409.

[217] Lieberman, A.F. & Van Horn, P. (2008) *Psychotherapy with Infants and Young Children*. New York: Guilford, p.11. Liberman would make the same point about Main's term 'disorganised attachment' (Chapter 3).

[218] E.g. Fearon, R.M.P., Bakermans-Kranenburg, M.J., & van IJzendoorn, M.H. (2010) Jealousy and attachment: the case of twins. In S.L. Hart & M. Legerstee (eds) *Handbook of Jealousy. Theory, Research, and Multidisciplinary Approaches* (pp.362–86). New York: Wiley, p.372.

[219] Ainsworth, M. (1969) CPA oral history of psychology in Canada interview. Unpublished. http://www.feministvoices.com/assets/Women-Past/Ainsworth/Mary-Ainsworth-CPA-Oral-History.pdf. Working on her thesis, in discussion with Bott: 'We came to the word "security" which I had defined in my own way, because it was a key concept, and I had defined it in a sort of Blatzian way. He said, "That is not the meaning of the word 'security'. Don't you know the original meaning of the word security?" And I shouted, "It doesn't matter what the original meaning was!" I was really angry at this point. He said, "It does matter." He implied that a word was a word and it never really lost that original meaning. And you know, he was right. He told me the word "security" had a Latin derivation and meant *sine cura* (without care).'

haven in the Strange Situation, but also this security seemed intelligible in the context of the sensitive caregiving the infants received at home, which would make them unconcerned or not worried about the caregiver's availability. As a consequence, these infants could implement the 'short version' of the expression of the attachment behavioural system, since the system was not complicated by inhibition, anger, or other forms of conflict or guardedness.

Looking back, researchers such as Sroufe and van IJzendoorn recalled that early reports of the strength of the association between Strange Situation behaviour and caregiver sensitivity reported in *Patterns of Attachment* contributed to an intense interest in attachment theory and to use of the Strange Situation among a generation of younger researchers.[220] It was, though, very rare for extensive naturalistic observations at home to take place; such an expenditure of resources would have been reckless for a developmental psychologist in a field increasingly focused from the 1970s onwards on quantification and rapid research. The naturalistic observations conducted by Ainsworth and colleagues were, perhaps in part as a result, treated as sufficient, especially since the association between secure attachment and caregiver sensitivity would replicate time and again through the 1980s. In the 1990s, Ainsworth's conclusions were also backed up by findings that naturalistic or intervention-based changes in caregiver sensitivity had significant effects on the frequency of secure attachment, supporting the idea of a close causal relationship.[221]

The relationship between caregiver sensitivity and infant attachment appeared to be well replicated. However, few studies found an association with anything like the strength of Ainsworth's original Baltimore study. A meta-analysis in 1997 by Wolff and van IJzendoorn found a much lower association than Ainsworth, with $r(835) = .24$ for mothers and $r(544) = .13$ for fathers.[222] Van IJzendoorn commented that it has been disheartening for younger researchers to find such modest effect sizes, when they had been led by Ainsworth's initial work to expect vast correlations.[223] Nonetheless, he emphasised that these are still very notable findings, reflecting processes that, over time, are threaded through thousands upon thousands of child–caregiver interactions. Furthermore, many of the studies included in the meta-analysis depended on very short periods of observation; the study with the second longest period of observation after the Baltimore study found associations between sensitivity and security similar to those of Ainsworth.[224] Recent work by Madigan and colleagues found that the association between caregiver sensitivity and infant Strange Situation classification was moderated by the measure used. The Maternal Behaviour Q-sort

[220] Sroufe, L.A. (1985) Attachment classification from the perspective of infant–caregiver relationships and infant temperament. *Child Development*, 56(1), 1–14, p.7; Wolff, M.S. & van IJzendoorn, M.H. (1997) Sensitivity and attachment: a meta-analysis on parental antecedents of infant attachment. *Child Development*, 68(4), 571–91, p.585. On the 'winner's curse' of unrepresentatively strong findings in early studies leaving a legacy for later research see Young, N.S., Ioannidis, J.P.A., & Al-Ubaydli, O. (2008) Why current publication practices may distort science. *PLoS Med*, 5 (10), e201.

[221] Van IJzendoorn, M., Juffer, F., & Duyvesteyn, M. (1995) Breaking the intergenerational cycle of insecure attachments: a review of attachment-based interventions on maternal sensitivity and infant security. *Journal of Child Psychology and Psychiatry*, 36, 225–48; Howes, C., Galinsky, E., & Kontos, S. (1998) Child care caregiver sensitivity and attachment. *Social Development*, 7(1), 25–36.

[222] Wolff, M. S. & van IJzendoorn, M.H. (1997) Sensitivity and attachment: a meta-analysis on parental antecedents of infant attachment. *Child Development*, 68(4), 571–91; Van IJzendoorn, M.H. & Wolff, M.S. (1997) In search of the absent father—meta-analyses of infant–father attachment: a rejoinder to our discussants. *Child Development*, 68(4), 604–609.

[223] Van IJzendoorn, M.H. (2019) Replication crisis lost in translation? Paper presented at International Attachment Conference, Vancouver, 20 July 2019.

[224] Pederson, D.R., Gleason, K.E., Moran, G., & Bento, S. (1998) Maternal attachment representations, maternal sensitivity, and the infant–mother attachment relationship. *Developmental Psychology*, 34(5), 925–33.

developed by David Pederson, Greg Moran, and Sandi Bento,[225] and the CARE-Index developed by Patricia Crittenden during graduate study with Ainsworth[226] had the strongest associations, whereas other assessments of sensitivity, including Ainsworth's original measure, had weaker associations.[227]

Researchers have generally not returned to Ainsworth's methodology of naturalistic observation to reconsider the sensitivity–attachment link inductively. Instead, the approach adopted by attachment researchers has generally been deductive identification of other factors. In subsequent years, other factors besides sensitivity have been identified deductively and then found to be important. One is the emotional climate of the home in higher-risk samples, which appears to exert direct influence on child security unmediated by the behaviour of the parent towards the child.[228] Researchers also found important moderators of the sensitivity–attachment link. Child genotype may play a role, with a gene × environment interaction proposed by Barry, Kochanska, and Philibert, though evidence to date has not consistently confirmed this proposal.[229] Another moderator of caregiver sensitivity for attachment security may be the extent and manner of parental involvement with the child, which have substantial gender differences in many samples.[230] Further study of moderators of the relationship between sensitivity and attachment has flourished recently, with the availability of large datasets permitting comparison of the correlates of sensitivity in low-risk and high-risk samples.[231]

Researchers such as Elizabeth Meins have proposed that at least some of the association between caregiver sensitivity and infant attachment can be explained by the caregiver's

[225] Pederson, D.R. & Moran, G. (1995) Appendix B: maternal behavior Q-set. *Monographs of the Society for Research in Child Development*, 60(2–3), 247–54.

[226] Crittenden, P.M. (1979) CARE Index: coding manual. Unpublished manual, Miami, FL. The CARE Index scales false positive affect and a construct of 'compulsivity'. It also differentiates insensitive intrusiveness from insensitive unresponsiveness. Madigan and colleagues reported a much larger range for the CARE Index than for other measures in terms of associations with sensitivity across studies. This may reflect the wider lens of the CARE Index, which can be anticipated to contribute to measurement variance between studies with populations characterized by different caregiving profiles.

[227] Madigan, S., Verhage, M.K., Schuengel, C., et al. (2019) Parental sensitivity and mentalization as predictors of attachment quality: a meta-analysis. Paper presented at International Attachment Conference, Vancouver, 20 July 2019. Length of of time of observation was not a moderator. But this was likely clouded by differences between the measures. Madigan and colleagues also reported that when coders of sensitivity and infant Strange Situations were not independent, $r = 1.08$. An important appraisal of the different measures of sensitivity, and an attempt to synthesize their strengths through differentiated subscales, has recently been published: Heinisch, C., Galeris, M.G., Gabler, S., et al. (2019) Mothers with postpartum psychiatric disorders: proposal for an adapted method to assess maternal sensitivity in interaction with the child. *Frontiers in Psychiatry*, 22 July, 10.

[228] Raikes, H.A. & Thompson, R.A. (2005) Links between risk and attachment security: models of influence. *Journal of Applied Developmental Psychology*, 26(4), 440–55. Raikes and Thompson contrasted the emotion climate of the home with the role of socioeconomic factors, which they found influenced the security of attachment as mediated by caregiver behaviour.

[229] Barry, R.A., Kochanska, G., & Philibert, R.A. (2008) G× E interaction in the organization of attachment: mothers' responsiveness as a moderator of children's genotypes. *Journal of Child Psychology and Psychiatry*, 49(12), 1313–20; Luijk, M.P., Roisman, G.I., Haltigan, J.D., et al. (2011) Dopaminergic, serotonergic, and oxytonergic candidate genes associated with infant attachment security and disorganization? In search of main and interaction effects. *Journal of Child Psychology and Psychiatry*, 52(12), 1295–307.

[230] Lamb, M.E. (2002) Infant–father attachments and their impact on child development. In C.S. Tamis-LeMonda & N. Cabrera (eds) *Handbook of Father Involvement: Multidisciplinary Perspective* (pp.93–117). Mahwah, NJ: Lawrence Erlbaum; Lucassen, N., Tharner, A., van IJzendoorn, M.H., et al. (2011) The association between paternal sensitivity and infant–father attachment security: a meta-analysis of three decades of research. *Journal of Family Psychology*, 25(6), 986–92.

[231] Verhage, M.L., Fearon, R.P., Schuengel, C., et al. (2019) Collaboration on attachment transmission synthesis. Does risk background affect intergenerational transmission of attachment? Testing a moderated mediation model with IPD. Paper presented at Biennial Meeting of Society for Research in Child Development, Baltimore, MD.

attention to and interest in the child's emotional experience.[232] Fonagy and colleagues even argued that this association is an artefact, with both caregiver sensitivity and individual differences in the Strange Situation reflecting the caregivers' capacity to imagine, perceive, and interpret their child's behaviour in terms of intentional mental states (e.g., needs, desires, feelings, beliefs, goals, and reasons), as well as their own behaviour towards the child in such terms. They have termed this general capacity 'mentalisation', and as 'reflective function' when it is applied within an attachment relationship.[233] Recently, Fonagy and colleagues proposed that individual differences in infant attachment reflect forms of trust or distrust in information given by caregivers about the environment and their own availability. Whereas Ainsworth argued that Bowlby missed the value of learning in thinking about the evolutionary function of attachment relationships, Fonagy and colleagues took this argument further. They speculated that the most important evolutionary function of attachment relationships is that young children learn from their caregiver whether trust or distrust is the safer response to personally relevant information.[234] Evaluating the criticisms of Ainsworth by Fonagy and colleagues, Zeegers and colleagues conducted a meta-analysis to investigate the relative contributions of sensitivity and mentalisation to infant attachment classifications. They found that together the two predictors accounted for 12% of variance in attachment classsifications. After controlling for sensitivity, the relationship between parental mentalisation and infant–caregiver security was $r = .24$. And after controlling for mentalisation, the relationship between parental sensitivity and infant–caregiver security was $r = .19$. Sensitivity also partially mediated the association between mentalisation and infant–caregiver security ($r = .07$).[235] Such findings suggest that Meins, Fonagy, and others were right to argue for the importance of mentalisation, but that sensitivity is not reducible to mentalisation.[236]

Besides her emphasis on the causal role of caregiver sensitivity, another source of later controversy lay in Ainsworth's description of Group B, and the prototypically secure B3 subgroup in particular, as 'normative':

Subgroup B3 is the largest in the sample, and accounts for 42% of the total sample. We consider it to be the normative group, not merely because it is the largest, but also because, as

[232] Meins, E., Fernyhough, C., Fradley, E., & Tuckey, M. (2001) Rethinking maternal sensitivity: mothers' comments on infants' mental processes predict security of attachment at 12 months. *Journal of Child Psychology and Psychiatry and Allied Disciplines*, 42(5), 637–48; Koren-Karie, N., Oppenheim, D., Dolev, S., Sher, E., & Etzion-Carasso, A. (2002) Mothers' insightfulness regarding their infants' internal experience: relations with maternal sensitivity and infant attachment. *Developmental Psychology*, 38(4), 534–42.

[233] Fonagy, P. Steele, H., Steele, M., & Holder, J. (1997) Attachment and theory of mind: overlapping constructs? *Association for Child Psychology and Psychiatry Occasional Papers*, 14, 31–40.

[234] Fonagy, P. & Allison, E. (2014) The role of mentalizing and epistemic trust in the therapeutic relationship. *Psychotherapy*, 51(3), 372–80.

[235] Zeegers, M.A., Colonnesi, C., Stams, G.J.J., & Meins, E. (2017) Mind matters: a meta-analysis on parental mentalization and sensitivity as predictors of infant–parent attachment. *Psychological Bulletin*, 143(12), 1245–72.

[236] On the interpretation of effect sizes in psychology see Funder, D.C. & Ozer, D.J. (2019) Evaluating effect size in psychological research: sense and nonsense. *Advances in Methods and Practices in Psychological Science*, 2(2) 156–68: 'An effect-size r of .05 indicates an effect that is very small for the explanation of single events but potentially consequential in the not-very-long run, an effect-size r of .10 indicates an effect that is still small at the level of single events but potentially more ultimately consequential, an effect-size r of .20 indicates a medium effect that is of some explanatory and practical use even in the short run and therefore even more important, and an effect-size r of .30 indicates a large effect that is potentially powerful in both the short and the long run. A very large effect size (r = .40 or greater) in the context of psychological research is likely to be a gross overestimate that will rarely be found in a large sample or in a replication' (156).

we subsequently show, it is the subgroup whose members have the most harmonious interaction with their mothers.[237]

'Normative' is a tricky word. As Cicchetti and Beeghly observed, the term confusingly hinges judgements about what differs from a constant or average with assumptions about deviance or defectiveness.[238] The frequency of B3, the fact that it seemed a prototypical expression of the attachment behavioural system, uncomplicated by avoidance or resistance, and the strong relationship between B3 and caregiver sensitivity led Ainsworth and colleagues to speculate that this is the natural state of mothers and infants. They argued that the human attachment behavioural system is 'adapted (in the evolutionary sense) to include a mother whose reciprocal maternal behaviours are sensitively turned to infant signals'.[239] Ainsworth and her group accepted Bowlby's dictum on this matter that 'natural is better' (Chapter 1),[240] and hence that sensitive caregiving was both evolutionarily expectable and had the best implications for a child's mental health, in both the short and long term. In Ainsworth's view, 'the ordinary expectable social environment for a young child is both responsive and protective. These assumptions imply a fundamental compatibility between man and society';[241] in contrast, Groups A and C were believed to represent "developmental anomalies".[242]

This is a conclusion that Robert Hinde contested on two counts.[243] In criticizing Ainsworth's position, Hinde drew upon developments in ethology in the 1970s that were subsequent to Bowlby's development of his theory of the evolutionary function of attachment. John Maynard Smith and Richard Dawkins introduced the idea that evolution may have selected for a repertoire of behavioural patterns for achieving reproductive success in diverse circumstances (Chapter 3).[244] The 'optimal strategy' would be the one preferred when circumstances were favourable, and would generally be the most direct way of achieving reproductive success. However, 'conditional strategies' would be available as alternatives that would have greater likelihood of success under less-favourable circumstances. On the basis of these developments in the theory of evolutionary biology, Hinde argued that just because

[237] Ainsworth, M., Blehar, M., Waters, E., & Wall, S. (1978, 2015) *Patterns of Attachment: A Psychological Study of the Strange Situation*. Bristol: Psychology Press, p.229.

[238] Cicchetti, D. & Beeghly, M. (1990) An organizational approach to the study of Down syndrome: contributions to an integrative theory of development. In D. Cicchetti & M. Beeghly (eds) *Children with Down syndrome: A Developmental Perspective* (pp.29–62). Cambridge: Cambridge University Press, p.32. See also Canguilhem, G. (1966, 1989) *The Normal and the Pathological*, trans. C.R. Fawcett & R.S. Cohen. New York: Zone Books.

[239] Ainsworth, M.D.S. (1976) Discussion of papers by Suomi and Bowlby. In: G. Serban (ed.) *Animal Models in Human Psychobiology* (pp.37–47). New York: Plenum Press, p.43.

[240] When Bob Marvin, a former student and close colleague of Ainsworth, wrote to raise with Bowlby the question of whether infants could be adapted to various forms of caregiving environment, the reply (copied to Mary Ainsworth) was uncompromising: 'I need a lot of convincing that all these variations optimise infants' chances of survival.' Bowlby, J. (1975) *Letter to Robert Marvin*, 5 November 1975. PP/Bow/J.9/132. Nonetheless, Bowlby would ultimately be convinced (Chapter 3).

[241] Stayton, D.J., Hogan, R., & Ainsworth, M. (1971) Infant obedience and maternal behavior: the origins of socialization reconsidered. *Child Development*, 42(4), 1057–69, p.1059. The term 'ordinary expectable social environment' may have meant ordinary expectable social environment for forming an attachment relationship, rather than expectable within human evolutionary history, or expectable for twentieth century mothers. Ultimately, Ainsworth's intentions with the term are difficult to identify from her writings.

[242] Ainsworth, M.D.S. (1979) Attachment as related to mother–infant interaction. In J.S. Rosenblatt, R.A. Hinde, C. Beer, & M. Busnel (eds) *Advances in the Study of Behavior*, Vol. 9. (pp.1–51). New York: Academic Press, p.44.

[243] Hinde, R.A. (1982) Attachment: some conceptual and biological issues. In J. Stevenson-Hinde & C. Murray Parkes (eds) *The Place of Attachment in Human Behavior* (pp.60–78). New York: Basic Books.

[244] Smith, J.M. (1979) Game theory and the evolution of behaviour. *Proceedings of the Royal Society London, B*, 205(1161), 475–88; Brockmann, H.J., Grafen, A., & Dawkins, R. (1979) Evolutionarily stable nesting strategy in a digger wasp. *Journal of Theoretical Biology*, 77(4), 473–96.

it was common, and a direct expression of the attachment behavioural system, B3 could not be treated as an ideal appropriate to all circumstances. Nor could sensitivity be assumed to be expectable for human infants in the environment within which humans evolved; quite the opposite. Even if the secure pattern of attachment might have the better long-term outcomes, the other patterns of attachment may offer short-term advantages for achieving caregiver availability. Ever cautious about presenting proposals about the evolutionary origins of behaviour, Hinde did not press on to discuss what the advantages might be of the non-secure patterns of attachment.[245] His point was primarily to offer caution regarding the assumption that security is always best, both in the short and long term. Ainsworth was displeased with Hinde's remarks.[246] However, as Chapter 3 shows, Main came to much the same conclusions as Hinde, and took these conclusions further.[247] Though the debate has continued, Hinde's position seems certainly the more common one today among attachment researchers.

Avoidant attachment

Avoidant behaviour on reunion with the caregiver in the Strange Situation may last just a few seconds. Nonetheless, Ainsworth thought that the behaviour seemed important. Comparing Group A behaviour in the Strange Situation with their home observation data, Ainsworth and colleagues found apparently paradoxical results. Though infants in Group A dyads were precisely those that did not show distress in the Strange Situation, at home they were the most frequently distressed and aggressive.[248] The avoidance shown in the Strange Situation was definitively not a stable trait between the laboratory and the home setting. Curiously this point was missed by many of the second generation of attachment researchers, who assumed that lack of distress would characterise Group A infants across contexts in their theory and even in their design of measurement instruments.[249]

---

[245] Griffiths, P.E. (2008) History of ethology comes of age. *Biology and Philosophy*, 23, 129–34: 'At some stage in the mid-50s Hinde and Tinbergen explicitly discussed a division of the "four questions" of ethology (Tinbergen 1963), with the Oxford program focusing on "survival value" and "evolution", and the Cambridge department on "development" and "causation" (Hinde, personal communication)' (132).

[246] Ainsworth offered a long and detailed critical discussion of Hinde's remarks in Ainsworth, M. (1983) *Letter to Klaus Grossmann*, 13 January 1983. Mary Ainsworth Archive, Box M3173, Folder 4. Her main counterarguments were as follows: (i) the language of 'adaptation' used to refer to the insecure strategies by Hinde risked implying that they are equally good, when in fact longer-term security surely tends to be better; (ii) 'I see no reason for arguing that it is part of that normal time-frame for human mothers to reject their infants in the interests of infant autonomy and/or maximisang their own reproductive potential at 6 months or even at 1 year of age'; 'my point is that in the human species efforts to foster independence through withholding close contact from a baby when he is upset and much wants contact do not foster a healthy kind of independence. Perhaps such efforts, if gradual rather than abrupt, may foster self-reliance without destroying the security of attachment when begun in the second year of life. But I think that any time in the first year is too soon'; (iii) 'to understand the relationship between a given parent and a particular child obviously attachment cannot be the sole focus of attention'.

[247] For a recent review of critiques of the 'normative' position assigned to security by Bowlby and Ainsworth see Simpson, J.A. & Belsky, J. (2016) Attachment theory within a modern evolutionary framework. In J. Cassidy & P.R. Shaver (eds) *Handbook of Attachment: Theory, Research, and Clinical Applications* (pp.91–116). New York: Guilford.

[248] Ainsworth, M.D.S. (1977) Social development in the first year of life: maternal influences on infant–mother attachment. In J.M. Tanner (ed.) *Developments in Psychiatric Research* (pp.1–20). London: Hodder & Stoughton, p.17. Ainsworth's initial findings were elaborated and further confirmed by a secondary analysis of Ainsworth's data by Main: Main, M. & Stadtman, J. (1981) Infant response to rejection of physical contact by the mother. *Journal of the American Academy of Child Psychiatry*, 20(2), 292–307.

[249] E.g. Pederson, D.R. & Moran, G. (1995) A categorical description of infant–mother relationships in the home and its relation to Q-sort measures of infant–mother interaction. *Monographs of the Society for Research in*

A secondary analysis conducted by Main revealed that Group A infants exceeded both the other groups in terms of the number of times contact was initiated at home.[250] However, this proximity-seeking tended to have a 'tentative' quality, 'making partial approaches followed by moving off, or by going the whole way and then merely touching her'.[251] Yet when they did achieve close physical contact, they did not show active contact behaviour such as sinking in or relaxing comfortably against the mother's body. 'When put down they were more likely than infants of other groups to protest or to signal to be picked up again', despite the fact that protesting on being put down was the Group C signature move in the Strange Situation.[252]

Group A behaviour in the Strange Situation was also associated with relatively less-sensitive behaviour by caregivers towards their infants at home. The strongest association between Group A and caregiver behaviour in the home observation data was 'picking the baby up in an abrupt and interfering manner'. There was also a substantial negative relationship between Group A classification in the Strange Situation and a measure of 'affectionate behaviour while holding the baby' by the mothers in the home environment over the first year.[253] For instance, Tracey and Ainsworth reported that the mothers in Group A dyads kissed their babies more frequently than other dyads, but cuddled their babies proportionately less.[254] Ainsworth noted, however, that the baby also contributed to these dynamics. Assessments of 'tender, careful holding' of the baby predicted positive infant response in subsequent quarters, whereas positive infant response to holding did not predict maternal careful holding going forward. That is, the mothers' tender holding seemed to be driving the infants' response to holding and not vice versa.[255] This profile of findings together suggested to Ainsworth and colleagues that Group A attachment, and perhaps all attachment patterns, could be regarded as partly the result of a spiral between caregiver and infant signals.

Whilst, in general, 'tender, careful holding' aligned with Ainsworth's measure of sensitivity, an exception was the B1 subgroup of dyads. These dyads were classified as secure since infants greeted their caregiver with joy on reunion in the Strange Situation. However, like Group A, the infants did not approach their caregiver. In the home observations, B1 caregivers were found to be relatively sensitive: the average score out of 9 on the sensitivity scale was 7.4 for B3 dyads and 4.5 for B1 and B2 dyads, compared to scores 2–3 for Group A and C dyads.[256] However, in contrast to the other Group B dyads, the caregivers in B1 dyads received high ratings on apparent aversion to physical contact with their infant, though

Child Development, 60(2–3), 111–32; Pederson, D.R. & Moran, G. (1996) Expressions of the attachment relationship outside of the strange situation. *Child Development*, 67(3), 915–27.

[250] Reported from Main's secondary analysis of Ainsworth's home observation data: Main, M. (1980) Avoidance of attachment figures: index of disturbance. PP/Bow/J.4/1.

[251] Ainsworth, M.D.S. (1977) Social development in the first year of life: maternal influences on infant–mother attachment. In: J.M. Tanner (ed.) *Developments in Psychiatric Research* (pp.1–20). London: Hodder & Stoughton, p.18.

[252] Ainsworth, M., Blehar, M., Waters, E., & Wall, S. (1978, 2015) *Patterns of Attachment: A Psychological Study of the Strange Situation*. Bristol: Psychology Press, p.127.

[253] Ibid. p.145; Ainsworth, M. (1979) Infant–mother attachment. *American Psychologist*, 34(10), 932–7. Note 1, citing unpublished data. The researchers did not explain how they operationalized 'affectionate behaviour while holding the baby'.

[254] Tracey, R.L. & Ainsworth, M. (1981) Maternal affectionate behaviour and infant–mother attachment patterns. *Child Development*, 52(4), 1341–3.

[255] Ainsworth, M.D.S. (1979) Attachment as related to mother–infant interaction. In J.S. Rosenblatt, R.A. Hinde, C. Beer, & M. Busnel (eds) *Advances in the Study of Behavior*, Vol. 9. (pp.1–51). New York: Academic Press, p.29.

[256] Ainsworth, M., Blehar, M., Waters, E., & Wall, S. (1978, 2015) *Patterns of Attachment: A Psychological Study of the Strange Situation*. Bristol: Psychology Press, p.230, Table 27.

caregiver aversion to physical contact in B1 dyads was still lower than that for caregivers of Group A dyads.[257]

Ainsworth sought to make sense of the profile of behaviours of Group A infants in the Strange Situation and their experience at home. It appeared at first sight very surprising that Group A infants were the most distressed and angry at home, and yet responded to the Strange Situation with attentional and behavioural avoidance of the caregiver on reunion. Yet this discrepancy made sense in light of findings that infants in Group A received relatively less sensitive care. What appeared to Ainsworth to be taking place was visible and predictable evidence of a psychological inhibition: the attachment behavioural system was being activated by the Strange Situation, but its expression was being suppressed. In a letter from 1967 with some early speculations, Ainsworth wrote to Bowlby:

> This makes me think that at the same time that the baby is developing attachment behaviour (and I think of this as being developed through a feed-back rather than a reinforcement model) he may well also be developing defensive reactions to bring into play when he doesn't get the feedback he has come to expect. So a baby at one-year who seems relatively little attached may merely be one who has already built up a primitive but fairly effective defensive system. The whole thing makes considerable sense to me—especially because the babies of A1 nearly all had some fragments of attachment behaviour.[258]

At a time when speculations about motivation and inner processes were still anathema in much of American psychology, in the context of a backlash against the speculative and untestable mechanisms posited by psychoanalysis, this was an electrifying finding. The priority given to scientific prediction, feedback, and passively learnt behaviour in behaviourism was achieved precisely through the characteristic concerns of psychoanalysis on family context, internal conflict, the active defensive strategies of the individual, and the role of invisible motivations in prompting and inhibiting behaviour. Ainsworth's distinction between Groups A and B integrated apparently irreconcilable trends within psychology: she was studying family context and defensive strategies precisely through a laboratory-based, replicable observational study. This made her work especially eye-catching to contemporaries. Ainsworth later recalled that 'the fact that the Strange Situation was not in the home environment, that it was in the lab, really helped. I only did it as an adjunct to my naturalistic research, but it was the thing that everyone could accept somehow. It was so *demonstrable*.'[259]

With new doctoral students entering the research group in the early 1970s, Ainsworth's team became interested in why infants from Group A dyads concentrated their attention on toys just at the moment when other infants showed distress. The quality of this attention to the toys was poor, 'showing no investigative interest in the objects that they were either manipulating or moving toward, but rather banging them about repeatedly or throwing and retrieving them repeatedly'.[260] It seemed that the toys were being used as a distraction to avoid attending to the caregiver and other cues for the activation of the attachment system. Group A was therefore termed 'avoidant' by Ainsworth.

---

[257] Ibid. p.232 and Table 28.

[258] Ainsworth, M. (1967) *Letter to John Bowlby*, 17 October 1967. PP/Bow/K.4/12.

[259] Interview with Mary Ainsworth by Robert Karen cited in Karen, R. (1998) *Becoming Attached: First Relationships and How They Shape Our Capacity to Love*. Oxford: Oxford University Press, p.163.

[260] Ainsworth, M., Blehar, M., Waters, E., & Wall, S. (1978, 2015) *Patterns of Attachment: A Psychological Study of the Strange Situation*. Bristol: Psychology Press, p.275.

Influenced by Main's emerging ideas (Chapter 3), Ainsworth came to believe that the avoidant behaviour 'protects the baby from experiencing the rebuff that he has come to expect when he seeks close contact with his mother. It thus somewhat lowers his level of anxiety (arousal). It also leads him to turn to the neutral world of things.'[261] Avoidance allows the infant to remain alongside the caregiver, even if closeness is not achieved, whilst also escaping the contradiction between a desire to approach the caregiver and concern about what has happened in the past when physical closeness has been sought. The attention and orientation to the toys are aspects of what from the 1980s Ainsworth would term, following Bowlby, the 'defensive exclusion' of the attachment behavioural system: 'It is suggested that Pattern A babies under stress systematically exclude from perception (i.e. from highest-level processing) information that might intensely activate attachment behaviour. Thus they tend not to be distressed when the mother leaves the room in the separation episodes of the strange situation and when she returns to the reunion episodes, resorting instead to diversionary activity, which in this situation commonly consists of what appears to be exploratory behaviour.'[262] Both distress and the desire for comfort are excluded, resulting, Ainsworth speculated, in the maintenance of equilibrium.

Subsequent researchers have taken from Ainsworth's findings and theory the conclusion that avoidant attachment results from caregiver insensitivity in the form of rebuff of attachment signals. Though showing weaker effects than Ainsworth, later research generally replicated Ainsworth's findings that caregivers of avoidant dyads show lower levels of sensitivity than securely attached dyads,[263] and that caretakers in avoidant dyads specifically display higher levels of intrusive behaviour towards their infants.[264] Until recently, there has been remarkably little discussion of alternative pathways to avoidant attachment besides rebuff of attachment signals.[265] This is despite the fact that researchers have, over the years, empirically documented that other caregiver behaviours in naturalistic settings are associated with avoidance in the Strange Situation. Main's own analysis of the Ainsworth home observation data revealed that not only maternal rejecting behaviours but also maternal angry

---

[261] Ibid. p.312.

[262] Ainsworth, M. (1984) Attachment. In N.S Endler & J. McVicker Hunt (eds) *Personality and the Behavioral Disorders* (pp.559–602). New York: Wiley, p.566.

[263] E.g. Grossmann, K., Grossmann, K.E., Spangler, G., Suess, G., & Unzner, L. (1985) Maternal sensitivity and newborns' orientation responses as related to quality of attachment in northern Germany. *Monographs of the Society for Research in Child Development*, 50(1–2), 233–56; Koren-Karie, N., Oppenheim, D., Dolev, S., Sher, E., & Etzion-Carasso, A. (2002) Mothers' insightfulness regarding their infants' internal experience: relations with maternal sensitivity and infant attachment. *Developmental Psychology*, 38(4), 534.

[264] E.g. Smith, P.B. & Pederson, D.R. (1988) Maternal sensitivity and patterns of infant–mother attachment. *Child Development*, 59(4), 1097–101; Isabella, R. & Belsky, J. (1991) Interactional synchrony and the origins of infant–mother attachment. *Child Development*, 62, 373–84.

[265] Early exceptions include Lamb, M., Thompson, R.A., Gardner, W., & Charnov, E.L. (1985) *Infant–Mother Attachment: The Origins and Developmental Significance of Individual Differences in the Strange Situation.* Hillsdale, NJ: Lawrence Erlbaum, p.96; Grossmann, K.E., Grossmann, K., & Schwan, A. (1986) Capturing the wider view of attachment: a reanalysis of Ainsworth's Strange Situation. In C.E. Izard & P.B. Read (eds) *Measuring Emotions in Infants and Children*, Vol. 2 (pp.124–71). New York: Cambridge University Press. More recently see Sroufe, L.A. (2013) The promise of developmental psychopathology: past and present. *Development & Psychopathology*, 25(4.2), 1215–24. 'We need studies that unpack the heterogeneity in current categories by examining differential antecedents and pathways' (1216); Waters, T.E.A. & Facompré, C.R. (in press) Measuring secure base script knowledge in the Adult Attachment Interview. In E. Waters, B.E. Vaughn, & H.S. Waters (eds) *Measuring Attachment.* New York: Guilford: 'Simply saying a child is avoidant tells us little about what specific parenting behaviors lead that child to lose trust in their caregiver.'

behaviours predicted infant avoidance in the Strange Situation.[266] And in her analysis of videos of mother–toddler free play from her dissertation sample, Main reported:

> Mothers of mother-avoidant infants mocked their infants, or spoke sarcastically to or about them; some stared them down. One expressed irritation when the infant spilled imaginary tea. Our ratings showed a strong association between avoidance and maternal anger.[267]

Grossmann and colleagues found that North German mothers' expectation of self-reliance from their infants meant that half their sample received an avoidant attachment classification in the Strange Situation. This was despite the fact that, for a proportion of these infants, the expectation of self-reliance was not linked to other forms of maternal rejection, or to the later outcomes measured by the Grossmanns.[268] In contrast, both maternal and paternal sensitivity to the infant as assessed in home observations made sizeable contributions to later outcomes. Such findings suggest that one pathway to an avoidant attachment classification lies in cultural values around the suppression of distress signals, but that this pathway is not necessarily one with the same implications as when avoidance stems from caregiver insensitive and rejecting care.[269] (The issue of the contribution of cultural differences in care to the distribution of Strange Situation classifications is discussed further in the section 'Cross-cultural applicability of the Strange Situation'.)

Ambivalent/resistant attachment

Comparing the Strange Situation behaviour of infants from Group C dyads to the home observation data on the sample, Ainsworth and colleagues found that these infants displayed more distress at home than the secure infants, and especially on occasions when the caregiver attempted to leave the room.[270] However, few other differences were noted in the children's behaviour at home. Ainsworth reported the qualitative impression of a mismatch between

---

[266] Main, M. (1978) Avoidance of the attachment figure under stress: ontogeny, function and immediate causation. PP/Bow/J.4/1; Main, M. & Stadtman, J. (1981) Infant response to rejection of physical contact by the mother. *Journal of the American Academy of Child Psychiatry*, 20(2), 292–307.

[267] Main, M. (1980) Avoidance of attachment figures: index of disturbance. PP/Bow/J.4/1.

[268] Grossmann, K., Grossmann, K.E., Spangler, G., Suess, G., & Unzner, L. (1985) Maternal sensitivity and newborns' orientation responses as related to quality of attachment in northern Germany. *Monographs of the Society for Research in Child Development*, 50(1–2), 233–56; Fremmer-Bombik, F. & Grossmann, K.E. (1993) Über die lebenslange Bedeutung früher Bindungserfahrungen. In: H. Petzold (ed.) *Frühe Schädigungen—späte Folgen? Psychotherapie und Babyforschung*, pp.83–110. Paderborn: Jungfermann; Grossmann, K., Grossmann, K.E., & Kindler, H. (2005) Early care and the roots of attachment and partnership representation. The Bielefeld and Regensburg Longitudinal studies. In K.E. Grossmann, K. Grossmann, and E. Waters (eds) *Attachment from Infancy to Adulthood: The Major Longitudinal Studies* (pp.98–136). New York: Guilford.

[269] For aligned qualitative observations in a different context see Otto, H. (2014) Don't show your emotions! Emotion regulation and attachment in the Cameroonian Nso. In H. Otto & H. Keller (eds) *Different Faces of Attachment: Cultural Variations of a Universal Human Need* (pp.215–29). Cambridge: Cambridge University Press. Another pathway to an avoidant attachment classification in the Strange Situation may be the mind-mindedness of the caregiver, distinct from their rejection of physical contact. Elizabeth Meins and colleagues found that caregivers in dyads classified as avoidantly attached made fewer comments relevant to their child's inner states during free play. Meins, E., Fernyhough, C., de Rosnay, M., Arnott, B., Leekam, S.R., & Turner, M. (2012) Mind-mindedness as a multidimensional construct: appropriate and nonattuned mind-related comments independently predict infant–mother attachment in a socially diverse sample. *Infancy*, 17(4), 393–415, Table 1.

[270] Ainsworth, M., Blehar, M., Waters, E., & Wall, S. (1978, 2015) *Patterns of Attachment: A Psychological Study of the Strange Situation*. Bristol: Psychology Press, p.121.

infant signals and caregiver response, which contributed to low sensitivity. Even in the face of queries regarding the integrity of the C classification, Ainsworth felt there was a defining characteristic that linked the otherwise diverse behaviour of C1 and C2 infants. This was the resistance and displays of ambivalence when the caregiver offered comfort, across contexts:

> The ambivalence of Pattern C babies, both at home and in the strange situation, is easily understood. Their mothers, who were very inconsistent in their responsiveness to signals, often failed to pick the baby up when he most wanted contact, and often put him down again long before he was ready to be put down. Consequently, when attachment behaviour is intensely activated the baby has no confident expectation that his mother will respond to his need for close contact. Having been frustrated in such situations often enough in the past, his desire for close contact is intermingled with anger, because he rather expects his mother to be unresponsive. He wants contact and is angry if his mother does not respond, or if she tries some other mode of interaction, and yet he is still angry if she picks him up and is difficult to soothe; indeed, he may struggle to be put down only to protest and seek to be picked up again.[271]

The term 'inconsistent' was a common one in Ainsworth's lexicon, and regularly used with a variety of non-overlapping meanings. For instance, 'inconsistent sensitivity' is actually the technical label for the mid-point (5) on her sensitivity scale; caregivers from ambivalent/resistant dyads had scores on sensitivity well below this.[272] Yet from the mid-1970s, 'inconsistency' was a term she frequently used to describe the caregivers of ambivalent/resistant dyads, and was subsequently picked up by later attachment researchers as *the* defining cause of ambivalent/resistant attachment in Ainsworth's account. On this basis, later researchers assumed a model in which inconsistent care creates a lack of contingency for the infant: infants know that they can have their attachment signals heeded, but it is not clear when. As such, the threshold for the activation of the attachment behavioural system is lowered, and the threshold for termination raised. When the infant's intensified attachment behaviours and distress are accurately interpreted by the caregiver, this reinforces the strategy.[273] Much about this pathway is plausible, but the idea that it is 'inconsistency', specifically, that is the key ingredient remains unevidenced.[274] In fact, Ainsworth offers no data to suggest that the caregivers of ambivalent/resistant infants are unpredictably sensitive: in *Patterns of Attachment*, the specific behaviours that distinguished these mothers were in fact 'delay in responding

---

[271] Ainsworth. M.D.S. (1983) Patterns of infant–mother attachment as related to maternal care: their early history and their contribution to continuity. In: D. Magnusson & V.L. Allen (eds) *Human Development: An Interactional Perspective* (pp.35–55). New York: Academic Press, p.42.

[272] Ainsworth, M., Blehar, M., Waters, E., & Wall, S. (1978, 2015) *Patterns of Attachment: A Psychological Study of the Strange Situation*. Bristol: Psychology Press, p.231.

[273] Ainsworth, M.D.S., Bell, S.M., & Stayton, D.J. (1974) Infant–mother attachment and social development: 'socialisation' as a product of reciprocal responsiveness to signals. In: M.J.M. Richards (ed.) *The Integration of a Child into a Social World* (pp.9–135). Cambridge: Cambridge University Press; Cassidy, J. & Berlin, L.J. (1994) The insecure/ambivalent pattern of attachment: theory and research. *Child Development*, 65(4), 971–91; Mayseless, O. (1996) Attachment patterns and their outcomes. *Human Development*, 39(4), 206–23; Crittenden, P.M. (1999) Danger and development: the organisation of self-protective strategies. In J.I. Vondra & D. Barnett (eds) *Atypical Attachment in Infancy and Early Childhood Among Children at Developmental Risk* (pp.145–71). Oxford: Blackwell.

[274] The predictive power of contextual indicators of caregiver unpredictability have been examined by Belsky and colleagues in the NICHD sample, but not considered in relation to infant attachment patterns. Belsky, J., Schlomer, G.L., & Ellis, B.J. (2012) Beyond cumulative risk: distinguishing harshness and unpredictability as determinants of parenting and early life history strategy. *Developmental Psychology*, 48(3), 662–73.

to cry signals and occupying the time when holding the baby with routines'.[275] Their mean scores for sensitivity were the same as those of avoidant dyads. Though Ainsworth and colleagues found that mothers in ambivalent/resistant dyads displayed somewhat fewer rejecting behaviours towards their babies, the difference was not marked.[276]

However, there appears to be a second model in Ainsworth's writings regarding caregiving in ambivalent/resistant dyads. The quantitative findings reported in *Patterns of Attachment* (1978) were of (i) delay in responding to cry signals and (ii) occupying the time when holding the baby with routines. Main later described unpublished data from Ainsworth's Baltimore study, showing that 'in the first 3 months of life, the mothers of the infants who would later be resistant were extraordinarily inept in holding their infants (inept in 41% of holding episodes) and almost never "tender and careful" (tender and careful in 2% of episodes). Their face-to-face interactions with their infants were marked by the absence of contingent pacing'.[277] This suggests a caregiver who is not adverse to closeness with their baby but who finds it difficult to hold them fully in mind—leading to a delay in responding and less full, satisfying, and well-judged responses when they do occur.

Indeed, Ainsworth herself specifically claimed that 'the mother of a Pattern C baby is likely to enjoy contact with him even though she is often imperceptive of his need for it'.[278] The idea that the caregivers of ambivalent/resistant dyads are less effective at tracking their infant's inner states is supported by findings that they make comments relevant to their child's inner states during free play, but these appear to observers to have little relationship with the child's actual states.[279] It would be this imperceptiveness that would lead to a lack of confidence on the part of the infant in the attentional availability of the caregiver, the reduced threshold for activation of the attachment behavioural system, and the intensification of attachment signals. Ainsworth's final word on the classification made no mention of 'inconsistent' care, and instead foregrounded any caregiver behaviour that would lead a child to be uncertain about availability.[280]

Overall, however, the relative infrequency of ambivalent/resistant dyads in most American and European samples, the absence of a scale for coding the passivity characteristic especially of the C2 infants, and the lack of a sharp theory of caregiving antecedents have all contributed to distinterest in the ambivalent/resistant classification over the decades. Even when researchers found distinct correlates of the ambivalent/resistant classification, there has been little support for interpreting them from a network of other findings

[275] Ainsworth, M., Blehar, M., Waters, E., & Wall, S. (1978, 2015) *Patterns of Attachment: A Psychological Study of the Strange Situation*. Bristol: Psychology Press, p.245.

[276] Ibid. p.230, Table 27.

[277] Main, M. (1995) Recent studies in attachment: overview, with selected implications for clinical work. In S. Goldberg, R. Muir, & J. Kerr (eds) *Attachment Theory: Social, Developmental and Clinical Perspectives* (pp.407–70). Hillsdale, NJ: Analytic Press, p.417.

[278] Ainsworth, M.D.S. (1983) Patterns of infant–mother attachment as related to maternal care: their early history and their contribution to continuity. In D. Magnusson & V.L. Allen (eds) *Human Development: An Interactional Perspective* (pp.35–55). New York: Academic Press, p.42.

[279] Meins, E., Fernyhough, C., de Rosnay, M., Arnott, B., Leekam, S.R., & Turner, M. (2012) Mind-mindedness as a multidimensional construct: appropriate and nonattuned mind-related comments independently predict infant–mother attachment in a socially diverse sample. *Infancy*, 17(4), 393–415, Table 1. See also Kelly, K., Slade, A., & Grienenberger, J.F. (2005) Maternal reflective functioning, mother–infant affective communication, and infant attachment: exploring the link between mental states and observed caregiving behavior in the intergenerational transmission of attachment. *Attachment & Human Development*, 7(3), 299–311.

[280] Ainsworth, M.D.S. & Eichberg, C.G. (1991) Effects on infant–mother attachment of mother's experience related to loss of an attachment figure. In: C.M. Parkes, J. Stevenson-Hinde, & P. Marris (eds) *Attachment Across the Life Cycle* (pp.160–83). London: Routledge, p.162.

and hypothesis-generating discussions.[281] Ambivalence/resistance retains a place in the system—17% of dyads received this classification according to a recent meta-analysis[282]— but without researchers finding much need to give it discussion, with exceptions such as Crittenden and Mayseless.[283] The weak network of theory and empirical findings around the ambivalent/resistant classification has led to significant problems for the field in pinning down the relationship between the C and D classifications (Chapter 4).

Conflict behaviours in the Strange Situation

Ainsworth was generally of the view that the classificatory system she had developed was open-ended. In *Patterns of Attachment*, she wrote 'it is inconceivable that any system based on a relatively small sample could comfortably accommodate all patterns represented in the total population'.[284] She wanted to ensure space to accommodate the unforeseen. One strategy Ainsworth used to keep her system open was to have an explicit residual category, to serve as a worksite for identifying further patterns. At the start of her work with the Strange Situation, she used Group C to encompass infants who did not fit the other two groups, especially on the basis of seeming 'disturbed'. This was still part of the function of the classification as late as *Patterns of Attachment*, though the classification came increasingly to be defined by resistance (C1) and passivity (C2)—and then, after Ainsworth, generally just by resistance. During her sabbatical at Stanford, Ainsworth wrote to Bell of the value of having an intense and critical relationship between theory and observation, where each could change a researcher's perception of the other:

> Even the most beautiful of theories is never as beautiful as truth or fact. To have destroyed a theory is therefore an excellent thing. It is a step forward. And one need not tremble lest a fact destroy a theory, even one's own. One must seek it. Underneath lies a discovery.[285]

One unexpected discovery occurred when Ainsworth attempted to assess the stability of her categories by bringing the dyads from one wave of her sample back two weeks later for a second Strange Situation. Whilst the response of the infants in dyads classified as secure was very largely the same, the response of the seven infants in avoidantly attached dyads was

---

[281] Exceptions include Luijk, M.P., Velders, F.P., Tharner, A., et al. (2010) FKBP5 and resistant attachment predict cortisol reactivity in infants: gene–environment interaction. *Psychoneuroendocrinology*, 35(10), 1454–61; Beebe, B. & Lachmann, F.M. (2014) Future resistant dyads. In *The Origins of Attachment: Infant Research and Adult Treatment* (pp.104–114). London: Routledge. However, it is probable that these latter findings will not be replicated by other laboratories: the coding system of Beebe and colleagues is not given in sufficient detail in their published works to permit replication, and no training is available for other laboratories to learn the system.

[282] Verhage, M.L., Schuengel, C., Madigan, S., et al. (2016) Narrowing the transmission gap: a synthesis of three decades of research on intergenerational transmission of attachment. *Psychological Bulletin*, 142(4), 337–66, Table 4.

[283] Among the few sustained discussions of the classification are Cassidy, J. & Berlin, L.J. (1994) The insecure/ambivalent pattern of attachment: theory and research. *Child Development*, 65(4), 971–91; Crittenden, P.M. (1999) Danger and development: the organisation of self-protective strategies. In J.I. Vondra & D. Barnett (eds) *Atypical Attachment in Infancy and Early Childhood Among Children at Developmental Risk* (pp.145–71). Oxford: Blackwell; Scher, A. & Mayseless, O. (2000) Mothers of anxious/ambivalent infants: maternal characteristics and child-care context. *Child Development*, 71(6), 1629–39.

[284] Ainsworth, M., Blehar, M., Waters, E., & Wall, S. (1978, 2015) *Patterns of Attachment: A Psychological Study of the Strange Situation*. Bristol: Psychology Press, p.229.

[285] Ainsworth, M. (1968) *Letter to Sylvia Bell*, 2 January 1968. Mary Ainsworth Archive, Box M3169, Folder 6.

quite different. Every one now approached the caregiver on reunion. But they did so whilst showing fragments of avoidant behaviour. Ainsworth concluded that the infants had been overstressed.[286] The approach to the caregiver shown by these infants did not reflect their expectation that the caregiver would be available, like the infants in secure dyads. Instead it reflected the extent of their distress and fear.[287] In this context, the avoidance was breaking down into the kinds of conflict behaviour that had been described by Hinde (Chapter 1), displaying wishes to both approach and avoid.

Between 1968 and 1973, Main undertook her doctoral research with Ainsworth. As well as the measures required for her doctoral research, Main instructed her coders 'to note each time that the toddler did anything which seemed odd to them'; this included 'hand-flapping; echolalia; inappropriate affect; and other behaviours appearing out of context'.[288] Five out of the forty-nine infants were found to display such odd behaviour that it was difficult to fit them within the Ainsworth classifications: two of these infants were force-classified as secure, whereas three 'were informally termed A–C infants within the laboratory' and classi-fied either as A or C.[289] Main noted that two of these 'A–C' infants showed reunion behaviour that combined an attempt to approach the caregiver with signs of fear and avoidance. One threw her hands in front of her face on reunion, whereas the other engaged in asymmetric handslapping whilst creeping forward. Main 'asked Mary Ainsworth as my dissertation ad-visor what to do. Characteristically cautious, but certain these infants were insecure, she re-commended that for the time being (until more samples were collected and studied) 'we place them in Group A'.[290] Main wrote wryly in a footnote to her doctoral thesis that, though this technique was pragmatically useful, 'Linnaeus might not approve'.[291]

From the 1970s, Ainsworth also took an interest in stereotypic and tension behaviours, though this interest was hampered by the fact that the set-up of her Strange Situations had only given observers a 'profile view (at best)' rather than a frontal view of the baby on re-union.[292] Ainsworth was also reliant on detailed written observations, rather than the full video recording used by the next generation of attachment researchers. Initially Ainsworth

[286] This finding would later be replicated, inadvertently, by researchers at Uppsala University: Granqvist, P., Hesse, E., Fransson, M., Main, M., Hagekull, B., & Bohlin, G. (2016) Prior participation in the strange situation and overstress jointly facilitate disorganized behaviours: implications for theory, research and practice. *Attachment & Human Development*, 18(3), 235–49.

[287] Ainsworth, M., Blehar, M., Waters, E., & Wall, S. (1978, 2015) *Patterns of Attachment: A Psychological Study of the Strange Situation*. Bristol: Psychology Press, p.218.

[288] Main, M. (1977) Analysis of a peculiar form of reunion behaviour seen in some day-care children. In R. Webb (ed.) *Social Development in Childhood* (pp.33–78). Baltimore: John Hopkins, pp.70–71.

[289] Main, M. & Solomon, J. (1990) Procedures for identifying infants as disorganised/disoriented during the Ainsworth Strange Situation. In M.T. Greenberg, D. Cicchetti, & E.M. Cummings (eds) *Attachment in the Preschool Years* (pp.121–60). Chicago: University of Chicago Press, p.126. On the A–C designation see Crittenden, P.M. & Ainsworth, M. (1989) Child maltreatment and attachment theory. In D. Cicchetti & Y. Carlson (eds) *Child Maltreatment: Theory and Research on the Causes and Consequences of Child Abuse and Neglect* (pp.432–63). Cambridge: Cambridge University Press. Also Lamb, M., Thompson, R.A., Gardner, W., & Charnov, E.L. (1985) *Infant–Mother Attachment: The Origins and Developmental Significance of Individual Differences in the Strange Situation*. Hillsdale, NJ: Lawrence Erlbaum. In a cluster analysis performed on four samples, there were seven clus-ters: one was 'a relatively rare group of infants displaying both avoidance and resistance' (217).

[290] Mary Main, personal communication, August 2012. See Duschinsky, R. (2015) The emergence of the disor-ganized/disoriented (d) attachment classification, 1979–1982. *History of Psychology*, 18(1), 32–46.

[291] Main, M. (1973) Exploration, play and cognitive functioning. Unpublished doctoral thesis, Johns Hopkins University, p.21.

[292] Ainsworth, M., Blehar, M., Waters, E., & Wall, S. (1978, 2015) *Patterns of Attachment: A Psychological Study of the Strange Situation*. Bristol: Psychology Press: Observers in Ainsworth's procedure 'had a good view of a baby's face as he approached either the mother's or stranger's chair, a profile view (at best) of a baby oriented to the door or to a person entering' (34).

associated stereotypic and tension behaviours with the B4 subclassification. B4 was introduced in 1969 to capture infants from Silvia Bell's sample who were very upset by the separation episodes, but who did manage to use their caregiver as a source of support and calm
before the end of the Strange Situation.[293] In *Patterns of Attachment*, one of the criteria used
to define B4 was that the subclassification included any 'other signs of disturbance, such as
inappropriate, stereotyped, repetitive gestures or motions'.[294] As a consequence, the B4 subtype was regarded by some as a rather unstable element within the system.[295] The inclusion
of other signs of disturbance as one of its criteria was later formally retracted as a criterion
for B4 by Ainsworth, with the introduction of the D classification (Chapter 3).[296]

In *Patterns of Attachment*, Ainsworth and colleagues explicitly considered the discrepant
behaviour they were seeing in the Strange Situation in terms of Hinde's concept of 'conflict
behaviour':

> When two antithetical systems are activated simultaneously, they may be said to be in con-
> flict … The other system may not become manifest in behaviour until either the overriding
> behaviour is terminated (or becomes less strongly activated) or some shift in the situation
> increases the activation of the system until it overrides the behaviour of the previously
> stronger system. When two conflicting systems are more nearly equal in level of activation
> there may be alternation of behaviours, 'compromise' behaviours in which behavioural
> elements of both systems are combined, or intention movements or other fragmentary be-
> havioural representatives of one or the other system. Furthermore, the behaviour activated
> by one stimulus object may be redirected towards another that is not involved in the con-
> flict … Finally, overt behaviour may be determined by a third system, which is also at a
> moderate level of activation, although not as high a level as the two conflicting systems that
> tend to block each other—a phenomenon the ethologists label 'displacement behaviour'.[297]

In an unpublished paper from around the period of composition of *Patterns of Attachment*,
Ainsworth and colleagues argued that there was a 'distress language' to be deciphered in
these odd behaviours, and that this language would be important for comprehending infant experience: 'Once one has gotten to know the distress language, these subtle signals
make the distress of the child who is trying with might and main to control it all the more
poignant'.[298] The final pages of *Patterns of Attachment* were dedicated to a strong call—which
has never been quoted by subsequent researchers—for study of the meaning of conflict

---

[293] Ainsworth, M., Bell, S.M., & Stayton, D.J. (1969) Individual differences in strange-situational behaviour
of one-year-olds. http://eric.ed.gov/?id=ED056742. Later version: Ainsworth, M.D.S., Bell, S.M., & Stayton, D.J.
(1971) Individual differences in strange-situation behavior of one-year-olds. In H.R. Schaffer (ed.) *The Origins of
Human Social Relations* (pp.17–58). New York: Academic Press.

[294] Ainsworth, M., Blehar, M., Waters, E., & Wall, S. (1978, 2015) *Patterns of Attachment: A Psychological Study
of the Strange Situation*. Bristol: Psychology Press, p.61.

[295] E.g. Van IJzendoorn, M.H., Tavecchio, L.W.C., Goossens, F.A., Vergeer, M.M., & Swaan, J. (1983) How B
is B4? Attachment and security of Dutch children in Ainsworth's Strange Situation and at home. *Psychological
Reports*, 52(3), 683–91.

[296] Personal communication from Mary Ainsworth to Mary Main, January 1985, cited in Main, M. & Solomon,
J. (1990) Procedures for identifying infants as disorganised/disoriented during the Ainsworth Strange Situation.
In M.T. Greenberg, D. Cicchetti, & E.M. Cummings (eds) *Attachment in the Preschool Years* (pp.121–60).
Chicago: University of Chicago Press, p.149.

[297] Ainsworth, M., Blehar, M., Waters, E., & Wall, S. (1978, 2015) *Patterns of Attachment: A Psychological Study
of the Strange Situation*. Bristol: Psychology Press, p.273.

[298] Ainsworth, M. (1976) *Attachment and Separation in Paediatric Settings*. Unpublished manuscript. PP/Bow/
J.1/40.

behaviours seen in the Strange Situation, and their different potential causes. In the early 1980s, Ainsworth wanted to hold a conference for Strange Situation coders, dedicated to exploration of anomalous behaviours. Ultimately, though, she decided that she lacked the time and money to host this event. Meanwhile, however, she encouraged her graduate students Mary Main and Patricia Crittenden in their study of infants who showed behaviours discrepant with her categories for coding the Strange Situation.[299] And she anticipated that research with clinical samples would ultimately lead to additions to her coding system, with particular relevance for coding clinical samples. After all, her three categories had been developed on the basis of a sample of participants recruited according to demographic characteristics that would reduce adversities.[300] In the meantime, the anomalies did not appear to threaten use of the Strange Situation as the basis for building a research programme. Bowlby's position seems to have been aligned with Ainsworth's. Bowlby was not reconciled to the idea that the three Ainsworth classifications were sufficient for work with clinical samples.[301] However, he did not pursue the matter in print, except in his remarks on the work of Ainsworth's students. The issue would ultimately be left for the next generation of attachment researchers (Chapter 3).

Everett Waters

Stability

Part of Ainsworth's legacy for the field of attachment research was her mentorship of a remarkable cohort of students, many of whom became leaders of the second generation of attachment research. Among the undergraduates she taught who would become colleagues in attachment-related research were Mark Cummings, Mark Greenberg, Robert Marvin, David Olds, and Everett Waters. Her graduate students at Johns Hopkins were Silvia Bell, Mary Blehar, Inge Bretherton, Alicia Lieberman, Mary Main, and Sally Wall. Michael Lamb was a student with her for a year at Johns Hopkins, before Ainsworth left for Virginia. Ainsworth's graduate students and mentees at Virginia included Jude Cassidy, Deborah Cohn, Virginia Colin, Patricia Crittenden, Rogers Kobak, Carolyn Eichberg, and Ulrike Wartner.[302] In later life, Ainsworth wrote fondly of her students as her 'academic family', a phrase that continues to be used by attachment researchers in the developmental tradition to describe their community.[303] The phrase has perhaps recurred in part because it captures the warmth, care, and

[299] Crittenden, P.M. & Ainsworth, M.D. (1989) Child maltreatment and attachment theory. In D. Cicchetti & V. Carlson (eds) *Child Maltreatment: Theory and Research on the Causes and Consequences of Child Abuse and Neglect* (pp.432–61). Cambridge: Cambridge University Press; Ainsworth, M. (1991) Past and future trends in attachment research. Film of the presentation made available by Avi Sagi-Schwartz (Chair), International Society for the Study of Behavioral Development, Minneapolis, July 1991.

[300] Ainsworth, M. (1985) Patterns of mother–infant attachments. *Bulletin of the New York Academy of Medicine* 61, 792–812, p.788.

[301] Solomon, J., Duschinsky, R., Bakkum, L., & Schuengel, C. (2017) Toward an architecture of attachment disorganization: John Bowlby's published and unpublished reflections. *Clinical Child Psychology and Psychiatry*, 22(4), 539–60. See also Bowlby, J. (1981) Clinical applications: material for lectures. PP/Bow/F.3/103: 'Patterns of attachment: Secure attachment; Anxious attachment; Compulsive self-reliance; Compulsive care-giving; Psychopathic detachment.'

[302] Bretherton, I. (2000) Mary Dinsmore Salter Ainsworth (1913–1999). *American Psychologist*, 55, 1148–9.

[303] E.g. Ainsworth, M. (1983, 2013) An autobiographical sketch. *Attachment & Human Development*, 15(5–6), 448–59, p.458.

loyalty of the field of attachment research, which matches well the common idea of family; and in part because it captures the conflict, compassion, and compromises of the field of attachment research, which matches the all-too-human, fumbling-at-times actuality of family.

One of Ainsworth's students who was important in shaping her legacy for developmental psychology was Everett Waters. Waters worked with Ainsworth for almost two years, taking courses and graduate seminars and acting as a research assistant. In addition, he joined graduate students Mary Blehar and Sally Wall helping Ainsworth prepare the book length report of her Baltimore project, *Patterns of Attachment*. Waters' roles included preparing the report on multivariate analysis of the ABC classification system and editing draft chapters.[304] In 1972, on the strength of Ainsworth's recommendation, Waters was admitted to the University of Minnesota's Institute of Child Development. Classmates soon directed him toward assistant professor Alan Sroufe and his work on the development of smiling and laughter. Sroufe's interests inclined toward a general theory of emotional development and he was eager to tap Waters' first-hand experience with attachment research. Mentoring led to collaboration and soon a fast friendship, and a series of influential papers.

An early paper by Sroufe and Waters was a turning point for acceptance of Ainsworth's Strange Situation classifications within the wider developmental science community.[305] In this paper 'Attachment as an organizational construct', published in 1977, Sroufe and Waters summarised the cornerstones and significance of the theoretical work of Bowlby and Ainsworth and discussed recent empirical results in a pointed response to several criticism rooted in temperament and learning theory paradigms.

A first criticism that Sroufe and Waters sought to combat was that Ainsworth's secure vs insecure distinction could be explained as temperamental differences in sensitivity to the stress of separation or in terms of how often mothers reinforced crying and dependency. The mistake was that the secure vs insecure distinction did not map onto crying vs non-crying in the separation episodes. In fact, half of secure one-year-olds protested separation in the Strange Situation (primarily B3 and B4) and half did not (B1, B2, and some B3). Thus, as Sroufe and Waters pointed out, classifications depended not on separation protest but on responses to mother's return. Moreover, Sroufe and Waters pointed to data showing that minimal separation protest in A infants was not simply a matter of temperament or reinforcement cycles. These explanations assumed that non-crying infants were indifferent to separation. Certainly research with American parents indicated that many regarded the infants who showed avoidant behaviour in the Strange Situation as the most competent, since they seemed to not be distressed by the separations.[306] In a piece of swift ingenuity, Sroufe and Waters reported evidence from concurrent heart-rate recordings that 'avoidant infants showed sustained heart-rate acceleration on reunion (in the absence of vigorous motor activity), suggesting clear affective response rather than indifference.'[307] Infants in dyads

[304] In 2015, Waters initiated a reissue of the now classic book with additional appendices and a new preface in which he, Inge Bretherton, and Brian Vaughn discussed the book's impact and its significance for current work.

[305] Sroufe, L.A. & Waters, E. (1977) Attachment as an organizational construct. *Child Development*, 1184–99. Goldberg, S. (2000) *Attachment and Development*. London: Routledge: 'Ainsworth's work was also subjected to heated criticism and, until the publication of Sroufe and Waters' 1977 paper on "attachment as an organisational construct" and the emergence of supporting data from other laboratories, it was neither understood nor accepted by the larger community of developmental psychologists' (236).

[306] E.g. Hubbs-Tait, L., Gray, D., Wierzbicki, M., & Englehart, R. (1994) Perceptions of infant boys' behavior and mental health: relation to infant attachment. *Infant Mental Health Journal*, 15(3), 307–15.

[307] Sroufe, L.A. & Waters, E. (1977) Attachment as an organizational construct. *Child Development*, 1184–99, p.1191. These findings are detailed further in Sroufe, L. & Waters, E. (1977) Heart-rate as a convergent measure in clinical and developmental research. *Merrill-Palmer Quarterly*, 23, 3–27. In later research using heart-rate

classified as avoidant were interpreted as inhibiting a display of attachment behaviour and keeping their distress secret from the caregiver, rather than having less desire for comfort than other infants in the Strange Situation.

A second criticism was that infant attachment behaviours do not intercorrelate highly, show weak stability over time, and are strongly influenced by context. This was taken by critics as an invalidation of the construct of infant attachment.[308] Of particular importance was a paper published in *Psychological Bulletin* by Masters and Wellman from 1974, which offered a detailed critique of attachment research, including a report that 'little stability of attachment behaviors was found if the intervening time was three minutes, one day, three months, four months, or longer'.[309] This was a potentially decisive criticism in light of the central role early experience plays in attachment theory. Ainsworth and her small group of collaborators experienced these critiques as a serious threat to the emerging paradigm. There was 'a real sense of emergency' in the small attachment research community.[310] One response to Masters and Wellman was theoretical counterargument and clarification. Sroufe and Waters argued that attachment is a behavioural system, not the particular behaviours selected to achieve the set-goal. Particular behaviours are of primary relevance only to the inferred inner organisation they are understood to express. If reaching works quickly to achieve contact with the caregiver, there might be no need to also engage crawling towards the caregiver. If fussing works, there might be no need to use crying. The selection of behaviours will be sensitive to context.[311]

A second response to Masters and Wellman was empirical. Waters undertook to demonstrate that the results Masters and Wellman had reported regarding the absence of stability stemmed from their focus on individual behaviours, rather than the organisation of behaviour. He collected Strange Situation assessments with 50 middle-class dyads at 12 months and 18 months of age. There was almost no continuity of attachment behaviours displayed towards the caregiver across the half-year period, as Masters and Wellman had predicted. Only

measures, there is some discrepancy between findings, suggesting that infants in avoidant dyads are more physiologically stressed than infants in secure dyads, and findings indicating comparability. Nonetheless, it has been taken for granted by researchers since Sroufe and Waters that most infants in avoidant dyads are indeed distressed by the separation, even after the widespread increase in daycare, and that their avoidant behaviour represents a masking and inhibition of a desire to seek the caregiver's availability, rather than an absence of this desire. On later findings see e.g. Spangler, G. & Grossmann, K.E. (1993) Biobehavioral organization in securely and insecurely attached infants. *Child Development*, 64(5), 1439–50; Hill-Soderlund, A.L., Mills-Koonce, W.R., Propper, C., et al. (2008) Parasympathetic and sympathetic responses to the strange situation in infants and mothers from avoidant and securely attached dyads. *Developmental Psychobiology*, 50(4), 361–76.

[308] E.g. Cairns, R.B. (1972) Attachment and dependency: a psychobiological and social learning synthesis. In J.L. Gewirtz (ed.) *Attachment and Dependency* (pp.29–80). Washington, DC: Winston; Gewirtz, J. (1972) On the selection and use of attachment and dependence indices. In J.L. Gewirtz (ed.) *Attachment and Dependency* (pp.179–215). Washington, DC: Winston; Rosenthal, M. (1973) Attachment and mother–infant interaction: some research impasses and a suggested change in orientation. *Journal of Child Psychology and Psychiatry and Allied Disciplines*, 14, 201–207.

[309] Masters, J. & Wellman, H. (1974) Human infant attachment: a procedural critique. *Psychological Bulletin*, 81, 218–37, p.224.

[310] Everett Waters, personal communication, August 2019

[311] Sroufe and Waters also showed that low correlations between individual attachment behaviors were also partly an artifact of inadequate sampling of these low frequency behaviors. Specifically, because the discrete behaviors were typically samples for as little as 3-minutes, they did not provide a reliable (reproducible) estimate of an infant's typical behavior. Indeed, for many of these behaviors, Sroufe and Waters determined that it would require hundreds of minutes of observation to obtain the reliable scores needed to correctly estimate stability. Waters then showed that Ainsworth's approach to scoring interactive behavior in terms of the organisation of multiple behaviors across Strange Situation episodes yielded more reliable scores on proximity seeking, contact, maintaining, avoidance and resistance scores that could be quite stable across a full six month test-retest interval.

smiling at the mother and touching the mother were stable across time; there was no continuity in other important behaviours such as proximity-seeking.[312] Yet using Ainsworth's more broadly defined proximity-seeking, contact-maintaining, avoidance, and resistance constructs, there was a consistent pattern of stability, particularly in the key reunion episodes (for example, .62 for avoidance and .58 for resistance, both significant < .01). This empirical result demonstrated more effectively than any narrative rebuttal the limitations of Masters and Wellman's critique as well as the strength and potential of the new attachment paradigm.

Forty-eight out of the fifty infants received the same classification at both 12 and 18 months. This confirmed Waters' expectation that more broadly defined and integrative assessments would yield even higher stability than even individual scales. At the same time, this result is much higher than in subsequent studies. Several factors could contribute to this. First, each case was scored on the basis of a consensus among several experienced independent coders. Moreover, the sample consisted of first-born infants from intact middle-class families. None of the infants had experienced regular out-of-home care. It is also important to note a methodological limitation of the study. At the time, the only trained scorers for the Strange Situation were Ainsworth and her students and the small Minnesota team. Consequently, the same experts coded both time-points. Though coding the two time-points six months apart, the overlap in coders may have unintentionally reduced the independence of their assessments and elevated the stability of the clasifications.

There are times when having an extreme statement made allows the deep truth within it to be released; and there are times when the extreme qualities end up skewing reception of a complex truth in ways that are difficult to subsequently get heard. The sheer strength of stability of attachment classifications over time reported by Waters reflects a little of both predicaments. This was the first independent test of the stability of Ainsworth's categories, and would prove critical to their acceptance by the wider community of developmental scientists. Indeed, Waters' study appeared as empirical support for an image—suggested at times by Bowlby and Ainsworth—of the results of early care as impervious to change, at least in the short term. This image was further supported by the use of continuity from the Strange Situation by Main and colleagues in the development and validation of new attachment measures (Chapter 3).[313]

Baldwin and Fehr suggest that a contributing factor to the birth of the social psychological tradition of attachment research in the 1980s (Chapter 5) was the impression, given by the reported findings of Waters, of individual differences in attachment as stable trait-like variables.[314] As well as among many researchers, the idea of attachment patterns as set in early childhood also became a pervasive part of the reception of Bowlby, Ainsworth, Waters, and Main among clinical and child welfare readers.[315] Aligned with Waters' findings, several

---

[312] Waters, E. (1978) The reliability and stability of individual differences in infant–mother attachment. *Child Development*, 49(2), 483–94, p.488, Table 3.

[313] For just one of many examples in which the Waters' stability study and Main's six-year follow-up are together taken to prove Bowlby's claims about continuity from early childhood see Lipps, A.J. (2009) Review of Klaus E. Grossman, Karin Grossman, and Everett Waters (eds): attachment from infancy to adulthood. *Child & Adolescent Social Work Journal*, 26, 379–82.

[314] Baldwin, M.W. & Fehr, B. (1995) On the instability of attachment style ratings. *Personal Relationships*, 2(3), 247–61.

[315] See critical discussions of assumptions among practitioners about the fixedness of early attachment patterns in Fraley, C.R. (2002) Attachment stability from infancy to adulthood: meta-analysis and dynamic modeling of developmental mechanisms. *Personality and Social Psychology Review*, 6(2), 123–51; Crittenden, P.M. (2016) *Raising Parents: Attachment, Representation, and Treatment*, 2nd edn. London: Routledge; Granqvist, P., Sroufe, L.A., Dozier, M., et al. (2017) Disorganized attachment in infancy: a review of the phenomenon and its implications for clinicians and policy-makers. *Attachment & Human Development*, 19(6), 534–58.

other samples in the 1980s similarly demonstrated high stability of the categories over time.[316] However, Waters was clearly concerned that such high levels of stability suggested a lack of environmental responsiveness, which seemed implausible. He was also worried that with only 50 infants in his original study, chance might have contributed to an overestimate of stability. He therefore sought to conduct further research with high-risk dyads in order to put boundaries on the previously reported stability before misapprehensions could arise about attachment classifications being fixed for good in infancy.

Studying 100 high-risk dyads in the Strange Situation, Vaughn, Waters, and colleagues found only 62 allocated to the same classification six months later. Discontinuities, however, were often logical: dyads that changed from a secure to an insecure classification tended to be those where the mother had experienced more stressful life-events in the meantime.[317] Vaughn, Waters, and colleagues argued that this implied that patterns of attachment could change if caregivers faced factors that would contribute to more or less sensitivity to their child: 'There is little room today for a construct that does not recognise the environmental responsiveness of individual differences. The validity of the attachment construct is greatly enhanced by our prediction and confirmation of stability in some cases and change in others.'[318] Ainsworth herself fully agreed that a child's experiences of changes in interaction with caregivers 'predictably lead to changes in patterns of attachment.'[319] She described herself as 'delighted that researchers are increasingly turning to an examination of exceptions to stability of attachment-pattern,'[320] and encouraged her students to explore such exceptions.[321] At the same time, Ainsworth cautiously anticipated that early experiences of secure base/safe haven availability or unavailability may have relevance for later development, even in the context of subsequent change (Chapter 4).[322]

It became a common finding that the Ainsworth classifications were generally less stable in studies with participants drawn from high-risk samples. However, in the 1980s, studies were also reported, even with low-risk samples, that found no short-term stability of the categories. Sociologically, it may be noted that this coincides with a sharp rise in use of day-care from the 1970s, which could be expected to loosen the association between maternal care and attachment classifications since less time would be spent together by mother and child.[323] The most influential study to show weak stability in the 1980s was a report

[316] Main, M. & Weston, D.R. (1981) The quality of the toddler's relationship to mother and to father: related to conflict behavior and the readiness to establish new relationships. *Child Development*, 52(3), 932–40; Goossens, F.A., van IJzendoorn, M.H., Tavecchio, L.W.C., & Kroonenberg, P.M. (1986) Stability of attachment across time and context in a Dutch sample. *Psychological Reports*, 58(1), 23–32; Kermoian, R. & Leiderman, P.H. (1986) Infant attachment to mother and child caretaker in an East African community. *International Journal of Behavioral Development*, 9(4), 455–69.

[317] Vaughn, B., Egeland, B., Sroufe, L.A., & Waters, E. (1979) Individual differences in infant–mother attachment at twelve and eighteen months: stability and change in families under stress. *Child Development*, 50(4), 971–5.

[318] Ibid. p.975.

[319] Ainsworth, M. (1991) Past and future trends in attachment research. Film of the presentation made available by Avi Sagi-Schwartz (Chair), International Society for the Study of Behavioral Development, Minneapolis, July 1991.

[320] Ainsworth, M. (1985) Patterns of infant–mother attachments: antecedents and effects on development. *Bulletin of the New York Academy of Medicine*, 61(9), 771–91, p.787.

[321] Main, M. (1999) Mary D. Salter Ainsworth: tribute and portrait. *Psychoanalytic Inquiry*, 19(5), 682–736; Bretherton, I. (2000) Mary Dinsmore Salter Ainsworth (1913–1999). *American Psychologist*, 55, 1148–9; Crittenden, P.M. (2017) Gifts from Mary Ainsworth and John Bowlby. *Clinical Child Psychology and Psychiatry*, 22(3), 436–42.

[322] Ainsworth, M. (1991) Past and future trends in attachment research. Film of the presentation made available by Avi Sagi-Schwartz (Chair), International Society for the Study of Behavioral Development, Minneapolis, July 1991. https://www.youtube.com/watch?v=TWS1XBA7vmk.

[323] https://www.census.gov/topics/families/child-care/data.html

by Thompson, Lamb, and Estes.[324] Like Vaughn and colleagues, they found that both continuity and discontinuity in attachment classifications was predictable in light of changes in care: over half of infants changed attachment classification with their mother when she entered full-time employment, and all the infants in the sample changed attachment classification if they began receiving over 15 hours a week of non-parental care. However, the relative instability of attachment classifications in the sample provided part of the staging platform for Lamb and colleagues' important early criticisms and qualifications of Ainsworth's Strange Situation procedure, which were published as a long article in *Behavioral and Brain Sciences* in 1984. Though it does not seem to have been the authors' intent, these criticisms were interpreted as a rejection, rather than qualification, of the validity of the Strange Situation procedure. The article by Lamb and colleagues in the journal was followed by responses from numerous researchers, mostly pouring scorn on the procedure and attachment theory in general.[325]

Lamb and colleagues' appraisal and qualification of every jutting aspect of the Strange Situation, utilizing the detailed knowledge of an insider, offered excellent ammunition to critics making general attacks on attachment as a research paradigm. Indeed, the observations of Lamb and colleagues are still cited today as clinching the 'methodological shortcomings and unsupported assumptions' of Ainsworth's research, and as making the attachment paradigm as a whole untenable.[326] Most importantly at the time, however, Lamb and colleagues struck a nerve in headlining the lack of stability of classifications of attachment in a low-risk sample, which appeared to contradict the claim by Bowlby and Ainsworth that 'this internalised something we call attachment' is a 'retentive inner mechanism which serves as a kind of filter for the reception and interpretation of interpersonal experience', and in this way shapes later behaviour.[327] Lamb and colleagues felt that this offered an important qualification to the paradigm, but by no means intended their stance as a rejection of attachment research. Nor did they intend their stance even as a rejection of the Strange Situation, a form of measurement that they subsequently continued to use.

The Lamb and colleagues article brought home to the attachment community the extent to which they were depending on tacit knowledge for organizing their research paradigm.

[324] Thompson, R.A., Lamb, M.E., & Estes, D. (1982) Stability of infant–mother attachment and its relationship to changing life circumstances in an unselected middle-class sample. *Child Development*, 53(1), 144–8.

[325] Lamb, M.E., Thompson, R.A., Gardner, W.P., Charnov, E.L., & Estes, D. (1984) Security of infantile attachment as assessed in the 'strange situation': its study and biological interpretation. *Behavioral and Brain Sciences*, 7(1), 127–47; Lamb, M.E., Gardner, W., Charnov, E.L., Thompson, R.A., & Estes, D. (1984) Studying the security of infant–adult attachment: a reprise. *Behavioral and Brain Sciences*, 7, 163–71.

[326] Vicedo, M. (2020) On the history, present, and future of attachment theory. Reply to Robbie Duschinsky, Marinus van IJzendoorn, Sarah Foster, Sophie Reijman & Francesca Lionetti 'attachment histories and futures'. *European Journal of Developmental Psychology*, 17(1), 147–55, p.148.

[327] Ainsworth, M. (1967) *Infancy in Uganda*. Baltimore: Johns Hopkins University Press, pp.429–30. In line with Lamb's concerns, researchers examined the respective contribution of infant attachment with mother and father as assessed with the Strange Situation to later child attachment representations. The general finding was that neither makes an especially strong contribution, and that the extent of caregiver involvement with the child is an important moderator. Grossmann, K., Grossmann, K.E., & Kindler, H. (2005) Early care and the roots of attachment and partnership representations. In K.E. Grossmann, K. Grossmann, & E. Waters (eds) *Attachment from Infancy to Adulthood: The Major Longitudinal Studies* (pp.98–36). New York: Guilford; Steele, H. & Steele, M. (2005) The construct of coherence as an indicator of attachment security in middle childhood. the friends and family interview. In K.A. Kerns & R.A. Richardson (eds) *Attachment in Middle Childhood* (pp.137–60). New York: Guilford. The continuity between infant–mother attachment in the Strange Situation and the six-year assessments in the Berkeley sample is higher than most other studies. In part this is because the six-year samples were developed semi-inductively from the infant data on the sample. See Chapter 3.

Most researchers at the time were using the Ainsworth scales in the absence of reliability checks against existing research groups, or any demonstration of cross-group agreement.[328] Ainsworth assumed that the scales and categories could be used without training or the construction of a manual.[329] The Thompson, Lamb, and Estes findings alerted Waters, Sroufe, and other early attachment researchers in Ainsworth's circle that the Strange Situation coding protocols were not self-sufficient.[330] Knowing how to code the Strange Situation in the manner of Ainsworth was, in fact, partly an oral culture held by a small number of researchers associated with Ainsworth's group (then at Virginia), and the Berkeley and Minnesota laboratories (Chapters 3 and 4). In response to the article by Lamb and colleagues, it was judged that inter-rater reliability between research groups and a formal process of certification were needed to ensure valid use of the assessment. This prompted the introduction of a training institute in coding the Strange Situation, which has been run yearly at Minnesota by Alan Sroufe (and later Elizabeth Carlson and Robert Weigand) for over three decades now.[331]

Curiously, the Ainsworth sensitivity scale was not subject to this formalisation of training and certification [332] Presumably, since the scale was not published it was in less danger of unrestricted use. Additionally, though central to the work of attachment researchers, this scale has had less of a flagship status for the field's critics and its defenders. By contrast, the Strange Situation was treated as the foundation of attachment research as an empirical paradigm, and so training to achieve scientific reliability was considered especially important. However, the role of the Strange Situation coding training institutes extended well beyond this, for instance in teaching relevant theory, providing opportunities for networking and wider processes of enculturation. As van IJzendoorn observed at the time, these dynamics of enculturation contributed to insularity in this community. In his view, a system of training institutes is ultimately necessary to ensure scientific reliability (though his laboratory, like others, would use the Ainsworth sensitivity scale without any such training). However, he expressed concern that training institutes may mean that researchers have to show their submission to specific coding systems and their logic before that researcher's voice is

---

[328] Ainsworth expressed dismay in a letter to Bowlby that Michael Lamb had written to the editor of *Child Development* to say that he had been a student of hers, as evidence of the validity of his coding. Though there was no formal training process or certification, Ainsworth personally did not regard him as sufficiently trained in coding the Strange Situation. Ainsworth, M. (1982) *Letter to John Bowlby*, 25 April 1982. PP/BOW/B.3/7. However, van IJzendoorn and Kroonenberg would later empirically compare Lamb's coding of a Swedish sample to coding of Strange Situations in other contexts, and found minimal differences in how the coding protocols had been interpreted. Van IJzendoorn, M.H. & Kroonenberg, P.M. (1990) Cross-cultural consistency of coding the strange situation. *Infant Behavior and Development*, 13(4), 469–85.

[329] Ainsworth, M. (1973) *Letter to Georgette Marie Psarras*, 9 July 1973. Mary Ainsworth Archive, Box M3176, Folder 2.

[330] One alternative to long training institutes was the development in the 1980s of an algorithm to turn scale scores into category classifications by Richters, Waters, and Vaughn. The algorithm was used at times in the early 1990s, but quickly fell out of favour. The reasons for this are never discussed in print, but may have included the introduction of the disorganized attachment classification (Chapter 3), and the social institutionalization of the Minnesota Strange Situation training as authoritative. Richters, J.E., Waters, E., & Vaughn, B.E. (1988) Empirical classification of infant–mother relationships from interactive behavior and crying during reunion. *Child Development*, 59(2), 512–22.

[331] Waters, E. (1983) The stability of individual differences in infant attachment: comments on the Thompson, Lamb, and Estes contribution. *Child Development*, 54(2), 516–20. See https://attachment-training.com/.

[332] This situation has only changed recently with training in the Ainsworth sensitivity scale offered by Marian Bakermans-Kranenburg in 2019.

acknowledged, leading to the exclusion of constructive disagreement and the insights that can come from it.[333]

Ultimately, later meta-analytic research appeared to significantly qualify the strong stability reported by the early studies—though whether this reflected the rise of daycare, methodological differences between early and later studies, or simply the assumulation of knowledge is difficult to unpick. In 2002, Fraley assembled findings from 23 papers using measures from the developmental tradition of attachment research (i.e., not self-report measures of attachment). Stability of a secure vs insecure attachment classification for assessments of up to a year would prove much lower in Fraley's meta-analysis than in the Waters study: $r = .32$ (compared to $r = .92$ in Waters).[334] Stability was higher in low-risk ($r = .48$) than high-risk ($r = .27$) samples.

In the influential Minnesota Longitudinal Study of Risk and Adaptation (Chapter 4) there was no continuity of secure vs insecure attachment classifications between infancy and the Adult Attachment Interview. Nonetheless, as in the paper by Thompson and colleagues, both continuity and discontinuity could be accounted for by a few specific factors, reflecting stressors and support experienced by the caregiver. In the case of the Minnesota study these were experiences of maltreatment after infancy, changes in family life stress, sensitivity in parent–child relationships at 13, and quality of romantic relationships in adolescence.[335] Such findings support the critics of Ainsworth and Waters: attachment classifications are substantially less stable in the short term than originally thought, and more responsive to context. However, it is critical to note that there is 'lawful discontinuity':[336] the reasons for the changes can be identified in factors that would certainly be expected to alter patterns of attachment.

Furthermore, even if stability is lower than suggested by Waters, there remains substantial evidence in support of the claim that attachment patterns have relevant continuity over time. In a 2013 meta-analysis of 127 papers, and 21,072 dyads seen in the Strange Situation, Pinquart and colleagues found equivalent findings to Fraley for short-term stability, and in fact showed that stability remained moderate throughout the first five years. They were also able to report that there were no significant differences between father–infant dyads and mother–infant dyads in terms of stability. Pinquart and colleagues also reported the valuable

---

[333] Van IJzendoorn, M.H. (1994) Process model of replication studies: on the relations between different types of replication. In R. van der Veer, M.H. van IJzendoorn, & J. Valsiner (eds) *On Reconstructing the Mind: Replicability in Research on Human Development* (pp.57–70). Norwood, NJ: Ablex: 'Until such enculturation has taken place, a researcher who cannot replicate a certain result may expect to be accused of being not competent enough to carry out the experiment ... A training of several weeks in one of the American research centers is considered necessary for the reliable and valid coding of the observations or interviews, and therefore for a plausible and persuasive contribution to the international discourse on attachment. When central theses of attachment theory are in danger of being falsified by "untrained" researchers, this "incompetence" and lack of enculturation will be explicitly used against the "dissident" (see, for an example, Waters, 1983)' (62).

[334] Fraley, C.R. (2002) Attachment stability from infancy to adulthood: meta-analysis and dynamic modeling of developmental mechanisms. *Personality and Social Psychology Review*, 6(2), 123–51.

[335] Weinfield, N.S., Sroufe, L.A., & Egeland, B. (2000) Attachment from infancy to early adulthood in a high-risk sample: continuity, discontinuity, and their correlates. *Child Development*, 71(3), 695–702; Carlivati, J. & Collins, W.A. (2007) Adolescent attachment representations and development in a risk sample. *New Directions for Child and Adolescent Development*, (117), 91–106; Sroufe, L.A., Coffino, B., & Carlson, E.A. (2010) Conceptualizing the role of early experience: lessons from the Minnesota Longitudinal Study. *Developmental Review*, 30(1), 36–51, pp.44–5.

[336] Belsky, J. & Pensky, E. (1988) Developmental history, personality and family relationships: toward an emergent family system. In R. Hinde & J. Stevenson-Hinde (eds) *Relationships Within Families* (pp.193–217). Oxford: Clarendon Press.

discovery that secure attachments were much more likely to be stable than insecure attachments (OR = 1.39), and that this effect was stronger in low-risk samples (OR = 1.73). Such findings suggest that children are more likely to keep a sense of their caregiver's availability once they have found it than they are to retain a sense of their caregiver's unavailability. They found that this effect is stronger when there are fewer contextual risks facing the dyad.[337] Pinquart and colleagues end on the optimistic note that the lower stability of insecure attachments suggests that, against the public image that Bowlby's popularizing writings helped foster of attachment patterns as fixed for life, there is substantial room for change especially among the families who may most need support. In these terms, there may be room for yet more optimism. In 2018, Opie reported a meta-analysis from 56 studies, with stability of $r = .26$. Accounting for differences between her findings and those of earlier studies, she had access to many more published papers, and identified significant evidence of publication bias, with studies reporting low stability less likely to have been published.[338]

Research on stability, initiated by Waters, overall raises two distinct points. First, contrary to the social learning theorists, that there is some stability suggests that the behaviour reflects more than the pushes and pulls of immediate caregiver reinforcement. This finding halted most, if not all, social learning critiques of attachment research, though the social learning theorists did not join the attachment enterprise. Links between attachment and social learning theory would have to be rediscovered by later researchers (see Chapter 6). Second, the question of longer-term stability addresses the theoretical concern of the extent to which early experience establishes a prototype for later interactions and/or are influenced by later developments. The central conclusion drawn by researchers was that attachment is influenced by later developments, and that this can be anticipated to be affected by changes in caregiving.[339] Use of language suggesting the fixedness of attachment patterns for most people can still be seen in the writings of some major attachment researchers.[340] However, perhaps a majority of writings on attachment now emphasise predictable movement between patterns of attachment, with continuity in substantial part the result of continuity of relationship qualities.[341]

---

[337] Pinquart, M., Feußner, C., & Ahnert, L. (2013) Meta-analytic evidence for stability in attachments from infancy to early adulthood. *Attachment & Human Development*, 15(2), 189–218. It should be mentioned, however, that poor short-term stability was demonstrated on the large NICHD sample. Groh, A.M., Roisman, G.I., Booth-LaForce, C., et al. (2014) IV. Stability of attachment security from infancy to late adolescence. *Monographs of the Society for Research in Child Development*, 79(3), 51–66.

[338] Opie, J. (2018) Attachment stability and change in early childhood and associated moderators. Unpublished doctoral thesis, Deakin University, Melbourne.

[339] An important work on this latter question, conducted by Waters and colleagues, was Waters, E., Merrick, S., Treboux, D., Crowell, J., & Albersheim, L. (2000) Attachment security in infancy and early adulthood: a twenty-year longitudinal study. *Child Development*, 71(3), 684–9. This study is not detailed here since it would require explanation of the Adult Attachment Interview, which is described in Chapter 3. In brief, the researchers found that 72% of the infants received a matching secure or insecure attachment classification in adulthood. However, 44% of the infants whose mothers reported negative life events change attachment classifications by the time the Adult Attachment Interview was conducted.

[340] For a recent description of early attachment patterns as generally consigned for life in the absence of intervention see Powell, B., Cooper, G., Hoffman, K., & Marvin, B. (2016) *The Circle of Security Intervention*. New York: Guilford, p.69.

[341] Besides Lamb, another early advocate for integrating discontinuity into the tenets of attachment theory was Crittenden, P.M. (1995) Attachment and psychopathology. In S. Goldberg, R. Muir, & J. Kerr (eds) *John Bowlby's Attachment Theory: Historical, Clinical and Social Significance*. New York: Analytical Press, pp.367–406. An emphasis on predicting discontinuity is also characteristic of the third generation of developmental researchers (Chapter 6).

Attachment Q-sort

As well as pursuing research on the stability of the Strange Situation classifications, Waters was a fierce advocate for the need for full construct validation for attachment measures. Following Cronbach and Meehl, he argued that any empirical findings take their meaning from the network of other related results, which provide the context for their interpretation.[342] Waters and Ainsworth discussed their alignment with this position in their correspondence.[343] In the case of the Strange Situation procedure, Waters and Deane expressed concern for a tendency within attachment research to search for associations between the infant classifications and various outcomes without any more general hypothesis than 'all good things go together'.[344] In their impression, with each such study, attachment research becomes less incisive, and the concept of attachment becomes increasingly debased into a general idea of close relationships in general (Chapter 5).[345]

Waters argued for a return to focus on what he termed 'the secure base phenomenon', which—confusingly for many readers—included for him both secure base and safe haven dynamics. He also argued that too much attention had been paid to the 'critical situations' of distress and reunion, designed to prompt the activation of the attachment system, with the Strange Situation providing visuals. Too little attention had been paid to the ordinary, incremental moments that form the basis for trust or distrust in the availability of the caregiver, especially contexts of non-distress, exploration, and quieter, ordinary feelings.[346] Whilst overt attachment behaviour would be less frequently seen in these circumstances, ordinary life in naturalistic settings was ultimately the substance that filled out and elaborated the attachment system, and especially expectations about the caregiver's availability as a secure base. Like Bowlby and Ainsworth in their final years,[347] and likely influenced by Ainsworth's stance directly, Sroufe and Waters were dismayed that attachment researchers had leapt upon the Strange Situation procedure at the expense of the naturalistic research. They felt that this direction of interest was due to a number of factor, including: poor general understanding among researchers of Bowlby and Ainsworth's specific characterisation of the attachment behavioural system; the resource costs associated with detailed home observations; the unusual observational acuity of Ainsworth for seeing patterns, which not all researchers possessed; and reification of the Group B classification as 'security' itself rather

---

[342] Cronbach, L. & Meehl, P. (1955) Construct validity in psychological tests. *Psychological Bulletin*, 52(4), 281–302; Waters, E. & Sroufe, L.A. (1983) Social competence as a developmental construct. *Developmental Review* 3, 79–97, p.80.

[343] Ainsworth, M. (1973) *Letter to Everett Waters*, 7 December 1973. Mary Ainsworth Archive, Box M3176, Folder 4.

[344] Waters, E. & Deane, K.E. (1985) Defining and assessing individual differences in attachment relationships: Q-methodology and the organization of behavior in infancy and early childhood. *Monographs of the Society for Research in Child Development*, 50(1/2), 41–65, p.42.

[345] Ibid. p.42.

[346] The point is developed in Waters, E. (2008) Live long and prosper: a note on attachment and evolution. http://www.psychology.sunysb.edu/attachment/gallery/live_long/live_long.html.

[347] Ainsworth, M. & Bowlby, J. (1991) 1989 APA award recipient addresses: an ethological approach to personality development. *American Psychologist*, 46(4), 333–41: The Strange Situation 'procedure soon became widely used, if not always wisely and well, and has quite overshadowed the findings of the research project that gave rise to it' (338).

than, as Ainsworth intended, a window into the child's experiences of care by an attachment figure and therefore a proxy for naturalistic observation.[348]

For any research paradigm truly loyal to Ainsworth's principles, Sroufe and Waters argued strongly that 'the strange situation is used only because it can stand in place of attachment as it would be observed in the home'.[349] It struck them as dangerous that so much work subsequent to the Baltimore study was predicated (whether researchers knew it or not) on the reliability of the link between Strange Situation assessments and secure base behaviour at home. To offer a means to replicate and further explore this essential finding, Waters and colleagues developed a new measure, the Attachment Q-Sort (AQS).[350] Waters recalls that several colleagues in the attachment community were resistant to the creation of an alternative to the Strange Situation.[351] Yet many colleagues, including Sroufe, supported this development and served as expert consultants on the development of the measure. Ainsworth stated her approval of the new measure.[352]

In the AQS, observers are asked to sort a set of behavioural descriptors of a child observed for a few hours in a naturalistic setting like the home. These descriptors, printed on pieces of card, are sifted into piles ranging from 'most descriptive of this child' to 'least descriptive of this child'. The set of descriptors covers a broad range of secure base and exploratory behaviour, affective response, social referencing, and other aspects of social cognition. Observers can then be kept unaware of the constructs that will be scored from the data they provide, whilst attachment phenomena can be picked out and distinguished from other aspects of behaviour. Like the Strange Situation, the measure is grounded in concretely observed behaviour. However, compared to the Strange Situation, the AQS can be used to assess ordinary interaction between a child and caregiver in naturalistic settings; it therefore has greater ecological validity than the dramatised prompts and interactions of the Strange Situation. For instance, it could have better cross-cultural validity than the Strange Situation, since the meaning of separation and reunion for young children likely differs by culture—though cultural values may still inflect the descriptors on the AQS cards.

Ainsworth emphasised that the developmental changes from infancy to toddlerhood entail nothing less than a 'recasting of attachment relationship, so that they now include perspective taking, include communication, negotiation and mutual plans'. Any adequate measure of attachment after infancy, she felt, needs above all to consider the way that 'seeing things from

[348] Waters, E., Kondo-Ikemura, K., Posada, G., and Richters, J.E. (1991) Learning to love. In M.R. Gunnar & L.A. Sroufe (eds) *Self Processes and Development* (pp.217–55). New York: Psychology Press, pp.241–2.

[349] Sroufe, L.A. & Waters, E. (1982) Issues of temperament and attachment. *American Journal of Orthopsychiatry*, 52(4), 743–6, p.743.

[350] On the history of Q methodology see Stephenson, W. (1953) *The Study of Behavior: Q-Technique and its Methodology*. Chicago: University of Chicago Press; Good, J.M. (2010) Introduction to William Stephenson's quest for a science of subjectivity. *Psychoanalysis and History*, 12(2), 211–43. Though Waters and colleagues cite Stephenson's legacy, the more proximal examples of Q methodology research cited as a predecessor for the Attachment Q-Sort were Baumrind, D. (1968) *Manual for the preschool behavior Q-Sort*. Berkeley: Institute of Human Development, University of California; and Block, J. (1978) *The Q-Sort Method in Personality Assessment and Psychiatric Research*. Palo Alto, CA: Consulting Psychologists Press.

[351] Waters, E., Posada, G., Crowell, J., & Lay, K.L. (1993) Is attachment theory ready to contribute to our understanding of disruptive behavior problems? *Development & Psychopathology*, 5(1–2), 215–24, p.222.

[352] Ainsworth, M. (1984) Attachment, adaptation and continuity. Paper presented at International Conference on Infant Studies, April 1984. PP/Bow/J.1/57: 'I am delighted with the extent to which this [Strange Situation] procedure has proved useful in research, but have repeatedly stated that its success should stimulate rather than discourage the development of other procedures ... It is paradoxical that the search for new procedures comes not from the critics of strange-situation research but from among those who have been most intimately involved in it. I mention here particularly Mary Main and Everett Waters.'

the partner's point of view' gets integrated with secure base/safe haven dynamics.[353] Whilst applications of the Strange Situation with toddlers and pre-schoolers have been developed, such extensions have been troubled by the dual pull to respond to such maturational differences and, simultaneously, retain the semblance of Ainsworth's infant system.[354] A special advantage of the AQS is that, with minor adaptions, it can be used with children of different ages.[355] The AQS could readily incorporate expected changes in the way that children:

- use their caregiver as a secure base and safe haven in the context of more sophisticated capacities for communication, negotiation, mutual planning, and perspective taking
- modulate the threshold for activation of the attachment behavioural system
- integrate cognition, affect, and behaviour as part of the system
- show attachment behaviour in interplay with other behavioural systems.

Q-methodology also has several psychometric advantages over Ainsworth's categories.[356] The primary output of the measure is the assessment of attachment security in terms of a continuous variable, based on the extent to which children can use their caregiver as a secure base and safe haven as needed within their everyday context. Waters did not, like Fraley and Spieker, provoke controversy by publicly opposing the statistical and theoretical advantages of a dimensional scale to a category-based approach. However, the way that the AQS was constructed quietly downplayed the importance of the avoidant and resistant classifications, focusing instead on how close or distant a case was from the paradigm of an infant using the caregiver as a secure base and safe haven.[357]

A recent meta-analysis by Cadman and colleagues, on the basis of 245 studies and 32,426 child–caregiver dyads, reported substantial convergent validity for the AQS. When children are assessed with the Ainsworth Strange Situation, and when the AQS is used for at least 180

[353] Ainsworth, M. (1991) Past and future trends in attachment research. Film of the presentation made available by Avi Sagi-Schwartz (Chair), International Society for the Study of Behavioral Development, Minneapolis, July 1991.

[354] For discussions of, and different approaches to, this problem see Cassidy, J., Marvin, R., with the Attachment Working Group of the John D. and Catherine T. MacArthur Network on the Transition from Infancy to Early Childhood (1992) Attachment organisation in preschool children: procedures and coding manual. Unpublished manual;Crittenden, P.M. (2017) Gifts from Mary Ainsworth and John Bowlby. *Clinical Child Psychology and Psychiatry*, 22(3), 436–42; Waters, E., Vaughn, B., & Waters, H.S. (eds) (in press) *Measuring Attachment*. New York: Guilford.

[355] Waters, E. & Deane, K.E. (1985) Defining and assessing individual differences in attachment relationships: Q-methodology and the organization of behavior in infancy and early childhood. *Monographs of the Society for Research in Child Development*, 50(1/2), 41–65.

[356] Waters, E. & Deane, K.E. (1985) Defining and assessing individual differences in attachment relationships: Q-methodology and the organization of behavior in infancy and early childhood. *Monographs of the Society for Research in Child Development*, 50(1/2), 41–65, p.53; Seifer, R. & Schiller, M. (1995) The role of parenting sensitivity, infant temperament, and dyadic interaction in attachment theory and assessment. *Monographs of the Society for Research in Child Development*, 60(2–3), 146–74.

[357] A supplement to the Attachment Q-Sort to scale disorganized attachment (Chapter 3) was developed in the 1990s by John Kirkland. However, the work was not published, or even discussed in print until recently. The only study to date to have used this supplement is Handley, E.D., Michl-Petzing, L.C., Rogosch, F.A., Cicchetti, D., & Toth, S.L. (2017) Developmental cascade effects of interpersonal psychotherapy for depressed mothers: longitudinal associations with toddler attachment, temperament, and maternal parenting efficacy. *Development & Psychopathology*, 29(2), 601–15. The authors report a strong association with disorganized attachment in the Strange Situation, though on a study using only 10% of their sample of 125 toddlers. On disorganized attachment and the Attachment Q-Sort measure see also the item analyses reported in Van Bakel, H.J. & Riksen-Walraven, J.M. (2004) AQS security scores: what do they represent? A study in construct validation. *Infant Mental Health Journal*, 25(3), 175–93.

minutes, agreement is substantial ($r = .39$), as are associations with measures of caregiver sensitivity ($r = .44$). Agreement is, however, reduced when a shorter period of observation is used ($r = .25$ with the Strange Situation; and .28 with caregiver sensitivity). The AQS assessed by observers is also able to predict later socioemotional outcomes for children ($r = .24$). One remarkable finding is that the AQS has an especially strong ability to predict later aggression and conduct problems symptoms ($d = .70$). Some of this effect may be explained by the fact that the AQS can be used with two-year-olds and this may be a developmental stage of particular importance for the development of conduct problems.[358] At times, researchers have also often asked parents themselves to complete the AQS. However, there are good reasons to suspect that this approach is less valid, since associations with the Strange Situation and sensitivity are much lower, and associations with caregiver report on the child temperament are substantial ($r = .33$).[359] It would seem that a child's own caregivers are less effective than unfamiliar observers at distinguishing a child's attachment behaviours from a global impression of their child's temperament.[360] Van IJzendoorn and colleagues praised the AQS, claiming that the availability of a second well-validated measure of child attachment alongside the Strange Situation helps 'separate the concept of attachment in young children from the way it is measured', a major contribution to the field.[361]

A recent development of potential importance has been the development of a brief version of the AQS by Fearon and colleagues.[362] Ainsworth fully acknowledged that the Strange Situation is far too laborious for screening purposes or regular use by clinicians and practitioners, and urged methodological innovation in this area.[363] To address this gap, the Brief Attachment Scale (BAS-16) is a pared-down version of the full Attachment Q-Sort, consisting of two scales: (i) harmonious interaction with the caregiver and (ii) proximity-seeking behaviours. Validated against the full AQS on a portion of the large NICHD sample, convergence between the measures was very good. The BAS-16 had associations with caregiver sensitivity ($r = .23$) and child externalizing behaviours at 24 months ($r = -.25$) equivalent to the full AQS, and there was no association with measures of infant temperament.

The NICHD sample also had classifications available for the Ainsworth Strange Situation—though in this sample there was no association between the Ainsworth classifications and the full AQS. As a result, the BAS-16 had all but no link with the Strange

[358] Fearon, R.P., Bakermans-Kranenburg, M.J., van IJzendoorn, M.H., Lapsley, A.M., & Roisman, G.I. (2010) The significance of insecure attachment and disorganization in the development of children's externalizing behavior: a meta-analytic study. *Child Development*, 81(2), 435–56, p.450.

[359] Cadman, T., Diamond, P.R., & Fearon, P. (2018) Reassessing the validity of the attachment Q-sort: an updated meta-analysis. *Infant and Child Development*, 27(1).

[360] See also Tarabulsy, G., Provost, M.A., Larose, S., et al. (2008) Similarities and differences in mothers' and observers' ratings of infant security on the attachment Q-sort. *Infant Behavior & Development*, 31(1), 10–22.

[361] Van IJzendoorn, M.H., Vereijken, C.M., Bakermans-Kranenburg, M.J., & Marianne Riksen-Walraven, J. (2004) Assessing attachment security with the attachment Q sort: meta-analytic evidence for the validity of the observer AQS. *Child Development*, 75(4), 1188–213, p.1207.

[362] Cadman, T., Belsky, J., & Fearon, R.M.P. (2018) The Brief Attachment Scale (BAS-16): a short measure of infant attachment. *Child: Care, Health and Development*, 44(5), 766–75. Independently of Fearon, Bakermans-Kranenburg and colleagues also developed a brief version of the AQS about 15 years earlier. Bakermans-Kranenburg, M.J., Willemsen-Swinkels, S.H.N., & van IJzendoorn, M.H. (2003) *Brief Attachment Screening Questionnaire*. Unpublished manuscript, Leiden University, Centre for Child and Family Studies. This was used as part of Rutgers, A.H., van IJzendoorn, M.H., Bakermans-Kranenburg, M.J., et al. (2007) Autism, attachment and parenting: a comparison of children with autism spectrum disorder, mental retardation, language disorder, and non-clinical children. *Journal of Abnormal Child Psychology*, 35(5), 859–70.

[363] Ainsworth, M.D.S. (1980) Attachment and child abuse. In G. Gerbner, C.J. Ross, & E. Zigler (eds) *Child abuse: an agenda for action* (pp.35–47). Oxford: Oxford University Press, p.45.

Situation. Fearon and colleagues suggest that greater convergence may be anticipated when the BAS-16 is used to assess responses to separation or some other mildly stressful event, when the attachment behavioural system will be activated. If so, this would offer important further validation of the new measure. Until then, what conclusions the field will draw regarding the usefulness of the BAS-16 as a brief measure of infant attachment are unclear, and will likely depend on the extent to which developmental attachment research is willing to rest weight on measures that do not agree with the Ainsworth Strange Situation.[364] For the second generation of attachment researchers, this would have been an anathema. For the third-generation leaders of the field, with a greater concern to sustain a dialogue with routine clinical practice, it may not only be possible but perhaps expectable.[365] The BAS-16 may also help facilitate cross-cultural attachment research in a way that has not been possible for the Strange Situation.

Secure base scripts

The Strange Situation, as a staged procedure requiring the semi-standardisation of caregiver behaviour, offers little insight into what caregivers actually do to support attachment and exploration in particular dyads. Yet Waters emphasised that the attachment behavioural system requires support to achieve coherence. This includes, for example, 'secure base/safe haven games' such as peek-a-boo, which dramatise the script of separation followed by reunion, and obstruction resolved into relational closeness and accessibility.[366] This teaching and learning of the secure base script is evident also in adolescent and adult relationships, when romantic relationships are invested with attachment components. In 'Bowlby's theory grown up', published in 1994, Crowell and Waters argued that 'commitment in secure-base terms is unlikely to be "hearts and flowers" responsiveness or "I want to marry you"; rather, we suggest it may be more like "I'm here, I will be here, I'm interested in what you do and what you think and feel, I will actively support your independent actions, I trust you and you can trust me to be here if you need me, et cetera".[367] All the small ways that adolescent or adult dyads repeatedly, across situations, affirm their availability to one another form the intricate little bones within the structure of the relationship and relationship-related expectations, giving strength and stability to its capacity to serve as a secure base and safe haven.

Everett and Harriet Waters observed that Bowlby's internal working model concept encompasses (i) how accessible or inaccessible attachment figures tend to be under ordinary situations, (ii) whether attachment behaviours are regarded as acceptable or unacceptable, and (iii) a forecast about how available and responsive these figures are when difficulties

---

[364] See Ziv, Y. & Hotam, Y. (2015) Theory and measure in the psychological field: the case of attachment theory and the strange situation procedure. *Theory & Psychology*, 25(3), 274–91.

[365] Compare, for instance, attempts to pare down established assessments of caregiving behaviour to develop a brief screening measure: Haltigan, J.D., Madigan, S., Bronfman, E., et al. (2019) Refining the assessment of disrupted maternal communication: using item response models to identify central indicators of disrupted behavior. *Development & Psychopathology*, 31(1), 261–77.

[366] Waters, E., Kondo-Ikemura, K., Posada, G., and Richters, J.E. (1991) Learning to love. In M.R. Gunnar & L.A. Sroufe (eds) *Self Processes and Development* (pp.217–55). New York: Psychology Press, p.236; Waters, E., Posada, G., Crowell, J.A., & Lay, K.L. (1994) The development of attachment: from control system to working models. *Psychiatry*, 57(1), 32–42, p.35.

[367] Crowell, J.A. & Waters, E. (1994) Bowlby's theory grown up: the role of attachment in adult love relationships. *Psychological Inquiry*, 5(1), 31–4, p.32.

are faced (Chapter 1).[368] Waters and Waters therefore argued that the idea of the internal working model is too clumsy and general a concept for developing specific testable hypotheses. They advocated instead the idea of 'scripts', sedimented in procedural memory by repetition and experience, which respond to particular cues with involuntary expectations about what tends to happen next and predispositions to behave in certain ways. Attention to attachment-related scripts therefore moves 'toward explaining what exactly the development of attachment representations is the development of'.[369] In fact, a similar point was proposed to Bowlby in the 1980s by John Byng-Hall; Bowlby was highly sympathetic, describing the specification of internal working models using the metaphor of a 'script' as 'a most valuable step'.[370]

Waters and Waters argued that at the heart of attachment theory are the secure base and safe haven responses, and of all the different content included within an 'internal working model' it is these that should be the focus of researchers' efforts.[371] This proposal has seen increasing acceptance among attachment researchers in recent years.[372] Such a script might include some source of distress for one member of a dyad; this prompts a signal for help; the signal is detected and help is offered; this help is accepted and proves effective; the interaction proves comforting; and matters are sufficiently resolved that other activities can be recommenced. Waters and Waters proposed that having a secure base script organizing the cognitive components of the attachment behavioural system is helpful for the expression of secure behaviour when exploration is called for, and for requesting and making use of support as needed if demands or threats arise. Waters and Waters developed methods for assessing the secure base script, both using narrative methodologies appropriate for children and in coding the Berkeley Adult Attachment Interview (Chapter 3). Such methods have demonstrated that secure base scripts in adolescence and adulthood are predicted by early experiences of sensitive care and early attachment patterns, are generally stable over time, and in turn predict adult caregiving behaviour to children and other aspects of functioning, including even adult physical health.[373]

---

[368] Waters, H.S. & Waters, E. (2006) The attachment working models concept: among other things, we build script-like representations of secure base experiences. *Attachment & Human Development*, 8(3), 185–97. They were influenced by earlier work by Schank, R. & Abelson, R. (1977) *Scripts, Plans, Goals, and Understanding: An Inquiry into Human Knowledge Structures*. New York: Lawrence Erlbaum; Bretherton, I. (1987) New perspectives on attachment relations: security, communication, and internal working models. In J.D. Osofsky (ed.) *Handbook of Infant Development*, 2nd edn (pp.1061–100). New York: Wiley. There was also other work in the 1990s that helped set the stage for the proposal of secure base scripts, e.g. Kirsh, S. & Cassidy, J. (1997) Preschoolers' attention to and memory for attachment relevant information. *Child Development*, 68, 1143–53.

[369] Waters, T.E.A. & Facompré, C.R (in press) Measuring secure base script knowledge in the Adult Attachment Interview. In E. Waters, B.E. Vaughn, & H.S. Waters (eds) *Measuring Attachment*. New York: Guilford.

[370] Bowlby, J. (1985) *Letter to John Byng-Hall*, 12 April 1985. PP/Bow/J.9/45, discussing Byng-Hall, J. (1985) The family script: a useful bridge between theory and practice. *Journal of Family Therapy*, 7(3), 301–305.

[371] Waters, H.S. & Waters, E. (2006) The attachment working models concept: among other things, we build script-like representations of secure base experiences. *Attachment & Human Development*, 8(3), 185–97.

[372] For instance, routine definitions of 'internal working models' have increasingly made appeal to the concept of script. E.g. Bakermans-Kranenburg, M.J., Juffer, F., & van IJzendoorn, M.H. (2019) Reflections on the mirror: on video-feedback to promote positive parenting and infant mental health. In C. Zeanah (ed.) *Handbook of Infant Mental Health*, 4th edn (pp.527–42). New York: Guilford.

[373] Waters, T.E., Brockmeyer, S.L., & Crowell, J.A. (2013) AAI coherence predicts caregiving and care seeking behavior: secure base script knowledge helps explain why. *Attachment & Human Development*, 15(3), 316–31; Waters, T.E., Ruiz, S.K., & Roisman, G.I. (2017) Origins of secure base script knowledge and the developmental construction of attachment representations. *Child Development*, 88(1), 198–209; Farrell, A.K., Waters, T.E.A., Young, E.S., et al. (2019) Early maternal sensitivity, attachment security in young adulthood, and cardiometabolic risk at midlife. *Attachment & Human Development*, 21(1), 70–86.

Waters and Waters conceptualised security as a single dimension, running counter to the central position of Ainsworth's three patterns of attachment in the research imagination of other attachment researchers. For them, the capacity to make effective use of others as a secure base and safe haven is much like a skill, and the effectiveness of skills is generally measured on continua. In support for this position, a taxometric study of secure base script knowledge in late adolescence and adulthood found a dimensional latent structure at both ages.[374] More generally, Waters and Waters also hold that the distinction between avoidant and ambivalent/resistant attachment is yet to have adequate substantion from home observations beyond those of Ainsworth, or empirical yield in decades of research. Nonetheless, over the coming years it can be anticipated that the conceptualisation and operationalisation of secure base scripts will be asked to incorporate some attention to the different ways that secure base scripts may be disrupted, given the characteristic interest in categories of socioemotional problems among attachment researchers (Chapter 3) and in clinical discourses (Chapter 6). This will no doubt include examination of associations with the different Strange Situation categories. Within the secure base script measures themselves, it may be that differences will be articulated and explored between the narratives of individuals who expect only instrumental support, those who expect insensitive care and partial access to a secure base/safe haven, and those who expect little or no secure base/safe haven availability at all.

Cross-cultural applicability of the Strange Situation

Two traditions of cross-cultural research

In evaluating the legacy of Ainsworth and the assessment measures she introduced, and important domain to consider is their application to cross-cultural research. Looking back in 2016 on the decades of research using Ainsworth's methods, Mesman, van IJzendoorn, and Sagi-Schwartz observed that 'the current cross-cultural database is almost absurdly small compared to the domain that should be covered'.[375] A central reason for this seems to have been that the early attachment researchers failed to secure an alliance with anthropology. Margaret Mead had famously been an early critic of Bowlby. The nub of their disagreement, from Bowlby's perspective, was that Mead seemed to be arguing that an infant cared for by interchangeable caregivers within a village would have the same prospects of healthy psychological development as an infant cared for by a small number of very familiar and cherished people. In direct discussion at the World Health Organisation in the 1950s, Mead put to Bowlby that the child would do fine with twenty different caregivers. Bowlby replied that in general he did not take the view that children would be harmed by having multiple caregivers; however, there were limits. Roughly equal care by twenty different caregivers would be unlikely to offer a young child the basis for discriminating, cherished relationships with

[374] Waters, T.E., Fraley, R., Groh, A., et al. (2015) The latent structure of secure base script knowledge. *Developmental Psychology*, 51(6), 823–30.
[375] Mesman, J., van IJzendoorn, M.H., & Sagi-Schwartz, S. (2016) Cross-cultural patterns of attachment: universal and contextual dimensions. In J. Cassidy & P. Shaver (eds) *Handbook of Attachment*. New York: Guilford (pp.790–815), p.809.

particular familiar figures.[376] This agrees with later findings from the anthropological litera-ture, summarised recently by the social anthropologist Sara Harkness as the conclusion that 'even in contexts of multiple caregiving, infants generally do not form close relationships with more than a few individuals'.[377]

Bowlby and Ainsworth held that care by more than one person was not anticipated to ne-cessarily disrupt the quality of the attachment relationships formed with these people. For example, 'a child cared for by several caregivers can, and frequently does, form as secure an attachment to one figure, his mother, as a child who has a more exclusive relationship with one figure'.[378] Unfortunately, however, Bowlby's impression of what was meant when anthro-pologists spoke of 'multiple caregiving arrangements' appears to have been frozen at Mead's characterisation of twenty interchangeable people. The result was a bizarre and quite specific blindspot. Bowlby was the consummate interdisciplinary researcher, drawing in knowledge from across disciplines including behavioural biology, cybernetics, linguistics, neurology, and epidemiology. Furthermore, in fact he read anthropological research regarding grief and mourning with great interest, and reported the benefit he had gained from reading an-thropological studies such as those by Raymond Firth, Geoffrey Gorer, David Mandelbaum, Phyllis Palgi, and Paul C. Rosenblatt. He also expressed appreciation for anthropological theory, such as the ideas of Durkheim and Malinowski.[379]

However, he tended to treat anthropologists who raised questions about his work as holding the same stance as Mead. So, for instance, when the Harvard anthropologists Sarah and Robert Levine came to talk to him in London about their research on multiple care-giving arrangements in Nigeria, he was apparently rude and dismissive.[380] He systemat-ically neglected discussion of the role of multiperson interactions in shaping attachment, since these were conflated with multiple caregiving.[381] With cross-cultural differences neglected, many relevant issues in his theory remained unresolved. For instance, despite reading much relevant ethnographic research, he left unaddressed in his writings the ques-tion of whether, if all human infants have the capacity for use of the caregiver as a secure base and safe haven, all cultures could be anticipated to scaffold and utilise this capacity. Sadly, Bowlby seems to have experienced anthropologists as insufficiently uninterested in the nuances of his work to make it worthwhile working out subtleties of his theory in dia-logue with anthropology.

---

[376] Tanner, J.M. & Inhelder, B. (eds) (1956) *Discussions on Child Development: Proceedings of the WTO Study Group of the Psychobiological Development of the Child*, Vol. 2. London: Tavistock, p.90. See also Bakermans-Kranenburg, M.J., Steele, H., Zeanah, C.H., et al. (2011) Attachment and emotional development in institutional care: characteristics and catch up. *Monographs of the Society for Research in Child Development*, 76(4), 62–91.

[377] Harkness, S. (2015) The Strange Situation of attachment research: a review of three books. *Reviews in Anthropology*, 44(3), 178–97, p.196.

[378] Ainsworth, M. (1963) The development of infant–mother interaction among the Ganda. In B.M. Foss (ed.) *Determinants of Infant Behaviour* (pp.67–104), Vol. 2. London: Methuen, p.95. Bowlby's annotations on this chapter are in an edition held by Richard and Xenia Bowlby.

[379] Bowlby, J. (1980) *Loss*. New York: Basic Books, p.126. W.H.R. Rivers was also an early influence. Van Dijken, S., van der Veer, R., van IJzendoorn, M., & Kuipers, H.J. (1998) Bowlby before Bowlby: the sources of an intellec-tual departure in psychoanalysis and psychology. *Journal of the History of the Behavioral Sciences*, 34(3), 247–69.

[380] LeVine, R.A. (2014) Attachment theory as cultural ideology. In H. Otto & H. Keller (eds) *Different Faces of Attachment: Cultural Variations on a Universal Human Need* (pp.50–65). Cambridge: Cambridge University Press.

[381] Bowlby's concerns fed Ainsworth's focus on dyadic interaction. In turn, Bowlby's antipathy to multi-person interactions and Ainsworth's focus on dyadic interaction together formed a serious obstacle to applications or extensions of attachment research beyond the dyad, including small group research—though see Ein-Dor's work discussed in Chapter 5. Likewise, though there are exceptions, multi-person caregiving arrangements have been comparatively underresearched by attachment researchers. Keller, H., Bard, K., Morelli, G., et al. (2018) The myth of universal sensitive responsiveness: comment on Mesman et al. (2017). *Child Development*, 89(5), 1921–8.

By contrast, both Bowlby and Ainsworth were very encouraging of anthropological study when they were confident that the researcher did not hold that twenty interchangeable carers would offer the basis for secure attachments. When Ainsworth's student Bob Marvin wrote reporting from his collaboration with Sarah and Robert LeVine, Bowlby described the work as 'interesting' and 'very valuable'.[382] No doubt a basis for Bowlby's different stance was that the LeVines took their observations of attachment behaviour shown by infants to multiple caregivers as a falsification of attachment theory. By contrast, Marvin emphasised observations, from the very same fieldwork, that when children were distressed, they nonetheless still generally sought their most familiar adult figure. For Ainsworth, such issues brought out a fundamental difference between anthropology and psychology as research paradigms: psychological research was grounded in the potential for quantitative assessment of inter-rater reliability in the study of behaviour, whereas anthropological research was based on meticulous ethnographic observations without attempts to achieve reliability with other observers. She was a stanch advocate for anthropological and qualitative observational methods within psychology.[383]

However, Ainsworth was also mindful that the standing of the emergent attachment paradigm in the positivist context of American academic psychology depended on assembling a body of quantitative findings. Immediacy's grip led the field away from precisely the tradition of mixed-methods research that had been fundamental to Ainsworth's own intellectual development until the mid-1960s.[384] As the Strange Situation classification became increasingly taken for granted, and developmental psychology moved towards an increased focus on large numbers as the basis for validity, it is now very rare even to find studies that investigate and report on the specific qualities of cases that run against the overall association.[385] Danziger referred to this phenomenon across academic psychology as the 'triumph of the aggregate'.[386] Insofar as it has been reflected in the priorities of researchers after Ainsworth, Klaus and Karin Grossmann described the triumph of the aggregate in the decline of mixed-methods inquiry as an inestimable loss to attachment research.[387]

However, in addition to differences in epistemology, a further factor hindering the development of an alliance with anthropology was the unattractiveness of Ainsworth's Strange Situation for ethnographic fieldwork.[388] It was laborious to train to code the measure. Any

[382] Bowlby, J. (1975) *Letter to Robert Marvin*, 5 November 1975. PP/Bow/J.9/132.

[383] Ainsworth, M. (1998) Harold Stevenson—SRCD oral history interview. http://srcd.org/sites/default/files/documents/ainsworth_mary_interview.pdf.

[384] A plea for mixed methods research on attachment has also been made by Rothbaum, F. & Morelli, G. (2005) Attachment and culture: bridging relativism and universalism. In W. Friedlmeier, P. Chakkarath, & B. Schwarz (eds) *Culture and Human Development: The Importance of Cross-Cultural Research to the Social Sciences*. Lisse: Swets & Zeitlinger; and by Keller, H. (2018) Parenting and socioemotional development in infancy and early childhood. *Developmental Review*, 50, 31–41. For a recent example of use of mixed-methods see Suchman, N., Berg, A., Abrahams, L., et al. (2019) Mothering from the inside out: adapting an evidence-based intervention for high-risk mothers in the Western Cape of South Africa. *Development & Psychopathology*, 32(1), 105–22.

[385] Exemplary contrary cases include Hobson, R.P., Patrick, M., Crandell, L., Garcia-Perez, R., & Lee, A. (2005) Personal relatedness and attachment in infants of mothers with borderline personality disorder. *Development & Psychopathology*, 17(2), 329–47; Kozlowska, K. (2010) Family-of-origin issues and the generation of childhood illness. *Australian and New Zealand Journal of Family Therapy*, 31, 73–91; Tharner, A., Verhage, M.L., Oosterman, M., & Schuengel, C. (2019) The case of attachment non-transmission: zooming in on the pathways through parental sensitivity. Paper presented at International Attachment Conference, Vancouver, 20 July 2019.

[386] Danziger, K. (1990) *Constructing the Subject: Historical Origins of Psychological Research*. Cambridge: Cambridge University Press, p.88.

[387] Grossmann, K. & Grossmann, K. (2012) *Bindungen—das Gefüge psychischer Sicherheit Gebundenes*. Stuttgart: Klett-Cotta.

[388] For a discussion of some of the requisites for successful alliance and collaboration between psychology and anthropology see Azuma, H. (1996) Cross-national research on child development: the Hess–Azuma collaboration

graduate students already needing to pursue fieldwork as part of their doctorate could quite reasonably be concerned by the additional time and uncertainty of seeking to gain reliability in Ainsworth's coding system. Furthermore, Ainsworth's tripartite division was regarded as rather crude as an attempt to capture infant experience and care practices in their particularity. The measure may have relevance to understanding individual differences within a culture, but this is only a minor goal within anthropology, which has generally been more concerned with interpreting social practices and meanings.[389] Anthropologists, often suspended between two worlds as individuals or with their families, were also specially aware from personal experience that separations and reunions have the potential for different meanings in different cultural contexts. Furthermore, social and cultural anthropology especially, at least since the 1980s, has had a general antipathy to claims that appear universalistic, and all the more so when this universalism appears value-laden.[390] To the extent that attachment discourses seemed to prize security above insecurity, with stakes for how children and families were evaluated, the paradigm appeared in conflict, quite fundamentally, with a premise of social and cultural anthropology.[391]

Practically, it was also truly cumbersome to conduct the Strange Situation outside of the laboratory.[392] Furthermore, in some cultures, it was regarded as potentially transgressive or, at least, quite rude for researchers to separate infants and caregivers.[393] The Ainsworth sensitivity scale might have been considered an alternative in the 1980s and 1990s. Ainsworth had reported such a strong correlation between maternal sensitivity and infant security that they could have been regarded as much the same construct. However, regrettably, the sensitivity scale remained unpublished. It was by far eclipsed by the Strange Situation, which as a standardised laboratory-based procedure was a more rhetorically useful source of credibility for the emergent attachment research paradigm than the sensitivity scale within the psychological research community in North America and Europe, even if it had reduced utility outside of it. With the sensitivity scale not even brought to market, researchers interested in examining the role of sensitivity in care across cultures were forced either to develop

in retrospect. In D.W. Shwalb & B.J. Shwalb (eds) *Japanese Childrearing: Two Generations of Scholarship* (pp.220–40). New York: Guilford.

[389] Keller, H. (2008) Attachment—past and present. But what about the future? *Integrative Psychological and Behavioral Science*, 42, 406–15. A good illustrative case of the use of the idea of 'attachment', but not attachment research, for interpreting social practices and meanings is Lowe, E.D. (2002) A widow, a child, and two lineages: exploring kinship and attachment in Chuuk. *American Anthropologist*, 104(1), 123–37. For reflection on the different aims of interpretive and experimental forms of research see Reddy, W.M. (2014) Humanists and the experimental study of emotion. In F. Biess & D.M. Gross (eds) *Science and Emotions after 1945: A Transatlantic Perspective* (pp.41–66). Chicago: University of Chicago Press. The social psychological tradition of attachment research (Chapter 5) has likewise seen little uptake within anthropology, sociology, human geography, or cognate social sciences concerned primarily with practices. An exception is Quinlan, R.J. & Quinlan, M.B. (2007) Parenting and cultures of risk: a comparative analysis of infidelity, aggression, and witchcraft. *American Anthropologist*, 109(1), 164–79. However, the social psychological tradition has also seen no critique from anthropologists. Presumably it has fallen under the blanket of 'developments after Ainsworth', which anthropologists have tended to ignore.

[390] Eriksen, T.H. & Nielsen, F.S. (2001) *A History of Anthropology*. London, Pluto Press.

[391] See e.g. Keller, H. (2018) Universality claim of attachment theory: children's socioemotional development across cultures. *Proceedings of the National Academy of Sciences*, 115(45), 11414–19; Keller, H., Bard, K., Morelli, G., et al. (2018) The myth of universal sensitive responsiveness: comment on Mesman et al. (2017). *Child Development*, 89(5), 1921–8.

[392] See e.g. Zevalkink, J., Riksen-Walraven, J.M., & Van Lieshout, C.F. (1999) Attachment in the Indonesian caregiving context. *Social Development*, 8(1), 21–40; True, M., Pisani, L., & Oumar, F. (2001) Infant–mother attachment among the Dogon of Mali. *Child Development*, 72(5), 1451–66.

[393] Otto, H. (2014) Don't show your emotions! Emotion regulation and attachment in the Cameroonian Nso. In H. Otto & H. Keller (eds) *Different Faces of Attachment: Cultural Variations of a Universal Human Need* (pp.215–29). Cambridge: Cambridge University Press.

their own scales, or to rely on dubious proxies for sensitivity such as household size. As a result, two research traditions developed in the 1980s and 1990s: developmental psychologists using measures developed in America in other countries; and qualitative ethnographic studies that eschewed these measures. Each represented a segregated part of Ainsworth's own biographical journey, which had traversed both ethnography and laboratory science.

Cross-cultural studies in the 1980s and 1990s using standardised attachment measures were generally conducted by attachment researchers or developmental psychologists with some personal contact with Ainsworth or her students—with the signal exception of the Japanese studies (discussed in the section 'The Strange Situation "abroad"').[394] An early example was Kermoian and Leiderman (1986), two psychological researchers who conducted a study of 26 Gusii infants from Kenya. The Strange Situation was adapted in several thoughtful ways, such as by taking place outside the mother's hut and by altering the reunion so that infants would be greeted with, as they would expect, the ritual handshake of greeting. The procedure was used both with the mother and with the person who most frequently cared for the infant during the day (generally a sibling). The coding was conducted by researchers trained by Main. Kermoian and Leiderman found that 61% of infants had a secure attachment classification with their mother, and 54% with their daycarer. Whereas security of attachment with mother was related to nutritional status, security of attachment with the daycarer was related to infant cognitive and motor development.[395] The researchers concluded that the pervasive association between infant–mother attachment and infant functioning which has been identified in American samples may be a reflection of the diversity of activities in which American infants and mothers jointly engage, in contrast to the Gusii where a high proportion of infant–mother interaction centres around feeding, and a high proportion of infant–daycarer interaction centred around exploration and daily tasks.

A significant limitation of the cross-cultural studies conducted by psychological researchers has been that only on rare occasions did these researchers accompany their research with ethnography, and generally only when the Strange Situation had not proved workable. A clear exception is Germán Posada and colleagues in their work on the sensitivity construct and secure base behaviour, but this has proved unusual.[396] Whilst attachment researchers may personally have read ethnographic research in situating their study, their write-up in psychology journals has rarely entered into dialogue with anthropologists. Nor would this have likely been rewarded by psychology journals or their reviewers. Ultimately, the ambition of these studies has been to demonstrate that the Strange Situation could tap meaningful variation in individual differences across different contexts, and to examine the role of culture in moderating the influence of caregiving on child attachment as represented by the distribution of Strange Situation classifications. The ambitions of attachment researchers in using the Strange Situation cross-culturally have been therefore, at best, only

[394] E.g. van IJzendoorn, M.H. & Kroonenberg, P.M. (1988) Cross-cultural patterns of attachment: a meta-analysis of the strange situation. *Child Development*, 59, 147–56; Grossmann, K.E., Grossmann, K., & Keppler, A. (2005) Universal and culture-specific aspects of human behavior: the case of attachment. In W. Friedlmeier, P. Chakkarth, & B. Schwarz (eds) *Culture and Human Development: The Importance of Cross-Cultural Research for the Social Sciences* (pp.75–97). New York: Psychology Press.

[395] Kermoian, R. & Leiderman, P.H. (1986) Infant attachment to mother and child caretaker in an East African community. *International Journal of Behavioral Development*, 9(4), 455–69.

[396] Posada, G., Carbonell, O.A., Alzate, G., & Plata, S.J. (2004) Through Colombian lenses: ethnographic and conventional analyses of maternal care and their associations with secure base behavior. *Developmental Psychology*, 40(4), 508–18; Posada, G. (2013) Piecing together the sensitivity construct: ethology and cross-cultural research. *Attachment & Human Development*, 15(5–6), 637–56.

marginally aligned with the aim of anthropology to understand cultural practices. There have been few discussions of how the Strange Situation and its coding might best be adapted to account for cultural context and to offer insight into cultures of caregiving.[397]

As such, the accusation by the anthropologist Heidi Keller that 'the only dimension that attachment researchers have recognised as cultural is the distribution of the attachment qualities'[398] has an unfortunate degree of truth. Cross-cultural research was not especially well aligned with developmental psychology as a disciplinary space in the 1980s and 1990s: there are few funders who support cross-cultural psychology, and few rewards within the academic community for the slower yield of publications this research strategy generally entails.[399] Ethnographic work ahead of a quantitative study would be possible, but would risk being penalised by developmental science journals, which look down on qualitative methods even for exploratory work. Attachment researchers have largely had to furnish their own evidence of cross-cultural relevance and, with few allies to take this work forward, the rate of publication has been slow. Furthermore, attachment researchers are not trained to conduct qualitative research or to draw on social and anthropological theories. Though there are certainly exceptions, this state of affairs contributes to a tendency for attachment researchers to use the Strange Situation and related measures without the empirical or conceptual work (at least in print) to examine whether or how these can be used in a valid way within a particular culture, or to develop testable hypotheses about the role of culture for variations in the functioning of the attachment and caregiving systems. This is precisely what collaboration with anthropology could have facilitated, if there had been appetite, funds, and/or satisfaction of mutual interests.

On the other hand, a second research tradition developed of qualitative studies engaging with issues of attachment. Sometimes this was conducted by developmental psychologists,[400] but by the 1990s the tradition was sustained almost exclusively by professional anthropologists. This anthropological literature has had three particular markers. A first is that it was cultural, not biological anthropology that took an interest in attachment. In fact, with James Chisholm as an exception,[401] there has been little sustained interest in attachment among biological anthropologists.[402] A second characteristic of this anthropological

---

[397] Exceptions include Marvin, R.S., VanDevender, T.L., Iwanaga, M.I., LeVine, S., & LeVine, R.A. (1977) Infant–caregiver attachment among the Hausa of Nigeria. In H.M. McGurk (ed.) *Ecological Factors in Human Development* (pp.247–60). Amsterdam: North-Holland; Crittenden, P.M. & Claussen, A.H. (eds) (2000) *The Organisation of Attachment Relationships*. Cambridge: Cambridge University Press; Thompson, R.A. (2017) Twenty-first century attachment theory. In H. Keller & K. Bard (eds) *The Cultural Nature of Attachment: Contextualizing Relationships and Development* (pp.301–19). Cambridge, MA: MIT Press.

[398] Keller, H. (2013) Attachment and culture. *Journal of Cross-Cultural Psychology*, 44(2), 175–94, p.180.

[399] The collaboration between Bob Marvin and the LeVines stands as an apparent exception to the division between these two traditions, even if it was not feasible to bridge the division completely through use of the Strange Situation. However, it is striking also as a somewhat isolated case, at least until the past decade. It also illustrates well the difficulties and lack of professional reward for such work. See Marvin, R.S., VanDevender, T.L., Iwanaga, M.I., LeVine, S., & LeVine, R.A. (1977) Infant–caregiver attachment among the Hausa of Nigeria. In H.M. McGurk (ed.) *Ecological Factors in Human Development* (pp.247–60). Amsterdam: North-Holland.

[400] E.g. Brazelton, T.B. (1972) Implications of infant development among the Mayan Indians of Mexico. *Human Development*, 15(2), 90–111; Tronick, E.Z., Morelli, G.A., & Ivey, P.K. (1992) The Efe forager infant and toddler's pattern of social relationships: multiple and simultaneous. *Developmental Psychology*, 28(4), 568.

[401] Chisholm, J.S. (1996) The evolutionary ecology of attachment organization. *Human Nature*, 7(1), 1–37; Chisholm, J. (2003) Uncertainty, contingency and attachment: a life history theory of theory of mind. In K. Sterelny & J. Fitness (eds) *From Mating to Mentality: Evaluating Evolutionary Psychology* (pp.125–54). Hove: Psychology Press.

[402] A signal exception is work by Belsky and colleagues on early attachment experiences as priming regarding the need for long-term or short-term focused reproductive strategies. This concept has generated substantial interest among biological anthropologists. Belsky, J., Steinberg, L., & Draper, P. (1991) Childhood experience,

literature was that the quality of the ethnography is high, and publications such as those of Nancy Scheper-Hughes have become classics of the anthropological literature in general. A third was that researchers have by and large displayed little knowledge of developments in attachment research since the 1980s; with some exceptions, their conversation has almost exclusively been with the ideas of Bowlby and Ainsworth, and especially Bowlby's writings.[403] And like Bowlby's earlier writings, they have tended—with exceptions[404]—to assume that care relationships are attachment relationships, without consideration of the attachment-specific qualities such as directional crying and preferential seeking suggested by the theory.

Researchers after Bowlby and Ainsworth are at times treated as mute followers of these founding figures by their anthropologist critics, rather than critical contributors to a living, branching tradition of theory and research. The work of Main, for example her discussion of conditional strategies, appears mostly unknown, or known only secondhand, in anthropological discussions of attachment.[405] Germán Posada's studies have likewise been ignored. In Scheper-Hughes' work, for example, 'attachment' was used to refer mostly to the caregiving system, and Bowlby was interpreted in caricature as an instinct theorist in part as a framing device through which the importance of economic and contextual factors can be highlighted in shaping care practice.[406] Bowlby was used rhetorically to represent 'biology', against anthropology's 'culture'. As a consequence, differences between the disciplines and their goals have combined with poor mutual impressions. Research psychologists seem to hold an impression of anthropologists who discuss attachment as ill-informed and apparently wilfully uninterested in contemporary attachment research—or as implacably hostile, without openings for discussion of how to better conduct research in developmental science.[407]

In a debate at the Leipzig Research Center for Early Child Development in November 2018, Ross Thompson argued that anthropologists have not recognised how the field has evolved since Bowlby and Ainsworth. Keller replied that this is essentially irrelevant, since

interpersonal development, and reproductive strategy: an evolutionary theory of socialization. *Child Development*, 62, 647–70.

[403] Though a critic of the tradition of attachment research located within developmental science, Heidi Keller has been an important figure in seeking bridges between disciplines, and in updating the 'working model' held of attachment researchers by anthropologists. See e.g. Otto, H. & Keller, H. (eds) (2014) *Different Faces of Attachment: Cultural Variations on a Universal Human Need*. Cambridge: Cambridge University Press. A heartening sign of a more serious interaction between developmental science and anthropology is the debate between Judy Mesman and Heidi Keller and colleagues, though the tendency towards talking past one another remains in evidence. See Keller, H., Bard, K., Morelli, G., et al. (2018) The myth of universal sensitive responsiveness: comment on Mesman et al. (2017). *Child Development*, 89(5), 1921–8.

[404] E.g. Meehan, C.L. & Hawks, S. (2015) Multiple attachments: allomothering, stranger anxiety, and intimacy. In H. Otto & H. Keller (eds) *Different Faces of Attachment: Cultural Variations on a Universal Human Need* (pp.113–40). Cambridge: Cambridge University Press.

[405] See e.g. Quinn, N. & Mageo, J. (eds) (2013) *Attachment Deconsidered: Cultural Perspectives on a Western Theory*. London: Palgrave; Morelli, G. (2015) The evolution of attachment theory and cultures of human attachment in infancy and early childhood. In L.E. Jensen (ed.) *The Oxford Handbook of Human Development and Culture: An Interdisciplinary Perspective* (pp.149–64). Oxford: Oxford University Press.

[406] Scheper-Hughes, N. (1993) *Death Without Weeping: The Violence of Everyday Life in Brazil*. Berkeley: University of California Press. Similar issues can be found in later anthropological works, even the otherwise excellent Gottlieb, A. (2004) *The Afterlife Is Where We Come From*. Chicago: University of Chicago Press.

[407] Though, unusually, collaboration and coauthorship between attachment researchers and anthropologists can be seen in Keller, H. (eds) (2017) *The Cultural Nature of Attachment: Contextualizing Relationships and Development*. Cambridge, MA: MIT Press.

the version of attachment theory in wider circulation is that of Bowlby and Ainsworth, and subsequent researchers have not raised their voices to correct this account:

> The real problem I have is that attachment theory in the applied field is really causing, to put it mildly, a lot of distress because children are evaluated according to attachment theory … I know that you would never subscribe to such a view. But what I'm missing is why attachment researchers don't form a louder voice in order to distance themselves from these appearances.[408]

Reflecting on a symposium on anthropology and attachment research held in Frankfurt the previous year, Thompson expressed dismay that the only alternative hypothesis the anthropologists seemed interested to present was that 'cultures vary'. Anthropologists' dismissal of so much of attachment research methodology and theory had, in Thompson's view, left nothing but critique. Thompson expressed the sincere wish that anthropologists had sought to be more constructive: 'That cultures vary is not a hypothesis; it is a truism'. He urged that critics seek to join the conversation with attachment researchers by making their criticisms relevant to hypothesis-generation, for instance about when sensitivity is and is not so relevant.[409] In this way, attention to universal processes and culturally specific processes could be brought together. Another example would be the Klaus and Karin Grossmann's reflections on forms of attachment avoidance that have a basis more in cultural factors than in insensitive care, and which may therefore have different correlates.

Keller, however, shot back at Thompson that attachment researchers only tend to recognise hypotheses if they relate narrowly to the 'gold standard' quantitative measures.[410] Furthermore, she alleged that hypotheses may not be recognised by attachment researchers unless they are made by an insider. Writing in a book co-edited by Keller, Weisner also observed that anthropologists feel deliberately ignored by developmental attachment research, which seems implacable in response to their concerns about Bowlby and Ainsworth's ideas, and the Strange Situation procedure in particular, contributing to a sense of frustration among anthropologists.[411] Whether this frustration is the anger of hope or the anger of despair is unclear. The overall result of interactions between attachment researchers and anthropologists from Bowlby to the present has been weak common ground or basis for mutual curiosity, as neither tradition treats the work of the other as engaging or valuable. Attachment researchers have mostly felt that they had to go it alone in pursuing cross-cultural quantitative research without support from anthropologists in adjusting or calibrating their measures, in the design of studies, or in interpreting results.

---

[408] Keller, H. & Thompson, R. (2018) Attachment theory: past, present & future. Recorded at the 2nd 'Wilhelm Wundt Dialogue', Leipzig University, 28 November 2018, hosted by the Leipzig Research Center for Early Child Development (LFE). https://www.youtube.com/watch?v=_nG5SelEj28.

[409] Cf. Aviezer, O., Sagi-Schwartz, A., & Koren-Karie, N. (2003) Ecological constraints on the formation of infant–mother attachment relations: when maternal sensitivity becomes ineffective. *Infant Behavior and Development*, 26(3), 285–99.

[410] Keller, H. & Thompson, R. (2018) Attachment theory: past, present & future. Recorded at the 2nd 'Wilhelm Wundt Dialogue', Leipzig University, 28 November 2018, hosted by the Leipzig Research Center for Early Child Development (LFE). https://www.youtube.com/watch?v=_nG5SelEj28.

[411] Weisner, T. (2014) The socialization of trust: plural caregiving and diverse pathways in human development across cultures. In H. Otto & H. Keller (eds) *Different Faces of Attachment* (pp.263–77). Cambridge: Cambridge University Press.

The Strange Situation 'abroad'

The founding work of cross-cultural research conducted by attachment researchers was the Bielefeld study by Klaus and Karin Grossmann, with results published in 1981. This study sent shockwaves through the small community of attachment researchers, as well as the wider community of developmental science researchers. The distribution of Strange Situation classifications differed markedly from those of Ainsworth, with more avoidant than secure dyads in the sample. This result was interpreted in terms of the aversion of German culture to displays of distress and the importance placed on independence, reflected in childcare practices that promoted infant self-reliance such as separate sleeping, and that penalised communication of anxiety by children.[412] The study became a conventional reference point, cited in reviews and textbooks, illustrating the limitations of the Strange Situation. In fact, however, subsequent studies in Germany have reported distributions that align well with both Ainsworth's distribution and other North American, European, and Australian samples. In a second sample, from Regensburg, the Grossmanns found that 62% of the dyads received a secure classification, 27.5% an avoidant classification, 5% an ambivalent/resistant classification, and a further 5% that could not be classified into the Ainsworth categories.[413] Another study in Berlin found that 77.5% of dyads in the sample were classified as secure, 17.5% were classified as avoidant, and 5% were classified as ambivalent/resistant.[414]

It has later been assumed that the Bielefeld findings could be explained by differences in caregiving practices characteristic of northern Germany.[415] Certainly, a subsequent analysis by the Grossmanns found that a proportion of the infants from avoidant dyads had received otherwise highly sensitive care from parents who experienced cultural pressure to encourage self-reliance in their children. In a later follow-up, these infants who had experienced sensitive care had outcomes equivalent to those from securely attached dyads, and unlike their fellow avoidantly attached dyads.[416] Such later findings, however, have generally

[412] Grossmann, K.E., Grossmann, K., Huber, F., & Watner, U. (1981) German children's behavior towards their mothers at 12 months and their fathers at 18 months in Ainsworth's Strange Situation. *International Journal of Behavioral Development*, 4(2), 157–81.

[413] Wartner, U.G., Grossmann, K., Fremmer-Bombik, E., & Suess, G. (1994) Attachment patterns at age six in south Germany: predictability from infancy and implications for preschool behavior. *Child Development*, 65(4), 1014–27. With the D classification included, the distributions were 50% B, 15% A, 4.5% C, and 30.5% D.

[414] Beller, E.K., & Pohl, A. (1986) The Strange Situation revisited. Paper presented at 4th International Conference on Infant Studies, Beverly Hills, April 1986. Distribution of attachment classifications reported in van IJzendoorn, M.H. & Kroonenberg, P.M. (1988) Cross-cultural patterns of attachment: a meta-analysis of the strange situation. *Child Development*, 59(1), 147–56. Even in a sample of German children known to social services for potential child abuse and neglect, rates of secure attachment have been found to be high at 24 months. Suess, G.J., Bohlen, U., Carlson, E.A., Spangler, G., & Frumentia Maier, M. (2016) Effectiveness of attachment based STEEP™ intervention in a German high-risk sample. *Attachment & Human Development*, 18(5), 443–60.

[415] However, empirical study of parents' perceptions of the appropriate attachment behaviour of young children showed few differences between north and south Germany: Scholmerich, A. (1996) Attachment security and maternal concepts of ideal children in northern and southern Germany. *International Journal of Behavioral Development*, 19(4), 725–38. An alternative explanation for the early independence encouraged in the Bielefeld infants might be found in war trauma experienced by the parents in the Bielefeld sample. Bielefeld was heavily bombed during World War II. By contrast, though the Messerschmitt aircraft factory and the oil refinery nearby were attacked, the town of Regensburg itself received little bombing. On German war trauma and attachment processes see the discussion in Kaiser, M., Kuwert, P., Braehler, E., & Glaesmer, H. (2018) Long-term effects on adult attachment in German occupation children born after World War II in comparison with a birth-cohort-matched representative sample of the German general population. *Aging & Mental Health*, 22(2), 197–207.

[416] Grossmann, K.E., Grossmann, K., & Schwan, A. (1986) Capturing the wider view of attachment: a reanalysis of Ainsworth's Strange Situation. In C.E. Izard & P.B. Read (eds) *Measuring Emotions in Infants and Children*, Vol. 2 (pp.124–71). Cambridge: Cambridge University Press.

been ignored, except among attachment researchers. The salience of the early Bielefeld findings, and their resonance with contemporary stereotypes about Germans as emotionally suppressed but secretly insecure, have held the imagination: the 'German' tendency towards avoidant attachment is still widely cited by both developmental psychologists[417] and critics of the attachment paradigm.[418]

The Grossmanns were trained to conduct the Strange Situation by Ainsworth, and were given support in coding the procedure by both Ainsworth and Main. By contrast, applications of the Strange Situation by Japanese researchers were the first to be conducted by a group without even distal ties to Ainsworth. A first study, published in 1984, was carried out in Tokyo by Durrett and colleagues. Of their 39 infant–caregiver dyads, 61% were classified as secure, 13% were classified as avoidant, 18% were classified as ambivalent/resistant, and 8% could not readily be classified into one of the Ainsworth classifications. The researchers found that rates of security were higher among dyads where the parent experienced more social support. These results generated little interest or discussion: they seemed merely to confirm the status of secure attachment behaviour as the most common pattern, and that it was associated with theoretically expectable antecedents. By contrast, a second Japanese study by Takahashi was conducted in Sapporo and published in 1986; 68% of the sample of 60 infant–mother dyads were classified as secure, 32% were classified as ambivalent/resistant, and not a single infant was classified as avoidant.[419]

In interpreting these findings, Takahashi drew a contrast between the common occurrence of minor infant–mother separations in the American context, and the rarity of such events in the lives of infants in traditional Japanese families, who generally experienced co-sleeping, co-bathing, and being carried on their mother's back. Takahashi emphasised that a three-minute separation is not a standardised experience, but one shaped by culture. For infants who have rarely, if ever, experienced separation from their mothers, the Strange Situation may induce panic rather than serve as a mild stressor, and so fail to reflect experiences in naturalistic settings. Considering these questions, Takahashi shared her cases with Sroufe at Minnesota (Chapter 4). Takahashi and Sroufe agreed that the Strange Situation was inappropriate for children who had so rarely experienced separations.[420] They also agreed

---

[417] E.g. Simonelli, A., De Palo, F., Moretti, M., Baratter, P.M., & Porreca, A. (2014) The Strange Situation procedure: the role of the attachment patterns in the Italian culture. *American Journal of Applied Psychology*, 3(3), 47–56.

[418] E.g. LeVine, R.A. (2014) Attachment theory as cultural ideology. In H. Otto & H. Keller (eds) *Different Faces of Attachment: Cultural Variations on a Universal Human Need* (pp.50–65). Cambridge: Cambridge University Press. See also Grossmann, K.E. & Grossmann, K. (1999) Mary Ainsworth: our guide to attachment research. *Attachment and Human Development*, 1, 224–8: 'Our study, though, became known more because of the high percentage of insecure-avoidantly attached infants (Grossmann, Grossmann, Huber, Wartner,1981) than for its many confirmations of Ainsworth's findings with a larger sample' (224). Another important early cross-cultural study of the 1980s was work by Sagi and Lamb exploring the attachment classifications of infants raised on Israeli kibbutzim with their mother, father, and communal caretakers. This research was of particular importance in highlighting the important contribution made by attachment figure overnight availability to security as assessed in the Strange Situation. Sagi, A., Lamb, M.E., Lewkowicz, K.S., Shoham, R., Dvir, R., & Estes, D. (1985) Security of infant–mother, –father, and –metapelet attachments among kibbutz-reared Israeli children. *Monographs of the Society for Research in Child Development*, 50(1/2), 257–75; Sagi, A., van IJzendoorn, M.H., Aviezer, O., Donnell, F., & Mayseless, O. (1994) Sleeping out of home in a kibbutz communal arrangement: it makes a difference for infant–mother attachment. *Child Development*, 65(4), 992–1004.

[419] Takahashi, K. (1986) Examining the Strange Situation procedure with Japanese mothers and 12-month-old infants. *Developmental Psychology*, 22(2), 265–70. In a later report on the same sample, 75% were classified as secure, 21% ambivalent/resistant, and 4% unclassifiable. Nakagawa, M., Lamb, M.E., & Miyake, K. (1992) Antecedents and correlates of the strange situation behavior of Japanese infants. *Journal of Cross-Cultural Psychology*, 23, 300–10.

[420] Alan Sroufe, personal communication, January 2019.

that the apparently high rate of ambivalent/resistant infants did not reflect the predomin-ance of this pattern of attachment, and was instead a misclassification of overdistressed in-fants. It was noteworthy that the play of these infants was not poor prior to the separations, as is the usual case for the anxious/resistant group. However, Sroufe states that Takahashi was placed under institutional pressure to claim that the findings cast doubt on the cross-cultural applicability of the Strange Situation in general. In her write-up she concluded that the Ainsworth Strange Situation was a culturally specific artefact, with poor cross-cultural applicability at least to traditional Japanese infant–caregiver dyads.[421] This finding stirred considerable attention. As Behrens subsequently observed, the Sapporo study findings res-onated with a trend in social scientific research in the 1980s to emphasise the uniqueness of Japan, and the lack of relevance of research paradigms developed on non-Japanese sam-ples.[422] Together with the Bielefeld study, the Sapporo study appeared to provide evidence of vast differences in caregiving practices, or of the lack of cross-cultural validity of the Strange Situation procedure, or both.

However, an additional option could be variance in how the Strange Situation procedure was applied. Takahashi stated in the methodology for her paper that 'as the original study (Ainsworth et al. 1978) didn't clearly describe when the episodes of distress were curtailed, we set the max-imum duration at 2 min. Thus the durations of distress in this study were longer than in most current studies in the United States.'[423] This statement illustrates the distance of the Sapporo researchers from Ainsworth: not only did they not consult with her, but also they had a weak grasp of Patterns of Attachment, since the instruction to curtail episodes if the child becomes dis-tressed is given clearly and repeatedly (on pages 35, 38, 39, 75, and 341). It is also mentioned in Ainsworth's other publications,[424] and in publications by other American and European attach-ment researchers in the 1970s.[425] Furthermore, the coders of the Sapporo Strange Situations had received no training or guidance from previous researchers who had used the coding protocols. In acknowledgement of the methodological flaws in the study, Klaus and Karin Grossmann were invited to Hokkaido University, Sapporo, and recoded the videos. Unfortunately, the results of this reanalysis were printed only in the Annual Report of the Center for Child Development at Hokkaido University, and so, in practice, were not in public circulation. The results of their re-analysis are, however, interesting and important.

On review of the recordings, the Grossmanns affirmed that the separations had been con-tinued too long. In line with Ainsworth's instructions in print, no child was permitted to cry for more than 30 seconds in either of the Grossmanns' samples. In the Sapporo sample, all infants were left to cry for at least 55 seconds and many for much longer: 'some infants cried as long as 4 minutes and 40 seconds in extreme despair'.[426] Many infants could do little

[421] Takahashi, K. (1990) Are the key assumptions of the 'Strange Situation' procedure universal? A view from Japanese research. Human Development, 33(1), 23–30.

[422] Behrens, K.Y. (2016) Reconsidering attachment in context of culture: review of attachment studies in Japan. Online Readings in Psychology and Culture, 6(1), 7.

[423] Takahashi, K. (1986) Examining the Strange Situation procedure with Japanese mothers and 12-month-old infants. Developmental Psychology, 22(2), 265–70, p.266.

[424] E.g. Ainsworth, M.D.S. & Bell, S.M. (1970) Attachment, exploration, and separation: illustrated by the be-havior of one-year-olds in a strange situation. Child Development, 41(1), 49–67.

[425] Serafica, F.C. & Cicchetti, D. (1976) Down's syndrome children in a strange situation: attachment and explor-ation behaviors. Merrill-Palmer, 22(2), 137–50; Smith, L. & Martinsen, H. (1977) The behavior of young children in a strange situation. Scandinavian Journal of Psychology, 18(1), 43–52.

[426] Grossmann, K.E. & Grossmann, K. (1989) Preliminary observation on Japanese infants' behavior in Ainsworth's strange situation. Hokkaido University Annual Report, Research and Clinical Center for Child Development, 11, 1–12.

but engage in exhausted sobbing through the second reunion rather than respond to the re-appearance of their mother. This behaviour characterised 76% of the whole Japanese sample left to cry intensely for more than two minutes.[427] Klaus and Karin Grossmann identified another factor that may have affected the distribution of classifications. Watching the videos, they observed that the mothers were shy and formal in the laboratory setting, and barely communicated with their infants while in the Strange Situation. A large minority rejected their infant's wish for contact, whereas this behaviour was shown by none of the German parents, precisely contrary to stereotype.[428] The Grossmanns observed that the Japanese in-fants seemed surprised by the inaccessibility of their caregiver, and this may have encour-aged the infants to intensify signals of distress and anger: 'the infants showed through their behaviour that they expected acceptance from their mothers', implying that the withdrawn behaviour was out of keeping with their usual expectations.[429] The Grossmanns concluded that the instructions given to the mothers had been interpreted by some as mandating with-drawn behaviour, when this was in fact uncharacteristic of these dyads.

Whereas Takahashi reported 68% of the sample as secure and 32% as ambivalent/re-sistant, the Grossmanns' blind recoding of the sample yielded a distribution of 76% secure, 11% ambivalent/resistant, 2% avoidant, and 11% unclassifiable dyads. They also observed conflict behaviours—what Main and Solomon would call indices of disorganised attach-ment (Chapter 3)—in a very substantial proportion of both the Group C and the Group B in-fants, but did not make a systematic report on this.[430] They agreed with the original coding in only 43% of cases originally coded as Group C. The Grossmanns suspected that the long sep-arations had blown out the avoidant conditional strategy, which requires the redirection of attention away from attachment-relevant stimuli. Such redirection is only possible at mod-erate arousal, not at the high arousal of the infants in the Sapporo study.[431] The first study using the Strange Situation in Japan, by Durrett and colleagues, had a distribution far closer to that of North American and European samples, though with somewhat fewer avoidant dyads and somewhat more ambivalent/resistant dyads. This suggested to the Grossmanns that cultural differences in caregiving might be playing a role in the distribution of condi-tional strategies over and above overstress caused by the procedural issues. In line with this assumption, they found that more Japanese Group C infants (50%) than German Group C infants (10%) cried immediately as separation began. However, complicating the picture, they also found that on average the Japanese sample cried less than the German sample as separations began, suggesting that the sample as a whole was not necessarily overwhelmed by separations per se.[432]

[427] Grossmann, K., Fremmer-Bombik, E., & Freitag, M. (1991) German and Japanese infants in the Strange Situation: are there differences in behavior beyond differences in the frequency of classes? Paper presented at meeting of International Society for the Study of Behavioral Development, Minneapolis, July 1991.Copy shared by Karin Grossmann.

[428] Ibid.

[429] Grossmann, K.E. & Grossmann, K. (1996) Kulturelle perspektiven der bindungsentwicklung Japan in und Deutschland. In G. Trommsdorff & H.-J. Konrad (eds) *Gesellschaftliche und individuelle Entwicklung Japan in und Deutschland* (pp.215–35). Konstanz: Universitätsverlag Konstanz.

[430] Grossmann, K.E. & Grossmann, K. (1989) Preliminary observation on Japanese infants' behavior in Ainsworth's strange situation. *Hokkaido University Annual Report, Research and Clinical Center for Child Development*, 11, 1–12.

[431] Grossmann, K., Fremmer-Bombik, E., & Grossmann, K.E. (1990) Familiar and unfamiliar patterns of attach-ment of Japanese infants. *Hokkaido University Annual Report, Research and Clinical Center for Child Development*, 2, 30–39.

[432] Grossmann, K., Fremmer-Bombik, E., & Freitag, M. (1991) German and Japanese infants in the Strange Situation: are there differences in behavior beyond differences in the frequency of classes? Paper presented at

Debate about the Sapporo study went quiet for a decade, until the matter was revived by Rothbaum, Miyake (one of the collaborators on the Sapporo study), and colleagues in 2000. In a high-profile paper in the *American Psychologist* they repeated Takahashi's earlier claims that the Sapporo data showed that the Strange Situation is not cross-culturally valid as an assessment of individual differences.[433] Like Takahashi, they pointed to the prolonged skin-to-skin contact and the pre-emption of needs experienced by Japanese infants compared to the distal interactions of western infants, which they supposed would make any separations unbearable for most Japanese infants. Rothbaum and colleagues also drew on the tradition of qualitative ethnographic research to propose that Japanese caregivers value signs of infant dependency over displays of autonomy, and that this would account for the higher numbers of ambivalent/resistant and the fewer avoidant dyads. They could point to no quantitative findings in support of this claim, however, and the only direct study showed the opposite: that Japanese caregivers value dependency far less than the infant using the caregiver as a safe base from which to explore.[434] Rothbaum and colleagues dismissed this study, however, since it was from Tokyo and they presumed that the findings therefore reflected the western values of a metropolitan capital city.[435]

To appraise the claims of Rothbaum and colleagues, Kondo-Ikemura and colleagues conducted another study in Sapporo in the 2010s. The Strange Situation procedure was carried out in line with Ainsworth's protocols. They found that 69% of dyads were classified as secure, 2% as avoidant, 16% as ambivalent/resistant, and 13% as disorganised. They found that the infant attachment classifications were strongly predicted by Adult Attachment Interviews with the parents, in line with research in other societies (Chapter 3).[436] And a sizeable proportion of mothers in the sample worked, suggesting that the infants were not unfamiliar with separations. Nonetheless, the number of avoidant dyads was low. Kondo-Ikemura and colleagues argued that the Strange Situation was generally a valid measure of individual differences in the Japanese context, associated with expectable covariates. They qualified that some aspect of Japanese childcare practice likely explains the low proportion of avoidant dyads, but they did not speculate on what this might be.

In a recent chapter, Mary True surveyed discussions of the cross-cultural validity of the Strange Situation.[437] She makes two points of particular relevance to appraising Ainsworth's legacy to cross-cultural developmental research. She reports from a meta-analysis comparing cultures that conventionally include prolonged skin-to-skin contact between infants and caregivers and cultures that conventionally use distal caregiving strategies. Rates

meeting of International Society for the Study of Behavioral Development, Minneapolis, July 1991. Copy shared by Karin Grossmann. However, curiously, the Japanese infants also seemed much less wary of the stranger than the German infants.

[433] Rothbaum, F., Weisz, J., Pott, M., Miyake, K., & Morelli, G. (2000) Attachment and culture: security in the United States and Japan. *American Psychologist*, 55(10), 1093–104.

[434] Vereijken, C.J.J.L., Riksen-Walraven, J.M., & Van Lieshout, C.F.M. (1997) Mother–infant relationships in Japan: attachment, dependency, and amae. *Journal of Cross-Cultural Psychology*, 28(4), 442–62

[435] Rothbaum, F. & Kakinuma, M. (2004) Amae and attachment: security in cultural context. *Human Development*, 47(1), 34–9. Cf. Posada, G., Lu, T., Trumbell, J., et al. (2013) Is the secure base phenomenon evident here, there, and anywhere? A cross-cultural study of child behavior and experts' definitions. *Child Development*, 84(6), 1896–905.

[436] Kondo-ikemura, K., Behrens, K.Y., Umemura, T., & Nakano, S. (2018) Japanese mothers' prebirth Adult Attachment Interview predicts their infants' response to the Strange Situation Procedure: the Strange Situation in Japan revisited three decades later. *Developmental Psychology*, 54(11), 2007–2015.

[437] True, M. (in press) Multiple pathways to infant disorganization: insights from an African dataset. In T. Forslund & R. Duschinsky (eds) *The Attachment Reader*. Oxford: Blackwell.

of secure attachment are the same between these two contexts. By contrast, rates of avoidance are lower and rates of ambivalent/resistance are higher when, as in the Japanese case, prolonged skin-to-skin contact is part of caregiving norms.[438] This accumulated evidence indicates systematic variation in the kind of conditional strategy used in the context of differences in caregiving cultures. However, True argues that such accumulated findings represent a denigration of Ainsworth's true legacy, since without articulation of the specific processes occurring within infant–caregiver interaction, any interpretation is recklessly speculative.

True states that attachment researchers have focused too much on supplying and then interminably discussing distributions in Strange Situation patterns. A limitation of Ainsworth's approach was the prominence she gave to the Strange Situation, when in fact the generative core of her insights came precisely from the combination of qualitative ethnography of general processes and quantitative assessment of dyadic processes. True observes that this potent combination has become fractured into the anthropological and developmental traditions of cross-cultural research on attachment. This has stalled efforts to pin down and operationalise the role of cultural factors in contributing to both adverse forms of care and the role of cultural protective factors, which may be of strong relevance to intervention science.[439]

Ainsworth's focus on the Strange Situation made sense in the context of the priorities and values of psychology as a discipline in the 1970s and 1980s. But it closed down conversation between psychology and anthropology, in a way that may well not have occurred had she headlined the sensitivity scale. In recent decades, attachment researchers have applied Ainsworth's sensitivity scale in measuring caregiving behaviour across various countries and contexts, where it has successfully predicted infant attachment behaviour and later socioemotional development.[440] It is certainly the case, as Röttger-Rössler among others has shown, that Ainsworth's language regarding 'appropriate' caregiver response is potentially ambiguous, depending heavily on training in order to clarify its meaning, and contributing to the potential for coders to judge appropriateness by specific cultural standards.[441] Much depends here on the design of studies that are thoughtful about cultural context and validity, and the work of coders to integrate the particularities of culture and childcare practices within the formal aspects of Ainsworth's system. This work is barely mentioned in the

[438] See also Mesman, J., van IJzendoorn, M.H., & Sagi-Schwartz, S. (2016) Cross-cultural patterns of attachment: universal and contextual dimensions. In J. Cassidy & P. Shaver (eds) *Handbook of Attachment* (pp.790–815). New York: Guilford, p.809.

[439] Exceptions include Posada, G., Carbonell, O.A., Alzate, G., & Plata, S.J. (2004) Through Colombian lenses: ethnographic and conventional analyses of maternal care and their associations with secure base behavior. *Developmental Psychology*, 40(4), 508–18; Howes, C. & Wishard Guerra, A.G. (2009) Networks of attachment relationships in low-income children of Mexican heritage: infancy through preschool. *Social Development*, 18(4), 896–914; Fuertes, M., Ribeiro, C., Gonçalves, J.L., et al. (2020) Maternal perinatal representations and their associations with mother–infant interaction and attachment: A longitudinal comparison of Portuguese and Brazilian dyads. *International Journal of Psychology*, 55(2), 224–33.

[440] Mesman, J., van IJzendoorn, M.H., & Sagi-Schwartz, A. (2016) Cross-cultural patterns of attachment. In J. Cassidy & P.R. Shaver (eds) *The Handbook of Attachment: Theory, Research, and Clinical Applications*, 3rd edn (pp.852–77). New York: Guilford; see also Posada, G. (2013) Piecing together the sensitivity construct: ethology and cross-cultural research. *Attachment & Human Development*, 15, 637–56.

[441] Röttger-Rössler, B. (2014) Bonding and belonging beyond WEIRD worlds: rethinking attachment theory on the basis of cross-cultural anthropological data. In H. Otto & H. Keller (eds) *Different Faces of Attachment: Cultural Variations on a Universal Human Need* (pp.141–68). Cambridge: Cambridge University Press. See also Carlson, V.J. & Harwood, R.L. (2003) Attachment, culture, and the caregiving system: the cultural patterning of everyday experiences among Anglo and Puerto Rican mother–infant pairs. *Infant Mental Health Journal*, 24(1), 53–73; LeVine, R.A., Gielen, U.P., & Roopnarine, J. (2004) Challenging expert knowledge: findings from an African study of infant care and development. In *Childhood and Adolescence: Cross-cultural Perspectives and Applications* (pp.149–65). Westport, CT: Praeger/Greenwood.

published literature, which means that the principles and processes through which it has been achieved are not transparent or available for discussion.[442] This is an issue that would likely have seen substantial resolution had anthropologists and developmental psychologists been able to listen to and learn from one another on the basis of more common ground.

Yet evidence in favour of the cross-cultural relevance of Ainsworth's construct is that differences from western cultural norms are not, in themselves, generally associated with lower scores for sensitivity. Rather, the majority of caregivers in most contexts around the world are characterised as showing sensitivity, except where families are facing conditions of social, economic, or political adversity, or where caregivers have themselves experienced trauma or maltreatment. And even then, the effects of adversity and trauma may in some instances be buffered by protective aspects of childcare practices.[443] Nonetheless, the gulf between attachment researchers and anthropologists has hindered the development of a global research agenda to explore these processes, and in turn the take-up of attachment research within the growing policy and research concern with child development and global public mental health.[444]

Some remaining questions

The crying question

Ainsworth and Bell's study of crying behaviour was the first analysis of the home observation data. They found that when mothers responded promptly to infants crying in the first quarter, they cry less in the final quarter of the first year.[445] This finding was a landmark report at the time, offering a symbolic victory for attachment theory.[446] It ran directly contrary to the behaviourist theory that if crying for a parent is heeded and brings about a positive outcome for the child, it will be repeated more often over time. Instead, the finding supported Bowlby's proposition that affection shown to children would not 'spoil' them and make them dependent, but in fact would help them feel confident in the availability of their caregiver or caregivers and less prone to distress.[447] Furthermore, Ainsworth and colleagues soon after

[442] Exceptions include Mesman, J., van IJzendoorn, M., Behrens, K., et al. (2016) Is the ideal mother a sensitive mother? Beliefs about early childhood parenting in mothers across the globe. *International Journal of Behavioral Development*, 40(5), 385–97; Posada, G., Trumbell, J., Noblega, M., et al. (2016) Maternal sensitivity and child secure base use in early childhood: studies in different cultural contexts. *Child Development*, 87(1), 297–311; Dawson, N.K. (2018) From Uganda to Baltimore to Alexandra Township: how far can Ainsworth's theory stretch? *South African Journal of Psychiatry*, 24, 8. Perhaps the only study to have examined the cross-cultural consistency of coding the Strange Situation is Van IJzendoorn, M. H. & Kroonenberg, P.M. (1990) Cross-cultural consistency of coding the strange situation. *Infant Behavior and Development*, 13(4), 469–85.

[443] E.g. Fourment, K., Nóblega, M., Conde, G., del Prado, J.N., & Mesman, J. (2018) Maternal sensitivity in rural Andean and Amazonian Peru. *Attachment & Human Development*, 27 March, 1–9.

[444] Kieling, C., Baker-Henningham, H., Belfer, M., et al. (2011) Child and adolescent mental health worldwide: evidence for action. *The Lancet*, 378(9801), 1515–25. However, see Bain, K. & Baradon, T. (2018) Interfacing infant mental health knowledge: perspectives of South African supervisors supporting lay mother–infant home visitors. *Infant Mental Health Journal*, 39(4), 371–84.

[445] Bell, S.M. & Ainsworth, M.D.S. (1972) Infant crying and maternal responsiveness. *Child Development*, 43(4), 1171–90.

[446] On the landmark status of this study see Lewis, M. (1997) *Altering Fate: Why the Past Does Not Predict the Future.* New York: Guilford, p.145.

[447] See the debate between attachment and behaviourist theorists over Ainsworth's findings: Gewirtz, J.L. & Boyd, E.F. (1977) Does maternal responding imply reduced infant crying? A critique of the 1972 Bell and

found that babies who reciprocated actively when held by their mother were less likely to protest when put down, and more likely to immediately turn to independent exploration.[448] Stayton and Ainsworth interpreted these findings by proposing that babies could accept cessation of contact because they are confident that the caregiver will be accessible if needed.[449]

That infant crying was reduced by the end of the first year rather than increased by prompt response by caregivers was a landmark finding, and one that Bowlby and Ainsworth continued to mention until the end of their careers with a passionate, steady insistence. The finding neatly encapsulated the empirical implications of attachment theory. Furthermore, in *Patterns of Attachment*, Ainsworth and colleagues reported that 'mothers who are promptly responsive to crying signals in the early months have babies who later become securely attached'.[450] The statistical procedures by which Ainsworth and Bell came to these conclusions were contested by her critics.[451] However, without any other longitudinal data available to help answer the question, the Baltimore findings were the only source of scientific information relevant to the heated question of whether babies should be left to cry.[452] In the 1980s, infant crying was also gaining in importance in the context of proposals, for instance by Michael Lamb and colleagues, that infant physical abuse may at times be triggered in parents as tiredness and emotional unrest and urgent cues meld together as hot frustration.[453]

The topic drew the attention of the young Marinus van IJzendoorn, then in his late twenties and newly appointed as full Professor at Leiden University. At the time, van IJzendoorn was immersed in reading attachment theory, writing the first Dutch book offering a detailed appraisal of Bowlby's ideas.[454] Van IJzendoorn had been asked to care for his six-month-old godson whilst the child's parents were away. He stood at the crib hour after hour, through the night, trying helplessly to quiet the baby, who cried without ceasing. Days became endless, and the nights even worse. By the time his godson's parents returned, van IJzendoorn had resolved to conduct a replication of Ainsworth and Bell's research, to understand more about how to reduce infant crying.[455] He worked with a doctoral student, Frans Hubbard, to collect

Ainsworth report. *Child Development*, 48, 1200–1207; Ainsworth, M.D.S. & Bell, S.M. (1977) Infant crying and maternal responsiveness: a rejoinder to Gewirtz and Boyd. *Child Development*, 48, 1208–16. For an example of Bowlby using Ainsworth's findings regarding crying as ammunition against social learning approaches see e.g. Bowlby, J. (1973) *Separation*. London: Pimlico, p.358.

[448] Ainsworth, M., Bell, S., & Stayton, D. (1972) Individual differences in the development of some attachment behaviors. *Merrill-Palmer*, 18(2), 123–43, p.136.

[449] Stayton, D. & Ainsworth, M. (1973) Individual differences in infant responses to brief, everyday separations as related to other infant and maternal behaviours. *Developmental Psychology* 9(2), 226–35, p.233.

[450] Ainsworth, M., Blehar, M., Waters, E., & Wall, S. (1978, 2015) *Patterns of Attachment: A Psychological Study of the Strange Situation*. Bristol: Psychology Press, p.146.

[451] E.g. Lamb, M., Thompson, R.A., Gardner, W., & Charnov, E.L. (1985) *Infant–Mother Attachment: The Origins and Developmental Significance of Individual Differences in the Strange Situation*. Hillsdale, NJ: Lawrence Erlbaum: 'A group difference in maternal unresponsiveness to crying in the first quarter led to the conclusion that "Mothers who are promptly responsive to crying signals in the early months have babies who later become securely attached" (Ainsworth et al. 1978, p.150). In fact, when the measure is expressed as a proportion (Maternal unresponsiveness per hour/Infant crying per hour), the proportion of A and B infants are equivalent, and the deviant group (C) contains only four dyads' (65).

[452] Newton, L.D. (1983) Helping parents cope with infant crying. *Journal of Obstetric, Gynecologic, & Neonatal Nursing*, 12(3), 199–204.

[453] Frodi, A.M. & Lamb, M.E. (1980) Child abusers' responses to infant smiles and cries. *Child Development*, 51(1), 238–41.

[454] Van IJzendoorn, M.H., Tavecchio, L.W.C., Goossens, F.A., & Vergeer, M.M. (1982) *Opvoeden in Geborgenheid. Een Kritische Analyse van Bowlby's Attachment Theorie*. Deventer: Van Loghum Slaterus.

[455] Van IJzendoorn, M.H. (2004) Roos. In H. Procee, H. Meijer, P. Timmerman, & R. Tuinsma (eds) *Bij die Wereld wil ik Horen! Zevenendertig Columns & Drie Essays over de Vorming tot Academicus* (pp.86–89). Amsterdam: Boom.

data on what would be a very intensive study. Data collection began in 1983 and took four years, using the new technology provided by an event recorder/FM audio registration unit.

The findings were clear-cut: when caregivers responded to fuss or cry signals, infants cried more often by the end of the first year. Yet journals were not keen to publish the results, and it took until the 1990s before the paper was finally in print.[456] Hubbard and van IJzendoorn realised that 'research on crying evolved into a "pièce de résistance" of attachment theory … It constituted a cornerstone of attachment theory and therefore was not really open to theoretical and empirical criticism.'[457] However, Hubbard and van IJzendoorn did not regard their results as representing an attack on attachment theory, but as criticism of specific aspects of Ainsworth and Bell's methodology. They argued that the Ainsworth and Bell paper adopted an inappropriate statistical approach, a crude strategy of measurement, and overconfidence in assertion of their findings on the basis of such a small sample. Hubbard and van IJzendoorn proposed that a distinction needed to be drawn between low-level fussing and loud and prolonged cries. They speculated that whereas their technology-enabled methodology allowed them to track the former, it is likely that only the latter would have been recorded every time by Ainsworth's live observers, even if fussing was sometimes noted.

Low-level fussing is not, Hubbard and van IJzendoorn argued, an attachment signal. Sensitive responsiveness to these behaviours may have little implication for informing the expectations that organise the attachment behavioural system; instead, they may encourage more fussing. This is in contrast to loud and prolonged cries by the infant, which are attachment signals. The term 'crying' was inherited by developmental psychology from ordinary language, but was not proving helpful since it hid this important distinction. Ainsworth herself would conclude: 'Even the most responsive mothers did not respond to a little cry that stopped spontaneously when a baby was put to sleep or a similar brief fuss when a baby was trying to turn over and could not manage by itself, however, succeeding next. But rarely did they fail to respond to a loud and prolonged cry.'[458] The Hubbard and van IJzendoorn findings have had little traction, however. Still today, the Ainsworth and Bell paper is widely cited to prove that prompt response to infant crying reduces subsequent crying. For instance, parents are taught about the finding to encourage nurturing care as part of Dozier and colleagues' influential Attachment and Biobehavioral Catch-up parenting intervention.[459]

Coding individuals

North American developmental psychology had long felt the tension between a stance that gave primacy to individuals and a stance that gave primacy to relationships.[460] Ainsworth's

[456] Hubbard, F.O. & van IJzendoorn, M.H. (1991) Maternal unresponsiveness and infant crying across the first 9 months: a naturalistic longitudinal study. *Infant Behavior and Development*, 14(3), 299–312.

[457] Hubbard, F.O.A. & van IJzendoorn, M.H. (1987) Maternal unresponsiveness and infant crying: a critical replication of the Bell & Ainsworth study. In L.W.C. Tavecchio & M.H. van IJzendoorn (eds) *Attachment in Social Networks. Contributions to the Bowlby–Ainsworth Attachment Theory* (pp.339–78). New York: Elsevier, p.344.

[458] Personal communication to Marinus van IJzendoorn, cited in ibid, p.368.

[459] Dozier, M. & Bernard, K. (2019) *Coaching Parents of Vulnerable Infants: The Attachment and Biobehavioral Catch-up Approach*. New York: Guilford, p.11.

[460] Sameroff, A. (2009) The transactional model. In A. Sameroff (ed.) *The Transactional Model of Development: How Children and Contexts Shape Each Other* (pp.3–21). Washington, DC: American Psychological Association. On the shift towards contextualism in developmental psychology in the 1970s see Lerner, R.M.,

group aligned themselves firmly with the latter perspective. The sensitivity measure is partly an assessment of individual differences between caregivers—responsiveness to crying perhaps more so, since it is a cruder measure. But in both cases there is no standardisation of infant behaviour: the measure assesses the way that particular infant signals are noticed and responded to by the caregiver, which is at least in part an assessment of the dyad in their interactive dance. There was one assessment in which this dance was not observed, however, and in which only individual behaviour was coded: the Strange Situation.

Ainsworth sought to semi-control the caregiver's behaviour in the Strange Situation in order to make the separations a standardised, ambiguous, but evocative stimulus. And the written coding system for the Strange Situation that she created was for individual infant behaviour only, an approach generally extrapolated by her students to the coding of patterns of attachment in separation–reunion procedures at later developmental stages.[461] In itself this is no problem. The behaviours of individual children in the Strange Situation are associated with interactions of the dyad at home, and can predict caregiver behaviour towards the child in other settings (Chapter 4). This is somewhat astonishing, profound even, and suggests that a coding system for individual behaviours can serve as a workable window on attachment as a dyadic property, since this behaviour reflects—even if imperfectly—infants' expectations about their caregiver's availability. Yet the methodological choice to code individual behaviours was not fully owned: Ainsworth did not accompany this de facto focus of the Strange Situation with any checklist to support its reliability as a measure of individual differences, as might have been expected. For instance, researchers using the procedure were not required to take note of whether a child was ill, was on relevant medication, or even had received regular care by the parent.[462] This is despite that fact that Ainsworth and later researchers readily acknowledged these factors as relevant to the reliability of a Strange Situation procedure. Klaus and Karin Grossmann believe that Ainsworth assumed that the Strange Situation would usually be accompanied by naturalistic observation of dyads, making a checklist for relevant individual differences superfluous.[463] However, as discussed, naturalistic observation fell away over time from attachment research, following the priorities of the wider discipline of developmental science.

This potential limitation on reliability has been accepted quietly by subsequent researchers. Perhaps it has been felt that the issue is minor, and that most infants in most samples will nonetheless respond to separation and reunion with a caregiver in ways that reflect to some extent the care they have received in that relationship. It may also have been felt by second-generation attachment researchers, and all the more by third generation, that it is now too late to add such reliability safeguards. Whereas such issues of reliability have generally been ignored, some attachment researchers have explicitly wondered whether it is

Hultsch, D.F., & Dixon, R.A. (1983) Contextualism and the character of developmental psychology in the 1970s. *Annals of the New York Academy of Sciences*, 412(1), 101–28.

[461] Cassidy, J., Marvin, R., with the Attachment Working Group of the John D. and Catherine T. MacArthur Network on the Transition from Infancy to Early Childhood (1992) Attachment organisation in preschool children: procedures and coding manual. Unpublished manual; Main, M. & Cassidy, J. (1988) Categories of response to reunion with the parent at age 6: predictable from infant attachment classifications and stable over a 1-month period. *Developmental Psychology*, 24(3), 415–26.

[462] Except when a sample has been specifically recruited with such factors in mind, e.g. Espinosa, M., Beckwith, L., Howard, J., Tyler, R., & Swanson, K. (2001) Maternal psychopathology and attachment in toddlers of heavy cocaine-using mothers. *Infant Mental Health Journal*, 22(3), 316–33.

[463] Grossmann, K. & Grossmann, K. (2012) *Bindungen—Das Gefüge psychischer Sicherheit Gebundenes*. Stuttgart: Klett-Cotta.

valid to assess attachment as a dyadic property with a focus on infant behaviours.[464] A few have sought to revise or create coding systems focused on dyadic interactions. The most direct attempt has been that of Crittenden, who elaborated coding systems for the Strange Situation and other assessment measures that explicitly assess caregiver–child interaction rather than the individual behaviour of the child.[465] One of the systems for coding behaviour at age six by the Berkeley group was the unpublished Strage and Main approach to coding reunions of verbal children; this was also a dyadic coding system.[466] And Lyons-Ruth and colleagues developed a dyadic-based coding system called the Goal-Corrected Partnership in Adolescence Coding System.[467] Nonetheless, the predominant approach to the assessment of child–caregiver attachment has certainly remained the coding of individual child behaviours following the protocol set out in Ainsworth and colleagues in *Patterns of Attachment*.

Main attempted to title a paper 'Security of attachment characterises relationships, not infants', with the running header of 'Relationships, not infants' (though the paper ended up with a different title in its published version as a concession to gruelling rounds of peer-review feedback).[468] Bowlby put matters starkly in *Attachment, Volume 1*: 'any statement about a child of twelve months himself showing a characteristic pattern of attachment behaviour, distinct from the interactional pattern of the couple of which he is a partner, and implying some degree of autonomous stability, is certainly mistaken'.[469] Yet one consequence of an individual-focused coding system for the Strange Situation has been that the predominant language used to discuss the categories of the Strange Situation is of secure, avoidant, and ambivalent/resistant infants. It is clear that a factor contributing to such language was that the coding system assessed individual behaviours. However, an additional factor has been that it is incredibly cumbersome to keep writing out 'behaviour shown in the Strange Situation by an infant in a dyad classified as avoidant, suggesting a certain history of infant–caregiver interactions'; it is easier to refer to an avoidant or A infant. Such terminology implied—or at the very least ceaselessly risked the implication—that attachment was a fixed individual trait and ultimate explanation. This is the kind of implication that, once everyone is asleep, creeps out and drinks the blood of a relationship-focused paradigm. Looking back

[464] E.g. Fonagy, P. (2000) *Attachment Theory and Psychoanalysis*. New York: Other Press.

[465] Crittenden, P.M. (1992) *Preschool Assessment of Attachment*. Miami: Family Relations Institute; Crittenden, P.M. (2016) *Raising Parents: Attachment, Representation, and Treatment*, 2nd edn. London: Routledge. The Cassidy/Marvin MacArthur preschool system has some elements of a dyadic focus, though these are not foregrounded. Cassidy, J., Marvin, R., with the ttachment Working Group of the John D. and Catherine T. MacArthur Network on the Transition from Infancy to Early Childhood (1992) Attachment organisation in preschool children: procedures and coding manual. Unpublished manual. Dyadic coding is more foregrounded in Marvin's later work: Britner, P.A., Marvin, R.S., & Pianta, R.C. (2005) Development and preliminary validation of the caregiving behavior system: association with child attachment classification in the preschool Strange Situation. *Attachment & Human Development*, 7(1), 83–102.

[466] Main, M., Kaplan, N., & Cassidy, J. (1985) Security in infancy, childhood, and adulthood: a move to the level of representation. *Monographs of the Society for Research in Child Development*, 50, 66–104; Strage, A. & Main, M. (1985) Attachment and parent–child discourse patterns. Paper presented at Biennial meeting of Society for Research in Child Development, Toronto. PP/Bow/J.4/4.

[467] Obsuth, I., Hennighausen, K., Brumariu, L.E., & Lyons-Ruth, K. (2014) Disorganized behavior in adolescent-parent interaction: relations to attachment state of mind, partner abuse, and psychopathology. *Child Development*, 85(1), 370–87.

[468] Main, M. & Weston, D. (1981) The independence of infant–mother and infant–father attachment relationships: security of attachment characterises relationships, not infants. PP/Bow/J.4/3. The paper was ultimately published under the title 'The quality of the toddler's relationship to mother and to father: related to conflict behavior and the readiness to establish new relationships'.

[469] Bowlby, J. (1969, 1982) *Attachment, Volume 1*. London: Penguin, p.349.

over three decades of research using the Strange Situation, and two decades of training coders, Sroufe acknowledges:

> We readily slip into describing cause in terms of individual traits rather than developmental systems. At the outset I want to adopt the curved finger of accusation and say that attachment theorists, such as myself, are equally vulnerable to this problem. Frequently, we slip into using terms such as 'securely attached child' when we know that attachment is really a relationship term, and the proper description would be 'a child with a history of a secure relationship with the primary caregiver'. We don't do it because this is unwieldy.[470]

Eagle proposed that this discourse has contributed to a focus on individual differences rather than relationships in attachment research more generally. He claimed that despite the theoretical acknowledgement of attachment as a relational construct, in practice the fact of the matter is that most attachment research is indistinguishable from a research programme that imagines individual differences as fixed traits.[471] There are certainly exceptions: an example is the attention of Sroufe and Egeland to continuities in security and insecurity that may be expressed as different forms of behaviour depending on the child's stage of development (Chapter 4). And Guy Bosmans and colleagues pursued innovative work examining attachment-relevant transitory states, contrasting them to more stable individual differences in attachment.[472] However, in general, Eagle's observation does have purchase. Fonagy and Campbell, taking the criticism further, recently argued that unless attachment research can move away from a spiritless obsession with categories for individual differences between humans, it will have no 'intellectual vigour and relevance', and likely no future (see Chapter 6).[473]

Early experiences vs continuity of care

Ainsworth and colleagues found that caregiver sensitivity in the home observation data predicted infant attachment in the Strange Situation. And a generation of subsequent researchers found a host of associations between the Strange Situation and later outcomes. However, Ainsworth and her team did not have the data to make claims about the implications of infant attachment for later development; and later researchers only very rarely undertook extensive home observations. Those that did, such as Klaus and Karin Grossmann, conducted their research with samples facing comparatively few adversities or sources of disruption. Given that caregiver sensitivity is quite stable over time unless specific changes intrude which alter the resources available to the caregiving system, it remained entirely unclear whether attachment as measured by the Strange Situation was functioning as an autonomous

---

[470] Sroufe, L.A. (2007) The place of development in developmental psychopathology. In A. Masten (ed.) *Multilevel Dynamics in Developmental Psychopathology: Pathways to the Future: The Minnesota Symposia on Child Psychology*, Vol. 34 (pp.285–99). Mahwah, NJ: Lawrence Erlbaum, p.291.

[471] Eagle, M. (2013) *Attachment and Psychoanalysis*. New York: Guilford, p.55. See also Kobak, R. & Bosmans, G. (2018) Attachment and psychopathology: a dynamic model of the insecure cycle. *Current Opinion in Psychology*, 25, 76–80, p.76.

[472] Bosmans, G., Van de Walle, M., Goossens, L., & Ceulemans, E. (2014) (In)variability of attachment in middle childhood: secure base script evidence in diary data. *Behavior Change*, 31, 225–42.

[473] Fonagy, P. & Campbell, C. (2015) Bad blood revisited: attachment and psychoanalysis. *British Journal of Psychotherapy*, 31(2), 229–50, p.236.

predictive variable, or whether maternal sensitivity or other aspects of the caregiving context were behind the scenes, doing the causal work. This question was raised by Michael Lamb and colleagues in their controversial criticisms of the Strange Situation. They argued that 'relationships between early experiences and later outcomes have been demonstrated only when there is continuity in the circumstances'.[474] It was not known, therefore, whether the causal factor for these later outcomes was early experiences of care in early childhood, early patterns of attachment, or experiences of care at the time of later outcomes. Or all three independently. Or an interaction. This question, left largely unexplored, has muddied uses of attachment theory to inform clinical and preventative work.

Ainsworth acknowledged the problem head-on in a paper delivered to the International Conference on Infant Studies in April 1984. She urged colleagues to accept that 'stability of patterns of attachment during infancy is influenced by the degree to which family interaction is stable, while still not making what I think is the error of attributing continuity wholly to such stability'.[475] Likewise, the prediction from early attachment to later child outcomes was argued to follow the same logic. Part of what was measured in the Strange Situation was the consequences of the caregiving the child had received. Change the caregiving, and these implications change. However, Ainsworth argued that the residue of experiences of caregiving do, over time, come to organise the attachment behavioural system in relatively durable ways. Yet this conference address by Ainsworth remained unpublished, and the position generally attributed to her has been that infant attachment is of special importance because of its major role in mediating early care and later development and mental health outcomes. By the early 1990s, Everett Waters was expressing deep concern that this assumption had come to function as 'dogma and doctrine'.[476] There were a few studies that examined the contributions of infant attachment and later caregiving, generally finding that both made a contribution to peer co-operativeness, language skills, school readiness, and behaviour problems.[477] In these, child outcomes were generally better when early insecure attachment in the Strange Situation was followed by sensitive care than when early secure attachment in the Strange Situation was followed by subsequent insensitive care. In 1998, Thompson observed that 'virtually all attachment theorists agree that the consequences of a secure or insecure attachment arise from an interaction between the emergent internal representations and personality processes that attachment security may initially influence, and the continuing quality of parental care that fosters later sociopersonality growth'.[478] However, no studies were conducted to see whether the Strange Situation added to prediction beyond early caregiver sensitivity.

[474] Lamb, M., Thompson, R.A., Gardner, W., & Charnov, E.L. (1985) *Infant–Mother Attachment: The Origins and Developmental Significance of Individual Differences in the Strange Situation*. Hillsdale, NJ: Lawrence Erlbaum, p.4.

[475] Ainsworth, M. (1984) Attachment, adaptation and continuity. Paper presented at International Conference on Infant Studies, April 1984. PP/Bow/J.1/57

[476] Waters, E., Posada, G., Crowell, J., & Lay, K.L. (1993) Is attachment theory ready to contribute to our understanding of disruptive behavior problems? *Development & Psychopathology*, 5(1–2), 215–24, p.217.

[477] E.g. Erickson, M., Sroufe, L.A., & Egeland, B. (1985) The relationship of quality of attachment and behavior problems in preschool in a high risk sample. *Monographs of the Society for Research in Child Development*, 50 (1–2), 147–86; Belsky, J. & Fearon, R.P. (2002) Early attachment security, subsequent maternal sensitivity, and later child development: does continuity in development depend upon continuity of caregiving? *Attachment & Human Development*, 4(3), 361–87.

[478] Thompson, R. (1998) Early sociopersonality development. In W. Damon & N. Eisenberg (eds) *Handbook of Child Psychology: Vol. 3. Social, Emotional, and Personality Development*, 5th edn (pp 25–104). New York: Wiley, p.58.

Sroufe and Egeland's Minnesota group was one of the few laboratories that had lon-gitudinal data on caregiver behaviour, infant attachment classifications, and later devel-opmental outcomes. But they only made separate reports of the relationship between sensitivity and the Strange Situation,[479] and the Strange Situation and later outcomes,[480] or folded caregiver sensitivity and infant Strange Situation classifications together into an 'early caregiving experiences composite'.[481] The position of Sroufe and Egeland appears to have been that neither sensitivity nor the Strange Situation is in itself 'attachment', which cannot be directly measured but must be inferred. As such, to Sroufe and Egeland, whether it was the sensitivity scale or the Strange Situation that was doing the predicting was rather irrelevant. Both measures were assumed to be only vantages on dyadic differences in the at-tachment relationship, scientific proxies for detailed observations of infant–caregiver inter-action in naturalistic settings. Sroufe and Egeland appeared to prefer the Strange Situation, however, when they had specific hypotheses about the correlates of the avoidant or ambiva-lent/resistant attachment classifications. Since the retirement of Sroufe and Egeland, the Minnesota group have tended to stop reporting analyses on the longitudinal correlates of the Strange Situation at all, and instead have generally reported longitudinal associations of caregiver sensitivity.[482]

However, it should not be thought that Minnesota alone had the data to examine the question of whether it is actually sensitivity that is behind associations between the Strange Situation and other correlates. After Minnesota, there have subsequently been other labora-tories with relevant data. One is the huge NICHD dataset, which has over a thousand dyads with assessments using the Strange Situation and of sensitivity at multiple time-points, including prior to the Strange Situation (though the measure of sensitivity had differences from Ainsworth's scale, since it included warmth and lack of intrusiveness).[483] This dataset has been available for three decades, and could have been used to see if the Strange Situation added to prediction after inclusion of prior caregiver sensitivity. An obstacle to tests of medi-ation, however, may have been norms and expertise in statistical analysis among the develop-mental science community. Attachment researchers tended to rely in the 1980s on one-way analyses of variance and other statistical tests that permitted examination of the implications of caregiving on attachment, or attachment on some other variable. Mediational path ana-lyses would only really enter into attachment research from the 1990s, despite earlier claims made for its relevance.[484] However, the issue was not simply methodological, but grounded

[479] E.g. Egeland, B. & Farber, E.A. (1984) Infant–mother attachment: factors related to its development and changes over time. *Child Development*, 55(3), 753–71 .

[480] E.g. Sroufe, L.A. (1983) Infant-caregiver attachment and patterns of adaptation in preschool: the roots of maladaptation and competence. In M. Perlmutter (ed.) *Development and Policy Concerning Children with Special Needs: The Minnesota Symposia on Child Psychology*, Vol. 16 (pp.41–83). Hillsdale, NJ: Lawrence Erlbaum.

[481] E.g. Jimerson, S., Egeland, B., Sroufe, L.A., & Carlson, B. (2000) A prospective longitudinal study of high school dropouts examining multiple predictors across development. *Journal of School Psychology*, 38(6), 525–49.

[482] See e.g. Farrell, A.K., Waters, T.E.A., Young, E.S., et al. (2019) Early maternal sensitivity, attachment security in young adulthood, and cardiometabolic risk at midlife. *Attachment & Human Development*, 21(1), 70–86.

[483] NICHD Early Child Care Research Network (1999) Child care and mother–child interaction in the first three years of life. *Developmental Psychology*, 35, 1399–413. Belsky and Fearon conducted an analysis of the relative contributions of attachment and sensitivity to later outcomes in this dataset, but only included measures of sensi-tivity subsequent to the Strange Situation. Belsky, J. & Fearon, R.P. (2002) Early attachment security, subsequent maternal sensitivity, and later child development: does continuity in development depend upon continuity of care-giving? *Attachment & Human Development*, 4(3), 361–87.

[484] Connell, J.P. (1987) Structural equation modeling and the study of child development: a question of good-ness of fit. *Child Development*, 58, 167–75

in a theoretical commitment to attachment patterns as developmentally causal. This is supported by the fact that multiple regression was used with increasing frequency through the 1980s by attachment researchers, in line with a broader trend in developmental psychology, but attachment and sensitivity were not examined together in an attempt to identify their respective contributions. When, in the 2000s, structural equation modelling was deployed by the Minnesota group to analyse their data, a composite variable containing both the Ainsworth infant attachment patterns and early caregiving experiences was used, rather than separating these out.[485]

In 1998, Elizabeth Carlson from the Minnesota group published an article addressing the disorganised attachment classification.[486] Though Carlson's work is addressed further in Chapter 3 and 4, it is important to mention this article here, as it was the first published work by the Minnesota group in which early caregiving and an infant attachment classification were entered into a mediational analysis. As an index of early caregiving, Carlson used a composite which included observer-assessed caretaking skill of the mother, the mother's sensitivity, and information about whether the caregiver had been abusive or engaged in suicide attempts. She found that the relationship between this early care composite and adolescent mental health problems was fully mediated by the disorganised attachment classification. She also found that avoidant attachment made an independent contribution to adolescent mental health problems. However, she did not include avoidant attachment within the mediational model.

The first full answer to Lamb's question about the predictive significance of sensitivity and attachment would wait for a study by Beijersbergen, Juffer, Bakermans-Kranenburg, and van IJzendoorn, reported in 2012.[487] Beijersbergen and colleagues conducted a follow-up with 125 adolescents who had been adopted early in their childhoods. Maternal sensitivity and infant attachment were assessed at 12 months of age. When the children were 14 years old, maternal sensitivity was assessed again during a discussion around difficult and conflict-evoking topics. The Adult Attachment Interview (Chapter 3) was used to assess the adolescents' state of mind regarding attachment. The researchers found no continuity of attachment between infant attachment in the Strange Situation and states of mind regarding attachment in the Adult Attachment Interview. However, maternal sensitivity in infancy and adolescence predicted continuity of secure attachment. Furthermore, a change from maternal insensitivity in infancy to sensitivity in adolescence predicted a change in attachment patterns from insecure to secure. The researchers concluded that continuity of attachment seems dependent on continuity of the caregiving context, as Lamb and Waters both predicted: 'We therefore submit that attachment theory should be a theory of sensitive parenting as much as it is a theory of attachment.'[488]

At age 23, the sample was asked to complete Waters and Waters' attachment script assessment. The same results appeared. There was no continuity of attachment from infancy to young adulthood. Sensitive care during childhood, but not adolescence, was a good predictor

---

[485] Carlson, E.A., Sroufe, L.A., & Egeland, B. (2004) The construction of experience: a longitudinal study of representation and behavior. *Child Development*, 75(1), 66–83.

[486] Carlson, E.A. (1998) A prospective longitudinal study of attachment disorganization/disorientation. *Child Development*, 69(4), 1107–28.

[487] Beijersbergen, M.D., Juffer, F., Bakermans-Kranenburg, M.J., & van IJzendoorn, M.H. (2012) Remaining or becoming secure: parental sensitive support predicts attachment continuity from infancy to adolescence in a longitudinal adoption study. *Developmental Psychology*, 48(5), 1277–82.

[488] Ibid. p.1281.

of secure base scripts at age 23.[489] This was a controversial finding, given the extent of prior emphasis on prediction from the Strange Situation. An informal network of quantitatively oriented attachment researchers including Bakermans-Kranenburg and van IJzendoorn made a call in 2014 for further work on this question. They asserted 'an urgent need for theory-driven studies that address mediating processes that account for such enduring effects, for example by addressing questions concerning whether such long-term continuities are due to the ongoing supportive function of attachment relationships and/or the early effects of attachment experiences on the construction of stable psychological structures'.[490]

However, the emphasis on sensitivity by many researchers since Ainsworth has been challenged by Ainsworth's former student Jude Cassidy and her colleagues. Just as Waters argued that amorphous measurements of 'attachment' should be superceded by precise attention to the availability of a secure base/safe haven script, Cassidy and colleagues argued that sensitivity should be superceded by the capacity of a caregiver to provide a secure base and safe haven.[491] Whilst in general this capacity will align with sensitivity, Cassidy and colleagues argued that they are entirely distinguishable. Sensitivity considers all of a caregiver's response to any infant cues, whereas secure base/safe haven provision is more specific about which infant cues are relevant and which caregiver responses. Sensitivity is also concerned with the caregiver's promptness of response, which is not necessarily as central for secure base/safe haven provision. These proposals have received initial support from a a recent study by Woodhouse and colleagues of 174 mother–infant dyads facing socioeconomic adversities.[492] The researchers found that observed secure base/safe haven provision was a much better predictor of Strange Situation classifications than observed sensitivity, and accounted for 16% of variance. The association between the two observational measures of caregiving was weak ($r = .11$). Woodhouse and colleagues also conclude that secure base/safe haven provision likely has greater cross-cultural applicability than the Ainsworth sensitivity construct.

Conclusion

See Table 2.2 in the Appendix to this chapter for consideration of key concepts discussed here.

Ainsworth's methodological innovations were a depth charge thrown into the water of developmental psychology: bubbles from the explosion are still coming to the surface today. The influence of Ainsworth's research programme on subsequent attachment research has been foundational, enduring, and profound. Ainsworth observed that 'research methods

[489] Schoenmaker, C., Juffer, F., van IJzendoorn, M.H., Linting, M., van der Voort, A., & Bakermans-Kranenburg, M.J. (2015) From maternal sensitivity in infancy to adult attachment representations: a longitudinal adoption study with secure base scripts. *Attachment & Human Development*, 17(3), 241–56.

[490] Groh, A.M., Fearon, R.P., Bakermans-Kranenburg, M.J., van IJzendoorn, M.H., Steele, R.D., & Roisman, G.I. (2014) The significance of attachment security for children's social competence with peers: a meta-analytic study. *Attachment & Human Development*, 16(2), 103–36, p.126.

[491] Cassidy, J., Woodhouse, S.S., Cooper, G., Hoffman, K., Powell, B., & Rodenberg, M. (2005) Examination of the precursors of infant attachment security: implications for early intervention and intervention research. In L.J. Berlin, Y. Ziv, L. Amaya-Jackson, & M.T. Greenberg (eds) *Enhancing Early Attachments: Theory, Research, Intervention, and Policy* (pp.34–60). New York: Guilford.

[492] Woodhouse, S.S., Scott, J.R., Hepworth, A.D., & Cassidy, J. (2020) Secure base provision: a new approach to examining links between maternal caregiving and infant attachment. *Child Development*, 91(1), 249–65.

influence the theoretical formulation associated with it. The reverse is also true.'[493] The Strange Situation is an extreme case. Rather than simply a tool for deployment in line with researchers' intentions, the Strange Situation extended the ambitions of an area of research, whilst also shaping the kinds of action and thought that subsequently seemed feasible or worthwhile.[494] On the one hand, the Strange Situation has provided the basis for a cumulative research paradigm for the study of early relationships for over 50 years—an astonishing feat. Over 15,000 child–caregiver dyads have been seen in the Strange Situation in the course of published research in this period. There will be many thousands more involved in unpublished research and clinical and forensic practice. Without the development of the Strange Situation, attachment theory would very likely have failed to take root within American developmental psychology.[495] By the same token, Granqvist suggested that if a measure had been developed for cognitive science or evolutionary psychology of equal importance as the Strange Situation for developmental psychology, it is quite possible that attachment theory would have put down roots in these disciplines too.[496]

On the other hand, to a degree that dismayed Ainsworth, the Strange Situation became the essence of attachment research at the expense of mixed methods research and naturalistic observation: 'I have been quite disappointed that so many attachment researchers have gone on to do research with the Strange Situation rather than looking at what happens in the home or in other natural settings—like I said before, it marks a turning away from "fieldwork", and I don't think it's wise.'[497] Ainsworth was proud of the Strange Situation and the way that it helped contribute to recognition for attachment theory. Nonetheless, Klaus and Karin Grossmann report that 'in our last encounter with Mary Ainsworth, she said that she regretted the Strange Situation book [*Patterns of Attachment*], which had really eclipsed what she had in mind. She said, sadly, that she rather would have written a book about sensitivity.'[498] The Strange Situation was constructed by Ainsworth as a heuristic, a means to further explore Bowlby's theory of behavioural systems. However, in general, the Baltimore longitudinal study was part-misrepresented and part-misinterpreted as a hypothesis-testing endeavour, giving findings the appearance of greater certainty and closure than they warranted.[499] And more specifically, the Strange Situation came to replace the interactions in the home that it had been intended to capture and preserve. Individual differences in the form of

[493] Ainsworth, M. (1969) Object relations, dependency and attachment. *Child Development*, 40, 969–1025, p.1003.

[494] Cf. Sayes, E. (2014) Actor–network theory and methodology. *Social Studies of Science*, 44(1), 134–49.

[495] For detailed argument on this point see van IJzendoorn, M.H., Tavecchio, L.W.C., Goossens, F.A., & Vergeer, M.M. (1982) *Opvoeden in Geborgenheid: Een Kritische Analyse van Bowlby's Attachment Theorie*. Amsterdam: Van Loghum Slaterus. By way of comparison, for discussion of a movement in psychoanalytic theory in the same period that failed to take root within academic psychology see McLaughlin, N.G. (1998) Why do schools of thought fail? Neo-Freudianism as a case study in the sociology of knowledge. *Journal of the History of the Behavioral Sciences*, 34(2), 113–34.

[496] Granqvist, P. (2020) *Attachment, Religion, and Spirituality: A Wider View*. New York: Guilford: 'That the placement of attachment theory and research within mainstream psychology is largely a historical coincidence, resulting from some skilled developmental psychologists' receptiveness to Bowlby's ideas. They adopted the theory, contributed to it, and made it a major part of psychology. However, attachment theory, originating in ethology, was among the first fully developed theories within what was later to become evolutionary approaches to human psychology. Similarly, as evidenced in Bowlby's use of a cybernetic model and his borrowing of the internal working model construct, attachment theory grew in the same soil that later produced cognitive science.'

[497] Ainsworth, M. (1995) On the shaping of attachment theory and research: an interview with Mary D.S. Ainsworth. *Monographs of the Society for Research in Child Development*, 60(2/3), 2–21, p.12.

[498] Klaus and Karin Grossmann, personal communication, November 2018.

[499] The Sroufe and Egeland Minnesota group were an exception here; core to their mission was an attempt to replicate and evaluate Ainsworth's findings, to test out their scientific standing (Chapter 4).

attachment categories became the focus of attention, even as Bowlby's behavioural systems model became part of the backdrop rather than an active concern.

The second generation of attachment researchers inherited from Bowlby and Ainsworth a theory with (i) apparently intuitive and accessible elements, including positions on normative child rearing, integrated with (ii) subtle, technical distinctions in the use of concepts and theory (e.g. between attachment behaviour and the attachment behavioural system), and (iii) complex observational measures. This facilitated the development of a division between an inner core of specialised developmental researchers and a wide popular constituency of practitioners, parents, and policy-makers interested in attachment theory and research, with terms like 'attachment' and 'security' offering switchers and relays between these different domains. Frequently, these groups have talked right past one another with the same words. Neither subtle, technical distinctions nor complex observational measures are easily transmitted through a print medium. It is also hard to effectively debate and discuss them in public, even when this can be acknowledged as a good use of time. One consequence is that attachment ideas, for all their accessibility to diverse audiences, have been continually at risk of being understood in ways that differ wildly from the understanding of researchers.

An important example has been the way that readers generally interpreted Ainsworth's construct of 'sensitivity' in line with the ordinary language connotations of the term. This is hardly surprising, since the coding system for sensitivity remained unpublished (until the 2015 reissue of *Patterns of Attachment* by Waters) and the operationalisation of the construct was little discussed in print. Chapter 1 describes how criticism of attachment theory has at times mistaken the ideas popularised by Bowlby in the 1950s for the commitments of subsequent researchers, leading attachment researchers to experience their paradigm as chronically misunderstood and somewhat maligned, and critics to regard attachment research as a heedless and arrogant enterprise.[500] This has proven an obstacle to effective dialogue between attachment research and anthropology. Furthermore, the gap between researchers and their publics left open space for entrepreneurs to enter the market as authorities. At times this has resulted in high-quality and well-informed popular texts and commercial trainings. However, at times these entrepreneurs have profited from the circulation of accounts of attachment theory and research that in important ways run contrary to available empirical evidence (Chapter 6).

A second consequence of the role of subtle, technical distinctions and complex observational measures has been obstacles to the diffusion of expert knowledge, expertise, and authority. It encouraged the development of an oral culture among developmental researchers based on lines of mentorship and attendance at lengthy training institutes, to permit the development and trained exercise of complex (and often implicit) skills of perception, thought, appreciation, and valuation[501]—the development of an 'attachment' eye.[502] Through the training institutes, researchers could become socialised in tacit skills of observation, conceptualisation, and judgement that offered access to the practical intricacies of relevant theory,

---

[500] See also White, S., Gibson, M., Wastell, D., & Walsh, P. (2019) *Reassessing Attachment Theory in Child Welfare*. Bristol: Psychology Press. Collins has offered the term 'alien science' to describe the reception of research in cases with such a sharp disparity. Collins, H.M. (1999) Tantalus and the aliens: publications, audiences and the search for gravitational waves. *Social Studies of Science*, 29(2), 163–97.

[501] Reijman, S., Foster, S., & Duschinsky, R. (2018) The infant disorganised attachment classification: 'patterning within the disturbance of coherence'. *Social Science & Medicine*, 200, 52–8.

[502] Cf. Bourdieu, P. (1989) The social genesis of the eye. In *The Rules of Art*, trans. S. Emanuel (pp.313–21). Cambridge: Polity Press.

such as the secure base concept. However, the requirements of this socialisation within an oral culture have made the reproduction of the field challenging, and the number of developmental attachment researchers has remained comparatively small. Reliance on an oral culture has, at times, made it relatively difficult even for other developmental psychologists to understand the details of the phenomena under discussion, for instance how the Strange Situation categories are actually operationalised. For example, researchers speculate about the meaning of differences in infant–caregiver behaviour in the Strange Situation in ways largely cut loose from how it is coded.[503]

The role of an oral culture has also made it difficult for researchers not centrally concerned with attachment to accurately take from and meaningfully contribute to the tradition of research. An effect was that research groups where the oral culture could be accessed—such as Berkeley (Mary Main; Chapter 3), Minnesota (Alan Sroufe and others; Chapter 4), Regensburg (Klaus and Karin Grossmann), and SUNY (Everett Waters and Judith Crowell) in the 1980s[504]—became centres of gravity for developmental attachment research and the training of future researchers. The leaders of these research groups gained the status of 'authorities of delimitation', with a certain capacity to set the terms of the developmental tradition.[505] These dynamics are not only apparent in retrospect. Even in the 1980s, attachment researchers were themselves offering analysis and commentary on these sociological processes in print, worrying that the result would be a dynamic of 'insiderness' among certain research groups, to the exclusion of non-members.[506]

There were major advantages of having such centres of gravity for the developmental tradition. One was the capacity to develop a centralised training and reliability test for the Strange Situation, which has supported interlaboratory agreement as well as providing a site with ritual as well as pragmatic functions, such as cultivating junior researchers and developing international solidarity and networks. Another advantage was the momentum that was generated around high-investment, high-yield longitudinal studies such as the Minnesota Longitudinal Study of Risk and Adaptation (Chapter 4). A third advantage was forms of collaboration and sharing of data for particular purposes, supported by strong interpersonal relationships, for instance in appraising cross-cultural differences.[507] The development of the disorganised attachment classification was, as Chapter 3 will show, based in part on the willingness of other laboratories to share their tapes of the Strange Situation with Main and the Berkeley group.

---

[503] E.g. Koós, O. & Gergely, G. (2001) A contingency-based approach to the etiology of 'disorganized' attachment: the 'flickering switch' hypothesis. *Bulletin of the Menninger Clinic*, 65(3), 397–410.

[504] By the 1990s, additional centres of gravity included—though were not limited to—Pennsylvania (Jay Belsky), Harvard (Karlen Lyons-Ruth), Leiden (Marinus van IJzendoorn), Maryland (Jude Cassidy, Doug Teti), Haifa (Avi Sagi-Schwartz), and London (Peter Fonagy, Miriam Steele, and Howard Steele). Berkeley and Minnesota especially, and Regesburg and SUNY to an extent, nonetheless appeared to retain particular significance and, in certain regards, social priority. This dynamic can be seen in the pattern of citation by the research groups of one another.

[505] For a discussion of the role of authorities of delimitation see Foucault, M. (1969, 1972) *The Archaeology of Knowledge*, trans. A.M. Sheridan Smith. London: Routledge, Chapter 3.

[506] E.g. Tavecchio, L.W. & van IJzendoorn, M.H. (eds) (1987) *Attachment in Social Networks: Contributions to the Bowlby–Ainsworth Attachment Theory*. New York: Elsevier; Emde, R.N. & Fonagy, P. (1997) An emerging culture for psychoanalytic research? *International Journal of Psychoanalysis*, 78(4), 643–51: 'Extensive training is often needed for coding and observation, which can lead not only to isolation but to shared assumptions that are unspecified among those doing the research' (649).

[507] E.g. van IJzendoorn, M.H. & Kroonenberg, P.M. (1990) Cross-cultural consistency of coding the strange situation. *Infant Behavior and Development*, 13(4), 469–85; Sagi, A., van IJzendoorn, M.H., & Koren-Karie, N. (1991) Primary appraisal of the Strange Situation: a cross-cultural analysis of preseparation episodes. *Developmental Psychology*, 27(4), 587–96.

However, one negative consequence of the manner in which the developmental tradition was transmitted was that some aspects of Ainsworth's approach were adopted with, in retrospect, too little explicit discussion. One aspect, emphasised by Roisman and van IJzendoorn, was the focus on intensive, small-scale work in distinct research groups.[508] A huge advantage was that this supported fidelity of measurement. In general, larger studies have tended to have poor associations between the Strange Situation and measures of sensitivity, which has raised questions in some quarters about whether coders rushed their task.[509] Roisman and van IJzendoorn suggest that an alternative might have been to build collaborative consortia, with data-sharing between the many small groups. Pursuing just such a strategy, the willingness of researchers in the developmental tradition of attachment research to share and pool data has reached its apex in forms of Individual Participant Data meta-analysis in recent years (Chapter 6).[510] The strong, somewhat 'familial' interpersonal connections of the developmental tradition may be supposed to have supported the development of such data-sharing initiatives.

Another less-advantageous aspect of Ainsworth's approach that was followed by the second generation, and which is interesting in retrospect, was her eschewal of popular media. Bowlby was keen to use television, radio, magazine articles, and books published by popular presses to influence clinicians, policy-makers, and the wider public.[511] These methods were not pursued by Ainsworth and they were not generally adopted by the subsequent generation of attachment researchers.[512] In fact, Ainsworth's correspondence time and again reveals her deep discomfort when she was approached with requests for prescriptive advice. The eschewal of popular media by Ainsworth and the vast majority of her confederates stands out as unusual among their peers. Child development researchers, in general, have been among the most active in public engagement among psychological researchers, in part due to the ready public and practitioner audience for knowledge in this area, and the growing policy problematisation of child development.[513] It should be acknowledged that

---

[508] See Roisman, G.I. & van IJzendoorn, M.H. (2018) Meta-analysis and individual participant data synthesis in child development: introduction to the special section. *Child Development*, 89(6), 1939–42.

[509] The particular object of contention here has been the NICHD sample: NICHD Early Child Care Research Network (1997) The effects of infant child care on infant–mother attachment security: results of the NICHD Study of Early Child Care NICHD Early Child Care Research Network. *Child Development*, 68(5), 860–79.

[510] Verhage, M.L., Fearon, R.P., Schuengel, C., et al. (2018) Examining ecological constraints on the intergenerational transmission of attachment via individual participant data meta-analysis. *Child Development*, 89(6), 2023–37.

[511] The disjuncture between the willingness to engage with public media between Bowlby and Ainsworth was already remarked upon by Karen, R. (1990) Becoming attached. *The Atlantic*, February 1990: 'Ainsworth is all but unknown to the public (and to many psychoanalysts and psychiatrists, who tend to be unfamiliar with trends in developmental psychology), and yet her fame in the world of infant development exceeds that of John Bowlby himself … Unlike Bowlby, who holds the light as if he were born to it, she doesn't seem at home.' Ainsworth, M. (1990) *Letter to John Bowlby*, 24 1990, PP/BOW/B.3/8.

[512] Some further limited exceptions can be identified. For instance, Sroufe was involved in writing a popular textbook, and composed a few newspaper articles. Marti Erickson led the Children, Youth & Family Consortium after finishing the STEEP intervention and the research, and worked directly in family policy. Generally, though, the difference in scale between Bowlby's public engagement activities and those of Ainsworth and the second generation of attachment researchers is profound. As will be discussed further in Chapter 6, the lack of public engagement by second-generation researchers stands in contrast to the extensive public-facing activities of third-generation attachment researchers such as Sheri Madigan. Madigan, S. (2019) Beyond the academic silo: collaboration and community partnerships in attachment research. Paper presented at International Attachment Conference, Vancouver, 20 July 2019: 'The public are looking for information, and will get misinformation unless we extend research findings to the public. I am taking it as a responsibility of mine to disseminate information to those who want it, often parents and clinicians.'

[513] See e.g. Britto, P.R., Lye, S.J., Proulx, K., et al., and the Early Childhood Development Interventions Review Group, for the Lancet Early Childhood Development Series Steering Committee (2017) Nurturing care: promoting early childhood development. *The Lancet*, 389(10064), 91–102; Leach, P. (ed.) (2017) *Transforming Infant Wellbeing: Research, Policy and Practice for the First 1001 Critical Days*. London: Routledge.

there are exceptions. Patricia Crittenden and Peter Fonagy have been energetic in communicating to public and professional constituencies about attachment theory.[514] And the Circle of Security graphic of the caregiver as a secure base and safe haven has circulated widely as a visual representation of Ainsworth's concepts.[515] Nonetheless, as Goldberg observed, after Bowlby 'many attachment researchers (myself included) have been reluctant to take on this responsibility' of knowledge exchange with non-researchers.[516]

Beyond the model provided by Ainsworth, several further reasons might be identified for the neglect of public engagement by the second generation of attachment researchers. One would surely be the lack of incentives for public engagement within American academic life in the 1980s and 1990s. The second generation also saw directly the problems and misunderstandings caused by Bowlby's popularizing texts; there may have been a sense of wanting to seal themselves off from what they felt unable to mend. A further reason for the lack of public engagement activities by Ainsworth and most of her successors is likely to have been the urgent priority felt for the development of attachment as a distinct and differentiated scientific paradigm, a 'field' for attachment research.[517] This was understood to entail efforts to test and secure the main aspects of what were judged Ainsworth's legacy: the Strange Situation and its expectable caregiving and behavioural correlates. In this regard, as we shall see in Chapter 3, Main was both the quintessential second-generation researcher and a marked exception. Few of the second generation were as deeply steeped in and committed to Ainsworth's ideas and methods, and most of Main's work focused on correlates of the Strange Situation in one way or another. Yet Main was also a radical innovator, introducing new theoretical ideas, changing the coding of the Strange Situation procedure, and creating assessments of attachment for later in the lifecourse. She also shaped interpretations of Ainsworth and Bowlby. These developments, discussed in Chapter 3, would establish the methodological and theoretical mainstream for the second generation of attachment researchers through the 1990s and 2000s.

[514] See e.g. Spieker, S.J. & Crittenden, P.M. (2018) Can attachment inform decision-making in child protection and forensic settings? *Infant Mental Health Journal*, 39(6), 625–41; Fonagy, P. & Higgitt, A. (2004) Early mental health intervention and prevention: the implications for government and the wider community. In B. Sklarew, S.W. Twemlow, & S.M. Wilkinson (eds) *Analysts in the Trenches: Streets, Schools, War Zones* (pp.257–309). Mahwah, NJ: Analytic Press; Fonagy, P. (2018) Evidence submitted to the Evidence-Based Early-Years Intervention Inquiry. Science and Technology Committee (Commons). http://data.parliament.uk/writtenevidence/committeeevidence.svc/evidencedocument/science-and-technology-committee/evidencebased-early-years-intervention/written/77644.pdf.

[515] Powell, B., Cooper, G., Hoffman, K., & Marvin, R.S. (2009) The circle of security. In C.H. Zeanah (ed.) *Handbook of Infant Mental Health* (pp.450–67). New York: Guilford.

[516] Goldberg, S. (2000) *Attachment and Development*. London: Routledge, p.248. By way of comparison, consider the use of popular forums even for scholarly debates between specialists in evolutionary psychology in the 1990s. Cassidy, A. (2005) Popular evolutionary psychology in the UK: an unusual case of science in the media? *Public Understanding of Science*, 14(2), 115–41. The marked contrast between attachment research and evolutionary psychology in this regard has been noted by Granqvist, P. (2020) *Attachment, Religion, and Spirituality: A Wider View*. New York: Guilford.

[517] Bourdieu, P. (1975) The specificity of the scientific field and the social conditions of the progress of reason. *Social Science Information*, 14(6), 19–47; Bourdieu, P. (2004) *The Science of Science and Reflexivity*, trans. R. Nice. Chicago: University of Chicago Press. For equivalent processes in another area of the social sciences see Turner, S.P. (2012) De-intellectualizing American sociology: a history, of sorts. *Journal of Sociology*, 48(4), 346–63.

Appendix

Table 2.2 Some key concepts in Ainsworth's writings

Concept	Mistaken for	Technical meaning
Security	Personal wellbeing and confidence	Ainsworth used the term 'security' to mean a person's confidence in their efficacy to access the people/resources to have their needs met. When this confidence is available, its source was described by Ainsworth as a 'secure base'.
		She also used the term as a category label for a group of infants in her Strange Situation procedure. These infants seek physical or distal contact, are readily comforted following separations, and are able to return to play. This implied to Ainsworth that they were confident in their caregiver's availability.
Attachment figure	Mother	An attachment figure is a familiar person who is sought or wished for under conditions of alarm (i.e. when the attachment system is activated).
Attachment in adulthood	Continuation of individual differences in attachment from early childhood across the lifespan	Ainsworth described separation anxiety and secure base and safe haven dynamics as aspects of relationships in both childhood and adulthood. And following Bowlby, she anticipated some elements of continuity in how individuals respond within relationships that have these attachment components.
		The role of these attachment components in adulthood have been measured very differently, and more or less directly, by different attachment researchers.
Strange Situation	Definitive test of individual differences in attachment	A structured laboratory-based observational procedure developed by Ainsworth. The Strange Situation was intended to provide a window into a child's expectations about their caregiver's availability based on the history of their prior interactions. It is a validated proxy for direct observations of those interactions.
Sensitivity	Warmth and tenderness	Though used more expansively in her early work, the term 'sensitivity' was a highly technical one for Ainsworth from the late 1960s. By this she meant the ability of a caregiver to (i) perceive and to (ii) interpret accurately the signals and communications implicit in an infant's behavior, and given this understanding, to (iii) respond to them appropriately and (iv) promptly. Ainsworth developed a scale, unpublished until recently, for assessing caregiver sensitivity.
		Various other measures of sensitivity have subsequently been developed by attachment researchers. Not all of them measure sensitivity as technically defined by Ainsworth.

Illustrative Statement: 'Ainsworth's Strange Situation procedure showed that sensitive care was associated with infant security with their attachment figure.'

Mistaken for: Ainsworth's Strange Situation functions as a definitive test of the extent that individual infants deviate from a standard of security, representing their state of wellbeing. This state of wellbeing is associated with the warmth and tenderness shown by their mother.

Technical meaning: Ainsworth's Strange Situation is a validated proxy for naturalistic observations of dyads containing an infant and someone who functions, at least to a material extent, as an attachment figure. It is an imperfect research instrument based on a small sampling of behaviour, and subject to measurement error. However, findings using the procedure can be supported by convergence with those from other approaches, such as observations of caregiver sensitivity.

3

Mary Main, Erik Hesse, and the Berkeley Social Development Study

Biographical sketch

Mary Main was one of Ainsworth's first graduate students at the Johns Hopkins University. However, her distinctive training prior to graduate work meant that she came to the study of child development from an unusual angle. As an undergraduate she studied classics and natural sciences at St John's College, Maryland. This included four years of courses in literature and philosophy. Since Main had married one of her philosophy professors, Alvin Main, if she wanted to continue to graduate school she would need to find a programme nearby. Following her lifelong interest in language, Main applied to Hopkins to study psycholinguistics.[1] However, her application was accepted by Ainsworth for graduate work on child–caregiver attachment. Main completed her doctorate under Ainsworth in 1973. Her project was the third study to use the Strange Situation, after Ainsworth and Sylvia Bell, and the results were part of the 106 cases analysed in *Patterns of Attachment*. In 1973 she was appointed to a faculty position at the University of California, Berkeley. Settling in at Berkeley was disrupted by the death of Alvin Main. However, during the 1970s she managed to begin a longitudinal study in the Bay Area, conducting the Strange Situation with both mothers and fathers. Already in her dissertation, Main's interest in the work of Robert Hinde had led her to study conflict behaviours observed in the Strange Situation. She pursued this inquiry in her Bay Area sample, which led to the introduction of the disorganised attachment classification. A subset of families from the sample were invited back to the laboratory when the child was aged six. Main and her group inductively identified associations between the infant Strange Situation classifications and assessments of the six-year-old's behaviour and family drawings. The Strange Situations also had associations with the form taken by a parent's autobiographical narrative. This latter finding led to the development of the Adult Attachment Interview (AAI).[2] The Berkeley study has been described as 'the most influential, in-depth, and complex study of intergenerational factors in attachment' of its era.[3] Together with her second husband and collaborator Erik Hesse, Main introduced the hypothesis that disorganised attachment may be caused by caregivers' behaviour that alarms their infant, and that this alarming behaviour can be predisposed by unresolved experiences of loss or trauma. Building on the work of Bowlby and Ainsworth, contributions

---

[1] Main, M., Hesse, E., & Kaplan, N. (2005) Predictability of attachment behavior and representational processes at 1, 6, and 19 years of age: the Berkeley longitudinal study. In K.E. Grossmann, K. Grossmann, & E. Waters (eds) *Attachment from Infancy to Adulthood: The Major Longitudinal Studies* (pp.245–304). New York: Guilford, p.248.

[2] Hesse, E. (2016) The adult attachment interview: protocol, method of analysis, and empirical studies: 1985–2015. In J. Cassidy & P.R. Shaver (eds) *Handbook of Attachment: Theory, Research, and Clinical Applications*, 3rd edn (pp.553–97). New York: Guilford.

[3] Karen, R. (1998) *Becoming Attached: First Relationships and How They Shape Our Capacity to Love.* Oxford: Oxford University Press, p.363.

by the Berkeley group revolutionised and redefined the methodology and theory of attachment research.

Introduction

Main was the first of Ainsworth's graduate students to receive a faculty position and establish an independent research group. As a result, the most pressing item of business was replication. Whereas Ainsworth's original study in the mid-1960s had 26 infant–mother dyads, and *Patterns of Attachment* could report 106 infant–mother dyads, Main submitted a proposal in the mid-1970s to the William T. Grant Foundation for a much larger study, including both mothers and fathers. The proposal was accepted and Main was able to hire research assistance to support the recruitment of 189 families in 1976–77. For this replication and extension of Ainsworth's study, Main's sample was selected precisely to be low risk. All the families were middle- or upper-middle class. No teenage mothers were included, and none of the parental couples were divorced. Families were screened out if the infant had been born prematurely or had a low birth weight, or if there had been problems with the delivery. Families were also screened out if infants had experienced a separation of two weeks or more from their attachment figures. And only Caucasian or Asian families were included, to exclude as a confound the adversities black families faced with stigma and oppression. Families were also screened out if the father was unemployed, or if infants were in more than 25 hours of daycare per week, though parents were not excluded on the grounds of mental illness.

Deliberately unrepresentative of US families, Main's sample was intended to be low risk, as a point of comparison against which later studies addressing specific risks or particular populations could be compared.[4] However, it was also anticipated to be large enough for further detailed study of the difference between secure and avoidant attachment, which was Main's central interest in the mid-1970s.[5] Main's inclusion of fathers in the Berkeley longitudinal study can be situated in the context of shifts in American public and academic discourse in the 1970s that urged recognition of the significance of the father as a parent and as an attachment figure.[6] However, Ainsworth's decision to focus on mothers was a pragmatic one based on her limited resources and the childcare practice of the time in Baltimore. A decade later, distal changes in discourses around the family combined with the better

---

[4] Main, M., Hesse, E., & Kaplan, N. (2005) Predictability of attachment behavior and representational processes at 1, 6, and 19 years of age: the Berkeley longitudinal study. In K.E. Grossmann, K. Grossmann, & E. Waters (eds) *Attachment from Infancy to Adulthood: The Major Longitudinal Studies* (pp.245–304). New York: Guilford: 'We believed that only after the sequelae "naturally" arising out of enduring differences in attachment relationships have been delineated can researchers begin to trace—as P.T. Medawar put it in another context—the "variations which depart"' (258).

[5] Main, M. (1978) Avoidance of the attachment figure under stress: ontogeny, function and immediate causation. PP/Bow/J.4/3: 'The principle aims of the project are a) to test the proposition that avoidance of attachment figures in infancy predicts restricted affective responsiveness, aggression, and avoidance of adults other than the parents in early childhood; b) to provide norms for infant behaviour in the Strange Situation and in play settings; c) to compare and contrast mother–infant and father–infant relationships and the influence these relationships have upon development; d) to relate the child's behaviour toward peers and caregivers in nursery school to "joint" classifications of relationships to parent in infancy and to conflict vs harmony in the parent–parent relationship.'

[6] Biller, H.B. (1974) *Paternal Deprivation: Family, School, Sexuality, and Society*. Lexington, MA: D.C. Heath; Lamb, M.E. (1975) Fathers: forgotten contributors to child development. *Human Development*, 18, 245–66.

resources of the Berkeley study, leading to an expanded lens on parenting as well as a larger sample.

However, in fact Main did not ultimately have the funds to arrange rigorous coding for all 378 Strange Situation recordings. A report was made by Main and Weston in 1981 from a subset of 46 families who were invited to take part in both the Strange Situation at 12 and 18 months, and in an additional assessment of prosocial behaviour.[7] Of the infants seen with mother at 12 months, 68% of the dyads were classified as secure, 28% avoidant, and 4% ambivalent/resistant. For these same infants seen with father at 18 months, 59% of dyads were classified as secure, 35% as avoidant, and 6% as ambivalent/resistant. The distribution was therefore 'highly compatible' with the distributions from Ainsworth's sample, and indeed are well aligned with subsequent distributions.[8] Main and Weston reported that the attachment classification of an infant with one parent had a very weak, statistically insignificant association with the attachment classification of an infant with the other parent.[9] Furthermore, there was no significant association on the proximity-seeking, contact-maintaining, avoidance, or resistance scales.[10]

Main and Weston also reported that the attachment classification with each parent made an independent contribution to prosocial behaviour. This was assessed in a rather unusual laboratory-based procedure at 12 and 18 months. With a parent in the room, infants were approached by a clown who sought to play with the child. The clown approached the child with a mask, then removed the mask, called to the infant, and somersaulted about. The clown was asked by an adult to leave, and began to protest wretchedly: 'Extremely realistic sobbing. The cry lasts 50 seconds. Its realism is so strong that many adults hearing this cry for the first time are somewhat shaken.'[11] Prosociality was rated if infants engaged positively with the

[7] Main, M. & Weston, D.R. (1981) The quality of the toddler's relationship to mother and to father: related to conflict behavior and the readiness to establish new relationships. *Child Development*, 52(3), 932–40.

[8] Ibid. p.938. The rate of ambivalent/resistant was lower and the rate of avoidant attachment was higher than the distributions reported in a recent international meta-analysis, but this has turned out to be quite usual for American low-risk samples. Verhage, M.L., Schuengel, C., Madigan, S., et al. (2016) Narrowing the transmission gap: a synthesis of three decades of research on intergenerational transmission of attachment. *Psychological Bulletin*, 142(4), 337–66, Table 4: 60.4% secure, 22.5% avoidant, 17.1% ambivalent/resistant. The meta-analysis included only those studies that conducted both the Strange Situation and the AAI.

[9] Later research debated possible reasons for the small positive association between infant attachment classifications with respective parents. Spangler emphasised the role of individual infant dispositions. Spangler, G. (2013) Individual dispositions as precursors of differences in attachment quality: why maternal sensitivity is nevertheless important. *Attachment & Human Development*, 15(5–6), 657–72. A recent meta-analysis found that interparental conflict in non-clinical samples was inversely associated with attachment security ($r = -.28$). Interparental conflict may affect the care provided by both partners, or may directly impact the ambient sense of threat or caregiver availability in the home for the baby in all relationships. Tan, E.S., McIntosh, J.E., Kothe, E.J., Opie, J.E., & Olsson, C.A. (2018) Couple relationship quality and offspring attachment security: a systematic review with meta-analysis. *Attachment & Human Development*, 20(4), 349–77. It should also be highlighted that in newer studies with preschoolers—a period marked by an increase in father involvement, especially more recently—concordance is much higher, e.g. Bureau, J.-F., Martin, J., Yurkowski, K., et al. (2017) Correlates of child–father and child–mother attachment in the preschool years. *Attachment & Human Development*, 19, 130–50.

[10] Relatively few longitudinal studies have conducted attachment measures with multiple caregivers. As a consequence, little is known about the implications of convergent or divergent patterns of attachment with different caregivers. The only reported data on this come from Fonagy and colleagues, who reported that—whilst there were no effects for infancy—discrepant attachment classifications at age five in a modified Strange Situation were associated with conduct problems. Fonagy, P., Target, M., Steele, M., et al. (1997) Morality, disruptive behavior, borderline personality disorder, crime, and their relationships to security of attachment. In L. Atkinson & K.J. Zucker (eds) *Attachment and Psychopathology* (pp.223–74). New York: Guilford, p.247. However, in subsequent decades there has been no attempt to replicate these findings.

[11] Main, M., Weston, D.R., & Wakeling, S. (1979) Concerned attention to the crying of an adult actor in infancy. Paper presented at Society for Research in Child Development, San Francisco, March 1979. PP/Bow/J.4/3.

clown when invited to play and seemed sympathetic to the clown's crying. Children with two secure attachment relationships scored highest on prosociality; those with two inse- cure attachment relationships scored lowest; and those with one secure and one insecure at- tachment were rated in the middle.[12] Children with avoidant attachment relationships were found to often remain impassive in response to the crying clown, and their mothers were more likely to show a derisive facial expression when the clown began crying.[13] The Clown procedure appeared to especially stress children in avoidantly attached dyads. Unable to seek their caregiver directly for support, around half showed a variety of 'conflict behaviours' such as 'rocking back and forth whilst staring into space; assuming odd postures; engaging in odd tension movements; sudden inappropriate or empty laughter; vocalising to the wall in a "social" manner; an odd "frozen" facial expression; lying on the floor in foetal position with eyes closed'.[14] These behaviours were especially common in those who were avoidantly attached with both parents. Main took this to signify that conflict behaviours were elicited especially when the child experienced the relative unavailability of both caregivers as a safe haven. In a later reflection, however, Main concluded that the association between avoidance in the Strange Situation and conflict behaviours in the clown study may have been caused by caregivers 'who were harsh or frightened in addition to simply displaying aversion to phys- ical contact'.[15] The implication is that the close relationship Main initially would perceive between avoidance and conflict behaviour was, in part, an artefact of a sample in which the antecedents of avoidant attachment and the antecedents of conflict behaviours happened to co-occur.

When participants were aged around six years old, in 1982, 40 families were invited back to the laboratory, stratified by infant attachment classification.[16] No families with parents who had divorced in the intervening years were included.[17] A small grant from the Society for Research in Child Development helped cover the costs of the study, and Main's lively and intriguing classes attracted a talented group of Berkeley graduate students to work on the project: Donna Weston, Carol George, Judith Solomon, Nancy Kaplan, and Ellen Richardson. Each family was first visited at home by a member of the team, to take consent and build rapport. On arrival in the laboratory, the family viewed excerpts together from one of the films made by James Robertson ('Thomas: ten days in fostercare'). Study of family responses to the distressing, evocative film of a 14-day separation and reunions with father

[12] For a review of developments and unanswered questions since Main and Weston's report see Dagan, O. & Sagi-Schwartz, A. (2018) Early attachment network with mother and father: an unsettled issue. *Child Development Perspectives*, 12(2), 115–21.

[13] Main, M. (1978) Avoidance of the attachment figure under stress: ontogeny, function and immediate caus- ation. PP/Bow/J.4/3.

[14] Main, M. & Weston, D. (1981) The independence of infant–mother and infant–father attachment relation- ships: security of attachment characterises relationships, not infants. PP/Bow/J.4/3.

[15] Main, M. (1999) *Disorganized Attachment in Infancy, Childhood, and Adulthood: An Introduction to the Phenomena*. Unpublished manuscript, Mary Main & Erik Hesse personal archive.

[16] There is a discrepancy regarding the number of families in the six-year follow-up. In 1985 Main states that 'forty mothers, fathers, and their 6-year-old children (24 male, 19 firstborn) formed the sample of participants in this 1982 study': Main, M., Kaplan, N., & Cassidy, J. (1985) Security in infancy, childhood, and adulthood: a move to the level of representation. *Monographs of the Society for Research in Child Development*, 50, 66–104, p.79. However, Main stated on several later occasions that she and Ruth Goldwyn initially developed the AAI in 1982– 83 on 36 transcripts and then tested it on the remaining 66. If interviews were conducted with both mother and father, then this would mean 51 families were called back. The likely resolution to this discrepancy is that further data collection took place in 1983.

[17] George, C. (1984) Individual differences in affective sensitivity: a study of five-year olds and their parents. Unpublished doctoral dissertation, University of California, Berkeley.

and mother was the basis of Carol George's doctoral dissertation with Main.[18] George found that the parents from insecure dyads and children from insecure dyads were more likely to show signs of anger, disgust, and sarcasm in response to viewing the child's behaviour in the film. Yet as well as a stimulus for George's study, the film served as a prime for the attachment behavioural system and caregiving behavioural systems ahead of subsequent assessments.[19] The parents then left the room for individually administered life-history interviews (the AAI). The children remained in the playroom with an examiner. For 15 minutes they were asked to make a drawing of their choice, then one of their family. Next, the examiner asked the child to respond to six pictures of child–caregiver separations, giving their thoughts on what the separated child might feel or do (the Separation Anxiety Test).[20] The child and parents were reunited after about an hour's separation; in half the cases the mother returned first, and in half the cases the father. The reunion was filmed.

Main's approach to the analysis of her six-year data was deeply influenced by the five years she had spent as a graduate student within Ainsworth's research group. Main had been drenched to the bone in Ainsworth's ideas at a point that attachment research as an empirical paradigm was little more than this single laboratory at Baltimore. Ainsworth's identification of three patterns of infant attachment was felt by Main with incredible force. Why three? Researchers outside of the little laboratory often simply drew the conclusion that the result was arbitrary, primarily an artificial construction of diversity into pragmatic categories.[21] But Main had conducted 50 Strange Situations as part of her dissertation research, and was therefore in a position to see the Ainsworth system from the inside and to identify something remarkable: it was astonishingly un-arbitrary. Naturally there were marginal cases between the three groups. Yet the categories themselves seemed to Main to work unnervingly, miraculously well in offering the three basic images to which all the infants approximated in her dissertation sample. There really did seem to be, beyond any reasonable expectation, three patterns of attachment displayed not just in the 26 middle-class Baltimore infant–mother dyads recruited by Ainsworth for her initial study, but by the 106 middle-class infant–mother dyads from the studies by Ainsworth, Bell, and from Main's doctoral work.

The effectiveness of the Ainsworth classifications seemed to Main to imply something about the fundamental reality of human emotional life. It is hardly unusual for a doctoral student to look out at the whole world through the lens of her supervisor's work. Chapter 2 discussed how Blatz's work on security played a foundational role for Ainsworth in her thinking about adult personality, the behaviour of infants in Uganda, and ultimately individual differences in the Strange Situation. However, when Main started to look at the world through

---

[18] Ibid. The role of an attachment prime (the video of separation and reunion of a child) prior to conducting the AAI in the Berkeley study is not generally known and has not been discussed in the published literature. It could be that this made no difference, but no study has addressed the question.

[19] The question of whether priming is beneficial for or contaminates measures such as the AAI and the Experiences in Close Relationships scale in their capacity to measure adult attachment remains an open one and is rarely discussed. It is to be hoped that the growth of priming research will help bring this matter to light, and to explicit examination (Chapter 6) No doubt part of the issue is that both the AAI and ECR have been interpreted as measuring a 'thing' called adult attachment, when in fact matters are more complicated.

[20] Hansburg, H.G. (1972) *Adolescent Separation Anxiety: A Method for the Study of Adolescent Separation Problems.* Springfield: Thomas; Klagsbrun, M. & Bowlby, J. (1976) Responses to separation from parents: a clinical test for children. *British Journal of Projective Psychology,* 21, 7–21; Kaplan, N. (1987) Individual differences in 6-year olds' thoughts about separation: predicted from attachment to mother at age 1. Unpublished doctoral dissertation, Department of Psychology, University of California, Berkeley, CA.

[21] A significant recent example of this view is Gaskins, S. (2013) The puzzle of attachment. In N. Quinn & J.M. Mageo (eds) *Attachment Reconsidered: Cultural Perspectives on a Western Theory* (pp.33–66). London: Palgrave.

the lens of the Ainsworth infant attachment classifications, two surprising things happened. First, Main came to the exhilarating conclusion that the Ainsworth patterns represented the three basic strategies used by all humans, whether infants or adults, for handling distress in interpersonal contexts. Second, exceptions to these patterns therefore took on special significance and interest. Main's own powers as an observer of all scruffy particularities became combined with a theoretical focus on exceptions, developing a fourth category for behaviour suggesting a disruption in strategy.[22] On this basis, Main developed an account of individual differences in attachment as reflecting strategies for the direction of attention with respect to attachment-related perceptions and memories.

These ideas are not widely understood, especially as several key texts by Main were ultimately not published. However, they shaped the development of the AAI and other measures developed by Main, Hesse, and collaborators in the Berkeley group in the 1980s and 1990s. The theory and research of Main and colleagues has repeatedly been situated as a 'revolutionary shift' in attachment research.[23] Allen and Miga described how the work 'permits and indeed forces a new conceptualization of attachment, and opens up important avenues for assessing the attachment system beyond childhood'.[24] Holmes described it as the start of attachment research 'Phase 2', and Toth observed that it brought about the interest in attachment theory among the clinical community that Bowlby had sought but not managed on his own.[25]

The work of Main and colleagues has offered innovative, persuasive methods and theory with great heuristic power and value for researchers, especially in allowing them to extend the applications of attachment theory beyond infancy. However, at times, the qualities of these methods and theory have led them to enter into circulation without fine-grained distinctions being drawn, especially in the use of concepts and categories. This concern has been widely recognised by developmental attachment researchers in recent years, including by Main and her collaborators themselves.[26] There are a variety of reasons for this, which are discussed in this chapter. Of course, matters such as terminological precision and the exact articulation of categories are not really the priorities of pragmatic researchers, for whom the essential concern is whether measurement and prediction can be pursued more effectively or persuasively.[27] Yet, looking over the decades in a historical perspective, the pragmatic concerns of individual researchers have at times led to collective problems. Misunderstandings and miscommunication that are only minor irritants or not particular priorities for any individual researcher may, for a field, cause wide-ranging issues, played out incrementally over

[22] Some of the indicators of disorganised attachment—such as asymmetric facial movements—are rarely, if ever coded. They seem to be, at least in part, a product of Main's unusual eye for observational detail.

[23] Van IJzendoorn, M.H. & Bakermans-Kranenburg, M.J. (1997) Intergenerational transmission of attachment. A move to the contextual level. In L. Atkinson & K.J. Zucker (eds) *Attachment and Psychopathology* (pp.135–70). New York: Guilford, p.138; see also Durham-Fowler, J. (2013) An interview with Arietta Slade. *DIVISION/Review*, 7, 39–40.

[24] Allen, J.P. & Miga, E.M. (2010) Attachment in adolescence: a move to the level of emotion regulation. *Journal of Social and Personal Relationships*, 27(2), 181–90, p.182.

[25] Holmes, J. (2009) *Exploring in Security: Towards an Attachment-Informed Psychoanalytic Psychotherapy*. London: Routledge, p.4; Toth, S.L., Rogosch, F.A., & Cicchetti, D. (2008) Attachment-theory informed intervention and reflective functioning in depressed mothers. In H. Steele & M. Steele (eds) *The Adult Attachment Interview in Clinical Context* (pp.154–72). New York: Guilford, p.154.

[26] E.g. Main, M., Hesse, E., & Hesse, S. (2011) Attachment theory and research: overview with suggested applications to child custody. *Family Court Review*, 49(3), 426–63.

[27] Lakatos, I. (1970) Falsification and the methodology of scientific research programmes. In I. Lakatos & A. Musgrave (eds) *Criticism and the Growth of Knowledge* (pp.91–196). Cambridge: Cambridge University Press.

decades, with costs mounting. In particular, researchers have tended to neglect or skip over the underpinning logic of the contributions of the Berkeley group, to talk past one another as different meanings are given to concepts, and to neglect questions with important consequences for theory, research, and clinical practice.

Conditional strategies

The primacy of attention

During the years that Main was completing her doctorate in the Ainsworth laboratory, a fundamental question was the meaning of the behaviour shown by infants in Type A dyads. In 1969 Bowlby published *Attachment*, situating proximity with the caregiver as the set-goal of the attachment system. Avoidance of the caregiver on reunion therefore seemed at first sight to falsify Bowlby's theory. In fact, Ainsworth's home observation data were beginning to reveal a context for this behaviour, in the less-sensitive caregiving received by infants in avoidantly attached dyads. A year into her doctorate, at Ainsworth's urging, in 1970 Main posted a manuscript to Bowlby for feedback. In a wide-ranging theoretical text entitled 'Infant play and maternal sensitivity in primate evolution', Main made a variety of gutsy points. One was to question Bowlby's assumption that the environment within which humans evolved would reward a single 'setting' for the attachment system. Main proposed that the attachment system would need to be capable of calibration to a variety of environments, favourable and adverse. Sensitive caregiving is optimal, and the provision of a secure base would help a child to explore and learn. However, less-sensitive caregiving could be expected to elicit responses that would support survival even in adverse conditions. The vigilance of infants in ambivalent/resistant dyads was readily explicable in this account, as it helped retain proximity to a caregiver in potentially dangerous environments.[28] Avoidant behaviour, however, remained a puzzle for which Main, as yet, had no explanation.

Main's 1973 doctoral research headlined results showing the higher scores on cognitive development of the children from secure dyads.[29] However, perhaps the most critical finding for Main's later thinking was the observation that infants in secure dyads in her sample had the longest attention spans during play as toddlers. This suggested to her that children in insecure dyads had other behavioural systems or responses active and sapping attention from exploration. During her doctorate, Main also served as a coder for Berry Brazelton in a micro-analysis of filmed interactions between five mother and infant dyads, which occurred weekly over the first months of life. The focus of the analysis was on 'cycles of looking and non-looking, or attention and nonattention'.[30] Though Brazelton had come into the study

[28] Main, M. (1970) Infant play and maternal sensitivity in primate evolution. PP/Bow/J.4/1: 'The strange situation behaviour of infants whose mothers are and are not sensitive suggests different probabilities of survival in the environment of evolutionary adaptedness. In novel conditions, certainly insofar as the mother is present, the infant who can explore is better off; in conditions of stress or alarm, the infant who seeks and maintains contact with his mother [is better off].'

[29] Main, M. (1973) Exploration, play and cognitive functioning. Unpublished doctoral thesis, Johns Hopkins University.

[30] Brazelton, T.B., Koslowski, B., & Main, M. (1974) The origins of reciprocity: the early mother–infant interaction. In M. Lewis & L. Rosenblum (eds) *The Effect of the Infant on its Caregiver* (pp.49–76). New York: Wiley, p.49.

with the assumption that the infant would display continuous attention within interactions, the stop-frame analysis conducted by Main revealed a flexible movement between looking at and away from the caregiver. The researchers concluded that 'looking away behaviour reflects the need of each infant to maintain some control over the amount of stimulation he can take in via the visual mode in such an intense period of interaction'.[31] This looking away strategy was adopted more frequently when the caregiver was insensitive in offering stimulation that was not well aligned with the infant's pacing. Drawing on contemporary ideas from ethology, the researchers called this an 'approach-withdrawal model', a term that had been used to describe the way that animals might flexibly use approach and withdrawal behaviours to modulate the intensity of stimulation, and in this way remain well regulated.[32] This conclusion was supported by the finding that infant looking away behaviours were less common when caregivers were alert to indications that the infant was becoming 'upset or disintegrated' or otherwise having difficulty regulating:[33]

> When the infant demonstrates unexpected random behaviour, such as the jerk of a leg or an arm, the mother responds by stroking or holding that extremity, or by making a directed use of that extremity to jog it gently up and down, thereby turning an interfering activity into one that serves their interaction. In these ways she might be seen to teach the infant how to suppress and channel his own behaviour into a communication system.[34]

The authors criticised Bowlby for focusing too strictly on behaviour, following his ethological models, and his neglect of the role of attentional processes as a flexible resource for maintaining regulation and coherently structured interaction. They speculated that the interdependency of rhythms of attention and inattention within the relationship between infant and caregiver 'seemed to be at the root of their attachment'.[35]

After Main finished her doctorate in 1973, she continued reflecting on avoidant attachment. Her assumption was that, in contravening the predicted set-goal of the attachment system so directly, it would be 'predictive of interactive and affective disturbance'.[36] She developed scales for analysing caregiver–infant touch in the Ainsworth home observation data. Main found that the mothers in dyads classified as avoidant in the Strange Situation rebuffed physical contact with their babies much more frequently at home. They often rejected their infants' attachment behaviour, and more frequently displayed anger and flat affect in response to displays of distress. Over time, this increased the frequency with which their infants made tentative or circuitous approaches. In February 1974, Ainsworth wrote to Bowlby that 'we have found plenty of evidence that the mothers of A babies dislike physical contact, and that it is through behaviour relevant to physical contact that they (at least in large

[31] Ibid. p.60.
[32] Ibid. The term 'approach/withdrawal' was drawn from Schnierla, T.C. (1965) Aspects of stimulation and organisation in approach/withdrawal processes underlying vertebrate behavioural development. In D. Lehrman, R. Hinde, & E. Shaw (eds) *Advances in the Study of Behaviour*, Vol. 1 (pp.1–74). New York: Academic Press. On Chance's ethological work on gaze aversion see Kirk, R.G. (2009) Between the clinic and the laboratory: ethology and pharmacology in the work of Michael Robin Alexander Chance, c. 1946–1964. *Medical History*, 53(4), 513–36.
[33] Brazelton, T.B., Koslowski, B., & Main, M. (1974) The origins of reciprocity: the early mother–infant interaction. In M. Lewis & L. Rosenblum (eds) *The Effect of the Infant on its Caregiver* (pp.49–76). New York: Wiley, p.64.
[34] Ibid. p.65.
[35] Ibid. p.74.
[36] Main, M. (1973) Exploration, play and cognitive functioning. Unpublished doctoral thesis, Johns Hopkins University.

part) express rejection. Mary's theory is that this puts babies in a double bind, for they are programmed to want contact and yet are rebuffed (or at least have unpleasant experiences) when they seek it.'[37]

Main's undergraduate background in liberal arts at St John's College made her aware that novelists such as Hardy and Dostoevsky had 'long been aware of the attraction irrationally implicit in rejection'.[38] Whilst at the College, she married her philosophy professor, Alvin Nye Main. In the early 1970s, Alvin Main drew Mary Main's notice to a potential evolutionary basis for the attraction that may be prompted even in the context of rejection.[39] In *The Voyage of the Beagle,* Darwin noted that the amphibious sea lizard, when frightened, would never flee towards the water. To test this further, Darwin repeatedly frightened sea lizards, and then threw them into the water. They repeatedly swam right back to him on the land, directly towards their 'attacker'. Darwin interpreted this otherwise strange and counterproductive behaviour in terms of the sea lizard's evolutionary history:

> Perhaps this singular piece of apparent stupidity may be accounted for by the circumstance, that this reptile has no natural enemy whatever on shore, whereas at sea it must often fall a prey to the numerous sharks. Hence, probably, urged by a fixed and hereditary instinct that the shore is its place of safety, whatever the emergency may be, it there takes refuge.[40]

Alvin and Mary Main discussed the analogy with the infant of a caregiver disposed to rejecting or angry behaviour. For the sea lizard, 'if the source of the attack is "the shore" itself, the shore is nonetheless returned to as a haven of safety'.[41] Similarly, according to Bowlby's theory of the attachment behavioural system, the infant would be disposed by an evolutionarily channelled mechanism to seek proximity with the caregiver when alarmed as the haven of safety, even if the caregiver is also experienced as rejecting or threatening.[42]—hence a 'double bind'.

Alvin Main died of cancer in the summer of 1974, just following the end of Mary Main's first year as an assistant professor at Berkeley. In the grief of this loss, Mary Main experienced a period of writer's block that lasted around two years.[43] One text written during the period was a paper presented by Main and her friend Everett Waters, delivered in July 1975 to the International Society for the Study of Behavioural Development at the University of Surrey. Waters had earlier studied gaze aversion shown by infants in relation to the stranger. He proposed that gaze aversion can best be understood as an attempt to 'cut off' the stimulus from

---

[37] Ainsworth, M. (1974) *Letter to John Bowlby,* 1 February 1974. PP/BOW/B.3/4. The 'double bind' would later be redubbed a 'paradoxical injunction' by Main and Hesse in the 1990s.

[38] Main, M. (1977) Analysis of a peculiar form of reunion behavior seen in some daycare children: its history and sequelae in children who are home-reared. In R. Webb (Ed.), *Social Development in Childhood* (pp.33–78). Baltimore: Johns Hopkins University Press, p.56.

[39] That Alvin Main first drew Mary Main's attention to the passage in Darwin is mentioned in the acknowledgements to Hesse, E. & Main, M. (2006) Frightened, threatening, and dissociative parental behavior in low-risk samples: description, discussion, and interpretations. *Development & Psychopathology,* 18(2), 309–43.

[40] Darwin, C. (1839, 1972) *The Voyage of the Beagle.* New York: Bantam, pp.334–5.

[41] Main, M. (1977) Analysis of a peculiar form of reunion behavior seen in some daycare children: its history and sequelae in children who are home-reared. In R. Webb (Ed.), *Social Development in Childhood* (pp.33–78). Baltimore: Johns Hopkins University Press, p.58.

[42] Cf. Ainsworth, M.D.S. (1977) Attachment theory and its utility in cross-cultural research. In P.H. Leiderman, S.R. Tulkin, & A. Rosenfeld (eds) *Culture and Infancy: Variations in the Human Experience* (pp.49–67). New York: Academic Press: 'Infants may become attached to mothers who are rejecting, punitive, or actually brutal' (52–3).

[43] Ainsworth, M. (1976) *Letter to John Bowlby,* 16 September 1976. PP/BOW/B.3/5.

perception, which serves to modulate tendencies that it might evoke.[44] This agreed with the conclusions of Main's work with Brazelton. Main and Waters applied this idea to the behaviour of infants in Type A dyads seen in the Strange Situation.[45] They speculated that, as well as modulating arousal, visual cut-off allows the infant to remain close to a rejecting or angry parent—without 'falling into "all or nothing" response patterns which cannot be terminated voluntarily such as approach for comfort, or crying'.[46] In Ainsworth's observations, the children from dyads classified as Group A were precisely, and apparently paradoxically, those who showed more distress and clinginess at home than other children (Chapter 2). In Main's only published work from this period, a book chapter in a volume dedicated to the memory of her late husband, she proposed that the child who shows avoidant behaviour turns to objects of attention in the environment that will not add to heartache, or that might even provide the relief of distraction. In this way the child may retain control and flexibility of response.[47] Main offered her qualitative impression, however, that infants in avoidantly attached dyads were still more disposed to show conflict behaviours in the home than infants in secure dyads.[48]

Ainsworth had repeated the Strange Situation with the first wave of her sample two weeks after the first administration (Chapter 2). All seven of the infants in avoidantly attached dyads displayed conflict behaviour as they broke from their avoidance in panicked approach to the caregiver. The intensified activation of the attachment system from yet more separations, Main supposed, made cut-off and therefore avoidance impossible. As a consequence, these infants were no longer able to stay well regulated and near to the caregiver. Instead they were thrown into the 'all or nothing' response of direct approach, despite their concerns about the rebuff their experiences of their caregiver had led them to expect. The infants' approach was mottled by conflict behaviours as markers of this concern.[49] These reflections were further developed when Main spent September 1977 to May 1978 as a Fellow at the Centre for Interdisciplinary Research in Bielefeld, West Germany. The focus that year was on the application of biological principles to observable behaviour, and the other Fellows represented future leaders across a wide variety of disciplines. Alongside Main, other attendees included the biologists Richard Dawkins and John Maynard Smith, Robert Hinde's student and collaborator Patrick Bateson, Harry Harlow's student and collaborator Stephen Suomi,

[44] Waters, E., Matas, L., & Sroufe, L.A. (1975) Infant's reactions to an approaching stranger: description, validation, and functional significance of wariness. *Child Development*, 46, 348–56.

[45] They also reference the work of Daniel Stern as an influence on their thinking about gaze aversion and regulation: Stern, D.N. (1974) Mother and infant at play: the dyadic interaction involving facial, vocal and gaze behaviours. In M. Lewis & L.A. Rosenblum (eds) *The Effect of the Infant on its Caregiver* (pp.187–213). New York: Wiley.

[46] Main, M. & Waters, E. (1975) Autism and adaptation. Paper presented at International Society for the Study of Behavioural Development, University of Surrey, July 1975. PP/Bow/J.4/1.

[47] Main, M. (1977) Analysis of a peculiar form of reunion behavior seen in some daycare children: its history and sequelae in children who are home-reared. In R. Webb (Ed.), *Social Development in Childhood* (pp.33–78). Baltimore: Johns Hopkins University Press, p.47.

[48] Main, M. (1977) Sicherheit und Wissen. In K.E. Grossmann (Ed.), *Entwicklung der Lernfahigheit in der Sozialen Umwel* (pp.47–95). Munich: Kindler: 'Behaviours indicative of conflict should be expected of such a baby—such behaviours as in fact are found' (68).

[49] Reflecting decades later on the Ainsworth readministration of the Strange Situation, as well as later data from the Uppsala Longitudinal Study, Main and colleagues concluded that 'the magnitude of stress invoked by the stressful re-encounter with the strange situation may be sufficient to break the pattern of defensive avoidance, yielding an increased necessity of approach and the appearance of "disorganized" approach/avoidance behaviors instead'. Granqvist, P., Hesse, E., Fransson, M., Main, M., Hagekull, B., & Bohlin, G. (2016) Prior participation in the strange situation and overstress jointly facilitate disorganized behaviours: implications for theory, research and practice. *Attachment & Human Development*, 18(3), 235–49, p.244.

and the child psychiatrist and psychoanalyst Robert Emde.[50] The Fellowships were coordinated by the ethologist Klaus Immelmann and by Klaus and Karin Grossmann, who were in the process of attempting the first replication of Ainsworth's study outside of America. Fellows engaged in structured and unstructured group conversations at least two or three times a week with biologists and ethologists.

During her Fellowship in Bielefeld, Main applied ethological principles to the interpretation of avoidant attachment behaviour as seen in the Strange Situation. Ethology asked four questions of behavioural sequences (Chapter 1): first, the contribution of the behaviour for species survival or reproduction; second, how the behaviour came about through natural selection; third, the behaviour's underpinning mechanisms; and fourth, how it develops over the lifespan. Putting these questions to avoidant behaviour in the Strange Situation set Main on a collision course with Bowlby. Bowlby, and following him Ainsworth, had presumed that the environment within which humans evolved would have predisposed infants to seek their caregiver when alarmed, as their ultimate source of protection. Other behaviours were therefore abnormal and pathological. However, Maynard Smith and Dawkins were in the process of introducing a new account of the evolutionary biology of mating and reproductive behaviour, based on game theory. In game theory, the actions of individuals are treated as moves in a game, responsive to the environment and its potential costs and benefits. Applied to evolutionary processes, game theory suggested that species may develop a repertoire of strategies that can be initiated in response to various expectable environments and their costs and benefits.

In papers from 1979, Maynard Smith and Dawkins argued that the diversity of successful mating strategies could be explained if it was assumed that natural selection had predisposed a repertoire of behavioural patterns for achieving reproductive success in diverse circumstances.[51] The direct achievement of mating would be sought when conditions were favourable. However, a range of more circuitous routes to mating success were also available when a direct approach was not readily feasible. The latter were termed 'conditional strategies' by Maynard Smith and Dawkins. The term is a technical one. It does not imply that the direct achievement of a function or goal is 'unconditional'; direct expression of a goal-oriented response is usually dependent on a facilitative environment. Rather, the term 'conditional' was intended to refer to expectable behavioural sequences oriented towards at least partial achievement of a function or goal that would be preferred if the direct strategy could be anticipated to be unsuccessful. Main took this model of reproductive strategies and applied it to the Strange Situation. Just as the environments for reproductive success varied for the insects, reptiles, and birds of interest to Dawkins and Maynard Smith, so the caregiving environments of infants was also one with expectable variation in human evolutionary history.

From Bielefeld, Main sent Bowlby a manuscript entitled 'Avoidance of the attachment figure under stress: ontogeny, function and immediate causation' towards the end of 1978. She started from the ethological premise that 'maternal investment varies. Some desert and all must wean their infants. There must be a strategy for survival under these conditions.'[52]

---

[50] A set of papers reporting reflections on the year was published as Immelmann, K., Barlow, G., Petrinovitch, L., & Main, M. (1981) *Behavioral Development: The Bielefeld Interdisciplinary Project*. Cambridge: Cambridge University Press.

[51] Smith, J. M. (1979) Game theory and the evolution of behaviour. *Proceedings of the Royal Society London, B*, 205(1161), 475–88; Brockmann, H.J. & Dawkins, R. (1979) Joint nesting in a digger wasp as an evolutionarily stable preadaptation to social life. *Behaviour*, 71(3), 203–44.

[52] Main, M. (1978) Avoidance of the attachment figure under stress: ontogeny, function and immediate causation. PP/Bow/J.4/3.

She acknowledged that, at first sight, avoidant behaviour seen in the Strange Situation appears to disprove Bowlby's position that proximity will be sought when the attachment system is activated. However, the observation can be reconciled with the theory if it is assumed that 'avoidance of the attachment figure may function as a kind of conditional strategy for proximity maintenance'. Conditional proximity supplies a stand-in for a relationship that would offer genuine welcome. The infant can remain close by to a caregiver who might rebuff them if they attempted a direct approach, a rebuff that would be emotionally painful and might further reduce the caregiver's availability. To set out the apparent paradox: the relinquishment of full proximity implied by avoidance is part of its effectiveness, part of its basis for a qualified hope of a qualified caregiver availability.

Main later developed these ideas in two groundbreaking publications: a short note from 1979 entitled 'The "ultimate" causation of some infant attachment phenomena', and the 1981 chapter 'Avoidance in the service of proximity: a working paper' published in a book of papers by the Fellows at Bielefeld and co-edited by Main. In both texts, Main criticised Michael Lamb and colleagues, who had stated that Bowlby's position implies that infant avoidant behaviour is maladaptive since proximity with the caregiver is the basis for protection.[53] Main countered with an alternative reading of Bowlby. Bowlby himself had referred in passing to 'insecure attachment' as a 'strategy' in *Separation*, though his discussion had been of the clinginess of the ambivalent/resistant pattern.[54] And Main highlighted Bowlby's emphasis on the evolutionary basis of behaviour. From an evolutionary perspective, avoidance could be interpreted as a proactive response by the infant that 'paradoxically permits whatever proximity is possible under conditions of maternal rejection'.[55] Evolutionary processes would have selected for avoidance as one part of the infant repertoire for responding to caregivers, since infants who are able to avoid antagonising their caregivers or making demands that their caregiver will rebuff are more likely to have survived. Infants successfully utilising an avoidant strategy maintain an indirect but real proximity to their caregiver, as well as the regulatory control to continue to be responsive to the environment.[56]

Main also considered the ethological question of the behaviour's underpinning mechanisms. She regarded the phenomenon as, essentially, 'active visual, physical and communicative avoidance' of the caregiver in the context of an activation of the attachment system.[57]

[53] Rajecki, D.W., Lamb, M.E., & Obmascher, P. (1978) Toward a general theory of infantile attachment: a comparative review of aspects of the social bond. *Behavioral and Brain Sciences*, 1(3), 417–36.

[54] Bowlby, J. (1973) *Separation*. New York: Basic Books: 'There are, however, persons of all ages who are prone to show unusually frequent and urgent attachment behaviour and who do so both persistently and without there being, apparently, any current conditions to account for it. When this propensity is present beyond a certain degree it is usually regarded as neurotic. When we come to know a person of this sort it soon becomes evident that he has no confidence that his attachment figures will be accessible and responsive to him when he wants them to be and that he has adopted a strategy of remaining in close proximity to them in order so far as possible to ensure that they will be available' (165).

[55] Main, M. (1979) The 'ultimate' causation of some infant attachment phenomena: further answers, further phenomena, further questions. *Behavioral and Brain Sciences*, 2, 640–43, p.643.

[56] Main, M. (1981) Avoidance in the service of proximity: a working paper. In K. Immelmann, B. Barlow, L. Petrovich, & M. Main (eds) (1981) *Behavioral Development: The Bielefeld Interdisciplinary Project* (pp.694–9). Cambridge: Cambridge University Press, p.686. Lamb would appear to later acknowledge the point: Lamb, M., Thompson, R.A., Gardner, W., & Charnov, E.L. (1985) *Infant–Mother Attachment: The Origins and Developmental Significance of Individual Differences in the Strange Situation*. Hillsdale, NJ: Lawrence Erlbaum: It is 'questionable whether it is wise to view infantile behaviour as preadapted to an evolutionary niche that consists primarily of a sensitively responsive adult ... Evolution typically does not equip individuals with a single ideal pattern of behaviour, but rather with a repertoire of responses that may be selectively applied in different circumstances' (49).

[57] Main, M. & Weston, D. (1982) Avoidance of the attachment figure in infancy: descriptions and interpretations. In C. Parkes & J. Stevenson-Hinde (eds) *The Place of Attachment in Human Behavior*, pp.31–59. New York: Basic Books, p.31.

Yet, drawing on her work with Brazelton and with Waters, the paradigmatic form of avoidance for Main was gaze aversion. In Bielefeld initially, and then to a greater extent in 1980 during a second visit to the Grossmanns after their move to Regensburg, Main gradually came to the conclusion that gaze aversion was the most potent external marker of a fundamental internal process underpinning the visual, physical, and communicative qualities alike. This internal process was the redirection of attention away from the caregiver. This would inhibit the activating conditions of the attachment behavioural system. Gaze aversion and other forms of avoidant behaviour were therefore not just keeping the wish to approach from the caregiver's notice. They were also keeping this wish from the baby itself.[58] A version of 'Avoidance in the service of proximity' was later published in a celebratory volume in honour of Bowlby called *The Place of Attachment in Human Behavior*, edited by Colin Parkes and Joan Stevenson-Hinde. Other than some sections cut for concision, the only substantive change came in the conclusion. There it was argued that in infant avoidance of an attachment figure, 'we might better conceive of thought and behaviour as becoming *actively* reorganised away from the parent and the memory of the parent'.[59]

However, in the reception of Main's ideas from this period, the idea of attachment behaviour as reflecting attentional processes was little noticed. Instead, her application of evolutionary game theory in conceptualising the Ainsworth classifications as 'strategies' took centre stage, without bringing the attentional model with it from the wings. Given that both ideas are emphasised across Main's writings in the 1980s and 1990s, the period in which the received image of her ideas was established, this reception is curious at first sight. Three suggestions can be offered for the greater popularity of the idea of attachment strategies to the exclusion of attentional processes in the reception of Main's ideas. First, attention seemed to already be encompassed by the concept of 'internal working models'. Main's emphasis on attention therefore did not seem salient or novel, even if, in practice, when internal working models were defined or operationalised the focus was rarely on attention. Second, the concept of attachment strategies addressed a problem with Bowlby's theory. Bowlby's presumption that the secure response was the one primed by evolution offered no basis for understanding why avoidant and ambivalent/resistant behaviour could be seen in sample after sample studied using the Strange Situation. By contrast, Main's account of

---

[58] Main, M. (1981) Avoidance in the service of proximity: a working paper. In In K. Immelmann, B. Barlow, L. Petrovich, & M. Main (eds) (1981) *Behavioral Development: The Bielefeld Interdisciplinary Project* (pp.694–9). Cambridge: Cambridge University Press: 'The infant may hide its own needs, wishes, or behavioural tendencies from its mother (as in the signal function of avoidance) or even (as in the cut-off function) from itself' (687).

[59] Main, M. & Weston, D. (1982) Avoidance of the attachment figure in infancy: descriptions and interpretations. In C. Parkes & J. Stevenson-Hinde (eds) *The Place of Attachment in Human Behavior* (pp.31–59). New York: Basic Books, p.56–7. Italics not in original but added at the request of Main in feedback on this chapter. The idea of avoidance as a stable organisation of attention away from the caregiver when the attachment system was activated, as opposed to an artefact of the Strange Situation, was provisionally supported when a small study conducted by Main found an association between avoidance shown in the Strange Situation and on reunion at daycare. Blanchard, M. & Main, M. (1979) Avoidance of the attachment figure and social–emotional adjustment in day-care infants. *Developmental Psychology*, 15(4), 445–6. However, this was not a presumption that she or the field of attachment research would follow-up. An exception is Bick, J., Dozier, M., & Perkins, E. (2012) Convergence between attachment classifications and natural reunion behavior among children and parents in a child care setting. *Attachment & Human Development*, 14(1), 1–10. This paper, again, generated little further discussion. Though seemingly not discussed by researchers, it is possible that one methodological complexity in using daycare reunions to assess attachment with parents is that the daycare providers could also be attachment figures, leading to proximity-seeking with them at times or brief conflict behaviour. Furthermore, naturalistic observations in daycare are messy from a scientific perspective—including variability in the length of time children have been in daycare, and other occurrences in the environment. This will have made the setting less attractive to researchers.

individual differences in attachment as underpinned by attentional processes solved no existing problem. Additionally, methodologies for the study of attentional processes in young children, such as eye-tracking technology, were still emerging.[60] A third reason for the predominant emphasis on 'strategies' in interpretations of Main's theory may have been the timeliness of the concept. A sudden burst of appeals to the idea of 'strategy' occurred across the human sciences in the late 1970s, especially in conceptualisations of the formation of family units.[61] It was a concept that allowed social scientists to model expectable, patterned responses by individuals to their social environment, whilst keeping open the possibility for change. The idea of 'strategies' permitted the explanation of patterns of social interaction within and by families, as well as offering a lens on the techniques, including self-regulation, used in order to maintain this stability.[62]

With her account of attentional processes underpinning attachment strategies, Main was developing a model of individual differences seen in the Strange Situation. The infant in a securely attached dyad could flexibly turn attention to the environment or the caregiver in a manner responsive to the changing situation. Main regarded this strategy as reflecting a lack of concern regarding access to proximity with the caregiver, permitting the child's focus to be responsive to the changing environment of the Strange Situation. The infant in an avoidantly attached dyad, by contrast, was conceptualised by Main as attempting a partial reorganisation of attention away from the caregiver and towards the environment, in order to raise the threshold for activating and lower the threshold for terminating the attachment system. Gaze aversion, turning attention to the toys, and facing away from the caregiver all served to keep the caregiver out of the infant's focal awareness, thinning the influx of perceptions that would otherwise activate the attachment system (and that might also activate anger). This then raised the question of the evolutionary basis and underpinning mechanisms of ambivalent/resistant behaviour in the Strange Situation.

Resistance and universality

As early as 1970 Main had come to conceptualise the proximity-seeking and clingy behaviour of infants in ambivalent/resistant dyads as explicable in an evolutionary sense: vigilance regarding the availability of the caregiver might be expectable and helpful in some environments.[63] Main's further reflections on ambivalent/resistant attachment in the late 1970s were informed by a groundbreaking paper by Robert Trivers.[64] Whereas Bowlby had typically treated the infant's caregiver in terms of the caregiving behavioural system, Trivers emphasised that caregiving was only one priority for a parent. Other demands include the parent's

---

[60] Rayner, K. (1978) Eye movements in reading and information processing. *Psychological Bulletin*, 85, 618–60.

[61] For a review see Viazzo, P.P. & Lynch, K.A. (2002) Anthropology, family history, and the concept of strategy. *International Review of Social History*, 47(3), 423–52.

[62] Influential cases include Bourdieu, P. (1976) Marriage strategies as strategies of social reproduction. In R. Forster & O. Ranum (eds) *Family and Society*. Baltimore: Johns Hopkins University Press; Tilly, L.A. (1979) Individual lives and family strategies in the French proletariat. *Journal of Family History* 4, 37–52; Becker, G. (1981) *A Treatise on the Family*. Cambridge, MA: Harvard University Press. For discussion relevant to this wider shift in the human sciences towards a concern with themes of strategy, family, emotion, and self-regulation see Reddy, W.M. (1999) Emotional liberty: politics and history in the anthropology of emotions. *Cultural Anthropology*, 14, 256–88; Repo, J. (2018) Gary Becker's economics of population: reproduction and neoliberal biopolitics. *Economy and Society*, 47(2), 234–56.

[63] Main, M. (1970) Infant play and maternal sensitivity in primate evolution. PP/Bow/J.4/1.

[64] Trivers, R.L. (1974) Parent–offspring conflict. *Integrative and Comparative Biology*, 14(1), 249–64.

own survival, maintenance of sexual and social relationships, and the care of other offspring. There was every potential for conflict between parents and offspring. In fact, Bowlby had already noted this in passing, in his observation of angry and distressed protest among human toddlers during weaning or when their mother turns attention to a new baby.[65] Bowlby's remarks were influenced by the observations of his friend and colleague Robert Hinde, whose research group had observed angry and distressed protest behaviour by young rhesus monkeys in response both to weaning and to short-term separations from their mother.[66] Trivers was fascinated by Hinde's findings, and especially the observation that the more frequently infants were pushed away by their mother prior to separation, the more distress, tantrums, and clinging the infants showed on reunion. Trivers interpreted these responses as indicating 'that the infant interprets its mother's disappearance in relation to her predeparture behavior in a logical way: the offspring should assume that a rejecting mother who temporarily disappears needs more offspring surveillance and intervention than does a nonrejecting mother who temporarily disappears'.[67] The clinging, protesting behaviour observed by Hinde and others was regarded by Trivers as serving to signal to the caregiver that the child needs more investment before they would be able to survive alone. He regarded such signalling as part of the primate behaviour repertoire, selected by evolutionary processes, since it may have contributed to infant survival under conditions where caregiver investment in the child might otherwise not be forthcoming.

Influenced by Trivers' ideas, in a paper from 1979 Main identified that Trivers' argument has strong relevance for thinking about ambivalent/resistant attachment.[68] A lowered threshold for activation of the attachment system, and the alternation of angry and distressed behaviours, could be regarded as a 'conditional strategy'. It may well serve to retain the attention of the caregiver and prompt the activation of the caregiving system. If the child feels invisible to the caregiver, displays of distress, anger, and proximity-seeking/contact-maintaining can be anticipated to increase the child's visibility. However, it is a conditional rather than a primary strategy, since it is unnecessary when the attachment system can be satisfied directly through proximity-seeking. Furthermore, as Bowlby noted in *Separation*, infant anger may coerce caregiver attention to attachment signals, but it also has the potential for backfiring by antagonising the caregiver.

In 1982, Jude Cassidy—then a doctoral student with Ainsworth—spent a year in Main's laboratory at Berkeley. Main and Cassidy reflected on what ambivalent/resistant attachment would look like after infancy, and concluded that it would appear as behaviour that attempted 'to exaggerate intimacy with the parent, dependency on the parent, and his or her relatively immature status' with at least some 'hostility or physical ambivalence' evident.[69]

[65] Bowlby, J. (1973) *Separation*. New York: Basic Books, p.213; Bowlby, J. (1984) Violence in the family as a disorder of the attachment and caregiving systems. *American Journal of Psychoanalysis*, 44, 9–27, p.11.

[66] Hinde, R.A. & Spencer-Booth, Y. (1971) Effects of brief separation from mother on rhesus monkeys. *Science*, 173(3992), 111–18; Spencer-Booth, Y. & Hinde, R.A. (1971) Effects of brief separations from mothers during infancy on behaviour of rhesus monkeys 6–24 months later. *Journal of Child Psychology and Psychiatry*, 12(3), 157–72.

[67] Trivers, R.L. (1974) Parent–offspring conflict. *Integrative and Comparative Biology*, 14(1), 249–64, p.257.

[68] Main, M. (1979) The 'ultimate' causation of some infant attachment phenomena: further answers, further phenomena, further questions. *Behavioral and Brain Sciences*, 2, 640–43.

[69] Main, M. & Cassidy, J. (1988) Categories of response to reunion with the parent at age 6: predictable from infant attachment classifications and stable over a 1-month period. *Developmental Psychology*, 24(3), 415–26, p.418. Though published in 1988, Cassidy's visit to Berkeley and discussions with Main about the meaning of ambivalent/resistant attachment after infancy occurred during 1982. The paper was submitted to *Developmental Psychology* in mid-1986.

Whereas avoidant attachment represented a conditional strategy premised on the minimisation of attachment signals, ambivalent/resistant attachment included an intensification of attachment signals as well as their punctuation by anger. This was an idea that Cassidy brought back to Ainsworth's group at Virginia, where it generated a great deal of discussion, and was considered in print by Cassidy and Roger Kobak in 1988.[70]

In a paper published in 1994, Cassidy offered an interpretation of avoidance and ambivalence/resistance in terms of emotion regulation, as 'minimising' or 'maximising' the attachment behavioural system *itself* (Chapter 5).[71] Cassidy's account aligned with Bowlby's discussion of defensive exclusion as inhibiting the activation of behavioural systems, without specification of what exactly was being excluded (Chapter 1). It also aligned with other voices, such as Schore, calling at the time for the reinterpretation of attachment as, in general, the process through which self-regulation is achieved within close relationships.[72] It should be noted though that in contrast to Cassidy's more diffuse position, Main emphasised that these observable differences in strategy are underpinned by differences in attentional processes.[73] It is unclear the extent to which Cassidy realised that her description of minimising and maximising departed from Main in this regard. However, Kobak astutely observed already at the time that two different models of 'minimising and maximising' seemed to be in play. For his part, he strongly aligned himself with the centrality of attentional processes, criticising Main for not doing more to highlight to readers the fundamental role of attention in her conceptualisation of conditional strategies.[74]

For Main, avoidance was based on the direction of attention away from the caregiver, as well as other perceptions and memories that may activate the attachment system.[75] The

[70] Cassidy, J. & Kobak, R. (1988) Avoidance and its relation to other defensive processes. In J. Belsky & T. Neworski (eds) *Clinical Implications of Attachment* (pp.300–23). Hillsdale, NJ: Lawrence Erlbaum.

[71] Cassidy, J. (1994) Emotion regulation: influences of attachment relationships. *Monographs of the Society for Research in Child Development*, 59(2–3), 228–49; Cassidy, J. & Berlin, L.J. (1994) The insecure/ambivalent pattern of attachment: theory and research. *Child Development*, 65(4), 971–91. The theory of ambivalence/resistance and avoidance as representing maximising and minimising strategies has been attributed by Cassidy to both Main and herself. See e.g. Berlin, L.J. & Cassidy, J. (2003) Mothers' self-reported control of their preschool children's emotional expressiveness: a longitudinal study of associations with infant–mother attachment and children's emotion regulation. *Social Development*, 12(4), 477–95.

[72] Cassidy drew the theme of emotion regulation from Thompson, R.A. (1994) Emotion regulation: a theme in search of definition. *Monographs of the Society for Research in Child Development*, 59(2–3), 25–52. However, Thompson did not address attachment strategies. Furthermore, in contrast to Cassidy, he was at greater pains to emphasise that emotion regulation was not a single thing, and could be underpinned by a variety of processes: this might include, but would not necessarily include, the manipulation of attention. An influential contemporary voice emphasising emotion regulation was Schore, A.N. (1994) *Affect Regulation and the Origin of the Self: Applications to Affect Regulatory Phenomena*. Mahwah, NJ: Lawrence Erlbaum Associates.

[73] It is difficult to trace the lines of influence and the exact positions of Main, Cassidy, and Kobak in the 1980s and early 1990s from the published record, as there was clearly a good deal of personal communication and sharing of ideas between Berkeley and Virginia. Though a co-author on Cassidy's 1988 chapter, it seems that it was Main's position, rather than Cassidy's, that was subsequently adopted by Kobak.

[74] Kobak, R.R., Cole, H.E., Ferenz-Gillies, R., Fleming, W.S., & Gamble, W. (1993) Attachment and emotion regulation during mother–teen problem solving: a control theory analysis. *Child Development*, 64(1), 231–45.

[75] The parameters of what Main intended by the idea of 'attention' fluctuate. At times it includes perception and memory, to the degree that these processes are scaffolded by attention. However, at other times and foremost, attention appears to mean the *prioritisation of information within working memory*, such that perception of the environment and memory fall out of the definition of attention, even if they all work in the same direction, e.g. 'Maintenance of "minimising" (avoidant) or "maximising" (resistant) behavioural strategy is therefore likely eventually not only to become dependent on the control or manipulation of attention but also eventually to necessitate overriding or altering aspects of memory, emotion and awareness of surrounding conditions': Main, M. (1995) Recent studies in attachment: overview, with selected implications for clinical work. In S. Goldberg, R. Muir, & J. Kerr (eds) *Attachment Theory: Social, Developmental and Clinical Perspectives* (pp.407–70). Hillsdale, NJ: Analytic Press, p.451. On the question of whether 'attention' refers to a single process see e.g. Taylor, J.H. (2015) Against unifying accounts of attention. *Erkenntnis*, 80(1), 39–56.

infant's behaviour seemed to Main to be oriented to maintain the caregiver's peripheral rather than focal attention, presumably since the caregiver tended actually to be most available when not directly concerned with the baby: 'if the mother picked them up, they turned away and, as though attempting to distract her attention from themselves, pointed to toys and other aspects of the environment'.[76] In pointing to a toy on reunion, a behaviour that had perplexed Ainsworth, Main saw a tactic through which the infant in an avoidant dyad could manage the caregiver's attention, so that the child remained in the caregiver's awareness but not directly the object of concern.[77] By contrast, according to Main, distress and anger were intensified for infants in ambivalent/resistant dyads by attentional vigilance towards the availability of the caregiver, as well as other possible perceptions and memories that might hold information relevant to the caregiver's availability. In turn, this strategy centred the caregiver's own attention on the child:

> The A and C patterns of infant attachment organisation involve the overriding or manipulation of the otherwise naturally occurring output of the attachment behavioural system. Avoidance is conceived as a behavioural mechanism that permits the infant to shift attention away from conditions normally eliciting attachment behaviour, a shift that serves to minimise the output of the attachment behavioural system … The focus upon the attachment figure that is the essence of the type C strategy may be maintained by heightening responsiveness to what would ordinarily be only minimally arousing cues to danger. Thus, the type C infant may interpret a quiescent environment as threatening, in order to maintain the attention of the parent.[78]

The term 'conditional strategy' was drawn from ethological reflection on alternative forms of adult sexual behaviour in non-human animals. Main similarly did not limit conditional strategies to childhood in her theory. She proposed that the same strategies could be observable in caregiving behaviour: either minimisation of attention to the child and reduced activation of caregiving, or intensification of concern with the child.[79] For instance, following Trivers, she acknowledged that caregivers' past experiences or present adversities may lead them to minimise activation of the caregiving system, for instance to avoid overwhelming feelings evoked by the child or to ensure resources remain available for other challenges.[80] The minimising conditional caregiving strategy, Main suspected, may also serve to prime an infant for an environment in which early independence might be beneficial. Conversely, the maximising conditional strategy may serve to prime an infant for an environment in which prolonged dependence on relationships would be especially salient and valuable. However, Main was at pains to emphasise that the adoption of one caregiving strategy or another need

---

[76] Main, M. & Goldwyn, R. (1983) Predicting rejection of an infant from mother's representation of her own experiences. National Conference on Infant Mental Health, Children's Institute International, Los Angeles, February 1983. PP/Bow/J.4/4.

[77] On infant declarative pointing as the direction of attention see also Tomasello, M., Carpenter, M., & Liszkowski, U. (2007) A new look at infant pointing. *Child Development*, 78(3), 705–22.

[78] Main, M. (1990) Cross-cultural studies of attachment organization: recent studies, changing methodologies, and the concept of conditional strategies. *Human Development*, 33, 48–61, p.57.

[79] Main, M. (1995) Recent studies in attachment: overview, with selected implications for clinical work. In S. Goldberg, R. Muir, & J. Kerr (eds) *Attachment Theory: Social, Developmental and Clinical Perspectives* (pp.407–70). Hillsdale, NJ: Analytic Press, p.465.

[80] This position has been elaborated in the recent anthropological literature on attachment, e.g. Seymour, S.C. (2013) 'It takes a village to raise a child': attachment theory and multiple child care in Alor, Indonesia, and in North India. In N. Quinn & J.M. Mageo (eds) *Attachment Reconsidered* (pp.115–39). London: Palgrave

not be conscious, and that it would be a category error to regard parents as motivated by the evolutionary function of a strategy.[81] Instead, the proximal cause will be the demands of the present.

In a paper from 1990, 'Cross-cultural studies of attachment organization', Main argued that 'the maintenance of differing conditional strategies entails the utilisation of similar cognitive mechanisms across individuals'.[82] This made clear that she was playing for grand stakes; her proposals amounted to no less than a global model of human emotional life. Elaborating on the 1990 claim in a later work, Main asserted that 'there exist species-wide abilities that are not part of the attachment system itself, but can, within limits, manipulate (either inhibit or increase) attachment behavior in response to differing environments'.[83] As described in Chapter 1, already in 1956 Bowlby, Ainsworth, and colleagues had written that 'the personality patterns of children who have experienced long separation tend to fall into one or other of these two opposite classes': either 'over-dependent' and 'ambivalent' or 'mother-rejecting ... having repressed their need for attachment'.[84] This was already a momentous claim. However, whereas Bowlby and Ainsworth discussed the two classes as responses to separation, in her 1990 paper Main resituated these classes as the fundamental alterations of the attachment system and caregiving system, or potentially any behavioural system.

Main's model of conditional strategies was not, therefore, merely a localised psychological theory to account for the Strange Situation, but a philosophy of human experience in general, with resonances of Plato and Kant. These resonances signal the important, if complex, role of philosophy on the development of Main's ideas. The only mention of Main's parents in her published works is the remark that 'philosophy was much admired by my parents, who had introduced me to Plato, Kant, and several Eastern philosophies by age 10'.[85] As an undergraduate, she re-encountered Plato and Kant at St John's College in Maryland in the classes of her future husband, Alvin Main.[86] Now, in her 1990 paper, she was proposing that behind

---

[81] Main can be seen here moving in the direction of what would later become the life-history model of attachment, where the interaction between caregiving and attachment system is interpreted as a means through which children receive signals about the strategies that will be best adapted for the degree of adversity that characterises their environment, and in particular the relative need to prioritise immediate survival or long-term growth and exploration. See Chisholm, J.S. (1996) The evolutionary ecology of attachment organization. *Human Nature*, 7(1), 1–37; Belsky, J. (1999) Modern evolutionary theory and patterns of attachment. In J. Cassidy & P.R. Shaver (eds) *Handbook of Attachment* (pp.141–61). New York: Guilford. Main was cited and discussed by Chisholm and Belsky in thinking about evolutionary trade-offs; the line of intellectual history is likely the influence of Trivers on all three attachment theorists. Main's discussions of the evolutionary basis of individual differences in attachment essentially ended in 1990. By contrast, this would become a central focus in the work of Belsky over subsequent decades.

[82] Main, M. (1990) Cross-cultural studies of attachment organization: recent studies, changing methodologies, and the concept of conditional strategies. *Human Development*, 33, 48–61, p.58.

[83] Main, M., Hesse, E., & Kaplan, N. (2005) Predictability of attachment behavior and representational processes at 1, 6, and 19 years of age: the Berkeley Longitudinal Study. In K.E. Grossmann, K. Grossmann, & E. Waters (eds) *Attachment from Infancy to Adulthood: The Major Longitudinal Studies* (pp.245–304). New York: Guilford, p.256.

[84] Bowlby, J., Ainsworth, M., Boston, M., & Rosenbluth, D. (1956) The effects of mother–child separation: a follow-up study. *British Journal of Medical Psychology*, 29, 211–47, p.238.

[85] Main, M., Hesse, E., & Kaplan, N. (2005) Predictability of attachment behavior and representational processes at 1, 6, and 19 years of age: the Berkeley Longitudinal Study. In K.E. Grossmann, K. Grossmann, & E. Waters (eds) *Attachment from Infancy to Adulthood: The Major Longitudinal Studies* (pp.245–304). New York: Guilford, p.248.

[86] The curriculum at St John's College used no textbooks and only provided students with primary texts. So Main read Plato, Kant, and other philosophical texts in the original during her four years of study of the subject. With wry humour, she recalled Ainsworth's difficulties in trying to turn her new philosophically trained graduate student into a proper developmentalist: 'I heard that she said (unfortunately aptly, but I refused to consider the truth-value of the statement at the time) that she dreaded sending me out on home visits to Baltimore mothers, because I was virtually unable to engage in small-talk, and would probably ask them what they thought of Spinoza

the diversity of apparent infant behaviours there lies three essential forms for responding to distressing and challenging situation (cf. Plato, Aristotle); the basis for these differences stems from the structure of human experience, which shape human perception, language, and behaviour (cf. Kant).

Though the three Ainsworth categories were identified using 23 middle-class infants in the mid-1960s in Baltimore, for Main the categories exceeded this particularity to express the three basic ways that humans can respond to distressing and challenging situations. In the context of worries or other troubling feelings, there are three basic approaches: we can communicate about our feelings to someone we anticipate or hope might help us; we can keep our feelings to ourselves; or we can make our distress and frustration someone else's problem. As we saw in Chapter 2, Ainsworth took from Blatz the idea that the people we may need to depend upon are independent of us in a deep sense, and this can be regarded as a source of worry or as a source of reassurance, depending on what this freedom has implied for us in the past. Main's conditional strategies were responses to this predicament, based on the selective exclusion of information that would risk reducing the availability of the caregiver as a secure base and safe haven:

> The conditional behavioral strategy (avoidance or preoccupation) is understood to be imposed on a still-active primary strategy, imposed on aspects of memory, and imposed on awareness of surrounding conditions. Maintenance of the 'minimizing' (A) or 'maximizing' (C) behavioral strategy is then dependent on the control or manipulation of attention—specifically, an organized shift of attention away from conditions activating attachment behavior in Group A infants, and a heightened vigilance maximizing responsiveness to even minimal clues to danger in Group C infants. It seems inevitable that a continuing 'minimization or maximization of the display of attachment behavior relative to the naturally occurring output of the behavioral system' (Main, 1990) will eventually also involve the defensive exclusion or defensive distortion of certain memories and perceptions.[87]

An infant in an ambivalent/resistant dyad directs attention away from potential information that might suggest that the environment is unthreatening and that the caregiver is available. This infant therefore sees clearly, indeed overclearly, the human predicament that attachment figures are independent of us in worrying ways. Infants in an avoidant dyad direct attention away from potential information that might elicit alarm, distress, or a tendency to approach the caregiver for comfort. They see clearly, indeed with a reductive clarity, that as humans we are partly independent of our attachment figures. Each of the conditional

---

or something.' Main, M. (1999) Mary D. Salter Ainsworth: tribute and portrait. *Psychoanalytic Inquiry,* 19(5), 682–736, p.690. The influence of Plato especially is visible throughout one of Main's earliest papers, where her focus is on how security can be achieved when humans cannot ultimately rest on knowledge gained from the apparent world: Main, M. (1977) Sicherheit und Wissen. In K.E. Grossmann (Ed.), *Entwicklung der Lernfahigheit in der Sozialen Umwel* (pp.47–95). Munich: Kindler. After the death of Alvin Main, it is not clear that Main continued further reading in Plato and Kant, though her later work shows familiarity with philosophers such as Hans-Georg Gadamer and her University of California colleague Paul Feyerabend. Kant's noumenal–phenomenal distinction is drawn upon in Main, M. (1991) Metacognitive knowledge, metacognitive monitoring, and singular (coherent) vs. multiple (incoherent) models of attachment: some findings and some directions for future research. In P. Marris, J. Stevenson-Hinde, & C. Parkes (eds) *Attachment Across the Life Cycle* (pp.127–59). London: Routledge.

[87] Main, M. (1993) Discourse, prediction and recent studies in attachment: implications for psychoanalysis. *Journal of the American Psychoanalytic Association,* 41, 209–44, p.233; Main, M. (1990) Cross-cultural studies of attachment organization: recent studies, changing methodologies, and the concept of conditional strategies. *Human Development,* 33, 48–61.

strategies is acutely and effectively attentive to some aspect of reality, and in this way enacts a method of responding to alarm that may be of survival value under conditions where that aspect is of special importance. This may provide important information for children about how to calibrate the demands they make on the world in order to achieve what nurturance and resources may be available. The conditional strategy may also be experienced as a kind of 'secondary felt security', despite being held in place by anxiety; the reason for this is that the conditional strategies nonetheless offer predictable and therefore reassuring access to some sense of closeness and regulation.[88] However, for Main, each conditional strategy must also depend upon selective exclusion of another aspect of reality.[89] There will be, she predicted, a price to be paid for the conditional strategy in the long run, to the degree that this information about attachment relationships and about their own affective life remains lost or relatively opaque to the individual.[90]

With Main's model of Group A and Group C as conditional strategies, attachment theory became a global account of human emotion and relationships.[91] For Main, two conditional strategies existed for the attachment and the caregiving systems, and potentially for other behavioural systems. Its output could be minimised or intensified, and the basic architecture for these strategies would lie in the direction of attentional processes.[92] The magnitude of the impact for subsequent attachment theory of the encompassing conditional strategy model of individual differences in attachment cannot be overestimated. It has had more sway for later attachment theory than even the theory of attachment as a behavioural system that it ostensibly modified. Few developmental attachment researchers in the twenty-first century have made more than token mention of behavioural systems, or developed specific hypotheses from this concept (though see Chapter 5). Since the 1990s, the idea of attachment as a 'behavioural system', grounded in human evolutionary history, has rather the status of a memento that the developmental tradition of attachment research is pleased to have, and

---

[88] Main, M. (1995) Recent studies in attachment: overview, with selected implications for clinical work. In S. Goldberg, R. Muir, & J. Kerr (eds) *Attachment Theory: Social, Developmental and Clinical Perspectives* (pp.407–70). Hillsdale, NJ: Analytic Press, p.409.

[89] Main, M. (1990) Cross-cultural studies of attachment organization: recent studies, changing methodologies, and the concept of conditional strategies. *Human Development*, 33, 48–61, p.59.

[90] Main has been criticised for this position at times by critics who argue that there may be ecological niches where conditional strategies are simply superior. The implication that they represent a second-best option would then be both overgeneralised and potentially ethnocentric: 'Despite her recognition of alternative or "conditional" attachment strategies, in referring to insecure attachment as a "secondary" strategy, Main (1990) may be clinging to the view that because secure attachment is "primary" it must also be "normal"'. Chisholm, J.S. (1996) The evolutionary ecology of attachment organization. *Human Nature*, 7(1), 1–37, p.24. However, Main's position has been defended by Granqvist, who points to the disparity between markers of hidden distress and calm appearance characteristic of attachment avoidance. Granqvist agrees that there will be ecological niches where this disparity may be helpful. But he defends Main's claim that this should be regarded as a back-up strategy, since it predictably occurs primarily when direct communication about distress to the caregiver proves unsuccessful. Granqvist, P. (2020) *Attachment, Religion, and Spirituality: A Wider View*. New York: Guilford.

[91] Kobak, R.R., Cole, H.E., Ferenz-Gillies, R., Fleming, W.S., & Gamble, W. (1993) Attachment and emotion regulation during mother–teen problem solving: a control theory analysis. *Child Development*, 64(1), 231–45.

[92] Mary Main and Erik Hesse, personal communication, August 2019: 'With developmental maturation, each conditional strategy has greater variegation. Additionally, development allows humans to override a behavioural system in other ways than the two conditional strategies, producing a wider variety of potential strategies than those available to infants. These might well not be conditional strategies in the technical sense of being a behavioural repertoire made available by human evolutionary history for solving problems of survival and reproduction. They could be described as "strategic" in the non-technical sense—but it depends on how the word is being used.' In fact, it is not clear the extent to which this argument holds for the controlling-caregiving and controlling-punitive behavioural repertoires identified by Main and Cassidy in the six-year reunion system (see section 'The Main and Cassidy reunion system'). It could be imagined that these were ethological repertoires made available by human evolutionary history. On 'tertiary' attachment strategies see Chapter 5.

without which they might feel bereft, but which never gets actually brought out for further examination, except perhaps when teaching.[93]

By contrast, the image of human difference as strung out along axes of minimising and maximising has been the beating heart of attachment research for three decades, and central to hypothesis generation and the interpretation of empirical findings regarding individual differences. It has formed the 'grid of specification' according to which kinds of attachment behaviour in infancy and beyond have been divided, contrasted, related, grouped, classified, and derived in relation to one another.[94] The idea of minimising and maximising strategies is frequently cited as originating with Main, sometimes with Cassidy and Kobak, and occasionally with Hinde.[95] However, most often the image has been taken as simply a timeless part of attachment research as a paradigm, implied by Ainsworth's introduction of three patterns of attachment. This interpretation has been supported by Main's tendency to attribute her own ideas to Ainsworth, where these grew out of the soil of Ainsworth's own thinking.[96] It has likely also been supported by the elegant simplicity, amounting to apparent obviousness, of the theory of individual differences divided into minimising and maximising.

[93] A few attachment theorists have, however, explicitly argued for the retirement or supersession of Bowlby's control systems theory, e.g. Cassidy, J., Ehrlich, K.B., & Sherman, L.J. (2013) Child–parent attachment and response to threat: a move from the level of representation. In M. Mikulincer & P.R. Shaver (eds) *Nature and Development of Social Connections: From Brain to Group* (pp.125–44). Washington, DC: American Psychological Association. However, such arguments have not led to any sustained public discussion. Most attachment researchers impatient with Bowlby's theory of behavioural systems simply bypass it, and focus instead on individual differences in perceptions of caregiver availability. One reason has been put forward by Granqvist, who observed that attachment researchers have tended to avoid outright criticisms of Bowlby's model of the function and workings of the attachment system as a matter of courtesy, even if they know that Bowlby himself would have been dismayed and scornful of any such nicety that held back theoretical development. Granqvist, P. (2020) *Attachment, Religion, and Spirituality: A Wider View*. New York: Guilford. By contrast, in applying attachment theory to adult relationships, the question of the nature of attachment at this later developmental stage became of critical concern to the social psychological tradition of attachment research (Chapter 5).

[94] Foucault, M. (1969, 1972) *The Archaeology of Knowledge*, trans. A.M. Sheridan Smith. London: Routledge, Chapter 3.

[95] Since the 1990s, the dominant position of Main's interpretation of the categories of attachment has made her work the standard reference point for the theory of conditional strategies. However, in the 1980s the concept of attachment patterns as conditional strategies was actually more frequently ascribed to Hinde, who at the time was the much more senior and well-known figure. This was despite the fact that Main was the first to present this theory, in a short and quite obscure paper: Main, M. (1979) The 'ultimate' causation of some infant attachment phenomena: further answers, further phenomena, further questions. *Behavioral and Brain Sciences*, 2, 640–43. The concept of attachment patterns as conditional strategies was also offered by Hinde in a 1982 chapter without reference to Main: Hinde, R.A. (1982) Attachment: some conceptual and biological issues. In J. Stevenson-Hinde & C. Murray Parkes (eds) *The Place of Attachment in Human Behavior* (pp.60–78). New York: Basic Books. The origins of Hinde's use of the term are not fully clear. He had read Maynard Smith's and Dawkins' 1979 papers on conditional strategies soon after they were published, and was soon citing them. Maynard Smith and Hinde were also in direct discussion of these issues in 1982. See e.g. Hinde, R. (1982) *Letter to Maynard Smith*, 14 June 1982. John Maynard Smith Archive, British Library, MS 86840/46. Hinde may also have been part of conversations about conditional strategies with his student and collaborator Pat Bateson, who had been with Maynard Smith, Dawkins, and Main at Bielefeld. In 1978, Main presented a paper on 'detachment' at a colloquium to Hinde's research group, and she may have mentioned her ideas about conditional strategies then. Given that Hinde was ordinarily quite careful in attributing ideas that were not his own, it seems probable that all of these pathways of influence operated simultaneously, giving Hinde the impression that the concept was simply a familiar one in contemporary ethological discussions. Certainly already in 1979, Brockmann, Grafen, and Dawkins described the notion as 'a fashionable idea in modern ethology': Brockmann, H.J., Grafen, A., & Dawkins, R. (1979) Evolutionarily stable nesting strategy in a digger wasp. *Journal of Theoretical Biology*, 77(4), 473–96, p.473.

[96] E.g. Main M. (1999) Mary D. Salter Ainsworth: tribute and portrait. *Psychoanalytic Inquiry*, 19, 682–776: 'Ainsworth, however, saw these rejected infants as responding to the increased stress imposed by the strange situation by actively (although, of course, not necessarily consciously) shifting their attention so as to inhibit the behavioral and emotional manifestations of attachment—notably, proximity-seeking, crying, and anger' (719).

Ainsworth was, understandably, rather astonished that Main transformed her categories for the Strange Situation into an encompassing philosophy of existence, applicable to all behavioural systems. In a letter to John Bowlby in March 1984 (embarrassingly posted by accident, in fact, to Main),[97] Ainsworth expressed 'unease' with Main's ambitious and universalising proposals:

> She is convinced that I have discovered the three patterns of attachment—that she believes to hold not only for one-year-olds but throughout the life span. This is very flattering. Also I must confess I think that they are indeed the three major patterns. But ... I cannot quite believe that apart from the groups and subgroups I have identified there are [not] other less frequent occurring patterns that may be impossible to comprehend within these three major groups (A/B/C). To say nothing of cross-cultural variations.[98]

However, as she learned about Main's theories over the course of 1985 and became increasingly impressed with the promise of Main's AAI, Ainsworth remarked to Bowlby: 'You were right that I am in a sense a student of Mary Main's.'[99] Ainsworth's support played a critical role in establishing Main's account of conditional strategies as the central image of individual differences within attachment theory, as a paradigm primarily concerned with individual differences. In particular, Ainsworth's late paper with Eichberg reporting an exceptionally strong relationship between the infant classifications and the new AAI was of great symbolic as well as scientific importance.[100] Ainsworth supported and encouraged her different graduate students; Inge Bretherton, Everett Waters, Patricia Crittenden, and Bob Marvin were all making both methodological and theoretical innovations at the turn of the 1990s that built on Ainsworth's contribution.[101] However, by then the Ainsworth and Eichberg paper was already in print, and quickly came to be widely interpreted as confirmation of Main's extension of the Ainsworth categories across the lifespan, passing the baton of Ainsworth's role as the field's method-giver.[102] In addition to Ainsworth's support, Main's characterisation of avoidance and ambivalence/resistance as conditional strategies was seen

---

[97] Main, M. (1999) Mary D. Salter Ainsworth: tribute and portrait. *Psychoanalytic Inquiry*, 19, 682–776.

[98] Ainsworth, M. (1984) *Letter to John Bowlby*, 10 March 1984. PP/BOW/B.3/7.

[99] Ainsworth, M. (1985) *Letter to John Bowlby*, 23 December 1985. PP/BOW/B.3/8.

[100] Ainsworth, M. & Eichberg, C. (1991) Effects on infant–mother attachment of mother's unresolved loss of an attachment figure, or other traumatic experience. In C. Parkes, J. Stevenson-Hinde, & P. Marris (eds) *Attachment Across the Lifespan* (pp.160–83). London: Routledge.

[101] E.g. Bretherton, I., Prentiss, C., & Ridgeway, D. (1990) Family relationships as represented in a story-completion task at thirty-seven and fifty-four months of age. *New Directions for Child and Adolescent Development*, 48, 85–105; Vaughn, B.E. & Waters, E. (1990) Attachment behavior at home and in the laboratory: Q-sort observations and strange situation classifications of one-year-olds. *Child Development*, 61(6), 1965–73; Crittenden, P.M. (1992) Quality of attachment in the preschool years. *Development & Psychopathology*, 4(2), 209–41; Cassidy, J., Marvin, R., with the Attachment Working Group of the John D. and Catherine T. MacArthur Network on the Transition from Infancy to Early Childhood (1992) Attachment organisation in preschool children: procedures and coding manual. Unpublished manual.

[102] See the discussions of Ainsworth and Main for instance in Fonagy, P., Steele, H., & Steele, M. (1991) Maternal representations of attachment during pregnancy predict the organization of infant–mother attachment at one year of age. *Child Development*, 62(5), 891–905; Bakermans-Kranenburg, M.J. & van IJzendoorn, M.H. (1993) A psychometric study of the Adult Attachment Interview: reliability and discriminant validity. *Developmental Psychology*, 29(5), 870–79; Bacciagaluppi, M. (1994) The relevance of attachment research to psychoanalysis and analytic social psychology. *Journal of the American Academy of Psychoanalysis*, 22(3), 465–79. On the role of consecration of an heir at the end of life, and the balance between preserving the integrity of an inheritance and retaining the loyalty to the family of non-selected heirs see Goody, J. (1973) Strategies of heirship. *Comparative Studies in Society and History*, 15(1), 3–20; Bourdieu, P (2002, 2008) *The Bachelors' Ball: The Crisis of Peasant Society in Béarn*. Chicago: University of Chicago Press.

as a powerful explanatory tool. And the AAI, the first trainings in which by Main were co-taught with Ainsworth, was regarded as an exciting methodological development. In her final writings, Ainsworth urged her successors to retain an open-ended system, and not to close either theory or method around her categories.[103] However, a central goal of the second generation of attachment researchers was the construction of a cumulative empirical research paradigm of replicated results, and for this a settled coding system, rather than further exploration, was treated as desirable.

Convincing Bowlby

The conventional reference for the theory of conditional strategies over the decades has been Main's 1990 paper 'Cross-cultural studies of attachment organization'.[104] It was more elaborate than 'The "ultimate" causation of some infant attachment phenomena' from 1979, which is more of a note than a full paper. Her 1981 book chapter 'Avoidance in the service of proximity' was, by its own admission, meandering. It was also published in an edited volume in a context in which journal articles, across the social sciences, were coming to receive comparatively greater prominence. However, as a consequence, readers have generally missed the role of attention as the architecture underpinning Main's conceptualisation of conditional strategies. This was mentioned to a greater or lesser extent in all her work of the period—except the 1990 paper.

Main observed that the conflict between anger and attachment could flood out and interrupt the smooth expression of the attachment system. However, most ambivalent/resistant infants used the oscillation between distress and anger in quite a smooth way to retain the attention of their caregiver: when they were put down they cried to be picked up; when they were picked up, they squirmed away. Just as avoidance was paradoxically in the service of proximity for Group A infants, the distress and conflict of Group C infants appeared to in the service of organisation via proximity. In Main's perspective, the ambivalent/resistant classification seemed 'much the least well organised' of the Ainsworth classifications.[105] And in some work under Main's supervision, the ambivalent/resistant and unclassifiable infants were grouped together for analysis on the basis that both displayed conflict.[106] Nonetheless, ultimately, Main concluded that 'like an avoidant baby, a resistant baby may be said to be "organized" in the sense of having *a singular attentional focus*', i.e. retaining the attention of their caregiver.[107]

[103] Ainsworth M. (1990) Epilogue. In M.T. Greenberg, D. Cicchetti, & E.M. Cummings (eds) *Attachment in the Preschool Years* (pp.463–88). Chicago: Chicago University Press.

[104] Main, M. (1990) Cross-cultural studies of attachment organization: recent studies, changing methodologies, and the concept of conditional strategies. *Human Development*, 33, 48–61.

[105] Main, M. & Hesse, E. (1990) Parents' unresolved traumatic experiences are related to infant disorganized attachment status: is frightened/frightening parental behavior the linking mechanism? In M. Greenberg, D. Cicchetti, & M. Cummings (eds) *Attachment in the Preschool Years* (pp.161–82). Chicago: University of Chicago Press, p.179.

[106] E.g. Weston, D.R. (1983) Implications of mother's personality for the infant–mother attachment relationship. Unpublished doctoral dissertation, University of California, Berkeley: 'The C's mix attachment behaviours with resistance; the U's [i.e. unclassifiable cases] mix attachment behaviours with resistance and avoidance. These mixed patterns support the rationale for combining these two groups.'

[107] Main, M. (1995) Recent studies in attachment: overview, with selected implications for clinical work. In S. Goldberg, R. Muir, & J. Kerr (eds) *Attachment Theory: Social, Developmental and Clinical Perspectives* (pp.407–70). Hillsdale, NJ: Analytic Press, p.420. Italics added. Main also offered another characterisation of the ambivalent/

Main went to visit Bowlby in March 1978, and they discussed these ideas. In the course of these discussions Bowlby was persuaded that the attachment system may have evolved with a repertoire of strategies.[108] They discussed early draft material towards his book *Loss,* and in the final version he cited Main's perspective with approval. Bowlby had already from 1977 taken an interest in caregiving and compliant behaviour shown by children towards parents when they might not receive adequate care (Chapter 1). Main's proposal seemed to fit with this, since avoidant, caregiving, and compliant behaviour had in common the substitution of direct attempts to seek the caregiver's support for an alternative strategy that would be more effective given parental behaviour.[109] The exclusion of information that might activate the attachment system for children in this situation would have the predictable outcome of increased caregiver responsiveness and so survival value within human evolutionary history.[110] In *Loss,* Bowlby therefore situated the avoidant conditional strategy within the broader observation that 'as children know in their bones, when mother is prone to be rejecting it may be better to placate her than to risk alienating her altogether'. However, he also acknowledged Main's emphasis on attention as the underpinning infrastructure of avoidance as a conditional strategy:

An infant of this sort, instead of showing attachment behaviour as infants of responsive mothers do, turns away from his mother and busies himself with a toy. In so doing he is effectively excluding any sensory inflow that would elicit his attachment behaviour and is thus avoiding any risk of being rebuffed and … in addition he is avoiding any risk of eliciting hostile behaviour from his mother. Yet he remains in her vicinity. This type of

resistant infant: 'Like the avoidant baby, and unlike the secure baby, however, her attention is not fluid, and she focuses upon only one aspect of her surround' (420).

[108] Bowlby, J. (1978) Notes following discussion with Mary Main in March 1978 about the draft of Vol. 3 Loss. PP/Bow/H.78: Main found a 'correlation between violent screaming and hitting mother in home and avoidance in strange situation. The more attachment behaviour is aroused the more likely is avoidance to be exhibited. The less attachment behaviour is aroused the more likely he is to show angry (e.g. hit) behaviour & also attachment behaviour. A conditional strategy.'

[109] Bowlby's emphasis in *Loss* on avoidance, caregiving, and compliant behaviour as reflecting different forms of a common strategy in which a child masked distress would be influential for Patricia Crittenden, who was pursuing a doctorate with Ainsworth at the time. Crittenden, P.M. (1983) Mother and infant patterns of attachment. Unpublished doctoral dissertation, University of Virginia, Charlottesville; Crittenden, P.M. (1988) Relationships at risk. In J. Belsky & T. Nezworski (eds) *Clinical Implications of Attachment* (pp.136–74). Hillsdale, NJ: Lawrence Erlbaum. Main and Solomon later distinguished child caregiving behaviour towards the parent from disorganisation; as a result it does not feature in the Main and Solomon (1990) indices. Main, M. & Solomon, J. (1990) Procedures for identifying infants as disorganised/disoriented during the Ainsworth Strange Situation. In M.T. Greenberg, D. Cicchetti, & E.M. Cummings (eds) *Attachment in the Preschool Years* (pp.121–60). Chicago: University of Chicago Press, p.147. However, it was not given its own place in their infant coding protocols, which became the dominant system not just for reporting studies of the Strange Situation but also for measuring conceptualising attachment in general across childhood and the lifespan. Despite the heavy emphasis on the importance of child caregiving behaviour by Bowlby in his later writings, this topic has therefore largely disappeared from attachment research after his death, except in the work of Moss, Bureau, and colleagues, e.g. Moss, E., Bureau, J.-F., Cyr, C., Mongeau, C., & St-Laurent, D. (2004) Correlates of attachment at age 3: construct validity of the preschool attachment classification system. *Developmental Psychology,* 40, 323–34; Meier, M., Martin, J., Bureau, J.-F., Speedy, M., Levesque, C., & Lafontaine, M.-F. (2014) Psychometric properties of the mother and father compulsive caregiving scales: a brief measure of current young adult caregiving behaviours toward parents. *Attachment and Human Development,* 16(2), 174–91. Controlling-caregiving behaviour is part of the Main and Cassidy six-year reunion system, and in this context is often mentioned in expositions of attachment theory for clinical audiences. But there have been no trainings available in this measure for decades.

[110] Bowlby, J. (1980) *Loss.* New York: Basic Books: 'Given certain adverse circumstances during childhood, the selective exclusion of information of certain sorts may be adaptive' (45).

response, Main suggests, may represent a strategy for survival alternative to seeking close proximity to mother.[111]

Against his earlier position and also the common image of his work still in circulation today (Chapter 1), Bowlby can be seen here in *Loss* following Main in turning away from an image of the display of attachment behaviour as natural and best, towards acknowledgement of the evolutionary function and the at least short- or medium-term benefits of diverse forms of infant behaviour. And Bowlby would continue to refer to avoidance as a 'strategy' in his subsequent writing, acknowledging both short-term advantages and potential survival value and the longer-term contribution the strategy might make to mental illness.[112] Such treatment of avoidance as a conditional strategy fitted with Bowlby's wider transition in his late work from regarding proximity as the set-goal of the attachment system to seeing this as the physical and attentional availability of the caregiver.

However, though recognised by Bowlby, fundamental aspects of Main's account of conditional strategies have been missed by the subsequent attachment literature. Klaus and Karin Grossmann suggested that a key reason for this is that attachment researchers have generally regarded Main's introduction of the 'disorganised attachment classification' as superseding any early reflections.[113] As a result, very few attachment researchers have read any of Main's papers from prior to 1990. Attachment researchers repeat—and repeat—the idea of 'minimising' and 'maximising' strategies in summaries of the paradigm and in interpreting empirical results. Yet the fact that the original idea was of minimising or maximising attentional processes, specifically, is essentially unknown. Main made several efforts to clarify the centrality of attention to her account of individual differences in attachment. The most strenuous was her decision to title a paper from 2000 'The organised categories of infant child and adult attachment: flexible vs inflexible attention under attachment-related stress'.[114] Yet besides her most immediate collaborators such as Erik Hesse and Marinus van IJzendoorn,[115] and a few others with personal links to Main at one period or another such as Roger Kobak, Pehr Granqvist, and Carlo Schuengel,[116] researchers generally interpret Main as describing the minimisation or maximisation of either attachment behaviour or of distress (or both), rather than recognising her proposal of a causal account with attentional

---

[111] Bowlby, J. (1980) *Loss*. New York: Basic Books, p.73.

[112] E.g. Bowlby, J. (1989) Foreword. In E. Gut, *Productive and Unproductive Depression* (pp.xiii–xv). London: Routledge: 'Emmy Gut examines why people grow up unable to cope with painful problems and instead become locked in some fruitless strategy of avoidance which, however successful it may be in the short term, leads them in the longer term to become prone to depressive moods with no useful outcome' (xiv).

[113] Klaus and Karin Grossmann, personal communication, August 2012.

[114] Main, M. (2000) The organized categories of infant, child, and adult attachment: flexible vs. inflexible attention under attachment-related stress. *Journal of the American Psychoanalytic Association*, 48(4), 1055–96.

[115] E.g. Hesse, E. (1996) Discourse, memory, and the Adult Attachment Interview: a note with emphasis on the emerging cannot classify category. *Infant Mental Health*, 17(1), 4–11.

[116] Kobak's writings on the AAI in the 1990s suggest he felt that Main had not gone far enough in emphasising the role of attention, since she also headlined the concept of internal working model. The idea of the internal working model connoted to Kobak a representational rather than attentional basis for individual differences. Kobak, R.R., Cole, H.E., Ferenz-Gillies, R., Fleming, W.S., & Gamble, W. (1993) Attachment and emotion regulation during mother–teen problem solving: a control theory analysis. *Child Development*, 64(1), 231–45. See also Schuengel, C., de Schipper, J.C., Sterkenburg, P.S., & Kef, S. (2013) Attachment, intellectual disabilities and mental health: research, assessment and intervention. *Journal of Applied Research in Intellectual Disabilities*, 26(1), 34–46; Granqvist, P. (2020) *Attachment, Religion, and Spirituality: A Wider View*. New York: Guilford. Another exception is Waters, T.E., Brockmeyer, S.L., & Crowell, J.A. (2013) AAI coherence predicts caregiving and care seeking behavior: secure base script knowledge helps explain why. *Attachment & Human Development*, 15(3), 316–31.

processes at the centre. This may have been facilitated by a lack of clarity regarding the relative overlap or differences between Main's specific concern with attentional process and Bowlby's descriptive concept of defensive exclusion, since in *Loss* Bowlby treated the two accounts as aligned (Chapter 1). Difficulties in identifying and understanding Main's position have also been facilitated by Cassidy's influential reinterpretation of minimising and maximising strategies in terms of 'emotion regulation' in the 1990s.[117] In any case, eclipse of the role of attentional processes in individual differences for Main has made for much more general and less parsimonious hypothesis-generation. It has additionally obscured the nature of the links Main perceived between infant behaviour and individual differences in later development.

The infant disorganised classification

Conflict behaviour

In her doctoral dissertation Main had documented various forms of conflict behaviour in the Strange Situation, including 'stereotypies; hand-flapping; echolalia; inappropriate affect (inexplicable fears, inappropriate laughter) and other behaviours appearing out of context.'[118] She had also been impressed by an incident during her doctoral research. She had been meeting with an infant, Sara, and her mother:

> During the office interview, a thunderstorm took place and a bolt of lightning struck very near the building. The event was frightening even for the adults present—and Sara, though equidistant between both, dashed whimpering to the unfamiliar interviewer rather than her mother.[119]

Sara received the highest score for avoidance in the sample in the Strange Situation, and her mother had the highest score for aversion to physical contact with her infant. Main concluded that Sara's approach-avoidance conflict caused by the lightning was too intense to permit an organised avoidant response. The result was a redirection of attachment behaviour towards Main herself. For a time, interested to see if this effect would be replicable, Main planned an empirical study in which ten infants avoidantly attached with both parents and a comparison group of infants would be placed equidistant between the experimenter and the

---

[117] Cassidy, J. (1994) Emotion regulation: influences of attachment relationships. *Monographs of the Society for Research in Child Development*, 59(2–3), 228–49. For the rise of emotion regulation approaches to attachment, important predecessors to Cassidy include Tronick, E. (1989) Emotions and emotional communication in infants. *American Psychologist*, 44(2), 112–19, and Stern, D.N. (1985) *The Interpersonal World of the Infant*. New York: Basic Books. Hofer's work, discussed in Chapter 1, was also an important influence. Another significant article of the period, somewhat later than Cassidy's, was Lyons-Ruth, K. (1999) The two-person unconscious: intersubjective dialogue, enactive relational representation, and the emergence of new forms of relational organization. *Psychoanalytic Inquiry*, 19(4), 576–617.

[118] Main, M. (1977) Analysis of a peculiar form of reunion behavior seen in some daycare children: its history and sequelae in children who are home-reared. In R. Webb (Ed.), *Social Development in Childhood* (pp.33–78). Baltimore: Johns Hopkins University Press, p.70.

[119] Main, M. (1980) Abusive and rejecting infants. In N. Frude (Ed.), *The Understanding and Prevention of Child Abuse: Psychological Approaches* (pp.19–38). London: Concord Press, p.27.

mother and exposed to a sudden, loud crashing noise and flickering lights.[120] Fortunately for the infants, this study was not carried out.[121]

One reason may have been that it was not necessary: Main found that she could reliably observe conflict behaviour in other contexts. One was among young children who had experienced abuse. Main's graduate student Carol George proposed that conflict behaviour was expectable when young children experienced physical maltreatment by their caregiver. George observed ten physically abused toddlers and ten matched controls in a San Francisco daycare. She conducted careful qualitative observations, making detailed narrative notes. Based on analysis of these notes, George and Main reported that 'all of the abused children but none of the controls were observed to respond to peer affiliations with approach-avoidance behaviour,' such as approaching a professional carer but with their head averted.[122]

Additionally, Main found that she could reliably elicit conflict behaviour in the laboratory. Conflict behaviour was frequent, especially among infants in avoidantly attached dyads, in response to the unnerving crying clown both in Main's Berkeley sample and in the Grossmanns' Regensburg sample where the Clown procedure was also applied. In 1981, Main, working together with her graduate student Donna Weston, formulated an unpublished 'Scale for Disordered/Disoriented Infant Behaviour' for the Clown study. The original version appears to be lost, but a version of the scale was typed up by Main for Karin Grossmann in June 1982.[123] The manuscript shared with Grossmann is a nine-point scale, indexing behaviours including 'stereotypies, episodes of immobilisation, disoriented behaviour, misdirected behaviour, sudden disordered outbursts of activity, and sudden uninterpretable noises or movements'. In the 1982 manuscript, behaviour is identified by Main as 'disordered' based on the 'extent to which such behaviour may be indicative of difficulties in functioning', for instance by virtue of lacking either 'orientation' or 'purpose'.

Main was startled and intrigued by the fact that so many of these odd behaviours in human infants resembled the conflict behaviours described by Hinde in animals (Chapter 1): simultaneous or sequential contradictions in approaching the caregiver, misdirected approaches, poorly coordinated combinations of movements, freezing in place, or signs of confusion, out-of-context anger, or tension on reunion with the caregiver. In some cases, a child's behaviour in the Strange Situation seemed interrupted or misshapen by conflict behaviours. However, in other cases, the infant's response on reunion with their caregiver was dominated by other behaviours, making an Ainsworth classification impossible. Hinde was in Berkeley for the year 1979–80 as the Hitchcock Professor at the University of California, so Main

[120] Main, M. (1978) Avoidance of the attachment figure under stress: ontogeny, function and immediate causation. PP/Bow/J.4/3.

[121] Later in her career, another relevant study designed but not conducted by Main was to administer the Strange Situation without any toys. Since avoidance is a redirection of attention from the caregiver to the environment, Main suspected that the absence of toys would foil the avoidant strategy, and result instead in intense distress. Main, M. (1999) Epilogue. Attachment theory: eighteen points with suggestions for future studies. In J. Cassidy & P. Shaver (eds) *Handbook of Attachment* (pp.845–87). New York: Guilford, p.858. Madigan and colleagues subsequently showed that parents are more likely to show anomalous or alarming behaviours towards their children when asked to play with them without toys, a more challenging demand. Madigan, S., Moran, G., & Pederson, D. (2006) Unresolved states of mind, disorganized attachment relationships, and disrupted interactions of adolescent mothers and their infants. *Developmental Psychology*, 42(2), 293–304.

[122] George, C. & Main, M. (1980) Abused children: their rejection of peers and caregivers. In T. Field, S. Goldberg, D. Stern, & A. Sostek (eds) *High-Risk Infants and Children: Adult and Peer Interactions* (pp.293–312). New York: Academic Press, p.304.

[123] Main, M. (1982) *Scale for Disordered, Disoriented and Undirected Behaviors—Developed for Clown Session.* Unpublished manuscript, made available by Klaus and Karin Grossmann.

was able to discuss her observations and ideas with him; she later described the influence of Hinde on her thinking about conflict behaviours shown in the Strange Situation as 'strong and direct'.[124]

A new category

In a paper from 1981, Main and Weston published an interim report on 46 families where the Strange Situation had been coded for both infant–mother and infant–father interaction. They reported that 12.5%[125] could not be classified using the Ainsworth system: 'infants were not judged unclassifiable if they merely showed conflicted behavior or behaved oddly during the strange situation: one infant stared, talked to the wall, and indeed seemed almost to hallucinate, but was nonetheless regarded as secure in relation to the parent. Infants were judged unclassifiable only if their social and emotional behavior toward the parent could not be encompassed by the present Ainsworth system.'[126] However, in fact the large majority of the unclassifiable infants did show conflicted, confused, or apprehensive behaviours.

Yet Main and Weston's report on 'unclassifiable' cases was only on the Strange Situation procedures they had coded by that point. This was a fraction of the hundreds of Strange Situations conducted by the research group. The others still needed to be coded. In 1977, Judith Solomon joined Main's lab following a graduate focus on ethology and comparative psychology, which included attention to conflict behaviours in animals. Yet Main left soon after Solomon's arrival for Bielefeld, returning to Berkeley only in 1978. In her absence, Main instructed Solomon to learn how to classify the Strange Situation guided by Donna Weston and by feedback that Main sent by post.[127] Solomon began to compile detailed notes on cases she found difficult to classify, for discussion with Main on her return. At the same time, Solomon began to study a sample of maltreated infants in the Strange Situation with Carol George—a research project that was ultimately not completed or published. In coding these two samples, Solomon observed a variety of behaviours discrepant with the Ainsworth coding protocols, though they were particularly common in the maltreated sample: apparent signs of depression in infants; indications that an infant was attempting to muster a coherent

---

[124] Bahm, N.I.G., Main, M., & Hesse, E. (2017) Unresolved/disorganized responses to the death of important persons: relations to frightening parental behavior and infant disorganization. In S. Gojman de Millan, C. Herreman, & L.A. Sroufe (eds) *Attachment Across Clinical and Cultural Perspectives: A Relational Psychoanalytic Approach* (pp.53–74). London: Routledge, p.56. The chapter also mentions that 'Mary Main discussed conflict behaviour during two visits to Niko Tinbergen', one of the founders of ethology and of the empirical study of conflict behaviours: p.71.

[125] The 12.5% figure is rather mysterious. Table 1 in Main and Weston has 12 Strange Situations unclassifiable with either father or mother, out of 61 Strange Situations with each of father or mother. However, this would give a proportion of 9.7% unclassifiable. The researchers' comparison of classification with mother and father was made on 46 infants, i.e. 92 strange situations; 12 of 92 is 13% which is much closer to the 12.5% figure, but then does not agree with Table 1. Main, M. & Weston, D.R. (1981) The quality of the toddler's relationship to mother and to father: related to conflict behavior and the readiness to establish new relationships. *Child Development*, 52(3), 932–40. In 1986, Main reported that '152 strange situations were reviewed; 19 of the strange situations (12.5%) were judged unclassifiable'. Yet 19 of 152 is 8%, not 12.5%. Main, M. & Solomon, J. (1986) Discovery of a new, insecure-disorganized/disoriented attachment pattern. In M. Yogman & T.B. Brazelton (eds) *Affective Development in Infancy* (pp.95–124). Norwood, NJ: Ablex, p.103.

[126] Main, M. & Weston, D.R. (1981) The quality of the toddler's relationship to mother and to father: related to conflict behavior and the readiness to establish new relationships. *Child Development*, 52(3), 932–40, p.934

[127] Duschinsky, R. (2015) The emergence of the disorganized/disoriented (D) attachment classification, 1979–1982. *History of Psychology*, 18(1), 32–46.

strategy of approach or avoidance but failing to achieve this; infants initially approaching the caregiver but then veering off; and disoriented behaviours (e.g. the child leaves its arm hanging in the air).

The first use of a 'D' classification in the Berkeley study occurred in August 1979.[128] This was a case coded by Solomon. The infant's behaviour on reunion displayed a whole variety of conflict behaviours. After attempting at length to work out a best-fit Ainsworth classification, Solomon eventually gave up: 'Well, it is not A and it is not B and it is not C. I'm going to call it D.' Solomon's first use of the 'D' label was in pique. However, from 1979 Solomon and Main began thinking about and discussing a 'D' category for the Strange Situation. It was in line with Hinde's emphasis on conflict behaviours and on Main and Weston's existing work on cases unclassifiable by the Ainsworth coding protocols. Additionally, the fact that such behaviours were more common in the maltreatment sample Solomon was also coding spurred interest in their meaning.

Though they encased their observations within a category, Main and Solomon did not assume that the various forms of discrepant behaviour all meant the same thing. They were thinking in terms of the work by ethologists on conflict behaviour (Chapter 1):

> Our continuing focus on conflict behavior as it related to disorganized attachment status was derived from the work of the ethologists Niko Tinbergen, Konrad Lorenz and Robert Hinde. Hinde (1966) noted that conflicting behavioral tendencies are present under many conditions, with the most frequent outcome being that only one of the tendencies is actually observed. In some situations, however, both of the conflicting tendencies do appear in an animal's behavior, for example, in the alternating exhibition of the opposing behavioral patterns. In other situations, a third, apparently unrelated behavior pattern appears, such as preening in birds caught between feeding and flight. There are, additionally, conflict situations in which an animal is observed to freeze, to exhibit abnormal postures, or to engage in anomalous movements.[129]

Based on observations across various species, Hinde articulated very clearly the different conditions that would lead to different forms of conflict behaviour. It would undoubtedly have been possible for Main and Solomon to develop scales for conflicted, confused, or apprehensive infant behaviours. The use of differentiated scales within an overarching category was precisely the solution that Main's research group later adopted in the 1990s when studying parental behaviour.[130] That some infants scored on more than one scale would hardly have been a problem. Yet in the 1980s, in a field of empirical inquiry grounded on Ainsworth's Strange Situation and her patterns of attachment, categories were currency; to a large extent, categories formed a horizon of how data could readily be conceptualised and discussed at the time by attachment researchers. The publication of the influential DSM-III in 1983 (Chapter 1), as a clinical system based on categories, may also have played a distal role in supporting category-based thinking.

---

[128] Judith Solomon, personal communication, September 2012.

[129] Main, M. (1999) *Disorganized Attachment in Infancy, Childhood, and Adulthood: An Introduction to the Phenomena.* Unpublished manuscript, Mary Main & Erik Hesse personal archive; Hinde, R. (1966, 1970) *Animal Behavior*, 2nd edn. New York: McGraw.

[130] Abrams, K.Y., Rifkin, A., & Hesse, E. (2006) Examining the role of parental frightened/frightening subtypes in predicting disorganized attachment within a brief observational procedure. *Development & Psychopathology*, 18(2), 345–61.

In characterising conflict behaviours seen in the Strange Situation as a category, Main and Solomon sought to support their attempts to win attention to a phenomenon—or inter-related phenomena—that they saw as important, despite obstacles to such recognition. The obstacles were substantial. There was intense resistance to making any change to the Ainsworth coding system for the Strange Situation. Additionally, many of the behaviours lasted only a few seconds, and could easily be discounted as simply babies doing odd things because they are figuring out motor coordination. To gather more data and to support a claim to wider relevance, Main's laboratory began to collect unclassifiable tapes from other researchers working with high-risk samples such as Mary J. O'Connor, Elizabeth Carlson, Leila Beckwith, and Susan Spieker. Drawing on an analysis of both the Berkeley Strange Situations and these additional recordings from other samples, in the winter of 1982 Main and Solomon began work on what would be their 1986 chapter announcing 'discovery of a new, insecure-disorganised/disoriented attachment pattern'. This represented a shift in ter-minology. In initial discussions with Solomon, Main used the terms 'disordered' and 'dis-oriented' as overarching labels for the forms of conflict behaviour, following on from the use of these terms in the coding system for the Clown study. However, the term 'disordered' was judged to sound pejorative. It was not clear what the different behaviours meant, and so it was regarded as premature to describe them as a mental disorder.

In looking for a more descriptive word, the term 'disorganised' was available to Main and Solomon. The term had entered common use in neurology in the 1940s and 1950s to refer to the potential for strong feelings to be experienced as overwhelming. Affects such as anxiety, anger, awe, and ecstasy could be so intense and absorbing they make a person lost in the affect and unable to respond to the cues of the situation they are in.[131] The neurological literature used 'disorganised' to refer to the state following such intense and absorbing affects. It essen-tially meant 'overcome' by the feeling. Bowlby introduced the term into attachment theory in his 1960 paper on 'Separation anxiety', in order to propose that, whether in childhood or adulthood, grief could also be a disorganising affect. Having emphasised the value of the concept of 'disorganization', Bowlby then promised that 'this is a concept to which we shall be returning in a paper to follow'.[132] The promise was left unfulfilled, eliciting letters from readers requesting more detail about this idea of 'disorganisation' and why Bowlby thought it so important.[133] In *Attachment, Volume 1*, Bowlby returned to the issue of disorganisation. He restated his earlier claim that behaviour can become uncoordinated in the context of cer-tain intense emotions: 'Above a certain level, however, efficiency may be diminished; and, when in an experimental situation total stimulation is very greatly increased, behaviour be-comes completely disorganised.'[134] Here he added, however, that such overwhelming inten-sity is specifically expected in the context of conflicts between strong motivational systems, and 'in some cases, indeed, the behaviour that results when two incompatible behavioural systems are active simultaneously is of a kind that suggests pathology'.[135] He then reviewed Hinde's discussion of the various forms of 'conflict behaviour' seen in animals when two competing behavioural tendencies were activated. These included rapid transition between

---

[131] Leeper, R.W. (1948) A motivational theory of emotion to replace 'emotion as disorganized response'. *Psychological Review*, 55(1), 5–21; Goldstein, K. (1951) On emotions. *Journal of Psychology*, 31, 37–59.

[132] Bowlby, J. (1960) Separation anxiety. *International Journal of Psychoanalysis*, 41, 89–113, p.110.

[133] E.g. Bastiaans, J. (1963) *Letter to John Bowlby on behalf of the Dutch Psychoanalytic Society*, 22 January 1963. PP/BOW/B.3/20.

[134] Bowlby, J. (1969) *Attachment*. London: Penguin, p.96–7.

[135] Ibid.

one tendency and the other, poorly coordinated combinations, freezing in place, misdirected movements, or signs of confusion or tension.[136]

Main's colleagues at Berkeley, Block and Block, also drew on this term 'disorganisation' from neurology. They used the word to mean 'immobilised, rigidly repetitive or behaviourally diffuse' flooding behaviours, which could be expected when a child was experiencing 'a difficulty in recouping' in the face of behavioural conflict and distress.[137] The concept of disorganisation may have also appealed to Main and Solomon in the context of a technical use of the term 'organisation' that had sprung up following Ainsworth, Sroufe, and Waters (Chapters 2 and 4), who had cut the term 'organisation' loose from its ordinary language meaning and given it a technical sense: behaviour coordinated to achieving the set-goal of the attachment system. Behaviour that did not seem oriented to the achievement of this set-goal was therefore described by Ainsworth as 'disorganised' as early as 1968 in correspondence[138] and 1972 in print.[139] These were, importantly, the exact years in which Main was Ainsworth's doctoral student. What the different forms of conflict behaviour observed by Main and Solomon had in common was that they did not seem like components of a coherent and coordinated attempt to achieve proximity. Avoidance could be interpreted as 'in the service of proximity', and therefore oriented to the achievement of the set-goal of the attachment system. By contrast, conflicted, confused, or apprehensive behaviours did not seem 'organised' to Main, in the technical sense of the word.[140] It may well have seemed logical, therefore, to call them disorganised.

At a four-day workshop in 1985 at the University of Washington, Ainsworth sat on the floor to be as close as possible to the screen as Main showed her tapes coded with the new disorganised classification. At the end of the event, Ainsworth wrote to Bowlby that she and 'everyone there was most impressed with the need for adding a new "D" or disorganised category to the classification system'.[141] Bowlby also became convinced that the behaviours identified by Main and Solomon were likely 'of great clinical concern', and he expressed pride in their work.[142] However, in the margins of his personal copy of Main and Solomon's 1986 chapter 'Discovery of an insecure-disorganized/disoriented attachment pattern', he wrote

---

[136] Hinde, R. (1970) *Animal Behavior*, 2nd edn. New York: McGraw-Hill, Chapter 13.

[137] Block, J. & Block, J. (1980) The role of ego-control and ego-resiliency in the organisation of behaviour. In W.A. Collins (ed.) *Development of Cognition, Affect, and Social Relations: The Minnesota Symposia on Child Psychology*, Vol. 13 (pp.39–101). Hillsdale, NJ: Lawrence Erlbaum, p.48.

[138] Ainsworth, M. (1968) *Letter to J.L. Gewirtz*, 5 August 1968. PP/Bow/K.4/12: 'I do agree that there are varied indices of attachment, and my data suggest that these are not necessarily highly correlated. I also tend to agree that the approach behaviours are more stable indices of attachment than are the "disorganization" responses—perhaps because there may be more diverse determiners of disorganization behaviour than there are for approach behaviour to specific persons. I think it will require much more research to ascertain how "disorganization" responses relate to the more "positive" components of attachment.'

[139] Ainsworth, M. (1972) Attachment and dependency: a comparison. In J. Gewirtz (Ed.), *Attachment and Dependency* (pp.97–137). Washington, DC: Winston: 'Gewirtz and Cairns (both in this volume) have also distinguished the "positive" indices from other indices of attachment. They characterise the behaviour activated by separation as disorganised, whether because of the emotional component contingent upon the frustration of separation or because of the disruption of other ongoing behavioural sequences' (114).

[140] Main, M. & Solomon, J. (1986) Discovery of a new, insecure-disorganized/disoriented attachment pattern. In M. Yogman & T.B. Brazelton (eds) *Affective Development in Infancy* (pp.95–124.) Norwood, NJ: Ablex: 'Infants who cannot be classified within the present "A, B, C" system do not appear to us to resemble one another in strange situation in coherent, organised ways' (97).

[141] Ainsworth, M. (1985) *Letter to John Bowlby*, 14 February 1985. PP/BOW/B.3/8.

[142] Bowlby, J. (1988) The role of attachment in personality development. In *A Secure Base* (pp.134–54). London: Routledge Press, p.124; Bowlby, J. (1990, 2015) John Bowlby: an interview by Virginia Hunter. *Attachment*, 9, 138–57: 'Mary Main, Inge Bretherton … very admirable, able people. So the field is now being explored by first class scientists doing first class research of high clinical relevance. That I'm very, very proud of' (151).

that the authors would have done better to call it a 'status' because the unitary term 'pattern' may result in confusion if readers interpret it in the Ainsworth sense. In this marginalia, he observed that Main would likely agree with this reasoning, since she had indicated to him in a discussion in March 1986 that, in her view, 'trauma to the attachment system causes disorganisation of behaviour but does not create a new category'.[143]

However, one key advantage of making a new classification was that it cleaned up the existing categories: many of the children who could now be classified as disorganised in at-risk samples had previously been classified as 'secure' because, despite manifest displays of conflict or confusion, they had protested the departure of their caregiver and been comforted on reunion. This was a particular problem, for instance, in the influential Minnesota Longitudinal Study of Risk and Adaptation (Chapter 4) and in clinical samples.[144] Ainsworth had also observed conflict behaviours in the samples reported in *Patterns of Attachment*, and had even entered them into the coding protocol as characteristic of the B4 subtype (Chapter 2). Main was able to demonstrate in Washington that conflicted, confused, or apprehensive behaviours were not limited to this subtype, but could be found across the Ainsworth patterns of attachment. In fact, Main could show examples of Strange Situation procedures where forms of conflict, confusion, or apprehension so disrupted reunions that it was the dominant response. As she wrote in a paper composed in 1986, the extent of conflict behaviour was in theory on a spectrum. In a small number of cases, though, the conflict was so pervasive that it drowned out other responses: 'disorganization operates as a category only in extreme cases, being otherwise ... a dimension'.[145]

The meaning of disorganisation

By the time of their 1990 chapter offering protocols for coding the new category, Main and Solomon had closely analysed 100 recordings of infants from low-risk samples and 100 recordings from high-risk samples.[146] They proposed certain infant behaviours to be indicative of a 'disorganised' attachment response. They clustered the identified behaviours into seven indices based on how they appeared:

    I. Sequential displays of contradictory behaviour;
   II. Simultaneous display of contradictory behaviour;
 III. Undirected, misdirected or incomplete movements;
 IV. Stereotypies, mistimed movements and anomalous postures;
   V. Freezing or stilling;

---

[143] Bowlby, J. (1986) Marginalia on Main and Solomon's 'Discovery of an insecure-disorganized/disoriented attachment pattern'. PP/BOW/J.7/6; see Reisz, S., Duschinsky, R., & Siegel, D.J. (2018) Disorganized attachment and defense: exploring John Bowlby's unpublished reflections. *Attachment & Human Development*, 20(2), 107–34.

[144] E.g. Gaensbauer, T.J. & Harmon, R.J. (1982) Attachment behavior in abused/neglected and premature infants. In R.N. Emde & R.J. Harmon (eds) *The Development of Attachment and Affiliative Systems* (pp.263–89). New York: Plenum Press.

[145] Main, M. & Cassidy, J. (1988) Categories of response to reunion with the parent at age 6: predictable from infant attachment classifications and stable over a 1-month period. *Developmental Psychology*, 24(3), 415–26, pp.423–4.

[146] Main, M. & Solomon, J. (1990) Procedures for identifying infants as disorganized/disoriented during the Ainsworth Strange Situation. In M.T. Greenberg, D. Cicchetti, & E.M. Cummings (eds) *Attachment in the Preschool Years* (pp.121–60). Chicago: University of Chicago Press.

    VI.   Display of apprehension of the caregiver;

    VII. Overt signs of disorientation.

To facilitate coding, Main and Solomon presented general guidelines and a nine-point scale.[147] This scale is partly a measure of the extent of inferred disorganisation of the attachment system, and partly a ranking of how certain a coder is that they are seeing behaviour suggesting disruption of the attachment behavioural system. A score above 5 is sufficient for placement of the dyad into a D classification.[148]

    As Main and Solomon acknowledged, behaviours pertaining to the first five indices were already discussed by Hinde and Bowlby as classic 'conflict behaviours' (Chapter 1). Main and Solomon introduced two further kinds of behaviour, based on their analysis of the recordings: apprehension directed towards the caregiver, and disorientation or confusion on reunion or in proximity with the caregiver. They knew that apprehension did not really fit under the term 'disorganisation', since the behaviour could well be behaviourally coherent and coordinated. However, at a more abstract level of analysis, apprehension of the caregiver nonetheless seemed in conflict with proximity, considered as the set-goal of the attachment system.[149] Unlike the Ainsworth patterns which tended to be more discrete, Main and Solomon found that infants who showed one kind of conflict, apprehension, or disorientation also regularly showed some other kind. This led them to regard the phenomena as highly related, even if not necessarily all of a piece. As a result, the different behaviours were grouped together as a 'disorganised' category.

    Yet their use of the term 'disorganised' differed from the dictionary definition. And they did not clarify this for the reader at the time, something both authors now regret. The dictionary, everyday meaning of the term 'disorganization' suggests randomness and a lack of predictable responsiveness to contingencies: 'to destroy the system or order of; to throw into confusion or disorder'.[150] According to the connotations of the word in ordinary language, what Main and Solomon appeared to be proposing was a category of undifferentiated chaos. The scientific concept was taken hostage by its ordinary language connotations.[151] In Spangler and Schieche, for instance, the authors wrote that 'as disorganized infants, by definition, do not have any coherent strategies, behavioral regulation is restricted or even not possible at all'.[152] Likewise, Wanaza and colleagues wrote that 'disorganization is defined as the

---

[147] Ibid. p.133.

[148] Technically, a score of 5 was given as the mid-point, and could be the basis for a D classification on the judgement of the coder. However, subsequent coders have tended to mark such cases as 5.5.

[149] Duschinsky, R. (2015) The emergence of the disorganized/disoriented (D) attachment classification, 1979–1982. *History of Psychology*, 18(1), 32–46.

[150] Oxford English Dictionary (1990) 'disorganize'. Oxford: Oxford University Press.

[151] Exceptions include Waters, E. & Crowell, J.A. (1999) Atypical attachment in atypical circumstances. *Monographs of the Society for Research in Child Development*, 64(3), 213–20; Rauh, H., Ziegenhain, U., Muller, B., & Wijnroks, L. (2000) Stability and change of infant–mother attachment in the second year of life: relations to parenting quality and varying degrees of daycare experience. In P.K. Crittenden & A.H. Claussen (eds) *The Organization of Attachment Relationships: Maturation, Culture and Context* (pp.251–76). Cambridge: Cambridge University Press; Slade, A. (2014) Imagining fear: attachment, threat, and psychic experience. *Psychoanalytic Dialogues*, 24(3), 253–66; Solomon, J. & George, C. (2016) The measurement of attachment security and related constructs in infancy and early childhood. In J. Cassidy & P.R. Shaver (eds) *The Handbook of Attachment*, 3rd edn (pp.366–98). New York: Guilford.

[152] Spangler, G. & Schieche, M. (1998) Emotional and adrenocortical responses of infants to the Strange Situation. *International Journal of Behavioral Development*, 22(4), 681–706, p.700. A further factor subsequently contributing to the image of disorganisation as chaos was findings in the early 1990s by Spangler and by Hertsgaard of elevated hypothalamic–pituitary–adrenal (HPA) reactivity following the Strange Situation among young children who received a disorganised attachment classification. Spangler and Grossmann had 9 D dyads,

collapse of attachment strategy under conditions of stress; under such conditions, disorganized individuals select a set of behaviors that are irrelevant to their need for downregulation of discomfort'.[153] Commentators at the research–practice interface have criticised the idea of attachment disorganisation as clinically evocative but unhelpful, since the concept means incomprehensibility and therefore offers no clues to clinicians about how to proceed.[154]

In fact, the term 'disorganisation' was used in three ways in Main and Solomon's 1986 and 1990 chapters—not one of which aligns well with the dictionary definition. The term was used by Main and Solomon to describe (i) observable behaviour that seemed to lack order or relevance to achieving proximity with the caregiver; (ii) a disruption of the attachment behavioural system, caused by past experiences of child–caregiver interaction and inferable from observed behaviour; (iii) and the label given to the category used for coding the Strange Situation.[155] In using the same term 'disorganised' to refer to both behaviour and/or psychological process and/or the overall category, Main and Solomon had a specific aim, though it was not well articulated at the time. 'Disorganisation' was used as a conceptual tool for picking out 'an observed contradiction in movement pattern, corresponding to an inferred contradiction in intention or plan'.[156] The theoretical stakes of using the term 'disorganized' to mean both behaviour and psychological process was the claim that the diverse behaviours picked up by the Main and Solomon indices could well have different antecedents and sequelae, but what they had in common was that they suggested disruption or breakdown at the level of the attachment system. This was the rationale for the 'radical notion that the many, highly diverse indices of disorganization and disorientation can be placed under one heading'.[157]

In the early 1990s, Main created a revised version of the Main and Solomon coding protocols, though she did not publish it. This version is distributed to trainees at the Minnesota Strange Situation training institute, run by Alan Sroufe and Betty Carlson.[158] Main's revisions predominantly entailed adding further forms of behaviour under the seven indices. For instance 'overbright greeting' was added to Direct Indices of Apprehension (Index VI), presumably as this was interpreted as an early form of caregiving or compliance by the child

and Hertsgaard had 11. However, in a later study by Luijk and colleagues with 57 D dyads, the earlier findings failed to replicate. Furthermore, in 1999, Spangler and Grossmann later acknowledged that the overwhelming majority of the association between D and HPA reactivity in their study was attributable to Index VII behaviour (direct indices of disorientation), and there was no association at all for conflict behaviours where confusion or apprehension were not also present. Spangler, G. & Grossmann, K.E. (1993) Biobehavioral organization in securely and insecurely attached infants. *Child Development*, 64, 1439–50. Hertsgaard, L., Gunnar, M., Erickson, M.F., & Nachmias, M. (1995) Adrenocortical responses to the strange situation in infants with disorganized/disoriented attachment relationships. *Child Development*, 66(4), 1100–106; Spangler, G. & Grossmann, K.E. (1999) Individual and physiological correlates of attachment disorganization in infancy. In J. Solomon & C. George (eds) *Attachment Disorganization* (pp.95–124). New York: Guilford; Luijk, M.P., Velders, F.P., Tharner, A., et al. (2010) FKBP5 and resistant attachment predict cortisol reactivity in infants: gene–environment interaction. *Psychoneuroendocrinology*, 35(10), 1454–61.

[153] Wazana, A., Moss, E., Jolicoeur-Martineau, A., et al. (2015) The interplay of birthweight, dopamine receptor D4 gene (DRD4), and early maternal care in the prediction of disorganized attachment at 36 months of age. *Development & Psychopathology*, 27, 1145–61, p.1157.

[154] E.g. Baim, C. & Morrison, T. (2014) *Attachment-Based Practice with Adults*. Brighton: Pavilion.

[155] Duschinsky, R. & Solomon, J. (2017) Infant disorganized attachment: clarifying levels of analysis. *Clinical Child Psychology and Psychiatry*, 22(4), 524–38.

[156] Main, M. & Solomon, J. (1990) Procedures for identifying infants as disorganized/disoriented during the Ainsworth Strange Situation. In M.T. Greenberg, D. Cicchetti, & E.M. Cummings (eds) *Attachment in the Preschool Years* (pp.121–60). Chicago: University of Chicago Press, p.133.

[157] Ibid. p.151.

[158] https://attachment-training.com/training/#1.

towards the caregiver. Main also added guidance to coders on 'Major Considerations' for coding disorganised attachment. The primary consideration was 'Is the behaviour inexplicable (no evidence of immediate goal or rationale) OR is the behaviour explicable only if we presume: a) The baby is afraid of the parent; b) The baby is inhibited from approach without being able to shift attention to the environment?'[159] Here we can see that disorganisation is operationalised as behaviours that seem confused, apprehensive, or conflicted. Also visible is the technical distinction for Main between avoidance and disorganised attachment, hinging on the fact that the former can direct attention to the environment in order to maintain regulation, whereas in the latter this conditional strategy of the use of attention to circumvent approach/avoidance conflict is not feasible. However, this manuscript remained unpublished, and generally available only to junior researchers who are tasked with coding. With exceptions, many senior researchers in the field of attachment research have therefore not known how the category is actually coded, for instance that only some infants will look apprehensive—others will look confused or conflicted (or a combination of the three). Senior researchers have tended to be unaware of the significant role coders must give to inferences about how the infant is directing attention in the Strange Situation.

In putting confused, apprehensive, and conflicted behaviours together, Main and Solomon did not intend to imply that they all meant the same thing. In fact, they stated in print that 'our discovery of the D category of infant Strange Situation behaviour rested on an unwillingness to adopt the "essentialist" or "realist" position regarding the classification of human relationships'.[160] Their epistemological position, like Bowlby's, treated categories as 'provisional, albeit nonarbitrary approximations',[161] and Main and Solomon end their 1990 chapter with an extended criticism of essentialist approaches to categorisation in the history of biology. Yet these remarks by Main and Solomon on the dangers of essentialism have never been cited or discussed. In general, the ensuing literature respectfully cites but gives little evidence of having directly read the book chapters introducing the classification. Main and Solomon were widely interpreted as introducing an exhaustive addition to the Ainsworth system. They have therefore been accused of being bent upon 'reducing complex human experience to typologies'.[162] Likewise, it has been assumed that their category aimed simply to soak up possible variation in human behaviour beyond the Ainsworth patterns and treat it all as evidence of dysfunction.

For instance, Gaskin argued that 'the category is really just a residual one': rather than itself designating any meaningful phenomena, the existence of the classification 'might be seen more productively as evidence of the inadequacy of the three attachment classifications' introduced by Ainsworth on the basis of her Baltimore middle-class sample.[163] This

---

[159] The other major considerations were: "2) Timing of the appearance of disorganized behaviour: a) stronger index of disorganisation if occurs at first moments of reunion; b) however, even D-like behaviour appearing only in Episode 3 may yield a D classification. 3) Consider what the baby does next, namely, if the baby goes to the parent as though for comfort after a bit of disorganisation (i.e. stereotypies then comforted). If they become organised quickly, discount the D behaviour). Main, M. (undated) *Disorganised/Disoriented Classification Scheme: Major Considerations*. Unpublished manuscript, received from Elizabeth Carlson, and cited with her permission.

[160] Main, M., Kaplan, N., & Cassidy, J. (1985) Security in infancy, childhood, and adulthood: a move to the level of representation. *Monographs of the Society for Research in Child Development*, 50, 66–104, p.99.

[161] Main, M. (1995) Recent studies in attachment: overview, with selected implications for clinical work. In S. Goldberg, R. Muir, & J. Kerr (eds) *Attachment Theory: Social, Developmental and Clinical Perspectives* (pp.407–70). Hillsdale, NJ: Analytic Press, p.422.

[162] O'Shaughnessy, R. & Dallos, R. (2009) Attachment research and eating disorders: a review of the literature. *Clinical Child Psychology & Psychiatry*, 14(4), 559–74, p.559.

[163] Gaskins, S. (2013) The puzzle of attachment. In N. Quinn & J.M. Mageo (eds) *Attachment Reconsidered* (pp.33–66). London: Palgrave, p.39.

misunderstanding has a history that goes back to the very introduction of the classification. Mark Cummings was one of the editors of the volume within which Main and Solomon's 1990 chapter was published. In his contribution to the volume, he argued that 'deviations from expected sequences do not constitute a sufficient criterion for classification'.[164] Against what he took to be Main and Solomon's perspective, he proposed that D behaviours could not all be expected to reflect the same process of breakdown of 'general functioning', and that therefore the category lacked coherence and meaning.[165] A better criterion for disorganisation, Cummings argued, would be behaviours that do not appear to function to achieve 'felt security', which Sroufe and Waters had proposed, as the set-goal of the infant's attachment system (Chapter 4).[166]

Psychological constructs are usually subjected to statistical analysis to see which elements cluster together and which among these clusters are especially involved in associations with other variables of interest. By contrast, though it is not uncommon to hear praise of the 'strong psychometric properties' of the Strange Situation procedure and its classification as a whole,[167] in fact no psychometric study has ever been reported on the infant disorganised attachment classification. Though perhaps less in social psychology than in developmental psychology (Chapter 5), psychological scientists are generally satisfied to work with instruments that have expectable correlates and fit with a conceptual framework, no matter that psychometric work is incomplete. Furthermore, psychometric work receives little professional reward for psychological researchers. Another potential obstacle is that a sample of adequate size for psychometric research is needed—though in the case of disorganised attachment this cannot have been the only factor in play, since a number of such samples have long been available now. Rather, it was simply assumed that disorganisation was best treated as a single category.

No assessment was made, for instance, of whether the one-to-nine scale would be more serviceable than the category. And no exploration was made of the component parts of disorganisation, for instance to economise the coding system. The underdeveloped and rather complicated coding protocol made application of the classification time-consuming and, beyond this, very hard to learn. The result has been a significant bottleneck for research using the Strange Situation due to the small number of reliable coders and the disincentives of investing time and resource in learning the system. It has also limited the circulation of important practical knowledge, leading to frequent speculative discussions about disorganisation among attachment researchers that have been wholly cut loose from how it is actually coded.[168] Yet prediction of negative outcomes was treated by researchers—and subsequently by clinicians and policy-makers—as validity. Indeed, the disorganised classification also quickly bore fruit in predictive significance.

---

[164] Cummings, E.M. (1990) Classification of attachment on a continuum of felt-security. In M.T. Greenberg, D. Cicchetti, & E.M. Cummings (eds) *Attachment in the Preschool Years* (pp.311–38). Chicago: University of Chicago Press, p.319.

[165] Ibid. p.316.

[166] Ibid. p.326.

[167] E.g. Bernard, K., Dozier, M., Bick, J., Lewis-Morrarty, E., Lindhiem, O., & Carlson, E. (2012) Enhancing attachment organization among maltreated children. *Child Development*, 83(2), 623–36, p.632.

[168] Reijman, S., Foster, S., & Duschinsky, R. (2018) The infant disorganised attachment classification: 'patterning within the disturbance of coherence'. *Social Science & Medicine*, 200, 52–8. See also van IJzendoorn, M.H. (1995) Adult attachment representations, parental responsiveness, and infant attachment: a meta-analysis on the predictive validity of the Adult Attachment Interview. *Psychological Bulletin*, 117(3), 387–403: 'Amount of training in coding the disorganized/disoriented category also appeared to be strongly related to differences in effect sizes; less training in the application of the complicated coding system was associated with smaller effect sizes' (394).

The short-term test-retest stability of disorganised attachment as assessed twice using the Strange Situation was $r = .35$. This was regarded as at least adequate to validate the measure, and potentially rather high considering that the classification was, at times, made on the basis of quite fleeting behaviours[169]—though stability between infancy and toddlerhood or preschool has been found to be much lower.[170] Incidence of the disorganised attachment classification was also discovered to be more common in clinical samples, samples known to social services, and in samples facing multiple adversities, suggesting that it reflected some adverse experience or process. In community samples with relatively few adversities, around 15% of infants show a sufficiently high degree of confused, disoriented, or apprehensive behaviours towards their caregiver in the Strange Situation for a disorganised classification to be assigned. However, this increases to a majority of infants from families drawn from samples facing multiple compounding adversities, or where maltreatment of the child has been documented.[171] Of particular importance for acceptance of the new classification, however, was the prediction of conduct problems. An early and influential study by Lyons-Ruth and colleagues, reported in 1991, found disorganised infant attachment associated with aggressive behaviour in preschool in a sample of dyads known to child protection services.[172]

The link between the infant disorganised attachment classification and later aggressive behaviour has been confirmed by numerous studies. By 2010, Fearon and colleagues could report from a meta-analysis of 69 studies a modest but material association ($d = .34$) between disorganisation and various externalising behaviours (including attentional problems).[173] The association was stronger in samples where families were known to clinical or professional services ($d = .43$) or facing low socioeconomic status ($d = .44$). Indeed, for many samples, disorganised infant attachment only predicted later externalising problems in conjunction with other forms of adversity.[174] For disorganised attachment, as for the Ainsworth avoidant classification (Chapter 2), the Strange Situation conducted with two-year-olds seemed to predict later externalising problems more effectively than when it was conducted with infants, perhaps because one of the particular developmental challenges of this age is

---

[169] Van IJzendoorn, M.H., Schuengel, C., & Bakermans-Kranenburg, M.J. (1999) Disorganized attachment in early childhood: meta-analysis of precursors, concomitants, and sequelae. *Development & Psychopathology*, 11(2), 225–50.

[170] The latest meta-analytic findings are reported by Opie, J. (2018) Attachment stability and change in early childhood and associated moderators. Unpublished doctoral thesis, Deakin University, Melbourne. Extracting results from 56 studies, stability from infancy to toddlerhood was $r = .10, p = .09, df = 7.12$. Stability from infancy to preschool age was $r = .19, p = .052, df = 6.81$. Stability of disorganisation assessed using the Cassidy–Marvin system was higher: $r = .32, p = .02, df = 3.30$.

[171] Cyr, C., Euser, E.M., Bakermans-Kranenburg, M., & van IJzendoorn, M. (2010) Attachment security and disorganization in maltreating and high-risk families: a series of meta-analyses. *Development & Psychopathology*, 22, 87–108.

[172] Lyons-Ruth, K., Repacholi, B., McLeod, S., & Silva, E. (1991) Disorganized attachment behavior in infancy: short-term stability, maternal and infant correlates, and risk-related subtypes. *Development & Psychopathology*, 3(4), 377–96. Another study of particular importance for acceptance of Main's methodological innovations as a whole was the finding by Fonagy, Steele, and Steele that four-way Strange Situation classifications could be predicted by four-way AAIs conducted prenatally with mothers. Fonagy, P., Steele, H., & Steele, M. (1991) Maternal representations of attachment during pregnancy predict the organization of infant–mother attachment at one year of age. *Child Development*, 62(5), 891–905.

[173] Fearon, R.P., Bakermans-Kranenburg, M.J., van IJzendoorn, M.H., Lapsley, A.M., & Roisman, G.I. (2010) The significance of insecure attachment and disorganization in the development of children's externalizing behavior: a meta-analytic study. *Child Development*, 81(2), 435–56. On the interpretation of effect sizes in psychology see Funder, D.C. & Ozer, D.J. (2019) Evaluating effect size in psychological research: sense and nonsense. *Advances in Methods and Practices in Psychological Science*, 2(2), 156–68.

[174] For a discussion see Tharner, A., Luijk, M.P., van IJzendoorn, M.H., et al. (2012) Infant attachment, parenting stress, and child emotional and behavioral problems at age 3 years. *Parenting*, 12(4), 261–81.

learning to regulate frustration in relationships.[175] Researchers have also documented other sequelae, including small-to-moderate associations with social competence and friendships ($d = .25$).[176]

A meta-analysis by Groh and colleagues found no association with later depression or anxiety.[177] But other mental health outcomes have been documented. For instance, a classification of disorganised/disoriented attachment in infancy predicts severity of later post-traumatic stress disorder (PTSD) symptoms following a trauma—an association that was found not to be attributable to the many co-occurring risk factors.[178] In her landmark 1998 paper, Carlson also documented associations in the Minnesota Longitudinal Study of Risk and Adaptation between infant disorganised attachment and general mental health in early adulthood, with a particularly strong association for dissociative symptoms.[179] The Carlson paper helped secure perceptions of disorganisation as, in Sroufe's words, an 'incredibly powerful construct, being among other things the strongest single predictor of later psychopathology'.[180] Yet Groh, Fearon, van IJzendoorn, Bakermans-Kranenburg, and Roisman have presented meta-analytic findings inconsistent with Carlson's apparent emphasis on the implications of infant disorganised attachment for general psychopathology, finding instead stronger links with externalising problems specifically.[181] The Minnesota findings are discussed further in Chapter 4.

Fear and causality

The Main and Solomon 1990 chapter laid out protocols for coding the classification. Each of the seven Index headings was followed by a variety of concrete examples of kinds of behaviour seen by Main and Solomon in their review. Some of the examples are italicised, which means that behaviour of this sort may, on its own, be sufficient for a D classification. Other examples are not italicised, which means that only when other kinds of conflicted, confused, or apprehensive behaviour is present should a D classification be considered. The rationale was not made explicit by Main and Solomon for the inclusion of particular examples, or for which examples are italicised, or how to weight observations that differ from the examples. This has contributed to the bottleneck in reliable coders. A careful

[175] Fearon, R.P., Bakermans-Kranenburg, M.J., Van IJzendoorn, M.H., Lapsley, A.M., & Roisman, G.I. (2010) The significance of insecure attachment and disorganization in the development of children's externalizing behavior: a meta-analytic study. *Child Development*, 81(2), 435–56, p.450.

[176] Groh, A.M., Fearon, R.P., Bakermans-Kranenburg, M.J., Van IJzendoorn, M.H., Steele, R.D., & Roisman, G.I. (2014) The significance of attachment security for children's social competence with peers: a meta-analytic study. *Attachment & Human Development*, 16(2), 103–36.

[177] Groh, A.M., Roisman, G.I., van IJzendoorn, M.H., Bakermans-Kranenburg, M.J., & Fearon, R.P. (2012) The significance of insecure and disorganized attachment for children's internalizing symptoms: a meta-analytic study. *Child Development*, 83(2), 591–610.

[178] MacDonald, H.Z., Beeghly, M., Grant-Knight, W., et al. (2008) Longitudinal association between infant disorganized attachment and childhood posttraumatic stress symptoms. *Development & Psychopathology*, 20(2), 493–508.

[179] Carlson, E.A. (1998) A prospective longitudinal study of attachment disorganization/disorientation. *Child Development*, 69(4), 1107–28.

[180] Sroufe, L.A. (2003) Attachment categories as reflections of multiple dimensions. *Developmental Psychology*, 39(3), 413–16, p.414.

[181] Groh, A.M., Fearon, R.M., IJzendoorn, M.H., Bakermans-Kranenburg, M.J., & Roisman, G.I. (2017) Attachment in the early life course: meta-analytic evidence for its role in socioemotional development. *Child Development Perspectives*, 11(1), 70–76, p.73.

retrospective examination of the protocol, conducted together with Solomon, reveals that behaviours are included when they are conflicted, confused, or apprehensive. And, again in retrospective examination, italicisation was based on six factors: (i) frequency of a behaviour, (ii) its pervasiveness or duration, (iii) its abruptness in behavioural sequence, (iv) the extent to which it occurs either close to reunion or in physical proximity with the caregiver, (v) whether it can be better explained as a reaction to the immediate environment, and (vi) the extent to which the infants' responses to their caregiver suggest the experience of apprehension.[182]

This latter item in the protocol reflects a theory that Main had been developing with her husband and collaborator Erik Hesse. Hesse entered undergraduate study in psychology at Berkeley as an adult, after studying to become a professional musician. Following completion of his studies in 1981, he worked as a research collaborator with Main, for instance as one of the coders for the Kaplan drawing system (discussed in the section 'The Kaplan and Main family drawing system'). At the start of her relationship with Hesse, Main had been thinking intensively about the role of avoidant behaviour in the Strange Situation. She concluded that a rejecting or angry parent would distress an infant, activating the attachment system and a desire for proximity, but simultaneously would evoke a tendency to withdraw from the parent. Avoidant behaviour would circumvent the ensuing approach–avoidance conflict.[183]

Hesse's ingenious proposal was that one cause of the conflicted, confused, and apprehensive behaviours that Main and Solomon were seeing in the Strange Situation would be experiences of alarming behaviour by the caregiver, the haven of safety sought by the attachment system. This would not permit the redirection of attention that, for Main, provided the infrastructure for a conditional strategy: 'the infant may at times be experiencing a fear or distress too intense to be deactivated through a shift in attention (the Ainsworth A pattern), yet at least momentarily cannot be ameliorated through approach to the attachment figure (the Ainsworth B and C patterns)'.[184] This predicament could be produced if 'the fear the infant experiences stems from the parent as its source', due to the injunction of the attachment system to approach the caregiver when alarmed.[185] Alarming behaviour by an attachment figure would cause an injunction to both approach and take flight, blocking the redirection of attention upon or away from the caregiver that underpins the two forms of infant conditional attachment strategy. Main and Hesse put forward this idea in a 1990 chapter that immediately followed the Main and Solomon protocols, establishing it essentially and fundamentally within reception of the D classification. In their writings of the period, and in personal communication with colleagues, they proposed that 'it is the interjection of fear into the caregiving experience that is essential to developing a disorganised/disoriented attachment'.[186]

[182] Duschinsky, R. & Solomon, J. (2017) Infant disorganized attachment: clarifying levels of analysis. *Clinical Child Psychology and Psychiatry*, 22(4), 524–38.

[183] Main, M. & Stadtman, J. (1981) Infant response to rejection of physical contact by the mother. *Journal of the American Academy of Child Psychiatry*, 20(2), 292–307.

[184] Main, M. & Hesse, E. (1990) Parents' unresolved traumatic experiences are related to infant disorganized attachment status. In M.T. Greenberg, D. Cicchetti, & E.M. Cummings (eds) *Attachment in the Preschool Years* (pp.161–81) Chicago: University of Chicago Press, p.163.

[185] Ibid. p.182.

[186] Cicchetti, D. & White, J. (1988) Emotional development and the affective disorders. In W. Damon (ed.) *Child Development: Today and Tomorrow* (pp.177–98). San Francisco: Jossey-Bass, citing a personal communication from Main, p.185.

Supporting evidence for association of the caregiver with fear as one pathway to disorganised infant attachment was already available by the time of Main and Hesse's 1990 chapter,
from Dante Cicchetti and his research group (Chapter 4). The Harvard Child Maltreatment
Project was initiated in 1979 by Cicchetti and Aber, as a large longitudinal study, modelled on
the Minnesota Longitudinal Study of Risk and Adaptation.[187] A small subsample were seen
in the Strange Situation and classified using the Ainsworth categories.[188] Twenty-two dyads
were known to child protection services for abuse and/or neglect of the child or an older
sibling; 21 were a matched comparison group. However, a third of the sample were classified as securely attached according to the Ainsworth coding protocols. There were a few different proposals available at the time for additions to Ainsworth's system for use with clinical
samples. One was that of Ainsworth's student Patricia Crittenden, who observed that some
abused infants show both avoidant and resistant attachment (A–C).[189] However, the Main
and Solomon disorganised attachment classification appealed to Cicchetti and colleagues
as more encompassing; it was assumed that finer-grained distinctions would be worked out
later. The disorganised classification also had emerging evidence of predictive validity.[190]
The data were recoded for disorganisation by Cicchetti and Barnett; Barnett was blind to the
children's maltreatment status; 82% of the infant–caregiver dyads known to child protection
services were classified as showing disorganised attachment and 14% classified as secure; in
the comparison group, 19% were classified as disorganised and 52% classified as secure. At
18 months, 61% of dyads known to child protection services were classified as showing disorganised attachment, compared to 29% in the comparison group.[191]

In the empirical developmental attachment tradition initiated by Ainsworth, it was widely
held that home observations were needed to validate new measures or the adaptation of existing measures. By the early 1990s, Ainsworth was expressing her dismay that 'so many attachment researchers have gone on to do research with the Strange Situation rather than
looking at what happens in the home ... in part it has to do with the "publish or perish"
realities of academic life'.[192] And Sroufe and Waters agreed that 'the strange situation is used
only because it can stand in place of attachment as it would be observed in the home'.[193] As
such, 'any procedure claiming to assess attachment (even variations or new applications of

---

[187] Another early, important study of a sample with substantial rates of maltreatment was conducted by Mary Jo
Ward. Ward was also a former student of Sroufe's, graduating a few years after Cicchetti: Ward, M.J. & Carlson, E.A.
(1995) Associations among adult attachment representations, maternal sensitivity, and infant–mother attachment
in a sample of adolescent mothers. *Child Development*, 66(1), 69–79.

[188] Schneider-Rosen, K., Braunwald, K.G., Carlson, V., & Cicchetti, D. (1985) Current perspectives in attachment theory: illustration from the study of maltreated infants. *Monographs of the Society for Research in Child
Development*, 50(1–2), 194–210.

[189] Crittenden, P.M. (1988) Relationships at risk. In J. Belsky & T. Nezworski (eds) *Clinical Implications of
Attachment Theory* (pp.136–74). Hillsdale, NJ: Lawrence Erlbaum. See also Radke-Yarrow, M., Cummings, E.M.,
Kuczynski, L., & Chapman, M. (1985) Patterns of attachment in two- and three-year-olds in normal families and
families with parental depression. *Child Development*, 56, 884–93.

[190] Carlson, V., Cicchetti, D., Barnett, D., & Braunwald, K. (1989) Finding order in disorganization: lessons
from research on maltreated infants' attachments to their caregivers. In D. Cicchetti & V. Carlson (eds) *Child
Maltreatment: Theory and Research on the Causes and Consequences of Child Abuse and Neglect* (pp.494–528).
Cambridge: Cambridge University Press, p.507.

[191] Barnett, D., Ganiban, J., & Cicchetti, D. (1999) Maltreatment, negative expressivity, and the development
of type D attachments from 12 to 24 months of age. *Monographs of the Society for Research in Child Development*,
64(3), 97–118.

[192] Ainsworth, M. (1995) On the shaping of attachment theory and research: an interview with Mary D.S.
Ainsworth. *Monographs of the Society for Research in Child Development*, 60(2–3), 2–21, p.12.

[193] Sroufe, L.A. & Waters, E. (1982) Issues of temperament and attachment. *American Journal of Orthopsychiatry*,
52(4), 743–6, p.743.

the Ainsworth procedure) must be anchored to observations of the attachment–exploration balance in the natural environment. That is the crucial criterion.'[194] Though the Strange Situation is often described as the 'gold standard', Sroufe and Waters characterised detailed naturalistic observations as the true 'standard' for assessing attachment. Cicchetti and colleagues revealed one kind of experience in the home environment that could substantially increase the likelihood of disorganised attachment. Yet Main and colleagues regarded it as implausible that in the low-risk Bay Area sample, all infants who received a disorganised attachment classification had received maltreatment from their caregiver. And, as mentioned in the section 'A new category', Main and Solomon found that apprehension of the caregiver and disorientation were more common in the tapes they reviewed from maltreatment or very high-risk samples, whereas these behaviours were uncommon in the infants classified as disorganised in the Bay Area sample.

Conversations between Main and Hesse led to the conclusion that there could be other forms of alarming caregiver behaviour besides abuse. Main's written notes from home observations during her doctorate offered too little detail to be the basis for a published study, and her group had not collected new observations of the child's behaviour at home for the Berkeley study. So she was not in a position to examine how disorganised attachment in the Strange Situation related to a child's behaviour at home in samples not specifically known to child protection services. Ainsworth regarded a home observation study as 'highly desirable' for the validation of the classification.[195] Likewise, van IJzendoorn alleged that 'since the D category has not been widely validated against home behavior, its meaning is not yet fully clear'.[196] To answer such concerns, Main, though she had no home observation recordings, did have observations of infant free-play sessions in the laboratory with both the child's mother and father. If alarming behaviour in playful and other more ordinary interactions was shown predominantly by parents in dyads classified as disorganised in the Strange Situation, then this would offer one form of ecological validation for the classification, and at the same time help shed light on its cause or causes.

---

[194] Sroufe, L.A. (1996) *Emotional Development*. Cambridge: Cambridge University Press, p.181.

[195] Ainsworth, M. & Eichberg, C. (1988) *Effects on Infant–Mother Attachment of Mother's Experience Related to Loss of an Attachment Figure or Other Traumatic Experience*. Unpublished manuscript. PP/Bow/J.1/62: 'It would be highly desirable for future research to undertake intensive observation of parent–infant interaction in the natural environment of the home in the case of infants classified as D' (40). Incredibly, in the three decades since the introduction of the classification, this 'crucial criterion' has never been systematically pursued; the only work on the question was the accidental observation of disorganised attachment behaviour at home in a few infants during Carlo Schuengel's doctoral study: Schuengel, C., van IJzendoorn M.H., Bakermans-kranenburg, M.J., & Blom, M. (1998) Frightening maternal behaviour, unresolved loss, and disorganized infant attachment: a pilot-study. *Journal of Reproductive and Infant Psychology*, 16(4), 277–83: 'Unexpectedly, as it was not an aim of our study, we observed disorganized attachment behaviour in two infants during the home observations. This behaviour qualified, if it had been observed in the context of the Strange Situation, for a D-classification. Surprisingly, the two infants who were disorganized at home were not disorganized in the Strange Situation' (282). Another study later examined the behaviour of dyads classified as disorganised, not at home, but in response to an injection at the doctors', yielding weak but interesting findings. Wolff, N.J., Darlington, A.S.E., Hunfeld, J.A., et al. (2011) The influence of attachment and temperament on venipuncture distress in 14-month-old infants: the generation R study. *Infant Behavior and Development*, 34(2), 293–302: 'The current study showed that there was a trend for attachment disorganization to predict higher levels of venepuncture distress in 14-month-old infants. Furthermore, the interaction of disorganized attachment and fearful temperament was significantly associated with distress; fear predicted an increase in distress only in infants with a disorganized attachment classification' (299).

[196] Van IJzendoorn, M.H., Goldberg, S., Kroonenberg, P.M., & Frenkel, O.J. (1992) The relative effects of maternal and child problems on the quality of attachment: a meta-analysis of attachment in clinical samples. *Child Development*, 63(4), 840–58, p.854.

From the early 1990s, Hesse undertook doctoral research at Leiden University, supervised by van IJzendoorn. As part of this research, Hesse and Main began to formulate a coding system for alarming caregiver behaviours, based initially on theory and then on review with their graduate students of 13 observations from the Berkeley sample of infant–mother or infant–father interaction during unstructured play from before the Clown session.[197] Many of the potentially alarming behaviours they observed were fleeting; the coding system developed by Hesse and Main to identify and capture these moments is penetrating, subtle, and extremely difficult to learn (even on the rare occasions on which training has been offered). It was dubbed the 'FR coding system', named after two central components: frightening and frightened caregiver behaviours. Examples of frightening behaviour provided by the coding manual were directly threatening or predatory behaviours, such as bared teeth, or lunging or looming at the infant without markers of play or prior warning. Merely angry behaviours by the caregiver, or ordinary forms of 'culturally sanctioned' discipline, were not included.[198] Frightened behaviours shown by the caregiver towards the infant were also identified, such as sudden withdrawal from the baby or a strong startle response in response to the infant's approach. Such displays were anticipated to alarm the infant when they sought the caregiver as a safe haven. A third kind of behaviour identified by Hesse and Main was apparently dissociative behaviours by the caregiver, which were assumed to potentially frighten an infant through the caregiver's inexplicable attentional unavailability.[199] The role of dissociative caregiver behaviours was proposed to Main and Hesse by their friend Giovanni Liotti, whom they had met at Bowlby's 80th birthday party in 1987 and then visited in Rome in 1990.[200]

In the course of the 1990s, Hesse and Main continued to scope potentially alarming caregiving behaviours through review of 62 further Berkeley recordings of caregiver–infant interaction and also recordings drawn from four diverse samples where Strange Situation data were also available. One was Karlen Lyons-Ruth's sample of families known to social services in Boston.[201] Another was a doctoral project by their student Mary True, who had recorded mother–infant interactions among the Dogon of Uganda.[202] A third sample was collected by Debby Jacobvitz in Texas; though a community sample, rates of alarming caregiver behaviours and of disorganised attachment were unusually high.[203] And a fourth

---

[197] This was a pilot study for part of Kelly Abrams' doctoral dissertation research: Abrams, K.Y. (2000) Pathways to disorganization: a study concerning varying types of parental frightened and frightening behaviors as related to infant disorganized attachment. Unpublished doctoral dissertation, University of California at Berkeley.

[198] Curiously, the scale did explicitly not include angry verbal threats by the caregiver to a child. This might have been simply an oversight, rather than a theoretically motived decision, given that verbal threats were included by Main in the traumatic abuse scale for the AAI composed around the same time. Additionally it is likely that, in practice, coders would code verbal threats as 'threatening' in any case.

[199] Hesse, E. & Main, M. (1999) Second-generation effects of unresolved trauma in nonmaltreating parents: dissociated, frightened, and threatening parental behavior. *Psychoanalytic Inquiry*, 19(4), 481–540.

[200] Main, M. & Hesse, E. (1992) Attaccamento disorganizzato/disorientato nell'infanzia e stati mentali dissociati dei genitori. In M. Ammaniti & D. Stern (1992) *Attaccamento e Psicoanalisi* (pp.80–140). Rome: Gius, Laterza & Figli; Liotti, G. (1992) Disorganized/disoriented attachment in the etiology of the dissociative disorders. *Dissociation: Progress in the Dissociative Disorders*, 5, 196–204.

[201] Lyons-Ruth, K., Bronfman, E., & Parsons, E. (1999) Chapter IV. Maternal frightened, frightening, or atypical behavior and disorganized infant attachment patterns. *Monographs of the Society for Research in Child Development*, 64(3), 67–96.

[202] True, M., Pisani, L., & Oumar, F. (2001) Infant-mother attachment among the Dogon of Mali. *Child Development*, 72(5), 1451–66.

[203] Jacobvitz, D.B., Hazen, N.L., & Riggs, S. (1997) Disorganized mental processes in mothers, frightening/frightened caregiving, and disoriented, disorganized behavior in infancy. Paper presented at Biennial meeting of Society for Research in Child Development, Washington, DC; Jacobvitz, D., Leon, K., & Hazen, N. (2006) Does expectant mothers' unresolved trauma predict frightened/frightening maternal behavior? Risk and protective factors. *Development & Psychopathology*, 18(2), 363–79.

sample of bereaved mothers was collected by Carlo Schuengel at Leiden for his doctoral research.[204] Both study of the Berkeley sample[205] and Schuengel's Leiden sample[206] revealed that in fact dissociative caregiver behaviours were the most predictive of disorganised attachment, more so even than directly frightening caregiver behaviours, though the two were intercorrelated.[207]

By 1995, Hesse and Main's work on the coding system had led to the addition of three further kinds of behaviour.[208] These were not in themselves assumed to be directly alarming, but were held to index the caregiver's potential for one of the three primary forms of alarming behaviour. These were: (i) behaving in a timid or deferential way toward the child;[209] (ii) sexualised behaviours toward the infant, suggesting confusion between the caregiving and sexual behavioural systems as well as a lack of capacity to monitor action; and (iii) behaviours by the caregiver that are coded in the Main and Solomon indices for infant disorganisation, such as misdirected behaviours or briefly moving in a stiff, asymmetrical manner. These latter behaviours were assumed to represent some significant disruption at the level of the caregiving system and therefore serve as distal markers of alarming caregiving. In the Berkeley sample, Hesse and colleagues found that these additional forms of FR caregiving behaviour were not associated with infant disorganised attachment; however, they suspected that this may have been a function of their low-risk cohort.[210]

[204] Schuengel, C., Bakermans-Kranenburg, M.J., & Van IJzendoorn, M.H. (1999) Frightening maternal behavior linking unresolved loss and disorganized infant attachment. *Journal of Consulting and Clinical Psychology*, 67(1), 54–63.

[205] Abrams, K.Y. (2000) Pathways to disorganization: a study concerning varying types of parental frightened and frightening behaviors as related to infant disorganized attachment. Unpublished doctoral dissertation, University of California at Berkeley.

[206] This finding is discussed in Out, D., Bakermans-Kranenburg, M.J., & van IJzendoorn, M.H. (2009) The role of disconnected and extremely insensitive parenting in the development of disorganized attachment: validation of a new measure. *Attachment & Human Development*, 11(5), 419–43, p.422.

[207] Neither study reported whether the range in the dissociation and frightening scales was equivalent. It was therefore unclear whether dissociation was more predictive because it was more frequently coded, or because it was indexing the more important cause. Anne Rifkin-Graboi, personal communication, July 2019.

[208] Hesse, E., Main, M., Abrams, K.Y., & Rifkin, A. (2003) Unresolved states regarding loss or abuse can have 'second-generation' effects: disorganized, role-inversion and frightening ideation in the offspring of traumatized non-maltreating parents. In D.J. Siegel & M.F. Solomon (eds) *Healing Trauma: Attachment, Mind, Body and Brain* (pp.57–106). New York: Norton.

[209] Hesse and colleagues identified that this behaviour was rare in the low-risk Berkeley sample and more frequently observed in high-risk samples: Abrams, K.Y., Rifkin, A., & Hesse, E. (2006) Examining the role of parental frightened/frightening subtypes in predicting disorganized attachment within a brief observational procedure. *Development & Psychopathology*, 18(2), 345–61, p.357. See also Lyons-Ruth, K., Bureau, J.F., Easterbrooks, M.A., Obsuth, I., Hennighausen, K., & Vulliez-Coady, L. (2013) Parsing the construct of maternal insensitivity: distinct longitudinal pathways associated with early maternal withdrawal. *Attachment & Human Development*, 15(5–6), 562–82.

[210] Abrams, K.Y., Rifkin, A., & Hesse, E. (2006) Examining the role of parental frightened/frightening subtypes in predicting disorganized attachment within a brief observational procedure. *Development & Psychopathology*, 18(2), 345–61. An expanded version of the FR coding system was developed by Lyons-Ruth, Bronfman, and Parsons (the Atypical Maternal Behavior Instrument for Assessment and Classification (AMBIANCE)). This assesses five dimensions of disrupted parental affective communication: negative-intrusive behaviour; role confusion; disorientation; affective communication errors; and withdrawal from the child. AMBIANCE is a more encompassing measure, with equivalent prediction of disorganised infant attachment to the FR system. Therefore, on the grounds of parsimony, some attachment researchers have expressed a preference for FR, e.g. Out, D., Bakermans-Kranenburg, M.J., & Van IJzendoorn, M.H. (2009) The role of disconnected and extremely insensitive parenting in the development of disorganized attachment: validation of a new measure. *Attachment & Human Development*, 11(5), 419–43. However, training is available annually in AMBIANCE, unlike the FR system. Efforts to economise AMBIANCE measure for use in routine clinical practice may also contribute to the popularity of the measure in the future, e.g. Haltigan, J.D., Madigan, S., Bronfman, E., et al. (2019) Refining the assessment of disrupted maternal communication: using item response models to identify central indicators of disrupted behavior. *Development & Psychopathology*, 31(1), 261–77.

Though only a tiny number of researchers have been trained by Main and Hesse to use it, the FR coding system itself has been widely praised. For instance, Rothbaum and Morelli, major critics of Ainsworth's work, praised the FR system as less prone to unacknowledged ethnocentric bias than Ainsworth's sensitivity scale.[211] Furthermore, empirical evidence has accumulated in support of the predicted association between infant disorganised attachment in the Strange Situation and caregiver behaviours coded with either the initial or the expanded version of the FR coding system. Madigan, Bakermans-Kranenburg, van IJzendoorn, and Moran reported from a meta-analysis that FR caregiver behaviour during observations accounts for 13% of the variance in attachment disorganisation.[212] Cassidy has criticised Main and Hesse for overclaiming the importance of the frightening/frightened pathway to disorganised attachment, since in fact 'the relation between frightening/frightened behaviour and infant disorganisation has been found to be relatively weak'.[213] There is certainly much unexplained variance, suggesting the role of factors besides frightening, frightened, or dissociative caregiving. Nonetheless, these are clearly causally important: the meta-analysis by Madigan and colleagues reveals that parents who displayed these behaviours were 3.7 times more likely to be part of dyads coded for disorganised attachment in the Strange Situation ($r = .34$, N = 851).[214]

An expanded version of the FR coding system was developed by Lyons-Ruth, Bronfman, and Parsons (the Atypical Maternal Behavior Instrument for Assessment and Classification (AMBIANCE)). This assesses five dimensions of disrupted parental affective communication: negative-intrusive behaviour; role confusion; disorientation; affective communication errors; and withdrawal from the child. AMBIANCE is a more encompassing measure, with equivalent prediction of disorganised infant attachment to the FR system.[215] Therefore, on the grounds of parsimony, some attachment researchers have expressed a preference for FR.[216] However, training is available annually in AMBIANCE, unlike the FR system. Efforts to economise AMBIANCE measure for use in routine clinical practice may contribute to the further popularity of the measure in the future.[217]

An important meta-analytic finding by van IJzendoorn and colleagues was that disorganised infant attachment was only weakly predicted by caregiver insensitive behaviours in general. Van IJzendoorn and colleagues concluded that the FR pathway was therefore

[211] Rothbaum, F. & Morelli, G. (2005) Attachment and culture: bridging relativism and universalism. In W. Friedlmeier, P. Chakkarath, & B. Schwarz (eds) *Culture and Human Development: The Importance of Cross-Cultural Research to the Social Sciences*. Lisse: Swets & Zeitlinger, p.110.

[212] Madigan, S., Bakermans-Kranenburg, M.J., Van Ijzendoorn, M.H., Moran, G., Pederson, D.R., & Benoit, D. (2006) Unresolved states of mind, anomalous parental behavior, and disorganized attachment: a review and meta-analysis of a transmission gap. *Attachment & Human Development*, 8(2), 89–111, p.102.

[213] Cassidy, J. & Mohr, J.J. (2001) Unsolvable fear, trauma, and psychopathology: theory, research, and clinical considerations related to disorganized attachment across the life span. *Clinical Psychology: Science and Practice*, 8(3), 275–98, p.283.

[214] Madigan, S., Bakermans-Kranenburg, M.J., Van IJzendoorn, M.H., Moran, G., Pederson, D.R., & Benoit, D. (2006) Unresolved states of mind, anomalous parental behavior, and disorganized attachment: a review and meta-analysis of a transmission gap. *Attachment & Human Development*, 8(2), 89–111.

[215] Bronfman, E., Madigan, S., & Lyons-Ruth, K. (2009–2014) *Disrupted Maternal Behavior Instrument for Assessment and Classification (AMBIANCE): Manual for Coding Disrupted Affective Communication*, 2nd edn. Unpublished manuscript, Harvard University Medical School.

[216] E.g. Out, D., Bakermans-Kranenburg, M.J., & Van IJzendoorn, M.H. (2009) The role of disconnected and extremely insensitive parenting in the development of disorganized attachment: validation of a new measure. *Attachment & Human Development*, 11(5), 419–43.

[217] Haltigan, J.D., Madigan, S., Bronfman, E., et al. (2019) Refining the assessment of disrupted maternal communication: using item response models to identify central indicators of disrupted behavior. *Development & Psychopathology*, 31(1), 261–77.

distinct from insensitivity.[218] Subsequently, however, Bailey and colleagues as well as other researchers provided evidence suggesting that the FR pathway and insensitivity overlap in high-risk families.[219] Proposals have also been put forward regarding the role of specific forms of insensitive care in disorganised attachment, including by Lyons-Ruth. Using AMBIANCE, Lyons-Ruth and collaborators identified a specific association between caregiver withdrawal from the child and disorganised attachment.[220] Another pathway to disorganised attachment has been suggested by researchers such as Spangler, who have argued that infant temperament or genetic factors may predispose at least some forms of disorganised attachment.[221] Main and Hesse have by and large been sceptical of such temperamental or genetic explanations and have pointed to the fact that classifications of disorganised attachment with different caregivers have little association, and that studies of temperamental or genetic antecedents have had a poor record of replication.[222] However, they have been intrigued by findings by van IJzendoorn and colleagues that suggest gene × environment interactions in the prediction of disorganised attachment.[223]

Yet, just as the ordinary language connotations of 'disorganisation' misled readers of Main and Solomon, so did the evocative connotations of the term 'fear' magnetise readers of Main and Hesse's chapter. Close examination of the Main and Hesse 1990 text from the vantage of the present suggests that the term 'fear' was used in a way that was insufficiently specified. The 1990 chapter fell subject to a danger already identified by Bowlby: 'unfortunately in colloquial English the word "fear" is used in many senses, often being synonymous with expectant anxiety and sometimes with fright'.[224] Main and Hesse meant to convey that one pathway to disorganised attachment may be when children come to associate their caregiver, for whatever reason, with feelings of alarm.[225] However, as a result of the way they used the term 'fear', it has been widely assumed by readers that Main and Hesse were proposing that disorganised

[218] Van IJzendoorn, M.H., Schuengel, C., & Bakermans-Kranenburg, M.J. (1999) Disorganized attachment in early childhood: meta-analysis of precursors, concomitants, and sequelae. *Development & Psychopathology*, 11(2), 225–50; Out, D., Bakermans-Kranenburg, M.J., & Van IJzendoorn, M.H. (2009) The role of disconnected and extremely insensitive parenting in the development of disorganized attachment: validation of a new measure. *Attachment & Human Development*, 11(5), 419–43.

[219] Bailey, H.N., Tarabulsy, G.M., Moran, G., Pederson, D.R., & Bento, S. (2017) New insight on intergenerational attachment from a relationship-based analysis. *Development & Psychopathology*, 29(2), 433–48. See also Gedaly, L.R. & Leerkes, E.M. (2016) The role of sociodemographic risk and maternal behavior in the prediction of infant attachment disorganization. *Attachment & Human Development*, 18(6), 554–69.

[220] Lyons-Ruth, K., Bronfman, E., & Parsons, E. (1999) Maternal frightened, frightening or disrupted behavior and disorganized infant attachment patterns. *Monographs of the Society for Research in Child Development*, 64(3), 67–96.

[221] Spangler, G., Johann, M., Ronai, Z., & Zimmermann, P. (2009) Genetic and environmental influence on attachment disorganization. *Journal of Child Psychology and Psychiatry*, 50(8), 952–61.

[222] Main's position was not, however, a full rejection of temperament-based explanations, e.g. 'I am inclined, however, to believe that researchers should still hold out the possibility of a small heritable component in disorganisation (e.g. overall fearfulness). This is an empirical question ... In my view, genetic differences may "get their innings" with respect to attachment organisation late rather than early in life.' Main, M. (1999) Epilogue. Attachment theory: eighteen points with suggestions for future studies. In J. Cassidy & P. Shaver (eds) *Handbook of Attachment* (pp.845–87). New York: Guilford, p.864–5. See also Groh, A.M., Narayan, A.J., Bakermans-Kranenburg, M.J., et al. (2017) Attachment and temperament in the early life course: a meta-analytic review. *Child Development*, 88(3), 770–95.

[223] Main, M., Hesse, E., & Hesse, S. (2011) Attachment theory and research: overview with suggested applications to child custody. *Family Court Review*, 49(3), 426–63, p.443; Bakermans-Kranenburg, M.J. & Van IJzendoorn, M.H. (2007) Research review: genetic vulnerability or differential susceptibility in child development: the case of attachment. *Journal of Child Psychology and Psychiatry*, 48(12), 1160–73.

[224] Bowlby, J. (1960) Separation anxiety. *International Journal of Psychoanalysis*, 41, 89–113, p.110.

[225] Duschinsky, R. (2018) Disorganization, fear and attachment: working towards clarification. *Infant Mental Health Journal*, 39(1), 17–29.

attachment represents a child afraid of their caregiver. It has been common to encounter statements even by authorities such as van IJzendoorn and Bakermans-Kranenburg referencing Main and Hesse as saying that, for instance, 'the essence of disorganized attachment is that the child is at times scared of the attachment figure'.[226]

To take further examples of the misapprehension of Main and Hesse's position, Paetzold and colleagues—the researchers in the social psychological tradition who have given most notice to disorganised attachment—stated that, according to Main and Hesse, 'infants in the disorganized category develop a fear of their attachment figures because these figures display frightening behaviors in their daily interactions with their children'.[227] Sinason wrote that 'disorganized attachment refers to grossly disorganized behavior on the part of the infant or child: apprehension in the presence of the mother or primary caretaker'.[228] And Rees wrote to fellow paediatricians that 'disorganized patterns arise if pervasive abuse leaves children ineffective both in self-sufficiency and in using relationships, lacking understanding of their own and others' feelings. Safe independence is unlikely and criminality in adulthood common without recovery'.[229] Reification of the fear–disorganisation relationship also appeared in proposals for National Institute for Health and Care Excellence guidelines on child attachment for clinicians in the UK.[230] However, following feedback from Main, Hesse, Lyons-Ruth, and others,[231] these guidelines were amended in the final version to avoid implying that frightening caregiver behaviour is the primary route to disorganised attachment.[232]

One contributing factor to misapprehensions regarding the role of fear in disorganized attachment may have been the illustrations in Main and Solomon's 1990 chapter.[233] This comes into relief if the illustrations in the original manuscript and the published chapter are compared. In both versions, pen drawings were presented of infants showing behaviour listed in the coding protocols. The drawings were tracings of the film negatives of video recordings of infants in the Strange Situation. In the original manuscript, the illustrations are of a variety of the behaviours. In the published version, the only set of illustrations is of explicit apprehension seen on reunion with the caregiver. There is a drawing of a child covering her mouth on reunion with her caregiver, which might also suggest confusion, but the drawing and Main and Solomon's commentary suggest that the behaviour should

---

[226] Van Rosmalen, L., van IJzendoorn, M.H., & Bakermans-Kranenburg, M.(2014) ABC+D of attachment theory. In P. Holmes & S. Farnfield (eds) *Routledge Handbook of Attachment: Theory* (pp.11–30). London: Routledge, p.21. See also Juffer, F., Struis, E., Werner, C., & Bakermans-Kranenburg, M.J. (2017) Effective preventive interventions to support parents of young children: illustrations from the Video-feedback Intervention to promote Positive Parenting and Sensitive Discipline (VIPP-SD). *Journal of Prevention & Intervention in the Community*, 45(3), 202–14: 'Disorganized attachment (Main & Solomon, 1990) is characterized by fear of the parent' (203).

[227] Paetzold, R.L., Rholes, W.S., & Kohn, J.L. (2015) Disorganized attachment in adulthood: theory, measurement, and implications for romantic relationships. *Review of General Psychology*, 19(2), 146–56, p.147.

[228] Sinason, V. (2016) The seeming absence of children with DID. In E. Howell & S. Itzkowitz (eds) *The Dissociative Mind in Psychoanalysis* (pp.221–8). London: Routledge, p.223.

[229] Rees, C. (2011) Children's attachments. *Paediatrics and Child Health*, 22(5), 186–92, p.187.

[230] National Institute for Health and Care Excellence (2015) First draft of *Children's Attachment: Attachment in Children and Young People Who Are Adopted from Care, in Care or at High Risk of Going into Care.* London: NICE. https://www.nice.org.uk/guidance/ng26/documents/childrens-attachment-full-guideline2.

[231] https://www.nice.org.uk/guidance/ng26/documents/consultation-comments-and-responses.

[232] NICE (2016) *Children's Attachment: Attachment in Children and Young People Who Are Adopted from Care, in Care or at High Risk of Going into Care.* London: NICE. https://www.ncbi.nlm.nih.gov/pubmed/26741018.

[233] Reijman, S., Foster, S., & Duschinsky, R. (2018) The infant disorganised attachment classification: 'patterning within the disturbance of coherence'. *Social Science & Medicine*, 200, 52–8.

be interpreted as indicating apprehension. In general, the facial expressions in the drawings convey terror and a crumpled misery. Though the drawings selected for inclusion in the published version are somewhat higher-quality drawings (less blotchy, more human-looking), their selection was also partly shaped by theory. They align much better with the Main and Hesse hypothesis that fear is implicated in at least some forms of disorganised attachment. Illustrations of visible fear of the caregiver served as a powerful encapsulation and expression of the process theorised to be underlying the diversity of disorganised behaviours. However, a disadvantage of privileging of illustrations of fear was that it was unrepresentative. There are a variety of behaviours used to classify disorganised attachment, including conflicted and confused behaviours without apparent apprehension of the caregiver.[234] And, in fact, visible apprehension of the caregiver in the manner of the drawings is very uncommon in community samples, and relatively rare even in samples facing significant adversities.[235] Incidence of clear apprehension of the caregiver in maltreatment samples has not been reported but is an outstanding question of the utmost significance, not least in terms of understanding the potential for measurement variance across samples among dyads who receive a disorganised attachment classification. As Padrón, Carlson, and Sroufe indicated, if one group of children show predominantly outright apprehension of the caregiver and another group predominantly non-frightened behaviours in the Main and Solomon indices, both might receive a disorganised attachment classification but have very different correlates.[236]

The choice of illustrations by Main and Solomon may well have had particular importance for the imagination of the disorganised infant by the readers of their chapter.[237] The image of fear on reunion is central, for example, to explanations of the category by researchers in papers,[238] discussion of disorganisation in textbooks for psychology students,[239] and guidance provided for social workers and other child-safeguarding practitioners in using disorganised attachment as an indicator of child maltreatment.[240] Waters criticised Main and Hesse for conveying an impression of disorganised attachment behaviours as always caused by

[234] Additionally, Solomon reported that the process of tracing the film negative lent the resulting drawings an overexpressed quality, which in her view conveyed even more of a sense of terror and misery than the films themselves. Personal communication, November 2016.

[235] E.g. adolescent parents: Forbes, L.M., Cox, A., Moran, G., & Pederson, D. (2006) Exploring expressions of disorganization in the Strange Situation in a high-risk sample. Poster presented at the World Association for Infant Mental Health, Paris, July 2006. https://ir.lib.uwo.ca/psychologypres/6/.

[236] Padrón, E., Carlson, E., & Sroufe, A. (2014) Frightened versus not frightened disorganized infant attachment: newborn characteristics and maternal caregiving. *American Journal of Orthopsychiatry*, 84(2), 201–208.

[237] The particular influence of visual representation for the interpretation of both new classificatory systems and the emotional state of others is well documented by sociologists of science: Coopmans, C., Vertesi, J., Lynch, M.E., and Woolgar, S. (eds) (2014) *Representation in Scientific Practice Revisited*. Cambridge, MA: MIT Press.

[238] E.g. Warren, S.L., Gunnar, M.R., Kagan, J., et al. (2003) Maternal panic disorder: infant temperament, neurophysiology, and parenting behaviors. *Journal of the American Academy of Child & Adolescent Psychiatry*, 42(7), 814–25: 'Infants who showed unusual behaviors such as fear of the mother, freezing, hitting, or running from the mother were classified as disorganized (group D)' (818). The selection of behaviours is heavily tilted towards those suggestive of fear, downplaying those suggestive of dissociation/confusion or conflict about approaching the caregiver but without obvious fear.

[239] Parke, R.D. & Clarke-Stewart, A. (2011) *Social Development*. New York: Wiley.

[240] Shemmings, D. & Shemmings, D. (2011) Indicators of disorganised attachment in children. http://www.communitycare.co.uk/2011/01/21/indicators-of-disorganised-attachment-in-children/; Wilkins, D. (2012) Disorganised attachment indicates child maltreatment: how is this link useful for child protection social workers? *Journal of Social Work Practice*, 26(1), 15–30. For critical appraisal of these statements see Granqvist, P., Sroufe, L.A., Dozier, M., et al. (2017) Disorganized attachment in infancy: a review of the phenomenon and its implications for clinicians and policy-makers. *Attachment & Human Development*, 19(6), 534–58.

fear, and all in the same way, blocking attention to the potential diversity of aetiological factors.[241] Lieberman criticised Main and Hesse on related grounds: for lack of clarity regarding whether disorganised attachment is essentially an expression of PTSD in children or an independent (or overlapping) construct.[242] And Bakermans-Kranenburg and van IJzendoorn drew attention to the potential 'heterogeneity of the mechanisms leading to disorganized attachment'.[243] In a 2006 article, Hesse and Main stated their wish that they had made it clearer that they intended their emphasis on frightened or frightening caregiver behaviour as 'one highly specific and sufficient, but not necessary, pathway to D attachment status'.[244] In this paper, Hesse and Main acknowledged that how their earlier work was framed and argued appears to have misled readers.[245]

Six-year systems

A move to the level of representation

When participants in the Berkeley study were six years old, 45 families were invited back to the laboratory, stratified by infant attachment classification. Whilst fathers and mothers went to be interviewed, the children were asked to do a drawing of their family. They were then asked to consider six pictured parent–child separations and offer their thoughts on what the pictured child might feel and do. They played in a sandbox for a quarter of an hour, before their parents returned—counterbalanced so that some fathers returned first and some mothers. In the early 1980s, the Berkeley group developed coding systems for these observational assessments. A coding system for the family drawings was developed by Main and her doctoral student Nancy Kaplan.[246] The response to the pictures of separation was analysed with an adaptation of a coding system developed by Klagsbrun and Bowlby.[247] And a coding system was developed for the reunion episodes by Cassidy and Main.[248] A coding system

---

[241] Waters, E. & Valenzuela, M. (1999) Explaining disorganized attachment: clues from research on mild-to-moderately undernourished children in Chile. In J. Solomon & C. George (eds) *Attachment Disorganization* (pp.265–90). New York: Guilford.

[242] Lieberman, A. & Amaya-Jackson, L. (2005) Reciprocal influences of attachment and trauma. In L. Berlin, Y. Ziv, L. Amaya-Jackson, & M. Greenberg (eds) *Enhancing Early Attachments* (pp.100–126). New York: Guilford. There seems to be extreme diversity of opinion between researchers today on this issue.

[243] Bakermans-Kranenburg, M.J. & van IJzendoorn, M.H. (2007) Research review: genetic vulnerability or differential susceptibility in child development: the case of attachment. *Journal of Child Psychology and Psychiatry*, 48(12), 1160–73, p.1164. See also Granqvist, P. (2020) *Attachment, Religion, and Spirituality: A Wider View.* New York: Guilford: 'while "fright without solution" sounds ominous, I have not yet seen persuasive evidence that the lion's share of D behaviors do in fact reflect fear of the caregiver. Granted, behaviors fitting to index 6 (direct indices of apprehension) yield converging evidence, but those behaviors tend to be quite rare in normal populations of infants. Also, for behaviors fitting the remaining six indices, a central role of fear remains hypothetical.'

[244] Hesse, E. & Main, M. (2006) Frightened, threatening, and dissociative parental behavior. *Development & Psychopathology*, 18(2), 309–343, pp.310–11.

[245] For further discussion of Main and Hesse's position on the fear–disorganisation relationship see Duschinsky, R. (2018) Disorganization, fear and attachment: working towards clarification. *Infant Mental Health Journal*, 39(1), 17–29.

[246] Kaplan, N. (1987) Individual differences in six-year-olds' thoughts about separation: predicted from attachment to mother at age one. Doctoral dissertation, University of California at Berkeley.

[247] Klagsbrun, M. & Bowlby, J. (1976) Responses to separation from parents: a clinical test for children. *British Journal of Projective Psychology*, 21, 7–21.

[248] Though Cassidy was Ainsworth's student at Johns Hopkins, she completed her dissertation on Main's data, given the close links between the two research groups. Main, M. & Cassidy, J. (1988) Categories of response to

specifically for the verbal interaction between child and caregiver on reunion was also developed by Amy Strage, a research associate in the group between 1983 and 1985.[249]

Findings from these analyses and those with the AAI were reported at a dedicated symposium in 1985 at the Society for Research in Child Development held in Toronto, and a summary published as the paper 'Security in infancy, childhood, and adulthood: a move to the level of representation' in a monograph for the Society, edited by Everett Waters and Inge Bretherton. New classifications for coding a mother's autobiographical discourse in the AAI had a strong correlation ($r = .62$) with the classification of that parent–child dyad in the Strange Situation five years earlier, and a marked correlation also for fathers ($r = .37$).[250] The prediction from infant attachment to responses at age six was an astonishing 68% to 85% in the case of the mother–child dyads. In the case of the father–child dyads, prediction from the Strange Situation to reunion behaviour was equivalent. But prediction was weak or non-significant for the other tasks. Main and colleagues supposed that, in contrast to a direct reunion with the parent, these latter measures were less effective at priming mental processes specific to the relationship with a particular parent. Their interpretation was that since almost all of the children in the subsample had their mother as their most familiar and primary caregiver, undifferentiated attachment primes such as a family drawing made children think about their mother rather than, or more than, for father.

In the early 1980s, even close collaborators and friends of Bowlby acknowledged that an inherent limitation of attachment research was that there was no way of measuring attachment after infancy.[251] Its relevance to other questions and concerns, such as therapeutic work with adults, seemed limited. Main and colleagues appeared to conclusively demonstrate that this was not so. Certainly the attachment behavioural system would change very dramatically with maturation. However, having conceptualised attentional processes as the underpinning architecture of individual differences in the Strange Situation, Main was in a position to extrapolate upwards and examine how attention was directed in relation to attachment figures in other contexts. For her, the Strange Situation procedure, children's drawings and discourse, and adult autobiographical discourse all had in common not any specific behaviour but a question about the direction of attention in relation to attachment figures. In 'A move to the level of representation', Main stated that across the different measures:

> In each of the insecure patterns of attachment, behavior and attention seem constricted in readily identifiable ways. Throughout the Strange Situation, for example, the insecure-avoidant infant attends to the environment and its features while actively directing attention away from the parent. The insecure-ambivalent infant, in contrast, seems unable to direct attention to the environment, expresses strong and sometimes continual fear and distress, and seems constantly directed toward the parent.[252]

reunion with the parent at age 6: predictable from infant attachment classifications and stable over a 1-month period. *Developmental Psychology*, 24(3), 415–26.

[249] Strage, A. & Main, M. (1985) Attachment and parent–child discourse patterns. Paper presented at Biennial meeting of Society for Research in Child Development, Toronto. PP/Bow/J.4/4.

[250] Main, M., Kaplan, N., & Cassidy, J. (1985) Security in infancy, childhood, and adulthood: a move to the level of representation. *Monographs of the Society for Research in Child Development*, 50, 66–104, p.91.

[251] E.g. Heard, D.H. (1981) The relevance of attachment theory to child psychiatric practice. *Journal of Child Psychology & Psychiatry* 22, 89–96.

[252] Main, M., Kaplan, N, & Cassidy, J. (1985) Security in infancy, childhood, and adulthood: a move to the level of representation. *Monographs of the Society for Research in Child Development*, 50, 66–104, p.74.

To situate and legitimate her ideas within the tradition of Bowlby's theory, on the first page of the 'A move to the level of representation' paper, Main described the individual differences characterised by her measures as based on differences in 'internal working models'.[253] She defined these, however, in a technical way to mean biases and filters in the processing of attachment-relevant information: 'We define the internal working model of attachment as a set of conscious and/or unconscious rules for the organization of information relevant to attachment and for obtaining or limiting access to that information, that is, to information regarding attachment-related experiences, feelings, and ideation'.[254] In terms of positioning within the academic field, claiming that the AAI assessed Bowlby's classic concept of 'internal working models' had clear symbolic advantages for gaining recognition and acceptance of Main's work.[255] However, the 'internal working model' was a problematic concept. Main did not mark for the reader that her technical definition departed from the way that the term had been used in Bowlby's work. There it could be used to mean almost anything cognitive. In particular, it could sometimes refer to mental representations of specific caregivers and sometimes to any cognitive process relevant to attachment (Chapter 1). One unfortunate result was that readers were led away from the fundamental logic through which Main extrapolated from the Strange Situation to coding systems for later in the lifespan, making this leap seem mysterious, and making the development of precise hypotheses for testing more difficult.[256]

In fact, for Main, the common thread linking the Strange Situation with her group's new measures was the 'rules for the direction and organisation of attention'.[257] Whereas in traditional psychoanalytic theory, defensive processes operate on mental content, in Main's account, attentional processes are used to exclude information that might result in patterns of attention and behaviour anticipated to be unhelpful based on representations of past experiences. Whilst representations might guide the direction of attention, for Main it was attentional processes that were ultimately what animated individual differences. So, for instance:

> In almost every assessment presented, children who had initially been judged insecure-avoidant [in infancy] showed an avoidant response pattern at 6 years of age. They directed attention away from the parent on reunion, attending to toys or to activities; responded minimally (although politely) when addressed; and sometimes subtly

[253] Zeanah and Barton reported that the concept of the internal working model, already by the end of the 1980s and thus even within Bowlby's lifetime, had all but become synonymous with Main's AAI categories. Zeanah, C.H. & Barton, M.L. (1989) Introduction: internal representations and parent–infant relationships. *Infant Mental Health Journal*, 10(3), 135–41, p.139.

[254] Main, M., Kaplan, N., & Cassidy, J. (1985) Security in infancy, childhood, and adulthood: a move to the level of representation. *Monographs of the Society for Research in Child Development*, 50, 66–104, p.66–7.

[255] On academic positioning see Baert, P. (2012) Positioning theory and intellectual interventions. *Journal for the Theory of Social Behaviour*, 42(3), 304–324.

[256] Santarelli, M. (2017) Security as completeness: a Peircean semiotic reading of the psychology of attachment. *European Journal of Pragmatism & American Philosophy*, 9(1). Attachment researchers such as Karlen Lyons-Ruth and Howard and Miriam Steele have debated the extent to which Main's ideas 'were creative achievements in their own right and were not contained in Bowlby's work'. This debate has been hampered by the fact that, in legitimising her methodological innovations, Main placed her work under the confused and confusing aegis of the 'internal working model' concept. Lyons-Ruth, K. (1998) Commentary on Steele and Steele: lexicons, eyes, and videotape. *Social Development*, 7(1), 127–31, p.128.

[257] Main, M., Kaplan, N., & Cassidy, J. (1985) Security in infancy, childhood, and adulthood: a move to the level of representation. *Monographs of the Society for Research in Child Development*, 50, 66–104, p.77.

moved away from the parent. They seemed ill at ease in discussing feelings regarding separation.[258]

The introduction of multiple new assessment methods was reported in the same chapter, alongside new reflections on Bowlby's concept of the 'internal working model'. As a consequence, all the explanations were highly compacted and their theoretical underpinnings are only sketched. Details of the six-year assessments remained obscure—with some measures, such as the family drawing, not reported at all. In the years after the 'A move to the level of representation' paper, these further details were not forthcoming. Kaplan did not publish the results from her dissertation. Strage did not write up her work. Cassidy published an analysis of the results of her dissertation work[259] but did not publish the coding system. The adaptation of the Separation Anxiety Test by the Berkeley group was also left unpublished, though it influenced work by Bretherton, Cassidy, George, and Solomon, and others on story-stem and doll-play approaches to the assessment of attachment, which have since flourished.[260] In 1986, Main completed a book manuscript with details of each of the coding systems, which was due to be published by Cambridge University Press. However, Main's sense that the systems were not yet adequately finished contributed to delays in the book's publication. One factor may have been that very few ambivalent/resistant dyads were available for the six-year follow-up, so the 'maximising' aspects of the coding systems was relatively underdeveloped. Main may also have had concerns that the coding system was 'overfitted' to her Berkeley sample, and wanted to see replications and take the chance to amend the systems before making them publicly available. Ultimately the book remained unpublished, though it circulated to several colleagues in manuscript form.

Over the decades, only a handful of individuals were ever trained in any of the six-year measures by Main.[261] Main also did not delegate the matter of training to any colleagues—until July 2019, when Naomi Gribneau Bahm, Kazuko Behrens, Anne Rifkin-Graboi, and Deborah Jacobvitz received certification to deliver trainings in the Main and Cassidy

---

[258] Main, M., Kaplan, N., & Cassidy, J. (1985) Security in infancy, childhood, and adulthood: a move to the level of representation. *Monographs of the Society for Research in Child Development*, 50, 66–104, p.96.

[259] Main, M. & Cassidy, J. (1988) Categories of response to reunion with the parent at age 6: predictable from infant attachment classifications and stable over a 1-month period. *Developmental Psychology*, 24(3), 415–26.

[260] Cassidy, J. (1988) Child–mother attachment and the self in six-year-olds. *Child Development*, 59, 121–34; Bretherton, I., Ridgeway, D., & Cassidy, J. (1990) Assessing internal working models of the attachment relationship: an attachment story completion task for 3-year-olds. In M. Greenberg, D. Cicchetti, & E.M. Cummings (eds) *Attachment in the Preschool Years: Theory, Research, and Intervention* (pp.273–308). Chicago: University of Chicago Press; Jacobsen, T., Edelstein, W., & Hofmann, V. (1994) A longitudinal study of the relation between representations of attachment in childhood and cognitive functioning in childhood and adolescence. *Developmental Psychology*, 30(1), 112–24; Emde, R.N., Wolf, D.P., & Oppenheim, D. (eds) (2003) *Revealing the Inner Worlds of Young Children. The MacArthur Story Stem Battery and Parent–Child Narratives*. Oxford: Oxford University Press.

[261] Ulrike Wartner received training from Main and achieved reliability with Main and with Ainsworth on the Main and Cassidy system: Wartner, U.G., Grossmann, K., Fremmer-Bombik, E., & Suess, G. (1994) Attachment patterns at age six in south Germany: predictability from infancy and implications for preschool behavior. *Child Development*, 65(4), 1014–27. Cohn stated that her group received training on the Main and Cassidy system in the 1980s, though no reliability test results were reported. Cohn, D.A. (1990) Child–mother attachment of six-year-olds and social competence at school. *Child Development*, 61(1), 152–62. Nancy Kaplan also trained a few colleagues to reliability: Pianta, R.C. & Longmaid, K. (1999) Attachment-based classifications of children's family drawings: psychometric properties and relations with children's adjustment in kindergarten. *Journal of Clinical Child Psychology*, 28(2), 244–55; Behrens, K.Y. & Kaplan, N. (2011) Japanese children's family drawings and their link to attachment. *Attachment & Human Development*, 13(5), 437–50; Granqvist, P., Forslund, T., Fransson, M., Springer, L., & Lindberg, L. (2014) Mothers with intellectual disability, their experiences of maltreatment, and their children's attachment representations: a small-group matched comparison study. *Attachment & Human Development*, 16(5), 417–36.

reunion system. (The same researchers will also be trained and certified to deliver training in the FR coding system from summer 2020.)[262] However, in the meantime, the lack of trained coders produced a gap in the availability of consecrated measures of attachment. For school-age children, alternatives such as the Manchester Child Attachment Story Task and the Child Attachment Interview have been developed.[263] Nonetheless, one consequence of the *de facto* unavailability of the Berkeley six-year measures has been that, with few studies being conducted, over time publications that have used these measures have become regarded as rather niche.[264] A second consequence has been that what research has been conducted with the Berkeley six-year measures has almost always occurred 'off the books', without training or a standardised test to confirm reliability against other research groups.[265] Researchers have been forced to proceed on the basis of the scanty information available in the public domain. A rather sad case is the work of Dallaire and colleagues, who describe their attempt to reconstruct a coding manual for the family drawing coding system, having carefully scoured the little information made publicly available by Main's research group.[266] Finally, a third consequence has been that new measures to address this gap have emerged only slowly, since they had to contend with the position of Main's six-year system as the orthodox and authoritative approach to assessment; as in the case of the Manchester Child Attachment Story Task, often researchers sought validation of new assessments against the Berkeley measures, treated as the gold standard.[267] They also often emulated the Berkeley four-category model. Lyons-Ruth, Bureau, and colleagues have been especially active in the

---

[262] Mary Main, personal communication, July 2019.

[263] Green, J., Stanley, C., Smith, V., & Goldwyn, R. (2000) A new method of evaluating attachment representations in young school-age children: the Manchester Child Attachment Story Task. *Attachment & Human Development*, 2(1), 48–70; Allen, B., Bendixsen, B., Babcock Fenerci, R. & Green, J. (2018) Assessing disorganized attachment representations: a systematic psychometric review and meta-analysis of the Manchester Child Attachment Story Task. *Attachment & Human Development*, 20(6), 553–77. See also the 'Security Scale', Kerns, K.A., Klepac, L., & Cole, A. (1996) Peer relationships and preadolescents' perceptions of security in the child–mother relationship. *Developmental Psychology*, 32, 457–66; the 'Child Attachment Interview', Target, M., Fonagy, P., & Shmueli-Goetz, Y. (2003) Attachment representations in school-age children: the development of the Child Attachment Interview (CAI). *Journal of Child Psychotherapy*, 29(2), 171–86; the 'Friends and Family Interview', Steele, H. & Steele, M. (2005) The construct of coherence as an indicator of attachment security in middle childhood: the Friends and Family Interview. In K.A. Kerns & R.A. Richardson (eds) *Attachment in Middle Childhood* (pp.137–60). New York: Guilford; the 'School-Age Assessment of Attachment', Crittenden, P.M., Kozlowska, K., & Landini, A. (2010) Assessing attachment in school-age children. *Child Clinical Psychology and Psychiatry*, 14, 185–208; and the 'School Attachment Monitor', Vo, D.-B., Rooksby, M., Tayarani, M., et al. (2017) SAM: The School Attachment Monitor. Paper presented at 2017 Conference on Interaction Design and Children (IDC '17), Stanford, CT, 27–30 June 2017, pp.671–4.

[264] It is striking that a high proportion of subsequent studies using the six-year systems have been published in *Attachment & Human Development*. The lack of formal interlaboratory reliability procedures may have contributed to the lack of wider interest in the results of findings using these measures, though this has not been a problem for the Ainsworth sensitivity scale.

[265] One route taken by some researchers has been to seek training in coding preschool Strange Situations from Bob Marvin, and then extrapolate upwards. E.g. Moss, E., Cyr, C., & Dubois-Comtois, K. (2004) Attachment at early school age and developmental risk: examining family contexts and behavior problems of controlling-caregiving, controlling-punitive, and behaviorally disorganized children. *Developmental Psychology*, 40(4), 519–32.

[266] Dallaire, D.H., Ciccone, A., & Wilson, L.C. (2012) The family drawings of at-risk children: concurrent relations with contact with incarcerated parents, caregiver behavior, and stress. *Attachment & Human Development*, 14(2), 161–83.

[267] E.g. Green, J., Stanley, C., Smith, V., & Goldwyn, R. (2000) A new method of evaluating attachment representations in young school-age children: the Manchester Child Attachment Story Task. *Attachment & Human Development*, 2(1), 48–70; Target, M., Fonagy, P., & Shmueli-Goetz, Y. (2003) Attachment representations in school-age children: the development of the Child Attachment Interview (CAI). *Journal of Child Psychotherapy*, 29(2), 171–86.

development of observational measures that offer equivalent categories to those identified by Main.[268] However, it is telling that they have tended to develop measures for alternative ages, such as middle childhood and seven- to eight-year-olds. This would appear partly motivated by a desire to make assessments available for these age groups, but also, implicitly, to avoid the appearance of competition with Main's six-year measures, which remain widely perceived as the 'gold standard' even if no training has been available and few studies conducted over the past decades.

Access to two unpublished books by Main offers a chance to flesh out the brief description of the reunion and family drawing measures in Main's 1985 'A move to the level of representation' paper. The first book is *Behaviour and the Development of Representational Models of Attachment* from 1986. In one of Bowlby's last pieces of professional correspondence, composed less than two months before his death in October 1990, he wrote to his Portuguese translator Sonia Monteiro de Barros: 'I wonder if you are following Mary Main's recent work? . . . She has a book in press with Cambridge University Press which will be very remarkable.'[269] This book essentially comprises the coding manuals for the Strange Situation; the AAI; the Strage and Main discourse system; the Kaplan family drawing system; and the Main and Cassidy reunion system.[270] The Kaplan adaptation to the Separation Anxiety Test was not described. The second book is *Four Patterns of Attachment Seen in Behaviour, Discourse and Narrative: An Abstract for Psychoanalysis* from 1995.[271] This book was written in honour of the psychoanalyst Joe Sandler; when he died just as the book was ready for submission, Main chose not to submit it to the publisher. The 1995 book contains a description and commentary on the measures from the 1986 book, together with a discussion of attachment and psychoanalytic theory and of epistemological aspects of Main's work. The six-year systems, little discussed in print, help reveal the logic of Main's approach to the more famous AAI, as well as her thinking about classification and method in developmental science. Together

[268] Bureau, J.-F., Easlerbrooks, M.A., & Lyons-Ruth, K. (2009) Attachment disorganization and controlling behavior in middle childhood: maternal and child precursors and correlates, *Attachment & Human Development*, 11(3), 265–84; Brumariu, L.E., Giuseppone, K.R., Kerns, K.A, et al. (2018) Middle childhood attachment strategies: validation of an observational measure. *Attachment & Human Development*, 20(5), 491–513

[269] Bowlby, J. (1990) *Letter to Sonia Monteiro de Barros*, 6 August 1990. PP/Bow/B.3/40;Main, M. (1986) *Behaviour and the Development of Representational Models of Attachment: Five Methods of Assessment*. Unpublished manuscript, Mary Main & Erik Hesse personal archive.

[270] Though it was adapted by Kaplan and Main, the Separation Anxiety Test was an already-existing measure. It was therefore not described in this book about new measurement systems. For reasons of space, and because there are no more than a handful of reliable coders, the measure will not be discussed in detail below. The most significant influence of the measure was on the rise of story-stem methods in attachment research: Bretherton, I. & Oppenheim, D. (2003) The MacArthur story stem battery. In R.N. Emde, D.P. Wolf, & D. Oppenheim (eds) *Revealing the Inner Worlds of Young Children: The MacArthur Story Stem Battery and Parent–Child Narratives* (pp.55–80). Oxford: Oxford University Press. Nonetheless, some important studies using the Kaplan and Main version of the Separation Anxiety Test include: Shouldice, A. & Stevenson-Hinde, J. (1992) Coping with security distress: the separation anxiety test and attachment classification at 4.5 years. *Journal of Child Psychology and Psychiatry*, 33(2), 331–48; Jacobsen, T., Edelstein, W., & Hofmann, V. (1994) A longitudinal study of the relation between representations of attachment in childhood and cognitive functioning in childhood and adolescence. *Developmental Psychology*, 30, 112–24; Granqvist, P., Forslund, T., Fransson, M., Springer, L., & Lindberg, L. (2014) Mothers with intellectual disability, their experiences of maltreatment, and their children's attachment representations: a small-group matched comparison study. *Attachment & Human Development*, 16(5), 417–36; Forslund, T., Brocki, K.C., Bohlin, G., Granqvist, P., & Eninger, L. (2016) The heterogeneity of attention-deficit/hyperactivity disorder symptoms and conduct problems: cognitive inhibition, emotion regulation, emotionality, and disorganized attachment. *British Journal of Developmental Psychology*, 34(3), 371–87.

[271] Main, M. (1995) *Four Patterns of Attachment Seen in Behaviour, Discourse and Narrative: An Abstract for Psychoanalysis*. Unpublished manuscript, Mary Main & Erik Hesse personal archive.

they offer deeper entry than the published record into Main's approach to the measurement of attachment and the theoretical commitments that organise this approach.

Guess and uncover

Central to Main's work in the 1980s was a new, inductive approach to the development of coding systems. Guess and uncover is a memory game for children. In the game, each player secretly writes a number pattern that follows a rule. For instance, 3, 6, 10, 15, 21, 28. They then cover all but two numbers from the right-hand-side. One player attempts to predict the third number in their friend's pattern. If they are correct (a 'hit'), they get to continue to guess the fourth number, and so on. If they do not guess correctly (a 'miss'), the number is revealed, but their opponent gets to take a turn. The game uses inductive processes in the identification of a pattern, forming the basis for a deductive system that can support further extrapolation. Main used this game as a methodology for developing new coding systems. This is only mentioned in print in any detail in Main and Cassidy's 1988 paper, and even there it appears with sufficient brevity that it was not clear how someone else might use guess and uncover in a scientific context.[272] The approach has almost never been mentioned again by subsequent attachment researchers,[273] who instead tend to chalk up Main's new coding systems to her genius, solely and unreplicably.[274] Yet there is no opposition between recognition of Main's creativity and consideration of the 'guess and uncover' methodology used in the development of her coding systems. Furthermore, inattention to or lack of awareness of Main's approach has stopped later researchers from either using or evaluating it.

Main first applied this methodology in guiding the work of a new, young research assistant in her group, Ruth Goldwyn. Edward Goldwyn had made a documentary film for the BBC in the early 1970s, depicting the work of Ainsworth at Baltimore.[275] During his time working on the project, Goldwyn became friends with Mary Main. Some years later, when he went to Berkeley to make another film, he and his 16-year-old daughter Ruth stayed

---

[272] Main, M. & Cassidy, J. (1988) Categories of response to reunion with the parent at age 6: predictable from infant attachment classifications and stable over a 1-month period. *Developmental Psychology*, 24(3), 415–26: 'A judge who was well-informed with respect to infant attachment classification in general, but who was blind to the infant attachment classifications for this sample, studied reunion responses across the sample as a whole and then (one by one) studied each child's reunion responses in an attempt to guess the probable infant attachment classification with a given parent. The sixth-year system was gradually developed from this case-by-case study. We used both rationales regarding a correct guess (match) and information regarding the actual infancy categories of sixth-year misses (mismatches) in developing the sixth-year system' (417).

[273] An exception is Goldberg, S. (2000) *Attachment and Development*. London: Routledge, p.63. The semi-dialectical method of scale development has, however, been used by former members of Main's laboratory, e.g. Solomon, J., George, C., & De Jong, A. (1995) Children classified as controlling at age six: evidence of disorganized representational strategies and aggression at home and at school. *Development & Psychopathology*, 7(3), 447–63; Cassidy, J., Marvin, R., with the Attachment Working Group of the John D. and Catherine T. MacArthur Network on the Transition from Infancy to Early Childhood (1992) Attachment organisation in preschool children: procedures and coding manual. Unpublished manual.

[274] E.g. Fonagy, P. & Campbell, C. (2015) Bad blood revisited: attachment and psychoanalysis. *British Journal of Psychotherapy*, 31(2), 229–50. For discussions of the concept of 'genius' in the history of psychology and alternative approaches that nonetheless recognise individual qualities and their influence on science see Ball, L.C. (2012) Genius without the 'Great Man': new possibilities for the historian of psychology. *History of Psychology*, 15(1), 72–83; Simonton, D.K. (2018) Creative genius as causal agent in history: William James's 1880 theory revisited and revitalized. *Review of General Psychology*, 22(4), 406–420.

[275] If at First You Don't Succeed … You Don't Succeed, released August 1972. https://genome.ch.bbc.co.uk/df74b910f3a64da5871107a126f61095.

with Main. By the time she finished secondary school, Ruth had no clear sense of her future plans. Therefore, as a gap-year, in 1981 she went to Berkeley and joined Main's group. Goldwyn was invited to read books by Bowlby and Hinde, and Darwin's book on the origin of emotions, and she audited Main's classes.[276] She also worked with Kaplan in recruiting and collecting data in the six-year follow-up, including conducting half of the interviews with parents. Once the data were collected, however, Goldwyn was not immediately needed for any other projects. Though study of events reported in the interview with the parents was part of George's doctoral project, George went on maternity leave after completing the interview transcriptions.[277]

Main was intrigued by a particular transcript: 'Although the speaker was clearly essentially coherent and collaborative, Main noted that he went to slightly unusual lengths in describing tender, emotionally affecting aspects of his life, lingering in somewhat lengthy descriptions of his loss of a beloved family member ... like a B4 infant, this speaker to a slightly unusual degree seemed to be attempting to draw and maintain the interviewer's attention, and (not untowardly) to evoke a sympathetic response.'[278] And, remarkably, this father was part of a dyad classified B4 five years earlier. Main set Goldwyn, her teenage research assistant, a 'guess and uncover' challenge. Could she match the transcripts of the parents' autobiographical interviews to their child's Strange Situation classification from five years earlier?

Ultimately the result was the basis for the AAI coding system, which is discussed later in the chapter in the section 'Adult Attachment Interview'. The system was based on 'guess and uncover' on a sample of 36 transcripts, and then applied to 66 further cases: 'Developing the system involved moving (blind) through each transcript in the development sample, and in each instance using feedback ("correct" or "incorrect") with respect to the infant's attachment classification to that adult) to refine and to further develop the rule system. This is a slow-moving but highly profitable method of rule development, and it was used in the creation of every succeeding system.'[279] Part of what made the method so powerful and creative compared to the standard hypothesis-testing tradition in psychology was that both 'hits' and 'misses' fed fine-grained inductive information into a theory-driven deductive system.[280] It was therefore exceptionally well adapted for discerning unexpected links in new data on the basis of a pre-existing frame of reference, in this case the infant attachment classifications which Main had come to regard as reflecting the basic forms of human emotional life. As Main put it, 'hypothesis-testing procedures were combined with inductive

---

[276] Ruth Goldwyn, personal communication, August 2013.

[277] The research strategy for George's dissertation had been to count incidents—such as losses—in the lives of participants, rather than to examine participants' interpretation of events: George, C. (1984) Individual differences in affective sensitivity: a study of five-year olds and their parents. Unpublished doctoral dissertation, University of California, Berkeley.

[278] Hesse, E. (2016) The Adult Attachment Interview: protocol, method of analysis, and empirical studies: 1985–2015. In J. Cassidy & P.R. Shaver (eds) Handbook of Attachment: Theory, Research, and Clinical Applications, 3rd edn (pp.553–97). New York: Guilford, p.554.

[279] Main, M. (1986) Behaviour and the Development of Representational Models of Attachment: Five Methods of Assessment. Unpublished manuscript, Mary Main & Erik Hesse personal archive.

[280] Main, M. (1995) Four Patterns of Attachment Seen in Behaviour, Discourse and Narrative: An Abstract for Psychoanalysis. Unpublished manuscript, Mary Main & Erik Hesse personal archive: 'Our approach to the development of methodologies for research in attachment has been at once dialectical and in keeping with the hypothesis-testing canons of natural science ... The reading of each transcript was informed by both our general knowledge of the meaning implicit in differing kinds of discourse or narrative, and our more specialized knowledge of processes influencing individual differences in attachment. On reading each transcript, we formed a hypothesis regarding likely infant Strange Situation response to that parent as a speaker, utilizing the existing background rules.'

processes'.[281] Assuming the accuracy of the infant classifications, the benefit would then be that 'this method maximises the likelihood of the discovery of new, attachment-associated patterns'.[282]

In her unpublished 1995 book *Four Patterns of Attachment Seen in Behaviour, Discourse and Narrative*, Main offered further reflection on the guess and uncover methodology.[283] She linked it to the idea of the 'hermeneutic circle' in the work of hermeneutic philosophers such as Heidegger, Jaspers, and Gadamer: 'In this circle, the relations between the whole and the part move forward with each repeatedly transforming and extending understanding of the other. Thus, each part contributes to the understanding of the whole which, transformed, then directs attention to new parts. These again alter the meaning of the whole'.[284] For Heidegger and later philosophers in this tradition, the hermeneutic circle was a description of how all human understanding operates. Mortal and mutable, each of us interprets new perceptions always in the context of our horizon of pre-existing assumptions, which in turn can be modified by the new perception.

Main regarded the guess and uncover method as a sharpening and intensification of this process of 'dialectic' between parts and wholes. The horizon of assumptions gets brought to an explicit point every time the researcher dares to extrapolate from their existing rules in guessing the next case, and the encounter with novelty is likewise sharpened as a source of inductive learning by the repeated feedback of both 'hits' and 'misses' and attempt to then revise existing rules. The process is then extended at a meta-level as the rules generated, ideally, on a sub-sample are applied to the sample as a whole. The system is then fine-tuned and subjected to attempts at replication on further samples. Through this process, the coding system is likely to be changed by learning from the first few additional samples.[285] Over time, the rate of learning slows, as the system is stabilised by a system of rules that are effective enough to deal with most novelty. Further refinements may occur, in principle. Without fail, *every one* of Main's coding systems identifies itself as unfinished and with future changes expected, though none has seen revision now for decades.

Main offered a characterisation of this hermeneutic circle within Ruth Goldwyn's 'guess and uncover' challenge on the AAI transcripts:

> Should a transcript predicted to belong to the parent of a secure infant then indeed be found to 'belong' to the parent of a secure infant, we continued forward with the sample utilizing the existing rules. A mis-match between our hypothesis regarding the way an infant would respond to a given speaker in the Strange Situation (e.g., secure) and the infant's actual Strange Situation behavior toward the speaker (e.g., avoidant) was regarded as an instance of real discordance if no theoretical explanation could be provided for the fact that the infant had been judged avoidant. In this case the 'rules' for identifying the parents of secure and avoidant infants would have been left unchanged. However, this same mis-match was

---

[281] Ibid.

[282] Main, M. (1986) *Behaviour and the Development of Representational Models of Attachment: Five Methods of Assessment*. Unpublished manuscript, Mary Main & Erik Hesse personal archive.

[283] Main, M. (1995) *Four Patterns of Attachment Seen in Behaviour, Discourse and Narrative: An Abstract for Psychoanalysis*. Unpublished manuscript, Mary Main & Erik Hesse personal archive.

[284] Ibid.

[285] Main, M. (1987) Project proposal to the Guggenheim Memorial Foundation, November 1987. PP/Bow/B.3/ 36/1: 'It is an elegant property of these methods that within any sample they can be almost exhaustively refined against the Strange Situation behaviour of the infant, so that even a review of this single Bay Area sample would no doubt lead to modification and improvement.'

used to tentatively refine the systems for identifying both the parents of secure and the parents of avoidant infants if a rationale for its appearance could be provided. In this case, aspects of the previous rule-systems would have been eliminated, extended or altered, and a tentative, modified system would have been devised. This modified system would then be tested as further transcripts were read and infant Strange Situation status 'uncovered'. Should the modified system fail to correctly identify the parents of other avoidant infants, it would likely be abandoned in favor of reversion to the earlier system, while success would tend to instantiate the modifications made. This semi-dialectical method of system development focuses initially upon the understanding of each individual dyad, and combines inductive and deductive strategies. Note that this method recognizes and retains genuine mis-matches between infant and parent.[286]

Reflecting on the 'guess and uncover' approach used by Main and colleagues in the development of their measures, this approach has some quite clear limitations. Main was well aware that the approach risked over-fitting coding systems to the data of the original sample. It also took continuity as a methodological assumption: this is no problem when recognised as an assumption. Yet with few details about 'guess and uncover' publicly available, attachment researchers and the wider community of readers naturally interpreted Main's identification of continuities as a research finding. This contributed to an expectation of continuity in subsequent research, and to publication bias against reports of discontinuity.[287]

With 'guess and uncover' interpreted as proof of continuity rather than as a technique for generating hypotheses, it was wholly to be expected that researchers in the 1990s would be concerned when findings showed a 'transmission gap' between AAI classifications and Strange Situation classifications.[288] However, it was also wholly to be expected that later researchers would face a growing weight of evidence suggesting much weaker continuity than in Main's findings, as they have done in the past few years (Chapter 6).[289] In the meantime, however, over decades the assumption of continuity, together with the dominance of the idea of minimising and maximising strategies, has powerfully shaped the imagination of attachment research. For instance, new measures developed for different age-groups have tended to retain the same categories used by Main. Few attachment measures have had their categories developed inductively, based on theory about age-appropriate tasks and naturalistic observation. They did not seem much need, since the relevant categories already seemed to have been set out in advance by Main. The Minnesota group are among the exceptions (Chapter 4), but their measures have had less theoretical influence, and uptake, than those of the Berkeley group.

At the same time, for the purposes of making novel observations and links, the particular strengths of 'guess and uncover' must be acknowledged. The integration of inductive and deductive strategies within the approach was central to Main's elaboration of her new methods,

---

[286] Main, M. (1995) *Four Patterns of Attachment Seen in Behaviour, Discourse and Narrative: An Abstract for Psychoanalysis.* Unpublished manuscript, Mary Main & Erik Hesse personal archive.

[287] Opie, J. (2018) Attachment stability and change in early childhood and associated moderators. Unpublished doctoral thesis, Deakin University, Melbourne.

[288] Van IJzendoorn, M. (1995) Adult attachment representations, parental responsiveness, and infant attachment. *Psychological Bulletin*, 117(3), 387–403.

[289] Verhage, M.L., Fearon, R.P., Schuengel, C., et al. (2018) Examining ecological constraints on the intergenerational transmission of attachment via individual participant data meta-analysis. *Child Development*, 89(6), 2023–37.

and to the novel hypotheses that they permitted. The hypothesis of a link between a dyad's attachment classification in the Strange Situation and qualities of the parent's discourse was perhaps the most remarkable, and is discussed further in the section 'Adult Attachment Interview'. However, 'guess and uncover' was also integral to Main and Cassidy's identification of the 'controlling' categories in the six-year reunion assessment.

The Main and Cassidy reunion system

Building on the success of Goldwyn's use of 'guess and uncover' on the AAI transcripts, the method was next applied by Cassidy during her visit to Berkeley in 1982. Several videotapes from the six-year reunion were stolen in a theft, and some tapes were unusable due to technical difficulties. There were 33 children available with reunions with both parents for Cassidy to analyse:

> As the system was first being developed, a number of correct guesses (matches) were readily made. For example, a child who craned her head around to smile at the mother, talked to mother about her experiences of the last hour, and invited the mother to play was correctly identified as having been secure with mother in infancy, and succeeding children who responded similarly to reunion with the parent were then correctly identified as having been secure with that parent in infancy. We also used misses (mismatches) in system development. For example, the first child seen to fail to speak in response to the parent's increasingly frantic conversational overtures was identified as a child who had been avoidant of the parent as an infant. When this guess proved incorrect (the child had been disorganized/disoriented), we reviewed the reunion behaviour of children who had correctly been identified as insecure-avoidant in infancy and discovered that avoidant children were at least minimally responsive to the parent when pressed, giving brief answers (e.g., 'What's that nice-looking set of toys you've been playing with?' 'Sandbox.'). Succeeding 6-year-olds who confrontationally refused response to a particular parent (e.g., 'Let me ask you again. What's that nice-looking set of toys you've been playing with?' ' … ') were considered more likely to have been disorganized/disoriented with that parent in infancy. A new, controlling-punitive response category was gradually developed and separated from the insecure-avoidant and secure response categories.[290]

The Main and Cassidy rule system was then given to an independent researcher to recode the whole sample including, it would appear, the development set. The independent researcher found 84% of child–mother reunions predictable from the infant attachment classification, and 62% of child–father reunions.[291]

Main and Cassidy classified dyads as secure if, on reunion at age six, the child remained calm and relaxed, but also expressed open pleasure on the parent's return, and initiated conversation or interaction with the parent (or seemed ready to communicate if he or she did not initiate interaction). Responsiveness to the parent was often displayed as a ready expansion

[290] Main, M. & Cassidy, J. (1988) Categories of response to reunion with the parent at age 6: predictable from infant attachment classifications and stable over a 1-month period. *Developmental Psychology*, 24(3), 415–26, p.417.
[291] Main, M. (1986) *Behaviour and the Development of Representational Models of Attachment: Five Methods of Assessment.* Unpublished manuscript, Mary Main & Erik Hesse personal archive.

of the parent's own remarks, continuing the conversation. In the Main and Cassidy system, dyads were classified as avoidant if the child responded only minimally. The six-year-old child did not turn away from the caregiver, or partially stonewall them, as might an avoidant infant (especially the A1 subgroup). Instead, the child turned down the intensity of interaction to simmer whenever opportunities arose. For instance several seemed very interested in examining the toys just as they saw their parent enter. Neither anger nor affection was much in evidence. Dyads were classified as resistant if on reunion there was 'exaggerative or maximizing of relatedness to the parent' by the child, for instance 'putting the arm around the parent and head-cocking while looking towards the camera (as though posing for a mother–child portrait), speaking in a baby-like voice, or sitting on the parent's lap.' There could be some signs of frustration with the parent, though this was much less in evidence than in the infant category.

Main and Cassidy created two categories of disorganised attachment for the six-year reunion system. In both cases the child's behaviour towards the caregiver was controlling. The first to be identified was behaviour that was punitive and directive: one previously disorganized child ordered the mother to 'Sit down and shut up, and keep your eyes closed! I said, keep them closed!'[292] Another form of punitive behaviour was rejection of the parent through a hostile and implacable silence, timed in such a way as to leave the parent humiliated or embarrassed. A further child from this group 'pushed the door shut as his mother tried to open it ... another said immediately and angrily on his mother's entrance, 'Don't bother me.'[293] In the other category the control was solicitous and caregiving. In one such dyad, the child asked the parent what she had been doing and how she was feeling, then carefully invited her to play, reassuring her that it would be fun for her. Another asked: 'Are you tired, Mommy? Would you like to sit down and I'll bring you some [pretend] tea?'[294] One form of solicitous behaviour that particularly interested Main was 'overbright' behaviour, in which the child showed a nervous, skipping cheerfulness on reunion. Main and Cassidy observed that 'brightness and caregiving of this kind do not merely alleviate the parent's present but temporary depression or anxiety, but ultimately are used to relieve or forestall the experience of anxiety by the child':

One child in the Berkeley sample had been in the playroom with the mother (with whom she was secure) when she heard the father returning. She said to the mother, in an unmistakably depressed and resigned tone, 'He's coming', but then immediately upon reunion gave an exceptionally bright greeting and smile, ("DAD!") and began immediately to attempt to direct and guide her father's attention ("See, this is a ...").[295]

[292] Hesse, E. & Main, M. (2000) Disorganized infant, child, and adult attachment: collapse in behavioral and attentional strategies. *Journal of the American Psychoanalytic Association*, 48(4), 1097–127, p.1107. That the punitive category was identified before the caregiving category is revealed by a handwritten note sent by Main to Bowlby in 1982, identifying six categories from Cassidy's work thus far: '1. Actively reestablishing relationship; 2. Responsive and confident in relationship. 3. Avoidant. 4. Punitive/rejecting. 5. Hesitant/confused. 6. Not yet classified': Main, M. & Cassidy, J. (1982) Handwritten note attached to 'Quality of attachment from infancy to early childhood: stability of classification, changes in behaviour', submitted to SRCD. PP/Bow/J.4/4.

[293] Main, M. & Cassidy, J. (1983) Secure attachment in infancy as a precursor of the ability to tolerate being left alone briefly at five years. Paper presented at 2nd World Congress of Infant Psychiatry, Cannes, March 1983. PP/Bow/J.4/4.

[294] Hesse, E. & Main, M. (2000) Disorganized infant, child, and adult attachment: collapse in behavioral and attentional strategies. *Journal of the American Psychoanalytic Association*, 48(4), 1097–127, p.1106.

[295] Main, M. (1986) *Behaviour and the Development of Representational Models of Attachment: Five Methods of Assessment*. Unpublished manuscript, Mary Main & Erik Hesse personal archive.

In the case of controlling-punitive behaviour, the anger system appeared to have been re-cruited in the service of attachment. Main and colleagues theorised that angry behaviour permitted the child to regulate the relationship, and ensured a conditional kind of proximity, even if it did not afford comfort.[296] In the case of controlling-caregiving behaviour, the care-giving system appeared to have been recruited in the service of attachment. As Bowlby had described in *Loss* just a few years earlier, caregiving behaviour displayed by a child to a care-giver might help keep the caregiver near and prop up the adult's own capacity to offer care (Chapter 1). The child was therefore also offered conditional access to proximity, even if this proximity was achieved at the expense of acknowledgement of the child's own attachment-related feelings.

Though there were too few instances for Main and Cassidy to make a third category, the researchers also noted that some children displayed sexual or romantic behaviours towards their parent. They described this as an 'emerging' category, which would probably achieve full category status after more cases had been seen.[297] Again, this could be regarded as the recruitment of components of what would later become the sexual system in adolescence, in the service of maintaining the potential for closeness with the attachment figure.[298] Some further six-year-olds displayed conflict behaviours or disorientation on reunion with their caregiver, with similar kinds of behaviours as those in the Main and Solomon infant system. Initially, Main and Cassidy also had a category for 'confused' behaviour on reunion; how-ever, this was not elaborated in later versions of the system.[299]

Ainsworth criticised Main and Cassidy for their use of the label 'disorganised attachment' to characterise controlling-punitive and controlling-caregiving behaviours in the six-year system. She did not think it was an appropriate description for behaviours that clearly seem environmentally responsive and coherently sequenced.[300] Controlling-caregiving behaviour (and perhaps controlling-punitive behaviour) could predictably offer access to conditional proximity with the caregiver, making it 'organised' by Main's own earlier definition. In the controlling-punitive and controlling-caregiving categories, attention may also be coherent, in being focused on the adult. Furthermore, the use of anger or caregiving (or sexuality) in the service of attachment could be a behavioural repertoire channelled by human evo-lutionary history, like the avoidant and ambivalent/resistant strategies. However, the term 'disorganised' was retained by Main and Cassidy to signal the longitudinal continuities with the infant category. It also served to mark two ideas held by Main and Cassidy regarding these children. A first was that the controlling behaviour suggested a chronic obstacle to the

[296] An alternative/additional hypothesis has been put forward by Bureau and colleagues. In a chaotic and threat-ening family context, it may not be wise to appear helpless; pre-emptive displays of threatening dominance may save you from trouble. Bureau and colleagues found more hostility from mother at home in infancy to be associ-ated with punitive behaviour at age 8 ($r = .40$). Punitive behaviour was also associated with severe physical abuse of the participant by mother as reported by mother when participant was age 19 ($r = .39$). Bureau, J.-F., Easterbrooks, A., & Lyons-Ruth, K. (2009) The association between middle childhood controlling and disorganized attachment and family correlates in young adulthood. Society for Research in Child Development Biennial Meeting, Denver, Colorado.

[297] Main, M. (1986) *Behaviour and the Development of Representational Models of Attachment: Five Methods of Assessment.* Unpublished manuscript, Mary Main & Erik Hesse personal archive.

[298] Main, M. & Cassidy, J. (1986) Categories of response to reunion with the parent at age six: predictable from infant attachment classifications and stable over a one-month period. PP/Bow/J.4/4.

[299] Main, M. & Cassidy, J. (1982) Handwritten note attached to 'Quality of attachment from infancy to early childhood: stability of classification, changes in behaviour', submitted to SRCD. PP/Bow/J.4/4.

[300] Ainsworth, M. (1991) Past and future trends in attachment research. International Society for the Study of Behavioral Development, Minneapolis, July 1991. Film of the presentation made available by Avi Sagi-Schwartz (Chair).

termination of the attachment system sometime earlier in the child's experience. Anger or caregiving would not have been pressed into service, they felt, if the child had received predictable access to proximity with their attachment figure in another way, whether through directly communicating distress and seeking care or through an avoidant or ambivalent/resistant conditional strategy. Secondly, a central aspect of the attachment system in childhood is that children seek care from someone stronger and/or wiser when they are distressed. However, controlling-punitive and controlling-caregiving behaviour involve an inversion of power between child and parent. There is therefore assumed to be a symbolic 'disorganisation' of the attachment system, even if behaviour is coherent, in the chronic confusion of roles.[301]

Controlling-punitive and controlling-caregiving behaviour may be smoothly sequenced and ultimately achieve a conditional proximity with the caregiver. Both punitive and caregiving behaviour allow children to approach, and their behaviour may help them retain the attention of the caregiver—understood to be a requisite to any successful functioning of the caregiving system. The fact that two main forms were found at age six, and that the evolutionary function of the controlling-punitive and controlling-caregiving behaviour could be inferred, suggests that they could be regarded as 'conditional strategies'. However, Main has never referred to the controlling-punitive and controlling-caregiving categories as 'conditional strategies'—even though this has become common usage among close collaborators such as Cassidy and Liotti.[302] She does not offer an explanation for this. The Main and Cassidy six-year system was an extrapolation from the infant system, so it is quite possible that simply by definition for Main any behaviour labelled 'disorganised' could not be a conditional strategy, with the connotations of the term itself shaping theory. Perhaps, however, it could also be that for Main a conditional strategy had to offer an alternative way of achieving the goal of the behavioural system. Other attachment researchers defined the goal of the attachment system more widely as the availability of the caregiver or the maintenance of 'organisation', and so the controlling behaviours seem to be strategic in this sense.[303]

[301] Cassidy, J., Marvin, R., with the Attachment Working Group of the John D. and Catherine T. MacArthur Network on the Transition from Infancy to Early Childhood (1992) Attachment organisation in preschool children: procedures and coding manual. Unpublished manual: 'Children who were formerly disorganized and/or disoriented have become quite organized—organized in controlling the parent. (It may be that it is the relationship that has become disorganized at age 6, in that the ordinary family structure, with the parent in control of the child, has become reversed; see Marvin & Stewart, 1990.) It is as if a child who cannot count on the parent for structure steps in and provides structure (takes control).' Comparing the infant Main and Solomon classification to the six-year controlling classifications, Cassidy and Marvin stated that 'in one, the child's behavior is disorganized; in the other, it is the usual hierarchical structuring, with parent in control of child, which has become disorganized—or at least seriously disordered'. This last qualification signals the slippage occurring as the term 'disorganised' is pressed into diverse non-overlapping usages. Acknowledging that the term disorganisation is operating at multiple levels of analysis, contributing to potential confusion, Moss and colleagues distinguished 'behaviourally-disorganized' forms of disorganisation, where apparent coherence is lacking, from controlling-caregiving and controlling-punitive behaviours. O'Connor, E., Bureau, J.F., Mccartney, K., & Lyons-Ruth, K. (2011) Risks and outcomes associated with disorganized/controlling patterns of attachment at age three years in the National Institute of Child Health & Human Development Study of Early Child Care and Youth Development. *Infant Mental Health Journal*, 32(4), 450–72.

[302] E.g. Cassidy, J., Marvin, R., with the Attachment Working Group of the John D. and Catherine T. MacArthur Network on the Transition from Infancy to Early Childhood (1992) Attachment organisation in preschool children: procedures and coding manual. Unpublished manual: 'the strategy of controlling the parent's behavior appears to have evolved from a lack of any consistent strategy for dealing with the attachment figure in infancy'; Liotti, G. (2006) A model of dissociation based on attachment theory and research. *Journal of Trauma & Dissociation*, 7(4), 55–73; Lyons-Ruth, K., Dutra, L., Schuder, M.R., & Bianchi, I. (2006) From infant attachment disorganization to adult dissociation: Relational adaptations or traumatic experiences? *Psychiatric Clinics*, 29(1), 63–86.

[303] See e.g Cassidy, J., Marvin, R., with the Attachment Working Group of the John D. and Catherine T. MacArthur Network on the Transition from Infancy to Early Childhood (1992) Attachment organisation in

By contrast, Main's model of the attachment system was formed by Bowlby's early control system model in which proximity terminated the system. The controlling-punitive and controlling-caregiving six-year-olds, even if they do achieve proximity to hit or settle their parent, do so primarily to the rhythms required for regulating the parent. Such behaviour can be inferred to ultimately benefit the attachment system in offering some proximity, but it is not clear that the system can be terminated if this rhythm is generally unrelated to the child's attachment needs.

Stability between infant attachment and the Main and Cassidy six-year system was high. All 12 infants classified as secure with mother in infancy were classified as secure five years later. Six out of the eight avoidant dyads received the same classification, as did eight out of twelve disorganised dyads.[304] This led Main and Cassidy to conclude that controlling-punitive and controlling-caregiving behaviour can be regarded as an attempt to organise and regulate the behaviour of a caregiver who might otherwise be alarming. For instance, both behaviours might retain the attention of a caregiver struggling with trauma, who might otherwise enter into episodes of abrupt unavailability. Cassidy recruited 50 dyads in Charlottesville for a replication of the six-year reunion study. Intercoder reliability was 90% ($\kappa = .84$) for the organised categories. However, eight of the twelve category disagreements involved the D category. In a reapplication of the procedure after one month in Charlottesville, stability for the disorganised classification was poor: only seven of fourteen (50%) children classified as controlling in Session 1 were controlling in Session 2.[305] This may be one reason why Main regarded the system as unfinished and has only offered training on it to a few researchers over the decades.[306]

An important later study using the Main and Cassidy system was conducted by Solomon and George, former doctoral students in Main's group. During the separation they had the children in their sample complete a doll-play procedure featuring story stems regarding getting hurt, a threatening monster, separation, and reunion; meanwhile, their mothers were asked to complete the AAI and an interview about their experiences as a parent.[307] The six-year reunions were coded by Cassidy. Solomon and George found that the mothers of

preschool children: procedures and coding manual. Unpublished manual: 'The concept of "strategies" refers to each individual's attempts to maintain a particular organization in relation to attachment.'

[304] Main, M. & Cassidy, J. (1988) Categories of response to reunion with the parent at age 6: predictable from infant attachment classifications and stable over a 1-month period. *Developmental Psychology*, 24(3), 415–26.

[305] Ibid. p.421.

[306] Another replication of the Main and Cassidy study was conducted by Wartner and colleagues, who managed to recall 40 of the Regensburg sample (92%) five years later. Wartner received training in the coding system from Main, and a number of videos were second coded by Main and Ainsworth for reliability. Prediction from infancy to the six-year reunion revealed 82% agreement ($\kappa = .723$). Wartner, U.G., Grossmann, K., Fremmer-Bombik, E., & Suess, G. (1994) Attachment patterns at age six in south Germany: predictability from infancy and implications for preschool behavior. *Child Development*, 65(4), 1014–27. Kazuko Behrens' doctoral thesis, supervised by Main and Hesse, was intended as a further attempt to replicate Main and Cassidy in the Japanese context. Behrens found a strong ($r = .60$) relationship between the AAI with parents and the six-year reunions. Behrens, K.Y., Hesse, E., & Main, M. (2007) Mothers' attachment status as determined by the Adult Attachment Interview predicts their 6-year-olds' reunion responses. *Developmental Psychology*, 43(6), 1553–67.

[307] The procedure resembles the Kaplan and Main Separation Anxiety Test, another projective measure used with the six-year participants in the Berkeley sample while the parents were taken for AAIs. The findings were also strikingly similar. However, details of the findings from Kaplan's Separation Anxiety Test were only briefly described in print at the time, with most of Kaplan's work remaining unpublished. For a subsequent summary of these findings see the discussion of the Separation Anxiety Test in Main, M., Hesse, E., & Kaplan, N. (2005) Predictability of attachment behavior and representational processes at 1, 6, and 19 years of age: the Berkeley Longitudinal Study. In K.E. Grossmann, K. Grossmann, & E. Waters (eds) *Attachment from Infancy to Adulthood: The Major Longitudinal Studies* (pp.245–304). New York: Guilford, p.256.

secure six-year-olds had a distinctive quality in offering a balanced and detailed provision of helping the child cope with worries. The mothers of avoidant six-year-olds had a distinctively rejecting quality both towards the child and towards the caregiver's own difficulties, with a pervasively negative attitude towards themselves and their child.[308] And the mothers of controlling six-year-olds described feeling helpless and out of control in their relationships with the child: 'Some children in the controlling group were described as wild or helpless and vulnerable (e.g., locking the mother out of the house, persistent bed-wetting, wild tantrums). Other children were described as precocious or powerful (e.g., comedian-like behavior, amazing acting abilities, caregiving skills, supernatural powers, special connections with the deceased).'[309] All of the caregivers classified as unresolved on the AAI were part of dyads classified as controlling on reunion; indeed, there was a match between six-year reunion and AAI classifications in 81% of cases ($\kappa = .74$).[310]

In their doll-play, the children classified as controlling demonstrated themes of fear and danger, in contrast to the rest of the sample: 'the narrative structure of these stories can best be described as chaotic and flooded. Catastrophe, sometimes multiple catastrophes, often arise without warning; dangerous people or events are vanquished, only to surface again and again. Objects float and have magical, malignant powers; punishments are abusive and unrelenting'; 'fantastic disasters frequently arose without warning. Further, children hastily gave post hoc explanations for these as though they were surprised and disturbed by the direction the story had taken.'[311] Five of the seven children classified as controlling-caregiving seemed 'extremely uncomfortable with the task and did not want to enact a story'. When given repeated prompts, their narratives were brimming with themes of 'chaos and disintegration'.[312] Solomon and George observed that for the controlling group as a whole, 'fears disrupted their doll-play by flooding the content in a chaotic and primitive way or were inflexibly contained through a brittle strategy of inhibition of play'.[313] Children from dyads classified as controlling were more likely to be judged as having behavioural problems by their teachers and by their parents, whereas there were no differences between the secure and organised-insecure dyads on these measures.

After her work on the six-year reunion system, Cassidy undertook a large project with another of Ainsworth's former students, Robert Marvin, in the development of a preschool system for coding the Strange Situation. These efforts were supported by a working group, including Ainsworth and Main, funded by the MacArthur Foundation.[314] Unlike the Ainsworth coding system, which developed inductively from naturalistic observation, the Cassidy and Marvin coding protocol elaborated 'up' from the infant coding system and

---

[308] George, C. & Solomon, J. (1996) Representational models of relationships: links between caregiving and attachment. *Infant Mental Health Journal*, 17(3), 198–216, p.210.

[309] Ibid. p.212.

[310] Ibid. Table 4.

[311] Solomon, J., George, C., & De Jong, A. (1995) Children classified as controlling at age six: evidence of disorganized representational strategies and aggression at home and at school. *Development & Psychopathology*, 7(3), 447–63, p.454, 460.

[312] Ibid. p.454.

[313] Ibid.

[314] The members of the working group who contributed to the Cassidy and Marvin system were Mary Ainsworth, Kathryn Barnard, Leila Beckwith, Marjorie Beeghly, Jay Belsky, Janet Blacher, Inge Bretherton, Wanda Bronson, Heather Carmichael-Olsen, Dante Cicchetti, Keith Crnic, Mark Cummings, Ann Easterbrooks, John Gottman, Mark Greenberg, Robert Harmon, Lyn LaGasse, Mary Main, Colleen Morisset, Janet Purcell, Doreen Ridgeway, Nancy Slough, Susan Spieker, Mathew Speltz, and Joan Stevenson-Hinde.

'down' from the six-year reunion system.[315] Main's 'guess and uncover' method was used with a set of 300 Strange Situations drawn from various American (and one British) research groups. The MacArthur preschool system is based in the first instance on common themes between the two systems. First, 'the pattern shown by infants classified insecure/avoidant (pattern A) is strikingly similar to that shown by six-year-olds classified insecure/avoidant: children at both ages avoid intimate interaction or contact, maintain an affective neutrality, and convey the impression that the parent's return is of no particular importance to them'. Second, 'the pattern shown by infants classified securely attached (pattern B) is strikingly similar to that shown by six-year-olds classified securely attached: children at both ages show interest in proximity or at least interaction with the attachment figure'. Third, the ambivalent preschool classification incorporates the resistance of the Ainsworth infant system and the intensified signalling of relatedness to the parent of the Main and Cassidy system. Immature behaviour contributes to a subclassification of ambivalence, on the analogy of passivity in the Ainsworth infant system. Fourth, disorganised attachment is coded on the basis of either Main and Solomon behaviours from the infant system or the controlling-caregiving or controlling-punitive behaviours from the Main and Cassidy system. In 2002 Cassidy and Marvin added some additional subclassifications, including a depressed subclassification and one for children who seemed overtly fearful of their caregiver.[316]

The Cassidy and Marvin system has been used very widely and, with annual training available, new studies using the approach continue to regularly appear. As such, in all likelihood it represents the most important legacy of the Main and Cassidy system, where training has not been available. There has been a severe bottleneck for relevant research in middle childhood over the decades. For instance, the only large randomised study of adoption after institutionalisation, the English and Romanian Adoptee project, conducted a separation-reunion procedure with their participants at age six. Due to the *de facto* lack of availability of the Main and Cassidy method, the researchers chose to code their data using the Cassidy and Marvin system. They found uninterpretable results.[317] The researchers concluded that the Cassidy and Marvin system was not appropriate for their study. Given the unique nature and global importance for policy of the English and Romanian Adoptee project, this was a wasted opportunity on a historic scale.

Given the lack of availability of training, the most—and potentially the only—especially influential study since the 1990s to have used the Main and Cassidy system was a longitudinal study by Ellen Moss and colleagues. With a community sample of 120 French Canadian children, they coded the Strange Situation at 2.5 years using the Cassidy and Marvin system and a separation-reunion procedure coded with the Main and Cassidy system at 5.5 years. Though trained in the Cassidy and Marvin system, it is not clear that Moss and colleagues were trained in the Main and Cassidy system, or sought (or could seek) interlaboratory reliability. The researchers found moderate stability of attachment classifications over the preschool years (secure: 72%, $z = 6.0$; avoidant: 44%, $z = 3.6$; ambivalent: 62%, $z = 5.0$; disorganized: 77%, $z = 5.6$). None of the dyads classified as disorganised at 2.5 years was classified

[315] Cassidy, J., Marvin, R., with the Attachment Working Group of the John D. and Catherine T. MacArthur Network on the Transition from Infancy to Early Childhood (1992) Attachment organisation in preschool children: procedures and coding manual. Unpublished manual.

[316] Ibid. Update September 2002.

[317] Kreppner, J., Rutter, M., Marvin, R., O'Connor, T., & Sonuga-Barke, E. (2011) Assessing the concept of the 'insecure-other'category in the Cassidy–Marvin scheme: changes between 4 and 6 years in the English and Romanian adoptee study. *Social Development*, 20(1), 1–16.

as secure at 5.5 years. Changes from secure to disorganised attachment were associated with changes in caregiver behaviour towards the child,[318] lower marital satisfaction, and events such as bereavement and parental hospitalisation. In addition to the separations associated with hospitalisation, Moss and colleagues offered the speculation that 'parental hospitalization is also likely to compromise the child's confidence in parents as a source of protection and security.'[319]

In an expansion of the sample by Moss and colleagues to include a number of five-year-olds, 68% of the children classified in the D group showed one of the controlling responses on reunion; 32% showed Main and Solomon-style disorganisation. Maternal report of marital conflict and unhappiness was associated with the display of Main and Solomon indices on reunion, but not with the Main and Cassidy controlling behaviours: 'The unpredictability and overwhelming nature of the family environment, which is disrupted by severe marital conflict, may compromise the possibility of the child's forming an organized integrated model of attachment, even one of a role-reversed controlling nature.'[320] The researchers did not include measures of exposure to violence, abuse, neglect, or other forms of adversity that might have shed further light on the experiences of these children. However, contrary to the researchers' expectation, Moss and colleagues found no association between maternal depression and any of the forms of disorganisation, including the controlling strategies. Though given that this was a community sample, they by no means ruled out that such an association would be seen in a population facing more adversities. Moss and colleagues did find, though, that families of children who developed a controlling-caregiving pattern were more likely to have experienced a major bereavement. Children who showed controlling-punitive behaviours on reunion with their parent were rated by teachers as displaying more conduct problems at school; children who showed controlling-caregiving behaviours were rated by teachers as displaying more anxiety and depression at school.

The Kaplan and Main family drawing system

Another of the six-year systems developed by the Berkeley group was a system for coding family drawings. The use of drawing tasks as a projective measure had roots in the work of both Bowlby and Ainsworth.[321] The children in the Berkeley six-year follow-up had been

---

[318] The Moss and colleagues observational measure of caregiver–child interaction includes scales for: Coordination, Communication, Partner Roles, Emotional Expression, Responsivity–Sensitivity, Tension, Mood, and Enjoyment. See Moss, E., Rousseau, D., Parent, S., St-Laurent, D., & Saintonge, J. (1998) Correlates of attachment at school age: maternal reported stress, mother–child interaction, and behavior problems. *Child Development*, 69, 1390–405.

[319] Moss, E., Cyr, C., Bureau, J. F., Tarabulsy, G.M., & Dubois-comtois, K. (2005) Stability of attachment during the preschool period. *Developmental Psychology*, 41(5), 773–83, p.781. Moss and colleagues also conducted the Solomon and George doll-play measure with their sample when the children were aged eight. Agreement between the Main and Cassidy system and the doll-play measure was 73% (κ = .45), Dubois-Comtois, K., Cyr, C., & Moss, E. (2011) Attachment behavior and mother–child conversations as predictors of attachment representations in middle childhood: a longitudinal study, *Attachment & Human Development*, 13(4), 335–57.

[320] Moss, E., Cyr, C., & Dubois-comtois, K. (2004) Attachment at early school age and developmental risk: examining family contexts and behavior problems of controlling-caregiving, pontrolling-punitive, and behaviorally disorganized children. *Developmental Psychology*, 40(4), 519–32, p.529.

[321] In his 'Forty-four thieves' paper, Bowlby reported on a case where he had used a drawing task to seek a sense of the child's inner life: 'Lily had always been a miserable and frightened child ... She spent most of her spare time in the streets just mooning about. She was very slow and dreamy and took hours to do things. Her mother described how she sometimes got "miles away" which made her feel "creepy" ... When asked to do a drawing she preferred an abstract design to a picture.' Bowlby, J. (1944) Forty-four juvenile thieves: their characters and home-life.

asked to complete a family drawing. Like Ainsworth's use of projective measures (Chapter 2), Kaplan and Main intended the family drawing task as a standardised, ambiguous, and evocative stimulus, to elicit individual differences based on past experiences in the family relationships. It was also well aligned with Kaplan's background in arts and humanities from her undergraduate studies at Sarah Lawrence College.[322] The 'guess and uncover' methodology was, once again, utilised in the development of the Kaplan and Main drawing system. However, rather than use a development sample and then apply the scheme to the rest of the data, the number of family drawings was judged too small for this approach. Kaplan and Main therefore performed no external test, but used the whole sample in the development on the scheme: 'Moving blind through the set of drawings while developing the rules for identifying the classifications, the two original judges independently obtained hit-rate [with the infant classifications] of close to 80%. The drawings and the rule-system were then given to a third blind judge who had not participated in the development of the system: this judge obtained an overall hit-rate of 76%.'[323]

Family drawings classified as secure by Kaplan and Main had the general quality of being 'rational and realistic'. Kaplan and Main found that figures tended to be complete, with eyes, nose, mouth, hair, hands, and feet. This was despite the fact that there was no relationship between an independent assessment of drawing skill and attachment classification at age six. Drawings classified as secure had figures that seemed well grounded, with legs planted in a way that suggested that the floor beneath them, even if invisible, was adequately stable. Figures appeared in the middle of the picture, and did not have their arms closed off from one another or seem to be in over-rigid postures. When height differences were characterised, no figure loomed over anyone else. Objects and houses might appear in the picture, but did not dominate the scene in a way suggesting that attention was being directed away from the attachment figures. A curious aspect of the secure classification in the Kaplan and Main system is that they specifically stated that the absence of the self from the picture is not relevant to the classification. This was partly the result of their inductive methodology, since the absence of the subject was seen in a number of pictures where the child had previously been classified secure in infancy. However, the conclusions also seems theoretically motivated. Whereas 'internal working models' are generally described by other attachment researchers as representations of the self and others (Chapters 1 and 5), the secure classification on the six-year drawing system shows that this was not Main's primary concern. Depictions of the self are not necessarily relevant: what mattered was the kind of attention directed towards or away from attachment figures and attachment-relevant experiences (Chapter 2).

International Journal of Psycho-Analysis, 25, 19–53, p.26. Bowlby, Ainsworth, and colleagues also asked children to complete projective drawing tasks after they returned from hospitalisation. Ainsworth, M.D. & Boston, M. (1952) Psychodiagnostic assessments of a child after prolonged separation in early childhood. *British Journal of Medical Psychology*, 25, 169–201, p.175.

[322] Karen, R. (1998) *Becoming Attached: First Relationships and How They Shape Our Capacity to Love.* Oxford: Oxford University Press, p.211.

[323] Main, M. (1986) *Behaviour and the Development of Representational Models of Attachment: Five Methods of Assessment.* Unpublished manuscript, Mary Main & Erik Hesse personal archive. No further information appears to be available regarding the breakdown of associations between the infant attachment classifications and the six-year drawing system, or the associations between the different six-year systems. The match between the infant classifications and the Kaplan drawing system for mothers was reported as 78% and as non-significant for fathers by Main, M. (1987) Project proposal to the Guggenheim Memorial Foundation, November 1987. PP/Bow/B.3/36/1.

Family drawings classified as avoidant by Kaplan and Main had many merry figures with little individuation. They also often lacked arms, or had their arms in postures not suitable for physical contact with others. Kaplan and Main found this especially interesting, since when asked to do a different drawing, of a bear, arms were then present and the apparently unwelcoming posture was absent. The figures also seemed rather isolated from one another on the page. The overriding characteristic was a picture of a family with attention directed away from the potential for the members' potential vulnerability to or intimacy with one another. Family drawings classified as resistant tended to draw out-of-scale family figures, placed very close together, sometimes even with overlapping arms or shoulders. Several features of the drawings emphasised vulnerability. For instance, some of the children drew themselves with round bellies; half of children in this category, and no other child in any other classification, drew an unusual slant to the neck and head relative to the shoulders and the rest of the body, a posture that suggested coy submission. However, there were relatively few ambivalent/resistant children in the sample, and the classification was somewhat unfinished.[324]

Drawings classified as disorganised had some disrupted or chaotic elements, such as the child having to redo and redo the task or being unable to attempt it effectively. Kaplan and Main also identified two elements that corresponded to the punitive and caregiving behaviours that had been observed by Cassidy in the reunion episodes. A first was the presence of ominous elements in the picture, such as black clouds looming over the figures, dismembered or floating body-parts, or rows of skeletons in the background.[325] A second was overbright elements 'which at first sight appear simply very sweet or very cheerful (e.g. a family standing on a row of hearts with a small sun drawn directly over the mother's head; a huge sun with a smiling face dominates the figures in the picture)'. This was different to the addition of hearts and flowers added by many other children, since here the cheerful elements seemed to dominate the image and to have a role in emotionally propping up the characters rather than expressing their inner state.

Though an unpublished system, the research community was intrigued by the Kaplan and Main coding system, since it seemed to offer a special access to the child's 'internal world'.[326] It was also the least resource-intensive measure to date produced by the developmental tradition of attachment research. An attempt to replicate the Kaplan and Main study was conducted by Fury, Carlson, and Sroufe using data from the Minnesota Longitudinal Study of Risk and Adaptation. No training by Kaplan or Main or attempt to achieve cross-laboratory

---

[324] Poor inter-rater reliability was reported by Pianta and Longmaid on the distinction between resistant and disorganised family drawings: Pianta, R.C. & Longmaid, K. (1999) Attachment-based classifications of children's family drawings: psychometric properties and relations with children's adjustment in kindergarten. *Journal of Clinical Child Psychology*, 28(2), 244–55.

[325] These ominous elements also seemed to resonate with Kaplan and Main's insecure/disorganized-fearful classification for the Separation Anxiety Test. In response to pictures of child–caregiver separations, functioning as story stems, children who received this classification showed behaviours suggestive of fear. These included extreme voicelessness occurring only in response to the test stimuli, lapses in discourse disorganization suggestive of segregated systems (e.g. 'yes-no-yes-no-yes-no'), accounts of events with an eerie quality in which there is no human cause, or worries that the caregiver might have died. Some children also became abruptly aggressive to the assessor or the test materials. Kaplan, N. (1987) Individual differences in 6-years olds' thoughts about separation: predicted from attachment to mother at age 1. Unpublished doctoral dissertation, Department of Psychology, University of California, Berkeley.

[326] E.g. Warren, S.L., Emde, R.N., & Sroufe, L.A. (2000) Internal representations: predicting anxiety from children's play narratives. *Journal of the American Academy of Child & Adolescent Psychiatry*, 39(1), 100–107.

reliability was reported.[327] The children in the study were eight- to nine-year-olds. Fury and colleagues had concerns about some aspects of the system. First, 'many of the Kaplan and Main signs that required a large measure of subjectivity (e.g., "faint ominousness"; "pained smile") were excluded'.[328] Second, some of the signs seemed overparticular, and a product of overfitting of the coding system to the Berkeley sample. Indeed, they found that only one of the indicators of avoidance from the Berkeley drawing study—the positioning of figures' arms—was associated with avoidant attachment in the infant Strange Situation in the Minnesota sample. Fury also alleged that the semi-inductive 'guess and uncover' methodology used by Kaplan and Main was overly scattershot in the identification of specific markers, and that Kaplan and Main offered too little in the way of principles regarding 'precisely how various descriptors were organised and distributed'.[329] In the Fury study, none of the individual markers of disorganised attachment in the drawing system was associated with disorganised attachment in the infant Strange Situation. However, when signs were combined into aggregate indices, the expectable associations appeared, though associations were weak or modest (avoidance, $r(168) = .15$, $p < .05$; resistance, $r(168) = .27$, $p < .001$).[330] The best association of the drawing system was not with the infant Strange Situation, but with a global measure of mental health: a .32 association with resistance in girls (though no association for boys) and a .36 association with avoidance in boys (though no association for girls).[331] Main was dismayed by these results, and in a 1995 chapter concluded that 'children's drawings should not be used in the assessment of attachment': at most, they should be 'regarded only as correlates of early attachment'.[332]

The Minnesota findings were replicated by Madigan and colleagues with 127 dyads drawn from a moderate-risk sample in Ontario, with a significant proportion of children diagnosed with forms of heart disease. Again, no training by Kaplan or Main or attempt to achieve cross-laboratory reliability was reported. These researchers found few links between infant attachment and specific markers in the drawings made by the seven-year-olds in their sample. However, they found that the match between the infant and the seven-year attachment classifications was 80%, with most of the mismatches occurring for the avoidant infant category: over half were classified as secure in the drawing system. The low stability in the high-risk Minnesota study and the high stability in the lower-risk Berkeley and Ontario samples is in line with findings regarding the stability of attachment classifications in general (Chapter 2). Madigan and colleagues speculated that a higher proportion of disorganised cases in the Minnesota study may also have played a role in the different results.[333]

---

[327] Inter-rater reliability was instead reported between Fury and an undergraduate student in Fury, G.S. (1996) The relation between infant attachment history and representations of relationships in school-aged family drawings. Unpublished doctoral dissertation, University of Minnesota.

[328] Fury, G., Carlson, E.A., & Sroufe, L.A. (1997) Children's representations of attachment relationships in family drawings. *Child Development*, 68(6), 1154–64, p.1115. A more detailed discussion of the excluded items is available in Fury, G.S. (1996) The relation between infant attachment history and representations of relationships in school-aged family drawings. Unpublished doctoral dissertation, University of Minnesota.

[329] Ibid.

[330] Fury, G., Carlson, E.A., & Sroufe, L.A. (1997) Children's representations of attachment relationships in family drawings. *Child Development*, 68(6), 1154–64, p.1161.

[331] Ibid. Table 1.

[332] Main, M. (1995) Recent studies in attachment: overview, with selected implications for clinical work. In S. Goldberg, R. Muir, & J Kerr (eds) *Attachment Theory: Social, Developmental and Clinical Perspectives* (pp.407–70). Hillsdale, NJ: Analytic Press, p.429.

[333] Madigan, S., Ladd, M., & Goldberg, S. (2003) A picture is worth a thousand words: children's representations of family as indicators of early attachment. *Attachment & Human Development*, 5(1), 19–37.

Running contrary to Main's 1995 claim that the drawing system should no longer be used as a measure of attachment, in a 2016 paper Gernhardt and colleagues observed that the system had, in fact, become increasingly popular over the subsequent decades. Suspicious of the measure, they wondered about its cross-cultural applicability. In their study, Gernhardt and colleagues used the drawing system—though without the disorganised classification—with 32 six-year-old children from Berlin and 21 six-year-old children from rural farming villages around Kumbo in Cameroon. Once again, no training by Kaplan or Main or attempt to achieve cross-laboratory reliability was reported. Their results showed that most of the pictoral markers of insecurity were dramatically more common in the Kumbo sample. For instance, neutral or negative facial affect characterised every drawing by the children from Kumbo, compared to a tiny fraction of the children from Berlin. Likewise, lack of individuation, arms downwards, and unusually small figures were common features in the Kumbo pictures, whereas they were rare in the Berlin pictures. Nearly half of the Kumbo drawings omitted the mother, whereas none of the Berlin drawings did so. Gernhardt concluded that the Kaplan and Main system is essentially a cultural artefact, without any cross-cultural validity. This conclusion is questionable since they did not examine whether the results of the drawing measure correlate with expectable individual differences in the children's lives or behaviour. Their view was that to do so would have been culturally inappropriate and potentially pathologising. Nonetheless, Gernhardt and colleagues do effectively make the point that many markers of insecurity identified by Kaplan and Main on the Berkeley sample need to be treated with caution when applied to contexts with different ways of thinking about, representing, and experiencing family life.[334] This caution is especially important since the underpinning principles for the Kaplan and Main system, which could have been used by researchers to responsively elaborate the specifics of the coding system to achieve greater cross-cultural applicability, remain unpublished and, additionally, underdescribed even in the unpublished texts.

Adult Attachment Interview

Semantic and episodic information

During the six-year follow-up at Berkeley, while their children were busy with tasks such as completing the family drawing, mothers and fathers were interviewed separately about their experiences relevant to attachment. Bowlby's 1980 book *Loss* had been shared with Main in draft a few years earlier. In this work Bowlby was interested in the variety of forms that memory can take, and especially the work of Tulving. According to Tulving, 'episodic' information comprises temporally dated episodes or events and of relations between such episodes or events, as experienced by an embodied subject; by contrast, 'semantic' information contains generalised propositions about the world.[335] Bowlby argued that whereas episodic information derives primarily from an individual's own embodied experience, semantic information is more explicit, linguistically encoded knowledge, in particular what others have

[334] Gernhardt, A., Keller, H., & Rübeling, H. (2016) Children's family drawings as expressions of attachment representations across cultures: possibilities and limitations. *Child Development*, 87(4), 1069–78.

[335] Tulving, E. (1985) How many memory systems are there? *American Psychologist*, 40, 385–98.

told the individual, especially as a child.[336] Kaplan, George, and Main therefore developed an interview protocol to include prompts for both descriptions of key attachment relationships and specific supportive memories.

The AAI began with a question, developed by Kaplan on the basis of her clinical interests,[337] asking speakers to describe their relationship with their parents. Main added a request that speakers choose five adjectives to describe each relationship, a prompt for semantic memory.[338] Speakers were then asked to explain what made them choose each adjective with reference to illustrative memories, a prompt for episodic memory. They were asked what they did when they were upset in childhood, a verbal analogue in the AAI for the separations and reunions experienced by a child in the Strange Situation procedure. Speakers were also asked whether they could remember being physically held by their parents for comfort as a child. This question was likewise a verbal analogue, this time for Main's 'Aversion to Physical Contact' scale for infants, which had proven singularly effective in discriminating caregivers in avoidant dyads in the Baltimore and Berkeley samples (Chapter 2). Another question asked by the interview protocol concerned whether speakers had any experiences of feeling rejected as a child, and if yes, why they now thought their parents had behaved as they did. Additionally, participants were asked whether they had undergone any major separations from their parents in childhood, building on Bowlby's classic concern (Chapter 1). They were also asked about occasions when parents might have been threatening to them, following on from Main's interest in the role of threatening behaviour in the aetiology of avoidant attachment. In line with a particular concern of Kaplan and Main's, and the topic of Bowlby's most recent book on *Loss*, participants were questioned about experiences of loss and bereavement. Participants were also asked about why their parents behaved as they did, and whether their early experiences of care have affected them as an adult.[339]

Any one of these questions might be asked of a person in certain contexts in ordinary life. However, the requirement to respond to this cumulative incision into speakers' experience of their attachment relationships was a demanding and potentially distressing challenge. It cut away the familiar, conventionalised rhythms of interaction that usually offer us mooring against memory. At the same time, a chance to talk to an interested person about personal experiences without interruption, exasperation, or contempt is something quite special. Amidst all its bustle, it is rare in ordinary life that we are freely given sustained and patient attention by another. Furthermore, the overall tone of exemplary incidents from our childhood is something that we have little reason to share as adults, and may have few prompts to consider in any structured way. There is a quality of matter-of-fact strangeness to the intimacy of delivering or receiving an AAI.

Applying the 'guess and uncover' approach, the first pattern identified by Goldwyn was that some parents described their childhoods in flatly glowing terms. There were no problems; everything was fine. Yet, intriguingly, rather than belonging to the accounts of parents from securely attached dyads, these accounts of perfect childhoods belonged to the parents from avoidantly attached dyads. Main and Goldwyn therefore termed this 'idealisation'. In a conference paper giving the first public report from this research, Main described a

---

[336] Bowlby, J. (1980) *Loss*. London: Pimlico, p.62–3.
[337] Kaplan's graduate work was part-funded by the National Center for Clinical Infancy Programs, and she subsequently became a clinician.
[338] George, C., Kaplan, N., Goldwyn, R., & Main, M. (1982–83) Attachment interview for parents. PP/Bow/J.4/4.
[339] Ibid.

'mother who stated initially that her mother "was a good one" and that they had "a fine relationship" later in the interview told us—as though spontaneously—that she had painfully broken her hand as a child. Although she had been in pain for weeks she had not told her mother because her mother would have been angry. This incident was recounted in almost the third person—i.e. "but one couldn't tell her". When this mother was seen in the Strange Situation with her infant, the behaviour of the child led to the dyad receiving top scores for avoidance.[340] Another facet of the transcripts of parents from avoidantly attached dyads was that though the parent asserted an ideal childhood, in fact they could supply few or no concrete memories of experiences of intimate and caring interactions. They often seemed to show little regard for "the need to depend on others" or "recognition of missing and needing others or being missed and needed by others".[341]

Furthermore, there were indications in the transcripts that at points speakers had experienced rejection in their attachment relationships. Yet this did not seem to inform the speaker's overall characterisation of the relationship, which was resolutely positive. Main ran an initial test on the first 26 transcripts and found a substantial association between idealisation of the parent and indications of early experiences of rejection ($r = .51$).[342] She also found a robust association between reports of early experiences of rejection in the AAI and displays of aversion to physical contact with the infant in the Clown session: $r = .56$ for mothers and $r = .63$ for fathers.[343] However, Main had the qualitative impression that this association was stronger for speakers where rejection was inferred by the coder, rather than consciously and clearly reported by the speaker.[344] Discussions between Goldwyn and Main identified what appeared to be the common thread: 'we may conceive of the AAI (like the Strange Situation) as creating conditions that arouse and direct attention toward attachment'.[345] Just as the infant in an avoidant attachment relationship directed attention and behaviour away from the caregiver on reunion in the Strange Situation, the parent in interview was directing attention and discourse away from the actual events of their childhood and associated feelings.[346] In

---

[340] Main, M. & Goldwyn, R. (1983) Predicting rejection of an infant from mother's representation of her own experiences. National Conference on Infant Mental Health, Children's Institute International, Los Angeles, February 1983. PP/Bow/J.4/4.

[341] George, C., Kaplan, N., Goldwyn, R., & Main, M. (1982–83) Attachment interview for parents. PP/Bow/J.4/4.

[342] Main, M. & Goldwyn, R. (1983) Predicting rejection of an infant from mother's representation of her own experiences. National Conference on Infant Mental Health, Children's Institute International, Los Angeles, February 1983. PP/Bow/J.4/4.

[343] Main, M. (1990) Parental aversion to infant-initiated contact is correlated with the parent's own rejection during childhood: the effects of experience on signals of security with respect to attachment. In T.B. Brazelton & K. Barnard (eds) *Touch* (pp.461–95). New York: International Universities Press, p.478.

[344] Ibid. p.485.

[345] This formulation is offered in unpublished texts from the 1980s, but eventually appeared in print in Main, M. (1995) Recent studies in attachment: overview, with selected implications for clinical work. In S. Goldberg, R. Muir, & J. Kerr (eds) *Attachment Theory: Social, Developmental and Clinical Perspectives* (pp.407–70). Hillsdale, NJ: Analytic Press, p.452.

[346] Main, M. & Goldwyn, R. (1984) Predicting rejection of her infant from mother's representation of her own experience: implications for the abused–abusing intergenerational cycle. *Child Abuse & Neglect*, 8(2), 203–17: 'Like the rejected infant, the rejected adult woman is expected to organize her attention away from attachment experiences and her feelings regarding those experiences, in an effort to preserve a certain type of mental organization' (210–11). From an earlier draft: Main, M. & Goldwyn, R. (1983) Predicting rejection of an infant from mother's representation of her own experiences. National Conference on Infant Mental Health, Children's Institute International, Los Angeles, February 1983. PP/Bow/J.4/4: 'In looking away from and ignoring the attachment figure, the infant is excluding attachment-relevant information from further processing. The rejected infant seems rather to resemble the rejected mother.'

both cases there is a swerve of the heart.[347] Main theorised that 'whether or not the move is conscious and deliberate, the experience of rejection by the mother in childhood has led to a shift of attention from attachment figures, experiences and feelings in adult life'.[348] Such experiences of rejection might include a parent's aversion to physical contact, but could also be produced by other forms of rebuff, incomprehension, or disparagement. In turn, infants of these caregivers show avoidant behaviour in the Strange Situation, keeping potential distress away from their own and their caregiver's attention. Main wrote to Bowlby, concluding that 'it appears that the infant does represent in its behaviour the parents' life, unconscious models and intentions'.[349]

During a visit to Berkeley in December 1982, Ainsworth looked at transcripts together with Main. They came to the conclusion that the idealised narratives of parents from avoidant dyads represented a reliance on semantic memory, at the expense of episodic memories that might have qualified such undifferentiated accounts.[350] This helped account for why speakers often reported a lack of memory for specific occasions when asked to substantiate the positive general account offered of their attachment relationships. Conversations with Ainsworth in 1982 revealed her qualitative impression that in the Baltimore sample, too, conversations with the mothers of avoidant dyads suggested idealising of their own childhoods.[351] Main and colleagues initially termed the speech of these caregivers 'detached', since its defining feature was a minimisation or disavowal of negative experiences, the feelings associated with these experiences, and of the value of relationships. However, this term from Bowlby was ambiguous, and Ainsworth thought that it risked connoting a lack of attachment (Chapter 1). Detached speech was therefore renamed 'dismissing' (labelled 'Ds').[352]

Another pattern identified by Goldwyn using 'guess and uncover' was that several speakers seemed highly concerned with grievances; they remained angry and preoccupied with their past and present relationships with attachment figures to such an extent that they often took long conversational turns and lost track of the question. They seemed focused on the vivid recollection of their childhood attachment relationships. Their goal at times seemed

---

[347] In early support for this conclusion, Dozier and Kobak reported that dismissing speakers distinctively showed increases in skin conductance levels from baseline in response to questions in the AAI about experiences of separation, rejection, and threat from attachment figures. Dozier, M. & Kobak, R.R. (1992) Psychophysiology in attachment interviews: converging evidence for deactivating strategies. *Child Development*, 63(6), 1473–80.

[348] Ibid.

[349] Main, M. (1983) *Letter to John Bowlby*, 15 January 1983. PP/Bow/J.4/4. Main's correspondence with Robert Hinde, John Crook, Mary Ainsworth, and John Bowlby is voluminous, as she was in continual contact with them by letter. She and Hesse are still collating her copy of these letters, so they are not considered in this chapter but will be the subject of a future article.

[350] Main, M. (1982) *Letter to John Bowlby*, 9 December 1982. PP/Bow/J.4/4: 'If you would like some transcripts to look over you would also be welcome. Mary Ainsworth had a wonderful time with them, and a splendid idea re: semantic vs episodic memory: the A's seem to have semantic memory.' On the wider context of attention to contradictions between forms of memory in the 1980s see Hacking I. (1995) *Rewriting the Soul: Multiple Personality and the Sciences of Memory*. Princeton, NJ: Princeton University Press; Danziger, K. (2008) *Marking the Mind: A History of Memory*. Cambridge: Cambridge University Press, Chapter 6.

[351] Reported as a personal communication in Main, M., Kaplan, N., & Cassidy, J. (1985) Security in infancy, childhood, and adulthood: a move to the level of representation. *Monographs of the Society for Research in Child Development*, 50, 66–104, p.97.

[352] One 'dismissing' subclassification, Ds2, has been criticised by later researchers as a poor fit for the category. Speakers in this classification derogate attachment relationships, though the classification can be made even on the basis of quite brief passages of speech rather than characterising a whole transcript. The subclassification has been found to fall with the preoccupied category in analyses on two large adult samples assessed using the AAI. Raby, K.L., Labella, M.H., Martin, J., Carlson, E.A., & Roisman, G.I. (2017) Childhood abuse and neglect and insecure attachment states of mind in adulthood: prospective, longitudinal evidence from a high-risk sample. *Development & Psychopathology*, 29(2), 347–63.

to become that of making a case against their parents, rather than responding precisely to the interviewer's questions. In the terms that Main had developed for thinking about the Strange Situation, these speakers were directing attention towards attachment-relevant cues, even if this was at the expense of cooperation with the interview. The speech of these caregivers was initially termed 'enmeshed-conflicted' (E); this was changed to 'preoccupied' as the first term was ultimately considered stigmatising, though the category label 'E' was retained. Preoccupied speech seemed to Main and Goldwyn to be analogous to the infant of an ambivalent/resistant dyad in the Strange Situation, who is anxious at even the prospect of separation, 'unable to direct attention to the environment, expresses strong and sometimes continual fear and distress, and seems constantly directed toward the parent'.[353] And indeed, some of the preoccupied speakers in the Berkeley sample had been part of such dyads five years earlier.

Goldwyn also discerned qualities that seemed to distinguish the speech of parents who had been part of securely attached dyads five years earlier. These speakers described both the positives and negatives of their early relationships with good balance, even if these relationships had been difficult. Conversations between Goldwyn, Main, and Hesse suggested that a central property of the transcripts of secure infants was that the speaker appeared to have ready access to both semantic and episodic memory and so could coordinate a response to both kinds of prompts.[354] Just like the secure infant in the Strange Situation could turn attention to the toys or the caregiver in response to changing environmental cues, the speakers seemed to be able to attend to both semantic and episodic memory, and positive and negative experiences, in a flexible way. In fact, the caregivers of dyads classified B3 in the Strange Situation in the Berkeley sample displayed these features most prototypically.[355] Main, Goldwyn, and Hesse therefore termed the speech of these caregivers 'secure-autonomous', not because the speaker seemed independently minded, but because the defining feature of the transcript was the absence of restrictions in the discussion of experiences. The category label given to these speakers was F, since they seemed 'freed through experience or thought to recognise the importance of attachment relationships, yet independent enough to evaluate them'.[356] This seemed to be in contrast to parents who had been part of avoidant and resistant dyads, where there seemed to be 'restrictions of varying types ... placed on attention and the flow of information with respect to attachment'.[357] In a handwritten annotation

[353] Main, M., Kaplan, N., & Cassidy, J. (1985) Security in infancy, childhood, and adulthood: a move to the level of representation. *Monographs of the Society for Research in Child Development*, 50, 66–104, p.74. Later research found greater physiological arousal in preoccupied speakers in response to questions about separation and threat: Beijersbergen, M.D., Bakermans-Kranenburg, M.J., van IJzendoorn, M.H., & Juffer, F. (2008) Stress regulation in adolescents: physiological reactivity during the Adult Attachment Interview and conflict interaction. *Child Development*, 79(6), 1707–20, p.1716.

[354] Main, M. & Goldwyn, R. (1983) Predicting rejection of an infant from mother's representation of her own experiences. National Conference on Infant Mental Health, Children's Institute International, Los Angeles, February 1983. PP/Bow/J.4/4.

[355] Main, M. (1991) Metacognitive knowledge, metacognitive monitoring, and singular (coherent) vs. multiple (incoherent) models of attachment: some findings and some directions for future research. In P. Marris, J. Stevenson-Hinde, & C. Parkes (eds) *Attachment Across the Life Cycle* (pp.127–59). New York: Routledge, p.142.

[356] George, C., Kaplan, N., Goldwyn, R., & Main, M. (1982–83) Attachment interview for parents. PP/Bow/J.4/4. Since A, B, and C were the Ainsworth classifications, Main termed her AAI classifications D, E, and F. D stood for "dismissing". By the mid-1980s, though, this was confusing since D was also the term used for the new Strange Situation classification, so dismissing discourse was relabelled 'Ds'.

[357] Main, M., Kaplan, N., & Cassidy, J. (1985) Security in infancy, childhood, and adulthood: a move to the level of representation. *Monographs of the Society for Research in Child Development*, 50, 66–104, p.100.

on a very early draft of the coding system, Main remarked that in the most prototypical of secure-autonomous speakers, 'there is a striking ability to integrate existing information'.[358]

This developing coding system was clearly unusual. Whereas most psychological measures for coding interviews focused on coding answers to particular questions, the developing Main, Goldwyn, and Hesse method for coding the AAI examined the transcript as a whole, across the dance and drift of spoken discourse. The questions induced speech about personal experiences without respite: 'in clinical terms, we would say that the objective of this interview is to "surprise the unconscious" with respect to attachment, through repeated, insistent probing' combined with a lack of reciprocity from the interviewer.[359] However, the most distinctive feature of the AAI as a scientific protocol, as well as perhaps its most audacious and uncanny feature, was its focus on apparent restrictions on information, which put the coder in the position of comparing 'the subject's own semantic categorisations of her experiences' with what 'we could discern [of] actual experience'.[360]

As such, the coding focused neither on the subject's stated opinions, nor on the individual's inferred actual history, since this is unknowable from an interview. The focus was instead on the manner in which the speaker attended to and communicated about attachment-related experiences. The coder was asked to consider both the internal consistency of the account and the extent to which the speaker's interpretation seemed plausible based on the episodic information provided.[361] In this, the coder had to consider the world from the speaker's point of view, and take a step back to evaluate the speaker's account of the world and appraise potential distortions of information. In this sense, the coding system had clear analogies to the clinical interviewing of the period in the USA, placing the coder in the position of clinician. Through the 1970s, under the influence of psychoanalysis, a dominant trend in clinical interviewing in the context of mental health was to seek to identify psychological defences or confusions expressed through speech and decipherable by the clinician.[362] However, from the 1980s, under the influence of the American Psychiatric Association's DSM-III, clinical interviewing increasingly sought to identify specifiable markers for categories of mental pathology out of the particularities of what and how individuals report their experiences.[363] The AAI had elements of both forms of clinical interview, which made it well suited and timely for clinicians with a psychoanalytic background in providing a scientific basis and

[358] George, C., Kaplan, N., Goldwyn, R., & Main, M. (1982–83) Attachment interview for parents. PP/Bow/J.4/4.

[359] George, C., Kaplan, N., & Main, M. (1985) Adult Attachment Interview, March 1985, 1st edn. PP/Bow/J.4/4.

[360] Main, M. & Goldwyn, R. (1983) Predicting rejection of an infant from mother's representation of her own experiences. National Conference on Infant Mental Health, Children's Institute International, Los Angeles, February 1983. PP/Bow/J.4/3.

[361] This was discussed by Main with reference to the debate in analytic philosophy between the coherence and correspondence theories of truth. Main, M. (1991) Metacognitive knowledge, metacognitive monitoring, and singular (coherent) vs. multiple (incoherent) models of attachment: some findings and some directions for future research. In P. Marris, J. Stevenson-Hinde, & C. Parkes (eds) *Attachment Across the Life Cycle* (pp.127–59). New York: Routledge, p.144; Main, M. (1993) Discourse, prediction and recent studies in attachment: implications for psychoanalysis. *Journal of the American Psycho-analytic Association*, 41, 209–44, p.237.

[362] E.g. Edinburg, G.M., Zinberg, N.E., & Kelman, W. (1975) *Clinical Interviewing and Counselling: Principles and Techniques*. New York: Appleton-Century-Crofts.

[363] Greco, M. (2016) What is the DSM? Diagnostic manual, cultural icon, political battleground: an overview with suggestions for a critical research agenda. *Psychology & Sexuality*, 7(1), 6–22. A wider context can be given also in the rise of assessment and classification of the speech of service-users as a mode of knowing and administrating within the professions from the 1970s to the 1980s, and with a particular concern with individuals able—or not able—to know and regulate themselves. The DSM contributed to this shift, but was also part of a wider process. Foucault, M. (2008) *The Birth of Biopolitics: Lectures at the College de France, 1978–1979*, trans. G. Burchell. New York: Palgrave MacMillan.

classifications for blockages or disruptions in how individuals are able to know or regulate themselves.

Main and colleagues felt that ultimately 'we were attempting to trace what could happen to information regarding negative or rejecting attachment experiences, other than their easy and coherent recognition and evaluation'.[364] On the one hand, it could be defensively excluded through lack of memory and/or idealisation. On the other hand, it could become a preoccupying focus of attention in a way that hindered evaluation.[365] Main described the object of the interview as the adult's state of mind with respect to attachment.[366] However, the phrase is quite misleading. Not least what is in question is not what psychological research generally means by a 'state': a transitory experience responding to an external prompt without the expectation of stability over time.[367] Unfortunately, the pivotal article in which Main set out and described the concept of 'state of mind' was accepted by the journal *Developmental Psychology* but then withdrawn by Main as ultimately unsatisfactory.[368] As such, the meaning of the term has often been unclear to her readers, contributing to misunderstanding of what the AAI actually measured, and fanned the flames of controversy regarding other forms of assessment (Chapter 5). Fonagy and colleagues, for instance, were left at a loss regarding the object of the AAI, wondering whether the coding system could actually be best considered as an indirect assessment of the caregiving system, rather than an assessment of anything attachment-related at all.[369] Fonagy and Campbell subsequently concluded that the AAI does assess something related to attachment, but that Main's own description of 'state of mind regarding attachment' in terms of internal working models has been confusing and, ultimately, a 'reductionist over-simplification'.[370] However, Fonagy and Campbell offered no further thoughts on what it is that the AAI does, in fact, measure.

In addressing this question, a first thing to note is that, despite its name, the AAI was not an assessment of individual differences in a unitary entity called 'attachment'.[371] This is despite the fact that, among developmental psychologists, 'adult attachment' has come to mean 'what the AAI assesses'. In fact, the name 'Adult Attachment Interview' appears to have

---

[364] Main, M. & Goldwyn, R. (1983) Predicting rejection of an infant from mother's representation of her own experiences. National Conference on Infant Mental Health, Children's Institute International, Los Angeles, February 1983. PP/Bow/J.4/3.

[365] George, C., Kaplan, N., Goldwyn, R., & Main, M. (1982–83) Attachment interview for parents. PP/Bow/J.4/4: 'The individual is not at all freed of the influence of early attachment relationships. He/she is unable to grow beyond them, and either accepts this state passively, or actively struggles against it without success. Although the individual may talk very readily and at length of the influence of early relationships, he/she is not independent enough to evaluate them and his/her place within them.'

[366] The underspecification of the concept of 'state of mind regarding attachment' might be seen as in part an effect of the importation of aspects of a clinical interview into the AAI methodology, but without the conventional aim of the interview—which was changing in any case in the period, from the identification of defences to the making of diagnoses.

[367] On the concept of 'state' in psychology see e.g. Chaplin, W.F., John, O.P., & Goldberg, L.R. (1988) Conceptions of states and traits: dimensional attributes with ideals as prototypes. *Journal of Personality and Social Psychology*, 54(4), 541–57.

[368] Main, M. & Goldwyn, R. (1989) *Interview Based Adult Attachment Classifications: Related to Infant–Mother and Infant–Father Attachment*. Unpublished manuscript, Developmental Psychology.

[369] Stein, H., Jacobs, N.J., Ferguson, K.S., Allen, J.G., & Fonagy, P. (1998) What do adult attachment scales measure? *Bulletin of the Menninger Clinic*, 62, 33–82, p.49. Worry about the object or objects of the AAI was also expressed by Stern, who reviewed various possibilities, but acknowledged that ultimately this remained an unsolved question. Stern, D.N. (1998) *The Motherhood Constellation: A Unified View of Parent–Infant Psychotherapy*. London: Karnac, p.38.

[370] Fonagy, P. & Campbell, C. (2015) Bad blood revisited: attachment and psychoanalysis. *British Journal of Psychotherapy*, 31(2), 229–50, p.234.

[371] Goldberg, S. (2000) *Attachment and Development*. London: Routledge, p.242.

originated from the interview's concern with attachment experiences. True, the demand to attend to and communicate about attachment-relevant experiences might well be alarming, and might therefore *also* activate the attachment system. But this was not tested or even discussed. In fact, the central focus of the coding system developed by Main, Goldwyn, and Hesse was on the capacity to attend to and communicate about attachment-relevant experiences and the feelings they evoke. Main referred to this, somewhat loosely, as individual differences in 'adult attachment', since this capacity seemed to her to have strong commonalities with the Ainsworth classifications at the level of attentional processes. The term 'adult attachment' was also a powerful assertion that the ideas of Ainsworth were relevant across the lifespan. However, use of the term generated confusion, as well as acrimony between developmental and social psychology researchers in which ownership over the capacity to measure something called 'attachment' became a central stake (Chapter 5). However, Main and Hesse's basic position is that 'there exist species-wide abilities that are not part of the attachment system itself, but can, within limits, manipulate (either inhibit or increase) attachment behavior in response to differing environments'.[372] In Main and Hesse's conceptualisation of the AAI, what is measured is the deployment of such abilities as applied to adult attention and communication regarding attachment-related matters, not the 'attachment system itself'.

Nor was the AAI developed primarily as an assessment of 'internal working models', if by this is meant representational content regarding attachment figures. (Admittedly, if 'internal working model' is taken to mean any cognitive components recruitable by the attachment system, then the AAI does tap these, but the claim does not tell us much.) Comparison of published with unpublished manuscripts suggests that Main's use of the concept of 'internal working model' in the mid-1980s in discussing the AAI was primarily a matter of tying her new methods to existing theory, rather than actually the basis on which she was conceptualising the measure. It was also a position she would drop already in the 1980s. At the meeting of the Society for Research in Child Development in Baltimore in June 1987, Main spent time with Hinde. Hinde had huge respect for Main's work, as well as a good deal of personal affection. However, underspecified causal claims about motivational processes seems to have been his personal *bête noire*. At the Baltimore conference he passionately chided Main for her appeal to the 'internal working model' concept.

Main wrote to Bowlby to report that she could see Hinde's point, and that she was planning to give the matter further thought.[373] From 1987 onwards, she ceased equating states of mind regarding attachment and internal working models. And in the late 1990s Main acknowledged in print Hinde's point that the characterisation of the AAI as an assessment of internal working models was, ultimately, 'misleading and unwarranted'.[374] Fonagy and Target agreed, arguing that Main's description of the AAI as assessing internal working models had prompted much 'futile' research and generally 'distracted attachment researchers'.[375]

---

[372] Main, M., Hesse, E., & Kaplan, N. (2005) Predictability of attachment behavior and representational processes at 1, 6, and 19 years of age: the Berkeley Longitudinal Study. In K.E. Grossmann, K.Grossmann, & E. Waters (eds) *Attachment from Infancy to Adulthood: The Major Longitudinal Studies* (pp.245–304). New York: Guilford, p.256.

[373] Main, M. (1987) *Letter to John Bowlby*, 3 June 1987. PP/Bow/B.3/36/1.

[374] Main, M. (1999) Epilogue. Attachment theory: eighteen points with suggestions for future studies. In J. Cassidy & P. Shaver (eds) *Handbook of Attachment* (pp.845–87). New York: Guilford, p.877.

[375] Fonagy, P. & Target, M. (2002) Early intervention and the development of self-regulation. *Psychoanalytic Inquiry*, 22(3), 307–35, p.328. For an example of confusion caused by Main's characterisation see, for instance, the widely cited paper Johnson, S.C., Dweck, C.S., & Chen, F.S. (2007) Evidence for infants' internal working models of attachment. *Psychological Science*, 18(6), 501–502. The authors found a difference in attentional processes between infants based on Strange Situation classifications. From this they conclude, in an unmonitored non sequitur, that

They were glad that she had altered her description of the AAI. However, this shift in Main's work has generally gone unnoticed and unheeded. Kobak and Esposito described how Main's appeal to internal working models inadvertently trained researchers' attention on personality trait-style qualities of individuals and their 'models' of others, rather than on attentional or communicative processes.[376] The characterisation of the AAI as an assessment of 'models' of attachment relationships led to the misleading characterisation of the measure as an assessment of 'attachment representations'. The AAI was not primarily an assessment of individual differences in representations held of particular parents, or even in representations of relationships in general, though both might influence classifications on the measure. Yet thanks to its initial characterisation in terms of internal working models, the AAI is still commonly described, including by trainers in the measure, as an assessment of 'attachment representations' in adults. This occurs even when researchers' own descriptions of what the AAI assesses—for instance, the processing of attachment-relevant information—actually do not agree with the usual meanings of the noun 'representations'.[377]

The term 'representations' essentially functions as a placeholder. But its use has unsurprisingly contributed to unwarranted assumptions about the measure. For instance, researchers have often wondered why adults are assigned a single classification, rather than a classification for each attachment relationship, as could be anticipated if the AAI was measuring representations of relationships.[378] The use of a single classification makes sense, however, if Main's focus on attentional and communicative processes in the years of its development is recognised: in her work, the AAI has been conceptualised as an assessment of individual differences prompted by the interview's demand on speakers to attend to and communicate regarding attachment-relevant experiences. The only researcher to have consistently highlighted the importance of Main's attentional model of states of mind regarding attachment has been van IJzendoorn. Van IJzendoorn had several advantages over other readers. For instance, in a paper from 1992, and citing his personal copy of the unpublished *Developmental Psychology* manuscript on the concept of 'states of mind', van IJzendoorn observed that generally in Main's writings 'the concepts of "internal representation," "state of mind," and "internal working model" of attachment are used interchangeably'. Nonetheless, he argued, the 'concept of "state of mind"' is in fact less about representational content and more about 'the direction and organization of attention and memory', as well as related affective and behavioural aspects.[379] Recognition of the importance assigned by Main to attention has gone on

---

this is proof of abstract mental representations of attachment figures: 'Secure infants looked relatively longer at the unresponsive outcome than the responsive outcome compared with the insecure infants. These results constitute direct positive evidence that infants' own personal attachment experiences are reflected in abstract mental representations of social interactions' (502).

[376] Kobak, R. & Esposito, A. (2004) Levels of processing in parent–child relationships: implications for clinical assessment and treatment. In L. Atkinson & S. Goldberg (eds) *Attachment Issues in Psychopathology and Interventions* (pp.139–66). Mahwah, NJ: Lawrence Erlbaum, p.143.

[377] Verhage, M.L., Fearon, R.P., C. Schuengel, et al. (2018) Examining ecological constraints on the intergenerational transmission of attachment via individual participant data meta-analysis. *Child Development*, 89(6), 2023–37; Messina, S., Reisz, S., Hazen, N., & Jacobvitz, D. (2019) Not just about food: attachments representations and maternal feeding practices in infancy. *Attachment & Human development*, 23 April, 1–20.

[378] It has sometimes been assumed that the AAI aimed to measure internal working models, but was faulty in its execution of this aim. For a later attempt to construct and validate such a measure see Miljkovitch, R., Moss, E., Bernier, A., Pascuzzo, K., & Sander, E. (2015) Refining the assessment of internal working models: the Attachment Multiple Model Interview. *Attachment & Human Development*, 17(5), 492–521.

[379] Van IJzendoorn, M.H. (1992) Intergenerational transmission of parenting: a review of studies in non-clinical populations. *Developmental Review*, 12(1), 76–99, p.80. Van IJzendoorn later even punned that the 'Move to the Level of Representation' was itself a 'revolutionary shift in attention' for the field of attachment

to guide van IJzendoorn's research using the Strange Situation and AAI, for instance his concern with genetic polymorphisms that influence the dopamine system, given the role of this system in attention and reward processing.[380]

Coherence

From early on in their examination of the transcripts, a central concept used by Main and Goldwyn to mark individual differences between the transcripts was 'coherence'. As van IJzendoorn and colleagues noted, however, the Main and Goldwyn usage was technical, and differed in potentially confusing ways from everyday English.[381] Indeed, a recent study by Lind and colleagues found an association of only $r = .37$ between Main and Goldwyn's scale for 'coherence' and a conventional measure of narrative coherence.[382] Main's first use of the term was in the first edition of the coding manual, in 1986, where they defined coherence as 'the extent to which the reader finds a unified, yet free-flowing picture of the subject's experiences, feelings and viewpoints within the interview, such that none of these require the reader to make her own, differing interpretation. In addition, the interview transcript is considered coherent when the subject seems able to easily point to the principle and rationale behind her responses; has thought or else seems ready to think about her past and its influences.'[383] In judging coherence, the manual urged the coder to look out for contradictions, especially between episodic and semantic memory, logical contradictions, and factual contradictions.

In the early 1990s, Main and Hesse continued to develop the concept of 'coherence' in reflecting on the question of what the coding system was capturing. In this, their thinking was influenced by the ideas of a colleague at Berkeley, the philosopher of language Paul Grice.[384] Grice had argued that cooperative discourse usually demands, except when permission is given by the partner, adherence to four conversational maxims:

---

research, away from behaviour and towards the manner in which attachment-relevant experiences are communicated: van IJzendoorn, M.H. (1995) Adult attachment representations, parental responsiveness, and infant attachment: a meta-analysis on the predictive validity of the Adult Attachment Interview. *Psychological Bulletin*, 117(3), 387–403, p.388. Other researchers close to Main and with access to her unpublished works have described 'state of mind' as referring to 'the way adults process attachment-related thoughts, memories and feelings'. Again, the difference from the ready connotations of the term 'attachment representations' is striking. Dozier, M. & Bates, B.C. (2004) Attachment state of mind and the treatment relationship. In L. Atkinson & S. Goldberg (eds) *Attachment Issues in Psychopathology and Intervention* (pp.167–80). London: Lawrence Erlbaum, p.167.

[380] E.g. Van IJzendoorn, M.H. & Bakermans-Kranenburg, M.J. (2006) DRD4 7-repeat polymorphism moderates the association between maternal unresolved loss or trauma and infant disorganization. *Attachment & Human Development*, 8(4), 291–307.

[381] Beijersbergen, M.D., Bakermans-Kranenburg, M.J., & van IJzendoorn, M.H. (2006) The concept of coherence in attachment interviews: comparing attachment experts, linguists, and non-experts. *Attachment & Human Development*, 8(4), 353–69. Morelli and Rothbaum also argued that the concept of coherence is defined in different ways in different cultures; it is not a cultural universal. Morelli, G. & Rothbaum, F. (2007) Situating the child in context: attachment relationships and self-regulation in different cultures. In S. Kitayama & D. Cohen (eds) *Handbook of Cultural Psychology* (pp.500–527). New York: Guilford.

[382] Lind, M., Vanwoerden, S., Penner, F., & Sharp, C. (2019) Narrative coherence in adolescence: relations with attachment, mentalization, and psychopathology. *Journal of Personality Assessment*, https://doi.org/10.1080/00223891.2019.1574805.

[383] Main, M. (1986) *Behaviour and the Development of Representational Models of Attachment: Five Methods of Assessment*. Unpublished manuscript, Mary Main & Erik Hesse personal archive.

[384] Grice, H.P. (1989) *Studies in the Way of Words*. Cambridge, MA: Harvard University Press.

Quality—'be truthful and have evidence for what you say'
Quantity—'be succinct, and yet complete'
Relation—'be relevant to the topic as presented'
Manner—'be clear and orderly'

Main partly retained her earlier definition of 'coherence', but also partly redefined it in terms of Grice's maxims.[385] Whereas initially the term had been defined as (i) the extent to which the reader finds a unified, yet free-flowing picture by the speaker that agrees with the reader's own account, the concept was tucked into (ii) the four dimensions identified by Grice. Characteristic of a secure-autonomous (F) transcript was that there was good episodic evidence for semantic generalisations; speakers could flexibly turn their attention to their past and to the interviewer in being succinct and yet complete and relevant: 'For these speakers, the focus of attention appears to shift fluidly between the interviewer's queries and the memories that are called upon. In this way, the speaker is able, regardless of the difficulty of the subject matter, to remain both truthful (consistent) and collaborative.'[386] Finally, the discourse of a secure-autonomous speaker was characteristically clear and orderly, often with a fresh quality to the speech. These qualities require a capacity to both turn genuine and curious attention to attachment-related memories and let go again in order to attend to the interviewer. Main and colleagues developed subscales to help coders in making a judgement about whether a transcript should be classified as secure, parallel to the function of Ainsworth's scales for the Strange Situation (Chapter 2). Of particular importance was a scale for the coherence of the transcript.[387]

Dismissing (Ds) interviewees tended to have poor episodic evidence for their semantic generalisations. They also tended to offer oversuccinct answers lacking the details of concrete experience, since they were not able to resource their responses through access to a richly populated and textured inscape of episodic information. Presumably this information had become defensively excluded. Relevance might also be weakly violated as the speaker deflected the conversation away from sensitive topics. In general, however, what is said is orderly. Preoccupied (E) interviewees tended to have poor alignment between episodic and semantic memory, as they were focused on the negative aspects of episodic memories even as they recounted events that could have other more balanced interpretations. However, the primary violations of coherence in a preoccupied transcript were excessive quantity of speech about topics that were not direct answers to the questions of the interview, often with poor orderliness in the communication of experiences caused by a focus on the memories themselves rather than on the comprehension of the interviewer. Their transcripts are a bit wild, marked by 'highly entangled, confusing, run-on sentences; failures to use past markers in quoting conversations with the parents; rapid oscillations of viewpoint within or between

[385] Main, M. (1991) Metacognitive knowledge, metacognitive monitoring, and singular (coherent) vs. multiple (incoherent) models of attachment: some findings and some directions for future research. In P. Marris, J. Stevenson-Hinde, & C. Parkes (eds) *Attachment Across the Life Cycle* (pp.127–59). New York: Routledge: 'Coherence appears both in an analysis based upon Grice's maxims with respect to coherence of discourse (Grice 1975), and in terms of overall plausibility' (129).

[386] Hesse, E. (1996) Discourse, memory, and the Adult Attachment Interview: a note with emphasis on the emerging cannot classify category. *Infant Mental Health Journal*, 17(1), 4–11, p.6.

[387] Secure-autonomous transcripts are also expected to demonstrate a range of feelings appropriate to the complexity of the autobiography being related. This was not developed as a scale by Main and colleagues, but does feature as a scale in a version of the AAI appropriate for young people: Steele, H., Steele, M., & Kriss, A. (2009) *The Friends and Family Interview (FFI) Coding Guidelines*. Unpublished manuscript.

sentences; unfinished sentences; insertion of extremely general terms into sentence frames ('sort of thing', 'and this and that'), and use of nonsense words or trailers as sentence endings ('dada-dada-dada').[388] Main and Hesse also created scales to help coders identify dismissing and preoccupied transcripts. To help distinguish dismissing states of mind regarding attachment, the researchers created scales including for idealisation of the parent and insistence on lack of recall. To help distinguish preoccupied states of mind regarding attachment, they created scales for involving/preoccupied anger and for passivity or vagueness of discourse. Like the Ainsworth scales, the scales for the AAI were initially given the primary role of supporting placement of cases within categories. As with the Strange Situation, coders were enjoined to record their scale scores, resulting in an archive of largely unpublished findings. These have become the target of great interest recently, especially in the context of Individual Participant Data meta-analysis (Chapter 6). However, from the 1990s onwards, the coherence score came to see use as a dimensional alternative, or complement, to the category-based coding system.[389]

Hesse reflected upon the meaning of coherence at an interpersonal level.[390] He conceptualised the AAI as constituting two tasks: to reflect on memories of attachment relevant experiences, and to communicate about these in a way that holds in mind the interviewer's specific questions. Transcripts classified as dismissing violate the first of these tasks; transcripts classified as preoccupied violate the second. In the same period, Main was reflecting on the meaning of coherence at a cognitive level. She proposed that the coherence of their discourse suggests that secure-autonomous speakers have a relatively unitary model of their experiences and how these influence their behaviour. She perceived that this integration of different sources of information and the lack of need to divert attention to the implementation of a conditional strategy might support a capacity to retain balance in the evaluation of

---

[388] Main, M. (1991) Metacognitive knowledge, metacognitive monitoring, and singular (coherent) vs. multiple (incoherent) models of attachment: some findings and some directions for future research. In P. Marris, J. Stevenson-Hinde, & C. Parkes (eds) *Attachment Across the Life Cycle* (pp.127–59). New York: Routledge, p.144. One group of transcripts showed substantial markers of splintering or incoherence. These speakers were preoccupied not so much by anger towards their caregiver, as by 'fearful attachment experiences—for example, experiences of physical or sexual abuse, traumatic loss, psychosis in a parent, or simple cruelty. There is evidence within the interview of active struggle with these experiences, but the subject is still implicitly fearful, confused or overwhelmed. The subject is not yet objective, or able to gather these chaotic and fearful episodes of experiences into a single abstract yet personally meaningful form.' Main gave these their own subclassification: 'fearful' (labelled E3). In some unpublished work, Main included E3 as a marker of unresolved/disorganised states of mind, e.g. Main, M., van IJzendoorn, M.H., & Hesse, E. (1993) *Unresolved/Unclassifiable Responses to the Adult Attachment Interview: Predictable from Unresolved States and Anomalous Beliefs in the Berkeley–Leiden Adult Attachment Questionnaire.* Unpublished manuscript. https://openaccess.leidenuniv.nl/dspace/bitstream/1887/1464/1/168_131.pdf. Several subsequent researchers criticised the inclusion of E3 as a form of preoccupation in the AAI system, e.g. George, C. & West, M.L. (2012) *The Adult Attachment Projective Picture System.* New York: Guilford, p.194. One interpretation would be that E3 speech, whilst not technically itself an unresolved/disorganised state of mind, meets the conditions that especially produce lapses: (i) extensive speech and (ii) about traumatic experiences, (iii) in a manner guided especially by the memories themselves rather than with relevance and order set by the interviewer's questions.

[389] E.g. Fonagy, P., Steele, H., & Steele, M. (1991) Maternal representations of attachment during pregnancy predict the organization of infant–mother attachment at one year of age. *Child Development,* 62, 891–905. A spur to use of the coherence score as an alternative to the category-based system came with a discriminant function analysis conducted by Crowell and colleagues, which found that the coherence score was of special importance for secure/insecure discrimination. Crowell, J.A., Treboux, D., Gao, Y., Fyffe, C., Pan, H., & Waters, E. (2002) Assessing secure base behavior in adulthood: development of a measure, links to adult attachment representations, and relations to couples' communication and reports of relationships. *Developmental Psychology,* 38(5), 679–93.

[390] Hesse, E. (1996) Discourse, memory, and the adult attachment interview: a note with emphasis on the emerging cannot classify category. *Infant Mental Health Journal,* 17(1), 4–11.

relationships, to perceive how the same reality could be seen in different ways, and to allocate attention as needed to different tasks.[391]

Main was also impressed by apparent differences in epistemology between speakers: secure-autonomous speakers 'adopted a more thoroughly constructivist view of their own knowledge-base than less secure adults', with more subtle forms of awareness of the appearance-reality distinction. Secure-autonomous speakers may acknowledge that their own perspective on an event may differ to that of a family member, or that their recall may be distorted by their regrets about the occurrence.[392] She believed that this constructivist view of knowledge served to support a speaker's capacity to examine their own experiences ('metacognition') when prompted by the environment, since there is less segregated information: 'more epistemic 'space" is available for such an individual 'because her thinking processes are not compartmentalised'.[393] Though Main acknowledged that it could be, in theory, that metacognitive capacities were facilitating secure-autonomous speech, or that there were bidirectional effects, her view was that secure attachment was the cause of metacognitive strengths such as clearsightedness in self-evaluation. A metacognitive monitoring scale was added to the AAI coding manual in 1991 to support coders in making a classification of secure-autonomous state of mind regarding attachment. (Nearly three decades later, however, the scale is still identified as unfinished in the AAI manual. The measurement of metacognitive monitoring would not be pursued further by Main, and would instead be taken up by Fonagy, Steele, and Steele in their work on reflective functioning and mentalisation.[394] Main's lack of further work on the metacognition scale has generally been interpreted as tacit endorsement of the approach of Fonagy and colleagues.)

Main conceptualised the reduced coherence of dismissing and preoccupied speakers as reflecting the conflict between segregated information, and thus conflict between different interpretations by speakers of their own past. Everyone has multiple models of reality, Main observed, but dismissing and preoccupied speakers seemed to have 'implicitly contradictory models of the same aspects of reality', segregated from one another perhaps without the speaker's awareness, but available to someone reading the transcript of their interview.[395] On this basis, Main criticised Bowlby's notion of the internal working model as too calm and settled a metaphor, to the point of actually being 'somewhat misleading'. Whilst perhaps applicable to secure-autonomous speakers, when asked to describe and evaluate their attachment experiences and relations, dismissing and especially preoccupied speakers present an array of 'contradictory thoughts, feelings, and intentions which can only loosely be described as a "model"'.[396] These speakers 'evidence difficulties in obtaining access to attachment-related

---

[391] Main reported unpublished data in support of this conclusion: in a study of 174 college students conducted in collaboration with Waters, 'self-reported difficulty dividing attention among several simultaneous tasks was found associated with lack of memory for childhood, with descriptions of the subject's mother as unforgiving, and with uncertainty that the subject could turn to one or both parents in times of trouble'. Main, M. (1991) Metacognitive knowledge, metacognitive monitoring, and singular (coherent) vs. multiple (incoherent) models of attachment: some findings and some directions for future research. In P. Marris, J. Stevenson-Hinde, & C. Parkes (eds) *Attachment Across the Life Cycle* (pp.127–59). New York: Routledge, p.155.

[392] Ibid. p.153.

[393] Ibid. pp.146–8 and Table 8.1.

[394] Fonagy, P., Steele, M., Steele, H., Moran, G.S., & Higgitt, A.C. (1991) The capacity for understanding mental states: the reflective self in parent and child and its significance for security of attachment. *Infant Mental Health Journal*, 12(3), 201–18.

[395] Main, M. (1991) Metacognitive knowledge, metacognitive monitoring, and singular (coherent) vs. multiple (incoherent) models of attachment: some findings and some directions for future research. In P. Marris, J. Stevenson-Hinde, & C. Parkes (eds) *Attachment Across the Life Cycle* (pp.127–59). New York: Routledge, p.132.

[396] Ibid. p.132.

information; in maintaining organisation in attachment-related information; and in preventing attachment-related information from undergoing distortion.[397] Whereas psychoanalytic theory might conceptualise such effects as evidencing the repression of mental contents relevant to past experiences, Main argued that what is 'defensively excluded in this conceptualisation is not the memory ... but rather an alternative attentional and behavioural patterning'.[398]

Just as Main conceptualised the infant showing avoidant behaviour in the Strange Situation as primarily avoiding disorganisation, and only secondarily the attachment figure, so dismissing speakers were conceptualised as primarily avoiding a breakdown in their conditional strategy and its attentional and behavioural architecture. And like the ambivalent/resistant infant, the preoccupied speaker was conceptualised as keeping attention and behaviour trained on attachment-relevant information, avoiding cues from the environment that might suggest other priorities for attention and behaviour. Whether in childhood or in adulthood, what conditional strategies have in common in Main and Hesse's thinking is that they 'follow upon alterations in the focus of attention'.[399] For it is attention that orchestrates what attachment-relevant information and cues are received from the environment or from memory. As such, these alterations in attachment-relevant information are topic specific. They were not anticipated to be carried over into the processing of matters irrelevant to secure base/safe haven availability.[400]

Yet alterations in attention to these specific matters were nonetheless anticipated by Main and colleagues to have wide-ranging implications for mental health. In line with this account, both dismissing and preoccupied states of mind have been found to be transdiagnostic. Though more prevalent in clinical samples, dismissing and preoccupied states of mind regarding attachment are not characteristic simply of any one form of mental illness (with the partial exception of a link between preoccupied states of mind and personality disorders). They are also remarkably stable during adulthood, though periods of developmental transition or changes in circumstances will often result in changes in states of mind regarding attachment.[401] However, contrary to Main's expectation, there has only been evidence of weak or moderate continuity from infant attachment classifications to AAI classifications, though infant disorganised attachment does generally predict a later insecure classification on the

[397] Ibid. p.143.

[398] Main, M. (1993) Discourse, prediction and recent studies in attachment: implications for psychoanalysis. *Journal of the American Psycho-analytic Association*, 41, 209–44, p.234.

[399] Main, M. & Hesse, E. (1992) Attaccamento disorganizzato/disorientato nell'infanzia e stati mentali dissociati dei genitori. In M. Ammaniti & D.N. Stern (eds) *Attaccamento e Psicoanalisi* (pp.80–140). Rome: Gius, Laterza & Figli, p.86.

[400] See Bakermans-Kranenburg, M.J. & van IJzendoorn, M.H. (1993) A psychometric study of the Adult Attachment Interview: reliability and discriminant validity. *Developmental Psychology*, 29(5), 870–79; Sagi, A., van IJzendoorn, M.H., Scharf, M., Koren-Karie, N., Joels, T., & Mayseless, O. (1994) Stability and discriminant validity of the Adult Attachment Interview: a psychometric study in young Israeli adults. *Developmental Psychology*, 30(5), 771–7; Crowell, J.A., Waters, E., Treboux, D., et al. (1996) Discriminant validity of the Adult Attachment Interview. *Child Development*, 67(5), 2584–99. The boundaries of 'attachment-relevant information' are not set out by Main and colleagues.

[401] Bakermans-Kranenburg, M.J. & Van IJzendoorn, M.H. (1993) A psychometric study of the Adult Attachment Interview: reliability and discriminant validity. *Developmental Psychology*, 29(5), 870–79; Crowell, J.A. & Hauser, S.T. (2008) AAIs in a high-risk sample: stability and relation to functioning from adolescence to 39 years. In H. Steele & M. Steele (eds) *Clinical Applications of the Adult Attachment Interview* (pp.341–70). New York: Guilford. There are ongoing discussions about the extent to which AAI classifications should be expected to be stable in the context of psychotherapy, e.g. Daniel, S.I.F., Poulsen, S., & Lunn, S. (2016) Client attachment in a randomized clinical trial of psychoanalytic and cognitive-behavioral psychotherapy for bulimia nervosa: outcome moderation and change. *Psychotherapy*, 53(2), 174.

AAI.[402] The question of the relationship between actual childhood experiences in attachment relationships and retrospective discourse in the AAI is one that remains debated, as the case of discussions of 'earned security' reveals especially clearly.

Earned security

In her use of 'guess and uncover' to identify forms of adult discourse associated with infant secure attachment, Goldwyn identified the importance of the speaker's ability, in the present, 'to take a balanced view of relationships'. However, the personal history recounted by such speakers seemed to have one of two forms. A first was 'a believable picture of one or both parents serving as a secure base or haven of safety in childhood, a picture which is not contradicted within the interview and which may even be illustrated by incidents of parental giving of comfort or support'.[403] Narrated in such accounts, it seemed to Main and colleagues, was secure-autonomous speech as a consequence of relatively unbruised and secure attachment relationships in childhood. Yet several transcripts in the development sample revealed speech that was about difficult childhoods, but marked by flexible attention to the good and the bad, to memories of the past and to communication with the interviewer in the present, and to their own perspective and that of others. For example, one mother who had experienced rejection by her family responded to the researchers' initial query regarding the nature of her early relationships: 'how many hours do you have? I have one of those families that they should write a whole book about. Okay, well to start with, my mother was not cheerful, and I could tell you right now the reason was that she was overworked.'[404] Though this mother had experienced rejecting caregiving, she seemed to Goldwyn and Main nonetheless able to acknowledge negative aspects of the relationship, with insight into both her own and her parents' experiences. When this mother and her infant had been seen in the Strange Situation five years earlier, they were classified as B3, and the dyad received the lowest possible score on the Ainsworth avoidance scale.[405]

In the first version of the coding system from 1982–83, Main and Goldwyn identified three trajectories that seemed to be linked, despite a caregiver's own difficult history of care, to secure-autonomous speech and a secure attachment relationship in the infant–caregiver relationship. A first was that some speakers seemed to have 'actively engaged in a period of rebellion and escape from the parents', moving away from these relationships as an opportunity to reorganise how they respond to distress in the context of relationships.[406] A second trajectory seemed to be that some speakers had 'forgiven the parents', holding in mind both their own perspective and feelings about events but also articulating a sense of the difficulties

[402] Grossmann, K.E., Grossmann, K., & Waters, E. (eds) (2005) *Attachment from Infancy to Adulthood: The Major Longitudinal Studies*. New York: Guilford; Pinquart, M., Feußner, C., & Ahnert, L. (2013) Meta-analytic evidence for stability in attachments from infancy to early adulthood. *Attachment & Human Development*, 15(2), 189–218.

[403] George, C., Kaplan, N., Goldwyn, R., & Main, M. (1982–83) Attachment interview for parents. PP/Bow/J.4/4.

[404] Main, M., Kaplan, N., & Cassidy, J. (1985) Security in infancy, childhood, and adulthood: a move to the level of representation. *Monographs of the Society for Research in Child Development*, 50, 66–104, p.96.

[405] Main, M. & Goldwyn, R. (1984) Predicting rejection of her infant from mother's representation of her own experience: implications for the abused–abusing intergenerational cycle. *Child Abuse & Neglect*, 8(2), 203–17, p.215–16.

[406] George, C., Kaplan, N., Goldwyn, R., & Main, M. (1982–83) Attachment interview for parents. PP/Bow/J.4/4.

their own parents had faced.[407] A third trajectory, perhaps predisposed by the fact that Main's sample was from near the University of California, Berkeley campus, was that some had 'engaged in a period of study undertaken with a view to understanding child–parent relationships and their influence'.[408] What all three trajectories seemed to have in common was the effortful achievement of a new perspective. By 1988, Main had come to refer to this as 'earned security'.

The first study to discuss earned security in print and to study it empirically was conducted by Main and Hesse's colleagues at the University of California, Carolyn and Philip Cowan, and published in 1994. The Cowans were conducting a longitudinal study of the transition to parenthood, and the AAI was administered to 40 adults when the first-born children in the study were 42 months. In the sample, 10 speakers were classified as insecure, 10 as 'continuous-secure', and 20 as 'earned secure'. Earned security was defined in practice by the Cowans as speakers who were classified as secure-autonomous in speech, but whose transcripts also indicated a high score for neglecting and rejecting behaviour by either caregiver, and a comparatively low score for loving behaviour by at least one caregiver. The Cowans found that the half of their sample who were judged to be continuous-secure speakers reported lower levels of depressive symptoms than the insecure or earned-secure speakers. However, observations of child–caregiver interaction indicated that the earned-secure speakers and continuous-secure speakers offered the same degree of warmth and structure as their children played, in contrast to a lower degree of warmth and structure offered by speakers who had been classified as insecure on the AAI.[409] The image of individuals able to 'earn' the benefits of secure early relationships through their own efforts in later childhood, adolescence, or adulthood has naturally been one with great appeal, especially in the American clinical community.[410] And indeed, researchers found that earned-secure speakers are more likely to have spent time in psychotherapy than continuous-secure, preoccupied, or dismissing speakers.[411] The classification also offered attachment researchers a powerful answer to accusations that attachment theory is concerned only with continuity from infancy to adult relationships. Moreover, it supported the application of the AAI as an outcome measure for evaluating psychotherapeutic interventions.[412]

Roisman and Sroufe, however, felt that there was a need to 'be cautious about retrospective reports'.[413] They cited Main and Goldwyn who had observed that it cannot be 'presumed

[407] Ibid.

[408] Ibid.

[409] Pearson, J.L., Cohn, D.A., Cowan, P.A., & Cowan, C.P. (1994) Earned-and continuous-security in adult attachment: relation to depressive symptomatology and parenting style. *Development & Psychopathology*, 6(2), 359–73.

[410] E.g. Guina, J. (2016) The talking cure of avoidant personality disorder: remission through earned-secure attachment. *American Journal of Psychotherapy*, 70(3), 233–50.

[411] Caspers, K.M., Yucuis, R., Troutman, B., & Spinks, R. (2006) Attachment as an organizer of behavior: implications for substance abuse problems and willingness to seek treatment. *Substance Abuse Treatment, Prevention, and Policy*, 1(1), 32; Saunders, R., Jacobvitz, D., Zaccagnino, M., Beverung, L.M., & Hazen, N. (2011) Pathways to earned-security: the role of alternative support figures. *Attachment & Human Development*, 13(4), 403–20.

[412] Levy, K.N., Meehan, K.B., Kelly, K.M., et al. (2006) Change in attachment patterns and reflective function in a randomized control trial of transference-focused psychotherapy for borderline personality disorder. *Journal of Consulting and Clinical Psychology*, 74(6), 1027–40.

[413] Roisman, G.I., Padrón, E., Sroufe, L.A., & Egeland, B. (2002) Earned-secure attachment status in retrospect and prospect. *Child Development*, 73(4), 1204–19, p.1205. Since the criticism of the earned-secure classification has become identified with Roisman, it is worth highlighting that Roisman and Sroufe are jointly the corresponding authors for the paper. The discussion is long, but the main section on p.1216 reads firmly as in Sroufe's voice and refers in the first person plural to other research not conducted by Roisman.

that these retrospective interviews can provide a veridical picture of early experience'.[414] In a paper published in 2002, Roisman and Sroufe set out to examine the earned-secure classification prospectively, drawing on the Minnesota Longitudinal Study of Risk and Adaptation (Chapter 4); 170 participants in the study completed the AAI at age 19. Since the Cowan's study, Main had also altered the coding manual to require that participants receive a score of lower than 2.5 on the scale for inferred loving parental behaviour in order to qualify as earned secure.[415] Roisman and Sroufe noted, however, that only three of the participants in their whole sample met this stringent standard, perhaps because they had conducted the AAI at age 19 so there had been only scant opportunity for individuals to achieve secure-autonomous status following such adverse care.[416] Roisman and Sroufe adopted an approach that resembled the Cowans, though with a few alterations based on methodological discussions in the intervening years.[417] On the basis of this approach, 24 participants were classified as earned secure.[418]

Roisman and Sroufe replicated the Cowans' finding that earned-secure speakers reported more current depressive symptoms. Prospective data also revealed that, a decade and a half earlier, their mothers had reported more symptoms of anxiety and depression in their children compared to both the continuous-secure speakers and those with a preoccupied or dismissing AAI classification. Findings were in the same direction in adolescence. Observations of the 19-year-old speakers in interactions with romantic partners revealed that earned-secure speakers scored much the same as continuous-secure speakers, and much more highly than dismissing and preoccupied speakers, on measures such as shared positive affect, provision of the partner with a secure base, and conflict resolution.

Yet, looking back in time, data from the prospective cohort study also revealed that there had been no difference between earned- and continuous-secure speakers in terms of their infant attachment classifications with either fathers or mothers. Additionally, in an observational assessment with their mothers at 24 months, earned-secure speakers had received the most supportive care of any of the children, more than the preoccupied, dismissing, and continuous-secure speakers. At age 13, the mother–child interactions of both earned-secure and continuous-secure speakers were much more supportive and positive than those of preoccupied and dismissing speakers. Roisman and Sroufe concluded that the 'earned-secures

[414] Main, M. & Goldwyn, R. (1998) *Adult Attachment Scoring and Classification Systems, Version 6.3.* Unpublished manuscript.

[415] This decision is discussed in Hesse, E. (2016) The Adult Attachment Interview: protocol, method of analysis, and selected empirical studies: 1985–2015. In J. Cassidy & P.R. Shaver (eds) *Handbook of Attachment: Theory, Research, and Clinical Applications,* 3rd edn (pp.553–97). New York: Guilford.

[416] Roisman, G.I., Padrón, E., Sroufe, L.A., & Egeland, B. (2002) Earned-secure attachment status in retrospect and prospect. *Child Development,* 73(4), 1204–19, p.1209. None of the 19-year-old participants in the Berkeley follow-up study was classified as 'earned secure' according to the stringent criteria either. Main, M., Hesse, E., & Kaplan, N. (2005) Predictability of attachment behavior and representational processes at 1, 6, and 19 years of age: the Berkeley longitudinal study. In K.E. Grossmann, K. Grossmann, & E. Waters (eds) *Attachment from Infancy to Adulthood: The Major Longitudinal Studies* (pp.245–304). New York: Guilford.

[417] This followed slight changes to the operationalisation of earned security made by Phelps and colleagues, and then by Paley and colleagues: Phelps, J.L., Belsky, J., & Crnic, K. (1997) Earned security, daily stress, and parenting: a comparison of five alternative models. *Development & Psychopathology,* 10, 21–38; Paley, B., Cox, M.J., Burchinal, M.R., & Payne, C.C. (1999) Attachment and marital functioning: comparison of spouses with continuous-secure, earned-secure, dismissing, and preoccupied attachment stances. *Journal of Family Psychology,* 13(4), 580–97.

[418] Examination of Table 1 in Roisman et al. (2002) reveals that distinguishing this group seems to have been more on the basis of reported difficult childhood relationships with fathers than with mothers. Roisman, G.I., Padrón, E., Sroufe, L.A., & Egeland, B. (2002) Earned-secure attachment status in retrospect and prospect. *Child Development,* 73(4), 1204–19.

were the beneficiaries of among the most supportive maternal care in a high-risk sample' and, as a consequence, 'we cannot rule out the possibility that self-described differences in early experience between retrospectively defined earned- and continuous-secures were primarily a function of positive and/or negative reporting biases (e.g. negative attentional biases associated with depression)'.[419]

Such findings underline the focus of the AAI on current states of mind regarding attachment: differences identified in the interview between subgroups of secure-autonomous speakers did pick out prospective differences in histories of care and relationships, such as more parent-reported symptoms of anxiety and depression in preschool among the earned-secure speakers. However, the findings seemed in some regards to also put into question the accounts of earned-secure speakers of adverse forms of care in childhood. Roisman and Sroufe interpreted their findings as suggesting that 'earned-secures did not rise above malevolent parenting through sheer will; rather, their success was scaffolded by caring adults, their security was a natural extension of a supportive (although not necessarily ideal) past'.[420] They therefore recommended that an alternative to the term 'earned security' might be considered. Hesse and Main subsequently agreed that 'the term earned-secure is not an ideal taxonomic label', and proposed the term 'evolved secure' as an alternative—though this proposal seems to have been ignored so far, or come too late in the day to change the presiding discourse.[421] And indeed, attachment researchers have generally continued to depict the childhoods of earned-evolved secure speakers as adverse, and secure-autonomous speech in the AAI as reflecting an individual achievement, something 'earned', in the face of this adversity.[422]

A further study by Roisman and colleagues has provided additional evidence relevant to appraisal of the 'earned-secure' classification. They found that speakers classified as earned/evolved secure, even on the basis of the stringent Main and Goldwyn criteria, experienced levels of maternal sensitivity comparable to dismissing and preoccupied speakers at between 5 and 64 months.[423] Their caregivers also had more financial difficulties and depressive symptoms. However, on other measures, these speakers appeared to have had more positive care. From middle childhood they experienced care that was around the sample average for sensitivity, and in adolescence observations of child–caregiver suggested that they received more sensitive care than preoccupied and dismissing speakers. They also received

[419] Ibid. p.1215. In support of attentional biases interpretation see Roisman, G.I., Fortuna, K., & Holland, A. (2006) An experimental manipulation of retrospectively defined earned and continuous attachment security. *Child Development*, 77(1), 59–71.

[420] Roisman, G.I., Padrón, E., Sroufe, L.A., & Egeland, B. (2002) Earned-secure attachment status in retrospect and prospect. *Child Development*, 73(4), 1204–19, p.1216. See also Roisman G. & Haydon K.C. (2011) Earned-security in retrospect: emerging insights from longitudinal, experimental, and taxometric investigations. In D. Cicchetti & G.I. Roisman (eds) *The Origins and Organization of Adaptation and Maladaptation: The Minnesota Symposia on Child Psychology*, Vol. 36 (pp.109–54). New York: Wiley.

[421] Hesse, E. (2016) The Adult Attachment Interview: protocol, method of analysis, and selected empirical studies: 1985–2015. In J. Cassidy & P.R. Shaver (eds) *Handbook of Attachment: Theory, Research, and Clinical Applications*, 3rd edn (pp.553–97). New York: Guilford, p.572. The term 'evolved' may also still carry over too many connotations from eugenics discourses to feel comfortable on the tongues of developmental researchers.

[422] E.g. Reiner, I. & Spangler, G. (2010) Adult attachment and gene polymorphisms of the dopamine D4 receptor and serotonin transporter (5-HTT). *Attachment & Human Development*, 12(3), 209–29. However, see recently Iyengar, U., Rajhans, P., Fonagy, P., Strathearn, L., & Kim, S. (2019) Unresolved trauma and reorganization in mothers: attachment and neuroscience perspectives. *Frontiers in Psychology*, 10, 110.

[423] Roisman, G.I., Haltigan, J.D., Haydon, K.C., & Booth-LaForce, C. (2014) Earned-security in retrospect: depressive symptoms, family stress, and maternal and paternal sensitivity from early childhood to mid-adolescence. *Monographs of the Society for Research in Child Development*, 79(3), 85–107, p.105.

much more positive paternal care than the preoccupied and dismissing speakers, with no differences from those classified continuous-secure. The study by Roisman and colleagues has been subject to theoretical and methodological criticism from Hesse, who remains unconvinced that earned-/evoked-secure speakers really did have more positive care.[424] In the context of such debates, the 'earned/evolved secure' classification will no doubt be subject to further research over the coming years by Roisman and other third-generation attachment researchers.[425] Nonetheless, all parties to the debate about 'earned security' agree that it should be emphasised that the AAI solicits a retrospective account: it is qualities in the speaker's discourse and reasoning about attachment-relevant experiences that form the basis of classification, not the nature of the events described. This is why attachment researchers have been especially intrigued by occasions when discourse or reasoning about attachment-relevant experiences appears to be disrupted.

Unresolved loss

An early observation made by Goldwyn was that at points some narratives became 'splintered and incoherent, so that ideas were lost, superficially unconnected ideas invaded one another, and the whole approach to the topic of attachment became disorganised'.[426] Goldwyn and Main documented occasions of varying degrees of such disrupted discourse—some extensive, some more momentary—across dismissing, preoccupied, and secure-autonomous transcripts, though they seemed somewhat predominant among preoccupied and dismissing speakers.[427] Goldwyn's application of 'guess and uncover' revealed that these transcripts frequently belonged to parents in dyads that had earlier been unclassifiable in the Strange Situation according to the Ainsworth categories. Furthermore, this semi-inductive method revealed that many of these speakers had experienced loss of attachment figures, especially before adolescence.[428] However, further examination of the transcripts in 1983 revealed that

---

[424] This finding is highlighted and discussed in Hesse, E. (2016) The Adult Attachment Interview: protocol, method of analysis, and selected empirical studies: 1985–2015. In J. Cassidy & P.R. Shaver (eds) *Handbook of Attachment: Theory, Research, and Clinical Applications*, 3rd edn (pp.553–97). New York: Guilford.

[425] A review of mood induction experiments to explore the meaning of earned/evolved security is presented in Roisman, G.I. & Haydon, K.C. (2011) Earned-security in retrospect: emerging insights from longitudinal, experimental, and taxometric investigations. In D. Cicchetti & G.I. Roisman (eds) *The Origins and Organization of Adaptation and Maladaptation: The Minnesota Symposia on Child Psychology*, Vol. 36 (pp.109–54). New York: Wiley.

[426] Main, M. & Goldwyn, R. (1983) Predicting rejection of an infant from mother's representation of her own experiences. National Conference on Infant Mental Health, Children's Institute International, Los Angeles, February 1983. PP/Bow/J.4/3.

[427] In the early 1980s, Main still regarded conflict behaviours as especially characteristic of avoidant infants under stress; likewise, in a conference presentation of 1983, Main proposed that splintered and incoherent elements would especially characterise discourse too, when a speaker adopting an avoidant strategy was faced with a procedure, like the AAI (or the Separation Anxiety Test), which asked them to contradict their characteristic conditional strategy and turn their attention to attachment-related experiences and feelings. However, by the mid-1980s and the 'Move to the level of representation' paper, Main had come to regard disorganisation as varying independently of the three Ainsworth classifications and their analogues in the AAI coding system. Main, M. & Goldwyn, R. (1983) Predicting rejection of an infant from mother's representation of her own experiences. National Conference on Infant Mental Health, Children's Institute International, Los Angeles, February 1983. PP/Bow/J.4/3.

[428] Main, M. (1982) *Letter to John Bowlby*, 9 December 1982. PP/Bow/J.4/4: 'There is a second-generation effect of early loss (through death) upon infant attachment behaviour. The infant whose parent lost a parent or other attachment figure before maturity becomes unclassifiable as A, B or C in the Ainsworth infant system.' Other speakers had experienced bizarre forms of early care, such as a mother whose obsessional symptoms meant that her children were regarded as too dirty to be allowed to touch her. By the end of 1982, Goldwyn and Main had

early loss in itself was not a good predictor of infant attachment classification. Rather, what seemed critical was that speakers seemed to show disruptions in their discourse, to be in a semantic sense 'at a loss', when discussing the dead attachment figure. The concept of 'unresolved grief' or 'unresolved mourning' had been gaining prominence in the clinical literature of the 1970s.[429] This development drew on earlier accounts by psychoanalysts, including Bowlby, of the way in which acknowledging and accepting a loss could contribute to mental health symptoms.[430] Building from both Bowlby and the contemporary clinical literature, Main and Hesse conceptualised the speakers as 'unresolved with respect to the mourning of an attachment figure'. These speakers were allocated an Unresolved/disorganised (U/d) classification.

In the late 1980s, Main and Hesse developed a 'Lack of Resolution for Mourning' scale, with support from a research assistant Anitra DeMoss. Most often markers of lack of resolution occurred in response to the direct question in the AAI about losses, but they could also be identified in other parts of the transcript that touch upon the relationship with the dead person. Main, Hesse, and Demoss distinguished two species of lapses in the transcripts.[431] Sometimes these co-occurred, especially in clinical or forensic samples, but mostly transcripts displayed one or the other as a characteristic form. A first species was *lapses in monitoring of reasoning* without recognition by the speaker, leading to breaches in 'coherence' through interruptions in the plausibility of the speaker's account.[432] For instance, such lapses were implied in a belief that the dead person remains alive and actively involved in the speaker's life (e.g. Mrs Q, Chapter 1). This includes statements in interview such as 'So I don't now what field I'm going to select, but my father [deceased 15 years ago in childhood] says that I should choose law'. Main and colleagues commented on 'this slip of the tongue to the present tense regarding a lost attachment figure. It is taken as an indication of disbelief that the person is dead and leads to U/d category placement because: a) the speaker is talking about something going on in his immediate surroundings; b) which is currently of vital import to him, and is c) actively bringing the long-deceased into a freshly constructed sentence; d) as though he or she continued to have input. However, slips to the present tense sometimes do not indicate serious disorientation/disorganisation. If, for example, a person says of a deceased father 'my father has been in banking for a number of years' the slip may be minor.[433]

developed two categories for transcripts containing splintered discourse. A first category was 'Lost: an attachment figure lost through death and parent has not mourned sufficiently'. A second category was 'Untouchable: the parents' parents were untouchable in a peculiar way, e.g. a mother whose mother always implied she was dirty, so that the children must not touch her'. George, C., Kaplan, N., Goldwyn, R., & Main, M. (1982–83) Attachment interview for parents. PP/Bow/J.4/4. This second category was not subsequently included in the coding system, presumably in part because it turned out to be rare.

[429] E.g. Lewis, E. (1979) Inhibition of mourning by pregnancy: psychopathology and management. *British Medical Journal*, 2(6181), 27–8; Fulmer, R.H. (1983) A structural approach to unresolved mourning in single parent family systems. *Journal of Marital and Family Therapy*, 9(3), 259–69.

[430] Deutsch, H. (1937) Absence of grief. *Psychoanalytic Quarterly*, 6, 12–22; Bowlby, J. (1963) Pathological mourning and childhood mourning. *Journal of the American Psychoanalytic Association*, 11(3), 500–541. See also Granek, L. (2010) Grief as pathology: the evolution of grief theory in psychology from Freud to the present. *History of Psychology*, 13(1), 46–73.

[431] That these were identified between 1987 and 1989 is suggested by the fact that the distinction is quite foreign to an earlier draft of the scale, sent to Bowlby as Main, M. & Hesse, E. (1987) Lack of resolution of mourning, 15 November 1987. PP/Bow/B.3/36/1.

[432] Main, M. (1991) Metacognitive knowledge, metacognitive monitoring, and singular (coherent) vs. multiple (incoherent) models of attachment: some findings and some directions for future research. In P. Marris, J. Stevenson-Hinde, & C. Parkes (eds) *Attachment Across the Life Cycle* (pp.127–59). New York: Routledge, p.144–5.

[433] Main, M., Goldwyn, R., & Hesse, E. (2002) *Adult Attachment Scoring and Classification System*. Unpublished manuscript, University of California at Berkeley, Department of Psychology.

The coding manual positioned lapses in reasoning about whether an attachment figure was dead or not dead as the paradigmatic case of unresolved loss. Other rarer lapses in reasoning around loss included confusion between the dead person and the speaker, and characterisations of events in time or space that are not possible—such as being present at a family tragedy and also, simultaneously, being absent from the event in another country. Lapses in reasoning were ultimately characterised as 'things which cannot be true in the external world',[434] though, anticipating problems with this definition, Main and colleagues advised coders as best they could to exclude statements that are grounded in a self-aware and integrated religious or cultural viewpoint.[435] An additional set of relatively common lapses of reasoning was identified by Main and Hesse as occurring when speakers stated that they have done something that cannot be true psychologically, such as using willpower to erase experience of a past event. These are claims that, as it were, cannot be true of the internal world.

A second type of lapse indicating unresolved states of mind was *lapses in the monitoring of discourse* without recognition by the speaker. Examples included: invasions of remarks about a death into apparently unrelated discussions; sudden use of eulogistic speech; exceptionally long blank pauses that the speaker does not him-/herself seem to notice; or apparent absorption in particular details surrounding the death.[436] Though there was no explicit statement in the AAI coding manual stating that lapses in reasoning are more important in making a classification than lapses in discourse, it is notable that only a few of the examples given of lapses in discourse are afforded a high score on the scale for unresolved loss, whereas many of the lapses in reasoning are given a high score. There may be more ambiguity regarding the cause of a lapse in the monitoring of discourse.[437] Additionally or as a consequence, it may be

[434] Ibid.

[435] Behrens, K.Y., Hesse, E., & Main, M. (2007) Mothers' attachment status as determined by the Adult Attachment Interview predicts their 6-year-olds' reunion responses: a study conducted in Japan. *Developmental Psychology*, 43(6), 1553–67: 'In Japan, it is a common, culturally polite practice in certain contexts to refer to deceased persons in the present tense. From early on, Japanese children are often encouraged to talk as if a deceased person is alive, as this is considered an act of respect for the deceased in a culture that traditionally has encouraged ancestral worship. Initially, speech usage of this kind was confusing for the AAI coder (Kazuko Y. Behrens) when attempting to score unresolved status. This was because guidelines in the AAI manual stipulate that present tense references to deceased persons can, when marked, imply a "lapse in reasoning" referred to as "dead/not-dead" (Hesse, 1999, p. 405). In other words, in English, some present tense slippages suggest that a speaker holds two incompatible belief systems, one in which the deceased person is understood to be dead, and a second in which he or she is considered to be alive (in the physical, not religious or meta-physical, sense). After studying a number of Japanese texts with present tense usage regarding deceased persons, however, it was possible (as it is in English) to distinguish normative from nonnormative forms. Thus, for example, when Japanese mothers discussed both talking to and/or instructing their child to talk to a deceased grandmother in the present tense at a portable shrine or altar before going to sleep, this could be considered analogous to a Western prayer. Hence, it is culturally sanctioned, and as such does not imply the frightening ideation that seems to often accompany anomalous dead/not-dead usages in English (see Hesse & Main, 2006). In contrast, Japanese normally uses the past tense when conveying factual information regarding deceased persons to a third party. Thus present tense usages in this latter context would be considered as potential slippages or lapses in speech, which could, depending on intensity, lead to a U placement' (1559).

[436] A third, rare form of lack of resolution was characterised as reports of extreme behavioural reactions to the death, such as of episodes of uncharacteristic violence or suicide attempts, where the speaker does not appear to realise in the present that the behaviour requires some remark to the interviewer to contextualise, explain it, or situate the action in relation to the speaker's present self. However, 'both our own experience and those of other investigators informally queried indicated that assignment to the unresolved-disorganised adult attachment category on the basis of reports of extreme behavioural reactions is very rare'. Main, M. & Morgan, H. (1996) Disorganization and disorientation in infant Strange Situation behavior: phenotypic resemblance to dissociative states. In L. Michelson & W. Ray (eds) *Handbook of Dissociation: Theoretical, Empirical and Clinical Perspectives* (pp.107–38). New York: Plenum Press, p.119.

[437] Though described as 'lapses', it is worth noting that markers of unresolved/disorganised states of mind are sometimes but not generally entirely out of the blue, as the term might suggest. There may often be a logic to their

inferred that lapses in discourse are less proximal markers than lapses in reasoning for what Main and colleagues were seeking to capture.

In line with this supposition, by the early 1990s, Main's work with Solomon on infant disorganisation had led to a re-evaluation of the concept of lack of resolution. In 1991, Main and colleagues wrote that 'as we have gained an increasing understanding of the nature of the link between the adult's and infant's state, unresolved/disorganised/disoriented has come to seem the best descriptor'.[438] Main and colleagues concluded that there could be various ways that a loss might be left unresolved over time but without contributing to a disorganised/ disoriented state of mind regarding the attachment-relevant cognition: 'thus, for example, effective dismissal of the import of a loss is certainly indicative of failure of resolution of mourning (and is often referred to as "failed mourning"), but is not considered disorganised/ disoriented'.[439] In such a case, attention has been effectively directed away from the potentially disorganising loss, much as Main conceptualised the Group A pattern in the Strange Situation as avoidance of conflict and loss of regulation.[440] A smooth surface is put in play by effective dismissal, against which grief and sorrow will ricochet.

Likewise, distressed pining after a lost attachment figure is often considered by clinicians as indicating that the work of mourning is not finished. And the term 'unresolved' would suggest that such cases would be included and coded. Indeed, several other researchers have advocated for the extension of the unresolved/disorganised classification to include this kind of response.[441] Again, however, Main and Hesse claimed that this 'distress is not considered evidence for a disorganised/disoriented state of mind', though they acknowledged that the boundary is less clear in this case since weeping does entail 'a very slight index of disorientation'.[442] The distinction between preoccupation with a loss and disorganisation/disorientation is real but somewhat permeable, just like in Main's thinking about C and D in the infant classification system, essentially since distress can be dysregulating. This implies a subtle but vital qualification. Though the category was named 'unresolved for loss', Main and colleagues specified in the manual that coders were *not* actually being instructed to identify lack of resolution. Rather, the coding protocols were situated as seeking to identify instances of the 'disorganised/disoriented state of mind' with regard to attachment that unresolved losses often seemed to occasion.[443] Discussions of an unresolved loss in the AAI seemed to be the

interruption of a state of mind regarding attachment. For instance, a dismissing speaker might close down to clipped replies even more in a discussion leading up to or following a lapse, in a strategy of avoidance of disorganisation; a preoccupied speaker might, derailed by a lapse, further lose track of the question and focus further on their feelings of grievance.

[438] Main, M., Demoss, A., & Hesse, E. (1991) Unresolved (disorganised/disoriented) states of mind with respect to experiences of loss. In M. Main, R. Goldwyn, & E. Hesse (2002) *Adult Attachment Scoring and Classification System*. Unpublished manuscript, University of California at Berkeley, Department of Psychology.

[439] Ibid.: 'One parent of a very secure child had been orphaned in traumatic circumstances. The parent described these circumstances briefly, adding firmly "topic closed". We did not consider this refusal indicative of an unresolved/disorganised response to the loss under discussion.'

[440] Ibid.: 'Whether the alternative being avoided is sorrow, fear, anger or some unwonted behaviour pattern, in failed mourning the subject avoids disorganisation by failing to focus on loss.'

[441] By way of contrast, Sagi-Schwartz and colleagues, and George and West, later argued that dismissal of a loss and distressed pining following a loss should have been regarded as unresolved states of mind. Sagi-Schwartz, A., Koren-Karie, N., & Joels, T. (2003) Failed mourning in the Adult Attachment Interview: the case of Holocaust child survivors. *Attachment & Human Development*, 5(4), 398–409; George, C. & West, M.L. (2012) *The Adult Attachment Projective Picture System: Attachment Theory and Assessment in Adults*. New York: Guilford.

[442] Main, M., Goldwyn, R., & Hesse, E. (2002) *Adult Attachment Scoring and Classification System*. Unpublished manuscript, University of California at Berkeley, Department of Psychology.

[443] Ibid.

frequent occasion of disruptions in attentional processes and the processing of information relevant to attachment. In Main and Solomon's work on the Strange Situation, the term 'disorganised' was used to refer to both behaviour and motivation. The term sought to laminate conflicting, confused, or apprehensive observable behaviour with inferences about the functioning of the (invisible) attachment system. So too in the AAI. The concept of 'unresolved' speech laminated observable lapses in reasoning or discourse in transcripts with inferences about the (invisible) integration and coherence of attentional processes in the retrieval and communication of information about attachment-relevant experiences.

Main and Hesse developed a nine-point scale for coding unresolved/disorganised/disoriented states of mind regarding attachment, which was based partly on the inferred extent of disruption to the retrieval and communication of information about attachment-relevant experiences, and partly on how certain the coder was that lapses of reasoning or discourse were what they were seeing in the transcript. As with the infant system, scores above 5 warranted a classification. In most instances, unresolved/disorganised/disoriented states of mind appeared as an interruption or splintering within the speaker's characteristic forms of reasoning and discourse when the topic of loss or abuse was raised, though in some cases it could be more pervasive across the transcript. Main and Hesse conjectured that frightening experiences or circumstances surrounding or following a loss or frightening ideas regarding the relationship with the lost figure would be one pathway to disorganised/disoriented states of mind. This idea was supported by the finding that unresolved states of mind regarding attachment are moderately associated with frightening, frightened, or dissociative behaviours by caregivers towards their infants ($r = .28$).[444] It was also supported by work by Beverung and Jacobvitz, which demonstrated that unresolved loss was twice as common when speakers perceived the loss as sudden.[445] However, to the researchers' surprise, there was no association in their sample between U/d following bereavement and age at loss, the nature of the relationship, the extent of emotional support, or the cause of death.

A fundamental study for the establishment of the U/d classification was conducted by Ainsworth and Eichberg. This was Ainsworth's final direct involvement in empirical research. The AAI and the Strange Situation were conducted with a sample of 45 Charlottesville mother–infant dyads. Ainsworth and Eichberg found that 30 dyads of the sample had experienced loss of an attachment figure, but 20 displayed few or no markers of unresolved/disorganised/disoriented state of mind regarding attachment. A qualitative review of these transcripts revealed that these speakers had experienced various forms of social connectedness following the bereavement, whether in terms of the availability of comfort from others or in terms of their own responsibility for other family members. Only two of the mothers classified as resolved for their loss were part of dyads classified as disorganised in the

[444] Madigan, S., Bakermans-Kranenburg, M.J., Van IJzendoorn, M.H., Moran, G., Pederson, D.R., & Benoit, D. (2006) Unresolved states of mind, anomalous parental behavior, and disorganized attachment: a review and meta-analysis of a transmission gap. *Attachment & Human Development*, 8(2), 89–111, Table 2.

[445] Beverung and Jacobvitz also speculated that the causal relationship may actually be reversed: U/d may subsequently make a loss feel like it took place more suddenly. However, their design was cross-sectional and a prospective study would be needed to examine which way causality runs, or whether there is a bidirectional relationship between U/d and perceived suddenness of the bereavement. Beverung, L.M. & Jacobvitz, D. (2016) Women's retrospective experiences of bereavement: predicting unresolved attachment. *OMEGA-Journal of Death and Dying*, 73(2), 126–40. In another study, Lyons-Ruth and colleagues found that retrospective report of parental death in childhood was only associated with unresolved loss at the level of a trend, and was not statistically significant ($r = 0.20$). Lyons-Ruth, K., Yellin, C., Melnick, S., & Atwood, G. (2003) Childhood experiences of trauma and loss have different relations to maternal unresolved and hostile-helpless states of mind on the AAI. *Attachment & Human Development*, 5(4), 330–52.

Strange Situation, showing clearly that loss in itself was not a powerful predictor of infant disorganised attachment.[446] In the final count, ten bereaved mothers received a U/d classification, and of these all were members of dyads classified by blind coders as disorganised/disoriented in the Strange Situation. The other five dyads who received a D classification had experienced frightening occurrences. Many of these were quite recent, such as a near-death experiences or a partner's severe drug dependency.[447] Half the mothers whose discourse received a U/d classification had a secondary classification as preoccupied. Ainsworth cited conversations with Main and Hesse that there can be a close relationship between preoccupation and unresolved states of mind. For instance, 'In the case of a mother who is preoccupied with her early attachments, it is reasonable to suppose that the memory of her fear of the parent might sometimes intrude into everyday life, and re-evoke the anxiety; as such times the infant might find his mother's behaviour especially frightening since there was no apparent occasion for it.'[448] Ainsworth and Eichberg also found a 90% match between the other classifications: secure-autonomous state of mind in the AAI was highly associated with infant secure attachment, and dismissing state of mind highly associated with avoidant attachment. There was no association between preoccupied state of mind and ambivalent/resistant attachment.

The strong association between the Strange Situation and the AAI, evidenced in a study coded by no less than Ainsworth herself, provided a powerful consecration of the later measure. However, the results for unresolved/disorganised states of mind from the Ainsworth and Eichberg study have subsequently had to be excluded from meta-analyses, since the study has been such an outlier in terms of the strength of the association between the AAI and the Strange Situation procedure.[449] Van IJzendoorn observed that, though generally regarded as a replication, the study should frankly be recognised as another exploratory work.[450] In fact, this was in no way masked by the authors. Ainsworth clearly stated in the paper that, after coding the sample a first time, she repeated her coding on the basis of changes made by Main to the coding manual, which led to the perfect correlation between unresolved loss and infant disorganised attachment.[451] However, there were no changes mentioned in the classification of secure-autonomous or dismissing states of mind regarding

[446] These findings were soon after replicated by Marian Bakermans-Kranenburg as part of her doctoral research: Bakermans-Kranenburg, M.J. & Van IJzendoorn, M.H. (1993) Gehechtheidsbiografie, verlieservaringen en beleving van het ouderschap. In J.R.M. Gerris (ed.) Opvoeding, Specifieke Groepen en Minderheden (pp.33–54). Lisse: Swets & Zeitlinger: 'We examined in a group of 75 mothers with loss experiences in which mothers with unresolved loss were distinguished from the others. The number of loss experiences that were experienced turned out to be of no importance to lack of resolution' (33). The researchers also reported that 'Unresolved loss is found in a minority (17%) of mothers with loss experiences' (48).

[447] Ainsworth, M.D.S. & Eichberg, C.G. (1991) Effects on infant–mother attachment of mother's experience related to loss of an attachment figure. In C.M. Parkes, J. Stevenson-Hinde, & P. Marris (eds) Attachment Across the Life Cycle (pp.160–83). New York: Routledge, p.164.

[448] Ibid. p.180.

[449] van IJzendoorn, M.H. (1995) Adult attachment representations, parental responsiveness, and infant attachment: a meta-analysis on the predictive validity of the Adult Attachment Interview. Psychological Bulletin, 117(3), 387–403; Verhage, M.L., Schuengel, C., Madigan, S., et al. (2016) Narrowing the transmission gap: a synthesis of three decades of research on intergenerational transmission of attachment. Psychological Bulletin, 142(4), 337–66.

[450] Van IJzendoorn, M.H. (2019) Replication crisis lost in translation? Paper presented at International Attachment Conference, Vancouver, 20 July 2019.

[451] Ainsworth, M.D.S. & Eichberg, C.G. (1991) Effects on infant–mother attachment of mother's experience related to loss of an attachment figure. In C.M. Parkes, J. Stevenson-Hinde, & P. Marris (eds) Attachment Across the Life cycle. New York: Routledge, p.164. This recoding and the discussions with Main that led to it are further described in Ainsworth, M. (1990) Letter to John Bowlby, 17 January 1990. PP/BOW/B.3/8.

attachment. It is therefore likely that Ainsworth's remarkable powers as an observer also contributed to the strength of the association.

In contrast to the 100% agreement reported by Ainsworth and Eichberg, the latest meta-analytic finding regarding the association between U/d parental discourse and the D classification in the Strange Situation based on three decades of research is $r = .21$. This is weaker than the associations between the other paired categories: secure-autonomous (F) discourse and secure (B) infant attachment have an association of $r = .31$; dismissing (Ds) discourse and avoidant (A) infant attachment have an association of $r = .29$; and preoccupied (E) discourse and ambivalent/resistant (C) attachment have an association of $r = .22$.[452] There has been much discussion of factors that may 'close the transmission gap' by mediating between a caregiver's state of mind regarding attachment and the classification of the caregiver–infant dyad in the Strange Situation.[453] A variety of proposals have been made including: caregiver perception of the child's behaviour in terms of intentional mental states (mentalisation); gene × environment interactions; caregivers' support for their child's exploration; caregivers' use of effective limit-setting; and the nature of the repair offered following mismatches between children's signals and their caregiver's responses.[454] However, a further proposal for the source of the transmission gap has had to do with the operation of the U/d classification, and especially in the way that unresolved traumatic experiences have been operationalised.

Unresolved traumatic abuse

Between 1987 and 1989, Main and Hesse ran three training institutes for the AAI: in London (organised by John Bowlby and John Byng-Hall), in Virginia (organised by Mary Ainsworth), and in Rome (organised by Nino Dazzi and Massimo Ammaniti).[455] During this time, Main and Hesse saw many new transcripts, especially those collected by clinical colleagues. These new transcripts clearly showed that disruptions of discourse suggestive of disorganised/disoriented states of mind regarding attachment could occur when speakers discussed memories besides bereavement. Besides bereavement, the other frequent occasion

---

[452] Verhage, M.L., Schuengel, C., Madigan, S., et al. (2016) Narrowing the transmission gap: a synthesis of three decades of research on intergenerational transmission of attachment. *Psychological Bulletin*, 142(4), 337–66. An additional recent meta-analytic finding work led by Madigan as part of the Collaboration on Attachment Transmission Synthesis (see Chapter 6) has been that parents with U/d classifications on the AAI are more likely to be part of dyads with disorganised attachment relationships, but not more or less likely to be part of dyads with avoidant or resistant attachment relationships than any other parents. Madigan, S. and the Collaboration on Attachment Transmission Synthesis (2019) *An Examination of the Cross-Transmission of Parent–Child Attachment Using an Individual Participant Data Meta-Analysis.* Unpublished manuscript, cited with permission of Sheri Madigan.

[453] van IJzendoorn, M.H. (1995) Adult attachment representations, parental responsiveness, and infant attachment: a meta-analysis on the predictive validity of the Adult Attachment Interview. *Psychological Bulletin*, 117(3), 387–403; IJzendoorn, M.H. & Bakermans-Kranenburg, M. (2019) Bridges across the intergenerational transmission of attachment gap. *Current Opinion in Psychology*, 25, 31–6.

[454] Fonagy, P. & Target, M. (2005) Bridging the transmission gap: an end to an important mystery of attachment research? *Attachment & Human Development*, 7(3), 333–43; Beebe, B. & Steele, M. (2013) How does microanalysis of mother–infant communication inform maternal sensitivity and infant attachment? *Attachment & Human Development*, 15(5–6), 583–602; Bernier, A., Matte-Gagné, C., Bélanger, M.È., & Whipple, N. (2014) Taking stock of two decades of attachment transmission gap: broadening the assessment of maternal behavior. *Child Development*, 85(5), 1852–65.

[455] Hesse, E. (1999) The Adult Attachment Interview: historical and current perspectives. In J. Cassidy & P. Shavers (eds) *Handbook of Attachment: Theory, Research, and Clinical Applications* (pp.395–433). New York: Guilford, p.406.

for lapses in discourse or reasoning seemed to be experiences of traumatic abuse. Main and Hesse's growing attention to traumatic abuse may also be placed in the context of the increased prominence of this topic within academic psychology and wider American cultural discourses by the late 1980s.[456] Until that point, Main and Hesse had advised coders to extend use of the 'unresolved loss' classification to encompass disorganised/disoriented states of mind about abuse: 'researchers were advised to use the indices of disorganisation and disorientation in thought processes during discussions of a loss in order to identify unresolved trauma of other kinds'.[457] One problem with this extension was that the standard AAI questions were not well adapted to exploring abuse, since the topic is only raised in quite a general way, in contrast to loss experiences which are extensively probed.[458] Nonetheless, the interview questions regularly elicited lapses in monitoring of reasoning and discourse in higher-risk samples, and occasionally in lower-risk samples too.[459] By the end of the 1980s, Main and Hesse had 'now completed a draft of a separate scale for assessing unresolved experiences of physical abuse'.[460] That bereavement and traumatic abuse could have the same kinds of consequences for attention and information-processing, and hence on discourse, seemed intuitive to Main and Hesse in light of their idea that the intrusion of fear in relation to an attachment figure might be a cause of both infant disorganised attachment and disorganised/disoriented states of mind. Traumatic abuse is, definitionally, frightening.

In fact the traumatic abuse scale, completed at the start of the 1990s, was not just for physical abuse but also included any experience where an attachment figure may have traumatised the child through frightening behaviour. Sexual abuse and threats to kill the child were therefore also included. Main and Hesse excluded cases where a 'parent was described as hostile or mean at times, but without being clearly highly frightening in the view of the judge'. They also advised that traumatic abuse should not be coded if the event was a one-off, even if a child was for instance hit in the face by a parent or touched sexually by a drunk parent through clothing, if this was not 'overwhelmingly frightening' or 'expected to escalate'. The coding manual suggested that an important factor in making this differentiation is the extent to which the speaker did or 'did not fear that the parent would go out of control'.[461] Main and colleagues advised that if the child was very frightened in the situation and/or afterwards, then it should be coded as traumatic abuse, even if the speaker does not now regard the behaviour as abusive.

[456] Hacking, I. (1995) *Rewriting the Soul*. Princeton, NJ: Princeton University Press; Fassin, D. & Rechtman, R. (2009) *The Empire of Trauma*. Princeton, NJ: Princeton University Press.

[457] Main, M. & Hesse, E. (1990) Parents' unresolved traumatic experiences are related to infant disorganized attachment status. In M.T. Greenberg, D. Cicchetti, & E.M. Cummings (eds) *Attachment in the Preschool Years* (pp.161–81). Chicago: University of Chicago Press, p.177.

[458] Bailey, H.N., Moran, G., & Pederson, D.R (2007) Childhood maltreatment, complex trauma symptoms, and unresolved attachment in an at-risk sample of adolescent mothers. *Attachment & Human Development*, 9(2), 139–61: 'In contrast to the extensive probes around loss experiences, abuse (in particular, sexual abuse) experiences are explored in less detail during the AAI in order to avoid distressing the participants' (143).

[459] The rarity of U/d for traumatic abuse in low-risk samples is discussed in Hesse, E. & van IJzendoorn, M. (1999) Propensities towards absorption are related to lapses in the monitoring of reasoning or discourse during the Adult Attachment Interview: a preliminary investigation. *Attachment & Human Development*, 1, 67–91. In a group of 190 Berkeley college students reported by the authors, only three were classified as U/d on the basis of unresolved states of mind regarding traumatic abuse (p.76).

[460] Main, M. & Hesse, E. (1990) Parents' unresolved traumatic experiences are related to infant disorganized attachment status. In M.T. Greenberg, D. Cicchetti, & E.M. Cummings (eds) *Attachment in the Preschool Years* (pp.161–81). Chicago: University of Chicago Press, p.177.

[461] Main, M., Goldwyn, R., & Hesse, E. (2002) *Adult Attachment Scoring and Classification System*. Unpublished manuscript, University of California at Berkeley, Department of Psychology.

Nonetheless, an unresolved/disorganised/disoriented (U/d) classification depended in part on how events were spoken about. Sexual or physical abuse by a parent, spoken about with 'continuing pain and regret' but without lapses in reasoning or discourse would not receive an unresolved/disorganised/disoriented classification.[462] An important example given in the coding system was 'alternating clear report of abuse with denial that it was abuse'. This had an important paradigmatic status in the manual, much like statements that imply that a dead person is still alive in scale for unresolved loss, since it suggested direct conflict between segregated accounts of reality.[463] Other markers of unresolved traumatic abuse given in the coding system included: feelings of having personally deserved abusive treatment by an attachment figure; confusion by speakers between themselves and the perpetrator; as well as other signs similar to unresolved mourning such as invasion of the topic of abuse into discussion of other matters.

In both the case of loss and abuse, Main and Hesse specified that the classification cannot be given if there is no specific and identifiable historical event mentioned in the transcript.[464] Additionally, in the case of abuse but not loss, the abuse described must be established as sufficiently severe and overwhelmingly frightening. Hence there may be experiences that, despite appearances, may not be coded as unresolved even if relevant disturbances of reasoning or discourse are present. These include: a parent leaving and never being seen again (but presumably remaining alive); anticipated bereavement in the case of a terminally ill attachment figure; experiences of chronic neglect in childhood; exposure to an atmosphere of emotional abuse between parents during childhood but without there being a stand-out 'event'; and fear of an intimidating current partner or ex-partner.[465] Similarly, it is not clear

[462] Ibid. However, the boundary can sometimes be unclear. For instance, in the AAI a traumatic event or terrible loss might be spoken about coherently, but then, shortly after, another subsequent event might be discussed with lapses in reasoning and/or discourse. It can be assumed that the demand to discuss the first traumatic event has depleted the attentional resources of the speaker, so that the second picks up some of the distress and confusion that had been held at bay. However, the result is that markers of U/d become attached to events that are neither bereavements nor traumatic. There seems to be a diversity of practice regarding how coders deal with such cases.

[463] Despite their paradigmatic status in the manual, alternations of reporting and denial of abuse suggestive of segregation may sometimes be difficult for coders to identify sharply in practice, given that cultural discourses on abuse are themselves quite confused and contradictory. What appears as alternation may simply be the implementation of a dismissing strategy as arousal increases in the course of the interview.

[464] Bakermans-Kranenburg and colleagues observed that part of what is at stake is the 'resolution' of trauma or loss, something that the AAI coding protocol only assesses, at best, implicitly: 'the classification system for unresolved loss or trauma identifies only positive markers for an unresolved state of mind. Markers for successful resolution of loss are not evaluated, so the classification system does not include a "resolved" category'. Bakermans-Kranenburg, M.J., Schuengel, C., & van IJzendoorn, M.H. (1999) Unresolved loss due to miscarriage: an addition to the Adult Attachment Interview. *Attachment & Human Development*, 1(2), 157–70, p.162. Cf. Iyengar, U., Kim, S., Martinez, S., Fonagy, P., & Strathearn, L. (2014) Unresolved trauma in mothers: intergenerational effects and the role of reorganization. *Frontiers in Psychology*, 5, 966.

[465] In practice, some of these cases may be treated by coders as if they were a frightening event, so that they can be classified as unresolved, though this was ultimately not the approach adopted, on the advice of Main and Hesse, in Goldwyn, R. & Hugh-Jones, S. (2011) Using the Adult Attachment Interview to understand reactive attachment disorder: findings from a 10-case adolescent sample. *Attachment & Human Development*, 13(2), 169–91. It is interesting that a study from the Leiden group found that reports of maltreatment in the AAI, but not U/d of maltreatment (or loss), were associated with hippocampal volume: Riem, M.M., Alink, L.R., Out, D., van IJzendoorn, M.H., & Bakermans-Kranenburg, M.J. (2015) Beating the brain about abuse: empirical and meta-analytic studies of the association between maltreatment and hippocampal volume across childhood and adolescence. *Development & Psychopathology*, 27(2), 507–520. Such findings suggest that the U/d for trauma construct may be excluding some relevant information. In support of this conclusion is the fact that the coding of maltreatment from the AAI used by Reim and colleagues *did* include several items, such as chronic neglect, that are excluded by Main, Goldwyn, and Hesse from the U/d classification. The question about the status of potentially traumatic experiences without a locatable single event in the AAI in part reflects a wider discussion about the meaning of the concept of 'trauma' in psychiatric nosology. Van der Kolk, B.A. (2017) Developmental trauma disorder: toward a rational diagnosis for children with complex trauma histories. *Psychiatric Annals*, 35(5), 401–408.

what status repeated hospitalisations has within the AAI coding system in terms of making an unresolved classification, even though hospitalisation was the foundational experience of trauma and loss in the emergence of attachment theory (Chapter 1). Pervasively frightening, frightened, or dissociative caregiving may contribute to a disorganised attachment classification in the Strange Situation and controlling behaviour on reunion at age six; but if the child from this dyad grows up without a specific bereavement or identifiable subsequent trauma that can be relayed discretely to the interviewer, it would be impossible for them to receive an unresolved classification on the AAI in adolescence or adulthood.[466]

In the coding manual, Main and colleagues advised coders to scale unresolved traumatic abuse and unresolved loss separately, and then to draw on both ratings in making a judgement regarding whether a transcript should be placed in the U/d category. Seen in wider context, this would appear a very surprising decision: abuse and bereavement are generally not treated as psychological experiences of a kind and of equivalent significance. However, from Main and Hesse's perspective, what abuse and loss have in common is that an experience of the attachment figure may make thinking about the attachment figure alarming and overwhelming, causing both the aversion and the intensification of attention. The scales for unresolved traumatic abuse and unresolved traumatic loss are therefore situated in the manual as means to the end of a categorical judgement regarding whether an unresolved/disorganised/disoriented state of mind regarding attachment is present to a marked degree. As such, following Main and Hesse's lead, the relative distribution of unresolved loss and unresolved traumatic abuse in studies is rarely available in published studies; only the overall U/d category is usually reported.[467]

However, a study by Fonagy and colleagues found that the association between unresolved traumatic abuse in a parent's AAI and infant disorganised attachment classification in the Strange Situation was higher than the usual association between U/d on the AAI and disorganised attachment in the Strange Situation.[468] Though acknowledging the need for further replication, on the basis of these findings Fonagy and colleagues suggest that the intrusion of unresolved traumatic experiences into everyday functioning may be a more potent cause of frightening or dissociative behaviours by caregivers towards their child than an unresolved loss.[469] These conclusions are in line with a little-discussed finding reported

[466] Lyons-Ruth, K., Yellin, C., Melnick, S., & Atwood, G. (2003) Childhood experiences of trauma and loss have different relations to maternal unresolved and hostile-helpless states of mind on the AAI. *Attachment & Human Development*, 5(4), 330–52. However, it is likely that such cases would, in practice, be placed by many coders as 'Cannot Classify', and included with the unresolved classification in analyses. See also Kisiel, C.L., Fehrenbach, T., Torgersen, E., et al. (2014) Constellations of interpersonal trauma and symptoms in child welfare: implications for a developmental trauma framework. *Journal of Family Violence*, 29(1), 1–14.

[467] One of the few studies to have done so is Weinfield, N.S., Whaley, G., & Egeland, B. (2004) Continuity, discontinuity, and coherence in attachment from infancy to late adolescence: sequelae of organization and disorganization. *Attachment & Human Development*, 6(1), 73–97. The researchers reported the important finding that, when examined prospectively in the Minnesota study, 'although maltreatment and disorganization share variance, only disorganization contributes unique variance to the prediction of unresolved abuse' (84).

[468] They also worried that there may be unacknowledged construct variance, such that the associations of the U/d classification (and their strength) may be different, depending on the relative proportion of trauma and loss in the sample. Berthelot, N., Ensink, K., Bernazzani, O., Normandin, L., Luyten, P., & Fonagy, P. (2015) Intergenerational transmission of attachment in abused and neglected mothers: the role of trauma-specific reflective functioning. *Infant Mental Health Journal*, 36(2), 200–212. See also Ballen, N., Demers, I., & Bernier, A. (2007) A differential analysis of the subtypes of unresolved states of mind in the adult attachment interview. *Journal of Trauma Practice*, 5(4), 69–93.

[469] Lyons-Ruth and Jacobvitz have commented that unresolved trauma and unresolved loss have materially different correlates in most of the studies that have reported them separately, even if they also share substantial variance. Lyons-Ruth, K. & Jacobvitz, D. (2016) Attachment disorganization from infancy to adulthood: neurobiological correlates, parenting contexts, and pathways to disorder. In J. Cassidy & P.R. Shaver (eds) *Handbook*

by Main and Hesse from their Berkeley sample that lapses in reasoning and discourse in the AAI occurred far more frequently in discussions of abuse experiences than in discussions of loss.[470] In 1995 Main also offered the provocative hypothesis that infant disorganised attachment will usually resolve by adulthood unless the basis of the disorganisation lies in traumatic abuse: 'So long as direct maltreatment is not involved, many, perhaps most, are expected to have become 'organised' by adulthood, being either secure, dismissing or preoccupied'.[471] A decade later, a follow-up conducted by Main and Hesse with 44 of the Berkeley sample at age 19 was consistent with this hypothesis. There was no association between infant disorganised attachment and an unresolved/disorganised classification on the AAI in this low-risk sample.[472] However, a more adequate appraisal of Main's hypothesis would require a cohort study including participants with abuse experiences.

Several criticisms of the operationalisation of unresolved traumatic abuse have been raised. George and Solomon, among others, criticised the coding system for unresolved/disorganised traumatic abuse as too limited. In their sample, most children who displayed controlling-punitive and controlling-caregiving behaviours on reunion had caregivers who were classified U/d on the AAI. However, examination of the cases where caregivers received a different classification revealed transcripts showing lapses in reasoning or discourse—but about kinds of events not included by the system, such as frightening occurrences in the immediate life of the speaker rather than in childhood. This was also observed by Ainsworth and Eichberg. George and Solomon concluded that 'our findings suggested that trauma should be defined as events that leave the individual feeling helpless and out of control, including current/recent traumatic events in the caregiving relationship'.[473]

Levinson and Fonagy also criticised the boundaries placed by Main and Hesse around the definition of traumatic abuse.[474] In a study in the 1990s of individuals incarcerated for violent crimes, they found that the prisoners reported histories of severe and appalling abuse in childhood. However, in the AAI their participants systematically dismissed the importance of these experiences, and so could not be coded as unresolved according to the coding protocols. Levinson and Fonagy argued that these experiences are, in fact, best regarded as indicating unresolved/disorganised states of mind regarding attachment, and that both unresolved and dismissed distress had contributed to the capacity of these speakers for callous

of Attachment: Theory, Research, and Clinical Applications, 3rd edn (pp.667–95). New York: Guilford; Byun, S., Brumariu, L.E., & Lyons-Ruth, K. (2016) Disorganized attachment in young adulthood as a partial mediator of relations between severity of childhood abuse and dissociation. Journal of Trauma & Dissociation, 17(4), 460–79.

[470] Main, M. & Hesse, E. (1992) Attaccamento disorganizzato/disorientato nell'infanzia e stati mentali dissociati dei genitori. In M. Ammaniti & D. Stern (1992) Attaccamento e Psicoanalisi (pp.80–140). Rome: Gius, Laterza & Figli.

[471] Main, M. (1995) Recent studies in attachment: overview, with selected implications for clinical work. In S. Goldberg, R. Muir, & J. Kerr (eds) Attachment Theory: Social, Developmental and Clinical Perspectives (pp.407–470). Hillsdale, NJ: Analytic Press, p.454.

[472] Main, M., Hesse, E., & Kaplan, N. (2005) Predictability of attachment behavior and representational processes at 1, 6, and 19 years of age: The Berkeley longitudinal study. In K.E. Grossmann, K. Grossmann, & E. Waters (eds) Attachment from Infancy to Adulthood: The Major Longitudinal Studies (pp.245–304). New York: Guilford, p.286. When Main and colleagues reworked their data so that participants with a primary unresolved or cannot classify status were separated from those with a predominant organised pattern and a secondary unresolved classification, the authors reported that there was a statistically significant relationship with infant disorganised attachment. However, they did not provide the strength of the association.

[473] George, C. & Solomon, J. (1996) Representational models of relationships: links between caregiving and attachment. Infant Mental Health Journal, 17(3), 198–216, p.213.

[474] Levinson, A. & Fonagy, P. (2004) Offending and attachment: the relationship between interpersonal awareness and offending in a prison population with psychiatric disorder. Canadian Journal of Psychoanalysis, 12(2), 225–51.

and violent behaviour.[475] (In practice, contemporary coding norms would now likely place the Levinson and Fonagy participants as 'Cannot Classify' rather than dismissing, since a truly dismissing transcript would not report abuse in a way that would seem severe and appalling. But this is an evolution in the culture of coding stemming from Hesse's work on the 'Cannot Classify' category, rather than reflecting a change to the manual.) Like Levinson and Fonagy, Lyons-Ruth and colleagues criticised the boundaries of the unresolved classification. They proposed that it should be extended to encompass discourse suggesting unresolved/disorganised states of mind where no bereavement or specific trauma is identifiable. They developed an additional 'Hostile/Helpless' coding system to identify unresolved/disorganised states apparent especially in the derogation of attachment figures or of speakers themselves, or in strong identification with a hostile or a helpless caregiver.[476] Fonagy, Target, Steele, and Steele likewise expanded the boundaries of the unresolved classification in their Reflective Functioning Scale, which includes assessment of 'unintegrated or bizarre statements, suggesting a lapse in reasoning, without this being around the topic of a bereavement or trauma'.[477]

However, Main and Hesse have been reluctant to alter the AAI coding system much in the past two decades. There are likely a few reasons for this. They perceived such changes as risking the capacity to commensurate empirical studies over time using the AAI. Furthermore, they clearly felt that it would be better to be overcautious in defining traumatic experiences, given that the concept of 'trauma' has seen such widespread and diffuse use, and their goal has ultimately been to pin down experiences that form the basis specifically for unresolved/disorganised/disoriented states of mind.[478] Bowlby's emphasis on the need to

[475] The preference of Fonagy and colleagues for Crittenden and Landini's amended version of the AAI in recent years may in part reflect the fact that one of these amendments was a more liberal definition of unresolved trauma, which did encompass dismissed trauma. Strathearn, L., Fonagy, P., Amico, J., & Montague, P.R. (2009) Adult attachment predicts maternal brain and oxytocin response to infant cues. *Neuropsychopharmacology*, 34(13), 2655; Fonagy, P. (2015) An honest day's work. *DMM News*, 18, p.2, September 2015. https://www.iasa-dmm.org/images/uploads/DMM%20News%20%2318-Sept%2015%20English.pdf. It should be noted, however, that rather than simply expanding the Main et al. system, available evidence suggests that the Crittenden and Landini coding system for the AAI appears to have a different object: Baldoni, F., Minghetti, M., Craparo, G., Facondini, E., Cena, L., & Schimmenti, A. (2018) Comparing Main, Goldwyn, and Hesse (Berkeley) and Crittenden (DMM) coding systems for classifying Adult Attachment Interview transcripts: an empirical report. *Attachment & Human Development*, 20(4), 423–38.

[476] In a sample of 45 high-risk mothers, around half of whom had been known to social services, Lyons-Ruth and colleagues reported that the 'Hostile/Helpless' system contributed additional prediction to disorganised attachment assessed in the Strange Situation, over and above the unresolved classification as coded using the Main et al. system. However, in interpreting these results it should be noted that, unusually, there was no association at all in this sample between U/d on the Main et al. system and infant disorganised attachment classifications. Lyons-Ruth, K., Yellin, C., Melnick, S., & Atwood, G. (2005) Expanding the concept of unresolved mental states: hostile/helpless states of mind on the Adult Attachment Interview are associated with disrupted mother–infant communication and infant disorganization. *Development & Psychopathology*, 17(1), 1–23; Melnick, S., Finger, B., Hans, S., Patrick, M., & Lyons Ruth, K. (2008) Hostile helpless states of mind in the AAI. A proposed additional AAI category with implications for identifying disorganised infant attachment in high risk samples. In H. Steele & M. Steele (eds) *Clinical Application of the Adult Attachment Interview* (pp.399–423). New York: Guilford. For further empirical comparison of the Main et al. and Lyons-Ruth et al. coding systems see Frigerio, A., Costantino, E., Ceppi, E., & Barone, L. (2013) Adult Attachment Interviews of women from low-risk, poverty, and maltreatment risk samples: comparisons between the hostile/helpless and traditional AAI coding systems. *Attachment & Human Development*, 15(4), 424–42.

[477] Fonagy, P., Target, M, Steele, H., & Steele, M. (1998) *Reflective Functioning Manual, Version 5*. London: UCL/Anna Freud Centre.

[478] One study presenting preliminary self-report associations between various forms of abuse, neglect, and adversity with bearing on this question is Thomson, P. & Jaque, S.V. (2017) Adverse childhood experiences (ACE) and Adult Attachment Interview (AAI) in a non-clinical population. *Child Abuse & Neglect*, 70, 255–63, Table 3.

attend to 'actual historical events' locatable in time and space (Chapter 1) also remained an influence in the background for Main and Hesse despite their assertion that the AAI is not a veridical representation of imputed historical experiences.[479] In practice, however, many but not all coders have circumvented the problem by coding cases with apparent unresolved states of mind but no locatable traumatic experiences as 'Cannot Classify'. This then allows classification 'by the back door' since, by convention, 'Cannot Classify' cases are folded in with Unresolved cases in statistical analyses.

Yet there has been some movement in the definition of the classification. For instance, throughout the 1990s unresolved/disorganised speech regarding miscarriage and stillbirth was classified with 'loss of pets' as not indicating a true trauma or bereavement. However, studies by Bakermans-Kranenburg and colleagues and by Hughes and colleagues found that infant disorganised attachment was predicted by lapses in reasoning or discourse relating to experiences of miscarriage and stillbirth, when this was probed in the interview.[480] Main and colleagues therefore acknowledged that these experiences 'may be rated using the same principles, although the nature of the loss should be marked on the coding form. At present such cases should be analysed separately.'[481] As a consequence, there has been some variation between laboratories in how such cases are handled, with some groups probing in interview and including unresolved trauma/loss regarding miscarriage and stillbirth as sufficient basis for a U/d classification, and others following the letter of the manual and not probing or including these experiences with the other cases in the U/d category.[482] In most samples, the number of cases is small enough that these variations are not critical. Rather, the instability reflects structural tensions faced by the AAI as an instrument in attempting to pin down the diffuse concept of trauma. It also reflects differences between Main/Hesse and their critics in conceptualising the idea of 'unresolved/disorganised/disoriented states of mind'.

---

[479] Mary Main, personal communication, August 2019.

[480] Bakermans-Kranenburg, M.J., Schuengel, C., & van IJzendoorn, M.H. (1999) Unresolved loss due to miscarriage: an addition to the Adult Attachment Interview. *Attachment & Human Development*, 1(2), 157–70; Hughes, P., Turton, P., Hopper, E., McGauley, G.A., & Fonagy, P. (2001) Disorganised attachment behaviour among infants born subsequent to stillbirth. *Journal of Child Psychology and Psychiatry*, 42(6), 791–801.

[481] Main, M., Goldwyn, R., & Hesse, E. (2002) *Adult Attachment Scoring and Classification System*. Unpublished manuscript, University of California at Berkeley, Department of Psychology. A recent self-report study found that when college student participants had no losses other than miscarriages within two years of their birth, this was not associated with higher scores on self-reported absorption. Self-reported absorption is, however, only a moderate correlate of U/d. Granqvist, P., Fransson, M., & Hagekull, B. (2009) Disorganized attachment, absorption, and new age spirituality: a mediational model. *Attachment & Human Development*, 11(4), 385–403; Bahm, N.I.G., Duschinsky, R., & Hesse, E. (2016) Parental loss of family members within two years of offspring birth predicts elevated absorption scores in college. *Attachment & Human Development*, 18(5), 429–42.

[482] Another ambiguous case may be unresolved states of mind regarding having a child with significant physical disabilities. The manual would not seem to include this as a possible instance of loss, since the parent has not been bereaved. However, a meta-analysis revealed that the unresolved classification was overrepresented among parents of physically disabled children. Bakermans-Kranenburg and van IJzendoorn offered their suspicion that coders were making U/d classifications on the basis of parents' 'unresolved mourning about the loss of their ideal child'. Bakermans-Kranenburg, M.J. & van IJzendoorn, M.H. (2009) The first 10,000 Adult Attachment Interviews: distributions of adult attachment representations in clinical and non-clinical groups, *Attachment & Human Development*, 11(3), 223–63, p.249. For theoretical discussion of unresolved mourning and disruption of the caregiving system see Pianta, R.C., Marvin, R.S., & Morog, M.C. (1999) Resolving the past and present: relations with attachment organization. In J. Solomon & C. George (eds) *Attachment Disorganization* (pp.379–98). New York: Guilford; Oppenheim, D., Koren-Karie, N., Dolev, S., & Yirmiya, N. (2009) Maternal insightfulness and resolution of the diagnosis are associated with secure attachment in preschoolers with autism spectrum disorders. *Child Development*, 80, 519–27.

Some remaining questions

Dissociation

Some attachment researchers, for instance Mary Target and several Italian colleagues, have accused Main and Hesse of self-contradiction and incoherence in theorising dissociation and fear.[483] They urge that there are significant outstanding questions for Main and Hesse in this area. This latter point is undoubtedly true. However, the accusation of self-contradiction and incoherence is overstated: fear, trauma, dissociation, and disorganisation have quite distinct and coherent places in Main and Hesse's theory. In 1992, Main and Hesse published a long and finely etched chapter discussing the mechanism that they saw as the basis for both infant disorganised attachment and unresolved/disorganised/disoriented states of mind regarding attachment. Central to their concerns in the chapter was the idea of 'dissociation', which had been gaining prominence in clinical and academic psychology through the previous decade, as well as public debates about 'recovered memories'.[484] Main and Hesse had their attention drawn to the concept by Giovanni Liotti, who argued for the potential value of the concept for interpreting seemingly contradictory, incomplete, or disrupted sequences of behaviour or speech.[485] The 1992 chapter by Main and Hesse offered an account of how dissociation related to other key concepts in their theory: fear, trauma, and attention. However, the work was only ever published in Italian.[486] Without an English translation, the chapter has not been widely known or discussed, contributing to a tendency for subsequent interpreters to treat fear, trauma, dissociation, and disorganisation as confused or as interchangeable elements in Main and Hesse's theory.[487]

In the model put forward in the 1992 chapter, the attachment system in childhood, the caregiving system in adulthood, and the retrieval and communication of attachment-related experiences in adulthood have something important in common. All three are underpinned

---

[483] Seganti, A., Carnevale, G., Mucelli, R., Solano, L., & Target, M. (2000) From sixty-two interviews on 'the worst and the best episode of your life': relationships between internal working models and a grammatical scale of subject–object affective connections. *International Journal of Psychoanalysis*, 81(3), 529–51, p.532.

[484] Kirshner, L.A. (1973) Dissociative reactions: an historical review and clinical study. *Acta Psychiatrica Scandinavica*, 49(6), 698–711; Van der Hart, O. & Dorahy, M.J. (2009) Dissociation: history of a concept. In P.F. Dell & J. O'Neill (eds) *Dissociation and the Dissociative Disorders: DSM-V and Beyond* (pp.3–26). London: Routledge. See also Itzkowitz, S., Chefetz, R.A., Hainer, M., Hopenwasser, K., & Howell, E.F. (2015) Exploring dissociation and dissociative identity disorder: a roundtable discussion. *Psychoanalytic Perspectives*, 12, 39–79.

[485] Liotti, G. (1992) Disorganized/disoriented attachment in the etiology of the dissociative disorders. *Dissociation*, 4, 196–204. See also Hacking, I. (1992) Multiple personality disorder and its hosts. *History of the Human Sciences*, 5(2), 3–31.

[486] Main, M. & Hesse, E. (1992) Attaccamento disorganizzato/disorientato nell'infanzia e stati mentali dissociati dei genitori. In M. Ammaniti & D. Stern (1992) *Attaccamento e Psicoanalisi* (pp.80–140). Rome: Gius, Laterza & Figli. This is a translation of the chapter 'Disorganized/disoriented attachment in infants as related to dissociative states of mind in their parents' from Hesse, E. (ed.) (1999) *Unclassifiable and Disorganized Responses in the Adult Attachment Interview and in the Infant Strange Situation Procedure: Theoretical Proposals and Empirical Findings.* Unpublished doctoral thesis, Leiden University. This English chapter is cited here rather than relying on a re-translation of the text back from the Italian. Some elements are repeated in the discussion in Hesse, E. & Main, M. (2006) Frightened, threatening, and dissociative parental behavior in low-risk samples: description, discussion, and interpretations. *Development & Psychopathology*, 18(2), 309–343. However, they are exceptionally compressed in the latter text, presumably given the challenges of the journal's word limit, to the point that the claims are not fully intelligible to a reader not already familiar with the 1992 chapter.

[487] E.g. Schore, A.N. (2009) Attachment trauma and the developing right brain: origins of pathological dissociation. In P.F. Dell & J.A. O'Neill (eds) *Dissociation and the Dissociative Disorders* (pp.107–41). London: Routledge.

by the coordination of attention, and individual differences 'follow upon alterations in the focus of attention' with respect to attachment-relevant information, including external perceptions and memories.[488] Attachment behaviour in infancy reflects these alterations in the focus of attention most directly, since the threshold for activation of the attachment system may be raised or lowered 'by focusing attention either away from or toward 1) the attachment figure and 2) any cues to danger implicit in the situation'.[489] Retrieval of information and communication with the interviewer in the AAI also reflects individual differences in the alteration of the focus of attention with respect to attachment-relevant information. Dismissing states of mind are underpinned by a tendency to direct attention away from attachment-relevant memories and perceptions in the past and in interaction with the interviewer. Preoccupied states of mind are underpinned by an intense focus on attachment-relevant memories and perceptions. Finally, the caregiving system is distinct from the attachment system. But the assemblage of the caregiving system incorporates some component elements from the attachment system, such as interpretations of the meanings of physical touch (Chapter 1). As such, individual differences in the alteration of the focus of attention with respect to attachment-relevant information may have some effect on the functioning of the caregiving system.

In 1990, Main and Hesse argued that an approach/avoidance conflict is produced in the Strange Situation for an infant with past experiences of a caregiver who displays alarming behaviour, since the same figure will elicit a disposition to both withdraw and approach as a safe haven, dispositions that are incompatible and mutually exacerbating. However, the behavioural account of an approach/avoidance conflict was the external face of a hypothesised mechanism occurring at the level of attention. In their 1992 chapter, the theory of this attentional mechanism was extended as a model of adult caregiving behaviour and autobiographical discourse. In all three cases, where attachment-relevant perceptions and memories are also experienced as alarming, Main and Hesse argued that attention cannot simply be turned away or turned to them since the other response intrudes. The result is a 'looping' of attention, and, if sustained or repeated over time, potential damage to the behavioural system itself is expectable.[490] This damage might be seen as weakened regulatory capacities, localised holes or blockages in the functioning of the system, or potentially even the development of relatively independent 'nets' of dispositional responses 'potentially organised with respect to one of the competing and incompatible goals'.[491] In the chapter, Main and Hesse appeared ambivalent as to whether dissociation represented a kind of defence or adaptation more extreme in kind than the conditional strategies (as for Bowlby), or essentially a kind of breakdown. In any case, in reducing environmental responsiveness and the integration of information, dissociation was anticipated to have repercussions for functioning and for mental health.

---

[488] Main, M. & Hesse, E. (1992) Disorganized/disoriented attachment in infants as related to dissociative states of mind in their parents. In E. Hesse (ed.) (1999) *Unclassifiable and Disorganized Responses in the Adult Attachment Interview and in the Infant Strange Situation Procedure: Theoretical Proposals and Empirical Findings.* Unpublished doctoral thesis, Leiden University.

[489] Ibid.: 'In contrast to Group B infants (whose attentional focus varies with circumstances) and Group A infants (who utilise an organised shift in attention away from the attachment figure and her whereabouts), Group C infants appear almost completely preoccupied with the attachment figure and her whereabouts throughout the situation.'

[490] Ibid.

[491] Ibid.

In the 1992 chapter, Main and Hesse proposed a new 'understanding of the qualitative structure of trauma' in the context of attachment.[492] Where an attachment-relevant experience is itself alarming and the looping of attention occurs, there are consequences for the encoding of the memory. The effective tagging and encoding of embodied memory, Main and Hesse supposed, requires the attentional process lost to the loop. The looping of attention inhibits the integration and semantic extraction of experiences, so that these memories may be accompanied by associations based on episodic rather than semantic resonances and may lack important contextual markers about time and place. This accounts for the unhoused, invasively intense quality of traumatic memories, and of the lapses in discourse and reasoning seen in the AAI. The common mechanism is also proposed as accounting for the fact that dissociation can be one consequence of such a wide variety of forms of trauma.

As van IJzendoorn and Schuengel among others have observed, 'the construct of dissociation can easily be overstretched to include almost every defense mechanism', and indeed Main and Hesse were rather unclear in their use of the term, sometimes intending a narrower 'prototypical' meaning and sometimes using the term loosely as a synonym for any form of mental segregation.[493] Nonetheless, it is quite possible to identify their key claims about dissociation through a close reading. Main and Hesse argued that the looping of attention can cause the most prototypically dissociated responses such as fugue states where a child or an adult is unresponsive to the environment, perhaps accompanied by 'blank, unseeing eyes' or 'upward rolls of the eyes' or a startle back to environmental alertness.[494] However, problems in the encoding of experience caused by past looping of attention can also produce segregation within behavioural systems, such that two incompatible responses may be activated without coordination in response to the same cue from memory or from the environment. This segregation was regarded by Main and Hesse as also supported by dissociative processes, even if in itself it is not reducible to dissociation and less prototypically dissociative than a fugue state.

In the chapter, Main and Hesse then applied their model one by one to frightening/frightened caregiver behaviour, to the infant Strange Situation, and to lapses in reasoning or discourse in the AAI. In relation to frightening/frightened caregiver behaviour, one of the three main categories is dissociative behaviours. Main and Hesse speculated that dissociative behaviours may occur when working memory—short-term perceptual and linguistic processing—is overwhelmed by the looping of attention around loss or abusive experiences relating to attachment figures. One potent cause of such looping is anticipated to be alarming memories of or associations with these figures. It may be prompted by unlikely objects

---

[492] Ibid.

[493] Van IJzendoorn, M.H. & Schuengel, C. (1996) The measurement of dissociation in normal and clinical populations: meta-analytic validation of the Dissociative Experiences Scale (DES). *Clinical Psychology Review*, 16(5), 365–82, p.375. Ambiguities in the history of the concept between broader and narrower uses go back to the nineteenth century. Middleton, W., Dorahy, M.J., & Moskowitz, A. (2008) Historical conceptions of dissociation and psychosis: nineteenth and early twentieth century perspectives on severe psychopathology. In A. Moskowitz, I. Schäfer, & M.J. Dorahy (eds) *Psychosis, Trauma and Dissociation. Emerging Perspectives on Severe Psychopathology* (pp.9–20). Oxford: Blackwell. An influential proposal was later made for detachment and mental segregation as distinct phenomena under the label of 'dissociation'. Holmes, E.A., Brown, R.J., Mansell, W., et al. (2005) Are there two qualitatively distinct forms of dissociation? A review and some clinical implications. *Clinical Psychology Review*, 25(1), 1–23.

[494] Main, M. & Hesse, E. (1992) Disorganized/disoriented attachment in infants as related to dissociative states of mind in their parents. In E. Hesse (ed.) (1999) *Unclassifiable and Disorganized Responses in the Adult Attachment Interview and in the Infant Strange Situation Procedure: Theoretical Proposals and Empirical Findings.* Unpublished doctoral thesis, Leiden University.

because it has been poorly encoded, so it takes an overexpansive field of reference. This then increases the circumstances that grant uncomfortable freedom to experiences of the past, and place memory's sharp edges up against the throat of the present. For instance, the touch of an infant may evoke poorly encoded and frightening memories for a caregiver of abusive touch by an attachment figure in childhood or adulthood.[495] This may then elicit dissociative, frightening, or frightened responses by the caregiver towards the child. Or again, the features of a child may recall those of a dead attachment figure, leading to loops of attention or activation of the fear behavioural system if the deceased attachment figure and/or their passing was in some way alarming.[496]

Even though they may co-occur, Main and Hesse were adamant, however, that not all frightening/frightened caregiver behaviours should be reduced to the effects of dissociation. There may be dissociative processes implicated in some or many of them, but not necessarily (i) to the same degree or (ii) in the same way. Though Main and Hesse do not elaborate the point, reasons for frightening behaviour by caregivers that do not require dissociation can readily be identified. One process is acknowledged by Dozier and Bernard, who observed in their work with at-risk dyads that 'frightening behaviours can be rewarding to parents because they are so powerful in eliciting reactions from children'.[497] Another case could be when a child's safe haven is regularly under attack in the context of domestic violence. These children may experience their caregiver's fear as frightening, without the caregiver's behaviour being dissociative. Main and Hesse's claim that dissociation may not always operate in the same way is also highlighted by their acknowledgement that other affects besides fear may be implicated in looping attention and anomalous caregiving behaviours. For instance, they later noted that if a loss has been profoundly confusing, the confusion may act in ways analogous to alarm in relation to the caregiver in producing attentional loops and overwhelming working memory.[498] Fonagy and colleagues suggested that other difficult feelings such as shame, guilt, anger, and disgust may be implicated in disrupting ordinary states of mind following trauma.[499] However, these are not matters considered by Main and Hesse.

[495] A related point was made by Enlow and colleagues, who argued that some kinds of trauma may be more likely to bring about frightening/frightened behaviour than others: Enlow, M.B., Egeland, B., Carlson, E., Blood, E., & Wright, R.J. (2014) Mother–infant attachment and the intergenerational transmission of posttraumatic stress disorder. *Development & Psychopathology*, 26(01), 41–65. 'For example, normative displays of infant helplessness, distress, and aggression may be especially threatening and triggering for mothers with PTSD resulting from intimate partner violence, particularly if the infant physically resembles the perpetrator' (59).

[496] Main, M. & Morgan, H. (1996) Disorganization and disorientation in infant Strange Situation behavior: phenotypic resemblance to dissociative states. In L. Michelson & W. Ray (eds) *Handbook of Dissociation: Theoretical, Empirical and Clinical Perspectives* (pp.107–138). New York: Plenum Press, p.126.

[497] Dozier, M. & Bernard, K. (2019) *Coaching Parents of Vulnerable Infants: The Attachment and Biobehavioral Catch-up Approach.* New York: Guilford, p.87.

[498] Bahm, N.I.G., Main, M., & Hesse, E. (2017) Unresolved/disorganized responses to the death of important persons: relations to frightening parental behavior and infant disorganization. In S. Gojman de Millan, C. Herreman, & L.A. Sroufe (eds) *Attachment Across Clinical and Cultural Perspectives: A Relational Psychoanalytic Approach* (pp.53–74). New York: Routledge, p.56.

[499] See e.g. Sharp, C., Fonagy, P., & Allen, J.G. (2012) Posttraumatic stress disorder: a social-cognitive perspective. *Clinical Psychology: Science and Practice*, 19(3), 229–40, pp.229–30. On guilt: in fact guilt appears alongside fear as implicated in U/d in an early version of the lack of resolution scale: Main, M. & Hesse, E. (1987) Lack of resolution of mourning, 15 November 1987. PP/Bow/B.3/36/1: 'The individual may indicate excessive fear, guilt or worry or regret regarding the previous relationship to the lost figure … guilt or fear may have become irrational.' However, guilt was subsequently removed, in line with Main and Hesse's increasing focus on fear from this period onwards. On disgust: as we have seen, Main found that the mother in one of the dyads classified as disorganised in her sample treated a child as too dirty to be allowed to touch her. And in the AAI there is already a classification for speakers who show derogating disgust towards close others, even in brief passages of the transcript (Ds2), though the classification system characterises Ds2 as dismissing rather than unresolved. The relationship between disgust and unresolved states of mind regarding attachment is also discussed in Buchheim, A. & George, A. (2011)

Appraising disorganised/disoriented attachment behaviour in the Strange Situation in light of their concern with dissociation, Main and Hesse observed that some of the behaviours used for coding infant disorganised attachment appear dissociated 'at a phenotypic level'. One category is 'freezing/stilling'. This, they suspected, directly reflects a lapse in serial processing in the context of looping attention. Another category Main and Hesse identified as phenotypically dissociative was 'direct indices of disorientation'. They regarded this kind of behaviour as caused by 'incompatible perceptions, experiences and impulses in which independent "nets" have developed and momentarily control behaviour'.[500] Some undirected behaviours could also have this basis, for instance when children approach the stranger with arms raised directly on reunion with their parent. Main and Hesse also argued that the most extreme and sharply defined 'sequential contradictory' and 'simultaneous contradictory' behaviours shown towards the caregiver on reunion may represent an expression of such independent 'nets' of responses. For instance, 'the infant may simultaneously scream for the parent and stretch as far out of the parent's arms as possible with eyes cast to the side'—this seems to entail fully developed behavioural dispositions in contradiction.[501] However, they identified two further kinds of behaviour listed in the Main and Solomon indices where a 'dissociative state need not be implied': direct apprehension of the caregiver, and forms of conflict about approach that remain environmentally responsive. They argued that 'not all disorganised-appearing behaviour listed by Main and Solomon need imply more than momentary experiences of conflict, and expressions of conflict between approach and avoidance behaviour towards the parent need not imply the intrusion of a dissociated secondary plan or system'.[502]

Having considered caregiving behaviour and the Strange Situation, Main and Hesse examined the potential relevance of dissociative processes in lapses of monitoring of reasoning or discourse in the AAI. In this case, they proposed that dissociation is the proximal mechanism of most, and perhaps 'virtually all', lapses in reasoning and discourse in the AAI.[503] In some cases, the lapses are minor and suggest merely absorption of attention

Attachment disorganisation in borderline personality disorder and anxiety disorder. In J. Solomon & C. George (eds) *Disorganised Attachment and Caregiving* (pp.343–82). New York: Guilford.

[500] Main, M. & Hesse, E. (1992) Disorganized/disoriented attachment in infants as related to dissociative states of mind in their parents. In E. Hesse. (ed.) (1999) *Unclassifiable and Disorganized Responses in the Adult Attachment Interview and in the Infant Strange Situation Procedure: Theoretical Proposals and Empirical Findings.* Unpublished doctoral thesis, Leiden University.

[501] Ibid. Main and Hesse report that a review of 300 Strange Situations from the Berkeley sample revealed only three such sharply defined cases where a child seemed to have fully developed behavioural dispositions to an avoidant conditional strategy and an ambivalent/resistant conditional strategy. In her doctoral project under Ainsworth, Crittenden found simultaneous or sequential display of the two conditional strategies much more frequently in maltreated children than in non-maltreated samples. Crittenden, P.M. (1988) Relationships at risk. In J. Belsky & T. Nezworski (eds) *Clinical Implications of Attachment* (p.136–74). Hillsdale, NJ: Lawrence Erlbaum.

[502] Main, M. & Hesse, E. (1992) Disorganized/disoriented attachment in infants as related to dissociative states of mind in their parents. In E. Hesse (1999) *Unclassifiable and Disorganized Responses in the Adult Attachment Interview and in the Infant Strange Situation Procedure: Theoretical Proposals and Empirical Findings.* Unpublished doctoral thesis, Leiden University. See also Main, M. & Morgan, H. (1996) Disorganization and disorientation in infant Strange Situation behavior: phenotypic resemblance to dissociative states. In L. Michelson & W. Ray (eds) *Handbook of Dissociation: Theoretical, Empirical and Clinical Perspectives* (pp.107–138). New York: Plenum Press: 'Not all disorganised-disoriented behaviours have a clear relation to dissociative phenomena' (108).

[503] This would be restated again later: 'Virtually all U/d lapses during the AAI appear to fit to a dissociative model.' Hesse, E. & Main, M. (2006) Frightened, threatening, and dissociative parental behavior in low-risk samples: description, discussion, and interpretations. *Development & Psychopathology,* 18(2), 309–343, p.311. This strengthens an earlier, more qualified position: 'Some lapses observed in the narratives of the parents of disorganised infants during discussions of traumatic events also appeared to fit to a dissociative model.' Main, M. & Morgan, H. (1996) Disorganization and disorientation in infant Strange Situation behavior: phenotypic resemblance to

during speech, conceptualised as a minor form of dissociation.[504] In other cases, the lapses are more major and suggest the operation of segregated processes, as when a speaker suffers from an 'intrusion of dissociated ideas, or holds two incompatible ideas regarding a loss or abuse experience in parallel'.[505] They gave out-of-context eulogistic speech about a lost attachment figure in the AAI as an example of absorption. Such discourse suggests that the question about losses evoked a memory which has been partially or wholly processed as an immediate perception.[506] The memory may have been encoded in such a way that it lacks cues for context, and/or frightening aspects of the information about the attachment figure are producing attentional loops that disturb working memory and the integration of remembering with the interpersonal demands of the present interview. By contrast, a more intense and potentially a qualitatively different form of dissociative processing may be seen in lapses in reasoning, when incompatible ideas regarding a loss or abuse experience appear to be held in parallel (e.g. dead/not dead). Usually such contradictions will be monitored and identified before they can appear in speech, or will be corrected after they occur. However, if attentional resources are tied up in loops, then monitoring can suffer as a result.[507]

In a 2006 article, Hesse and Main argued that future investigators should attempt to discriminate between the degree of 'dissociative components' in lapses of discourse and reasoning, and examine their distinct antecedents and associations with anomalous caregiving behaviours.[508] More of the 'transmission gap' between caregiver states of mind regarding

dissociative states. In L. Michelson & W. Ray (eds) *Handbook of Dissociation: Theoretical, Empirical and Clinical Perspectives* (pp.107–138). New York: Plenum Press, p.130.

[504] Psychological absorption has been defined as 'episodes of single ("total") attention that fully engage one's representational (i.e. perceptual, enactive, imaginative and ideational) resources'. Tellegen, A. & Atkinson, G. (1974) Openness to absorbing and self-altering experiences ('absorption'), a trait related to hypnotic susceptibility. *Journal of Abnormal Psychology*, 83, 268–77, p.268. This definition would later be the one cited in Hesse, E. & van IJzendoorn, M.H. (1999) Propensities towards absorption are related to lapses in the monitoring of reasoning or discourse during the Adult Attachment Interview. *Attachment & Human Development*, 1(1), 67–91.

[505] Main, M. & Hesse, E. (1992) Disorganized/disoriented attachment in infants as related to dissociative states of mind in their parents. In E. Hesse (ed.) (1999) *Unclassifiable and Disorganized Responses in the Adult Attachment Interview and in the Infant Strange Situation Procedure: Theoretical Proposals and Empirical Findings.* Unpublished doctoral thesis, Leiden University.

[506] See also Hesse, E. & Main, M. (2006) Frightened, threatening, and dissociative parental behavior in low-risk samples: description, discussion, and interpretations. *Development & Psychopathology*, 18(2), 309–343: 'As is clear from the above, not all U/d lapses are indicative of extreme dissociation. For example, the use of funereal speech, or unusual attention to detail, merely suggest elevated levels of the most "normative" component of dissociation, absorption. In contrast, most of those cited under section c) above, suggest the presence of real dissociative phenomena such as "segregated systems," although in most cases we assume these are unlikely to involve multiple executors capable of guiding action' (333).

[507] Later in the 1990s, Main and Hesse also proposed a dissociative basis when speakers in the AAI show 'no single attentional strategy' with respect to attachment, and instead 'the subject changes category in mid-interview in a shocking manner, as though completely shifting state of mind with respect to attachment mid-interview'. Transcripts showing this shift in states of mind regarding attachment would form one basis for the 'Cannot Classify' classification in the 1990s. Hesse, E. (1996) Discourse, memory, and the Adult Attachment Interview: a note with emphasis on the emerging cannot classify category. *Infant Mental Health Journal* 17(1), 4–11, p.5. Another form of Cannot Classify discourse is when low coherence scores make placement in the secure-autonomous category impossible, but there are no elevated scores for dismissing or preoccupied speech. Main and Hesse did not specifically suggest a dissociative basis for this form of discourse, but stated they anticipate that frightening and/or overwhelming historical experiences are implicated in derailing states of mind regarding attachment.

[508] Hesse, E. & Main, M. (2006) Frightened, threatening, and dissociative parental behavior in low-risk samples: description, discussion, and interpretations. *Development & Psychopathology*, 18(2), 309–343, p.333. One line of investigation pursued by Hesse has been examination of the role of absorption of attention. A self-report measure of a tendency towards absorption of attention has been found to be associated with the U/d classification in the AAI, which is in line with theory. However, associations have been moderate. See Hesse, E. & Van IJzendoorn, M.H. (1999) Propensities towards absorption are related to lapses in the monitoring of reasoning or discourse during the Adult Attachment Interview: a preliminary investigation. *Attachment & Human*

attachment and infant disorganised attachment might be closed, they argued, if the specific contribution of dissociative processes was unpicked. Furthermore, the prediction of sequelae such as later dissociative symptoms (Chapter 4) might be sharpened 'through an examination of subtypes of disorganisation and disorientation. Among the likeliest candidates to be predictive of the dissociative disorders are trance-like stilling and freezing, dissociated actions, and simultaneous or rapid alternation of avoidance and resistance.'[509] However, this call has not been noted by researchers in part because, in the absence of the 1992 chapter, the conceptual relationship between the U/d classification, dissociation, and fear has remained blurry. Main and Hesse hoped that the 2006 article would make their position clear, and regret that there appears to be little awareness of their account of how exactly U/d, dissociation, and fear interrelate.[510] In particular, few attachment researchers seem to know that Main and Hesse argued that lapses in reasoning or discourse in the AAI have varying degrees of a dissociative basis, but that only some forms of frightening/frightened caregiver behaviour are regarded as especially dissociative. Likewise, few know that Main and Hesse signal distinctions among more dissociative, apprehensive, and conflict behaviours (and a potential difference with stereotypic behaviours) within infant disorganised attachment. As a consequence, too few studies of attachment have included measures of dissociation, in part due to lack of recognition that the relationship between dissociation, trauma, and unresolved/disorganised states rather urgently requires empirical disentanglement.

One major exception has been van IJzendoorn, Bakermans-Kranenburg, and colleagues. Hesse's doctorate was completed under van IJzendoorn's supervision during the 1990s, and there were regular reciprocal visits by the researchers between Berkeley and Leiden. A study by Schuengel, van IJzendoorn, and Bakermans-Kranenburg provided data to examine Main and Hesse's proposal that the unresolved/disorganised/disoriented classification on the AAI would have a more intimate and consistent relationship with adult dissociative processes than frightening/frightened behaviour or the dyad's classification in the Strange Situation procedure. Following a review of measures of dissociation, the researchers selected a self-report measure—the Dissociative Experiences Scale—with strong evidence of validity and reliability.[511] The measure captures dimensions of depersonalisation, derealisation, and selective amnesia, in addition to absorption. In agreement with Main and Hesse's proposal, they found that reports of dissociative experiences are more common in speakers classified as unresolved/disorganised/disoriented in the AAI.

Later research has in general terms supported this link between the Dissociative Experiences Scale and unresolved/disorganised/disoriented speech in the AAI, but found that it may hold only for unresolved traumatic abuse, not unresolved loss.[512] On

Development, 1, 67–91; Granqvist, P., Fransson, M., & Hagekull, B. (2009) Disorganized attachment, absorption, and new age spirituality: a mediational model. *Attachment & Human Development*, 11(4), 385–403.

[509] Main, M. & Morgan, H. (1996) Disorganization and disorientation in infant Strange Situation behavior: phenotypic resemblance to dissociative states. In L. Michelson & W. Ray (eds) *Handbook of Dissociation: Theoretical, Empirical and Clinical Perspectives* (pp.107–138). New York: Plenum Press, p.131.

[510] Mary Main and Erik Hesse, personal communication, August 2019.

[511] Van IJzendoorn, M.H. & Schuengel, C. (1996) The measurement of dissociation in normal and clinical populations: meta-analytic validation of the Dissociative Experiences Scale (DES). *Clinical Psychology Review*, 16(5), 365–82.

[512] E.g. Zajac, K. & Kobak, R. (2009) Caregiver unresolved loss and abuse and child behavior problems: intergenerational effects in a high-risk sample. *Development & Psychopathology*, 21(1), 173–87; Madigan, S., Vaillancourt, K., McKibbon, A., & Benoit, D. (2012) The reporting of maltreatment experiences during the Adult Attachment Interview in a sample of pregnant adolescents. *Attachment & Human Development*, 14(2), 119–43. No association was found by Stovall-McClough, K. & Cloitre, M. (2006) Unresolved attachment, PTSD, and dissociation

the other hand, Schuengel and colleagues found no significant association between the self-report measure of dissociation and either frightening/frightened behaviours or with infant disorganised attachment.[513] Such findings suggest that more heterogeneous processes are in play in these latter two assessments, or that self-report cannot capture the forms of dissociation relevant to frightening/frightened behaviours or the kinds of caregiving linked to infant disorganised attachment. With so few trained coders of the frightening/frightened (FR) coding system, it is unsurprising there has been no later study to have used both this coding system and a measure of dissociation. However, it is a mark of the poor reception of Main and Hesse's ideas about fear, trauma, dissociation, and disorganisation that no later study has used a measure of caregiver dissociation alongside the Strange Situation.[514]

Further interrogation of the relationship between unresolved/disorganised/disoriented states of mind regarding attachment and the construct of trauma has been pursued by van IJzendoorn and colleagues. They conducted the AAI and a clinical assessment for posttraumatic stress disorder (PTSD) with 31 combat veterans in treatment for PTSD and 29 veterans not in treatment for PTSD. The researchers added a specific probe about combat experiences to the AAI schedule, and coded both combat-related lapses in reasoning or discourse and the non-combat-related lapses that are usually coded in other samples. Rates of secure-autonomous attachment did not differ between the groups. However, lapses in reasoning or discourse on the AAI in discussions of combat were found to be so strongly associated with PTSD symptoms that it was almost as if they were the same construct ($r = .80$):

> The convergence between AAI unresolved state of mind and PTSD symptomatology is remarkable as AAI unresolved state of mind and PTSD differ in severity of presentation, in prevalence in general populations and in the theoretical perspective from which they were constructed. These findings support the view that AAI unresolved state of mind and PTSD symptomatology share lack of integration as a common core phenomenon. This core phenomenon consists of the occurrence of discrete trauma-related disruptions of thought, speech, and action.[515]

in women with childhood abuse histories. *Journal of Consulting and Clinical Psychology*, 74(2), 219–28; or by Marcusson-Clavertz, D., Gušić, S., Bengtsson, H., Jacobsen, H., & Cardeña, E. (2017) The relation of dissociation and mind wandering to unresolved/disorganized attachment: an experience sampling study. *Attachment & Human Development*, 19(2), 170–90. Thomson and Jaque found an association between U/d and pathological forms of dissociation, but not absorption. Thomson, P. & Jaque, S.V. (2014) Unresolved mourning, supernatural beliefs and dissociation: a mediation analysis, *Attachment & Human Development*, 16(5), 499–514. However, the relationship with U/d is clouded by the diversity of measures of dissociation used across studies.

[513] Schuengel, C., Bakermans-Kranenburg, M.J., & van IJzendoorn, M.H. (1999) Frightening maternal behavior linking unresolved loss and disorganized infant attachment. *Journal of Consulting and Clinical Psychology*, 67(1), 54–63, p.59.

[514] The only other relevant study was contemporaneous with the work of Schuengel and colleagues, and is now over 20 years old. Lyons-Ruth and colleagues used both the Dissociative Experiences Scale and the Mississippi Scale for Post Traumatic Stress Disorder in a study of 45 mother–infant dyads from low-income families. They found that 'most mothers of disorganized infants fell into the low symptom group (64%), while the remaining third fell into the polysymptomatic group (36%)'. Such findings again suggest that dissociation in the context of trauma may be only one process implicated in infant disorganised attachment. Lyons-Ruth, K. & Block, D. (1996) The disturbed caregiving system: relations among childhood trauma, maternal caregiving, and infant affect and attachment. *Infant Mental Health Journal*, 17(3), 257–75, p.268.

[515] Harari, D., Bakermans-Kranenburg, M.J., De Kloet, C.S., et al. (2009) Attachment representations in Dutch veterans with and without deployment-related PTSD. *Attachment & Human Development*, 11(6), 515–36, p.350.

Bakermans-Kranenburg and van IJzendoorn also reported meta-analytic findings that almost all adults with PTSD across different samples are classified as unresolved (U/d).[516] They aligned these findings with Main and Hesse's proposal that some forms of unresolved/disorganised discourse are caused by the intrusion of poorly processed perceptions which 'may disrupt attention … in the form of absorption and unmonitored intrusions of memories, affects and sensory perceptions concerning the trauma'.[517] However, they warned that 'there may be an asymmetric relation in the sense that not all AAI unresolved trauma involves PTSD, while PTSD would almost always involve AAI unresolved trauma', at least when the trauma is probed for and coded.[518]

Van IJzendoorn and colleagues also examined lapses of reasoning or discourse appearing in discussion of experiences unrelated to combat. Whereas in the control group 7% displayed lapses in reasoning or discourse relating to these other experiences, 42% of the group in treatment for PTSD displayed U/d markers.[519] This finding was interpreted as suggesting that an unresolved state of mind regarding non-combat traumas may have predisposed vulnerability to lack of integration in mental processing of combat experiences. Traumas and losses may layer on top of one another, with each contributing to greater vulnerability to unresolved/disorganised states of mind. However, the researchers were led to reflect further on the image of segregated processing or dissociation solely as a risk factor by their later research. In a study of Holocaust survivors and a group of rigorously matched control participants, they found, as expected, that dissociative symptoms were more common among the Holocaust survivors. Yet there were no differences in the physical, psychological, or cognitive functioning in the children of the survivors compared to the control. Van IJzendoorn and colleagues proposed that some form of dissociation may here be serving, actually, as a

[516] Bakermans-Kranenburg, M.J. & van IJzendoorn, M.H. (2009) The first 10,000 Adult Attachment Interviews: distributions of adult attachment representations in clinical and non-clinical groups. *Attachment & Human Development*, 11(3), 223–63, p.249. The 'almost perfect' classification of participants with PTSD as showing U/d would likely have been yet higher if other researchers had, like the Leiden researchers in the Harari study of combat veterans, included probes specific to relevant forms of trauma and loss, rather than relying on the general questions in the interview protocol. Bailey and colleagues reported from their study of adolescent mothers that '71% of women with a history of sexual abuse, as reported on either the AAI or the trauma interview, were classified as Unresolved. This association may have been even stronger if a specific sexual abuse probe were included on the AAI.' Bailey, H.N., Moran, G., & Pederson, D.R. (2007) Childhood maltreatment, complex trauma symptoms, and unresolved attachment in an at-risk sample of adolescent mothers. *Attachment & Human Development*, 9(2), 139–61, p.153.

[517] Out, D., Bakermans-Kranenburg, M.J., & van IJzendoorn, M.H. (2009) The role of disconnected and extremely insensitive parenting in the development of disorganized attachment: validation of a new measure. *Attachment & Human Development*, 11(5), 419–43, p.435.

[518] Harari, D., Bakermans-Kranenburg, M.J., De Kloet, C.S., et al. (2009) Attachment representations in Dutch veterans with and without deployment-related PTSD. *Attachment & Human Development*, 11(6), 515–36, p.351. In fact, later research with involvement by van IJzendoorn qualified this picture, finding that only half of adolescent patients who had experienced child sexual abuse and met clinical criteria for PTSD were classified U/d on the AAI. See van Hoof, M.J., van Lang, N.D., Speekenbrink, S., van IJzendoorn, M.H., & Vermeiren, R.R. (2015) Adult Attachment Interview differentiates adolescents with childhood sexual abuse from those with clinical depression and non-clinical controls. *Attachment & Human Development*, 17(4), 354–75. In this sample, unresolved state of mind had no association with dissociative symptoms.

[519] These findings align with those of Nye and colleagues, who found that 50% of a group of Vietnam veterans identified as disabled by PTSD received a U/d classification, compared to 16% in a control sample. The researchers reported that U/d classification was associated with greater probability of a comorbid anxiety disorder. Nye, E.C., Katzman, J., Bell, J.B., Kilpatrick, J., Brainard, M., & Haaland, K.Y. (2008) Attachment organization in Vietnam combat veterans with posttraumatic stress disorder. *Attachment & Human Development*, 10(1), 41–57. Parallel findings are reported for other forms of trauma: 70% of those with U/d for trauma in a sample of women with histories of childhood sexual and/or physical abuse were also identified by clinical interview as showing PTSD by -Stovall McClough, K. & Cloitre, M. (2006) Unresolved attachment, PTSD, and dissociation in women with childhood abuse histories. *Journal of Consulting and Clinical Psychology*, 74(2), 219–28.

protective factor: 'Removing traumatic memories from one's mind may result in reduced hyper vigilance, normal cortisol levels, and reduced fight or flight responses, all of which might be adaptive', and indeed may reduce the display of frightened/frightening behaviours towards children.[520] This conclusion is supported by recent work on the Dozier and colleagues Attachment and Biobehavioural Catch-up intervention, in which dissociative behaviour by caregivers towards their infants was strongly *negatively* associated with emotional dysregulation in response to frustrating tasks when the children were aged three and four.[521]

In another later paper, van IJzendoorn and collaborators added a further qualification to the image of early unresolved loss or trauma predisposing U/d for combat experiences. A study of 184 twins revealed that genetic factors accounted for around half of variance in dissociative symptoms, suggesting a role for genetic factors; however, the contribution of genes associated with dissociation was intensified for individuals who had experienced trauma.[522] This suggests a complex gene × environment interplay in the activation of dissociative processes. Genetic contributions to dissociation may then be implicated in the higher rates of lapses of reasoning and discourse among both combat and non-combat experiences in veterans with PTSD. However, an alternative/additional explanation could be that the traumatic combat experiences activated a latent predisposition towards dissociation, undermining the retrieval of and communication about earlier non-combat-related experiences in the AAI.

Van IJzendoorn and Bakermans-Kranenburg punned that the relationship between trauma, dissociation, and the unresolved classification is an 'unresolved issue' for the field.[523] Like an unresolved loss or trauma, the issue is barely recognised among researchers and the audiences of attachment research, if at all, and reflects a lack of integration of different kinds of information. Yet despite their punning, van IJzendoorn and Bakermans-Kranenburg clearly regarded this as a serious problem. Unless matters are clarified by further research, they even wondered whether lack of resolution for trauma on the AAI 'shows sufficient incremental validity beyond established measures for posttraumatic stress symptomatology' to be worth continuing to use.[524] The appearance of unresolved discourse in the AAI could be an expression of PTSD, or—more likely—of some part of this somewhat heterogenous phenomenon.[525] Furthermore, van IJzendoorn and Bakermans-Kranenburg anticipate that

[520] Fridman, A., Bakermans-Kranenburg, M.J., Sagi-Schwartz, A., & van IJzendoorn, M.H. (2011) Coping in old age with extreme childhood trauma: aging Holocaust survivors and their offspring facing new challenges. *Aging & Mental Health*, 15(2), 232–42, p.240.

[521] Yarger, H.A. (2018) Investigating longitudinal pathways to dysregulation: the role of anomalous parenting behaviour. Unpublished doctoral dissertation, University of Delaware.

[522] Pieper, S., Out, D., Bakermans-Kranenburg, M.J., & van IJzendoorn, M.H. (2011) Behavioral and molecular genetics of dissociation: the role of the serotonin transporter gene promoter polymorphism (5-HTTLPR). *Journal of Traumatic Stress*, 24(4), 373–80.

[523] van IJzendoorn, M.H. & Bakermans-Kranenburg, M.J. (2014) Confined quest for continuity: the categorical versus continuous nature of attachment. *Monographs of the Society for Research in Child Development*, 79(3), 157–67, p.165.

[524] Ibid. One approach to this question would be to see whether markers of U/d decline in AAI discourse following treatment for PTSD. Evidence from other fields to support the plausibility of this hypothesis was surveyed by Stovall-McClough, K. & Cloitre, M. (2006) Unresolved attachment, PTSD, and dissociation in women with childhood abuse histories. *Journal of Consulting and Clinical Psychology*, 74(2), 219–28.

[525] Dutra, S.J. & Wolf, E.J. (2017) Perspectives on the conceptualization of the dissociative subtype of PTSD and implications for treatment. *Current Opinion in Psychology*, 14, 35–9; Horwitz, A.V. (2018) *PTSD: A Short History*. Baltimore: Johns Hopkins University Press. The exact relationship between U/d and PTSD, as an umbrella diagnosis, was queried already two decades ago by Cole-Detke, H. & Kobak, R. (1998) The effects of multiple abuse in interpersonal relationships. *Journal of Aggression, Maltreatment & Trauma*, 2(1), 189–205. Several interpretations of the AAI have assumed that the U/d classification was, in fact, intended as a measure of PTSD, e.g. Wilkins, D., Shemmings, D., & Shemmings, Y. (2015) *A–Z of Attachment*. London: Palgrave, pp.164–5.

clarification of the relationship between the AAI and PTSD will be hindered by the fact that the AAI protocol does not adequately probe the topic of trauma. This is a point likewise made by Riber, and by Bailey, Moran, and Pederson.[526] Van IJzendoorn and Bakermans-Kranenburg, Riber, and Bailey and colleagues have all responded to this predicament by making adaptations to the questions asked in the AAI. Other researchers have not, or at least have not reported doing so. This is likely to have contributed to variability in reports of the association between the AAI and PTSD symptoms.

Another finding relevant here is that in a study of patients with a personality disorder diagnosis, Fonagy and colleagues documented that whilst participants have a more difficult time identifying their own unresolved losses, 87% of participants who regarded themselves as traumatised were rated as unresolved/disorganised/disoriented on the AAI.[527] If replicated by other studies, this high level of agreement between self-report of post-traumatic stress and unresolved trauma in the AAI would align with van IJzendoorn and Bakermans-Kranenburg's question about incremental validity.[528] One forthcoming study offers relevant findings. Whereas childhood PTSD is usually associated with lower hippocampal volume, Cortes Hidalgo and colleagues found that infant disorganised attachment was associated with larger hippocampal volume ($d = .21$) compared to other participants.[529] However, this is as yet only limited and preliminary evidence. The questions raised by van IJzendoorn, Bakermans-Kranenburg, Pederson, and others regarding how the U/d classification for the AAI relates or adds to existing assessments of PTSD remain an area for future research.

The status of depression

Another outstanding question left by the work of the Berkeley group has been the status of depression in relation to the Berkeley assessments of attachment. Depression has mostly been considered in relation to the AAI or in the mothers in dyads seen in the Strange

---

[526] Bailey, H.N., Moran, G., & Pederson, D.R. (2007) Childhood maltreatment, complex trauma symptoms, and unresolved attachment in an at-risk sample of adolescent mothers. *Attachment & Human Development*, 9(2), 139–61; Riber, K. (2016) Attachment organization in Arabic-speaking refugees with post traumatic stress disorder. *Attachment & Human Development*, 18(2), 154–75.

[527] Cirasola, A., Hillman, S., Fonagy, P., & Chiesa, M. (2017) Mapping the road from childhood adversity to personality disorder: the role of unresolved states of mind. *Personality and Mental Health*, 11(2), 77–90: '61.1% (n = 23) of those who had reported experiences of early loss were coded as U/d for loss, and 87.0% of participants with a history of abuse were rated as U/d for abuse' (82).

[528] Though certainly not an exact replication, another study has bearing: Howard and Miriam Steele and colleagues studied the relationship between the unresolved classification on the AAI and self-report of the 'Adverse Childhood Experiences' measure of early trauma. This differed from the Carasola study in that participants were not asked whether they considered themselves traumatised, but nonetheless it has some conceptual similarities since several of the 'Adverse Childhood Experiences' are explicitly various forms of experiences of abuse and neglect. The researchers found a dose-response relationship, gradiated up to four or more discrete indices of childhood trauma, at which point 65% of participants received an unresolved AAI classification. Murphy, A., Steele, M., Dube, S.R., et al. (2014) Adverse Childhood Experiences (ACEs) questionnaire and Adult Attachment Interview (AAI): implications for parent child relationships. *Child Abuse & Neglect*, 38(2), 224–33. See also Thomson, P. & Jaque, S.V. (2017) Adverse Childhood Experiences (ACE) and Adult Attachment Interview (AAI) in a non-clinical population. *Child Abuse & Neglect*, 70, 255–63.

[529] Reported in Van IJzendoorn, M.H. (2019) Replication crisis lost in translation? Paper presented at International Attachment Conference, Vancouver, 20 July 2019. Additionally, van Hoof and colleagues recently showed that unresolved status on the AAI is correlated with atypical amygdala resting-state functional connectivity even adjusting for mental health: van Hoof, M.J., Riem, M.M., Garrett, A.S., et al. (2019) Unresolved–disorganized attachment adjusted for a general psychopathology factor associated with atypical amygdala resting-state functional connectivity. *European Journal of Psychotraumatology*, 10(1), 1583525

Situation. Given that few infants or toddlers receive a diagnosis of depression, there has been little pressure for Main and colleagues or the wider field of attachment research to consider how depression in a young child might interact with or reflect disruption to the attachment system. In general, apparent symptoms of depression in children under three have been regarded by the scientific community as reflecting parental mental health rather than a quality or property of the child.[530] The Berkeley six-year measures have not been in wide circulation, so there has been almost no study of their relationship with depression in middle childhood.[531] One of the few such studies was conducted by Gullone and colleagues, who used the family drawing system with 326 children aged eight to ten. The researchers found a weak but material association between attachment insecurity and the child's report of depressive symptoms ($r = .25$).[532]

Whereas the contribution of child depression to disruption of the child's attachment system has been understudied, there have, by contrast, been numerous studies examining the association between maternal depression and infant attachment in the Strange Situation. This was a topic of special and widespread interest, since Bowlby's emphasis on caregiver unavailability was readily extrapolated to maternal depression as a potential source of major disruption to the infant–caregiver attachment relationship.[533] Several attachment researchers from diverse traditions—ranging from Hazan and Shaver to Cicchetti, Toth, and Rogosch—claimed that disorganised attachment was an expectable result of caregiver depression.[534] Studies set out to examine the question empirically. By 1999, van IJzendoorn and colleagues could report findings from a meta-analysis of 1053 dyads seen in the Strange Situation where the mother had been identified, either by clinicians or by the researchers, as showing symptoms of depression. To the surprise of the researchers, the percentage of dyads receiving a disorganised attachment classification was only 21%, not significantly different to incidence in the general population.[535] Van IJzendoorn and colleagues tried separating

[530] Joan Luby has been an important figure driving attention to depressive symptoms in children under three. Luby demonstrated that depressive symptoms in early childhood predict a later diagnosis of depression. Luby, J.L., Si, X., Belden, A.C., Tandon, M., & Spitznagel, E. (2009) Preschool depression: homotypic continuity and course over 24 months. *Archives of General Psychiatry*, 66(8), 897–905; Whalen, D.J., Sylvester, C.M., & Luby, J.L. (2017) Depression and anxiety in preschoolers: a review of the past 7 years. *Child and Adolescent Psychiatric Clinics*, 26(3), 503–522.

[531] In attachment research, the potential for child contributions to parental depression have generally been ignored. For instance, attachment strategies—for instance controlling-punitive behaviour—may make a reciprocal contribution to parental mental health once they have solidified. See Raposa, E.B., Hammen, C.L., & Brennan, P.A. (2011) Effects of child psychopathology on maternal depression: the mediating role of child-related acute and chronic stressors. *Journal of Abnormal Child Psychology*, 39(8), 1177–86.

[532] Gullone, E., Ollendick, T.H., & King, N.J. (2006) The role of attachment representation in the relationship between depressive symptomatology and social withdrawal in middle childhood. *Journal of Child and Family Studies*, 15(3), 263–77.

[533] Pound, A. (1982) Attachment and maternal depression. In C.M. Parkes & J. Stevenson-Hinde (eds) *The Place of Attachment in Human Behavior* (pp.118–30). Oxford: Oxford University Press; Lyons-Ruth, K., Connell, D.B., Grunebaum, H.U., & Botein, S. (1990) Infants at social risk: maternal depression and family support services as mediators of infant development and security of attachment. *Child Development*, 61(1), 85–98; DeMulder, E.K. & Radke-Yarrow, M. (1991) Attachment with affectively ill and well mothers: concurrent behavioral correlates. *Development & Psychopathology*, 3(3), 227–42.

[534] Hazan, C. & Shaver, P.R. (1994) Attachment as an organizational framework for research on close relationships. *Psychological Inquiry*, 5(1), 1–22, p.6; Cicchetti, D., Toth, S.L., & Rogosch, F.A. (1999) The efficacy of toddler–parent psychotherapy to increase attachment security in offspring of depressed mothers. *Attachment & Human Development*, 1(1), 34–66, p.36.

[535] Van IJzendoorn, M.H., Schuengel, C., & Bakermans-Kranenburg, M.J. (1999) Disorganized attachment in early childhood: meta-analysis of precursors, concomitants, and sequelae. *Development & Psychopathology*, 11(2), 225–50.

the seven studies of caregivers recruited from community samples from the nine studies recruited specifically on the basis of a diagnosis of clinical depression. In the former group there was no association with disorganised attachment, even at trend level. In the latter group there was a very weak ($r = .13$) association with disorganised attachment.[536]

One interpretation of these findings was that the severity of depressive symptoms may play a role. However, severity of depressive symptoms has not generally been found to moderate the relationship between maternal depression and infant disorganised attachment,[537] though one study reported that intermittent symptoms have a weaker effect than continuous symptoms of depression.[538] Comorbidity with other mental health issues has likewise generally not been found to strengthen the link between depression and disorganised attachment.[539] Tharner and colleagues hypothesised that the association between maternal depression and child disorganised attachment seen in clinical samples may be due to an interaction with environmental adversities such as poverty that might contribute to feelings of despair or overloading of demands on cognitive resources.[540] Equally, however, it is possible to use the same argument to suggest that clinical status is here serving as a weak index of other factors—for instance Hofer's 'hidden regulators' (Chapter 1)—with relevance to differences in infant–caregiver attachment, without depression itself making an independent contribution. Bigelow, Beebe, and colleagues have provided evidence suggesting an additional hypothesis: that the caregiver's capacity to hold the child in mind may account for what association there is between parental depression and infant disorganised attachment.[541]

As mentioned earlier, a meta-analysis by Groh and colleagues found that avoidant attachment in infancy predicted later depression and anxiety symptoms. But contrary to previous narrative reviews and the expectations of attachment researchers in general, there was no association between infant disorganised attachment and later symptoms of depression.[542]

---

[536] Ibid. p.237. See also Atkinson, L., Paglia, A., Coolbear, J., Niccols, A., Parker, K.C., & Guger, S. (2000) Attachment security: a meta-analysis of maternal mental health correlates. *Clinical Psychology Review*, 20(8), 1019–40.

[537] McMahon, C.A., Barnett, B., Kowalenko, N.M., & Tennant, C.C. (2006) Maternal attachment state of mind moderates the impact of postnatal depression on infant attachment. *Journal of Child Psychology and Psychiatry*, 47(7), 660–69; Tharner, A., Luijk, M.P., Van IJzendoorn, M.H., et al. (2012) Maternal lifetime history of depression and depressive symptoms in the prenatal and early postnatal period do not predict infant–mother attachment quality in a large, population-based Dutch cohort study. *Attachment & Human Development*, 14(1), 63–81; Flowers, A.G., McGillivray, J.A., Galbally, M., & Lewis, A.J. (2018) Perinatal maternal mental health and disorganised attachment: a critical systematic review. *Clinical Psychologist*, 22(3), 300–316.

[538] Campbell, S.B., Brownell, C.A., Hungerford, A., Spieker, S.J., Mohan, R., & Blessing, J.S. (2004) The course of maternal depressive symptoms and maternal sensitivity as predictors of attachment security at 36 months. *Development & Psychopathology*, 16(2), 231–52.

[539] The relationship between maternal depression and insecure-organised attachment was, however, moderated by comorbid personality disorder. Smith-Nielsen, J., Tharner, A., Steele, H., Cordes, K., Mehlhase, H., & Vaever, M.S. (2016) Postpartum depression and infant–mother attachment security at one year: the impact of co-morbid maternal personality disorders. *Infant Behavior and Development*, 44, 148–58.

[540] Tharner, A., Luijk, M.P., Van IJzendoorn, M.H., et al. (2012) Maternal lifetime history of depression and depressive symptoms in the prenatal and early postnatal period do not predict infant–mother attachment quality in a large, population-based Dutch cohort study. *Attachment & Human Development*, 14(1), 63–81, p.75.

[541] Bigelow, A.E., Beebe, B., Power, M., et al. (2018) Longitudinal relations among maternal depressive symptoms, maternal mind-mindedness, and infant attachment behavior. *Infant Behavior and Development*, 51, 33–44.

[542] Groh, A.M., Roisman, G.I., van IJzendoorn, M.H., Bakermans-Kranenburg, M.J., & Fearon, R.P. (2012) The significance of insecure and disorganized attachment for children's internalizing symptoms: a meta-analytic study. *Child Development*, 83(2), 591–610. Also of relevance here are findings from intervention research that suggest that a video-feedback intervention with caregivers reduces disorganised attachment, but has no effect on children's symptoms of depression. Klein Velderman, M., Bakermans-Kranenburg, M.J., Juffer, F., Van IJzendoorn, M.H., Mangelsdorf, S.C., & Zevalkink, J. (2006) Preventing preschool externalizing behavior problems through video-feedback intervention in infancy. *Infant Mental Health Journal*, 27(5), 466–93.

Groh and colleagues identified a critical mismatch between theory and empirical findings. Bowlby's primary discussions of depression, at least in print, suggested that depression occurs when a behavioural system cannot be terminated. From this account it would be expectable for unresolved loss and, probably, unresolved trauma to be associated with depression. Since the 1990s, Main's ideas have served as the field's dominant source of theory; though her expressive range is astonishing for a research scientist, she barely ever mentions depression. The result has been a gap in explanatory resources for considering why disorganised attachment has so little relationship with depressive symptoms, but has well-replicated associations with externalising symptoms.[543] Groh and colleagues glumly conclude that 'given the current state of the literature on attachment and internalizing symptoms, relatively little can currently be concluded with confidence'.[544] Perhaps something about the attachment system or attachment-relevant information can overcome many aspects of depression and nonetheless function sufficiently effectively. Attachment researchers have generally conceptualised depression as a kind of parental unavailability, but maybe this assumption is too quick or oversimple in some way. Or perhaps only some aspects of depression interact with the attachment system and the processing of attachment-relevant information; this might be suggested by Bowlby's distinctions between levels of defensive exclusion (Chapter 1). It seems likely that a requisite of further theory development in this area will be close attention to the constructs of disorganised attachment and unresolved/disorganised/disoriented states of mind, in order to better understand why they would have little association with depression.

Conclusion

See Table 3.1 in the Appendix to this chapter for consideration of key concepts discussed here. The theory, methodology, and even the basic conceptualisation of the research object of attachment research entered a new era with the innovations introduced by Main and colleagues in the 1980s. Yet criticisms of attachment theory and research, for example by anthropologists (Chapter 2), take Bowlby and Ainsworth as their targets and rarely demonstrate direct knowledge of the work of Main and colleagues. Indeed, the ideas and approaches of the Berkeley group are surprisingly unknown in the wider academic community and among the general public, and much of what is circulated has been cut-price, simplified versions mistaken for the technical form ('allodoxia'; Chapter 1).

---

[543] Unresolved/disorganised states of mind are associated with depression. But it is not clear how much this is driven by preoccupied states of mind. See Dagan, O., Facompré, C.R., & Bernard, K. (2018) Adult attachment representations and depressive symptoms: a meta-analysis. *Journal of Affective Disorders*, 236, 274–90.

[544] Groh, A.M., Roisman, G.I., van IJzendoorn, M.H., Bakermans-Kranenburg, M.J., & Fearon, R.P. (2012) The significance of insecure and disorganized attachment for children's internalizing symptoms: a meta-analytic study. *Child Development*, 83(2), 591–610. More recently, Bakermans-Kranenburg and van IJzendoorn issued a call to examine subtypes of depression, to support finer-grained hypothesis generation and testing regarding the mechanisms that link or do not link unresolved/disorganised attachment and depression. Reiner, I., Bakermans-Kranenburg, M.J., van IJzendoorn, M.H., Fremmer-Bombik, E., & Beutel, M. (2016) Adult attachment representation moderates psychotherapy treatment efficacy in clinically depressed inpatients. *Journal of Affective Disorders*, 195, 163–71, p.169.The call arises from a study conducted with 43 clinically depressed adults in an inpatient unit. The researchers found that patients with higher scores for security-autonomy on the AAI at admission to the inpatient unit saw greater improvements in their depression than other patients. No association was found with U/d on the AAI. Bakermans-Kranenburg and colleagues also highlighted the heterogeneity of the category of depression in Cao, C., Rijlaarsdam, J., van der Voort, A., Ji, L., Zhang, W., & Bakermans-Kranenburg, M.J. (2017) Associations between dopamine D2 receptor (DRD2) gene, maternal positive parenting and trajectories of depressive symptoms from early to mid-adolescence. *Journal of Abnormal Child Psychology*, 46(2), 365–79.

One contributing factor has been Main's approach to disseminating her work. Main has pursued little public engagement. Though she has sometimes delivered public lectures, she has never given interviews to the popular media or written articles for popular venues.[545] Key ideas in print are often to be found as book chapters in now-obscure volumes (e.g. 'Avoidance in the service of proximity'), or were not published in English (e.g. 'Attaccamento disorganizzato/disorientato nell'infanzia e stati mentali dissociati dei genitori', 'Sicherheit und Wissen'). Main's two most comprehensive statements of her perspective and methodological innovations were not published at all (*Behaviour and the Development of Representational Models of Attachment*, 1986; *Four Patterns of Attachment Seen in Behaviour, Discourse and Narrative*, 1995). Pivotal statements on the meaning of the 'state of mind regarding attachment' construct also remained unpublished (e.g. the AAI coding manual; 'Interview based adult attachment classifications: Related to infant–mother and infant–father attachment'). The Berkeley–Leiden Adult Attachment Questionnaire Unresolved States of Mind scale and several empirical studies using it (Chapter 5) all remained unpublished. Main's amendments to the protocol manual for the Strange Situation are only available in manuscript to those attending training institutes. The manuals for the FR coding system and the six year old systems remain unpublished. In accepting the criticisms raised in the present chapter, Main and Hesse have pledged that they will attempt to get more of these texts into print, to reduce their contribution to misapprehensions about their work.[546] This will include the AAI coding manual, which is currently 304 pages (though no doubt will be longer by the time it hits print).

Over the past 30 years or so, the restricted circulation of the work of Main and colleagues has made it difficult for the developmental research community drawing on the theory and measures originating in Berkeley to access, understand, and scrutinise their own constructs. Over the decades, the most direct access to the ideas and methods of developmental attachment research as oriented by Main has not been through published papers, but through fortnight-long in-person trainings in the AAI and Strange Situation which serve as opportunities for enculturation in an oral culture and its interpretive framework.[547] As we saw in Chapter 2, van IJzendoorn had already identified the potential risks of inaccessibility and insularity associated with an oral culture as one of the legacies of Ainsworth. One of the legacies of Main and colleagues has been an intensified reliance on an oral culture among researchers in the developmental tradition, such that full social citizenship of the community has been partly based on graduation from methods training institutes. This worked against integration between attachment researchers and the wider discipline of psychology: publications in journals such as *Child Development* or *Psychological Bulletin* by attachment researchers time and again reported results from Main's measures, but without the space in methods sections and discussion to elaborate fully what these actually meant. Even the basic explanation of measures like the AAI already requires an unusual amount of space for empirical science journals. It has been difficult to justify yet more exposition of technical detail in order to convey the concepts and theory held within the baroque coding systems.

---

[545] Main's acute concern with detail has likely made the compromises and simplifications of popularising discourse especially unappealing. A partial exception is an interview with Main and Hesse conducted by Dan Siegal, available on YouTube: https://www.youtube.com/watch?v=YJTGbVc7EJY.

[546] Mary Main and Erik Hesse, personal communication, August 2019.

[547] For details of the availability of training in the coding systems of Main and colleagues for the AAI and Strange Situation procedure see https://attachment-training.com/.

The limited circulation of detail about the Berkeley measures reduced—though certainly did not halt—their exposure to technical criticism, and to attempts at psychometric appraisal or modification, by researchers outside of Main's personal network.[548] It also left concepts such as 'state of mind regarding attachment' and 'disorganised attachment' circulating widely through the discipline of psychology severed from the context that would have clarified their sense.[549] Neither concept, for instance, has been well understood by social psychological attachment researchers (Chapter 5), since few—if any—social psychologists have received socialisation into the oral culture of the developmentalists or gained reliability in coding their measures. The restricted circulation of Main's texts and full detail on her ideas and measures also limited their effective reception beyond psychology. In particular, it has made it difficult for attachment assessments in the developmental tradition to enter cognate and applied areas, such as social work research and empirical inquiry in family law.[550] The measures were not built or adapted for travel, and so therefore generally did not, except in simplified, summary form.

There was one significant exception to the restricted circulation of the ideas of Main and colleagues. Main published several of her important publications in clinical journals, contributing to an exceptionally warm reception for her work, especially among psychoanalytic clinicians, and more recently among social workers. Her work was also advocated to the clinical community by popularisers such as Dan Siegel and David Shemmings.[551] The narrative of infant disorganised attachment as caused by frightening caregiver behaviour, and as leading to controlling-caregiving or controlling-punitive behaviour and to a wide range of mental health problems, has circulated very widely.[552] The AAI has also seen some clinical application, especially among clinicians with a background in psychoanalytic practice.[553] The contributions of Main and her colleagues have played a significant role, alongside the

[548] An early example was the elaboration of Main's incomplete metacognition scale into the reflective functioning scale by Fonagy, Howard and Miriam Steele, and colleagues. Fonagy, P., Steele, M., Steele, H., Moran, G.S., & Higgitt, A.C. (1991) The capacity for understanding mental states: the reflective self in parent and child and its significance for security of attachment. *Infant Mental Health Journal*, 12(3), 201–218. There have also been modifications by researchers who attended AAI training with Main, but who are more distant from her personal networks. These include Lyons-Ruth, K, Yellin, C., Melnick, S., & Atwood, G. (2005) Expanding the concept of unresolved mental states: hostile/helpless states of mind on the Adult Attachment Interview are associated with disrupted mother–infant communication and infant disorganization. *Development & Psychopathology*, 17(1), 1–23; Roisman, G., Fraley, R., & Belsky, J. (2007) A taxometric study of the Adult Attachment Interview. *Developmental Psychology*, 43(3), 675–86; Crittenden, P.M. & Landini, A. (2011) *Assessing Adult Attachment: A Dynamic-Maturational Approach to Discourse Analysis*. New York: Norton. For discussion of recent psychometric evaluation of the AAI see Chapters 4 and 6.

[549] Reijman, S., Foster, S., & Duschinsky, R. (2018) The infant disorganised attachment classification: 'patterning within the disturbance of coherence'. *Social Science & Medicine*, 200, 52–8.

[550] Nina Koren-Karie is one of very few senior academics based in a social work department to regularly use assessments of attachment from the developmental tradition. Koren-Karie was mentored by Sagi-Schwartz in the psychology department at Haifa and has a doctorate in psychology, which helped this movement of knowledge from developmental psychology into social work research.

[551] Siegel, D.J. (1999) *The Developing Mind*. New York: Guilford; Shemmings, D. & Shemmings, Y. (2011) *Understanding Disorganized Attachment: Theory and Practice for Working with Children and Adults*. London: Jessica Kingsley; Shemmings, D. (2016) Making sense of disorganised attachment behaviour in preschool children. *International Journal of Birth and Parent Education*, 4(1).

[552] See e.g. Howe, D., Brandon, M., Hinings, D., & Schofield, G. (1999) *Attachment Theory, Child Maltreatment and Family Support: A Practice and Assessment Model*. London: Macmillan; Golding, K.S. (2014) *Nurturing Attachments Training Resource: Running Parenting Groups for Adoptive Parents and Foster or Kinship Carers*. London: Jessica Kingsley.

[553] Steele, H. & Steele, M. (eds) (2008) *Clinical Applications of the Adult Attachment Interview*. New York: Guilford; Crowell, J.A. (2014) The Adult Attachment Interview. In S. Farnfield & P. Holmes (eds) *The Routledge Handbook of Attachment: Assessment* (pp.144–55). London: Routledge.

contribution of others such as Fonagy and Holmes,[554] in persuading the clinical community to attend to attachment research, something Bowlby himself felt that he had failed to achieve. Chefetz, for instance, described Main and Hesse's work as an 'explanatory godsend' for clinicians, offering a 'brilliant glow' to difficult clinical phenomena.[555]

Among the second generation of developmental attachment research, the work of Main and colleagues has had as much influence as that of Bowlby and Ainsworth. The Berkeley group have been described as having 'unprecedented resonance and influence'.[556] In his final years, Bowlby described Main's contributions to attachment theory as 'impressive', 'clinically sophisticated', and 'striking'.[557] When a critic spoke out at a conference against the complexity of the descriptions of children and adults that Main was compacting within categories of infant, child, and adult attachment, Bowlby replied 'it is a language of its own, and one wellworth learning'.[558] Alongside such support from Bowlby, Main has widely been regarded as receiving the baton of method-giver from Ainsworth, who used the Berkeley innovations in theory and methodology in her final publications (Chapter 2). As such, positions assumed to be held by Main have had a powerful authority for the second generation of attachment researchers, delimiting the parameters of methodology, and therefore to an extent the parameters of theory.[559] Unfortunately, the stances ascribed to Main frequently differ from, flatten, or petrify into cliché the beliefs of an actual individual, Mary Main, whose ideas have an underpinning architecture that is not widely understood.

Michael Rutter ascribed to Main and colleagues two of the five great advances in psychology contributed by research in attachment on the basis of their introduction of the infant disorganised attachment classification for the Strange Situation procedure, and the AAI.[560] However, these two methodological innovations were not wholly distinct. They both reflected Main's universal model of human emotion regulation, with special primacy given to the role of attentional processes in the formation of individual differences. As discussed in Chapter 2, the idea of behavioural systems was the basis for the Strange Situation procedure but then became interred within it. Likewise, the theory of attentional processes, the 'guess and uncover' approach, and the approach to evolutionary theory which formed the platform for Main's methodological innovations were all buried inside them. It might be thought that the notion of minimising and maximising strategies has been enormously popular among

---

[554] Holmes, J. (1996) Psychotherapy and memory—an attachment perspective. *British Journal of Psychotherapy*, 13(2), 204–218; Fonagy, P. (2000) *Attachment Theory and Psychoanalysis*. London: Karnac.

[555] Chefetz, R.A. (2004) Re-associating psychoanalysis and dissociation: a review of Ira Brenner's 'Dissociation of Trauma: Theory, Phenomenology, and Technique'. *Contemporary Psychoanalysis*, 40(1), 123–33, p.130.

[556] University of Haifa (2011) Honorary doctorate awarded to Prof. Mary Main. https://web.archive.org/web/20160602061335/http://newmedia-eng.haifa.ac.il/?p=5107.

[557] Bowlby, J. (1988) The role of attachment in personality development. In *A Secure Base* (pp.134–54). London: Routledge. The quotes are from, respectively, p.138, p.139, and p.147.

[558] Bowlby, cited in Steele, H. & Steele, M. (1998) Response to Cassidy, Lyons-Ruth and Bretherton: a return to exploration. *Social Development*, 7(1), 137–41, p.141.

[559] Bourdieu, P. (1971, 1991) Genesis and structure of the religious field. *Comparative Social Research*, 13, 1–45; Bourdieu, P. (1971, 1993) The market of symbolic goods. In R. Johnson (ed.) *The Field of Cultural Production*. New York: Columbia University Press, pp.112–42; Bourdieu, P. (1999, 2011) With Weber against Weber, trans. S. Susen. In S, Susen & B.S. Turner (eds) *The Legacy of Pierre Bourdieu: Critical Essays*. London: Anthem Press, pp.111–24; Bourdieu, P. (2004) *The Science of Science and Reflexivity*, trans. R. Nice. Chicago: University of Chicago Press.

[560] The other three were John Bowlby's abandonment of the notion of 'love' in favour of finer-grained concepts, the Ainsworth Strange Situation, and the introduction of the attachment disorder diagnosis within the DSM. See Rutter, M., Kreppner, J., & Sonuga-Barke, E. (2009) Emanuel Miller Lecture: attachment insecurity, disinhibited attachment, and attachment disorders: where do research findings leave the concepts? *Journal of Child Psychology and Psychiatry*, 50, 529–43.

attachment researchers. But—seemingly without realising that there is a distinction—the version that has come into use has been Cassidy's notion as minimising or maximising of attachment as individual strategies, rather than Main's version as minimising or maximising attention to attachment-relevant information as part of a repertoire of behaviours granted by human evolutionary history. Main's attentional theory has been little recognised, and has seen almost no use, no critical scrutiny, and no operationalisation.

A long-time collaborator of Cassidy's, Yair Ziv has considered the legacy of Ainsworth and Main, and appraised the overarching authority given to the four-category Strange Situation and AAI within the developmental tradition of attachment research. Ziv and Hotam argued that in the wider context of academic psychology, overarching theories have become rare, increasingly looked down on as departing or even distracting from the empirical task of psychological research.[561] They observed that, within the field of attachment research, 'scholars use the research tool as their guide, and, probably unintentionally, as the theory's 'surrogate', authorised by the predictive power of the methods.'[562] Ziv and Hotam alleged that attachment research has become largely a hunt for the correlates of the Strange Situation and AAI: further theoretical developments have been blocked by the identification of methodological tools with theoretical constructs, combined with the conviction that the methodology cannot be refined without undermining the basis for a cumulative research paradigm.[563] They express scepticism that methodological innovation—they give the example of the use of Ainsworth's dimensional scales advocated by Fraley and Spieker—would really represent a threat to the possibility of cumulative attachment research, though they know that others would disagree.[564]

It is plausible, as Ziv and Hotam argued, that attachment research has partially circumvented the decline of theory in academic psychology by embodying theory within methodology, protecting theoretical propositions whilst supplanting the need to explicitly acknowledge or discuss them.[565] However, other factors may be mentioned as having obstructed understanding of the position of Main and colleagues. These include confusions regarding the use of terminology, the complexity and gestalt-like quality to the coding of observational measures of attachment, and restrictions on the accessibility of Main and colleagues' texts containing details of methods and theory.

---

[561] Some similar proposals have been made in Flis, I. (2018) Discipline through method: recent history and philosophy of scientific psychology (1950–2018). Unpublished doctoral thesis, University of Utrecht. In a corpus analysis of the 2,046 psychology articles published to date in *Frontiers in Psychology*, Beller and Bender found that only 8.3% feature reference to a specific theory. A small number of theories were cited in more than three articles among the 2,046, suggesting their ongoing relevance and durability. Among these were, unsurprisingly, 'probability theory' and 'evolutionary theory' as underpinning aspects of any contemporary life science. There were also some domain theories such as the 'theory of planned behaviour'. However, the most frequent of all theories mentioned in at least three articles was 'attachment theory'. It was also the only theory from developmental psychology mentioned by at least three articles in the corpus. Beller, S. & Bender, A. (2017) Theory, the final frontier? A corpus-based analysis of the role of theory in psychological articles. *Frontiers in Psychology*, 8, 951.

[562] Ziv, Y. & Hotam, Y. (2015) Theory and measure in the psychological field: the case of attachment theory and the strange situation procedure. *Theory & Psychology*, 25(3), 274–91, p.278.

[563] Ibid. p.283.

[564] Researchers will likely differ on the extent to which they believe that there can be innovations that would add value, reward the resource investment, and still be plugged into the same meta-analyses. Kuhn, T.S. (1977) *The Essential Tension: Selected Studies in Scientific Tradition and Change*. Chicago: University of Chicago Press.

[565] The claims of Ziv and Hotam are restricted to the developmental tradition of attachment research, within which they were trained. However, the argument that method has incorporated and supplanted theorising can be applied to the social psychological tradition, where the two dimensions of anxiety and avoidance have formed the central theoretical framework over the past two decades, stabilised and protected by the Experiences of Close Relationships measure (Chapter 5).

The movement of Main's ideas across disciplinary spaces has occurred at the price of a mangled and simplified image of the methods and theory of the Berkeley group. Much like the Strange Situation was misadministered in Japan by researchers without the social links or deep theoretical knowledge to scaffold its appropriate use (Chapter 2), Main and colleagues have seen misapplications of their work in child welfare contexts.[566] This predicament can be regarded at least in part as resulting from a combination of the compelling, magnetic, and absorbative quality of the ideas such as attachment, fear, disorganisation, trauma, and dissociation—combined with problems in the effective circulation of the technical ideas and methods of Main and colleagues outside the communities of academic and psychoanalytic psychology. The characterisation of disorganisation as a category may also have inadvertently helped it meld with the diagnosis-focused infrastructures of clinical and welfare investigations of families. Third-generation attachment researchers have tended to avoid categories in their adaptations of attachment measures for use by practitioners, not only because dimensions often have better psychometric properties, but also to try to avoid the problems they have seen with the reception of Main and Solomon's disorganised classification.[567]

Main has had health difficulties at times which have reduced her capacity to write, to respond to questions and clarify ambiguities, as well as—until recently—to offer trainings (or train a trainer) in the six-year systems or the frightening/frightened coding system. This has been compounded by her perfectionism and concern with detail, which has made it extremely difficult for Main to judge a coding system or a piece of writing finished enough to go into circulation. As a result, over the decades vast swathes of her writing has remained unpublished, misunderstandings have abounded, and there have been barely a handful of accredited coders in any of the six-year systems or the frightening/frightened coding system. The infant disorganised coding system was also left in an underdeveloped state that contributes to it being difficult to learn; again, there are now remarkably few active, accredited coders.[568] Though dedicated researchers have found workarounds, such as the use of alternative assessments, the lack of training and reliable coders have obstructed lines of empirical inquiry in the developmental tradition of attachment research. For example, though Main and Hesse's work is cited as an inspiration in many attachment-based interventions, none has used frightened/frightening caregiving as an outcome measure.[569] (Main and Hesse have said that they will soon be certifying four trainers, contributing to the future availability of the FR coding system.)

---

[566] Main, M., Hesse, E., & Hesse, S. (2011) Attachment theory and research: overview with suggested applications to child custody. *Family Court Review*, 49(3), 426–63, p.441. See also Granqvist, P. (2016) Observations of disorganized behaviour yield no magic wand: response to Shemmings. *Attachment & Human Development*, 18(6), 529–33. For examples of the garbled reception and understanding of Main's work in policy discourse see e.g. Moullin, S., Waldfogel, J., & Washbrook, E. (2014) *Baby Bonds: Parenting, Attachment and a Secure Base for Children*. London: Sutton Trust; All Party Parliamentary Group for Conception to Age 2 (2015) *Building Great Britons*. London: Wave Foundation.

[567] Madigan, S. (2019) Beyond the academic silo: collaboration and community partnerships in attachment research. Paper presented at International Attachment Conference, Vancouver, 20 July 2019.

[568] Reijman, S., Foster, S., & Duschinsky, R. (2018) The infant disorganised attachment classification: 'patterning within the disturbance of coherence'. *Social Science & Medicine*, 200, 52–8.

[569] Dozier's group repeatedly described the central influence of Main and Hesse's work on their Attachment and Biobehavioural Catch-up intervention. However, in the absence of training in the FR system, they used an alternative assessment of caregiving behaviour in evaluating it: the Bronfman, Parsons, and Lyons-Ruth AMBIANCE coding system. Yarger, H.A. (2018) Investigating longitudinal pathways to dysregulation: the role of anomalous parenting behaviour. Unpublished doctoral dissertation, University of Delaware.

Restricted circulation of knowledge of the Berkeley measures has fuelled misunder-standings of Main's theoretical position, which is closely tied to understanding the meaning of the assessments she and colleagues developed. There are vast discrepancies between the assumed positions generally ascribed to 'Mary Main' regarding the four-category mode of individual differences, and the theoretical positions available on a close reading of Main's texts and coding manuals. These discrepancies are especially located around the unrecognised technical meanings given to key elements of Main's conceptual vocabulary, including 'disorganisation', 'fear', 'coherence', 'preoccupation', 'unresolved', and 'dissociation'. Yet there have been some researchers aware of Main's position and trained in use of her measures. One set of researchers with strong understanding and close per-sonal ties to Main and Hesse has been the Minnesota group. The work of Sroufe, Egeland, and colleagues with the Minnesota Longitudinal Study of Risk and Adaptation would prove just as influential as the Berkeley study for shaping the second generation of attach-ment research, providing independent validation of the measures developed in Baltimore and Berkeley, and reporting findings to support and to qualify the claims by Bowlby, Ainsworth, Main, and Hesse.

Appendix

Table 3.1 Some key concepts in Main and Hesse's writings

Concept	Mistaken for	Explanation in longhand
Categories for coding individual differences in attachment	Four boxes representing different 'kinds' of attachment	Ainsworth identified differences in the responses of infants in the Strange Situation to separation from and reunion with their familiar caregiver. These differences were characterised through various means, including a variety of interactive rating scales, two latent dimensions in a discriminant function analysis, and eight subtypes. These eight subtypes were pragmatically grouped into three categories. However, Ainsworth anticipated that more categories would be identified on the basis of further research.
		Main, however, proposed that the Ainsworth
		Strange Situation categories were a local form of a wider phenomenon. This was that the output of any behavioural system—including the attachment system and the caregiving system—could be increased or decreased based on how individuals direct their attention. Where individuals direct their attention away from the cues that might otherwise activate the behavioural system, the system is difficult to initiate and its output minimised. When individuals are vigilant to cues that would activate the behavioural system, the output of that system is maximised and the system difficult to terminate. She termed these 'conditional strategies' to highlight that these responses may not directly express the behavioural system, but would nonetheless likely have evolved because they helped an individual survive under certain kinds of adverse circumstances.

(continued)

Table 3.1 Continued

Concept	Mistaken for	Explanation in longhand
		Main presumed there would be three forms of expression of a behavioural system: a direct expression, its minimisation, or its maximisation. Where the expression of a behavioural system appeared to be undermined by conflict or confusion, Main characterised this with a fourth classification—'disorganisation'. However, no psychometric analysis was conducted to assess whether disorganisation was best considered as a category. The attachment categories are therefore best regarded as pragmatic tools for describing individual differences observed when using attachment measures, and embodying Main's thesis of minimising and maximising strategies.
		In unpublished written guidance provided to those learning to code the Strange Situation at Minnesota, Main advises that secure attachment in the Strange Situation is coded on the basis of behaviours that appear to flexibly direct attention to the caregiver or the environment depending on the situation. Avoidant attachment is coded on the basis of behaviours that direct attention away from the caregiver and towards the environment. Ambivalent/resistant attachment is coded on the basis of behaviours that direct attention away from the environment and vigilance is maintained about the caregiver's availability. Disorganised attachment is coded on the basis of behaviours that suggest conflict or confusion in the direction of attention either towards the caregiver or to the environment.
Avoidance (for children) Dismissing (for adults)	Ainsworth's attachment classification for infants who physically avoid their mother on reunion. Extrapolated metaphorically to characterise speakers in the AAI who 'avoid' the topic of attachment relationships	Ainsworth identified that some infants in the Strange Situation avoided approaching their caregiver on reunion; many turned away from the caregiver towards the toys, or drew the caregiver's attention to a toy.
		Main developed a theory that these infants were directing their attention away from cues to the activation of the attachment system. In doing so, these infants were not just physically avoiding the caregiver. They were also avoiding the conflict that would be evoked by expectations about rebuff from the caregiver based on past experiences, and the activation of the attachment system which would prompt proximity-seeking.
		Main drew on this account in developing the AAI coding system. With colleagues, she developed a 'dismissing' classification for speakers who, in an autobiographical interview, appeared to be directing attention away from attachment-relevant information about their past.
		Both avoidant behaviour in the Strange Situation and dismissing discourse in the AAI were understood to represent use of a strategy that cuts off attention to environmental cues that would otherwise feed information to a behavioural system—thereby avoiding disruption of this system and the ensuing reduced responsiveness to the environment.

Table 3.1 Continued

Concept	Mistaken for	Explanation in longhand
Ambivalence/ resistance (for children) Preoccupation (for adults)	Ainsworth's attachment classification for infants who show anger towards their mother on reunion. Extrapolated metaphorically to characterise speakers in the AAI who remain angry with their childhood attachment figures	Ainsworth identified that some infants in the Strange Situation showed distress and frustration with their caregivers on reunion, and were not readily able to be comforted by their caregiver.
		Main developed a theory that these infants were directing their attention vigilantly towards potential cues to the activation of the attachment system, and away from cues to the termination of the system. The continual activation of the system was regarded as prompting frustration. In turn, frustration was seen as helping to maintain vigilance, and also to maintain the attention of the caregiver.
		Main drew on this account in developing the AAI coding system. With colleagues, she developed a 'preoccupied' classification for speakers who, in an autobiographical interview, appeared to be directing attention and frustration towards attachment-relevant information about their past at the expense of cooperation with the interviewer in answering their exact questions.
		Both ambivalence/resistance in the Strange Situation and preoccupied discourse in the AAI were understood to represent a strategy that intensifies attention to environmental cues that would feed information to initiate a behavioural system, and the cutting off of attention from cues that would terminate the system. The unsatisfied system prompts frustration; at the same time, frustration may help maintain attention on relevant cues and attracting the attention of attachment figures.
Disorganisation	Random, chaotic behaviour and mental states characteristic of certain infants in the Strange Situation. The effect of child maltreatment	The term 'disorganisation' has regularly been used in five different ways by Main. She did so to draw links between behaviour and mental processes, and to identify potential similarities in mental processes across the life course.
		A first use of the term has been as an umbrella term for three different kinds of behaviour shown towards the object of a behavioural system: conflict, confusion, and/ or apprehension. These behaviours may, for instance, be shown by infants towards their caregiver in the Strange Situation, where the attachment system is presumed to be activated by the separations and reunions.
		A second use of the term has been to characterise a significant disruption of a behavioural system. It is this (invisible) disruption at the level of motivation that is presumed to cause the visible conflicted, confused, or apprehensive behaviour seen, for instance, in the Strange Situation.
		A third use of the term has been as a category label for infant–caregiver dyads seen in the Strange Situation, where conflicted, confused, and/or apprehensive behaviour is seen to a significant degree.

(continued)

Table 3.1 Continued

Concept	Mistaken for	Explanation in longhand
		A fourth use of the term was as the category label for controlling-punitive and controlling-caregiving behaviour in the Main and Cassidy six-year reunion system. The behaviour was generally smoothly sequenced and goal-oriented, and often resulted in some form of caregiver availability—so it was not technically disorganised at a behavioural level. However, Main and Cassidy used the term 'disorganised' to signal developmental continuities from infancy, and to highlight that controlling-punitive and controlling-caregiving behaviour likely arises in the context of disruption to the child–caregiver relationship and its usual hierarchies.
		A fifth use of the term has been to characterise the psychological process indicated by unresolved loss and trauma in the AAI. In their 1992 paper, Main and Hesse conceptualised this state as representing an overloading of working memory, as attention cannot be directed coherently either away from or towards attachment-relevant information.
Disorganised attachment behaviour	Random, chaotic behaviour and mental states characteristic of certain infants in the Strange Situation	Main and Solomon defined seven indices of disorganised attachment for coding the Strange Situation in their 1990 chapter. The first five were drawn from Hinde's 1966 discussion of 'conflict behaviours': behaviours shown when an organism experiences strong, conflicting motivations. The sixth was apprehension of the caregiver. The seventh was behaviours suggestive of confusion or disorientation. It was not assumed that all of these would mean the same thing. In Main and Hesse's later work, they suggested that many of the behaviours would to varying degrees reflect a history of alarming behaviours by caregivers. They also suggested that some, though certainly not all, may entail dissociative processes.
Attachment-related fear	A child scared of a frightening or abusive parent	The term 'fear' has a variety of connotations. Main and Hesse used the term in a technical sense, to describe the situation in which an attachment figure, their behaviour, or their absence in a major separation has been a source of alarm for a child. When they use the phrase 'fright without solution', this was intended to highlight that if a child is alarmed, the attachment system would prompt them to approach their caregiver. However, if the caregiver is themselves associated with alarm, then the child is placed in a conflict situation.
		In characterising 'fear without solution' as one pathway to disorganised attachment, Main and Hesse were not intending to imply that the caregiver has necessarily frightened the child directly. A situation in which a child observed violence perpetuated by their father towards their mother might also lead them to associate their mother with feelings of alarm.

Table 3.1 Continued

Concept	Mistaken for	Explanation in longhand
Attachment representations	Stable images held by people about their attachment figures	Main regarded the AAI as assessing the speaker's capacity for flexibility in organising information relevant to attachment and for obtaining or limiting access to that information. Secure-autonomous speakers could answer questions about their childhood fluently whilst also cooperating with their interviewer, paying attention to what is relevant for them, what level of detail is helpful and not overwhelming or confusing, etc. Dismissing speakers directed attention away from attachment-relevant experiences. Preoccupied speakers directed attention towards their dissatisfaction with attachment-relevant experiences at the expense of cooperation with the interviewer.
		Over time, Main characterised these individual differences in various ways: sometimes as 'internal working models', sometimes as 'attachment representations', and sometimes as 'states of mind regarding attachment'. None of these terms is an especially effective characterisation of what Main thought she had identified, and there remains a good deal of confusion about their meaning today. Generally, attachment researchers today use the terms 'attachment representations' and 'state of mind regarding attachment' to mean individual differences as measured by the AAI.
Coherence of discourse	Ordered and meaningful speech	Coherence represents an individual's presentation of a plausible, unified, yet free-flowing picture of experiences, feelings, and viewpoints—as well as their potential causes—within the AAI.
		Main anticipated that individuals whose speech displayed these characteristics would also meet Grice's maxims for cooperative discourse with the interviewer:
		Quality—'be truthful and have evidence for what you say'
		Quantity—'be succinct, and yet complete'
		Relation—'be relevant to the topic as presented'
		Manner—'be clear and orderly'
Lack of resolution	A trauma or loss that still preys on the mind of a speaker, for instance causing denial or distress when it is raised	Lack of resolution is a technical term used by Main, Goldwyn, and Hesse to characterise a particular phenomenon in the AAI. There are many ways in which a past loss or trauma might influence the present. For instance, individuals may block all thoughts of it. Or they may become distressed just thinking about it. Neither of these is lack of resolution in Main and colleagues' technical sense. In both cases, attention has been directed in an effective way away from, or towards, the loss or trauma. The loss or trauma is not resolved. But it is not technically 'unresolved' in the meaning intended by Main and colleagues.

(continued)

Table 3.1 Continued

Concept	Mistaken for	Explanation in longhand
		Lack of resolution occurs when the speaker's response when discussing a bereavement or a determinate traumatic event suggests disorganisation or disorientation in the capacity to attend to it. It is coded primarily on the basis of lapses in reasoning or discourse in discussions of childhood attachment relationships, from which a coder is able to infer this disorganisation or disorientation in mental processing around the loss or trauma.
		There are further technical qualifications on what is meant by lack of resolution. The most important is that the loss or trauma has to be a historically locatable event. Hence there may be experiences that, despite appearances, are not technically considered unresolved even if relevant disturbances of reasoning or discourse are present. These include: anticipated bereavement in the case of a terminally ill attachment figure; experiences of chronic neglect in childhood; exposure to an atmosphere of emotional abuse between parents during childhood but without there being a stand-out 'event'; and fear of an intimidating current partner or ex-partner.
Earned security	Individuals' 'earned' achievement of the benefits of secure early relationships through their own efforts in later childhood, adolescence, or adulthood	Early in their work on the AAI Main and colleagues found that participants who could speak coherently about their early attachment relationships tended towards two types. A first group had experienced positive early relationships. A second group had experienced difficult childhoods; nonetheless, they spoke with flexible attention to the good and the bad, and could turn fluently from considering memories of the past to communication with the interviewer in the present, taking stock of their own perspective and that of others. Main and colleagues termed these latter speakers 'earned secure'. The term is misleading, since it may seem to imply that individuals were able to rise above their early adversities through force of will. It also assumes that the earned-secure speakers did, indeed, have a more difficult childhood than non-earned-secure speakers; in fact, the AAI cannot assure this. Roisman and colleagues have been especially active in exploring whether an earned-secure classification in the AAI is actually associated with greater childhood adversity than other speakers classified as 'autonomous-secure'.
		As a consequence, Main and Hesse have renamed the classification 'evolved secure', to avoid the implication that it is the achievement of individual willpower. To date, attachment researchers have, however, largely ignored this rechristening, perhaps due to concerns about the term 'evolved'. Main and Hesse have also placed stringent criteria on the classification (a score of lower than 2.5 on the scale for inferred loving parental behaviour). So only speakers with credible evidence of extremely adverse caregiving who nonetheless show coherent speech can be considered as 'evolved secure'. However, these criteria are so stringent that few individuals can be identified in most samples.

Table 3.1 Continued

Concept	Mistaken for	Explanation in longhand
		Beyond its exact operationalisation, the functional meaning of the earned/evolved secure status in the AAI for attachment researchers has been to signal acknowledgement that states of mind regarding attachment can change over time, and that these changes themselves are potentially important.
Dissociation	Blocked communication between parts of the self	The term 'dissociation' is one with various meanings in discussions of mental health. Main has tended to use the term to mean one of two things. Either it has been used to mean much the same as 'segregation' (see Bowlby's use of the term). Or it has been used to mean specific behaviours suggestive of the segregation of perception, such as fugue states.

Note: The table has been confirmed by Mary Main and Erik Hesse.

Illustrative statement: 'Whereas avoidant attachment is associated with caregiver insensitivity and rebuff, Main's disorganised attachment classification is associated with frightening experiences of the caregiver. The caregivers of infants with this classification often have attachment representations characterised by lack of resolution of loss or trauma. An important mechanism underpinning this lack of resolution is proposed to be dissociation.'

Mistaken for: Main provided an exhaustive four-category system. Some infants, classified as avoidant, experienced less warm care. There is another category, comprising of ambivalent infants who also resist their caregiver's attempts to comfort them. A further category, disorganised infants, experienced abusive care, breaking their attachment system and causing random, chaotic behaviour in the Strange Situation. The behaviour of these caregivers can be explained by their own adverse experiences, which still disturb them, and which cause them to behave irrationally and dangerously towards their child.

Technical meaning: Some caregivers struggle to perceive and to interpret accurately the signals and communications implicit in an infant's behaviour, and given this understanding, to respond to them appropriately and promptly (i.e. sensitive care). For instance, caregivers may rebuff their infants' attachment behaviour. Main supposed that such behaviour by caregivers will expectably prompt a conditional strategy from the infant, in which attention is directed away from the caregiver in the Strange Situation so as to maintain regulation and environmental responsiveness. This is in contrast to another conditional strategy (ambivalent/resistant attachment) in which attention is directed vigilantly towards potential cues to the activation of the attachment system and away from cues to the termination of the system. However, both the primary (secure) strategy and the conditional strategies can be disrupted—for instance by conflicting affects. There may be a variety of causes of such disruption and a variety of forms of conflict, as Hinde had already shown. Main and Hesse identified that an especially important case is conflict between the disposition to approach the caregiver when alarmed and experiences of the caregiver as themselves in some way alarming. One potential cause of such experiences is when caregivers are abusive. However, other forms of caregiver behaviour can be alarming for infants, such as sudden and inexplicable lapses in a caregiver's attentional availability. Main and Hesse found that forms of alarming caregiving behaviour are more common among caregivers who show marked lapses in discourse or reasoning in the AAI, as defined by a technical set of criteria that identifies in these lapses indications of disrupted attentional processing of attachment-relevant information when discussing specific alarming events in their history.

4

Alan Sroufe, Byron Egeland, and the Minnesota Longitudinal Study of Risk and Adaptation

Biographical sketch

The Minnesota Longitudinal Study of Risk and Adaptation began in the early 1970s, initiated by Byron Egeland as a study of a large cohort of mothers living in poverty. In the 1970s and early 1980s, empirical attachment research had been primarily pursued by Ainsworth and her students. The research group led by Alan Sroufe and Egeland was important in providing a second pillar to hold up the paradigm from the 1970s to the present. The Strange Situation was conducted with the sample by Sroufe and his graduate students Everett Waters and Brian Vaughn. Early work by the research group documented the role of caregiving in shaping patterns of attachment in the Strange Situation, and also the capacity of infant attachment patterns to predict later social competence and mental health. Sroufe and Egeland created an 'electric atmosphere' in their research group, as they provided the first longitudinal evidence of the implications of attachment relationships.[1] Students described their 'imperturbable optimism', 'wisdom about human nature', and 'compassion' as important qualities in the creation of the atmosphere, along with the sense of contributing to meaningful and cutting-edge developmental science.[2] They were a great stabilising and integrative presence for the field of attachment research. Though Egeland and Sroufe have now retired, research with the Minnesota Longitudinal Study of Risk and Adaptation has continued.

Introduction

The Minnesota research group has been of critical importance to the establishment and development of attachment research. Whilst to the general public Bowlby remains the most visible and prominent representative of attachment research, within the American developmental science community this role has arguably been held by Sroufe and Egeland. Mary Ainsworth wrote to Sroufe in 1982, expressing her deep gratitude: 'One of the very best things that ever happened to attachment research was your decision to participate in it!'[3] In the introduction to their six-volume edited work on attachment theory, Slade and Holmes described the contribution of the Minnesota group as no less than a 'revolution,' one that 'brought attachment theory into mainstream academic psychology'.[4] In part as a consequence, attachment theory has at times been referred to as the Bowlby–Ainsworth–Sroufe

---

[1] Dante Cicchetti interviewed by Robert Karen, cited in Karen, R. (1998) *Becoming Attached: First Relationships and How They Shape Our Capacity to Love*. Oxford: Oxford University Press, p.167.

[2] Marvinney, D. (1988) Sibling relationships in middle childhood: implications for social-emotional development. Unpublished doctoral dissertation, University of Minnesota, p.i.

[3] Ainsworth, M. (1982) *Letter to Alan Sroufe*, 27 March 1982. Mary Ainsworth papers, Box M3173, Folder 3.

[4] Slade, A. & Holmes, J. (2014) Introduction. In *Attachment Theory*, Vol. 1 (pp.5–37). London: Sage, p.13.

tradition.[5] The primary scientific contribution of the Minnesota group under the leadership of Sroufe and Egeland has been to show the developmental implications of early caregiving and attachment. This was of essential importance for consolidating Ainsworth's findings and for showing why they mattered for development. Furthermore, on the basis of their empirical research, Sroufe, Egeland, and colleagues made important theoretical contributions to the conceptualisation of the role of attachment within development as a whole. Fonagy would describe Sroufe and the Minnesota group as having played a 'seminal role in extending the scope of attachment theory from an account of the developmental emergence of a set of social expectations to a far broader conception of attachment as an organizer of physiological and brain regulation.'[6]

In the 1940s, Bowlby felt unable to report on his clinical observations of child abuse (Chapter 1). By the 1970s, however, the clinical community had come to acknowledge the potential for parents to abuse and neglect their children.[7] There was growing policy interest in the role of abuse and neglect in contributing to later mental illness, aggressive behaviour, and social difficulties. There was also growing interest in the lives of single-parent families living in poverty, in the context of both changing family demography in America and the political problematisation of these families.[8] The Minnesota Longitudinal Study of Risk and Adaptation began in the 1970s as the world's first attempt to conduct a prospective study of child abuse. Until that point, all research on child abuse had been pursued retrospectively. This raised questions of validity, especially given the significant potential stigma for adults in revealing experiences of childhood abuse. Egeland, Amos Deinard, and Ellen Elkin wrote a proposal to the Centre of Maternal and Child Health to initiate a longitudinal cohort study. Funding was provided in 1975 for three years in the first instance. The researchers' belief in the value of prospective research exploring abuse and neglect proved well founded: decades later, only half of the adults in their sample with prospectively documented histories of childhood abuse self-reported that they had experienced maltreatment.[9]

Shortly before the study began, Arnold Sameroff visited the department at Minnesota and shared a draft of his classic paper proposing an 'ecological' model in which human development is shaped by the interaction between risk factors and environmental supports.[10] This model had a profound influence on the methodology of the study, which sought to identify and capture various risk and protective factors in line with Sameroff's idea of development

[5] E.g. Belsky, J. (2002) Developmental origins of attachment styles. *Attachment & Human Development*, 4(2), 166–70.

[6] Fonagy, P. (2015) Mutual regulation, mentalization, and therapeutic action. *Psychoanalytic Inquiry*, 35(4), 355–69, p.358.

[7] Hacking, I. (1991) The making and molding of child abuse. *Critical Inquiry*, 17(2), 253–88; Ferguson, H. (2004) *Protecting Children in Time: Child Abuse, Child Protection and the Consequences of Modernity*. London: Palgrave.

[8] Jones, J.P. & Kodras, J.E. (1990) Restructured regions and families: the feminization of poverty in the US. *Annals of the Association of American Geographers*, 80(2), 163–83; Hancock, A.M. (2004) *The Politics of Disgust: The Public Identity of the Welfare Queen*. New York: NYU Press.

[9] Shaffer, A., Huston, L., & Egeland, B. (2008) Identification of child maltreatment using prospective and self-report methodologies: a comparison of maltreatment incidence and relation to later psychopathology. *Child Abuse & Neglect*, 32(7), 682–92. These results agree with later meta-analytic findings: Baldwin J.R., Reuben, A., Newbury, J.B., & Danese, A. (2019) Agreement between prospective and retrospective measures of childhood maltreatment: a systematic review and meta-analysis. *JAMA Psychiatry*, 76(6), 584–93.

[10] The term 'risk' is multivalent and potentially obfuscating, as noted by Lupton, D. (1999) *Risk*. London: Routledge. However, Sroufe's usage has been clear and consistent throughout his career: Sroufe, L.A., Egeland, B., Carlson, E.A., & Collins, W.A. (2005) *The Development of the Person*. New York: Guilford: 'A risk factor is anything that increments the probability of some negative outcome' for individuals or families within a given population (28).

as multiply determined.[11] Particular attention was given to risk and protective factors in the life of the child's caregiver or caregivers. Egeland and colleagues recruited 267 women in the third trimester of pregnancy and living in poverty.[12] However, in line with Sameroff's ideas, Egeland and colleagues were intent on assessing the multiple adversities faced by the families, documenting the widespread prevalence of domestic violence, mental health problems, and drug and alcohol use. Forty-one percent of the mothers had not finished high-school education;[13] 86% of the pregnancies were unplanned, with a third of families having obtained no equipment necessary for the baby or made arrangements for somewhere for the baby to sleep;[14] the mothers were often socially isolated, with very low average levels of social support;[15] 59% were single at the time of their baby's birth, compared to a 13% national average in 1975;[16] and only 13% of the fathers were living in the same home as their children by the time they had reached 18 months of age. Soon after the study began, Egeland contacted Sroufe, a colleague at Minnesota, and together they conducted the Ainsworth Strange Situation with the sample, with input from two graduate students—Everett Waters and Brian Vaughn.[17] The Strange Situation was attractive as a procedure offering a window into the experiences of care and emotional development of the children in the sample. And the classifications for the procedure had the initial basis for construct validity through Ainsworth's Baltimore study (Chapter 2). For his dissertation Waters also conducted a parallel study of 50 mother–infant dyads from Minnesota who were not living in poverty. This allowed the Minnesota group to draw some comparisons to explore the role of socioeconomic adversity in predicting outcomes of interest, such as distribution of classifications in the Ainsworth Strange Situation.[18]

Egeland, Sroufe, and colleagues in the Minnesota group were sensitive to the cultural and moral context of developmental research with a sample facing such adversities.[19] One such factor was acrimonious debates at the time over whether abuse was in fact harmful to children's development, or whether associations between abuse and with negative outcomes could better be attributed to poverty.[20] One measure the Minnesota group took to respond to these controversies was to expend every effort to carefully measure both abuse and adversity

[11] Sameroff, A.J. & Chandler, M.J. (1975) Reproductive risk and the continuum of caretaking casualty. *Review of Child Development Research*, 4, 187–244; Mangelsdorf, S.C. (2011) The early history and legacy of the Minnesota Parent–Child Longitudinal Study. In D. Cicchetti & G.I. Roisman (eds) *The Minnesota Symposia on Child Psychology, Volume 36: The Origins and Organization of Adaptation and Maladaptation* (pp.1–12). Hoboken, NJ: Wiley.

[12] Egeland, B. & Sroufe, L.A. (1981) Attachment and early maltreatment. *Child Development*, 52(1), 44–52.

[13] Pianta, R.C., Sroufe, L.A., & Egeland, B. (1989) Continuity and discontinuity in maternal sensitivity at 6, 24, and 42 months in a high-risk sample. *Child Development*, 60, 481–7.

[14] Egeland, B., Jacobvitz, D., & Papatola, K. (1987) Intergenerational continuity of abuse. In R.J. Gelles & J.B. Lancaster (eds) *Child Abuse and Neglect: Biosocial Dimensions*. New York: Aldine De Gruyter, 255–76, p.259.

[15] Appleyard, K., Egeland, B., & Sroufe, L.A. (2007) Direct social support for young high risk children: relations with behavioral and emotional outcomes across time. *Journal of Abnormal Child Psychology*, 35(3), 443–57: '27% of the sample had only one or two individuals in their network' (447).

[16] US Bureau of the Census (1975) *Marital Status and Living Arrangements: March 1995 Update*. Washington, DC: US Government Printing Office. https://www.census.gov/library/publications/1975/demo/p20-287.html.

[17] The coders of the Strange Situations conducted at 12 months were Waters and Vaughn; the coders of the 18-month procedures were Sroufe and Lyle S. Joffe.

[18] Vaughn, B., Egeland, B., Sroufe, L.A., & Waters, E. (1979) Individual differences in infant–mother attachment at twelve and eighteen months: stability and change in families under stress. *Child Development*, 50(4), 971–5.

[19] Sroufe, L.A. (1970) A methodological and philosophical critique of intervention-oriented research. *Developmental Psychology*, 2(1), 140–45.

[20] Elmer, E. (1977) *Fragile Families, Troubled Children: The Aftermath of Infant Trauma*. Pittsburgh: University of Pittsburgh Press, discussed in Sroufe, L.A., Egeland, B., Carlson, E.A., & Collins, W.A. (2005) *The Development of the Person*. New York: Guilford, p.51.

in a variety of ways, building convergent validity piece by piece out of multiple sources of information. These included researcher observation, parent report, and professional assessments.[21] Such an approach allowed the Minnesota group to distinguish the shared and non-shared contribution of abuse and other adversities to later outcomes. Shaffer, Huston, and Egeland later reported that 40% of the non-maltreated child participants in their sample met diagnostic criteria for at least one mental disorder in late adolescence. Reports from abuse from one source made an additional contribution to later mental health, with an additional 20% of participants diagnosed with at least one mental disorder. There was, however, an additional 32% where abuse was validated by more than one source.[22]

A sense of the serious ethical commitment of Egeland, Sroufe, and colleagues in commencing a longitudinal study with a large sample recruited on the basis of low income and adversity, and the value of making sense of parents' experiences, comes through with special clarity in their early publications. In examining the antecedents of abusive caregiving, this did not imply that they ascribed blame to the caregivers.[23] Egeland and colleagues had specifically chosen a sample in poverty because deprivation of resources was so predictable as an antecedent of abuse. Responsibility for the care of children did not reside solely with their parent or parents: 'As a member of society one shares a responsibility with respect to the quality of care available to all children', wrote Sroufe in 1985, and 'if responsibility for the child's well-being does not reside in his or her inborn variation, then it is ours'.[24]

At the time the longitudinal study was beginning, there was a great deal of scepticism regarding claims, such as those of Bowlby, that early experience has a lasting role in human development. In the 1960s, researchers such as Jerome Kagan and Howard Moss had found little continuity in children's behaviour or cognitive responses over time.[25] However, these researchers assumed that continuity meant that the same behaviour or cognitive responses would be seen. The Minnesota group did not assume mimetic (homotypic) continuity in the forms of cognition, behaviour, or emotion shown by children in the context of maturation.[26] In this, they differed from Bowlby who tended to expect early adversities to be mirrored in later behaviour (Chapter 1). All development builds on itself, they believed, but straightforward continuity should not be expected. Even if the present is heavy with the past, this legacy is always altered by the need to respond to present circumstances.[27] In this perspective, the likelihood and extent of behaviours like abusive parenting are influenced by the interaction of risk and protective factors over time. Continuity would lie in the prediction of

---

[21] Egeland, B. & Sroufe, L.A. (1981) Attachment and early maltreatment. *Child Development*, 52(1), 44–52.

[22] Shaffer, A., Huston, L., & Egeland, B. (2008) Identification of child maltreatment using prospective and self-report methodologies: a comparison of maltreatment incidence and relation to later psychopathology. *Child Abuse & Neglect*, 32(7), 682–92, Table 3. As well as careful work to ensure the convergent and predictive validity of their quantitative measures, the Minnesota group made particular efforts to understand the perspectives of their participants. They therefore conducted extensive interviews with their participants. The interviews were used to create rating scales, though it is a shame that qualitative analyses of these interviews were never reported.

[23] Alan Sroufe interviewed in Karen, R. (1998) *Becoming Attached: First Relationships and How They Shape Our Capacity to Love*. Oxford: Oxford University Press: 'The poor single mothers in our study all want the best for their kids. They maybe can't do it. They may be so beaten down by their histories and their circumstances that they're doing a terrible job, but I've never seen one that didn't want to do it right' (378).

[24] Sroufe, L.A. (1985) Attachment classification from the perspective of infant–caregiver relationships and infant temperament. *Child Development*, 56(1), 1–14, p.12.

[25] Kagan, J. & Moss, H.A. (1962) *Birth to Maturity: A Study in Psychological Development*. New York: Wiley.

[26] Described in the historical section of Sroufe, L.A., Coffino, B., & Carlson, E.A. (2010) Conceptualizing the role of early experience: lessons from the Minnesota Longitudinal Study. *Developmental Review*, 30(1), 36–51, p.36.

[27] Sroufe, L.A. (1979) The coherence of individual development: early care, attachment, and subsequent developmental issues. *American Psychologist*, 34(10), 834–41.

later maladaptation by earlier maladaptation, even if these forms of maladaptation were conditioned by quite different developmental challenges. Such difficulties would be held in place not only by individual-level factors, but also by the insistent compounding of environmental risks and the paucity of forms of support over time, which provides poor soil for anything but problems to grow. The Minnesota group therefore focused their attention on factors that could contribute to change and stability, and the role of family life as a contributory to these processes.

A multigeneration longitudinal study was the necessary testing-ground for many of the ideas that Bowlby and Ainsworth had sketched about attachment. For Ainsworth, 'longitudinal research deals with the very stuff of life and human development, with all its consequent complexities and difficulties'.[28] The participant is sought and attended to in the round. In her time it was a general consensus among developmental researchers that 'long-term longitudinal studies have proved unmanageable', which was a good part of why she had limited herself to a study of the first year of infant–caregiver interaction.[29] Yet the importance assigned to early attachment relationship could only be accepted if it predicted later outcomes anticipated by the theory, and the most valid way to do this was through a prospective study rather than retrospective recall, with all its ensuing biases.[30] Sroufe, Egeland, and colleagues regarded the construct validation of infant attachment as demanding two tasks. One was already sufficiently available from the work of Bowlby and Ainsworth: 'a rich, interwoven network of interconnected theoretical proposition'. However, secondly, 'this structure must be secured through observation'.[31] A set of observations linking infant attachment not only to caregiving behaviour, but also to relevant developmental sequelae provided a protective belt for the emergent paradigm.[32]

Ultimately, 'the validity of the attachment concept, as with any construct, hinges on the network of empirical relations built up around it and its power in yielding a coherent picture of individual adaptation'.[33]

In line with Ainsworth's approach, the Minnesota group adopted two priorities in judging their methodology, oriented by a holism that aimed to train attention on the 'whole person',

[28] Ainsworth, M. (1962) The effects of maternal deprivation: a review of findings and controversy in the context of research strategy. In *Deprivation of Maternal Care: A Reassessment of its Effects* (pp.87–195). Geneva: WHO, p.106.

[29] Ainsworth, M. (1962) *Letter to John Bowlby*, 11 December 1962. Mary Ainsworth papers, Box M3168, Folder 1.

[30] Waters, E., Wippman, J., & Sroufe, L.A. (1979) Attachment, positive affect, and competence in the peer group: two studies in construct validation. *Child Development*, 50(3), 821–29: 'As a developmental construct, security of attachment can be validated only by confirming predicted external correlates' (822).

[31] Carlson, E.A., Sroufe, L.A., & Egeland, B. (2004) The construction of experience: a longitudinal study of representation and behavior. *Child Development*, 75(1), 66–83, p.77.

[32] On the concept of the protective belt for a scientific paradigm see Lakatos, I. (1978) *The Methodology of Scientific Research Programmes*. J. Worrall & G. Currie (eds). Cambridge: Cambridge University Press.

[33] Sroufe, L.A., Fox, N.E., & Pancake, V.R. (1983) Attachment and dependency in developmental perspective. *Child Development*, 54(6), 1615–27, p.1616. See also Main M. (1999) Mary D. Salter Ainsworth: tribute and portrait. *Psychoanalytic Inquiry*, 19, 682–776: 'if the links found in Ainsworth's small Baltimore sample were to endure the test of time, a number of vital empirical questions would have to be addressed. Perhaps the most central and enduring leader in this initial quest was Alan Sroufe of the Institute of Child Development at the University of Minnesota ... Sroufe's pioneering work made an immeasurable difference to Mary Ainsworth's acceptance in the empirically oriented psychological circles of the 1970's, since the Institute at the University of Minnesota was considered to be "hardheaded", and psychometrically sophisticated. As soon as Sroufe (shortly to be joined by Byron Egeland) began his investigations of infant–mother interaction, infant strange situation behavior, and the child's later development (the study with Egeland is presently continuing into young adulthood), Mary Ainsworth felt secured on two sides: in England, by her mentor, John Bowlby, and within the United States, by the much younger Alan Sroufe and his new student Everett Waters' (731).

not just cut-up aspects of the person's behaviour.[34] One was to seek opportunities for nat-uralistic observation, where possible, especially in the early years of the study. Whereas video technology was just becoming available to researchers in the late 1960s, for use by Ainsworth's doctoral students but not in her home observations, the Minnesota group made extensive use of video observations as well as observer report in order to capture the behav-iour of their families in detail, and in a way that permitted repeated coding and inter-rater reliability.[35] Critics alleged that Ainsworth's observational data by no means amounted to science. This criticism has been often repeated over the decades.[36] By contrast, use of video technology and multiple observers helped the Minnesota group combine the naturalistic observation valued by Ainsworth with a strengthened apparatus of scientific reliability and replication.

A second priority of the Minnesota group was to focus on broad-band competencies, rather than discrete measures.[37] Egeland, Sroufe, and colleagues tended to create 'com-posite' variables out of their measures. For instance, attachment classifications and maternal sensitivity and intrusiveness were often, though not always, folded together into an 'early caregiving composite'. The fact that sometimes they reported attachment classifications in-dependently and sometimes as part of a composite, and sometimes the 12- and 18-month assessments independently and sometimes within the composite, led critics to accuse the Minnesota group of a lack of transparency. Lamb and colleagues, for instance, accused the Minnesota team of privately running the analysis for all the permutations and reporting those that had the best prediction.[38] Certainly it is true that the choice of the use of the com-posite or attachment measures is generally left unjustified, which has at times proven an obs-tacle for attempts at replication or meta-analysis. However, on review of the publications of the Minnesota group, recourse to composite measures does not seem arbitrary. It occurs more often when the researchers were interested in broad-band or diffuse psychological pro-cesses. Additionally, for many of the investigations they wished to conduct, for instance in exploring the relative contribution of different adversities and of early care and attachment to later adaption, the Minnesota group had no precedents to follow. To an extent, they had to feel their way, trying out different approaches, hoping to hear the general trends in their data through composite measures, as well as to capture developmental processes anticipated

---

[34] Sroufe, L.A., Egeland, B., Carlson, E.A., & Collins, W.A. (2005) *The Development of the Person*. New York: Guilford, p.30.

[35] Duschinsky, R. & Reijman, S. (2016) Filming disorganized attachment. *Screen*, 57(4), 397–413.

[36] Most recently, on review of the notes in the Ainsworth archive, Vicedo expressed scorn that 'I do not believe any scholar would consider the notes taken by the diverse observers during home visits reliable scientific data'. Vicedo, M. (2018) On the history, present, and future of attachment theory. *European Journal of Developmental Psychology*, 17(1).

[37] Elicker, J., Englund, M., & Sroufe, L.A. (1992) Predicting peer competence and peer relationships in child-hood from early parent–child relationships. In R. Parke & G. Ladd (eds) *Family–Peer Relationships: Modes of Linkage* (pp.77–106). Hillsdale, NJ: Lawrence Erlbaum: 'There can be multiple pathways to adaptive success (see Sroufe & Jacobvitz 1989). Discrete measures, such as social participation or sharing, are used to provide concur-rent validity for the broad band competence measures, or in follow up analyses to examine specific aspects of overall competence. Additional assessment strategies compatible with the organizational perspective include: em-phasis on naturalistic observation, rather than on highly structured laboratory tasks, especially in the early stages of research; emphasis on situations in which there is a clear need for the individual to coordinate affect, condition and behaviour; and special attention to situations that tax the adaptive capacity of the individual' (83).

[38] A detailed evaluation and critique of all the Minnesota papers published by the early 1980s is presented as Chapter 9 of Lamb, M., Thompson, R.A., Gardner, W., & Charnov, E.L. (1985) *Infant–Mother Attachment: The Origins and Developmental Significance of Individual Differences in the Strange Situation*. Hillsdale, NJ: Lawrence Erlbaum. The issue of lack of transparency and the potential for cherry-picking strong results through compos-iting variables is, however, perhaps the primary criticism.

to be diffuse and pervasive rather than localised. Many of the assessment measures originally developed in Minnesota were used in subsequent cohort studies.

The concern with observation and with assessing broad-band competencies led the Minnesota group to utilise the laboratory as a site for 'critical situations' (Chapter 2), where aspects of ordinary experience could be dramatised. They designed and set tasks that required the child or dyad to coordinate affect, cognition, and behaviour—the components of a behavioural system—to solve the problem. The laboratory-based challenge might differ in degree from those encountered within the rich, obscuring colour and camouflage of everyday life. Nonetheless it was anticipated to present a broad-band demand upon the resources, expectations, and capacities of the individual or dyad, and in this way offer a window into their history and present-day functioning. The paradigmatic example of such a challenge for the Minnesota group was the Ainsworth Strange Situation, which taxed children's regulatory capacities and their trust in the availability of their caregiver, thereby offering some window into the dyad's history of secure base and safe haven provision (Chapter 2).[39] A later example was the 'friendship interview', a measure designed by the Minnesota group, which asked participants in sixth grade to describe their relationship with a close friend. Again, this was a broad-band demand relevant to the tasks characteristic of children's developmental stage. Not all such measures were equally successful, however. The friendship interview had excellent associations with social competence in girls, and was predicted well by early infant–caregiver interactions. However, the assessment did not work as well with boys in the sample: 'Minnesota males, and perhaps even more among our subpopulation of youth, are "men of few words".'[40]

The Minnesota Longitudinal Study of Risk and Adaptation has now been running for over 40 years, and is rightly regarded as a masterpiece of developmental scientific research and the 'gold standard in prospective studies of neglect and abuse'.[41] Even decades later, the sample has retained 163 out of the original 267 participants, an astonishing achievement and a testament to the commitment of the participants and researchers. The Minnesota Longitudinal Study of Risk and Adaptation has provided a special opportunity to explore the lives of the grandchildren of the parents originally recruited to the sample, and to trace developmental processes across generations. This multigenerational research has revealed both substantial change and marked continuities in parenting practices between the generations, with stability calculated at $r = .43$, controlling for a variety of covariates. In a regression analysis with all the correlates of second-generation caregiving, the care that these adults had themselves received accounted for 12% of variance.[42] This is far from the deterministic rhetoric sometimes deployed by Bowlby, especially in his populist writings (Chapter 1). However, a 12% difference in day-in-day-out parenting and care represents a very substantial difference in the family life of a young person. This finding exemplifies the contribution of the Minnesota study: considering a large range of risk and protective factors, following participants over

[39] Elicker, J., Englund, M., & Sroufe, L.A. (1992) Predicting peer competence and peer relationships in childhood from early parent–child relationships. In R. Parke & G. Ladd (eds) *Family–Peer Relationships: Modes of Linkage* (pp.77–106). Hillsdale, NJ: Lawrence Erlbaum, p.83.

[40] Sroufe, L.A., Egeland, B., Carlson, E.A., & Collins, W.A. (2005) *The Development of the Person.* New York: Guilford, p.185.

[41] Brown, D. (2009) Assessment of attachment and abuse history, and adult attachment style. In C.A. Courtois & J.D. Ford (eds) *Treating Complex Traumatic Stress Disorders: An Evidence-Based Guide* (pp.124–44). New York: Guilford, p.126.

[42] Kovan, N.M., Chung, A.L., & Sroufe, L.A. (2009) The intergenerational continuity of observed early parenting: a prospective, longitudinal study. *Developmental Psychology*, 45(5), 1205–13.

long periods, pursuing multivariate analyses, and making powerful empirical contributions that in turn have implications for theory and child welfare practice.

In this, one area of particular contribution to the field of attachment research was in the conceptualisation and study of emotions. In order to situate the findings regarding attachment from the Minnesota study, this chapter will begin by outlining Sroufe's general model of emotion. The selection of measures and the interpretation of findings by the Minnesota group were determined by a variety of factors which could vary from study to study. Nonetheless nearly all studies by the research group draw on Sroufe's theory in the justification for their research design or in making sense of their results. It is therefore important to consider this contribution before describing the major empirical reports from the cohort study. And whilst Sroufe's headline ideas are familiar and well cited, the development of his ideas, and their full depth, are less well known as they are often scattered across a variety of texts. As a result, many important aspects of Sroufe's theory of human emotional life have been surprisingly untapped by later researchers.

Theory of affect

Emotional development

Bowlby identified three components to behavioural systems: behavioural components, cognitive components, and affective components (Chapter 1). In the 1960s and 1970s he gave special attention to behaviour. This left its mark in many ways on the theory, not least in the name 'behavioural' systems. Though already present from the 1960s in his concept of 'internal working models', from the 1980s Bowlby focused attention on the cognitive aspects of behavioural systems. By contrast, the affective component of behavioural systems was always acknowledged but never elaborated by Bowlby. In his private notes, he observed this tendency in his writings, and attributed it to a desire to backlight the importance of phenomena downplayed by psychoanalytic theory. However, the result was a hole in attachment theory where an account of affect, motivation, and development should have been. For studies on other topics, this hole might have been of less consequence. For conceptualising the results of a longitudinal study with a central focus on child maltreatment, it was unsustainable. Sroufe felt that 'emotions and motivation are downplayed despite the fact that Bowlby's observations led him to describe attachment as an "affective" bond'.[43]

The neglect of emotion in Bowlby's work, in part an attempt to distance his approach from psychoanalysis, mirrored a trend in developmental psychology more generally. Though attention to emotion was on the rise, the main protagonist in the story of psychology in the late 1970s was cognition. Psychoanalytic theory retained a strong interest in emotion, but came into disrepute in American academic psychology departments, and there were few effective bridges between psychoanalytic theory and the empirical psychology of the period.[44] Yet

---

[43] Sroufe, L.A. (1996) *Emotional Development*. Cambridge: Cambridge University Press, p.177.

[44] For discussion of the standing of emotion within the psychological science of this period see Cicchetti, D. & Schneider-Rosen, K. (1984) Theoretical and empirical considerations in the investigation of the relationship between affect and cognition in atypical populations of infants: contributions to the formulation of an integrative theory of development. In C. Izard, J. Kagan, & R. Zajonc (eds) *Emotions, Cognition, and Behavior* (pp.366–406). Cambridge: Cambridge University Press. There were some exceptions and attempts at bridge-building, e.g. James, A.E. (1976) Freud, Piaget, and human knowledge. *Annual Review of Psychoanalysis*, 4, 253–77; Schlesinger, H.J.

through the 1970s, across the social sciences, attention to emotional life, emotion regulation, and the social situatedness of emotions was growing, reflecting rising attention to these topics in wider society and politics.[45] In a landmark book chapter from 1979, Sroufe argued that 'the child grows not as a perceptive being, not as a cognitive being, but as a human being who experiences anxiety, joy, and anger, and who is connected to its world in an emotional way'.[46] Together with Minnesota colleagues, Sroufe highlighted the flexibility of human behavioural systems, in contrast to reflexes, and the role of psychosocial challenges such as trust, autonomy, and control as providing the context of their progressive elaboration. Many behavioural systems include reflex or relatively inbuilt components, but become elaborated as they are fed by social and cultural experiences. For instance, the laugh response is predisposed for human infants by particular kinds of situation, such as incongruity in the context of mid–high arousal, but also by the availability of a caregiver who gives a positive appraisal to the incongruity.[47] Sroufe narrated infant development in terms of the gradual differentiation of arousal into various, initially quite general affects, and from there into more refined emotions that are differentiated by their specificity and directedness.[48]

These refinements are based partly on the social support the child receives in identifying and modulating affects when they arise in different contexts. Sroufe ascribed an important role to the provision of a safe haven when a child is distressed for the modulation of affect. However, he also elaborated on an expanded role for exploration. For Bowlby, the exploratory system has the function of learning about new and/or complex phenomena. Sroufe added to this that play, especially in the context of a secure base and stable routines, helps the infant learn, over time, to remain regulated in the context of higher levels of arousal: 'As caregiver and infant play, tension is escalated and de-escalated, to the edge of overstimulation and back again, commonly ending in the bursts of positive affect so rewarding for caregivers. Episode by episode, day by day, the infant's own capacity to modulate (and tolerate) tension is developed, and a reservoir of shared positive affect is created.'[49]

This reservoir, which Sroufe largely identified with the attachment system, is nestled initially within the relationship. However, over time it becomes in part the property of the child, as a sense of confidence and fluency in accessing, modulating, and expressing feelings, as well as recouping or finding relief afterwards. This becomes a skill, one that can help make for successful family and peer interactions. Frustration and conflicts can be experienced

(1971) Clinical-cognitive psychology: models and integrations. *Psychoanalytic Quarterly*, 40, 366–68. However, these had little traction.

[45] For psychological science see e.g. Izard, C. (1977) *Human Emotions*. New York: Plenum; Lewis, M. & Rosenblum, L. (1978) Introduction: issues in affect development. In M. Lewis & L. Rosenblum (eds) *The Development of Affect: The Genesis of Behavior*, Vol. 1 (pp.1–10). New York: Plenum. As a point of comparison, see the growing attention to emotions in anthropology. Rosaldo, M.Z. (1980) *Knowledge and Passion: Ilongot Notions of Self and Social Life*. Cambridge: Cambridge University Press. On the wider context of emotional citizenship in the late 1970s and early 1980s see Berlant, L. (2008) *The Female Complaint*. Durham, NC: Duke University Press.

[46] Sroufe, L.A. (1979) Socioemotional development. In J. Osofsky (ed.) *Handbook of Infant Development* (pp.462–515). New York: John Wiley, p.462.

[47] Ibid. p.502; Sroufe, L.A. & Wunsch, J.P. (1972) The development of laughter in the first year of life. *Child Development*, 43(4), 1326–44; Sroufe, L.A. & Waters, E. (1976) The ontogenesis of smiling and laughter: a perspective on the organization of development in infancy. *Psychological Review*, 83(3), 173–89.

[48] In general, though without full consistency, Sroufe used the term 'affect' to refer to the embodied reaction to a salient event, and 'emotion' to refer to the subjective experience of this reaction, including awareness of its source. An affect seems to have more of the early, embodied prototype in play, whereas an emotion seems to be more inflected by contemporary cognitive resources. However, this contrast is only elaborated implicitly by Sroufe.

[49] Sroufe, L.A. (1996) *Emotional Development*. Cambridge: Cambridge University Press, p.144.

without feeling unacceptable, dangerous, or spiralling into persistent activation or diffusion into other nearby emotions such as distress, fear, or despair:

> Resolving conflicts is an important building block of the child's emerging sense of competence at problem solving, and as Erikson argues, it also deepens the child's trust in the caregiving relationship. Such prototypical conflict experiences within the security of the caregiving relationship can also represent a model for later close relationships, providing an abiding confidence that relationships may be sustained despite strife, which allows a person to risk conflict in relationships and, ultimately, to even see its value.[50]

However, as well as social scaffolding by caregivers, the refinements of emotional development of young childhood depend on cognitive maturation. Unlike Bowlby for whom emphasis on emotional processes was felt to risk underplaying the cognitive components of behavioural systems, Sroufe emphasised that the two are intertwined. Cognitive achievements are spurred and textured by affects. In turn, the registering and differentiation of emotions is scaffolded by cognitive development:

> Cognitive factors underlie the unfolding of emotions: only with recognition is there pleasure and disappointment; only with some development of causality, object permanence, intentionality and meaning are there joy, anger, and fear; only with self-awareness is there shame. Also, distinctions among affects and their precursors call upon cognitive achievements—for example, fear, as reflected in more immediate distress upon a second exposure to a stranger, has been referred to as a categorical reaction, dependent upon assimilation to a negative scheme. Finally, the effects of sequence, setting, and other aspects of context on emotion are obviously mediated by cognition.[51]

Certain emotions, such as shame, pride, and guilt, are only possible once sufficient cognitive infrastructure is available, since, together with high arousal, they require identification of discrepancies between behaviour and the representation of our value from the perspective of others. Think, for instance, of the development over childhood of shame in what we have drawn with pencil and paper, or in our bodies, to the point that it is to an extent typical in adults. Sroufe observed that since toddlers are only just piecing together the representation of their value in the eyes of others, this impression may still be especially fragile. A consequence is that 'the toddler is vulnerable to a global feeling of dissolution when being punished for a specific behaviour (especially if done harshly or in a degrading way).'[52] Whereas in the first year of life, anxiety in relationships is associated particularly with separation, Sroufe argued that over the second year, cognitive advances allow psychological separations, such as scolding, to be pierced by as much anxiety as physical separations.[53]

In his account of emotional development, Sroufe took particular interest in the basic smile reflex, highlighting the critical role of social interaction. He wrote beautifully of the social smile as the 'crowning achievement' of the first three months of life, initiating the use

---

[50] Ibid. p.206.

[51] Sroufe, L.A. (1979) Socioemotional development. In J. Osofsky (ed.) *Handbook of Infant Development* (pp.462–515). New York: John Wiley, p.491.

[52] Sroufe, L.A. (1996) *Emotional Development*. Cambridge: Cambridge University Press, p.199.

[53] Ibid. p.126.

of positive affects within communication: 'the infant smiles and coos at its own feet, at its toy giraffe, and especially at the caregiver. For the first time it laughs in response to vigorous stimulation. "Pleasure has become an excitatory phenomenon", associated with high states of excitation (Escalona, 1968, p.159). With eyes sparking, caregiver and infant set out upon the task of establishing reciprocal exchanges.'[54] The infant does not yet have a 'representation' of the relationship—that will only come later, along with language—but they do have 'action schemes' which allow for procedure-level memories and expectation of how the caregiver will respond, coordinated recognition, and sharing of differentiated emotions, and some basic forms of independent emotion regulation.[55] Action schemes are encoded in a preverbal way that is qualitatively different to semantic memory, and that makes them more difficult to verbally analyse and re-evaluate.

With cognitive development, more complex and differentiated emotions are possible. Yet 'The more mature emotions do not displace precursor emotions. The smooth execution of behaviour can still produce pleasure, unfathomability and vague threat can produce wariness, and diffuse frustration can lead to intense distress at any age.'[56] Within the mature anger behavioural system of a one- or two-year-old remains the earlier more global, intense, and diffuse form, which becomes vocally evident in children's tantrums. The same, Sroufe argued, was true of other behavioural systems like fear: abject fear loses specificity and directedness, as well as its differentiation from nearby emotions such as distress.[57] The process of emotional maturation exemplified the broader commitment of Sroufe and the Minnesota group to the principle that all development is built on itself, with earlier forms remaining operative even if reforged by new opportunities, capabilities, and demands: 'Development is a dynamic process wherein what evolves derives from what was there before in a logical way, while, at the same time, prior experience or prior adaptation has a fundamentally new meaning in the now more complex system.'[58] Even if early experiences of support and care are supplanted by later adversity, they remain a resource that may be reactivated by a facilitative later context. Likewise, early vulnerability in the context of adversity can be reactivated, even many years later, when someone is faced with depriving or traumatic conditions.[59]

Within emotional maturation, Sroufe gave an important place to attachment processes. His stance was that 'attachment is critical and has a central place in the hierarchy

---

[54] Sroufe, L.A. (1979) Socioemotional development. In J. Osofsky (ed.) *Handbook of Infant Development* (pp.462–515). New York: John Wiley, p.478; Escalona, S.K. (1969) *The Roots of Individuality: Normal Patterns of Development In Infancy.* Oxford: Aldine.

[55] Sroufe, L.A. (1989) Relationships, self, and individual adaptation. In A.J. Sameroff & R.N. Emde (eds) *Relationship Disturbances in Early Childhood: A Developmental Approach* (pp.70–94). New York: Basic Books, p.76. The term 'emotion regulation' remains undefined in the writings of Sroufe and Egeland. However, in practice their usage resembles Thompson, R.A., Flood, M.F., & Lundquist, L. (1995) Emotional regulation and developmental psychopathology. In D. Cicchetti & S. Toth (eds) *Rochester Symposium on Developmental Psychopathology, Volume 6: Emotion, Cognition, and Representation* (pp.261–99). Rochester, NY: University of Rochester Press: 'emotional regulation consists of the extrinsic and intrinsic processes responsible for monitoring, evaluating and modifying emotional reactions, especially their intensive and temporal features, to accomplish ones goals ... this definition of emotion regulation includes maintaining and enhancing emotional arousal as well as inhibiting it' (265).

[56] Sroufe, L.A. (1996) *Emotional Development.* Cambridge: Cambridge University Press, p.64–5.

[57] Sroufe, L.A. (1979) Socioemotional development. In J. Osofsky (ed.) *Handbook of Infant Development*, (pp.462–515). New York: John Wiley, p.488; see also Sroufe, L.A. (1996) *Emotional Development.* Cambridge: Cambridge University Press, p.55.

[58] Sroufe, L.A., Egeland, B., Carlson, E.A., & Collins, W.A. (2005) *The Development of the Person.* New York: Guilford, p.11.

[59] See also Sroufe, L.A., Egeland, B., & Kreutzer, T. (1990) The fate of early experience following developmental change: longitudinal approaches to individual adaptation in childhood. *Child Development*, 61(5), 1363–73.

of development because of its primacy. The infant–caregiver attachment relationship is the core, around which all other experience is structured, whatever impact it may have.'[60] However, in occupying this central place, Sroufe held that attachment processes are nonetheless dependent on an infrastructure of various factors that stretch beyond them. One is the dependence of the attachment system on cognitive maturation. He assigned a particular role to cognitive anticipation and expectation, which is reflected in the partly innate capacity for joyous greeting of attachment figures. He proposed that 'bouncing, smiling, arms-raised gestures are differential to attachment figures, reflecting the positive value of the special scheme to which the attachment figures are immediately assimilated'.[61] Cognitive anticipation is also reflected in the capacity to hold an angry mood, even with a caregiver, or to inhibit the activation of a behavioural system that will result in disapproval or punishment. The infant begins to include his or her own potential feelings within the field of awareness, influencing responses. For instance, the knowledge that punishment and sadness will ensue may help hold the inhibition of a behavioural system in place.

Sroufe proposed that the infant's emerging sense of self is organised especially around 'patterns of behavioural and affective regulation, which grant continuity to experience despite development and changes in context'.[62] This is a good part of why attachment relationships are central to socioemotional development, and why the recognition, communication and modulation of emotion is central to the quality of attachment relationships. On the basis of this account, Sroufe offered rebuttal to Kagan's strongly worded accusation that temperament was a sufficient explanation for apparent differences in the quality of attachment relationship.[63] Sroufe argued that findings, such as those of Main and Weston (Chapter 3), showing barely any overlap between attachment classifications with different caregivers are important evidence here. They indicate that differences in attachment lie in the history of infant–caregiver interaction, and have no basis in differences in temperament.[64] Over time, Behrens observed that 'the attachment–temperament debate has subsided because most attachment researchers today incorporate some temperamental or biological assessment of children, recognizing the potential biological contribution in forming relationships'.[65] Van IJzendoorn and Bakermans-Kranenburg later criticised Sroufe and Kagan as partially responsible for the 'deadly war over dominance and territory' between attachment and temperament researchers, sustaining a polemic that obscured the way that parenting,

[60] Sroufe, L.A. (2005) Attachment and development: a prospective, longitudinal study from birth to adulthood. *Attachment & Human Development*, 7(4), 349–67, p.353.

[61] Sroufe, L.A. (1979) Socioemotional development. In J. Osofsky (ed.), *Handbook of Infant Development* (pp.462–515). New York: John Wiley, p.488.

[62] Sroufe, L.A. (1989) Relationships, self, and individual adaptation. In A.J. Sameroff & R.N. Emde (eds) *Relationship Disturbances in Early Childhood: A Developmental Approach* (pp.70–94). New York: Basic Books, p.83.

[63] Kagan, J. (1982) *Psychological Research on the Human Infant: An Evaluative Summary*. New York: W.T. Grant Foundation. See also Kagan, J. (1995) On attachment. *Harvard Review of Psychiatry*, 3(2), 104–106; Kagan, J. (1996) Three pleasing ideas. *American Psychologist*, 51(9), 901–908. On Kagan's role as a 'spokesperson' for critics of attachment research see Karen, R. (1998) *Becoming Attached: First Relationships and How They Shape Our Capacity to Love*. Oxford: Oxford University Press, p.253.

[64] Sroufe, L.A. (1985) Attachment classification from the perspective of infant–caregiver relationships and infant temperament. *Child Development*, 56(1), 1–14.

[65] Behrens, K.Y. (2016) Reconsidering attachment in context of culture: review of attachment studies in Japan. *Online Readings in Psychology and Culture*, 6(1), 7, p.25. See Vaughn, B.E. & Bost, K.K. (2016) Attachment and temperament as intersecting developmental products and interacting developmental contexts throughout infancy and childhood. In J. Cassidy & P.R. Shaver (eds) *Handbook of Attachment: Theory, Research, and Clinical Applications*, 3rd edn (pp.202–22). New York: Guilford.

attachment, and temperament interrelate (Chapter 7).[66] If, as Karen has suggested, Kagan intentionally helped to block access to key potential funders for attachment research through the 1980s, the war becomes quite intelligible.[67] Yet with Kagan's relevance for attachment research receding into the past, the opposition between attachment and temperament has lost some of its necessity. In an article from 2000, Sroufe and colleagues accepted that the majority of variance in internalising and anxiety symptoms in middle childhood is likely accounted for by temperamental and genetic factors.[68] And in a 2005 article, Sroufe highlighted the interaction between infant temperament and caregiving sensitivity in predicting infant ambivalent/resistant attachment in the Strange Situation in the Minnesota Longitudinal Study of Risk and Adaptation.[69] Nonetheless, with the exception of the ambivalent/resistant classification, a meta-analysis by Groh found little evidence for main effects of temperamental variation in the development of differences in infant attachment.[70] Exciting examinations of potential interactions between temperament and caregiving experiences are ongoing, but on the basis of a scientific consensus that ascribes an irreducibly important place to caregiving.[71]

Felt security

Attention to the behavioural, cognitive, *and* emotional components of behavioural systems led Sroufe to a different position to Bowlby regarding the set-goal of the attachment system. In his writings for a psychoanalytic audience, Bowlby identified important emotional components related to the set-goal of the attachment system. He specified that the desire to achieve the set-goal would be felt as 'anxiety'; when the caregiver is accessible if the child feels frightened, he or she will feel 'secure'; when the caregiver is accessible after the child has felt frightened, he or she will feel 'comforted'.[72] Yet, in *Attachment, Volume 1*, Bowlby gave

---

[66] Van IJzendoorn, M.H. & Bakermans-Kranenburg, M.J. (2012) Integrating temperament and attachment. The differential susceptibility paradigm. In M. Zentner & R.L. Shiner (eds) *Handbook of Temperament* (pp.403–24). New York: Guilford, p.409.

[67] Karen, R. (1998) *Becoming Attached: First Relationships and How They Shape Our Capacity to Love.* Oxford: Oxford University Press, p.256.

[68] Warren, S.L., Emde, R.N., & Sroufe, L.A. (2000) Internal representations: predicting anxiety from children's play narratives. *Journal of the American Academy of Child & Adolescent Psychiatry*, 39(1), 100–107: 'The variance accounted for by our variables in the prediction from 5-year-old narratives to 6-year-old internalizing and anxiety symptoms was substantial for this kind of research (20%), [and] there is a strong likelihood that genetic predisposition and temperament account for much of the remaining variance' (106).

[69] Sroufe, L.A. (2005) Attachment and development: a prospective, longitudinal study from birth to adulthood. *Attachment & Human Development*, 7(4), 349–67. These results were earlier reported in Susman-Stillman, A., Kalkoske, M., Egeland, B., & Waldman, I. (1996) Infant temperament and maternal sensitivity as predictors of attachment security. *Infant Behavior and Development*, 19(1), 33–47.

[70] Groh, A.M., Narayan, A.J., Bakermans-Kranenburg, M.J., et al. (2017) Attachment and temperament in the early life course: a meta-analytic review. *Child Development*, 88(3), 770–95.

[71] Spangler, G. (2013) Individual dispositions as precursors of differences in attachment quality: why maternal sensitivity is nevertheless important. *Attachment & Human Development*, 15(5–6), 657–72.

[72] Bowlby, J. (1960) Separation anxiety. *International Journal of Psycho-Analysis*, 41, 89–113, pp.93–4. In fact, use of the term 'comfort' to describe the set-goal of the attachment system in infancy led a subterranean existence over decades. For example, the concept of comfort can be seen dodging in and out of view in *Separation*: 'accessibility in itself is not enough. Not only must an attachment figure be accessible but he, or she, must be willing to respond in an appropriate way; in regard to someone who is afraid this means willingness to act as comforter and protector. Only when an attachment figure is both accessible and potentially responsive can he, or she, be said to be truly available. In what follows, therefore, the word "available" is to be understood as implying that an attachment figure is both accessible and responsive.' Bowlby, J. (1973) *Separation*. New York: Basic Books, p.234. Following Bowlby, Ainsworth tended to use 'availability' in descriptions of the set-goal in infancy in written presentations. However, in oral presentations she tended to use the term 'comfort'.

these subjective states primarily the role of concomitants to the set-goal of the attachment system, which he positioned as 'proximity' (Chapter 1). In the 1970s, however, there were growing concerns that the attachment paradigm was being hindered by a lack of precision in situating the subjective, felt aspects of the phenomena under discussion. The German ethologist and systems theorist Norbert Bischof, for example, observed that 'authors dealing with attachment quite commonly talk about the mother as a source of infantile "security". It should be noted, however, that this term does not clearly distinguish between an emotional state (feeling more or less secure) and an environmental fact.'[73] Sroufe and Waters likewise argued that Bowlby's neglect of emotion obscured, and even distorted, his account of the attachment behavioural system.

In 'Attachment as an organizational construct', published in 1977, Sroufe and Waters raised several objections to the sidekick role allocated to emotion.[74] They noted that some infants, such as those in dyads classified B1 by Ainsworth, appeared to have had their attachment system terminated by merely the return of the caregiver and distance interaction, without physical proximity-seeking. The ambivalent/resistant infant also achieved proximity in the Strange Situation, and yet the attachment system remains activated. Sroufe and Waters argued that emotions not only are important parts of the motivational system of attachment, but also condition its terminating conditions. In contrast to Bowlby, who offered a behavioural set-goal for the attachment system, Sroufe and Waters broadened this out. They proposed that the attachment system would be terminated when infants 'feel secure'. Proximity is one facilitating and sometimes a necessary contributor to this affective state. But it is the affective state that is the set-goal.[75]

Elsewhere, Sroufe proposed that 'the infant secure in his or her attachment has experienced the caregiver as a reliable source of comforting, as responsive to his or her signals, and as available and sensitive. The infant has learned that stimulation in the context of the caregiver will generally not be overwhelming and that when arousal threatens to exceed the infant's organizational capacity, the caregiver will intervene.'[76] Indeed, Sroufe was one of the very few researchers who, following Ainsworth, highlighted that the capacity to feel secure in attachment relationships would be influenced by feelings of security or insecurity in other domains (Chapter 2). Furthermore, 'the availability of cues associated with security (familiar procedures or objects, predictability, control) and a generalised expectancy concerning likely outcomes when tension is high' were assumed to feed into felt security within attachment relationships,[77] perhaps contributing to the small overlap in variance in attachment relationships with different caregivers.

Ainsworth did not appear to regard the broader emphasis on felt security as discrepant with the orthodox position represented by Bowlby. She initially reported reading the Sroufe and Waters paper with approval. However, over the years, she began to feel uncomfortable. Many second-generation attachment researchers began to rally to 'felt security', against what was increasingly regarded in the 1980s as the somewhat wooden quality to Bowlby's account

---

[73] Bischof, N. (1975) A systems approach toward the functional connections of attachment and fear. *Child Development*, 46(4), 801–17, p.802.

[74] Sroufe, L.A. & Waters, E. (1977) Attachment as an organizational construct. *Child Development*, 48(4), 1184–99.

[75] Ibid. p.1191.

[76] Sroufe, L.A. (1979) The coherence of individual development: early care, attachment, and subsequent developmental issues. *American Psychologist*, 34(10), 834–41, p.837.

[77] Sroufe, L.A. (1996) *Emotional Development*. Cambridge: Cambridge University Press, p.147.

of attachment relationships in terms of activating and terminating conditions.[78] Ainsworth's former student Mark Cummings was even developing a new coding system for the Strange Situation focused on felt security, as an alternative to coding proximity-seeking and contact maintaining.[79] Ainsworth brought the matter to Bowlby's attention in 1987, and the collaborators reflected together.[80] They were worried, justifiably as it turned out (Chapter 5), that the term 'felt security' left ambiguity regarding whether an individual would be consciously aware of whether or not they had a secure attachment. They were sure that individuals would not. However, they also registered that the set-goal of the attachment system, even in infancy, was not merely proximity. That early proposal of Bowlby's became rather battered as time passed since the 1960s.

Ultimately, Bowlby and Ainsworth came to the conclusion that the set-goal of the caregiver is the feeling of the caregiver's availability when called upon, which includes the possibility of proximity as needed:

> I am in agreement with you … I have for my part referred to 'availability' as the set-goal in the case of children and adults. It requires belief in the effectiveness of communication & belief that the attach figure will respond if called upon & that physical proximity is readily attainable when desired.[81]

The set-goal of the attachment system in infancy was revised by Ainsworth to be caregiver 'availability', assumed to incorporate behavioural, cognitive, and emotional components. In this, access to proximity was maintained as one of the proximal goals of the attachment system at high levels of activation, but not the ultimate set-goal regardless of level of activation. Unfortunately there was only one book chapter in which Ainsworth explicitly flagged the shift in position, and it was framed as a rejection rather than partial acceptance of Sroufe and Waters' position.[82] Furthermore, most readers assumed that when Bowlby and Ainsworth were referring to availability, they meant exclusively older children.[83] Attachment researchers still today have generally not integrated the different positions, and the set-goal of the attachment system remains variously defined as 'proximity', 'availability', 'accessibility', and 'felt security'.[84] Ainsworth's student Roger Kobak, recognising this problem, roundly

---

[78] E.g. Cicchetti, D. & Pogge-Hesse, P. (1981) The relation between emotion and cognition in infant development. In M. Lamb & L. Sherrod (eds) *Infant Social Cognition* (pp.205–72). Hillsdale, NJ: Lawrence Erlbaum; Erickson, M.F., Korfmacher, J., & Egeland, B. (1992) Attachments past and present: implications for therapeutic intervention with mother–infant dyads. *Development & Psychopathology*, 4(4), 495–507, p.496. In fact, Erickson and colleagues appear to have regarded Bowlby's behavioural system model as superseded already by his own notion of internal working models.

[79] Cummings, M.E. & El-Sheikh, M. (1986) *An Organizational Scheme for the Classification of Attachments on a Continuum of Felt-Security*. Morgantown: West Virginia University. https://files.eric.ed.gov/fulltext/ED288653. pdf.

[80] Ainsworth, M. (1987) *Letter to John Bowlby*, 28 November 1987. PP/BOW/B.3/8.

[81] Ainsworth, M. (1987) *Letter to John Bowlby*, 30 December 1987. PP/BOW/B.3/8.

[82] Ainsworth, M.D.S. (1990) Some considerations regarding theory and assessment relevant to attachments beyond infancy. In M.T. Greenberg, D. Cicchetti, & E.M. Cummings (eds) *Attachment in the Preschool Years: Theory, Research, and Intervention* (pp.463–88). Chicago: University of Chicago Press.

[83] See e.g. Kerns, K.A. & Brumariu, L.E. (2016) Attachment in middle childhood. In J. Cassidy & P. Shaver (eds) *Handbook of Attachment*, 3rd edn (pp.349–65). New York: Guilford.

[84] In the first and second editions of Cassidy and Shaver's *Handbook of Attachment*, a chapter by Kobak attempted to adjudicate the issue in favour of 'availability' as the set-goal of the attachment behavioural system. This section was removed from the chapter for the third edition. Besides Kobak's chapter, there has been little attempt to adjudicate the issue, except where it has caused problems on the borders between the developmental and the social psychology attachment traditions (Chapter 5). An early exception is Greenberg, M.T., Siegel, J.M., & Leitch, C.J. (1983) The nature and importance of attachment relationships to parents and peers during adolescence. *Journal of*

criticised everyone. Bowlby and Ainsworth were criticised for recognising so late in the day that caregiver availability, even in infancy, was broader than proximity. And Sroufe and Waters were criticised for underspecifying the role of physical proximity, and for defining felt security too loosely. Not least, Kobak was concerned that a whole host of factors could contribute to feeling secure, not all of which would be based in attachment processes.[85]

Kobak reserved particular criticism, however, for the way that Sroufe and Waters' proposal contributed to the split in attachment theory between the developmental tradition and the social psychology tradition (Chapter 5). Kobak regarded the split as based in part on a lack of clarity about how the attachment system actually works in adulthood, caused in part by Sroufe and Waters's overencompassing and subjective notion of felt security.[86] More recently, Kobak has moderated his criticisms, likely in the context of increased rapprochement between the developmental and social psychological traditions of attachment research. He has allowed that the shift from a focus on proximity to availability helped support a shift in 'the focus of attachment research from the study of young children's separations from caregivers to investigations of the quality of emotional communication in maintaining attachment bonds', a shift that he regards as overall a positive development for the field.[87]

Social affects

In the 1980s, Sroufe's theoretical reflections on attachment and emotional development were elaborated by the Minnesota group's empirical research. An important early study was 'The role of affect in social competence', published in 1984 by Sroufe, Fox, and Pancake, reporting a mixed methods study of the experiences of children in the sample in preschool.[88] Two preschool classes (15 children and 25 children) were constituted out of children in the sample who had received the same attachment classification at 12 and 18 months, stratified to include children from each of the Ainsworth classifications. The preschool lasted for 20 weeks.

Youth and Aolescence, 12(5), 373–86. Greenberg and colleagues retain proximity and felt security as two different set-goals of the attachment system, one or both of which may be met. For instance, the ambivalent/resistant infant was conceptualised as achieving proximity but not felt security.

[85] This criticism of Sroufe and Waters has recently been made again in a book chapter collectively written by a group of anthropologists and developmental psychologists: Gaskins, S., Beeghly, M., Bard, K.A., et al. (2017) Meaning and methods in the study and assessment of attachment. In H. Keller & K.A. Bard (eds) *Contextualizing Attachment: The Cultural Nature of Attachment* (pp.321–33). Cambridge, MA: MIT Press.

[86] Kobak, R. (1994) Adult attachment: a personality or relationship construct? *Psychological Inquiry*, 5(1), 42–4; Kobak, R. (1999) The emotional dynamics of disruptions in attachment relationships: implications for theory, research, and clinical intervention In J. Cassidy & P.R. Shaver (eds) *Handbook of Attachment: Theory, Research, and Application* (pp.21–43). New York: Guilford, p.31.

[87] Kobak, R., Zajac, K., & Madsen, S.D. (2016) Attachment disruptions, reparative processes, and psychopathology: theoretical and clinical implications. In P.R. Shaver & J. Cassidy (eds) *Handbook of Attachment*, 3rd edn (pp.25–39). New York: Guilford.

[88] Sroufe, L.A., ???Schork, E., Motti, F., Lawroski, N., & LaFreniere, P. (1984) The role of affect in social competence. In C. E. Izard, J. Kagan, & R. B. Zajonc (Eds.), *Emotion, cognition, and behavior* (pp. 289-319). Cambridge: Cambridge University Press. Mary Jo Ward later recalled this period: 'My fondest memories of Alan are from the year of the preschool project. He was in his element: choosing just the right subjects to compose a class, working daily with some very gifted teachers, supervising grad students, planning assessments and coming up with methods to capture the richness of what we were observing each day. But he was most happy about getting to know each of the precious children. His insights into each child's coping, his joy in their accomplishments, his concern for their trials gave us an amazing opportunity to experience the human side of developmental science. It's an example that we'll never forget.' Ward, M.J. (2009) *Tribute to L. Alan Sroufe on the Occasion of his Retirement*, 17 October 2009, Minneapolis. Unpublished manuscript shared by the author.

Based on detailed ethnographic observations, Sroufe and colleagues were struck by the role of positive emotion, which seemed to serve as the major currency of social interaction.

The children in the sample who found it difficult to socialise seemed often those who were unable to resource positive emotions to serve this role of currency.[89] From childhood onwards, Sroufe and colleagues theorised, something has to be shared in order to make or sustain a relationship. Emotion offers potent forms of sharing, and indeed of not sharing.[90] Relative access to shared positive affect therefore contributes to the creation and stabilisation of social hierarchies, which in turn channel the expression and acceptance of emotion between the preschool students. In the two different classes, Sroufe and colleagues asked the teachers to rank the students in order of social competence. They found a strong association between competence ranking and the frequency of affectively positive social interaction ($\rho = .70$, $p < .002$). Notably, however, the frequency of social interaction with a negative affective tone made no additional contribution, once shared positive emotions were taken into account. This suggests that the emotional tone of peer interactions was not simply a product of social competence, but that positive social interaction was linked, likely bidirectionally, to social success.[91] The researchers also documented that positive affect in itself was not critical for success with peers at the school, but shared positive social interaction specifically: 'the sharing of good feelings and the rewarding of other's overtures with positive affect'.[92]

Sroufe worked with his partner June Fleeson (later June Sroufe) in reflecting further on the social quality of affects. They made two key claims. A first was that if the relationship depends on sharing, then all partners in a relationship have to learn one another's roles in order to understand their own. As such, children learn all the 'parts' of a relationship with an attachment figure, not just their own role. There is no sense of determinism in Sroufe and Fleeson's reflection. Individuals may develop thoughts, feelings, or behaviours in relationships that develop out of earlier roles only in the most non-linear way.[93] However, early roles may press themselves forward at times, particularly when an adult is exhausted, bored, depleted, and/or poorly resourced. Across our lives, Sroufe and Fleeson argued, when we respond in ways that are intuitive and unreflective, this may be especially coloured by our history, and especially our experiences of attachment and of trauma. Bowlby had argued that children who have experienced abuse may find it hard to find and sustain the role of adequate caregiver because their representations in adulthood mirror those of their childhood. By contrast, Sroufe and Fleeson proposed that children who have experienced abuse not only have the abusive role available, but also may have relative difficulties accessing procedural components of sensitive caregiving—for instance, gentle, non-intrusive touch and the accurate recognition and modulation of affects. Children who have experienced abuse may also have comparatively less access, even into adulthood, to social relationships that help them sustain the caregiving role. In fact, in some cases, they may only have access to

[89] Sroufe, L.A., Schork, E., Motti, E., Lawroski, N., & LaFreniere, P. (1984) The role of affect in social competence. In C. Izard, J. Kagan, & R. Zajonc (eds) *Emotion, Cognition and Behavior* (pp.289–319). New York: Plenum, p.290.

[90] Sroufe, L.A. (1996) *Emotional Development*. Cambridge: Cambridge University Press: 'Emotion is part of all critical transactions with the environment. It guides, directs, and sometimes disrupts action. And it is the currency of personal relationships' (12).

[91] Sroufe, L.A., Schork, E., Motti, E., Lawroski, N., & LaFreniere, P. (1984) The role of affect in social competence. In C. Izard, J. Kagan, & R. Zajonc (eds) *Emotion, Cognition and Behavior* (pp.289–319). New York: Plenum, p.298–9.

[92] Ibid. p.305.

[93] Sroufe, L.A. & Fleeson, J. (1986) Attachment and the construction of relationships. In W. Hartup & Z. Rubin (eds) *Relationships and Development* (pp.51–71). Hillsdale, NJ: Lawrence Erlbaum.

relationships with individuals who have some investment in maintaining earlier patterns of power and identity. So efforts these children undertake as adults to avoid the abusive role may still leave them disadvantaged in attempting to parent well, especially when contextual demands elicit intuitive and unreflective responses.

A second key claim made by Sroufe and Fleeson was that the organisation of life within the family and the psychological coherence and emotional life of its members influence one another. If the integration of behaviour, thought, and emotion within the family over time is fragile or punctuated by crises, the members of the family will find emotion regulation difficult. Likewise, if a member of the family has difficulty organising behaviour, thinking, and emotions in coherent ways, this makes integration at the level of the family a greater challenge.[94] At both the individual and the family level, the integration of emotion with thoughts and feelings permits the modulation and direction of emotional expression. In turn this allows emotional experiences to inform and guide action but without threatening to overwhelm or disrupt its effectiveness.[95] Families regularly face external stresses and developmental change—some especially. This means that the organisation of family life is never a fully stable achievement, and for some families is under constant bombardment and active attempts at repair. Nonetheless, when integrative processes are linking behaviour, thinking, and emotions well, experiences shared by families, even difficult ones, can help inform the actions of its members in ways that help them respond to the present; likewise, experiences by individual members contribute to action at a family level.

By contrast, when family members find integration behaviour, thinking, and affect confusing or difficult, there will often be patterns to the fallout and response. Two broad possible 'strategies for adaptation' were highlighted by Sroufe and Fleeson, corresponding to the 'two primary patterns of anxious attachment'. A first is for the family to treat a wide array of situations as potentially combustable or distressing, and to seek continual emotional contact with one another around these troubles. A second is for the family to cut themselves off from interaction or communication when this might raise potentially troubling or distressing experiences for individuals.[96] Families adopting the latter strategy, who experience one another as unreachable or threatening under certain conditions, may outlaw those conditions rather than feel confident in their capacity to modulate and be informed by them. For instance, any expression of anger may be completely forbidden, with tense situations evoking 'ritualist (repetitive) patterns of avoidance'.[97] Sroufe and Fleeson observed that it is quite usual for one or even both of the strategies to be deployed by families handling the fallout from disruption or challenges, before a new organisation has been re-established. What signals a pathway towards problems for the family and its members, and may predispose or contribute to mental health problems, is if such strategies become rigid to the point that they block opportunities for repair, learning, or development.

From her doctoral research, a study of family relationships, Fleeson reported supportive findings.[98] Children were likely to display a tight and rigid control over their emotions when

[94] Sroufe, L.A. & Fleeson, J. (1988) The coherence of family relationships. In R.A. Hinde & J. Stevenson-Hinde (eds) *Relationships within Families: Mutual Influences* (pp.27–47). Oxford: Oxford University Press.

[95] See also Sroufe, L.A., Cooper, R.G., DeHart, G.B., & Marshall, M.E. (1996) *Child Development: Its Nature and Course*, 3rd edn. New York: McGraw-Hill, p.381.

[96] Sroufe, L.A. (1996) *Emotional Development*. Cambridge: Cambridge University Press, p.221.

[97] Sroufe, L.A. (1989) Relationships and relationship disturbances. In A.J. Sameroff & R.N. Emde (eds) *Relationship Disturbances in Early Childhood* (pp.97–124). New York: Basic Books, p.107.

[98] Sroufe, J.W. (1991) Assessment of parent–adolescent relationships: implications for adolescent development. *Journal of Family Psychology*, 5(1), 21–45.

raised in families where anger was disguised or distorted and in which members of the family did not feel able to communicate safely. Conversely, children were likely to display dysregulation of emotion under two conditions, which could occur separately or together. One was when integration was hindered by intrusive sharing of emotions by the parents. The other was when the roles in the family were distorted, with the opposite-sex parent seeking a closer relationship with the child than with his or her partner. In either case, intimacy occurs primarily to the parent's pacing, without modulation for the child's needs. Both situations were theorised by Fleeson to contribute to a feeling of lack of control for the child. The child's attachment relationship with the parent means that insulation against intrusive parental intimacy is a complex task at best. It may, in fact, be 'essentially impossible' for many younger children and early adolescents.[99] At that age, especially, our parents' concerns can be all but inescapable.

Intrusive intimacy

Pursuing the implications of intrusive intimacy with the parent as a distortion of the attachment relationship, Sroufe and Ward filmed mothers' behaviour during a toy cleanup task in the laboratory with the Minnesota sample when the children were toddlers. The researchers measured the extent to which the mothers showed sensual physical contact, sexual teasing, or requests for affection in the course of trying to persuade their toddler to put away the toys. Of the 173 participants who attended the toddler call-back, 16 showed one or more of these behaviours.

Sroufe and Ward distinguished forms of boundary dissolution from warmth or affection on a number of grounds: the behaviours were directed almost exclusively by the mothers towards their male toddlers; they were associated with more, not less, physical punishment and threats of punishment; they were not associated with measures of cooperative, encouraging, supportive, or affectionate behaviour; and they tended to interrupt the child's behaviour putting away the toys rather than facilitate this goal.[100] In fact, half of the punishing behaviours shown in the entire sample were displayed in these 16 dyads; this suggests a lack of monitoring of the environment by the mothers, as they knew they were being filmed.[101] Mothers who showed seductive behaviour towards their son did not display the same behaviour towards their daughter; instead they showed derision.[102] Eight of the 16 mothers were included in a subsample of 36 participants given a full family history interview, and assessed independently for indicators of abuse, including incest. Seven of the eight had histories suggesting that they had been required to supply emotional or sexual intimacy to their father or stepfather during childhood in ways that were 'suggestive of an incestuous-type

---

[99] Ibid. p.34. Reflecting on Sroufe and Fleeson's work in his private notes, Bowlby considered it a brilliant contribution, showing that 'it looks as though "self" is one pole of a relationship and so cannot be conceptualised except in terms of a relationship'. Bowlby, J. (1983) Concept of self . PP/Bow/H.8.

[100] Sroufe, L.A. & Ward, M.J. (1980) Seductive behavior of mothers of toddlers: occurrence, correlates, and family origins. *Child Development*, 51(4), 1222–9.

[101] Ibid. p.225.

[102] At age 13, the relationship between mother and daughter was also more peer-like than the rest of the sample, and the mothers displayed more child-like and needy behaviours towards their daughters: Sroufe, L.A. (1989) Relationships and relationship disturbances. In A.J. Sameroff & R.N. Emde (eds) *Relationship Disturbances in Early Childhood* (pp.97–124). New York: Basic Books, pp.77–8.

relationship'.[103] In a follow-up at 42 months, nearly half of the women reported experiences of intrafamilial sexual abuse (compared to 8% of the total sample).

The behaviours shown by adults displaying intimately intrusive behaviours should not be regarded as imitations of their own caregivers, as anticipated by a simple learning approach to intergenerational transmission of abuse—as for instance held by Bowlby (Chapter 1). Instead, Sroufe and colleagues argued that children learn both roles within attachment relationships, and that aspects of both can appear within adult behaviour:

> These mothers do not simply show deferred imitation of their parents' previous behaviour. For example, those who were exploited by their fathers do not literally do what their fathers did to them. Rather, they engage in the culturally specified adult female form of cross-gender child exploitation. They have internalised a relationship and not simply a set of behaviours.[104]

For this reason, the fact that some of the mothers were doing well with their children in other regards was not a surprise to the Minnesota group. The problem in some instances was quite localised: the attachment system may inform the caregiving system, and they will share some components, but they are distinct. The adult caregiving system is influenced in powerful ways, for instance, by contemporaneous social support. Therefore a parent's behaviour towards his or her child would not necessarily be expected to mirror the parent's past. For instance, if other relationships are available to provide a secure base and safe haven, children would be less likely to be treated as objects of the attachment system and elicit the sexuality and derision that had been woven into it by these mothers' childhood experiences. In support of the protective role of contemporaneous support, the Minnesota group found that only 9% of the mothers who engaged in boundary dissolution behaviours had a stable relationship with a partner, compared to 25% of the rest of the sample.[105]

The construct of boundary-dissolving behaviours was later found to have substantial predictive value. There was also substantial stability over time. In observations made at age 13 of dyads who had earlier shown seductive behaviours, boundary-dissolving behaviour was displayed by both adolescents and their parent.[106] It had become an organisational quality of the relationship involving both members of the dyad. A decade later, the Minnesota group reported a strong association between early boundary-dissolving behaviours by mothers and their child's number of sexual partners in adolescence.[107] Boundary dissolution in the age 13 assessment was also found to predict conduct and attention problems at age 16,

[103] Sroufe, L.A., Jacobvitz, D., Mangelsdorf, S., DeAngelo, E., & Ward, M.J. (1985) Generational boundary dissolution between mothers and their preschool children: a relationship systems approach. *Child Development*, 56(2), 317–25, p.322.

[104] Sroufe, L.A. (1989) Relationships and relationship disturbances. In A.J. Sameroff & R.N. Emde (eds) *Relationship Disturbances in Early Childhood* (pp.97–124). New York: Basic Books, p.103.

[105] Sroufe, L.A., Jacobvitz, D., Mangelsdorf, S., DeAngelo, E., & Ward, M.J. (1985) Generational boundary dissolution between mothers and their preschool children: a relationship systems approach. *Child Development*, 56(2), 317–25, p.324.

[106] Additionally, mothers with substance abusing partners were more likely to show peer-like or spouse-like behaviour with their 13-year-old sons; they were also more likely to have daughters who showed caregiving behaviour towards them. Hiester, M. (1993) Generational boundary dissolution between mothers and children in early childhood and early adolescence. Unpublished doctoral dissertation, University of Minnesota.

[107] Sroufe, L.A., Egeland, B., Carlson, E.A., & Collins, W.A. (2005) *The Development of the Person*. New York: Guilford, p.194.

over and above behavioural problems shown at age 13 and other measures of family functioning.[108] Such predictive validity offered support for the construct of boundary dissolution, though the measure has not subsequently seen use in later research by developmental scientists. One reason may have been that the idea of mothers behaving seductively towards their toddlers was simply too controversial and unthinkable an idea to be taken up by researchers. A broader trend may have been the decline of reference to family systems theory within developmental science over the subsequent decades. Furthermore, ideas of 'child abuse and exploitation' and the 'parentification of children' were increasingly salient in clinical discourses during the 1980s and 1990s: these covered some of the same ground as Sroufe and colleagues' work on boundary dissolution, but in both cases trained attention more on older children and on dyadic interaction.[109] Nonetheless, the fact that Sroufe's approach to thinking about affects and relationships contributed to the novel finding of the importance of boundary dissolution offered demonstration of its value. And the finding also highlighted the importance of caregiving experienced within attachment relationships for children's development.[110] Exploration of the antecedents and sequelae of early care was central to the concerns of the Minnesota group, with particular interest in measures of individual differences in infant attachment.

Correlates of attachment

Antecedents of attachment

Sroufe, Waters, and Vaughn conducted the Strange Situation with the sample of 267 mothers when their infants were 12 and 18 months. Sixty percent of the sample had stable attachment classifications over the six-month period. Of the 267 mothers, there were 31 cases of infant maltreatment, confirmed scrupulously through multiple methods.[111] Of these 31 mother–infant dyads, at 12 months, 62% were classified as insecurely attached, compared to 45% in the total Minnesota sample and 34% of the combined middle-class samples reported in Ainsworth and colleagues' *Patterns of Attachment*.[112]

---

[108] Nelson, N.N. (1994) Predicting adolescent behavior problems in late adolescence from parent–child interactions in early adolescence. Unpublished doctoral dissertation, University of Minnesota; Shaffer, A. & Sroufe, L.A. (2005) The developmental and adaptational implications of generational boundary dissolution: findings from a prospective, longitudinal study. *Journal of Emotional Abuse*, 5(2–3), 67–84.

[109] If intimately intrusive behaviours by parents towards their child had been framed as child abuse, then researchers would have been obliged to report the families to child protective services. This may have been a disincentive to include measure of such behaviours within a research study, given the ethical and administrative issues it would have raised.

[110] The research on boundary-dissolving behaviour at Minnesota also likely influenced the development of a scale for role-reversing behaviour in Main and Hesse's work on the Adult Attachment Interview (AAI).

[111] Egeland, B. & Sroufe, L.A. (1981) Attachment and early maltreatment. *Child Development*, 52(1), 44–52. According to a later report, using slightly different criteria to Egeland and Sroufe's 1981 paper, 47 children were abused and/or neglected by their caregivers in infancy (of 211 with adequate data; 22%), 66 in early childhood and in middle childhood (of 185 in early childhood and 190 in middle childhood; 35–36%), and 21 in adolescence (of 179; 12%). Johnson, W.F., Huelsnitz, C.O., Carlson, E.A., et al. (2017) Childhood abuse and neglect and physical health at midlife: prospective, longitudinal evidence. *Development & Psychopathology*, 29(5), 1935–46. The reasons for the change in definition of infant maltreatment from those used by Egeland and Sroufe are not fully provided by these later researchers.

[112] Egeland, B. & Sroufe, L.A. (1981) Attachment and early maltreatment. *Child Development*, 52(1), 44–52. Of studies using the Ainsworth classifications, there has been a very substantial association between maltreatment

In the total Minnesota sample, 21% of the dyads were classified as ambivalent/resistant. This was substantially higher than the 13% seen by Ainsworth.[113] The Minnesota group found that there was a powerful overlap between ambivalent/resistant attachment in the Strange Situation and the nurse's report on the regulatory capacities of the child as a newborn ($r = .46$), including their startle response ($r = .20$).[114] However, these findings, suggestive of a role for temperament, were reported in an undertone by the Minnesota group in their publications of the 1980s and 1990s, and were rarely mentioned in their review or theoretical works. (The field would have to wait for a recent meta-analysis by Groh and colleagues for the resistance–temperament link to resurface for discussion.)[115] Instead, the Minnesota group focused on the portion of the variance in ambivalent/resistant attachment that appeared to be environmental. Ainsworth had situated the broad notion of 'inconsistent care' as the origin of ambivalent/resistant attachment, though her more specific theory seemed to be that these children had caregivers who struggled to hold them in mind (Chapter 2). Egeland and Sroufe argued that inconsistent care may have been made more likely by the poverty and other adversities faced by their sample.[116] This interpretation was buttressed by their finding that half the cases of neglect were in dyads receiving a classification of ambivalent/resistant attachment. And a qualitative examination of the cases indicated a high level of drug use, which contributed to leaving the infant unattended for long stretches.[117]

A puzzle in the findings from this study was that 12 of the 31 abused infants were classified as securely attached, using Ainsworth's coding protocols. They displayed protest on separation, proximity-seeking, and some contact-maintenance on reunion, but could be comforted and were able to return to play. Yet they also displayed other behaviours that seemed to interrupt or contradict the secure pattern described by Ainsworth. Informally, the Minnesota group called these 12 cases 'unhealthy Bs': though they met the Ainsworth criteria for Group B, their behaviour in the Strange Situation did not seem secure.[118] In watching the tapes closely, Egeland and Sroufe identified behaviour that was 'neither avoidant nor resistant', but which nonetheless suggested insecurity, for instance responses to the caregiver that were 'apathetic or disorganized'.[119] Rather than disregarding these cases as

and insecure attachment. Baer, J.C. & Martinez, C.D. (2006) Child maltreatment and insecure attachment: a meta-analysis, *Journal of Reproductive and Infant Psychology*, 24(3), 187–97.

[113] This is only somewhat higher than the 17% reported in a recent meta-analysis: Verhage, M.L., Schuengel, C., Madigan, S., et al. (2016) Narrowing the transmission gap: a synthesis of three decades of research on intergenerational transmission of attachment. *Psychological Bulletin*, 142(4), 337–66, Table 4.

[114] Warren, S.L., Huston, L., Egeland, B., & Sroufe, L.A. (1997) Child and adolescent anxiety disorders and early attachment. *Journal of the American Academy of Child & Adolescent Psychiatry*, 36(5), 637–44, p.640. See also Waters, E., Vaughn, B.E., & Egeland, B.R. (1980) Individual differences in infant–mother attachment relationships at age one: antecedents in neonatal behavior in an urban, economically disadvantaged sample. *Child Development*, 51(1), 208–16.

[115] Groh, A.M., Narayan, A.J., Bakermans-Kranenburg, M.J., et al. (2017) Attachment and temperament in the early life course: a meta-analytic review. *Child Development*, 88(3), 770–95.

[116] Egeland, B. & Sroufe, L.A. (1981) Attachment and early maltreatment. *Child Development*, 52(1), 44–52, p.50. The same factors would also, however, have reduced the caregivers' attentional availability to their infant, increasing the relevance of a strategy that increased attachment signals in order to have their caregiver heed and respond to their desire for felt security. See Chapter 2 for criticism of the attribution of 'inconsistent care' as the ultimate cause of ambivalent/resistant attachment behaviour.

[117] A relationship between parental drug use and ambivalent/resistant attachment was also later documented by Seifer, R., LaGasse, L.L., Lester, B., et al. (2004) Attachment status in children prenatally exposed to cocaine and other substances. *Child Development*, 75(3), 850–68.

[118] Alan Sroufe and Byron Egeland, personal communication, July 2012.

[119] Egeland, B. & Sroufe, L.A. (1981) Developmental sequelae of maltreatment in infancy. *New Directions for Child and Adolescent Development*, 1981(11), 77–92, p.84.

'noise' produced by imprecision in the Strange Situation procedure, they suspected that the cases represented an attachment-relevant process of some significance. However, because Sroufe was coding the 18-month Strange Situations, he needed to be 'blind' as to which recordings were those of maltreated children. He therefore went rigorously out of his way to avoid speculating about the aetiology of this behaviour until data analysis was complete. Instead, Sroufe gave copies of these recordings to Main to examine (Chapter 3).

The Minnesota group were interested in the antecedents of the Ainsworth patterns of attachment, to see whether their findings aligned with those of the Baltimore study. Confirming Ainsworth's conclusions, Egeland and Farber reported that caregivers in secure dyads were more likely to display sensitivity during feeding episodes with their infants at three and six months and free play at six months. Though the association between sensitivity and security in the Minnesota study was much less strong than in Ainsworth's data, it was in the expected direction. The Minnesota group identified other variables that might suggest a more favourable and settled caregiving environment for infants in securely attached dyads. Mothers who lived with their partner for the first 12 months of the child's life were more likely to be part of a secure dyad.[120] It was also noted that mothers who reported fewer current adversities or stressors were more likely to have a child with a secure attachment relationship, a finding that 'shows the foolishness of blaming parents for developmental problems of the child. As life stress is reduced, quality of care improves, as does the quality of the child's attachment relationship.'[121]

Egeland and Farber examined nurses' ratings of the mothers' interest in their newborn baby. They found that infants in dyads later classified as avoidant had mothers who were reported to show less interest. Three months after the birth, caregivers in ambivalent/resistant dyads also scored lower on the Maternal Attitude Scale. This was a self-report measure with three scales: appropriate vs inappropriate control of child's aggression, encouragement vs discouragement of reciprocity, and acceptance vs denial of emotional complexity in child care. Furthermore, they found that infants in ambivalent/resistant dyads scored lower on scales of motor and mental development at nine months. The researchers suspected that if the infants had been easier to care for, or had caregivers who accepted the complexity of child care and could adapt to their child's needs, many of these dyads would have developed secure attachment relationships.[122] They found no difference between groups in the amount of warmth demonstrated to the infants by their caregivers. However, the mothers of infants who changed from secure to anxious over the six months were rated by observers as showing less delight in their baby than other caregivers at six months. Self-report measures of maternal personality, such as aggression and impulsivity, had little relationship with caregiving behaviours or Strange Situation classifications.[123]

One potential form of adverse caregiving that especially interested the Minnesota group was emotional neglect. This was a relatively new concept. An early advocate of the category of emotional neglect had been John Bowlby. Though he tended to ignore the role of emotion

[120] Egeland, B. & Farber, E.A. (1984) Infant–mother attachment: factors related to its development and changes over time. *Child Development*, 55(3), 753–71.

[121] Sroufe, L.A. & Waters, E. (1982) Issues of temperament and attachment. *American Journal of Orthopsychiatry*, 52(4), 743–6, p.744.

[122] Egeland, B. & Farber, E.A. (1984) Infant–mother attachment: factors related to its development and changes over time. *Child Development*, 55(3), 753–71, p.767.

[123] Egeland, B. & Brunnquell, D. (1979) An at-risk approach to the study of child abuse: some preliminary findings. *Journal of the American Academy of Child Psychiatry*, 18(2), 219–35.

as a cause or process in psychological life in his theorising, he was highly attentive to child emotion as an index of problems with the availability of adequate care. Already in 1971, Bowlby was arguing to the Home Office select committee on the adoption of children that there is an 'urgent need' for 'a really adequate research study of emotional neglect'.[124] The use of emotional life in the identification of abuse and neglect was a matter of contention in the early 1980s, as it seemed to involve an even stronger value judgement by social workers than physical or sexual abuse or physical neglect.[125] Yet emotional abuse and neglect swiftly grew into the primary basis for referrals to child protection services.[126] In 1985, Sroufe reported on the antecedents of emotional neglect/psychological unavailability in the Minnesota sample.[127] Though the infants who received this form of care received typical scores for mental and motor development at ten days and three months, by six months their development was impeded, and they departed more and more from the rest of the cohort with each further assessment of their development. At 12 months, 42% of the infant–caregiver dyads were classified as avoidant, and at 18 months 86% received this classification.[128] Much later, at age 17, Egeland reported that the large majority met diagnostic criteria for a psychiatric disorder: 53% met criteria for an anxiety disorder compared to 34% of the rest of the sample; 53% met criteria for a conduct disorder compared to 19% in the wider sample; and 25% met criteria for PTSD compared to 12% in the cohort as a whole.[129]

In the 1990s, after the introduction of the disorganised/disoriented attachment classification by Main and colleagues (Chapter 3), Elizabeth Carlson recoded the Minnesota Strange Situation recordings for disorganised attachment and examined caregiving antecedents. In her analyses she used the highest rating at either 12 or 18 months to represent a score for disorganisation. Examining antecedents of disorganised attachment, she found that the best predictor was a composite variable comprised of intrusive and insensitive caregiving ($r = .38$), and that various forms of neglect and maltreatment made a modest additional contribution (overall abuse/neglect $r = .29$; physical abuse $r = .20$; emotional neglect/psychological unavailability $r = .23$). She found no association between disorganised attachment and maternal mental health or drug and/or alcohol abuse.[130] This last finding, however, differs from later studies. A meta-analysis by Cyr and colleagues found that parental drug and/

[124] Bowlby, J. (1971) Evidence presented on 6/4/1971 to the Committee on the Adoption of Children, Home Office and Department of Health and Social Security, The National Archives, Kew, BN 29/2340.

[125] Rohner, R.P. & Rohner, E.C. (1980) Antecedents and consequences of parental rejection: a theory of emotional abuse. *Child Abuse & Neglect*, 4(3), 189–98; Trowell, J. (1983) Emotional abuse of children. *Health Visitor*, 56(7), 252–5.

[126] Cicchetti, D. & Manly, J.T. (1990) A personal perspective on conducting research with maltreating families: problems and solutions. In G. Brody & I. Sigel (eds) *Methods of Family Research: Families at Risk*, Vol. 2 (pp.87–133). Hillsdale, NJ: Lawrence Erlbaum. More recently, see Bilson, A., Featherstone, B., & Martin, K. (2017) How child protection's 'investigative turn' impacts on poor and deprived communities. *Family Law*, 47, 316–19.

[127] Sroufe, L.A. (1985) Attachment classification from the perspective of infant–caregiver relationships and infant temperament. *Child Development* 56(1), 1–14. An early report on findings from this analysis was covered in the *New York Times*:Brody, J.E. (1983) Emotional deprivation seen as devastating form of child abuse. *New York Times*, 20 December 1983. This was unusual: over the decades there has been relatively little press coverage of the Minnesota Longitudinal Study of Risk and Adaptation, as compared with other large longitudinal studies. Egeland and Sroufe did not much seek out media appearances.

[128] Sroufe, L.A. (1985) Attachment classification from the perspective of infant–caregiver relationships and infant temperament. *Child Development* 56(1), 1–14, p.9.

[129] Egeland, B. (1997) Mediators of the effects of child maltreatment on developmental adaptation in adolescence. In D. Cicchetti & S. Toth (eds) *Rochester Symposium on Developmental Psychopathology, Volume VIII: The Effects of Trauma on the Developmental Process* (pp.403–34). Rochester, NY: University of Rochester Press, Table 5.

[130] Carlson, E.A. (1998) A prospective longitudinal study of attachment disorganization/disorientation. *Child Development*, 69(4), 1107–28, Table 4.

or alcohol abuse did predict disorganised infant attachment, especially when compounded by other risk factors.[131] Likewise, some aspects of maternal mental health has been found to be relevant to the prediction of infant insecure and insecure-disorganised attachment, such as PTSD.[132] (On the relationship between caregiver depression and infant attachment see Chapter 3.)

Early social competence

Sroufe, Egeland, and colleagues did not regard secure attachment as any guarantee of positive later outcomes, but as a promotive or protective factor. Nonetheless, the Minnesota Longitudinal Study of Risk and Adaptation demonstrated a number of important and valuable findings regarding the later positive correlates of infant secure attachment. In a follow-up when the children were two years old, the dyads were invited to the laboratory; 190 families attended, of the 267 who started the study. Mother–child dyads were observed as they completed a series of tool-based problem-solving tasks together, several of which were more demanding than most two year olds would find comfortable. The reason for this was that assessments of behaviour or cognition alone would risk being confounded with other variables like IQ. Completion of a problem-solving task with a caregiver was assumed to represent a developmentally appropriate challenge to a toddler, requiring the integration of affect, cognition, and behaviour in order to stay on task and coordinate together effectively. This meant that the task could serve as an assessment of the ability of the children to mobilise and coordinate personal and social resources to realise the opportunities and potentials of the environment.[133]

This capacity was termed by Waters and Sroufe 'social competence'. The term was drawn from scholars such as Diana Baumrind, for whom social competence signified the 'social responsibility, independence, achievement orientation, and vigor' required of citizens of American capitalism.[134] Waters and Sroufe appreciated the metaphor of individual possibilities as shaped by the resources available to them. However, they departed from Baumrind and other individualising competency discourses in emphasising that qualities such as social responsibility and independence are not best thought of as individual properties, and certainly not in children. Rather, they should be regarded as transactional effects of individual–environment interactions, shaped by experiences of early care. The importance of early care for Waters and Sroufe lay in the fact that it shapes both the inner and external resources available to the child, and also influences how these resources are interpreted and used. In line with this emphasis on early experiences of care, the Minnesota group found that, according to the parent-report, children from dyads who had previously been classified as insecure attached showed more behaviour problems at home. Those caregivers from previously

[131] Cyr, C., Euser, E.M., Bakermans-Kranenburg, M.J., & Van Ijzendoorn, M.H. (2010) Attachment security and disorganization in maltreating and high-risk families: a series of meta-analyses. *Development & Psychopathology*, 22(1), 87–108, Table 4.

[132] E.g. Enlow, M.B., Egeland, B., Carlson, E., Blood, E., & Wright, R.J. (2014) Mother–infant attachment and the intergenerational transmission of posttraumatic stress disorder. *Development & Psychopathology*, 26(1), 41–65.

[133] Waters, E. & Sroufe, L.A. (1983) Social competence as a developmental construct. *Developmental Review*, 3, 79–97, p.81.

[134] Baumrind, D. (1978) Parental disciplinary patterns and social competence in children. *Youth & Society*, 9(3), 239–67, p.249. See also White, R. (1959) Motivation reconsidered: the concept of competence. *Psychological Review*, 66, 297–333.

insecure dyads who reported that their children showed fewer behavioural problems were observed to be respectful of their autonomy, offered more support, provided clearer structure, and were less hostile during the problem-solving tasks. These were also mothers who reported greater access to family support and friendship networks.[135] This suggested that the capacities of the caregiver were likewise shaped integrally by the availability of supportive provisions, and should not be regarded merely as an individual quality.

In later assessments at preschool age, the Minnesota group found that an interaction between supportive maternal care and secure attachment predicted stronger capacity for managing and delaying behaviour and wishes in order to flexibly achieve an overarching goal ('executive function').[136] In the two preschool classes constituted from children from the sample, there were also distinct sequelae of infant attachment. Children who so infuriated the teacher that they were sent to the corner were, on every occasion, those who had been classified as having an avoidant attachment relationship with their caregiver in infancy.[137] Sroufe and colleagues found that the children who were identified by observers—unaware of the attachment classification—as unable to engage effectively in independent activities were those who had earlier been in dyads classified as insecurely attached. The children from ambivalent/resistant dyads were observed to exhibit chronic, low-level contact seeking and attention seeking. By contrast, the children who had earlier been classified as part of avoidant dyads did not seek contact from the teacher, except when the intimacy of the contact would be reduced, such as in large-group time.[138] The preschoolers from insecure dyads were in general less socially competent than their peers, and found making and retaining friends more difficult.[139]

In the preschool classroom, the children were assigned into pairs and observed for a series of free-play interactions. The researchers found that only children with histories of avoidant attachment with their caregiver were seen to attempt to bully or victimise the other children. When children ended up in a sustained role of bullied or victimised, these were always children who had earlier received an insecure classification with their caregiver in the Strange Situation.[140] Sroufe and colleagues were interested in the fact that children with experience of an avoidant attachment relationship could assume either role, victimiser or victim. They interpreted this as evidence that, in receiving rejection or rebuff from their caregiver in response to their attachment behaviour, the infant in an avoidantly attached dyad is learning both how to reject and how to be rejected by others. Later researchers confirmed the link between infant avoidant attachment relationships and later aggressive behaviour, with meta-analytic research reporting an association of $d = .58$ for observation-based studies.[141] Sroufe

[135] Erickson, M., Sroufe, L.A., & Egeland, B. (1985) The relationship of quality of attachment and behavior problems in preschool in a high risk sample. *Monographs of the Society for Research in Child Development*, 50(1–2), 147–86, p.157, 164.

[136] Meuwissen, A.S. & Englund, M.M. (2016) Executive function in at-risk children: importance of father-figure support and mother parenting. *Journal of Applied Developmental Psychology*, 44, 72–80.

[137] Sroufe, L.A. (1983) Infant–caregiver attachment and patterns of adaptation in preschool: the roots of maladaptation and competence. In M. Perlmutter (ed.) *Minnesota Symposium in Child Psychology*, Vol. 16 (pp.41–83). Hillsdale, NJ: Lawrence Erlbaum, p.76.

[138] Sroufe, L.A., Fox, N.E., & Pancake, V.R. (1983) Attachment and dependency in developmental perspective. *Child Development*, 54(6), 1615–27.

[139] Sroufe, L.A. (1989) Relationships, self, and individual adaptation. In A.J. Sameroff & R.N. Emde (eds) *Relationship Disturbances in Early Childhood: A Developmental Approach* (pp.70–94). New York: Basic Books.

[140] Troy, M. & Sroufe, L.A. (1987) Victimization among preschoolers: the role of attachment relationship history. *Journal of the American Academy of Child and Adolescent Psychiatry*, 26(2), 166–72.

[141] Fearon, R.P., Bakermans-Kranenburg, M.J., Van IJzendoorn, M.H., Lapsley, A.M., & Roisman, G.I. (2010) The significance of insecure attachment and disorganization in the development of children's externalizing

and colleagues put forward a hypothesis to account for the association between avoidant attachment relationships and later aggressive behaviour.[142] They argued that the attachment relationship serves as a non-linear prototype for later relationships, with avoidant attachment based on a history of unavailability, disappointment, and frustration. Viewing others as hostile and remote, children with avoidant attachment relationships may respond with aggression fed by their frustration, leading in turn to further rejection,[143] and selective association with aggressive peers.[144]

Curiously, three decades later, this remains one of the only hypotheses proposed for the association between avoidant attachment and aggressive behaviour, and no test of the hypothesis has ever been specifically conducted.[145] Writing with Michael Rutter, Sroufe later acknowledged that the exact mechanism leading to conduct problems remains unclear: 'Avoidant attachment in infancy is associated with later conduct problems, but avoidant attachment is associated with low self-esteem, negative attributional biases, and rejection by peers and teachers, all of which may predispose to conduct problems. We are only beginning to understand how these chain effects operate.'[146] One factor that may have inhibited the generation and testing of hypotheses in this area has been the growth of findings that suggest that disorganised infant attachment is a somewhat better predictor of later externalising behaviours than avoidant attachment.[147]

In their study of preschool behaviour, the Minnesota team additionally found differences in the play of the children, in pairs, and also in other contexts. Preschoolers who had been classified as secure had narratives to the stories and games they made that routinely assumed a positive resolution to dangers, sickness, or other serious problems. If someone was hurt, they were taken to hospital and made better. This follows what Waters and Waters later called the 'secure base script' (Chapter 2). Children from avoidantly attached dyads were less likely to create such secure base stories. In fact, 'what is more noteworthy is the almost complete

behavior: a meta-analytic study. *Child Development*, 81(2), 435–56. Questionnaires of parents revealed an association of d = .22. Questionnaires of teachers revealed an association of d = .30.

[142] The hypothesis put forward later by Sroufe regarding the link between disorganised attachment and conduct problems could equally be applied as an alternative hypothesis in the case of avoidant attachment, given that both showed substantial prospective links to dissociative tendencies in Carlson's 1998 report. Sroufe, L.A. (2005) Attachment and development: a prospective, longitudinal study from birth to adulthood. *Attachment & Human Development*, 7(4), 349–67: 'Disorganized attachment also predicts conduct disorder, we believe, because of the dissociative tendencies and attendant problems with impulse control' (361).

[143] Renken, B., Egeland, B., Marvinney, D., Mangelsdorf, S., & Sroufe, L.A. (1989) Early childhood antecedents of aggression and passive-withdrawal in early elementary school. *Journal of Personality*, 57(2), 257–81.

[144] Sroufe, L.A. (2007) The place of development in developmental psychopathology. In A. Masten (ed.) *Multilevel Dynamics in Developmental Psychopathology: Pathways to the future. The Minnesota Symposia on Child Psychology*, Vol. 34 (pp.285–99). Mahwah, NJ: Lawrence Erlbaum, p.287.

[145] The matter has been examined in a meta-analytic treatment by Fearon, R.P., Bakermans-Kranenburg, M.J., Van IJzendoorn, M.H., Lapsley, A.M., & Roisman, G.I. (2010) The significance of insecure attachment and disorganization in the development of children's externalizing behavior: a meta-analytic study. *Child Development*, 81(2), 435–56. An alternative/additional hypotheses for the association between avoidant attachment and externalising behaviours is the idea that when an avoidant strategy fails or is disrupted, anger may be evoked. This may be as the intrusion of a segregated system, as proposed for example by Crittenden, P.M. (2016) *Raising Parents: Attachment, Representation, and Treatment*, 2nd edn. London: Routledge. Mikulincer and Shaver also suggested the idea of a dominance behavioural system, which may be engaged to supplement or replace a conditional strategy (Chapter 5).

[146] Rutter, M. & Sroufe, L.A. (2000) Developmental psychopathology: concepts and challenges. *Development & Psychopathology*, 12(3), 265–96, p.271.

[147] Fearon, R.P., Bakermans-Kranenburg, M.J., van IJzendoorn, M.H., Lapsley, A.M., & Roisman, G.I. (2010) The significance of insecure attachment and disorganization in the development of children's externalizing behavior: a meta-analytic study. *Child Development*, 81(2), 435–56.

absence of fantasy play concerning people. Such fantasies dominate the play of almost all preschool children and were well represented in the play of those with secure histories in our sample. These data reveal sharp contrasts in the working models of the two groups—one world is richly peopled, the other is not.'[148] This finding was partially supported by later research with the sample. As discussed in Chapter 3, when participants were asked to complete a family drawing, the drawings of children from avoidantly attached dyads were not found to be less populated than those of other children. However, adult figures were assessed by coders blind to the infant attachment classifications as showing more emotional distance between figures, more tension or anger, and figures were more likely to have their arms rigidly held at their sides rather than offering contact (e.g. holding hands).[149]

When the children in the sample were aged either five or eight, thirty families who also had another child no more than three years younger were called back to the lab. The parent was asked to leave and the siblings were given a set of games to complete together. For instance, in one game the siblings had to build a house out of blocks; in another the siblings had to work together to write using a stylus. The Minnesota group found that in sibling dyads where the elder sibling took on the role of guide in an effective way, this elder sibling was more likely to have had a history of secure attachment as assessed in earlier Strange Situations ($r = .37$).[150] Furthermore, the extent to which the elder sibling took the role of guide, and the extent to which they treated their sibling with sensitivity, independently predicted observer and teacher assessments of their social competence at school, over and above attachment relationships. There was no association between attachment classifications and measures of how much fun the siblings seemed to be having together or their cooperativeness. As such, the Strange Situation seemed to predict, not a positive relationship in general, but specifically secure base provision by older siblings to their younger brother or sister. This aligned with Sroufe's idea that children learn both roles in their relationships with attachment figures. This quality of the sibling relationship, even accounting for parent–child attachment, was found in turn to predict the elder sibling's peer competence at school. Sroufe and colleagues observed that such findings offer evidence for the potential importance of the attachment components of the relationships with siblings in the development of peer competence.[151]

Overall, the Minnesota Longitudinal Study of Risk and Adaptation was able to offer ample evidence that early attachment experiences are associated with early social competence. This provided suggestive evidence towards a transactional model of individual–environment interactions, in which experiences in relationships with attachment components contribute to forms of social competence, perhaps especially through the availability of secure base scripts. Slade and Holmes observed that the preschool findings at Minnesota were of particular importance for establishing attachment research as a paradigm within developmental psychology.[152] Sroufe, Egeland, and colleagues situated their findings as demonstrating the predictive validity of the Ainsworth Strange Situation, for instance in the finding

[148] Sroufe, L.A. (1989) Relationships, self, and individual adaptation. In A.J. Sameroff & R.N. Emde (eds) *Relationship Disturbances in Early Childhood: A Developmental Approach* (pp.70–94). New York: Basic Books, p.89.

[149] Fury, G., Carlson, E.A., & Sroufe, L.A. (1997) Children's representations of attachment relationships in family drawings. *Child Development*, 68(6), 1154–64.

[150] Marvinney, D. (1988) Sibling relationships in middle childhood: implications for social-emotional development. Unpublished doctoral dissertation, University of Minnesota. This relationship did not, however, hold when the elder sibling was themselves secondborn.

[151] Sroufe, L.A., Egeland, B., Carlson, E.A., & Collins, W.A. (2005) *The Development of the Person*. New York: Guilford, p.170.

[152] Slade, A. & Holmes, J. (eds) (2014) *Attachment Theory*. London: Sage.

of an association between avoidant attachment and later conduct problems. Indeed, this association has gone on to be well replicated. In retrospect, however, it is interesting that in their analyses the Minnesota group did not quite treat the Strange Situation as the priviledged measure of early attachment that it would become subsequently.[153] For instance, the Minnesota researchers would at times composite the Strange Situation with, or study its interactions with, other measures of early care. Sroufe and Egeland appear to have felt that 'attachment' itself cannot be directly measured, even by the Strange Situation, but must be inferred from the network of correlations that link early care to a child's later behaviour in theoretically expectable ways (Chapter 2). Having established correlations in early childhood, a next step in appraising the influence of early attachment relationships would be to see whether associations could still be found as the cohort matured into late childhood and adolescence.

Adolescence

When the sample reached 11 years old, in 1986, 48 children were recruited to attend a summer camp lasting four weeks. At this point, research on adolescence within academic psychology was on the cusp on becoming established: empirical study of adolescence barely existed in the late 1970s, and yet would be a central concern of developmental psychology by the early 1990s. The Society for Research on Adolescence was founded in the winter of 1984, and its first meeting was held in in Madison, Wisconsin, in 1986.[154] Adolescence was an object of increasing public and policy concern. However, more proximally, the attention given to the topic in developmental psychology can also be situated in the context of the maturing of a number of longitudinal cohort studies established in the 1970s. The Minnesota Longitudinal Study of Risk and Adaptation was a few years ahead of this general curve.

In the mid- to late 1980s, a central concern in the research literature was with how to achieve the psychological measurement of aspects of adolescent social development in an ecologically valid way.[155] The use of three summer camps with members of the cohort study was an ingenious solution. Most of the children were drawn from the subsample who had been studied in the preschool and who were already therefore stratified by attachment classification. Each of the three camps had 16 children. The programme of activities included group games, singing, swimming, art and craft projects, and sports. Weekly day trips were taken to recreation parks, and there was also one overnight camp-out.[156] During the camp, the children were observed, and in the last week each child was interviewed twice about his or her experiences of the camp and relationships with other campers.

Sroufe and colleagues examined the maintenance of appropriate gender boundaries at the summer camp as one particular index of social competence at 11 years of age. The construct of 'gender boundary violations' encompassed two rather different kinds of

[153] Ziv, Y. & Hotam, Y. (2015) Theory and measure in the psychological field: the case of attachment theory and the strange situation procedure. *Theory & Psychology*, 25(3), 274–91.

[154] See Steinberg, L. & Lerner, R.M. (2004) The scientific study of adolescence: a brief history. *Journal of Early Adolescence*, 24(1), 45–54.

[155] See e.g. Petersen, A.C. (1988) Adolescent development. *Annual Review of Psychology*, 39, 583–607.

[156] Elicker, J., Englund, M., & Sroufe, L.A. (1992) Predicting peer competence and peer relationships in childhood from early parent–child relationships. In R. Parke & G. Ladd (eds) *Family–Peer Relationships: Modes of Linkage* (pp.77–106). Hillsdale, NJ: Lawrence Erlbaum, p.92.

behaviour. One was hovering near opposite-sex groups or joining in their activities. The other was forms of sexual harassment or cross-gender aggression. No report was made on whether these behaviours were correlated. These two kinds of behaviours were aggregated by the researchers, though the way that the scale was constructed gave more weight to sexual harassment or cross-gender aggression than cross-gender interaction in general.[157] Elicker, Englund, and Sroufe found that there were marked negative associations between gender boundary violations and peers' ratings of campers social skill ($r = -.33$).[158] Children with a history of ambivalent/resistant relationships engaged in gender boundary violations much more frequently. They also sat next to opposite-gender children during large-group circle times more often. Gender boundary violations were predicted by earlier intergenerational boundary dissolution in early childhood.[159] Gender boundary violation would turn out to be an important variable in the Minnesota study, with strong predictive value for later outcomes. For instance, gender boundary violations at age 11 had a negative association with contemporary ($r = .58$) and later ($r = .31$) competence with peers in social situations,[160] lower satisfaction in adolescent dating relationships ($r = .47$),[161] and a dramatic association with age of commencement of sexual activity for girls ($r = .75$).[162]

During the summer camps, the 11-year-olds with histories of avoidant attachment relationships were indistinguishable from those with secure relationships when the tasks and challenges of the camp related to physical tasks or the inanimate environment. They also appeared confident in the first day of the camp, with less of the ordinary clumsy vulnerability and reserve of the other early adolescents. However, difficulties in social situations became more apparent over time.[163] For example, they were less effective when given tasks that required inferences about the thoughts and feelings of others, and they displayed a higher level of negative bias in their evaluations of their own group when asked to engage

[157] Sroufe, L.A., Bennett, C., Englund, M., Urban, J., & Shulman, S. (1993) The significance of gender boundaries in preadolescence: contemporary correlates and antecedents of boundary violation and maintenance. *Child Development*, 64(2), 455–66.

[158] Elicker, J., Englund, M., & Sroufe, L.A. (1992) Predicting peer competence and peer relationships in childhood from early parent–child relationships. In R. Parke & G. Ladd (eds) *Family–Peer Relationships: Modes of Linkage* (pp.77–106). Hillsdale, NJ: Lawrence Erlbaum, p.97.

[159] Sroufe, L.A., Bennett, C., Englund, M., Urban, J., & Shulman, S. (1993) The significance of gender boundaries in preadolescence: contemporary correlates and antecedents of boundary violation and maintenance. *Child Development*, 64, 455–66.

[160] Sroufe, L.A., Egeland, B., & Carlson, E.A. (1999) One social world: the integrated development of parent–child and peer relationships. In W. . Collins & B. Laursen (eds) *Relationships as Developmental Contexts: The Minnesota Symposia on Child Psychology*, Vol. 30 (pp.241–61). Mahwah, NJ: Lawrence Erlbaum, Table 11.4.

[161] Collins, W.A., Hennighausen, K.H., Schmit, D.T., & Sroufe, L.A. (1997) Developmental precursors of romantic relationships: a longitudinal analysis. In S. Shulman (ed.) *New Directions for Child Development*. San Francisco: Jossey-Bass (pp.69–84), p.78; Sroufe, L.A., Egeland, B., Carlson, E.A., & Collins, W.A. (2005) *The Development of the Person*. New York: Guilford, p.186.

[162] Ibid. p.194. Despite these intriguing results, in the two decades since the study took place, no further research has been done using the gender violations scale. It might be suspected that the amalgamation of cross-gender sociality and sexual harassment folded together phenomena that were of interest to two rather different communities of researchers; both have subsequently been considered in the literature on gender and education, but generally not together. An exception is research in qualitative feminist sociology, e.g. Renold, E. (2002) Presumed innocence: (hetero) sexual, heterosexist and homophobic harassment among primary school girls and boys. *Childhood*, 9(4), 415–34.

[163] Sroufe, L.A. & Egeland, B. (1991) Illustrations of person and environment interaction from a longitudinal study. In T. Wachs & R. Plomin (eds) *Conceptualization and Measurement of Organism–Environment Interaction* (pp.68–84). Washington, DC: American Psychological Association, p.76.

in groupwork.[164] Kagan argued that the unruffled behaviour of infants in avoidant dyads in the Strange Situation did not represent any kind of problem. He suggested that it may just reflect infants with a bold temperament, or infants who had been socialised by their parents to healthy independence.[165] Elicker, Englund, and Sroufe argued that the sequelae of infant avoidant attachment showed that neither interpretation was especially plausible. Instead, the behaviours shown at the summer camp by participants who had been in avoidant attachment relationships as infants could better be regarded as an effect of their experience of less caregiver availability as a safe haven to help develop successful emotion regulation and social competence.[166]

However, even if attachment does not begin as a trait, the Minnesota group concluded that individual differences related to attachment may become stable with development. When the children were recruited back for a summer camp reunion weekend at age 15, assessments of peer interaction were conducted. Whereas there was little stability in individual behaviours, global assessments of peer competence were very stable between the summer camp and the reunion.[167] A curious finding reported by Sroufe, Egeland, and Carlson was that peer competence at the reunion was predicted well by Strange Situation classifications and preschool behaviour a decade earlier, with little additional prediction accounted for by observations of social skills in the intervening years. The researchers were led to conclude that 'by age 5, much of the variance in adolescent social competence can be accounted for. Even though numerous capacities are only nascent or not at all apparent in the preschool period (e.g. coordinated group activities, intimacy).'[168] Soufe and colleagues highlighted that since preschool social competence was itself predicted by infant Strange Situation classifications, there seemed to be both a direct and an indirect effect of attachment on peer competence through childhood and adolescence. The researchers attributed this especially to the role that secure base and safe haven availability have for the modulation of emotion. Such capacity for modulation can contribute to skills in handling closeness in the face of potential peer conflicts and to tolerating the stimulation of group activities.[169] The emphasis on early attachment was also supported by another finding from the reunion weekend, reported by Englund, Levy, Hyson, and Sroufe in 2000. Within the group task at the reunion, the groups were asked to elect a spokesperson to report back to the wider group. The long-term implications of early experiences within attachment relationships were suggested by the fact that 'out of a total of 16 adolescents named spokesperson, 3 were

---

[164] Elicker, J., Englund, M., & Sroufe, L.A. (1992) Predicting peer competence and peer relationships in childhood from early parent–child relationships. In R. Parke & G. Ladd (eds) *Family–Peer Relationships: Modes of Linkage* (pp.77–106). Hillsdale, NJ: Lawrence Erlbaum, p.97.

[165] Kagan, J. (1984) *The Nature of the Child.* New York: Basic Books; Jerome Kagan interviewed by Robert Karen, 1 January 1989, cited in Karen, R. (1998) *Becoming Attached: First Relationships and How They Shape Our Capacity to Love.* Oxford: Oxford University Press: 'My view is, if you're attached, you are motivated to adopt the values of your parents. If your parent values autonomy, you'll be autonomous; if your parent values dependency, you'll be dependent' (151).

[166] Elicker, J., Englund, M., & Sroufe, L.A. (1992) Predicting peer competence and peer relationships in childhood from early parent–child relationships. In R. Parke & G. Ladd (eds) *Family–Peer Relationships: Modes of Linkage* (pp.77–106). Hillsdale, NJ: Lawrence Erlbaum, p.100.

[167] Englund, M.M., Levy, A.K., Hyson, D.M., & Sroufe, L.A. (2000) Adolescent social competence: effectiveness in a group setting. *Child Development*, 71(4), 1049–60.

[168] Sroufe, L.A., Egeland, B., & Carlson, E. (1999) One social world: the integrated development of parent–child and peer relationships. In W.A. Collins & B. Laursen (eds) *Relationships as Developmental Context: The 30th Minnesota Symposium on Child Psychology* (pp.241–62). Hillsdale, NJ: Lawrence Erlbaum, 241–62, p.256.

[169] Ibid. p.258.

classified as insecurely attached in infancy and 13 were classified as securely attached in infancy'.[170]

W. Andrew (Andy) Collins was the Director of the Minnesota Institute of Child Development from 1982. One of his particular research interests was the psychology of teenagers, and when the sample of the Minnesota Longitudinal Study of Risk and Adaptation reached this age he became heavily involved with the cohort study. At age 16 years, participants were invited back to the laboratory and participated in interviews about their dating and social lives, considered by the researchers to be key developmental challenges of midadolescence. Participants who had been in dyads classified as ambivalent/resistant in the Strange Situation were less likely than other participants to have dated, a finding Collins and Sroufe attributed to the relative emotional and social immaturity of this group. Participants who had been in dyads classified as securely attached in infancy were more likely to have had a romantic relationship that lasted at least three months.[171]

When the sample were 20–21 years old, 78 participants who were in a romantic relationship were invited to the laboratory along with their partner. Each member filled out a battery of self-report assessments of their relationship, and were also observed completing a collaborative task and discussing a touchy subject for their relationship. First publications from analysis of these data began to appear in 2001.[172] Study of the observations of the callback at 20–21 years was supported by the appointment of Jeff Simpson as a new professor at Minnesota in 2004. Simpson's background as a social psychologist in the self-report tradition of attachment research meant that he was well equipped for the study of adult romantic relationships.[173] The Minnesota group reported that infant attachment as assessed by the Strange Situation predicted several aspects of adult relationship functioning, including a robust association between infant disorganised attachment and the couple's hostility with one another ($r = .42$).[174] They found that secure infant attachment assessed by the Strange Situation was also associated with twice the rate of effective resolution of conflict among the young adults regarding the touchy subject.[175]

Other variables were also found to be very important. One concurrent factor was gender. Associations between Strange Situation classifications in infancy and the behaviour of the couple were generally stronger for men than for women. The researchers observed that male participants tended to set the tone in the collaborative task, even when female participants

[170] Englund, M.M., Levy, A.K., Hyson, D.M., & Sroufe, L.A. (2000) Adolescent social competence: effectiveness in a group setting. *Child Development*, 71(4), 1049–60, p.1056.

[171] Collins, A. & Sroufe, L.A. (1999) Capacity for intimate relationships: a developmental construction. In W. Furman, B.B. Brown, & C. Feiring (eds) (1999) *The Development of Romantic Relationships in Adolescence* (pp.125–47). New York: Cambridge University Press, p.135.

[172] Roisman, G.I., Madsen, S.D., Hennighausen, K.H., Sroufe, L.A., & Andrew Collins, W. (2001) The coherence of dyadic behavior across parent–child and romantic relationships as mediated by the internalized representation of experience. *Attachment & Human Development*, 3(2), 156–72.

[173] In historical perspective, Simpson's appointment can be regarded as an important moment for the social psychological tradition (Chapter 5) which has held substantial sway at Minnesota since the retirement of Egeland and Sroufe. Subsequently, the leaders of the Minnesota Longitudinal Study of Risk and Adaptation have been Jeff Simpson—a social psychologist—and Glenn Roisman, whose time with Chris Fraley at Illinois was influential for his attitude towards attachment methodology and theory (Chapter 3).

[174] Sroufe, L.A., Egeland, B., Carlson, E.A., & Collins, W.A. (2005) *The Development of the Person.* New York: Guilford, p.203.

[175] Salvatore, J.E., Kuo, S.I.C., Steele, R.D., Simpson, J.A., & Collins, W.A. (2011) Recovering from conflict in romantic relationships: a developmental perspective. *Psychological Science*, 22(3), 376–83.

had been confident and forthright in individual interviews.[176] Other antecedent variables were also highlighted.[177] Of particular importance was the finding by Simpson, Collins, Trans, and Haydon that the link between Strange Situation classifications and interaction with the romantic partner was partially mediated by the quality of peer relationships at school age.[178] Though their findings qualified the emphasis on continuity of Bowlby's early and populist writings, the researchers regarded their findings as confirmation of the proposal of developmental pathways from Bowlby's late theoretical writings (Chapter 1).[179] Aspects of early care remained relevant to some aspects of adult functioning, even after decades.[180] The factors proposed by the Minnesota group were of particular importance for these developmental pathways, such as emotion regulation and effective social relationships, and were also those that would suggest links to mental health. Following the centrality of mental health to Bowlby's conceptualisation of attachment and its implications, the Minnesota group gave this topic special attention.

Mental and physical health

When child participants in the cohort study reached 17 years of age, they were brought back for a detailed psychiatric interview. Other assessments were conducted at the time, including a holistic interview with the young people about their school, work, living situation, and dating life—and a parallel interview about participants with their mother.[181] If, as Slade and Holmes argued, the preschool study at Minnesota provided important support for attachment research as a paradigm in the 1990s, a parallel role was played by the findings from the psychiatric interview at age 17 in the 2000s, reported by Carlson.[182] In general, Kobak and Bosmans observed that infant attachment has ultimately been disappointing as a predictor

[176] Hennighausen, K.H. (1999) Developmental antecedents of young adult romantic relationships. Unpublished doctoral dissertation, University of Minnesota.

[177] See e.g. Madsen, S.D. & Collins, W.A. (2011) The salience of adolescent romantic experiences for romantic relationship qualities in young adulthood. *Journal of Research on Adolescence*, 21(4), 789–801; Labella, M.H., Johnson, W.F., Martin, J., et al. (2018) Multiple dimensions of childhood abuse and neglect prospectively predict poorer adult romantic functioning. *Personality and Social Psychology Bulletin*, 44(2), 238–51.

[178] Simpson, J.A., Collins, W.A., Tran, S., & Haydon, K.C. (2007) Attachment and the experience and expression of emotions in romantic relationships: a developmental perspective. *Journal of Personality and Social Psychology*, 92(2), 355–67. The mediational account has, however, later been criticised by Gillath and colleagues. Reviewing findings from other cohort studies, they argued that the model presented by Simpson and colleagues underestimates the extent to which early attachment experiences provide scaffolding for the quality of peer relationships. The quality of peer relationships is therefore not an independent intervening variable. Gillath, O., Karantzas, G.C., & Fraley, R.C. (2016) *Adult Attachment: A Concise Introduction to Theory and Research*. London: Academic Press, p.69.

[179] Van Ryzin, M.J., Carlson, E.A., & Sroufe, L.A (2011) Attachment discontinuity in a high-risk sample. *Attachment & Human Development*, 13(4), 381–401, p.397.

[180] In a later meta-analysis based on 80 independent samples (N = 4441), Groh and colleagues found a robust association between attachment security with mother and peer competence (d = .39). The association was of the same strength no matter how long after the attachment assessment peer competence was measured: there was no moderation by age, suggesting effects were enduring. Groh, A.M., Fearon, R.P., Bakermans-Kranenburg, M.J., van IJzendoorn, M.H., Steele, R.D., & Roisman, G.I. (2014) The significance of attachment security for children's social competence with peers: a meta-analytic study. *Attachment & Human Development*, 16(2), 103–136, p.128.

[181] https://innovation.umn.edu/parent-child/wp-content/uploads/sites/35/2018/08/M001-List-of-Measures.pdf.

[182] Carlson, E.A. (1998) A prospective longitudinal study of attachment disorganization/disorientation. *Child Development*, 69(4), 1107–28.

of adult mental health, with 'lack of specificity and relatively small effect sizes'.[183] However, Carlson's report helped to support the idea that early attachment as measured by the Strange Situation does play a distinct and important role, even if this role is of less magnitude than Bowlby tended to suggest. In line with the general preference at Minnesota for composite measures, Carlson treated the psychiatric interview as a measure of overall mental health, coded on a seven-point scale. She did not differentiate by kind of mental health problem. She found that infant avoidant attachment, infant disorganised attachment, middle childhood behaviour problems, and poor observed child–parent boundaries at age 13 each made an independent contribution to total mental health problems at age 17, together accounting for a third of the variance.

In the past few years, meta-analytic research has led several senior figures in the developmental tradition of attachment research to query the conclusion drawn by Carlson, and taken by her readers, that Strange Situation classifications are associated with general mental health problems. Meta-analytic work indicated that infant avoidant and disorganised attachment in the Strange Situation tended to be much more associated with externalising problems, and less with internalising problems such as anxiety or depression.[184] In fact, Carlson was not actually *intending* to make the specific claim that avoidant and disorganised attachment would be generally associated with all mental ill health[185]—though technically this is what she reported and what readers naturally understood. Instead, her report was based on the Minnesota creed of using composite measures, especially for pioneering work, with the expectation that later researchers would pursue differentiation.[186] Today, the question of whether the Strange Situation predicts primarily externalising problems remains an area of ongoing discussion among researchers, not least since several phenomena of clinical concern (e.g. PTSD, ADHD) are poorly captured by the division between externalising and internalising mental health issues.[187]

As well as studying prospective links between the Strange Situation and general mental health at age 17, building on the ideas of Main and colleagues (Chapter 3) Carlson conducted a hypothesis-driven analysis of associations with dissociative symptoms. She found that infant avoidant attachment, infant disorganised attachment, and middle childhood behaviour problems made independent contributions, and together accounted for 17% of the symptoms. Infant disorganised attachment and child abuse also made independent contributions to later self-injurious behaviour and other symptoms of borderline personality disorder. The association between the Strange Situation classifications and later borderline symptoms was

[183] Kobak, R. & Bosmans, G. (2018) Attachment and psychopathology: a dynamic model of the insecure cycle, *Current Opinion in Psychology*, 25, 76–80, p.76.

[184] Groh, A.M., Fearon, R.P., van IJzendoorn, M.H., Bakermans-Kranenburg, M.J., & Roisman, G.I. (2017) Attachment in the early life course: meta-analytic evidence for its role in socioemotional development. *Child Development Perspectives*, 11(1), 70–76.

[185] Betty Carlson, personal communication, May 2019.

[186] Though not discussed in the paper, in Table 5 Carlson presented findings from teacher report of participants suggesting that disorganised attachment was associated weakly with internalising problems in elementary and high school ($r = .19, .18$), and had no association with externalising problems. Carlson, E.A. (1998) A prospective longitudinal study of attachment disorganization/disorientation. *Child Development*, 69(4), 1107–28, Table 5. The findings may be the product of chance. However, it is conceivable that the distinctive predominance of child neglect in the Minnesota sample compared to other studies may have played a role in these results running contrary to later meta-analyses of samples.

[187] See e.g. Jacobvitz, D., Hazen, N., Zaccagnino, M., Messina, S., & Beverung, L. (2011) Frightening maternal behavior, infant disorganization, and risks for psychopathology. In D. Cicchetti & G.I. Roisman (eds) *The Origins and Organization of Adaptation and Maladaptation: The Minnesota Symposia on Child Psychology*, Vol. 36 (pp.283–322). Hoboken, NJ: Wiley.

mediated by responses to the family drawing task at age eight and interview measures of representations of the self and key relationships (including the 'friendship interview') in early adolescence.[188]

Another paper by the Minnesota group reported findings that infant ambivalent/resistant attachment was distinctively associated with anxiety problems in adolescence ($r = .26$), even controlling for maternal anxiety and child temperament, but had no other links to mental illness.[189] This was important in providing a source of prospective validity for the category. Following Main (Chapter 3), Sroufe proposed that the infant ambivalent/resistant attachment pattern entails a strategy of hypervigilance and hyperattentiveness regarding the availability of the caregiver: 'Such a stance may be adaptive in insuring contact with the caregiver when there is a genuine threat, but a price is paid for such chronic wariness and vigilance.'[190] However, attempts to replicate the finding of a link between infant ambivalent/resistant attachment and later anxiety problems have failed, at least when observational and interview measures have been used.[191]

Another finding that ran contrary to expectations was a report by the Minnesota group using a composite of Strange Situation classifications and measures of early caregiving. The researchers examined the association of this composite with depression at age 17, anticipating based on available theory that insecure attachment and early care would both be robust predictors of later depression.[192] Yet Duggal, Carlson, Sroufe, and Egeland reported in 2001 that in the Minnesota study the composite accounted for only 3% of variance, controlling for maternal depression. Furthermore, it lost significance entirely in a regression once account was taken of the amount of support from family and friends the mother received in the child's first five years. By contrast, prospectively documented child abuse remained significant in predicting depression: together, maternal social support and documented child abuse accounted for 19% of variance in adolescent depression.[193] However, intriguingly,

[188] Carlson, E.A., Egeland, B., & Sroufe, L.A. (2009) A prospective investigation of the development of borderline personality symptoms. *Development & Psychopathology*, 21(4), 1311–34. A later study by Lyons-Ruth and colleagues found only a marginal association between infant disorganised attachment and later self-injurious behaviours, but there was a marked relationship between maternal withdrawing behaviours in response to child distress, forms of disorganised attachment that entailed approaching the caregiver, and suicidality in early adulthood. Lyons-Ruth, K., Bureau, J.F., Holmes, B., Easterbrooks, A., & Brooks, N.H. (2013) Borderline symptoms and suicidality/self-injury in late adolescence: prospectively observed relationship correlates in infancy and childhood. *Psychiatry Research*, 206(2–3), 273–81.

[189] Warren, S.L., Huston, L., Egeland, B., & Sroufe, L.A. (1997) Child and adolescent anxiety disorders and early attachment. *Journal of the American Academy of Child & Adolescent Psychiatry*, 36(5), 637–44.

[190] Sroufe, L.A. (2005) Attachment and development: a prospective, longitudinal study from birth to adulthood. *Attachment & Human Development*, 7(4), 349–67, p.361.

[191] Groh, A.M., Roisman, G.I., van IJzendoorn, M.H., Bakermans-Kranenburg, M.J., & Fearon, R.P. (2012) The significance of insecure and disorganized attachment for children's internalizing symptoms: a meta-analytic study. *Child Development*, 83(2), 591–610; Madigan, S., Atkinson, L., Laurin, K., & Benoit, D. (2013) Attachment and internalizing behavior in early childhood: a meta-analysis. *Developmental Psychology*, 49(4), 672–89. In contrast, a positive association ($r = .37$) between resistant attachment and anxiety has been reported when self-report measures of anxiety are included in the meta-analysis: Colonnesi, C., Draijer, E.M., Jan, J.M., et al. (2011) The relation between insecure attachment and child anxiety: a meta-analytic review. *Journal of Clinical Child and Adolescent Psychology*, 40, 630–45. This would suggest that one of the distinct sequelae of resistant attachment is participant *report* of anxiety symptoms on self-report measures, perhaps as a consequence of a maximising strategy (Chapter 5).

[192] E.g. Cicchetti, D. & Schneider-Rosen, K. (1986) An organizational approach to childhood depression. In M. Rutter, C. Izard, & P. Read (eds) *Depression in Young People: Clinical and Developmental Perspectives* (pp.71–134). New York: Guilford.

[193] Duggal, S., Carlson, E.A., Sroufe, L.A., & Egeland, B. (2001) Depressive symptomatology in childhood and adolescence. *Development & Psychopathology*, 13(1), 143–64. The finding that insecure attachment does not predict later depression after taking into account maternal social support ran too far contrary to expectations, and has generally been ignored by subsequent researchers who have continued to treat insecure childhood attachment as a

more recently when the sample were followed up to adulthood, symptoms of depression were more likely to remit among those participants who had been in a secure attachment relationship as infants.[194] Early attachment relationships may play less of a role in predisposing or triggering depression than in stabilising symptoms.

Somewhat better specificity and greater effect sizes were seen with respect to responses to trauma. Enlow, Egeland, and colleagues reported an analysis of PTSD symptoms in data from the adolescent psychiatric interview. Rates of PTSD were doubled for dyads where mothers were assessed as showing emotional neglect/psychological unavailability.[195] There was no association between Strange Situation classifications and later traumatic experiences per se.[196] However, for those participants with insecure attachment relationships who did experience later trauma, there was a dose-response relationship with PTSD symptoms: 12% of infants in dyads classified as secure at both 12 and 18 months in the Strange Situation developed PTSD following trauma exposure; 28% received the diagnosis when assessed as belonging to an insecure dyad in either the 12- or 18-month Strange Situation; and 46% had PTSD in adolescence following trauma exposure if they had an insecure attachment relationship at both 12 and 18 months.[197] Disorganised infant attachment appeared to make no additional contribution beyond insecurity.

Sroufe, Carlson, Levy, and Egeland also reported findings regarding the respective contribution of Strange Situation classifications and middle childhood behaviour problems to later mental health. Children with a history of secure attachment relationships who showed few conduct problems at school had the lowest scores for mental illness. Children with a history of insecure attachment relationships who showed significant conduct problems at school had the very highest scores for mental illness, and the lowest scores for their education and social relationships. The researchers reported, however, that children with a mixed history (secure attachment and later behaviour problems; or insecure attachment and later positive functioning) had equivalent scores. They were likewise functioning at an equivalent level in their education and social relationships. Sroufe and colleagues concluded that children who were struggling in middle childhood but who had a secure attachment relationship in infancy 'drew upon a more positive foundation', which accounted for their better outcomes than their peers with insecure infant attachment relationships.[198]

In educational research in the 1990s, adolescent conduct problems and poor achievement were identified as cardinal predictors of young people dropping out of school. The Minnesota Longitudinal Study of Risk and Adaptation was unusual in being able to examine

---

cause of depression in adult caregiers. See e.g. Toth, S.L., Rogosch, F.A., & Cicchetti, D. (2008) Attachment-theory informed intervention and reflective functioning in depressed mothers. In H. Steele & M. Steele (eds) *The Adult Attachment Interview in Clinical Context* (pp.154–72). New York: Guilford: 'Retrospective studies have found that depressed adults report histories replete with inadequate or abusive care. Thus insecure childhood attachment relationships may contribute to mothers' depression' (155). It is possible, however, that there are two different diagnostic entities in play. Duggal and colleagues were reporting on depressive symptoms; Toth and colleagues were discussing major depressive disorder.

[194] Sroufe, L.A., Coffino, B., & Carlson, E.A. (2010) Conceptualizing the role of early experience: lessons from the Minnesota longitudinal study. *Developmental Review*, 30(1), 36–51, p.45.

[195] Sroufe, L.A., Egeland, B., Carlson, E.A., & Collins, W. A. (2005) *The Development of the Person.* New York: Guilford, p.249.

[196] Enlow, M.B., Egeland, B., Carlson, E., Blood, E., & Wright, R.J. (2014) Mother–infant attachment and the intergenerational transmission of posttraumatic stress disorder. *Development & Psychopathology*, 26(01), 41–65.

[197] Ibid. p.54.

[198] Sroufe, L.A., Carlson, E.A., Levy, A.K., & Egeland, B. (1999) Implications of attachment theory for developmental psychopathology. *Development & Psychopathology*, 11(1), 1–13, p.8.

this question prospectively, including variables from early childhood. A regression analysis indicated that the child's gender, the degree of chaos in the early home environment, and a composite of infant attachment and caregiver sensitivity could predict 77% of children who had dropped out of school by age 16. When these variables were included, more proximal variables such as truancy, disciplinary problems, and failing grades in high school were no longer significant. The same was true for peer rejection, conduct problems, and low school achievement. As such, Jimerson, Egeland, Sroufe, and Carlson concluded that 'many established "predictors" may be better conceptualized as markers of presence on the pathway', leading from early caregiving to dropping out of school. The reason for this, they argued, is that 'success in school calls upon numerous capacities for self-regulation that begin to be formed in the early years'.[199] Raby and colleagues, in fact, later documented that early maternal sensitivity predicted academic achievement by adulthood at least as well as it predicted social competence, controlling for covariates such as maternal education and socioeconomic status.[200] The picture is complicated, unsurprisingly, by the fact that experiences of education have a bidirectional relationship with development. Englund, Egeland, and Collins elsewhere documented that developmental outcomes could be altered, for some children, by their experience of the school itself.[201] As we saw in Chapter 2, Ainsworth anticipated that feelings of security in different domains would influence each other. And Bowlby specifically identified that a school may serve attachment functions for a young person.[202]

Though social psychologists had pursued research on the topic for over a decade,[203] in the 2010s the relationship between attachment and physical health outcomes was heralded as a 'new frontier' for developmental attachment research.[204] Puig, Englund, Simpson, and Collins examined the links between early attachment and later medically unexplained or 'non-specific' symptoms at age 32, controlling for a variety of covariates including adult socioeconomic status, life stress, and social support. Individuals who had been part of ambivalent/resistant dyads in infancy as assessed in the Strange Situation were three times more likely to report symptoms such as dizzy spells, headaches, skin trouble, back ache, and indigestion than those adults who had been part of secure dyads. They were also six times more likely to report physical health conditions. Individuals who had been part of avoidantly attached dyads in infancy were three times more likely than those from secure dyads to report inflammation-related illnesses such as heart disease, high blood pressure, and asthma. Participants who were part of dyads classified as secure at both 12 months and 18 months reported the fewest physical illnesses in adulthood compared to those who were part of dyads classified as insecure at one or both assessments.

---

[199] Jimerson, S., Egeland, B., Sroufe, L.A., & Carlson, B. (2000) A prospective longitudinal study of high school dropouts examining multiple predictors across development. *Journal of School Psychology*, 38(6), 525–49, p.544.

[200] Raby, K.L., Roisman, G.I., Fraley, R.C., & Simpson, J.A. (2015) The enduring predictive significance of early maternal sensitivity: social and academic competence through age 32 years. *Child Development*, 86(3), 695–708.

[201] Englund, M.M., Egeland, B., & Collins, W.A. (2008) Exceptions to high school dropout predictions in a low-income sample: do adults make a difference? *Journal of Social Issues*, 64(1), 77–94.

[202] Bowlby, J. (1969, 1982) *Attachment*. London: Penguin, p.207. The potential for school to serve as a secure base has been elaborated by Geddes, H. (2006) *Attachment in the Classroom: A Practical Guide for Schools*. London: Worth Publishing.

[203] For a review see Pietromonaco, P.R. & Beck, L.A. (2019) Adult attachment and physical health. *Current Opinion in Psychology*, 25, 115–20.

[204] Cassidy, J. (2015) Early relationships, later functioning: why and how a secure base matters. Keynote address presented at 7th International Attachment Conference, New York; Ehrlich, K.B. & Cassidy, J. (2019) Attachment and physical health: introduction to the special issue. *Attachment & Human Development*, 21(1), 1–4.

The researchers proposed that caregiver provision of a secure base and safe haven in the context of stable routines offers an external source of biological, as well as psychological, regulation. Insensitive care may heighten stress reactivity across the lifespan, inscribed on the body in the form of 'non-specific' symptoms like headaches, skin trouble, and back ache, where physical and psychological stress together may contribute to symptom development and maintenance over time. Conversely, sensitive care may reduce stress reactivity across the lifespan, leading to fewer non-specific symptoms and fewer symptoms relating to the human inflammatory response, which is activated by alarming or threatening experiences.[205] This hypothesis has been confirmed by other findings from the Minnesota group showing that assessments of maternal sensitivity blocked the association between stressful life events and physical ill health, and also predicted a lower body-mass index and fewer physical symptoms for participants with fewer stressful life events.[206] Also relevant to this hypothesis were findings that child neglect contributed to adult physical health according to both self-report measures of physical symptoms and biomarkers of cardiometabolic risk.[207]

The study of attachment and health has been an exciting area of research in the social psychological tradition over the past decade.[208] It seems likely that investigation of the implications of attachment for physical health is likely to be a growth area over the coming years in the developmental tradition, pursuing the pioneering and striking findings from Minnesota.[209] This will be facilitated by the collection of genetic data from the cohort. It will also be facilitated by the fact that a number of new large cohort studies were initiated in the 2000s in Europe with a rich array of measures of physical health. For example, the Generation R cohort study in the Netherlands includes Strange Situation procedures with 900 infants, a number of observational measures of parent and child behaviour, and a vast array of assessments of physical health over the subsequent decade, as well as genetic information on the sample.[210] The prospect of new integrations between attachment research and biological and medical research using the Minnesota Longitudinal Study of Risk and Adaptation and other cohort studies seems not only possible, but likely.

Another area where future reports are to be expected is on three-generational processes. The Minnesota group recently followed up the grandchildren of the original women recruited to the sample. Strange Situation procedures were conducted with these grandchildren. Raby, Steele, Carlson, and Sroufe found little evidence of intergenerational continuities in attachment security. One pattern in the data was that mothers who had themselves had insecure attachment relationships in the 1970s but who formed secure attachment relationships with their own infant had higher-quality concurrent support from family and friends. Though

---

[205] Puig, J., Englund, M.M., Simpson, J.A., & Collins, W.A. (2013) Predicting adult physical illness from infant attachment: a prospective longitudinal study. *Health Psychology*, 32(4), 409–417.

[206] Farrell, A.K., Simpson, J.A., Carlson, E.A., Englund, M.M., & Sung, S. (2017) The impact of stress at different life stages on physical health and the buffering effects of maternal sensitivity. *Health Psychology*, 36(1), 35–44; see also Farrell, A.K., Waters, T.E.A., Young, E.S., et al. (2019) Early maternal sensitivity, attachment security in young adulthood, and cardiometabolic risk at midlife. *Attachment & Human Development*, 21(1), 70–86.

[207] Johnson, W.F., Huelsnitz, C.O., Carlson, E.A., et al. (2017) Childhood abuse and neglect and physical health at midlife: prospective, longitudinal evidence. *Development & Psychopathology*, 29(5), 1935–46.

[208] Pietromonaco, P.R. & Beck, L.A. (2019) Adult attachment and physical health. *Current Opinion in Psychology*, 25, 115–20.

[209] Ehrlich, K.B. & Cassidy, J. (2019) Attachment and physical health: introduction to the special issue. *Attachment & Human Development*, 21(1), 1–4.

[210] E.g. Windhorst, D.A., Mileva-Seitz, V.R., Linting, M., et al. (2015) Differential susceptibility in a developmental perspective: DRD4 and maternal sensitivity predicting externalizing behavior. *Developmental Psychobiology*, 57(1), 35–49.

there was little continuity between generations in security or insecurity in general, there was specifically substantial continuity in disorganised infant attachment: half of the mothers who had been part of dyads that received a classification of disorganised attachment in the 1970s had children who received the same classification. This was in contrast to only 20% of dyads where the mother had no history of an infant disorganised attachment classification.[211]

Dissociation

For Sroufe, an individual's experience of 'self' was best conceptualised as an emergent organisation, constituted through the routine integration of cognition, emotion, and behaviour. Within this organisation, the whirring clockwork that sustains ordinary adaptation is assembled out of both historical and contemporary machinery. Earlier components are incorporated into later behavioural systems and may remain accessible. This produces the strange and uneven inner space of thoughts and feelings characteristic of human experience, as well as contributing to the way that our own behaviour has the capacity to surprise or disconcert us. Sroufe's emphasis, however, was above all on the coherence of the assemblage of components, an expression of his methodological principle of holism.[212] He regarded this constituted organisation as experientially stabilised by memory processes, which register continuities in an individual's qualities and capacities across contexts and relationships.[213] Nonetheless, memory, expectations, and images of the value of the self in the eyes of others can become a facet of self-monitoring and a guide for behaviour, filtering the meaning of later social experiences. Experiences in relationships, in turn, contribute to the further stabilisation or reorganisation of the inner organisation: 'the self was forged within vital relationships; within such relationships, it continues to evolve'.[214]

The identification of selfhood with organisation over the course of development contributed to the special attention given by Sroufe and colleagues to dissociative symptoms. In *Defences that Follow Loss,* Bowlby had situated dissociation as a form of defensive exclusion, a psychological process that blocked episodic information about the perception of events in time and space from reaching and activating a behavioural system (Chapter 1). It was a 'particular sort of segregating process', and in this had elements in common with attachment avoidance, even if Bowlby believed that the two were distinguishable.[215] However, Bowlby did not publish his speculations on dissociation. Though he had Robertson's qualitative observations, he lacked the data to press further. Writing in 1996, Egeland and Susman-Stillman

---

[211] Raby, K.L., Steele, R.D., Carlson, E.A., & Sroufe, L.A. (2015) Continuities and changes in infant attachment patterns across two generations. *Attachment & Human Development,* 17(4), 414–28.

[212] Sroufe, L.A. & Rutter, M. (1984) The domain of developmental psychopathology. *Child Development,* 17–29, p.20. Holism is listed top of the list of principles governing any true developmental perspective; Sroufe, L.A. (1996) *Emotional Development.* Cambridge: Cambridge University Press, p.8. On the history of holism within psychology see Shelley, C. (2008) Jan Smuts and personality theory: the problem of holism in psychology. In R. Diriwächter & J. Valsiner (eds) *Striving for the Whole: Creating Theoretical Syntheses* (pp.89–109). New Brunswick: Transaction Publishers.

[213] Sroufe, L.A. (1990) An organizational perspective on the self. In D. Cicchetti & M. Beeghly (eds) *The Self in Transition: Infancy to Childhood* (pp.281–307). Chicago: University of Chicago Press: 'The self should be conceived as an inner *organisation* of attitudes, feelings, expectations and meanings, which arises itself from an *organised* caregiving matrix (a dyadic *organisation* that exists prior to the emergence of the self) and which has *organisational* significance for ongoing adaptation and experience. The self is *organisation.* It arises from *organisation.* It influences ongoing *organisation* of experience' (281).

[214] Ibid. p.303.

[215] Bowlby, J. (1962) Defences that follow loss: causation and function. PP/Bow/D.3/78.

acknowledged that, in the wake of Bowlby's threadbare published comments, 'there is some confusion over the relation of attachment and dissociation'.[216]

The Minnesota group included questions relevant to child dissociative symptoms in twelve different assessments made by mothers and teachers, the first in kindergarten and the last at 16 years. At age 19, the 168 participants remaining in the study provided self-report of their own experiences of dissociative symptoms on the Carlson and Putnam Dissociative Experiences Scale.[217] Mothers were asked about potential traumatic life events experienced by their child during the 12, 18, 30, 42, 48, 54, and 64 month assessments and when their child was 19 years old. At 19 years, participants themselves were also asked to complete this assessment. Ogawa, Sroufe, and colleagues found that in preschool, dissociative symptoms were predicted well by neglect in infancy.[218] In elementary school, 27% of variance in children's dissociative symptoms was predicted by their mother's experience of abuse as a child, physical abuse experienced by the child, and avoidant attachment in the Strange Situation. In both preschool and elementary school, the child's IQ made a small negative contribution to the score. In adolescence, the best predictor of dissociative symptoms was avoidant attachment assessed in the Strange Situation. Additional contributions were made by exposure to domestic violence in infancy, disorganised attachment as assessed in the Strange Situation, and experiences of physical abuse in adolescence. Together these variables accounted for 19% of variance in dissociative symptoms. At age 19, 30% of variance in dissociation could be accounted for by only three variables, all from infancy: caregiver psychological unavailability, infant disorganised attachment, and maternal-report measures of infant distractibility and attention-span. Psychological unavailability in infancy alone accounted for 19% of variance. It was curious that, besides infant attachment, the 19-year assessment was predicted so powerfully by two variables that had previously not proven relevant, both from infancy. However, it should be noted that the 19-year assessment was a self-report of dissociative symptoms by the young persons themselves, whereas previous waves had been maternal or teacher report.

Ogawa, Sroufe, and colleagues also examined factors that predicted dissociative symptoms in the clinical range, participants with high but not clinical levels of symptoms, and participants with few symptoms. In preschool, they found that infant neglect predicted symptoms in the clinical range, whereas witnessing domestic violence and parental psychological unavailability predicted high but not clinical levels of symptoms. The two groups were quite distinct in terms of their antecedents. Witnessing domestic violence was also associated with high but not clinical levels of symptoms in elementary school. Symptoms in the clinical range were differentially predicted by neglect in infancy, infant disorganised attachment in the Strange Situation, and concurrent physical abuse experienced by the school-aged child. In adolescence, the clinical group was distinguished strongly by infant avoidant and infant disorganised attachment in infancy. High but not clinical levels of symptoms were predicted by concurrent physical abuse. In early adulthood, the clinical group was distinguished from the others on the basis of maternal psychological unavailability in infancy and

[216] Egeland, B. & Susman-Stillman, A. (1996) Dissociation as a mediator of child abuse across generations. *Child Abuse & Neglect*, 20(11), 1123–32, p.1129. The work by Main and Hesse offering the most sustained attention to these issues remained published only in Italian (Chapter 3).

[217] Carlson, E.B. & Putnam, F.W. (1993) An update on the Dissociative Experiences Scale. *Dissociation*, 6, 16–27.

[218] Ogawa, J.R., Sroufe, L.A., Weinfield, N.S., Carlson, E.A., & Egeland, B. (1997) Development and the fragmented self: longitudinal study of dissociative symptomatology in a nonclinical sample. *Development & Psychopathology*, 9(4), 855–79, p.874.

disorganised attachment in the Strange Situation. The authors interpreted their data as suggesting two pathways. A first pathway was to clinical levels of dissociation, based to a surprising degree on experiences in infancy. These include experiences of neglect in infancy, and of avoidant and disorganised attachment. In fact, 'an examination of the zero-order correlations between disorganized attachment and dissociation at each time period reveals a linear trend with a positive slope (Time 2 $r = .14$, n.s.; Time 3 $r = .20$ $p < .05$; Time 4 $r = .25$ $p < .01$; Time 5 $r = .35$ $p < .001$)'.[219] A separate analysis was run which found that disorganised infant attachment alone marginally elevated dissociative symptoms in early adulthood, but that disorganised attachment and the experience of at least one form of trauma had a strong link to dissociative symptoms ($F[2, 125] = 12.0, p < .001$).[220]

The second pathway was to subclinical but substantial levels of dissociative symptoms. This pathway was predicted by concurrent physical abuse, and tended to stop once the participants reached the greater independence of young adulthood. Ogawa, Sroufe, and colleagues concluded that 'psychopathological dissociation should not be viewed as the top end of a continuum of dissociative symptomatology, but as a separate taxon'.[221] However, they highlighted that avoidant attachment appeared to make an independent and robust contribution to dissociative symptoms, except to the participant self-report measure. Whereas dissociation reduces environmental responsiveness by blocking a form of perception, avoidance retains awareness of the environment whilst bracing against the attachment system, directing attention away from cues that might activate it (Chapter 1). Nonetheless, Ogawa, Sroufe, and colleagues reflected that the contribution of infant attachment to later observed dissociative symptoms perhaps lies in the fact that avoidance may at times shade into dissociative processes, or may predispose a vulnerability to dissociation. Nonetheless, the lack of correlation between avoidance and self-report of dissociation required explanation. The Minnesota group drew on Bowlby's published reflections to speculate that avoidant attachment as a strategy of defensive exclusion may be more mature in young adulthood, in the context of cognitive maturation and social independence, allowing the strategy to work more effectively, with less 'leakage' in the form of dissociation. It might also be supposed that avoidant attachment strategies could suppress awareness and/or reporting of dissociative symptoms.

Giovanni Liotti had proposed that infant neglect and avoidant and disorganised attachment may all have in common that they disrupt the early integrative processes that pull together behavioural systems (Chapter 3).[222] Building on these ideas from Liotti, Carlson, Yates, and Sroufe suggested that dissociation may be regarded as a strategy of self-regulation in the face of threat, where such integration has been poor, and where the caregiver cannot be approached directly to offer a safe haven and an external source of integration.[223] Experiences of domestic violence and physical abuse that a child cannot escape are liable to cause some dissociative symptoms, as a strategy developed for the purposes of

[219] Ibid.
[220] Ibid. p.868.
[221] Ibid. p.855.
[222] Liotti, G. (1992) Disorganized/disoriented attachment in the etiology of the dissociative disorders. *Dissociation*, 5, 196–204.
[223] Carlson, E.A., Yates, T.M., & Sroufe, L.A. (2009) Development of dissociation and development of the self. In P.F. Dell & J.A. O'Neil (eds) *Dissociation and the Dissociative Disorders: DSM-V and Beyond* (pp.39–52). New York: Routledge: 'The process of dissociation, which begins as a protective mechanism to promote the integrity of the self in the face of trauma, may directly threaten optimal functioning when employed routinely or pervasively' (47).

self-regulation. However, clinical levels of symptoms are more likely when the need for this strategy occurs in infancy, since it may be used pervasively in the absence of other strategies and because infancy may be a period of special importance for the formation of behavioural systems and psychological coherence. This might account for the interaction between trauma and disorganised attachment. Traumatic events are those that can be anticipated to overwhelm established coping strategies. They may therefore be a catalyst for dissociative symptoms for those children who were unable to lay a solid foundation for integration and emotion regulation in infancy.[224]

More recently, Haltigan and Roisman reported findings from the NICHD Study of Early Child Care and Youth Development of 1,149 families.[225] Dissociative symptoms were assessed by mothers at six time-points and by teachers at three time-points between age 4 and age 15. Participants themselves reported symptoms at age 15. The researchers found no evidence that infants from dyads classified as disorganised in the Strange Situation later showed dissociative symptoms. Infants from dyads classified as avoidant did have elevated dissociative symptoms as rated by their teachers and mothers, though not in their self-report. Haltigan and Roisman commented that 'the claim that infant attachment disorganization represents a unique risk factor for the development of dissociative symptomatology has been given much attention and cachet in the literature, perhaps because of a theoretical account that provides an especially compelling rationale for this association. That said, the bedrock of science is the replicability of its findings.'[226] Given that the NICHD study is a community-risk sample, and the Minnesota sample was selected specifically on the basis of adversities, Haltigan and Roisman raised the prospect that infant disorganised attachment may contribute to later dissociative symptoms in interaction with severe or chronic trauma. A link might be drawn here with Main's prediction (Chapter 3) that infant disorganised attachment will usually resolve by adulthood unless the basis of the disorganisation lies directly in child maltreatment.[227] Most researchers have, however, responded by ignoring the Haltigan and Roisman study, which remains relatively comparatively cited four years after its publication. There has been informal discussion of whether the NICHD sample was coded effectively for disorganisation, given that the classification does not predict well in this cohort study. However, a further possibility, one with quite serious implications for attachment research, is that the forms of disorganised attachment may differ between high-risk and low-risk samples (Chapter 3). These questions will likely be resolved over the coming years as more recent cohort studies enter adolescence and adulthood, if funds can be secured for later follow-up and measures are used to assess dissociative symptoms.

[224] Ibid. p.43. For aligned reflections by other attachment researchers see also Schuder, M. & Lyons-Ruth, K. (2004) 'Hidden trauma' in infancy: attachment, fearful arousal, and early dysfunction of the stress response system. In J. Osofsky (ed.) *Young Children and Trauma* (pp.69–104). New York: Guilford; Liotti, G. (2004) Trauma, dissociation, and disorganized attachment: three strands of a single braid. *Psychotherapy: Theory, Research, Practice, Training*, 41(4), 472.

[225] Haltigan, J.D. & Roisman, G.I. (2015) Infant attachment insecurity and dissociative symptomatology: findings from the NICHD Study of Early Child Care and Youth Development. *Infant Mental Health Journal*, 36(1), 30–41.

[226] Ibid. p.8.

[227] Main, M. (1995) Recent studies in attachment: overview, with selected implications for clinical work. In S. Goldberg, R. Muir, & J. Kerr (eds) *Attachment Theory: Social, Developmental and Clinical Perspectives* (pp.407–470). Hillsdale, NJ: Analytic Press: 'So long as direct maltreatment is not involved, many, perhaps most, are expected to have become "organised" by adulthood, being either secure, dismissing or preoccupied' (454).

Developmental psychopathology

The domain of developmental psychopathology

The work of Sroufe and Egeland was fundamental to the emergence of developmental psychopathology, as a movement within developmental psychology.[228] In turn, developmental psychopathology has supported the continuation of attachment theory as a significant reference-point within contemporary developmental psychology. An important part of the legacy of the Minnesota Longitudinal Study and of Sroufe and Egeland as attachment researchers is therefore revealed through consideration of the rise of developmental psychopathology.

Though based on earlier ideas,[229] the movement was initiated primarily by a conference hosted by Norman Garmezy and Michael Rutter at the Center for Advanced Study in Behavioral Sciences at Stanford from 1979 to 1980.[230] The conference was sponsored by the William T. Grant Foundation, as part of a growing public and policy concern about child abuse and maltreatment, contributing to an increased availability of research funds in this area.[231] The meeting was prompted especially by findings from high-risk longitudinal studies set up around specific diagnostic entities such as schizophrenia that nonetheless highlighted the role of poverty, contextual risks and conflictual family relationships in the prediction of a variety of mental health outcomes for individuals and across generations.[232] The compounding of adversities seemed to be much more predictive than any 'main effect' from imputed single causes. The researchers' concerns were also galvanised by interest in the potential role of individual and social protective factors in buffering risks faced by individuals and families.[233] Garmezy and Rutter drew on the term 'resilience' in conceptualising

---

[228] Masten, A.S. (2006) Developmental psychopathology: pathways to the future. *International Journal of Behavioral Development*, 30(1), 47–54; Cicchetti, D. (2013) An overview of developmental psychopathology. In P. Zelazo (ed.) *Oxford Handbook of Developmental Psychology* (pp.455–80). Oxford: Oxford University Press.

[229] The movement took its name from Achenbach's 1974 book *Developmental Psychopathology* (New York: Ronald Press). A former trainee of Norman Garmezy at Minnesota, in his book Achenbach argued that classifications of adult mental disorder should not be imposed backward on childhood. Achenbach called for a new paradigm thinking about mental health in a way commensurate with developmental processes. Cicchetti reviewed other precursors in Cicchetti, D. (1990) A historical perspective on the discipline of developmental psychopathology. In J. Rolf, A. Masten, D. Cicchetti, K. Nuechterlein, & S. Weintraub (eds) *Risk and Protective Factors in the Development of Psychopathology* (pp.2–28). New York: Cambridge University Press.

[230] There were a number of other relevant meetings at the time, such as the High Risk Consortium, San Juan, Puerto Rico, 11–13 March 1980; and the 15th Annual Minnesota Symposium on Child Development, Minneapolis, 30 October–1 November 1980. See W.A. Collins (ed.) *The Concept of Development: The Minnesota Symposia on Child Psychology*, Vol. 15. Hillsdale, NJ: Lawrence Erlbaum. In-person meetings of the movement would be supported by subsequent annual Minnesota Symposia, and also the Rochester Symposia on Developmental Psychopathology which were initiated in 1987 by Cicchetti.

[231] Other key sources of funding that supported the emergence of developmental psychopathology included the National Center on Child Abuse and Neglect, which was founded in 1974, and the National Institute of Mental Health in the 1980s.

[232] Garmezy, N. (1971) Vulnerability research and the issue of primary prevention. *American Journal of Orthopsychiatry*, 41, 101–116; Garmezy, N. (1974) Children at risk: the search for the antecedents of schizophrenia. Part I. Conceptual models and research methods. *Schizophrenia Bulletin*, 1(8), 14–90; Rutter, M. & Quinton, D. (1984) Parental psychiatric disorder: effects on children. *Psychological Medicine*, 14(4), 853–80.

[233] Rutter, M. (1979) Protective factors in children's responses to stress and disadvantage. In M.W. Kent & J.E. Rolf (eds) *Primary Prevention of Psychopathology, Vol. 3: Social Competence in Children*. Hanover: University Press of New England.

this process.[234] The proceedings of the Stanford conference were published by Garmezy and Rutter as *Stress, Coping, and Development in Children* in 1983.[235]

Also in 1983, Sameroff proposed the dual-risk model of psychopathology, in which the particular role of multicausal models of cumulative risk factors was highlighted in the role of mental illness.[236] Emergent longitudinal findings appeared to show that any one risk factor had little association with later disturbance. What seemed to be critical was the combination of liabilities and supports. Additionally, in his 1983 chapter, Sameroff began to sketch the ideas that would later form his distinction between 'protective' supports and 'promotive' support for development, the former contributing to beneficial stability and the latter contributing to thriving.[237] Overall, this account firmly emphasised the contextual embeddedness of mental health, and the transactional relationship between different obstacles and difficulties individuals face in their lives. As mentioned above, a presentation by Sameroff of his emerging ideas prior to this publication proven influential in the choice of initial measures in the Minnesota Longitudinal Study of Risk and Adaptation.

Garmezy and Sroufe were colleagues and friends, and taught classes together at Minnesota, where there had been growing momentum around developmental approaches to mental health since the 1970s.[238] Sroufe and Rutter's 1984 article 'The domain of developmental psychopathology' was a turning-point for developmental psychopathology, as the movement resolved into an explicit and self-identified alternative paradigm for the study of mental health. Whereas the dominant medical model started from adult diagnostic

---

[234] This term was introduced to psychology from ecology by Jack Block in the 1950s to refer to a quality of individual children that allows some to flexibly return to adaptive functioning after a disturbance; 'resilience' was then transferred to the wider literature on adversity and development by Emmy Werner in the early 1970s. Block J. & Thomas, H. (1955) Is satisfaction with self a measure of adjustment? *Journal of Abnormal and Social Psychology*, 51(2), 254–9; Werner, E.E., Bierman, J.M., & French, F.E. (1971) *The Children of Kauai Honolulu*. Hawaii: University of Hawaii Press; Werner, E. & Smith, R. (1988) *Vulnerable but Invincible: A Longitudinal Study of Resilient Children and Youth*. New York, Adams, Bannister & Cox; Masten, A.S. & Garmezy, N. (1985) Risk, vulnerability, and protective factors in the developmental psychopathology. In B.B. Lahey & A.E. Kazdin (eds) *Advances in Clinical Child Psychology*, Vol. 8 (pp.1–51). New York: Plenum.

[235] Garmezy, N. & Rutter, M. (eds) (1983) *Stress, Coping, and Development in Children*. Baltimore: Johns Hopkins University Press. The influence of Garmezy on the emergence of developmental psychopathology in the 1980s is addressed in a festschrift from 1990: Rolf, J., Masten, A.S., Cicchetti, D., Nuechterlein, K., & Weintraub, S. (eds) (1990) *Risk and Protective Factors in the Development of Psychopathology*. Cambridge: Cambridge University Press. Meanwhile, another important development was the Social Science Research Council's Committee on Social and Affective Development during Childhood, which held a symposium in 1982. Members included Michael Rutter, Carroll Izard, and Carol Dweck and the committee was chaired by Martin Hoffman. A further development in 1983 was the first meeting of the MacArthur Working Group on the study of Attachment in the Transition Period, which was concerned with the application of attachment theory and methods beyond infancy (Chapter 3). The Network met twice yearly between 1983 and 1987. Members of the network included Mary Ainsworth and several of her former students including Inge Bretherton, Jude Cassidy, Mark Cummings, Mark Greenberg, Mary Main, and Robert Marvin. The group also included other researchers who would play an important role in the subsequent development of attachment theory including Jay Belsky, Dante Cicchetti, and Susan Spieker.

[236] Sameroff, A.J. (1983) Developmental systems: contexts and evolution. In P. Mussen (ed.) *Handbook of Child Psychology*, Vol. 1 (pp.237–94). New York: Wiley.

[237] The concept of 'promotive factors' to describe processes that enhance the likelihood of adaptation (in contrast to protective factors, which buffer the likelihood that adversities will have an effect) was introduced by Sameroff, A.J. (1999) Ecological perspectives on developmental risk. In J.D. Osofsky & H.E. Fitzgerald (eds) *WAIMH Handbook of Infant Mental Health: Vol. 4. Infant Mental Health Groups at Risk* (pp.223–48). New York: Wiley. The terms 'protective-stabilising' and 'protective-enhancing' were also introduced by Luthar in making this distinction: Luthar, S.S. (1993) Annotation: methodological and conceptual issues in the study of resilience. *Journal of Child Psychology and Psychiatry*, 34, 441–53.

[238] Garmezy later attributed the influence of both Sroufe and Rutter to his reorientation away from research on adult schizophrenia and towards the study of child and adolescent development. Masten, A.S. (1995) Interview with Norman Garmezy. SRCD oral history interview. http://srcd.org/sites/default/files/documents/garmezy_norman_interviewweb.pdf.

categories and explored precursors, developmental psychopathology was defined by a concern to study 'the origins and time course of a given disorder, its varying manifestation with development, its precursors and sequelae, and its relation to nondisordered patterns of behaviour. Thus, developmental psychopathologists may be just as interested in a group of children showing precursors of a disordered behavior pattern, but not developing the disorder proper, as the group that in time manifested the complete pathology.'[239]

Sroufe and Rutter highlighted that the distinction between adaptation and pathology was context-dependent. They give the example of an avoidant response to an abusive attachment figure, which might include not only physical avoidance but also 'blunting or controlling emotional experiences'. This response is 'adaptive' in the sense of being intelligible and helpful for a young child, for whom proximity or displays of distress or desire for comfort may not be safe. However, the very same adaptation 'may later compromise the child's ability to maximally draw upon the environment'.[240] Even stereotypic behaviour (Chapter 3) could be seen in this light: these odd, seemingly purposeless behaviours can best be regarded as 'meaningful' responses that at some point helped modulate arousal, and which have therefore been retained as a response to stress.[241] Sroufe and Rutter argued that adult mental health should be understood as, in part, the residue of the history of ways in which an individual responded to earlier challenges, and in part a new, inventive attempt to turn existing expectations, skills, and strategies towards contemporary problems and opportunities.[242] Where continuities are seen across periods of development these will rarely be in the display of identical forms of behaviour, but rather in the meaning of the behaviours as a way of engaging with the environment. For instance, there are vast differences between weeping and clinging in infancy, on the one hand, and impulsivity, jealousy, and continual dramas in adulthood, on the other. But both profiles may serve similar interpersonal functions and have their basis in a low threshold of activation of the attachment system.

As such, Sroufe and Rutter made a plea for broad-band indices of adaptation, whether in peer-relations or mental health. In line with Sroufe and Waters' earlier 'Attachment as an organizational construct' (Chapter 2), Sroufe and Rutter argued that little stability of behaviour would be expected in the context of an individual's changing developmental challenges and environment. By contrast, broader indices would predict well to later adaptation in general, since they would capture the extent to which adaptation had required significant compromise or even led to failures in meeting challenges in earlier life. In this, their argument lay the ground for proposals by Rutter's former collaborator Avshalom Caspi and colleagues in 2014 for a general 'p-factor' representing general mental ill-health, rather than the division of symptoms into specific diagnoses.[243]

---

[239] Sroufe, L.A. & Rutter, M. (1984) The domain of developmental psychopathology. *Child Development*, 55(1), 17–29, p.18.

[240] Ibid. p.23.

[241] Sroufe, L.A. (1990) Considering normal and abnormal together: the essence of developmental psychopathology. *Development & Psychopathology*, 2(4), 335–47: 'Stereotypy increased in frequency and intensity during demanding tasks, was preceded by heart rate acceleration, and was followed by a pronounced heart rate deceleration … We suggested that both stereotypies and behavioural negativism were serving the purpose of modulating arousal' (337).

[242] Sroufe, L.A. & Rutter, M. (1984) The domain of developmental psychopathology. *Child Development*, 55(1), 17–29, p.21.

[243] Caspi, A., Houts, R.M., Belsky, D.W., et al. (2014) The p factor: one general psychopathology factor in the structure of psychiatric disorders? *Clinical Psychological Science*, 2(2), 119–37. The debt to developmental psychopathology is clear in this paper: Rutter's work is cited as an 'initial motivation', and 'developmental psychopathology' is one of the article's three keywords.

Though Sroufe tended to regard positive internal working models of self and relationships as characteristic of mental health,[244] in his writings on developmental psychopathology he was keen to argue that there is no content of internal working models that is itself adaptive. Positive models are primarily beneficial when combined with environments in which expressions of positive models such as self-esteem or a capacity to trust can generate opportunities and rewards, which is not always the case. Against essentialism about either adaptation or pathology, in their 1984 article Sroufe and Rutter argued that it is the interaction with context that is critical for the meaning of even patterns of attachment.[245] For example, though generally a protective factor over time in the wider context of development, secure attachment may in theory function variously as a vulnerability, protective or a risk factor, depending on local circumstances.[246] Indeed, attachment was a central concern for developmental psychopathology, since it provided both theory and empirical results supporting the role of transdiagnostic, developmental processes for mental health, with any factor compounded by the network of other risk and protective factors experienced by a group or population.[247]

Though an outspoken critic of Bowlby's notion of 'maternal deprivation', Rutter nonetheless praised Bowlby's work as having 'ushered in the era' in which the developmental psychopathology perspective was possible, especially through his adoption of the concept of 'developmental pathways' from embryology (Chapter 1).[248] Rutter also observed that 'Bowlby's (1951) World Health Organization monograph had raised expectations of the power of prediction from experiences in infancy and on the preventive value of psychosocial interventions, but also it had run into a storm of academic criticism. Both proved only half-right. The over-riding potency of infantile experiences has not been supported by subsequent research, but the focus on children's attachments to their parents has paid off richly.'[249] Sroufe, perhaps, if forced to give proportions, would likely have said that Bowlby was three-quarters right.[250] Even if the direct effects of early attachment have been smaller

---

[244] Elicker, J., Englund, M., & Sroufe, L.A. (1992) Predicting peer competence and peer relationships in childhood from early parent–child relationships. In R. Parke & G. Ladd (eds) *Family-Peer Relationships: Modes of Linkage* (pp.77–106). Hillsdale, NJ: Lawrence Erlbaum, p.80.

[245] Sroufe, L. & Rutter, M. (1984) The domain of developmental psychopathology. *Child Development*, 55(1), 17–29, p.23.

[246] Egeland, B., Carlson, E., & Sroufe, L.A. (1993) Resilience as process. *Development & Psychopathology*, 5(4), 517–28: 'Any constitutional or environmental factors may serve as vulnerability, protective, or risk variables' (517).

[247] Rutter, M. (1983) Stress, coping and development: some issues and some questions. In N. Garmezy & M. Rutter (eds) *Stress, Coping, and Development in Children* (pp.1–42). Baltimore: Johns Hopkins University Press, p.23.

[248] Rutter, M. (1985) Resilience in the face of adversity: protective factors and resistance to psychiatric disorder. *British Journal of Psychiatry*, 147(6), 598–611, p.598.

[249] Rutter, M. (1986) Child psychiatry: looking 30 years ahead. *Journal of Child Psychology and Psychiatry*, 27(6), 803–840, p.803. See also Rutter, M.L. (1999) Psychosocial adversity and child psychopathology. *British Journal of Psychiatry*, 174(6), 480–93: 'Bowlby's 1951 monograph, although overstating the case in some respects, led to a major change in the approach to experiences during the preschool years' (482).

[250] Sroufe, L.A. (1986) Appraisal: Bowlby's contribution to psychoanalytic theory and developmental psychology; attachment: separation: loss. *Journal of Child Psychology and Psychiatry*, 27(6), 841–9. Regarding the debate between Bowlby and Rutter over what priority to assign to early experience, the Minnesota group argued that no global position was acceptable, or in line with evidence from embryology. Sroufe, L.A., Coffino, B., & Carlson, E.A. (2010) Conceptualizing the role of early experience: lessons from the Minnesota longitudinal study. *Developmental Review*, 30(1), 36–51: 'It is clearly not always the case that early experience is most critical … Maternal nutrition during pregnancy is a dramatic contrary example. While certain nutrients like folic acid are critically important in the early embryonic period, poor general maternal nutrition has almost no demonstrable effects in the first trimester, because the tiny developing organism can simply take many of the nutrients it needs from maternal stores. However, in the third trimester, when rapid fetal size and weight gain is occurring, adequate maternal nutrition is crucial' (37–8).

than anticipated by Bowlby, the Minnesota Longitudinal Study of Risk and Adaptation provided ample evidence of the continuing importance of early experiences in some areas of life, such as enduring associations between early experiences of abuse and later relationships with peers and romantic partners.[251] Looking back on the results of the study, Sroufe, Coffino, and Carlson concluded that 'early experience can be conceptualized in terms of creating vulnerabilities or strengths with regard to later experience, including what experiences are sought and how they are interpreted, rather than as directly producing particular outcomes'.[252]

This emphasis on the power of prediction, for which Bowlby was a forerunner, was central to developmental psychopathology as a domain of inquiry. It was assumed that reasonable certainties were possible regarding the probabilities entailed by developmental pathways. In particular, hypotheses could be developed for testing against prospective data, to explore the 'characteristics or histories that buffer individuals against stress or that provide them with attitudes, orientations, and skills that promote successful coping with stress, and … factors that produce vulnerability to stress or coping failures'.[253] In wider social and political context, the emergence of developmental psychopathology can be regarded as aligned with a rise of public health and primary prevention approaches to mental health.[254] It was also supported by a broader trend in social and policy science towards a concern with the capacities of individuals to handle the potential fallout of societal and economic uncertainties and problems.[255] In turn, the prominence and credibility given to 'resilience' by the emergent field of developmental psychopathology helped contribute to its resonance and deployment across contexts in the 1990s—albeit generally completely shorn of developmental concerns, and formulated instead as a quality of individual 'invulnerability'.[256] In their contribution to Anthony and Cohler's influential book on *The Invulnerable Child*, Farer and Egeland castigated the editors and other authors for what they regarded as a false and unethical framing of the question of adaptation in the context of adversity.[257]

Though considered one of the 'founders' of developmental psychopathology, Sroufe was also regarded as a distinct voice. He was known for his characteristic criticisms of medical models of diagnosis; his emphasis on lifespan development and intergenerational processes;

[251] Sroufe, L.A., Egeland, B., Carlson, E.A., & Collins, W.A. (2005) *The Development of the Person.* New York: Guilford: 'We may think of early experience as the foundation for the building. The foundation cannot be more important than solid supporting beams or a sturdy roof; without these, the house will not last. But at the same time, a house cannot be stronger than its foundations' (11). For a recent and comprehensive report see Raby, K. L., Roisman, G.I., Labella, M.H., Martin, J., Fraley, R.C., & Simpson, J.A. (2019) The legacy of early abuse and neglect for social and academic competence from childhood to adulthood. *Child Development*, 90(5), 1684–701.

[252] Sroufe, L.A., Coffino, B., & Carlson, E.A. (2010) Conceptualizing the role of early experience: lessons from the Minnesota longitudinal study. *Developmental Review*, 30(1), 36–51, p.38.

[253] Sroufe, L.A. & Rutter, M. (1984) The domain of developmental psychopathology. *Child Development*, 55(1), 17–29, p.19.

[254] Spaulding, J. & Balch, P. (1983) A brief history of primary prevention in the twentieth century: 1908 to 1980. *American Journal of Community Psychology*, 11, 59–80; Cowen, E. L. (1983) Primary prevention in mental health: past present and future. In R.D. Felner, L.A. Jason, J.N. Montsugu, & S.S. Farber (eds) *Prevention Psychology: Theory, Research and Practice* (pp.290–97). New York: Pergammon Press.

[255] E.g. Rose, N. & Lentzos, F. (2017) Making us resilient: responsible citizens for uncertain times. In S. Trnka & C. Trundle (eds) *Competing Responsibilities: The Ethics and Politics of Contemporary Life* (pp.27–48). Durham, NC: Duke University Press.

[256] Bourbeau, P. (2018) A genealogy of resilience. *International Political Sociology*, 12(1), 19–35. See e.g. Howard, D.E. (1996) Searching for resilience among African-American youth exposed to community violence. *Journal of Adolescent Health*, 18(4), 254–62.

[257] Farber, E. & Egeland, B. (1987) Abused children: can they be invulnerable? In J. Anthony & B. Cohler (eds) *The Invulnerable Child*. New York: Guilford, 253–88, p.286.

his concern with the interdependence of different family relationships; his hostility to temperament researchers where they neglected the role of caregiving factors; and his dismay at images of 'resilience' that constructed it as an individual quality rather than a social effect.[258] He and Egeland were also among the strongest advocates for the value of considering typical and atypical forms of development within the same frame, based on the assumption that the processes involved would be mutually revealing. Sroufe and Egeland argued that the role of many social factors in ordinary life is best revealed when they are absent or intensified to an unusual degree. They pointed, for instance, to the importance of the family and friendship networks available to the mothers in their sample: when there were improvements of social support to mothers who had otherwise been especially isolated, their children's mental health and conduct in school saw dramatic improvements. However, in the sample in general, social support had only a modest overall relationship with child behaviour.[259]

Furthermore, the Minnesota Longitudinal Study of Risk and Adaptation led Sroufe, Egeland, and colleagues to a distinctive position on the role of risk factors across the lifespan. They agreed with the consensus in developmental psychopathology that risk factors were cumulative. However, they were unusual in offering some qualifications to this position. Kaufman and Zigler had argued that various risks were interchangeable, and what mattered was their number: for instance, various forms of child abuse were argued to have the same implications.[260] The Minnesota group were definitely interested in the use of summary variables and the study of cumulative effects: they generally found stronger effects when multiple forms of abuse compounded. However, they held that risk factors would often interact in specific ways. Egeland reported that two-thirds of participants who had been physically abused showed oppositional defiant disorder. This was in line with other research groups who had found that physical abuse predicted clinically significant levels of conduct problems. However, the multi-assessment and longitudinal nature of the Minnesota data allowed Egeland to show that this association was, at least in his sample, a secondary effect of the links between physical abuse and other forms of maltreatment and inadequate care.[261] Conduct problems were in fact best predicted by the co-occurrence of caregiver psychological unavailability, neglect, and sexual abuse. The Minnesota group also reported findings showing the implications of specific forms of abuse. Berzenski, Yates, and Egeland reported that emotional abuse, whether alone or in combination with other forms of abuse, made a particularly powerful contribution to anxiety and depression, while the combination of physical and emotional abuse was especially strongly associated with conduct problems.[262] They also

[258] These positions can already be seen in comparing Sroufe's chapter to others in Ciccheti, D. (1989) (ed.) *The Emergence of a Discipline: Rochester Symposium on Developmental Psychopathology*, Vol. 1. Hillsdale, NJ: Lawrence Erlbaum. Some of these differences would also later be remarked upon by Michael Rutter, looking back on the period: Rutter, M. (2008) Developing concepts in developmental psychopathology. In J.J. Hudziak (ed.) *Developmental Psychopathology and Wellness: Genetic and Environmental Influences* (pp.3–22). New York: American Psychiatric Publications.

[259] Sroufe, L.A. & Egeland, B. (1991) Illustrations of person and environment interaction from a longitudinal study. In T. Wachs & R. Plomin (eds) *Conceptualization and Measurement of Organism-Environment Interaction* (pp.68–84). Washington, DC: American Psychological Association, p.69.

[260] Kaufman, J. & Zigler, E. (1989) The intergenerational transmission of child abuse. In D. Cicchetti & V. Carlson (eds) *Child Maltreatment: Theory and Research on the Causes and Consequences of Child Abuse and Neglect* (pp.129–50). Cambridge: Cambridge University Press.

[261] Egeland, B. (1997) Mediators of the effects of child maltreatment on developmental adaptation in adolescence. In D. Cicchetti & S. Toth (eds) *Rochester Symposium on Developmental Psychopathology: Vol. VIII. The Effects of Trauma on the Developmental Process* (pp.403–434). Rochester, NY: University of Rochester Press.

[262] Berzenski, S.R., Yates, T.M., & Egeland, B. (2014) A multidimensional view of continuity in intergenerational transmission of child maltreatment. In J.E. Korbin & R.D. Krugman (eds) *Handbook of Child Maltreatment*, Vol.

highlighted research findings from other groups that indicated that parental depression reduces the likelihood of physical abuse, but increases the likelihood of sexual abuse.[263]

The Minnesota group were distinctive among developmental psychopathologists for their interest in the capacity of risk factors at one stage to go dormant until the developmental challenges of a later stage made them salient again: 'Even following change, early patterns of attachment retain a potential for reactivation ... Certain issues and certain arenas of functioning—those tapping anxiety about the availability of others or apprehension regarding emotional closeness—will be especially likely to reveal the legacy of early attachment, even during periods of generally adequate functioning.'[264] For instance, Yates, Dodds, Sroufe, and Egeland found that exposure to interpartner violence in the preschool years reappeared as a powerful predictive factor in contributing to behavioural problems at age 16, at a time when the key developmental challenges are forming intimate relationships, handling commitment and its conflicts, establishing boundaries with peers, and coordinating same- and cross-gender relationships.[265] The Minnesota group later reported that exposure to interpartner violence in the preschool years predicted later partner violence perpetration and victimisation for both male and female participants. Participants who initiated partner violence perpetration and/or victimisation between age 26 and age 32 had greater exposure to partner violence in the preschool years than participants who showed no or declining domestic violence over these years.[266] Collins, LaFreniere, and Simpson argued that such findings confirm that 'one must understand the trajectory of an individual's relationship history to fully appreciate, situate, and comprehend his or her

2 (pp.115–29). New York: Springer. Another example from the Minnesota group was work by Jeff Simpson and colleagues examining the implications of early environmental unpredictability—operationalised as changes in residence, cohabitatio, and parental occupation that occur before a child is five years old. These early experiences have been found to predict later aggressive behaviour, more substance use at age 16, and more sexually risky behaviour at age 23. This is in contrast to changes in residence, cohabitation, and parental occupation after the age of five, which have barely any effect. Furthermore, the combination of these factors and harsh maternal caregiving additionally predicted adolescent risk-taking behaviours. See Simpson, J.A., Griskevicius, V., & Kuo, S.I. (2012) Evolution, stress, and sensitive periods: the influence of unpredictability in early versus late childhood on sex and risky behavior. *Developmental Psychology*, 48(3), 674–86; Doom, J.R., Vanzomeren-Dohm, A.A., & Simpson, J.A. (2016) Early unpredictability predicts increased adolescent externalizing behaviors and substance use: a life history perspective. *Development & Psychopathology*, 28(4), 1505–16.

[263] Berzenski, S.R., Yates, T.M., & Egeland, B. (2014) A multidimensional view of continuity in intergenerational transmission of child maltreatment. In J.E. Korbin & R.D. Krugman (eds) *Handbook of Child Maltreatment*, Vol. 2 (pp.115–29). Dordrecht: Springer. For parental depression reducing the likelihood of physical abuse see Pears, K.C. & Capaldi, D.M. (2001) Intergenerational transmission of abuse: a two-generational prospective study of an at-risk sample. *Child Abuse & Neglect*, 25(11), 1439–61. For parental depression increasing the likelihood of sexual abuse see Leifer, M., Kilbane, T., & Kalick, S. (2004) Vulnerability or resilience to intergenerational sexual abuse: the role of maternal factors. *Child Maltreatment*, 9(1), 78–91.

[264] Sroufe, L.A., Carlson, E.A., Levy, A.K., & Egeland, B. (1999) Implications of attachment theory for developmental psychopathology. *Development & Psychopathology*, 11(1), 1–13, p.6; see also Sroufe, L. & Rutter, M. (1984) The domain of developmental psychopathology. *Child Development*, 55(1), 17–29, p.20.

[265] Yates, T.M., Dodds, M.F., Sroufe, L.A., & Egeland, B. (2003) Exposure to partner violence and child behavior problems: a prospective study controlling for child physical abuse and neglect, child cognitive ability, socioeconomic status, and life stress. *Development & Psychopathology*, 15(1), 199–218, p.209; Sroufe, L.A., Egeland, B., Carlson, E.A., & Collins, W.A. (2005) *The Development of the Person*. New York: Guilford, Table 4.2.

[266] Narayan, A.J., Labella, M.H., Englund, M.M., Carlson, E.A., & Egeland, B. (2017) The legacy of early childhood violence exposure to adulthood intimate partner violence: variable- and person-oriented evidence. *Journal of Family Psychology*, 31(7), 833–43. On the direct and indirect pathways between exposure to domestic violence in childhood and perpetration or victimisation in adulthood see also Narayan, A.J., Englund, M.M., Carlson, E.A., & Egeland, B. (2014) Adolescent conflict as a developmental process in the prospective pathway from exposure to interparental violence to dating violence. *Journal of Abnormal Child Psychology*, 42(2), 239–50; Zamir, O., Szepsenwol, O., Englund, M.M., & Simpson, J.A. (2018) The role of dissociation in revictimization across the lifespan: a 32-year prospective study. *Child Abuse & Neglect*, 79, 144–53.

adult relationships. This view of how development and relationships continually intersect across the lifespan is one of the major and lasting legacies of Sroufe and Egeland's work on the entire field of psychology.[267]

Another finding illustrates the ongoing role of early experience as a 'resource' to later adaptation.[268] A clinical interview was conducted when participants in the Minnesota study were aged 28, assessing 'global adaptive functioning'. This scale was based on the clinician's impression of the individual's overall psychological, social, and occupational functioning, and scored on a continuous scale. This measure is not just an assessment of mental illness or difficulties, then, but also positive adaptation and thriving. Infant Strange Situation attachment classifications had a very substantial association with this measure of adaptation and thriving several decades later (r = .41). Path analysis revealed that this association was partly direct (r = .26), even taking into account a large variety of mediators. Infant attachment appeared to remain, even after so many years, directly entangled in the coping and thriving of the Minnesota study participants at the most general level. The remainder of the association between Strange Situation classification and global adaptive functioning was mediated through a complex path including peer relationships at age 16, effectiveness in handling issues in romantic relationships in early adulthood, and total experience of life stress. Englund and colleagues within the Minnesota group characterised infant attachment as a species of 'social capital', and cumulative with other forms of social capital such as supportive friendships and romantic relationships in contributing to psychological, social, and occupational functioning.

Developmental pathways

The journal *Development and Psychopathology* was established in 1989 by Dante Cicchetti. The initial idea for the journal had come to Cicchetti during his years teaching seminars on developmental psychopathology for Sroufe's classes, and then coteaching with Sroufe in his final year of graduate school.[269] Sroufe's articles for *Development and Psychopathology* in the 1990s are magisterial and programmatic. In particular, they set out his particular problems with medical models of diagnosis. The 'essence of developmental psychopathology', Sroufe argued, was attention to developmental processes that span both mental health and illness.[270] He agreed with Egeland that developmental psychopathology needed to have an operational definition of targets of inquiry and intervention, like child abuse or conduct disorders.[271] A collectively agreed definition would permit convergent validity in measurement, stability in theory-building, and clarity of message in communicating with policy-makers. However,

[267] Collins, W.A., LaFreniere, P., & Simpson, J.A. (2011) Relationships across the lifespan: the benefits of a theoretically based longitudinal-developmental perspective. In D. Cicchetti & G.I. Roisman (eds) *The Origins and Organization of Adaptation and Maladaption: The Minnesota Symposium on Child Psychology*, Vol. 36 (pp.155–83). New York: Wiley, p.177.

[268] Englund, M.M., Kuo, S.I.C., Puig, J., & Collins, W.A. (2011) Early roots of adult competence: the significance of close relationships from infancy to early adulthood. *International Journal of Behavioral Development*, 35(6), 490–96.

[269] Cicchetti, D. (2013) The legacy of development and psychopathology. *Development & Psychopathology*, 25(4.2), 1199–200, p.1200.

[270] Sroufe, L.A. (1990) Considering normal and abnormal together: the essence of developmental psychopathology. *Development & Psychopathology*, 2(4), 335–47, p.335.

[271] Egeland, B. (1991) From data to definition. *Development & Psychopathology*, 3(1), 37–43.

Sroufe argued that too much research to date had assumed that medical diagnoses could serve to define these targets of interest:

> The disease model requires syndromic integrity. If the disease model is apt for children's behavioral and emotional problems, children generally should manifest tight clusters of symptoms, with unique indicators of other syndromes being absent. But in reality children commonly manifest problems that cut across established categories. To be sure, one disorder may potentiate another in medicine as well, but not nearly to the extent implied by the prevalence of co-morbidity of childhood disturbances ... Comorbidity is the rule, not the exception. Moreover, broad classes of problems such as externalizing behaviors are predictive of a myriad of later conditions, including depression.[272]

Sroufe, Carlson, Levy, and Egeland argued that these concerns should be approached through the lens of Bowlby's metaphor of developmental pathways, which implies a series of specific hypotheses:

> (a) At any age, current quality of care will add to early attachment history in predicting pathology, given that adaptation is always the joint product of current circumstances and early history. (b) Likewise, broader aspects of current contexts, including relationships outside of the family and stresses and challenges of the period, also will increase prediction beyond early attachment; (c) a cumulative history of maladaptation will be more pathogenic than a single early period of poor functioning with pathology ever more likely the longer a maladaptive pathway has been followed, and (d) change itself will be predictable in light of changes in stress and/or support.[273]

This approach led Sroufe and colleagues to highlighted three ways that a developmental psychopathology perspective was a necessary counterweight to the disease model that dominates medicine.

1. Sroufe and colleagues argued that a diagnosis-focused science would end up missing broad causal factors that cross-cut and precede mental health and illness. Though ignored by a focus on diagnostic categories, attention to subclinical symptoms is critically important, both for understanding how clinical conditions develop and for understanding how mental health can be maintained. In this regard, Sroufe and colleagues claimed that family relationships are not a risk factor like any other, but play a fundamental role in shaping patterns of emotion regulation. This means that family relationships are especially important for the initiation and prolongation of most mental health symptoms.[274] For instance, Carlson, Jacobvitz, and Sroufe found that relationship stability and social support for the mothers in

---

[272] Sroufe, L.A. (1997) Psychopathology as an outcome of development. *Development & Psychopathology*, 9(2), 251–68, p.257. See also Rutter, M. & Sroufe, L.A. (2000) Developmental psychopathology: concepts and challenges. *Development & Psychopathology*, 12(3), 265–96.

[273] Sroufe, L.A., Carlson, E.A., Levy, A.K., & Egeland, B. (1999) Implications of attachment theory for developmental psychopathology. *Development & Psychopathology*, 11(1), 1–13, p.3.

[274] Sroufe, L.A., Duggal, S., Weinfield, N.S., & Carlson, E. (2000) Relationships, development, and psychopathology. In M. Lewis & A. Sameroff (eds) *Handbook of Developmental Psychopathology*, 2nd edn (pp.75–92). New York: Kluwer Academic/Plenum Press, p.84.

their sample emerged as a powerful predictor of ADHD symptoms in their child participants.[275]

2. Second, they highlighted that the same diagnosis could reflect various diverse developmental pathways, with varying implications for treatment. ADHD was a clear example: Sroufe and colleagues felt that problems around attention and the integration of affect, cognition, and behaviour were best regarded as common signals of a developmental pathway rocked by adversities, rather than primarily a diagnostic entity in themselves.[276] Supporting the idea that the same diagnosis could reflect different pathways, Aguilar, Sroufe, Egeland, and Carlson found two quite distinct routes to conduct problems and aggression in adolescence: one based on factors beginning in early childhood and leading to early-onset and persistent symptoms, another beginning in adolescence and associated with concurrent life stress and internalising symptoms.[277] Sroufe and colleagues expressed concern that a diagnosis called 'attachment disorder', applicable only to a tiny proportion of children who had not formed a stable selective attachment, would magnetise attention away from the broader relevance of patterns of attachment to developmental pathways.[278]

3. Third, Sroufe and colleagues suggested that developmental pathways could result in various diagnoses. A pathway beginning from an avoidant attachment relationship in infancy could help predispose various forms of mental illness, depending on what then ensued in that child's life and what other coping tactics were elaborated.[279] Avoidant attachment suggests that key matters of concern cannot be brought to the attention of the caregiver, that the child must suppress or redirect distress, and that they may receive less support from caregivers in handling difficult feelings when they do unavoidably arise. Whilst not a clinical pathology in themselves, these aspects of avoidant attachment might contribute to the initiation of mental health symptoms and/or their prolongation. Clinical interventions and support focused on particular diagnosis could well, Sroufe and colleagues argued, miss the underlying developmental trajectory and hence the causal processes in play. This would reduce the effectiveness of the clinical work.[280] In an important paper from 2005, Appleyard, Egeland, Dulmen, and Sroufe examined the impact of six risk factors in childhood (child maltreatment, interparental violence, family disruption, low socioeconomic status, and high parental stress) on symptoms relating to conduct problems and aggression in adolescence. The study showed that the number of risks in early childhood predicted the extent

---

[275] Carlson, E.A., Jacobvitz, D., & Sroufe, L.A. (1995) A developmental investigation of inattentiveness and hyperactivity. *Child Development*, 66(1), 37–54, p.52.

[276] E.g. Sroufe, L.A. (2007) The place of development in developmental psychopathology. In A. Masten (ed.) *Multilevel Dynamics in Developmental Psychopathology: Pathways to the Future: The Minnesota Symposia on Child Psychology*, Vol. 34 (pp.285–99). Mahwah, NJ: Lawrence Erlbaum, p.297.

[277] Aguilar, B., Sroufe, L.A., Egeland, B., & Carlson, E. (2000) Distinguishing the early-onset/persistent and adolescence-onset antisocial behavior types: from birth to 16 years. *Development & Psychopathology*, 12(2), 109–132.

[278] Rutter, M. & Sroufe, L.A. (2000) Developmental psychopathology: concepts and challenges. *Development & Psychopathology*, 12(3), 265–96, pp.273–4; Sroufe, L.A., Duggal, S., Weinfield, N., & Carlson, E. (2000) Relationships, development, and psychopathology. In A.J. Sameroff, M. Lewis, & S.M. Miller (eds) *Handbook of Developmental Psychopathology* (pp.75–91). New York: Kluwer Academic/Plenum Publishers, p.83.

[279] Cicchetti, D. & Sroufe, L.A. (2000) Editorial: the past as prologue to the future: the times, they've been a'changin'. *Development & Psychopathology*, 12, 255–64.

[280] See also Sroufe, L.A. & Jacobvitz, D. (1989) Diverging pathways, developmental transformations, multiple etiologies and the problem of continuity in development. *Human Development*, 32(3–4), 196–203.

of symptoms in adolescence in a linear fashion. The authors therefore concluded that 'the experience of an additional risk factor does not increase the odds of problems in a multiplicative way. For interventionists, such information might imply that there does not appear to be a "point of no return" beyond which services for children are hopeless, and that every risk factor we can reduce matters.' The implication was that 'interventions should be designed as comprehensive programs that enhance as many aspects of family life as possible'.[281]

The approach to developmental psychopathology of Sroufe, Egeland, and colleagues is well illustrated by their study of dissociative symptoms, discussed earlier. It was characteristic that the starting point of the Minnesota group was inquiry into dissociative processes in a population-based perspective. Rather than contrasting a group of patients with a diagnosis of a dissociative condition with healthy controls, Sroufe and colleagues explored the factors that can contribute to clinically significant and subclinical levels of dissociative symptoms. They leveraged the collection of data at multiple time-points, from multiple informants, to provide a rich picture of developmental pathways. The factors explored ranged from what may be individual-level factors such as infant distractibility, to relational factors such as infant attachment or present-day physical abuse, to the mother's own childhood experiences—which her child might not even know. The researchers found that relational factors, more than individual factors, were important for predicting dissociative symptoms, which supported the researchers' broader conceptualisation of risk and resilience.

The report on the antecedents of dissociative symptoms, however, also illustrates a limitation of the approach adopted by Sroufe and colleagues. Their analysis was solely within-sample. Without justifying the exclusion, they did not include structural factors such as socioeconomic disadvantage as a possible predictor within their analyses of dissociation. Socioeconomic disadvantage was characteristic of their whole sample as a consequence of the original recruitment strategy, which reduced relevant variance. Nonetheless, Sroufe and colleagues included socioeconomic disadvantage as an independent variable in other analyses, such as the sequelae of abuse and antecedents of ADHD, and found that it contributed to prediction.[282] It was not as if the Minnesota group were uninterested in socioeconomic disadvantage, even if they regarded it as a distal risk factor and always mediated by proximal factors such as family behaviours and social support.[283] As Egeland observed, 'even in

[281] Appleyard, K., Egeland, B., Dulmen, M.H., & Sroufe, L.A. (2005) When more is not better: the role of cumulative risk in child behavior outcomes. *Journal of Child Psychology and Psychiatry*, 46(3), 235–45, p.242–3. This stance would be contested by researchers such as Bakermans-Kranenburg, as we shall see.

[282] Carlson, E.A., Jacobvitz, D., & Sroufe, L.A. (1995) A developmental investigation of inattentiveness and hyperactivity. *Child Development*, 66, 37–54; Egeland, B. (1997) Mediators of the effects of child maltreatment on developmental adaptation in adolescence. In D. Cicchetti & S. Toth (eds) *Rochester Symposium on Developmental Psychopathology: Vol. 8. The Effects of Trauma on the Developmental Process* (pp.403–434). Rochester, NY: University of Rochester Press. Similarly socioeconomic status has been used by other researchers conducting analyses of the dataset, e.g. Raby, K.L., Roisman, G.I., Fraley, R.C., & Simpson, J.A. (2015) The enduring predictive significance of early maternal sensitivity: social and academic competence through age 32 years. *Child Development*, 86(3), 695–708.

[283] Yates, T.M., Egeland, B., & Sroufe, A. (2003) Rethinking resilience. In S. Luthar (ed.) *Resilience and Vulnerability: Adaptation in the Context of Childhood Adversities* (pp.243–66). Cambridge: Cambridge University Press: 'Poverty is a distal risk factor whose effects are mediated by proximal risk factors such as parenting behaviors, family structure, community variables, and the broader social networks within which the child and her or his family are embedded' (245).

our poverty sample, socioeconomic status was a confound'.[284] Many of the findings from the the Minnesota Longitudinal Study of Risk and Adaptation have replicated with low-risk samples.[285] However, Haltigan and Roisman found that infant avoidant attachment, but not disorganisation, was associated with later dissociative symptoms in the NICHD study. In cases such as this, where findings differ, the exclusion of socioeconomic factors as a potential confound by the Minnesota group has contributed to difficulty in interpreting results.[286]

Resilience

'Resilience' was one of the headline concepts from the emergence of developmental psychopathology as a movement within developmental science. Colleagues of Sroufe and Egeland at Minnesota, such as Ann Masten, Norm Garmezy, and Auke Tellegan, played especially important roles in fostering this discourse.[287] Some members of the developmental psychopathology movement were interested in examining individual-level factors that could lead research participants to do better than expected in response to adversity.[288] This is the concept of resilience that would generally get absorbed by cognate disciplines, and by public and policy discourses.[289] Sroufe and Egeland regretted this interpretation of the concept. In what became the dominant interpretation within developmental psychopathology over time, they took an opposing stance, emphasising that resilience is a relational process.[290] They demonstrated that many of the studies that have shown links between temperamental robustness and positive outcomes in the face of adversity have had significant methodological flaws. For instance, a key work in the characterisation of resilience as a form of individual 'invulnerability' was Werner and Smith's cohort study of 505 men and women who were born in 1955

[284] Egeland, B. (1997) Mediators of the effects of child maltreatment on developmental adaptation in adolescence. In D. Cicchetti & S. Toth (eds) *Rochester Symposium on Developmental Psychopathology: Vol. 8. The Effects of Trauma on the Developmental Process* (pp.403–434). Rochester, NY: University of Rochester Press, p.428.

[285] Fraley, R.C. & Roisman, G.I. (2015) Do early caregiving experiences leave an enduring or transient mark on developmental adaptation? *Current Opinion in Psychology*, 1, 101–106.

[286] Lyons-Ruth and colleagues reported findings from a high-risk sample of 76 families, comprising 41 referred to child protective services and 35 matched comparisons. Data were available on 56 families who remained in the sample 20 years later. Lyons-Ruth and colleagues reported that observed lack of responsiveness of parents at home and in the laboratory to their infants accounted for half of the variance in participants' self-report of dissociative symptoms at age 19 on the Carlson and Putnam Dissociative Experiences Scale. The researchers did not find that either disorganised attachment or trauma predicted later dissociative symptoms; no analysis appears to have been conducted for avoidant attachment. However, verbal abuse by parents, which was not assessed by the Minnesota study, made an additional contribution to dissociative symptoms in adolescence, over and above caregiver emotional neglect/psychological unavailability. Dutra, L., Bureau, J.F., Holmes, B., Lyubchik, A., & Lyons-Ruth, K. (2009) Quality of early care and childhood trauma: a prospective study of developmental pathways to dissociation. *Journal of Nervous and Mental Disease*, 197(6), 383–90.

[287] Garmezy, N., Masten, A.S., & Tellegen, A. (1984) The study of stress and competence in children: a building block for developmental psychopathology. *Child Development*, 55(1), 97–111.

[288] E.g. Anthony, E.J. (1974) Introduction: the syndrome of the psychologically vulnerable child. In E.J. Anthony & C. Koupernik (eds) *The Child in his Family: Children at Psychiatric Risk*, Vol. 3 (pp.3–10). New York: Wiley.

[289] Harper, D. & Speed, E. (2012) Uncovering recovery: the resistible rise of recovery and resilience. *Studies in Social Justice*, 6, 9–25; Joseph, J. (2013) Resilience as embedded neoliberalism: a governmentality approach. *Resilience*, 1(1), 38–52.

[290] On later regret among developmental psychopathologists regarding the widespread popular interpretation of the concept of resilience, and the role of some of their members in contributing to this interpretation see Luthar, S.S., Cicchetti, D., & Becker, B. (2000) The construct of resilience: a critical evaluation and guidelines for future work. *Child Development*, 71(3), 543–62.

on the Hawaiian island of Kauai.[291] Sroufe and Egeland noted, however, that only one temperamental variable in childhood was linked to positive outcomes, and this was the mother's description of her child as 'loveable' at two years old. They expressed doubt that this can confidently be regarded as reflecting inherent child variation.[292]

The term 'resiliency' implies an individual trait, and was therefore regarded by the Minnesota group as unacceptably misleading. But the term 'resilience' may more readily imply a process, even if often it has been used to refer to a trait. In 2003, Yates, Egeland, and Sroufe set out their definition of 'resilience' as a description of the capacity of children to garner resources that allow them to negotiate the present effectively and set up internal and external resources for future challenges.[293] The emphasis on both internal and external resources provided a place for individual-level factors. However, the placement of these factors in developmental perspective suggested that it is 'as supports accumulate' that an individual develops the 'acquired attitudes, expectations, and capacities to marshal resources [to] enable them to cope better with the additional challenge they may face'.[294]

The characteristics usually ascribed to 'resilient individuals', such as a calm temperament or optimism, were firmly regarded by Yates, Egeland, and Sroufe as developmental and social outcomes, mediated through the inner calibration of behavioural systems and by ongoing family and peer relationships. This made their position a profoundly destigmatising one, since it emphasised that mental health symptoms are an ordinary and expectable response to the accumulation of adversities, especially through childhood and adolescence, in the context of inadequate support. They were also early critics of a unidimensional concept of resilience, and urged recognition that positive outcomes despite adversities in one domain of life may in fact corrode opportunities in another domain that requires quite a different set of resources and capacities to the first. The paradigmatic case for Yates, Egeland, and Sroufe was avoidant attachment, which was conceptualised as an intelligible and likely helpful response to a less-sensitive caregiving context, but as making later emotion regulation and peer relationships more difficult in certain regards.[295] Yates and colleagues suggested that keeping our worries and desires to ourselves reduces our exposure to hurt and disappointment, but if we lack the capacity to do otherwise then this saps something from us that might have otherwise been used elsewhere in building a richer and more stable life, as we lose heart in the prospects of attaining or sharing anything more than what we can muster alone. This then may fuse the avoidance into place, as we miss the opportunities that may arise for recognition and response to our worries and desires by others.[296]

---

[291] Werner, E.E. & Smith, R.S. (1982) *Vulnerable but Invincible: A Study of Resilient Children.* New York: McGraw-Hill; Werner, E.E. & Smith, R.S. (1992) *Overcoming the Odds: High Risk Children from Birth to Adulthood.* Ithaca, NY: Cornell University Press.

[292] Sroufe, L.A. (2007) The place of development in developmental psychopathology. In A. Masten (ed.) *Multilevel Dynamics in Developmental Psychopathology: Pathways to the Future: The Minnesota Symposia on Child Psychology*, Vol. 34 (pp.285–99). Mahwah, NJ: Lawrence Erlbaum, p.293.

[293] Yates, T.M., Egeland, B., & Sroufe, A. (2003) Rethinking resilience. In S. Luthar (ed.) *Resilience and Vulnerability: Adaptation in the Context of Childhood Adversities* (pp.243–66). Cambridge: Cambridge University Press, pp.249–50.

[294] Supkoff, L., Puig, J., & Sroufe, L.A. (2013) Situating resilience in developmental context. In M. Ungar (ed.) *The Social Ecology of Resilience* (pp.127–42). New York: Springer, p.128.

[295] Egeland, B., Carlson, E., & Sroufe, L.A. (1993) Resilience as process. *Development & Psychopathology*, 5(4), 517–28. See also Luthar, S.S., Doernberger, C.H., & Zigler, E. (1993) Resilience is not a unidimensional construct: insights from a prospective study of inner-city adolescents. *Development & Psychopathology*, 5(4), 703–717.

[296] Sroufe, L.A., Coffino, B., & Carlson, E.A. (2010) Conceptualizing the role of early experience: lessons from the Minnesota longitudinal study. *Developmental Review*, 30(1), 36–51, p.39.

Yates, Egeland, and Sroufe illustrated their argument by pointing to the developmental tra-jectories of children who displayed substantial behavioural problems at school. Causadias, Salvatore, and Sroufe found that, of children showing conduct problems, those who had experi-enced the most favourable early care showed the fewest mental health problems and had more supportive friendships in adolescence.[297] Yates, Egeland, and Sroufe argued that a positive foun-dation had served as a resource for meeting the challenges of adolescence. The early foundation may have proven a 'promotive factor', enhancing the probability of later adaptation, not merely buffering the effects of contemporary adversity. Such findings were taken as showing that re-silience is a description of the availability and utilisation of resources, rather than an inherent quality of individuals: 'Consider the alternative interpretation that an early history of positive adaptation reflects an underlying individual trait called resilience. In this view, some of these children were resilient, then were not, and then were again.'[298] Had the longitudinal study begun in preschool, the fact that some of the children had better outcomes than others would have seemed to be an effect of their individual characteristics; viewed in developmental context, these differences in fact were predictable from their experiences of early care.[299]

Perhaps the single most famous finding regarding resilience of the Minnesota Longitudinal Study of Risk and Adaptation was the identification of factors that could 'break the cycle of abuse', the transmission of abusive caregiving from one generation to the next. When parents who were abused as children were asked whether they would raise their child differently, all but four said yes, vowing that they would not repeat their own maltreatment. Yet based on interviews with the mothers in their sample, and multimethod assessments of child wellbeing and safety, the Minnesota group found that some mothers were not able to fulfil these vows. They found that about a third of caregivers who reported that they had been abused went on to abuse their own child: a much higher proportion than matched controls but overall a minority of cases. There was a substantial gap in intergenerational transmis-sion, a finding that has subsequently been well replicated.[300] Egeland, Jacobvitz, and Sroufe reported that depression was exceptionally prevalent among the abusing mothers, and they 'tended to view their children in an entirely negative or positive light and failed to recognize the ambivalence, which, of necessity, accompanies child care'.[301]

---

[297] See also Causadias, J.M., Salvatore, J.E., & Sroufe, L.A. (2012) Early patterns of self-regulation as risk and promotive factors in development: a longitudinal study from childhood to adulthood in a high-risk sample. *International Journal of Behavioral Development*, 36(4), 293–302.

[298] Yates, T.M., Egeland, B., & Sroufe, A. (2003) Rethinking resilience. In S. Luthar (ed.) *Resilience and Vulnerability: Adaptation in the Context of Childhood Adversities* (pp.243–66). Cambridge: Cambridge University Press, p.251.

[299] Another illustration is Supkoff, L., Puig, J., & Sroufe, L.A. (2013) Situating resilience in developmental con-text. In M. Ungar (ed.) *The Social Ecology of Resilience* (pp.127–42). New York: Springer: 'We found that we could distinguish between those who recovered from depression in adulthood following formation of a romantic part-nership from those who did not recover after partnering on the basis of different histories of infant attachment (Sroufe, Corffino & Carlson 2010)' (138). In fact, however, these findings are not reported in Sroufe, Corffino, and Carlson (2010). Some analogous results are reported in Salvatore, J.E. (2011) Moderating processes in the link be-tween early caregiving and adult individual and romantic functioning: the distinctive contributions of early adult romantic relationships. Unpublished doctoral dissertation, University of Minnesota. However the interaction is between the early childhood composite variable, not attachment, and adult relationships, in predicting depressive symptoms at age 23.

[300] E.g. Widom, C.S., Czaja, C.J., & DuMont, K.A. (2015) Intergenerational transmission of child abuse and neg-lect *Science*, 347(6229), 1480–85; Ben-David, V., Jonson-Reid, M., Drake, B., & Kohl, P.O. (2015) The association between childhood maltreatment experiences and the onset of maltreatment perpetration in young adulthood controlling for proximal and distal risk factors. *Child Abuse & Neglect*, 46, 132–41.

[301] Egeland, B., Jacobvitz, D., & Sroufe, L.A. (1988) Breaking the cycle of abuse. *Child Development*, 59(4), 1080–1088, p.1087.

Egeland, Jacobvitz, and Sroufe reported that the abused mothers who did not go on to abuse their child were distinguished by one or more of three experiences. First, some had emotional support from a non-abusive adult during their childhood. Second, some had participated in therapy. Third, some had a stable and emotionally supportive relationship with their adult partner. Egeland and colleagues observed that what these three experiences have in common is that they are experiences in which a secure base and safe haven has been provided, a 'basis for developing alternative or transformed models of relationship'.[302] One of the case studies they provide is of a mother 'VF'.[303] VF grew up in a family of ten children, all of whom ended up in foster care. Her mother would regularly beat the children, and as an adult VF still had scars from the physical abuse. Scared of being taken away from her mother like her older siblings, VF lied repeatedly at school to account for her bruises and cuts. However, when she was 11 years old, her mother asked child protection services to take VF. At the point that she left her mother's care she had never been to a doctor or dentist—and did not know what these were. She spent two years in a first foster home, then two more foster homes. She then spent two years in a centre for treatment of substance dependency. During this time, she had psychotherapy. At age 18 she moved into an apartment with another girl, and very shortly after that became pregnant. When her son was a year old, she entered into a long-term relationship and eventually married. She and her husband both found work and had three more children together. Egeland and colleagues reported that 'VF seems particularly aware of her past', and was able to use this awareness to consider how it affects her caregiving. VF regarded her period of therapy and the support of her husband as important for helping her care for her children.

The researchers were powerfully struck that certain social experiences helped some mothers interrupt the continuities in abusive caregiving between generations.[304] However, a later report by Enlow, Englund, and Egeland found that maternal experiences of child maltreatment predicted behavioural problems in their children at age seven, even if the mothers were not maltreating. This pathway was mediated by social isolation and negative life events such as financial difficulties, bereavements, and illness. The researchers concluded that 'mothers able to "break the intergenerational cycle of maltreatment" may still be at risk for creating a negative caregiving context through increased stress exposures and reduced social support, part of the developmental sequelae of their maltreatment histories'.[305] In a review chapter, Egeland and colleagues drew attention to research from other laboratories showing that, when abused parents do abuse their children, the kinds of abuse can be quite dissimilar.[306]

[302] Ibid. p.1082.

[303] Egeland, B., Jacobvitz, D., & Papatola, K. (1987) Intergenerational continuity of abuse. In R.J. Gelles & J.B. Lancaster (eds) *Child Abuse and Neglect: Biosocial Dimensions* (pp.255–76). New York: Aldine De Gruyter, p.269.

[304] Subsequent research has suggested that it is concrete ecological and financial supports that especially predict the interruption of the transmission of abusive care, more than individual psychological factors. St-Laurent, D., Dubois-Comtois, K., Milot, T., & Cantinotti, M. (2019) Intergenerational continuity/discontinuity of child maltreatment among low-income mother–child dyads: the roles of childhood maltreatment characteristics, maternal psychological functioning, and family ecology. *Development & Psychopathology*, 31(1), 189–202.

[305] Bosquet Enlow, M., Englund, M.M., & Egeland, B. (2018) Maternal childhood maltreatment history and child mental health: mechanisms in intergenerational effects. *Journal of Clinical Child & Adolescent Psychology*, 47(1), 47–62. Later research with the sample also indicated competence in romantic relationships as a potent mediator of the association between experiences of abuse and neglect in childhood and parenting identified as maltreating. Labella, M.H., Raby, K.L., Martin, J., & Roisman, G.I. (2019) Romantic functioning mediates prospective associations between childhood abuse and neglect and parenting outcomes in adulthood. *Development & Psychopathology*, 31(1), 95–111.

[306] Berzenski, S.R., Yates, T.M., & Egeland, B. (2014) A multidimensional view of continuity in intergenerational transmission of child maltreatment. In J.E. Korbin & R.D. Krugman (eds) *Handbook of Child Maltreatment*, Vol. 2 (pp.115–29). New York: Springer.

For instance, Thompson and colleagues found that mothers who had experienced sexual or physical violence as children were substantially more likely to have a child subject to inquiry from child protective services. Yet 75% of these referrals were for neglect.[307] The movement of abuse between the generations appears not to be mimetic, as Bowlby had assumed (Chapter 1).

The Minnesota group emphasised that resilience is not a singular entity. Individuals can do well in one area of their life, but less well in others, as a result of the internal and external resources available to them—as well as the cut and colour of the challenges they face. The availability of a secure base as a form of social support helped promote non-abusive caregiving behaviours in mothers in their sample who had themselves experienced abuse. However, the early life stress these mothers experienced in receiving abuse nonetheless had implications for the mental health of their children. Sroufe and Egeland emphasised the importance of both life stress and social support in developmental perspective. When individuals responded to adversity with more positive outcomes, Sroufe and colleagues claimed that in regression analyses—not reported in print—the combination of life stress at different points and social support at different points could account for 80% of variance in outcomes: 'Thus, little is left to mystery with adequate developmental data. Our research has found, time and time again, that resilience is not simply a function of good outcomes despite bad experience, but also an example of prior good experience facilitating the mobilisation of resources.'[308] However, the analyses that lead to the 80% figure are not described in the text or in other published work.

Gender

In 'The domain of developmental psychopathology', Sroufe and Rutter proposed that gender is an important category to investigate.[309] Both researchers found in their longitudinal studies that after puberty males facing risk factors were more likely to display aggression, conduct problems, and other 'externalising' forms of mental health problems, whereas girls were more likely to display depression, anxiety, and other 'internalising' symptoms. Sroufe and Rutter acknowledged that biological factors play a role, but overall their emphasis fell on social and cultural causes of this difference. This conclusion was later reinforced by Bakermans-Kranenburg and colleagues, who found no such gender differences in the distribution or trajectory of depressive symptoms in a Chinese sample, in contrast to European and American samples.[310] Sroufe and Rutter pointed to the role of powerful cultural norms

---

[307] Thompson, R. (2006) Exploring the link between maternal history of childhood victimization and child risk of maltreatment. *Journal of Trauma Practice*, 5(2), 57–72. A recent meta-anlysis of 142 studies showed modest intergenerational transmission of abuse (k = 80; d = .45), and of kind of abuse (neglect: d = .24; physical abuse: d = .41; emotional abuse: d = .57; sexual abuse: d = .39). See Madigan, S., Cyr, C., Eirich, R., et al. (2019) Testing the cycle of maltreatment hypothesis: meta-analytic evidence of the intergenerational transmission of child maltreatment. *Development & Psychopathology*, 31(1), 23–51.

[308] Supkoff, L., Puig, J., & Sroufe, L.A. (2013) Situating resilience in developmental context. In M. Ungar (ed.) *The Social Ecology of Resilience* (pp.127–42). New York: Springer, p.134. It is not clear, however, what outcome measures were used.

[309] Sroufe, L. & Rutter, M. (1984) The domain of developmental psychopathology. *Child Development*, 55(1), 17–29.

[310] Cao, C., Rijlaarsdam, J., van der Voort, A., Ji, L., Zhang, W., & Bakermans-Kranenburg, M.J. (2017) Associations between dopamine D2 receptor (DRD2) gene, maternal positive parenting and trajectories of depressive symptoms from early to mid-adolescence. *Journal of Abnormal Child Psychology*, 46(2), 365–79.

around gender that shape the expression of emotions, the activation of the caregiving system, the modulation of closeness and intimacy, and acceptable bases for self-esteem. They give particular emphasis to gender socialisation, since 'girls in our culture are socialized toward compliance, inhibition, passivity, and reliance on others'. Depression and anxiety are congruent with these forms of socialisation in European and American societies. Sroufe and Rutter also refer to the experience of girls of sexual vulnerability, harassment, and the threat of rape.[311]

In the Minnesota Longitudinal Study of Risk and Adaptation, Pianta, Sroufe, Egeland, and colleagues observed aspects of gender socialisation. For instance, boys who were rated by observers and by their mothers as less socially skilled received more sensitive care at later follow-up, whereas this compensation by mothers was not provided to girls. In fact, girls who were more self-controlled received more sensitive care, which the researchers suspect may have been a form of reward and reinforcement.[312] Gender also played a role in shaping the context of mental health symptoms. For instance, Pianta, Sroufe, and Egeland found profound effects of the kind of role model provided by mothers to their daughters, both as a potential risk and a potential protective factor for internalising symptoms. There was no such effect for boys.[313]

Sroufe and colleagues argued that 'gender is a key aspect of the preschooler's emerging self concept. Being a boy or a girl is central to the definition of the self. Development of a gender-based self-concept involves three steps. First, children gradually adopt sex-typed behaviour—actions that conform to cultural expectations regarding what is appropriate for boys or for girls. Second, children simultaneously acquire a gender-role concept—a beginning knowledge of the cultural stereotypes regarding males and females. Finally, children develop an emotional commitment to their particular gender.'[314] Pursuing this reasoning, the Minnesota group conducted research to examine antecedents of the extent to which children regarded gender as a permanent characteristic.[315] They asked preschool participants whether someone's gender could change in different situations, such as if they put on different clothes. They found that maternal tendencies towards angry or depressive mood reduced girls' perception of gender as a permanent characteristic. By contrast, mothers' support and guidance for problem-solving and their responsiveness at home predicted greater gender concept stability for boys. There was no effect for attachment classification in the Strange Situation.

Indeed, it appeared to Sroufe and Egeland that gender and the attachment system were mostly unrelated phenomena. Given the importance of gender for so many aspects of life, the relatively modest role of gender differences in attachment research is

[311] Sroufe, L. & Rutter, M. (1984) The domain of developmental psychopathology. *Child Development*, 55(1), 17–29, p.26.

[312] Pianta, R.C., Sroufe, L.A., & Egeland, B. (1989) Continuity and discontinuity in maternal sensitivity at 6, 24, and 42 months in a high-risk sample. *Child Development*, 60(2), 481–7, p.486.

[313] Pianta, R.C., Egeland, B., & Sroufe, L.A. (1990) Maternal stress in childrens' development: predictions of school outcomes and identification of protective factors. In J.E. Rolf, A. Masten, D. Cicchetti, K. Neuchterlen, & S. Weintraub (eds) *Risk and Protective Factors in the Development of Psychopathology* (pp.215–35). Cambridge, MA: Cambridge University Press.

[314] Sroufe, L.A., Cooper, R.G., DeHart, G.B., & Marshall, M.E. (1996) *Child Development: Its Nature and Course*, 3rd edn. New York: McGraw-Hill, p.373.

[315] Sroufe, L.A. & Egeland, B. (1991) Illustrations of person and environment interaction from a longitudinal study. In T. Wachs & R. Plomin (eds) *Conceptualization and Measurement of Organism–Environment Interaction* (pp.68–84). Washington, DC: American Psychological Association.

curious.[316] This was already remarked upon by Ainsworth. In correspondence with Bowlby, Ainsworth wrote:

> I believe that the main reason why the issue of sex differences has been so neglected in regard to attachment is that such differences seem to be absent in infancy. Certainly, the three main attachment patterns (strategies) do not differ in incidence among males and females. That makes sense, because in infancy protection is just as important for males as for females, and the kind of protection that is needed is essentially the same for both sexes.[317]

Yet gender would similarly prove of relatively little relevance to the distribution of attachment classifications in middle childhood or adolescence, at least when observational measures were used.[318] Whilst developmental psychopathology has generally been concerned with the interaction of risk and protective factors, there is no implication that all aspects of life will interact to the same extent. Gender and attachment were regarded by Sroufe and Egeland as both important aspects of a child's experience and relevant to their developmental outcomes. In particular, both gender socialisation and attachment were regarded as contributing to the elaboration and calibration of the caregiving and sexual behavioural systems. However, they considered these contributions as largely independent, rather than in interaction—though this was not formally tested. After Sroufe and Egeland's retirement, some small associations were found by Raby, Roisman, and colleagues on the Adult Attachment Interview (AAI) when this was coded dimensionally rather than categorically: dismissing is slightly more common in male participants ($r = .17$), and preoccupation in female participants ($r = .22$).[319] However, such associations are not large enough to imply a need to substantially renegotiate Sroufe and Egeland's position on gender and attachment.

Two case studies

Case descriptions are woven in elegantly to the reports of the Minnesota group, particularly in Sroufe's early book chapters.[320] However, it was rare for the group to describe in detail the result of the assessments that had taken place over the years with particular dyads. Two case studies, however, were reported in substantial depth at the end of the 1990s. One was the case

---

[316] Sroufe, L.A., Cooper, R.G., DeHart, G.B., & Marshall, M.E. (1996) *Child Development: Its Nature and Course*, 3rd edn. New York: McGraw-Hill: 'Gender is a central organising theme in development. It plays a key role in the way people define and experience their worlds. In all societies, parents and others treat boys and girls differently and expect different things from them. Because of this, children learn cultural stereotypes regarding male and female behaviours and characteristics. This learning begins early and is pervasive. It manifests itself in children's activities, preferences, and social styles. Even among preschoolers, gender is so salient that a child's most advanced thinking is often applied to it. Preschoolers label and categorise different activities in terms of gender (Fagot et al. 1992); they remember modelled behaviours better when they are "gender appropriate" (Bauer 1993); and in general they use gender as a basis for organising information (Serbin et al. 1993)' (372–3).

[317] Ainsworth, M. (1989) *Letter to John Bowlby*, 16 November 1989. PP/BOW/B.3/8.

[318] Bakermans-Kranenburg, M.J. & van IJzendoorn, M.H. (2009) No reliable gender differences in attachment across the lifespan. *Behavioral and Brain Sciences*, 32(1), 22–3.

[319] Raby, K.L., Labella, M.H., Martin, J., Carlson, E.A., & Roisman, G.I. (2017) Childhood abuse and neglect and insecure attachment states of mind in adulthood: prospective, longitudinal evidence from a high-risk sample. *Development & Psychopathology*, 29(2), 347–63, Table 4.

[320] E.g. Sroufe, L.A. (1983) Infant–caregiver attachment and patterns of adaptation in preschool: the roots of maladaptation and competence. In M. Perlmutter (ed.) *Development and Policy Concerning Children with Special Needs: The Minnesota Symposium in Child Psychology*, Vol. 16 (pp.41–83). Hillsdale, NJ: Lawrence Erlbaum.

of Beth. At 12 months, Beth and her mother received a classification of ambivalent/resistant attachment, and at 18 months a classification of secure attachment. Beth's father was killed in a car crash, but at 24 months Beth and her mother both seemed to be doing well under the circumstances. Beth was able to cooperate effectively with her mother in the 24-month tool-use situation, and at 42 months was persistent and enthusiastic in attempting the difficult Barrier Box task.[321] At the end of first grade, Beth's mother had remarried. Her teacher described Beth as a bit of a loner, but doing quite well academically. In an interview during second grade, the interviewer noticed that Beth seemed afraid of her stepfather, who was regularly drunk. A year later, Beth and her mother moved into a women's shelter. In the sixth grade follow-up, Beth and her mother were living with the stepfather again.

At the follow-up when participants were 17 years old, it took some time for the researchers to locate Beth. In interview, she described that her stepfather had been subjecting her to multiple forms of maltreatment since she was 12 years old. Child protection services inquiries had been deflected by her mother and father, who presented Beth herself as the problem and disengaged when this narrative was questioned. She had left home at 16, and her parents left the state in order to avoid a court order that the stepfather leave the home to protect the younger siblings. Beth first lived with a foster family, then a boyfriend, then her grandparents. She had remained in school throughout this period. The clinical interview at age 17 revealed no current psychiatric diagnosis. The interview documented depression in early adolescence, and a subclinical phobia of small spaces. She also reported one past suicide attempt. At age 19, Beth had been awarded a scholarship to attend college and had completed one semester. She had recently withdrawn due to problems with her boyfriend, including abuse. However, she planned to return to school, had a part-time job, and seemed to be doing very well in other areas of her life. She was in the process of seeking counselling.

A second detailed case study offered by the Minnesota group was that of Laura Miller (a pseudonym). In the 1990s, a furious controversy raged regarding whether adult 'recovered memories' of child sexual abuse were fabulations or truthful recollections of previously repressed experience.[322] In 1998, the journal *Development and Psychopathology* dedicated a special issue to this concern, which highlighted the need for thinking about how memory processes following trauma might be drawn upon for coping and for other adaptive challenges.[323] In line with this interest, in an article from the same year, Duggal and Sroufe reported the first ever prospective report in which sexual abuse was documented by multiple sources, and the young person subsequently reported no recall of the abuse for a time, and then 'recovered' the memory. Data for the case study were drawn from the longitudinal study, from a follow-up interview with Laura and her mother, from the records of a

---

[321] Egeland, B. (1997) Mediators of the effects of child maltreatment on developmental adaptation in adolescence. In D. Cicchetti & S. Toth (eds) *Rochester Symposium on Developmental Psychopathology: Vol. VIII. The Effects of Trauma on the Developmental Process* (pp.403–434). Rochester, NY: University of Rochester Press, p.417.

[322] E.g. Herman, J.L. (1992) *Trauma and Recovery*. New York: Basic Books; Ceci, S.J. & Loftus, E.F. (1994) 'Memory work': a royal road to false memories? *Applied Cognitive Psychology*, 8, 351–64. For professionals' views on recovered memories see Ost, J., Wright, D.B., Easton, S., Hope, L., & French, C.C. (2013) Recovered memories, satanic abuse, dissociative identity disorder and false memories in the UK: a survey of clinical psychologists and hypnotherapists. *Psychology, Crime & Law*, 19(1), 1–19. For discussions of this debate in historical context see e.g. Hult, J. (2005) The re-emergence of memory recovery: return of seduction theory and birth of survivorship. *History of the Human Sciences*, 18(1), 127–42.

[323] Toth, S. L. & Cicchetti, D. (1998) Remembering, forgetting, and the effects of trauma on memory: a developmental psychopathology perspective. *Development & Psychopathology*, 10(4), 589–605.

therapist who worked with the family after child protection services became involved when Laura was four years old, and from interviews with Laura's child protection worker and her therapist.

A first sign of sexual trauma was documented in preschool. Laura was one of the children who was part of the preschool class made up of members of the sample. The head teacher of the preschool reported sexual behaviours shown by Laura in the preschool classroom. In the interview with mothers when their children were 54 months, Ms Miller (Laura's mother) stated that Laura had described a dream in which her father, who had some limited custody, had come into her bed while she was sleeping and touched her, while she pleaded with him to stop. When confronted, Laura's father denied sexually abusing Laura, but agreed to see Laura for only three hours per week and only with a third party present. Ms Miller asked child protection services if visitation could be prevented entirely, but physical examination for penetration was negative and by this time Laura would not talk any further about the incident, so it would have been difficult to evidence by the legal standards of the time. However, Laura was referred for therapy. The therapist notes from the period agree with Ms Miller's account. They also state that Laura spontaneously announced to the therapist, a month after intake, that 'Daddy knows he did it, he's just scared'. The notes included record of Laura's anxiety and anger towards her father.[324] The father was interviewed by the therapist and said that he had no memory of sexually abusing his daughter, and that if it occurred it would have been while he was on drugs. At the end of first grade, Laura's teacher related that Laura had told her that the reason her parents had divorced was that her father had abused her, but that he was not doing it any more. Duggal and Sroufe concluded that 'Multiple sources of evidence discussed in this section consistently support the conclusion that Laura experienced trauma of a sexual nature during early childhood'.[325] The last record in which Laura evidenced knowledge of abuse was at age eight, in the therapist notes.

In her engagements with mental health services in seventh and ninth grade, she did not mention childhood sexual abuse as a presenting issue. At age 16, participants in the study were asked to complete a broad-ranging written health interview. One of the items was the question: 'Have you ever been sexually abused? Sexual abuse is when someone in your family or someone else touches you in a place you did not want to be touched, or does something to you sexually which they shouldn't have done.' Laura indicated that she had not been sexually abused. The interviewer noted that Laura appeared unguarded in her replies, and disclosed various other personal information with candour. At age 17, in a clinical interview to assess symptoms of post-traumatic stress disorder, Laura was asked whether she had ever had any terrible and unusual experiences. She reported, without hesitation, that she had experienced nothing of this kind. In response to a query regarding experiences of abuse, including sexual abuse, Laura replied that this had not happened to her. She was again candid in discussing other difficult past and present experiences, including contemporary mental health problems. Ms Miller recalled that during adolescence, Laura reported being happy to spend time with her father and wanted to see him more. Ms Miller did not bring up the issue of abuse or ask direct questions because she felt that she had been warned by child protection services to avoid 'putting words in Laura's mouth'.[326]

[324] Duggal, S. & Sroufe, L.A. (1998) Recovered memory of childhood sexual trauma: a documented case from a longitudinal study. *Journal of Traumatic Stress*, 11(2), 301–321, p.306.

[325] Ibid. p.311.

[326] Ibid. p.313.

When Laura was 18, she took part in an AAI (Chapter 3), which includes a question about experiences of abuse. In response to this question, Laura described a recent conversation with her boyfriend about her first memories of her parents. This triggered a 'really overwhelming feeling', and led Laura to seek out a trusted teacher. During the conversation with the teacher, she reportedly recovered memories of her father kissing her while she was in bed, with a sense that there was a sexual component to the interaction:

> I told her this first memory and then it just came to me. Like, it just was so clear in my mind, um, you know he like did this to me, whatever. And um, and I like went into complete shock ... I just felt like I was really dizzy and, and I couldn't really see very well and, and there was like all these noises going on, but I didn't know what they were, and and it wa- I was really confused and, like I couldn't cry but I felt like I should be.[327]

She added: 'You know he bent, he was like walking over to me and he bent down and kissed me. And there's something after that and I don't know what it is.'[328] Following the conversation with the teacher, Laura's relationship with her father changed strikingly. She felt scared of him most of the time, interspersed with missing him terribly. Duggal and Sroufe argued that exclusion of memory of the event made sense if Laura was forced to see her father during her childhood. There was a logic to the memory resurfacing at age 18, since this was the threshold of Laura's independence from her parents and the need for visitation. Duggal and Sroufe situated Laura's case as illustrating the role of defensive processes as adaptive responses to situations that cannot be controlled or escaped. They conjectured that it seemed a good sign for Laura's later development that she could release the exclusion of the painful memory at the point that she was no longer required to see her father.

There is no sense that the two published case studies are representative of the sample as a whole. They nonetheless offer a valuable window into the way that the multiple assessments of the Minnesota Longitudinal Study of Risk and Adaptation together offered the research group an encompassing picture of human lives, each hard-won and remarkable. The cases illustrate the approach to child development that framed Egeland and Sroufe's work on the Minnesota study. The assessments conducted by the Minnesota group allowed lines of continuity and discontinuity in development to be examined, alongside exploration of the interdependence and lurching along of different social relationships. Comparison of the two cases illustrates the important role of changing adversities and social supports for the kinds of resilience they could muster. For instance, the cases of Beth and Laura illustrate disinhibiting parental drug and alcohol use as a risk factor for the children, which compounded with other adversities and forms of unforgiving isolation they faced.

Both case studies were reported in the late 1990s. There have subsequently been several further waves of data collection. The field has also seen a 'changing of the guards' with the retirement of Sroufe and Egeland. Such a significant developmental transition has come with new challenges, and, as could be anticipated, has required the elaboration and change in the field's inner organisation. One angle on the lines of developmental continuity between past and present is to consider one of Sroufe and Egeland's former students, Dante Cicchetti, who now holds Sroufe's William Harris Professorship in Child Development at the University of

---

Minnesota. Cicchetti did not primarily regard himself as an attachment researcher. However, the approach of Sroufe and Egeland and the findings of the Minnesota Longitudinal Study of Risk and Adaptation have been a central component of his influential approach to developmental psychology. Consideration of Cicchetti's work offers an illustration of one way that the legacy of the study of attachment at Minnesota has been inherited by subsequent researchers.

Two former students

Dante Cicchetti

Part of Mary Ainsworth's achievement was to have translated a new and exciting methodological innovation into a new generation of attachment researchers in the 1970s and 1980s, including many important future leaders (Chapter 2). The other primary hub of attachment research during the period was the Minnesota group, which was also critical for mentoring a second generation of attachment researchers. Sroufe commented that his proudest achievement has been the contribution made by his former students to the field.[329] One of Sroufe's last doctoral students was Glenn Roisman, whose work was discussed in Chapter 3. At the other end of his career, one of his first doctoral students was Dante Cicchetti. Cicchetti had a drive to examine experiences of risk and improve outcomes for families rooted in his own childhood. As he later recalled in interview, 'much of my research has been influenced by my own experiences. Early encounters with poverty and harsh conditions played a major role in fuelling my research interest in child maltreatment.'[330] He later dedicated his Award from the American Psychological Association for Distinguished Senior Career Contribution to Psychology in the Public Interest to his younger sister 'Candace, who died in the fall of 2000. She represents one of all too many individuals who unfortunately lose battles due to adverse circumstances and mental illness.'[331] Cicchetti has also written about his own struggles around mental health.[332]

Cicchetti's doctoral thesis examined the affective and cognitive development of infants with Down syndrome.[333] Cicchetti badged his work as an application of the organisational perspective, announced in the Sroufe and Waters 1977 paper 'Attachment as an organizational construct' (Chapter 2).[334] Over four decades there is an explanation of this

---

[329] Alan Sroufe, personal communication to Dante Cicchetti, cited in Cicchetti, D. (2011) Champions of psychology: Dante Cicchetti—an interview with APS Student Caucus. *Association for Psychological Science Observer*, 24(9). http://www.psychologicalscience.org/index.php/publications/observer/champions-ofpsychology-dante-cicchetti.html.

[330] Ibid.

[331] Cicchetti, D. (2004) Biography. *American Psychologist*, 59(8), 1–4 p.728–31.

[332] Cicchetti, D. (2015) Reflections on Carroll Izard's contributions: influences on diverse scientific disciplines and personal recollections. *Emotion Review*, 7(2), 104–109.

[333] Cicchetti, D. & Sroufe, L.A. (1976) The relationship between affective and cognitive development in Down's syndrome infants. *Child Development*, 47, 920–29.

[334] Several other later researchers in developmental psychopathology situated themselves as under the banner of Sroufe's 'organisational perspective'. See for instance Wyman, P.A., Cowen, E.L., Work, W.C., & Kerley, J.H. (1993) The role of children's future expectations in self-system functioning and adjustment to life stress: a prospective study of urban at-risk children. *Development & Psychopathology*, 5(4), 649–61. However, Cicchetti has been the most consistent advocate for this as an explicit approach to and model of developmental psychopathology.

perspective in nearly every first-author article and book chapter he has written. Following Sroufe, Cicchetti emphasised that individual behaviours should not be the unit of analysis in the study of child development. Instead, researchers should focus on the integration of resources in responding to the most important challenges from the environment relevant to a person at that time in their lives.[335] Bowlby's concept of probabilistic developmental pathways had just been introduced during Cicchetti's time as a graduate student, and this proved an important influence on his exploration of the interaction of factors in both risk and resilience, and the reciprocal interpretation of typical and atypical development in light of one another.[336] As a graduate student at Minnesota, Cicchetti co-authored a review paper with Egeland on antecedents of child maltreatment, with particular attention paid to the role of poverty, family conflict, and alcohol and substance use.[337] He documented that parents who maltreat their children show no single set of personality traits or fit into specific psychiatric diagnostic categories. Instead there are a wide variety of factors that together contribute to the likelihood of maltreatment, as well as other potential difficulties for children and families. The fact that a diversity of pathways could lead to the same outcome would be dubbed by Cicchetti as 'equifinality'; the fact that a single pathway could contribute to diverse outcomes would be dubbed 'multifinality'.[338]

After leaving Minnesota in 1977, his central focus in the 1980s was basic research on child maltreatment. Cicchetti took up a faculty position at Harvard, where he won a grant for over $2 million from the National Center on Child Abuse and Neglect for a study of the etiology, intergenerational transmission, and developmental sequelae of children. Funding for follow-up research with the sample was provided by the National Institute of Mental Health and the William T. Grant Foundation. He became Director of the Mt. Hope Family Center at the University of Rochester in 1985. During the 1980s, Cicchetti played a pivotal role in the initiation of developmental psychopathology as a movement within developmental science. He sustained a punishing schedule of productive work during the decade as the movement was established. One metric is his work as an editor: as well as initiating the journal *Development and Psychopathology* and the annual *Rochester Symposium on Developmental Psychopathology*, Cicchetti co-edited 10 books through the 1980s. He also published 26 articles as first author.

By the end of the decade, the National Academy of Sciences had embraced developmental psychopathology as the overarching framework for its report *Research on Children*

---

[335] Cicchetti, D. & Sroufe, L.A. (1978) An organizational view of affect: illustration from the study of Down's syndrome infants. In M. Lewis & L. Rosenblum (eds) *The Development of Affect* (pp.309–350). New York: Plenum Press; Cicchetti, D. & Schneider-Rosen, K. (1986) An organisational approach to childhood depression. In M. Rutter, C. Izard, & P. Read (eds) *Depression in Young People: Clinical and Developmental Perspectives*. New York: Guilford.

[336] Cicchetti, D. & Greenberg, M.T. (1991) The legacy of John Bowlby. *Development & Psychopathology*, 3(4), 347–50.

[337] Cicchetti, D., Taraldson, B., & Egeland, B. (1978) Perspectives in the treatment and understanding of child abuse. In A. Goldstein (ed.) *Prescriptions for Child Mental Health and Education* (pp.301–378). New York: Pergamon.

[338] Cicchetti, D., Cummings, E.M., Greenberg, M.T., & Marvin, R.S. (1990) An organisational perspective on attachment beyond infancy: implications for theory, measurement and research. In M.T. Greenberg, D. Cicchetti, & E.M. Cummings (eds) *Attachment in the Preschool Years* (pp.1–50). Chicago: University of Chicago Press, p.35; Cicchetti, D. & Rogosch, F.A. (1996) Equifinality and multifinality in developmental psychopathology. *Development & Psychopathology*, 8, 597–600. These terms were drawn from general systems theory and embryology: see von Bertalanffy, L. (1968) *General System Theory*. New York: Braziller; Weiss, P. (1969) *Principles of Development*. New York: Hafner.

and *Adolescents with Mental, Behavioural, and Developmental Disorders*,[339] and the National Institute of Mental Health had situated developmental psychopathology as the organising framework for future research funding priorities for child and adolescent mental health.[340] In 1990, the eminent developmental researcher Robert Emde described the work of Cicchetti, Mary Main, and others as commencing the 'third phase of attachment research'.[341] If Bowlby's initiation of attachment theory had represented the first phase, and the validation of the Strange Situation by Ainsworth, Sroufe, Egeland, and others in the late 1970s and 1980s had represented the second phrase, the third phase was characterised by innovations in methodology to examine attachment beyond infancy and new insights into risk and protective factors for mental illness.

Yet the continuities between the work of Cicchetti and Sroufe were strong and fundamental. Cicchetti picked up from Sroufe and colleagues an abiding concern for the implications of early attachment relationships, even if this concern would be integrated within a broader frame. For instance, he argued for greater attention to the implications of cultural differences in constituting and shaping risk and promotive factors, and individual and group responses to challenges.[342] However, the prime extension of Sroufe's model was the inclusion of biological factors. Cicchetti was led to a concern with biological differences from the start of his career in making sense of the experiences of families with an infant with Down syndrome. However, he was also part of a generation of researchers with much more ready access to a diversifying array of biomedical measures. Cicchetti argued that the account of resilience provided by Sroufe and colleagues could be expanded and enhanced through attention to biological factors, such as neurological, endocrinal, genetic, and immunological processes, as sources of stability and change in developmental pathways.[343]

Behavioural systems such as attachment were reconceived as having affective, cognitive, behavioural, cultural, and neuroendocrinal components. Cicchetti therefore argued that assessments of maltreated children by child protective services as well as researchers should include both biological and psychological measures. However, for Cicchetti, this was only as a more fiercely realised version, not different in kind, from Sroufe's stance that the development of the 'whole person' must be kept in view.[344] It was also an extension of Sroufe's focus on the emotional components of behavioural systems. Cicchetti regarded emotions as having four components: non-verbal components, verbal components, experiential components,

[339] National Academy of Sciences (1989) *Research on Children and Adolescents with Mental, Behavioral, and Developmental Disorders.* Washington, DC: National Academy Press.

[340] US Department of Health and Human Services (1990) *National Plan for Research on Child and Adolescent Mental Disorders.* Rockville, MD: US Department of Health and Human Services, National Institute on Mental Health.

[341] Emde, R. (1990) Preface. In M.T. Greenberg, D. Cicchetti, & E.M. Cummings (eds) *Attachment in the Preschool Years* (pp.ix–xii). Chicago: University of Chicago Press, p.x.

[342] Coll, C.G., Akerman, A., & Cicchetti, D. (2000) Cultural influences on developmental processes and outcomes: implications for the study of development and psychopathology. *Development & Psychopathology*, 12(3), 333–56. On the role of cultural components within the organisation of the attachment behavioural system see also Morelli, G., Chaudhary, N., Gottlieb, A., et al. (2017) Taking culture seriously: a pluralistic approach to attachment. In H. Keller & K.A. Bard (eds) *The Cultural Nature of Attachment* (pp.139–69). Cambridge, MA: MIT Press.

[343] Cicchetti, D. (2002) How a child builds a brain: insights from normality and psychopathology. In W. Hartup & R. Weinberg (eds) *Child Psychology in Retrospect and Prospect: The Minnesota Symposia on Child Psychology*, Vol. 32 (pp.23–71). Mahwah, NJ: Lawrence Erlbaum.

[344] Curtis, W.J. & Cicchetti, D. (2003) Moving research on resilience into the 21st century: theoretical and methodological considerations in examining the biological contributors to resilience. *Development & Psychopathology*, 15(3), 773–810.

and biological components.[345] For instance Cicchetti and colleagues utilised the Egeland and Sroufe methodology of inviting their child participants to take part in summer camps in order to see how individuals form and respond to the developmental challenge of peer relationships. However, unlike Egeland and Sroufe, Cicchetti and colleagues interpreted the behaviour of the individuals and the interactions of the groups in light of neuroendocrinal data, as well as self-report and observation.[346]

Egeland and Sroufe did not have available such neurological and hormonal measures and did not give biological processes a specific place in their thinking about behavioural systems.[347] However, to some extent both researchers were attentive to biological factors. For instance, Sroufe and Waters pioneered the use of physiological measures of cardiac response to show the distress of the apparently unruffled infants in avoidant dyads. And there is every reason to assume that if other physiological measures of sympathetic nervous system response had been available, for instance saliva cortisol, Sroufe and Waters would have measured these too.[348] Nonetheless, of the two principal investigators, Egeland appears to have been the more sympathetic to biological assessments. He drew on assessments of puberty development in elaborating structural equation models of the antecedents of teenage sexual behaviour and alcohol use. Attentive to the multicausal processes involved in puberty timing, Egeland and colleagues regarded physical maturity as a 'combined effect of hormones and social interactions'.[349] He also offered speculations on the neurophysiological processes that provide the infrastructure for avoidant and resistant attachment.[350] Cicchetti and Egeland have subsequently worked together on a study of contribution of genotype to insecure attachment in the Minnesota sample. The researchers found that variance in the serotonin-transporter-linked polymorphic region (5-HTTLPR) had no association with whether a child was classified as secure or insecure. However, for those classified as insecure, it contributed to the prediction of an ambivalent/resistant or avoidant attachment classification, through children's emotional reactivity.[351] 5-HTTLPR also predicted the subtype of secure attachment, contributing to the more distressed (B3 and B4) or less distressed (B1 and B2) form of security. The effect seemed to be independent of the contribution made to

[345] Cicchetti, D. & White, J. (1988) Emotional development and the affective disorders. In W. Damon (ed.) *Child Development: Today and Tomorrow* (pp.177–98). San Francisco: Jossey-Bass.

[346] Cicchetti, D. & Rogosch, F.A. (2001) The impact of child maltreatment and psychopathology upon neuroendocrine functioning. *Development & Psychopathology*, 13, 783–804.

[347] Egeland, B. (1983) Book review: the second year: the emergence of self awareness by J. Kagan. *Journal of Orthopsychiatry*, 53, 365–7: 'Most of us tend to ignore the issue of inheritance and the biological basis of behavior' (366).

[348] Sroufe had a career-long concern with medications given to children, and this concern was generally a sense of dismay at how social and family relationships got sidelined by the hunt for neuroendocrinal solutions to developmental problems. See e.g. Sroufe, L.A. & Stewart, M.A. (1973) Treating problem children with stimulant drugs. *New England Journal of Medicine*, 209, 407–413; Sroufe, L.A. (2012) The 'other' drug dilemma. *USA Today*, May 2012, p.21.

[349] Siebenbruner, J., Zimmer-Gembeck, M.J., & Egeland, B. (2007) Sexual partners and contraceptive use: a 16-year prospective study predicting abstinence and risk behavior. *Journal of Research on Adolescence*, 17(1), 179–206, p.184.

[350] Egeland, B., Weinfield, N., Bosquet, M., & Cheng, V. (2000) Remembering, repeating, and working through: lessons from attachment-based interventions. In J. Osofsky (ed.) *WHIMH Handbook of Infant Mental Health, Vol. 4* (pp.35–89). New York: Wiley: 'Suboptimal social environments tend to promote physiological systems that are dominated by the parasympathetic branch of the autonomic nervous system (avoidant histories) or the sympathetic branch of the autonomic nervous system (resistant histories)' (42).

[351] Raby, K.L., Cicchetti, D., Carlson, E.A., Cutuli, J.J., Englund, M.M., & Egeland, B. (2012) Genetic and caregiving-based contributions to infant attachment: unique associations with distress reactivity and attachment security. *Psychological Science*, 23(9), 1016–23.

attachment classification by caregiver sensitivity: there was no interaction effect between the variables. On the basis of such findings, Raby, Cicchetti, Egeland, and colleagues have called for 'reconciliation' between Sroufe's focus on attachment and Kagan's focus on temperament, arguing that both can make a contribution.[352] However, it should be noted that Raby's later work on the NICHD sample has not offered support for the role of molecular genetic factors in predicting attachment classifications.[353]

In agreement with Sroufe and Egeland, Cicchetti viewed it as an important intervention against the stigma attached to mental illness to view symptoms as ordinary and statistically expectable responses to a dynamic accumulation of adversities, and relative lack of supports, in the course of development.[354] Whilst less adverse to use of diagnostic categories in assessments than Sroufe, Cicchetti has been mindful of the sociological processes that led to the dominant role of diagnoses within psychology, and in his own work on children and adolescents has focused much more on cross-diagnostic developmental and relational processes.[355] Cicchetti and Toth have been extensively involved, for example, in studies that measure traumatic experiences, but have expressed doubts about the criteria used to diagnose trauma in clinical practice, for instance the need for a precipitating single event.[356] They have also expressed concern regarding the varied connotations of the term 'trauma', which can lead to miscommunication between researchers, for instance in discussion of the implications of trauma across developmental periods.

The decision to not intervene with the families in the Minnesota study, even the maltreating families not known to child protective services, in their study, but to watch and try to understand was one that weighed heavily on Sroufe and colleagues.[357] They felt that their participants had signed up for a cohort study, not an intervention study, and that it was also important to understand the naturalistic antecedents and implications of child maltreatment in order to inform future intervention efforts. By contrast, Egeland was actively involved in the creation of the STEEP intervention (which is discussed in the section 'Holism in interventions'). Like Egeland, Cicchetti was concerned with both epidemiology and clinical intervention, a position he and Toth described as 'Bowlby's dream come full circle' in contributing to clinical practice.[358] However, Cicchetti and Toth argued that Bowlby's attention to psychological unavailability must be elaborated into a more multicausal model, capable of acknowledging factors such as economic, medical and housing difficulties, without

---

[352] Ibid. p.1017.

[353] Raby, K.L., Roisman, G.I., & Booth-LaForce, C. (2015) Genetic moderation of stability in attachment security from early childhood to age 18 years: a replication study. Developmental Psychology, 51(11), 1645–9.

[354] Hinshaw, S.P. & Cicchetti, D. (2000) Stigma and mental disorder: conceptions of illness, public attitudes, personal disclosure, and social policy. Development & Psychopathology, 12(4), 555–98.

[355] E.g. Richers, J.E. & Cicchetti, D. (1993) Mark Twain meets DSM-III-R: conduct disorder, development, and the concept of harmful dysfunction. Development & Psychopathology, 5(1–2), 5–29.

[356] Cicchetti, D. & Toth, S.L. (1997) Preface. In D. Cicchetti & S.L. Toth (eds) Rochester Symposium on Developmental Psychopathology: Trauma: Perspectives on Theory, Research, and Intervention, Vol. 8 (pp.xi–xvi). Rochester, NY: University of Rochester Press.

[357] Sroufe, L.A., Egeland, B., Carlson, E.A., & Collins, W.A. (2005) The Development of the Person. New York: Guilford, p.84.

[358] Cicchetti, D., Toth, S.L., & Lynch, M. (1995) Bowlby's dream comes full circle. In Advances in Clinical Child Psychology (pp.1–75). Boston: Springer. Cf. Bowlby, J. (1988) A Secure Base. London: Routledge: It was 'unexpected that, whereas attachment theory was formulated by a clinician for use in the diagnosis and treatment of emotionally disturbed patients and families, its usage ... has been mainly to promote research in developmental psychology' (ix).

collapsing levels of analysis.[359] Cicchetti and Toth also supplemented Bowlby's approach with Sroufe's more fine-grained attention to different developmental challenges across the lifecourse. For instance, Cicchetti and Toth argued that it follows from an organisational perspective that even when a child has been supported to achieve good outcomes following maltreatment, developmental reorganisations—such as the transition to parenthood—could result in vulnerabilities. The reorganisation may well draw upon earlier affective, cognitive, behavioural, and neuroendocrine components that had previously not been much in evidence.[360] On the other hand, Cicchetti and Toth emphasised that developmental transitions such as adolescence, and their ensuing shifts in challenges and relevant resources, can also represent opportunities for reorganisation away from pathology, especially if there are resources available on the basis of past experience or present support.[361]

Additionally, intervention research offered the prospect of experimental rather than naturalistic evidence for theoretical hypotheses. Intervention studies allow mechanisms of change and stability for families to be specified, and causation more readily distinguished from correlation.[362] Cicchetti, Toth, and colleagues were early adopters of the use of randomised control trials to evaluate interventions with families and the use of attachment measures as intervention outcomes.[363] Even as attachment theory has seen a decline in authority and acceptance within the developmental science community, Cicchetti has remained supportive of research in this area. In his role as a prominent and influential editor, he has allocated space to attachment theory as a key paradigm within developmental psychopathology. From his perspective, the preferential attachment relationships with a caregiver or caregivers established in infancy 'provide a context for children's emerging bio-behavioral organization', influencing the integration of 'neurobiological, cognitive, affective, and behavioral capacities that influence ongoing and future relationships, as well as the understanding of self'.[364] Stating their agreement with Sroufe, Egeland and colleagues, Cicchetti, and Boyle have argued that 'variations in early attachment are not considered to be pathology, or as directly causing pathology. However, they do lay the foundation for disturbances in developmental processes which can eventuate in psychopathology'.[365] For instance, the researchers

[359] Cicchetti, D. & Toth, S.L. (1995) Child maltreatment and attachment organization: implications for intervention. In S. Goldberg, R. Muir, & J. Kerr (eds) *Attachment Theory: Social, Developmental, and Clinical Perspectives* (pp.279–308). Hillsdale, NJ: The Analytic Press, p.280.

[360] Cicchetti and colleagues termed this 'hierarchic motility': the way that early components may be incorporated into later behavioural systems and remain accessible to be activated, especially during periods of extreme stress. This can be an asset, if earlier resources can be made available and repurposed for new tasks. However, it can also be a liability if these earlier components are called upon but not well suited to contemporary challenges. See Cicchetti, D. (1994) Integrating developmental risk factors: perspectives from developmental psychopathology. In C. Nelson (ed.) *Threats to Optimal Development: Integrating Biological, Psychological, and Social Risk Factors: The Minnesota Symposia on Child Psychology*, Vol. 27 (pp.229–72). Hillsdale, NJ: Lawrence Erlbaum.

[361] Cicchetti, D. & Toth, S.L. (eds) (1996) *Rochester Symposium on Developmental Psychopathology: Adolescence : Opportunities and Challenges*, Vol. 7. Rochester, NY: University of Rochester Press.

[362] Cicchetti, D. & Hinshaw, S.P. (2002) Prevention and intervention science: contributions to developmental theory. *Development & Psychopathology*, 14(4), 667–71; Toth, S.L., Sturge-Apple, M.L., Rogosch, F.A., & Cicchetti, D. (2015) Mechanisms of change: testing how preventative interventions impact psychological and physiological stress functioning in mothers in neglectful families. *Development & Psychopathology*, 27(4), 1661–74.

[363] Cicchetti, D., Toth, S.L., & Rogosch, F.A. (1999) The efficacy of toddler–parent psychotherapy to increase attachment security in offspring of depressed mothers. *Attachment & Human Development*, 1(1), 34–66; Toth, S.L., Rogosch, F.A., & Cicchetti, D. (2008) Attachment-theory informed intervention and reflective functioning in depressed mothers. In H. Steele & M. Steele (eds) *The Adult Attachment Interview in Clinical Context* (pp.154–72). New York: Guilford.

[364] Cicchetti, D. & Doyle, C. (2016) Child maltreatment, attachment and psychopathology: mediating relations. *World Psychiatry*, 15(2), 89–90, p.89.

[365] Ibid. p.90.

found that secure attachment at 26 months fully mediated the association between a psycho-therapy intervention for parents suffering from depression and their child's display of con-duct problems at school eight years later.[366]

Cicchetti and colleagues were the first researchers to use the Main and Solomon dis-organised attachment classification in a sample of maltreated children.[367] The Harvard Child Maltreatment Project was initiated in 1979 by Cicchetti and Aber, as a large longi-tudinal study, modelled on the Minnesota Longitudinal Study of Risk and Adaptation.[368] A small subsample were seen in the Strange Situation and classified using the Ainsworth categories.[369] Twenty-two dyads were known to child protection services for abuse and/or neglect of the child or an older sibling; 21 were a matched comparison group. However, a third of the sample were classified as securely attached, which was an unexpected and concerning finding. Like Egeland and Sroufe, the infants in these dyads displayed dis-rupted behaviour that seemed to interrupt or contradict their use of the caregiver as a secure base. There were a few different proposals available for additions to Ainsworth's system. One was that of Ainsworth's student Patricia Crittenden, who observed that many abused infants show both avoidant and resistant attachment (A–C).[370] Another was the Main and Solomon disorganised attachment classification, which appealed to Cicchetti and colleagues as more encompassing; it was assumed that finer-grained dis-tinctions could be worked out later. The disorganised classification also had the advan-tage of evidence from Main's laboratory of relevant correlations with interviews with the caregivers and with the child's later behaviour, offering a source of predictive validity.[371] The analysis used a coding of the data conducted by Cicchetti and Barnett; Barnett was blind to the children's maltreatment status: 82% of the infant–caregiver dyads known to child protection services were classified as showing disorganised attachment and 14% classified as secure; in the comparison group 19% were classified as disorganised and 52% classified as secure. At 18 months, 61% of dyads known to child protection services were classified as showing disorganised attachment compared to 29% in the comparison group.[372]

[366] Guild, D.J., Toth, S.L., Handley, E.D., Rogosch, F.A., & Cicchetti, D. (2017) Attachment security mediates the longitudinal association between child–parent psychotherapy and peer relations for toddlers of depressed moth-ers. *Development & Psychopathology*, 29(2), 587–600.

[367] Carlson, V., Cicchetti, D., Barnett, D., & Braunwald, K. (1989) Finding order in disorganization: lessons from research on maltreated infants' attachments to their caregivers. In D. Cicchetti & V. Carlson (eds) *Child Maltreatment: Theory and Research on the Causes and Consequences of Child Abuse and Neglect* (pp.494–528). Cambridge: Cambridge University Press.

[368] Another early, important study of a sample with substantial rates of maltreatment was conducted by Mary Jo Ward, also a former student of Sroufe: Ward, M.J. & Carlson, E.A. (1995) Associations among adult attachment representations, maternal sensitivity, and infant–mother attachment in a sample of adolescent mothers. *Child Development*, 66(1), 69–79.

[369] Schneider-Rosen, K., Braunwald, K.G., Carlson, V., & Cicchetti, D. (1985) Current perspectives in attach-ment theory: illustration from the study of maltreated infants. *Monographs of the Society for Research in Child Development*, 50(1–2), 194–210.

[370] Crittenden, P.M. (1988) Relationships at risk. In J. Belsky & T. Nezworski (eds) *Clinical Implications of Attachment Theory* (pp.136–74). Hillsdale, NJ: Lawrence Erlbaum.

[371] Carlson, V., Cicchetti, D., Barnett, D., & Braunwald, K. (1989) Finding order in disorganization: lessons from research on maltreated infants' attachments to their caregivers. In D. Cicchetti & V. Carlson (eds) *Child Maltreatment: Theory and Research on the Causes and Consequences of Child Abuse and Neglect* (pp.494–528). Cambridge: Cambridge University Press, p.507.

[372] Barnett, D., Ganiban, J., & Cicchetti, D. (1999) Maltreatment, negative expressivity, and the development of type D attachments from 12 to 24 months of age. *Monographs of the Society for Research in Child Development*, 64(3), 97–118.

In a later study, Cicchetti, Rogosch, and Toth used the Strange Situation as part of the evaluation of two different forms of intervention with 137 families known to child protection services for infant abuse and/or neglect.[373] They also included 52 matched families as a non-maltreating comparison sample. The maltreating families were allocated to one of three conditions. In the first condition, they received usual social work support. In the second condition, they received an intervention that focused on teaching parents about infants' needs. In the third condition, the mother–child dyad received once-a-week psychotherapy, using the model of child–parent psychotherapy developed by Selma Fraiberg[374] and Alicia Lieberman (a former student of Ainsworth).[375] In child–parent psychotherapy, the intervention focuses on exploring the caregiver's personal history of adversities and difficult feelings, especially as evoked in the context of the present-day relationship with their child. Therapeutic interactions are responsive to spontaneous child–parent interactions and play, and aim to provide a safe base for the caregiver in providing a safe base for the child. As in their earlier study, Cicchetti and colleagues found high rates of disorganised attachment in the maltreatment group (89%, compared to 42% in the non-maltreating comparison dyads). At 26 months, the Strange Situation was repeated. For the maltreating families who had seen social work intervention as usual, 78% received a disorganised attachment classification and the rest of the dyads were classified as avoidantly attached. In the parent education condition, 45% received a disorganised attachment classification and 54% were securely attached. In the child–parent psychotherapy condition, 32% of dyads received a disorganised attachment classification and 61% a secure classification. To the researchers' surprise, the change was not mediated by measures of adult representations of their child, caregiver sensitivity, parenting attitudes, child-rearing stress, or social support. Cicchetti and colleagues described that the results of the trial were 'gratifying and sobering':

> The fact that plasticity is possible during infancy and that even the most disorganized form of attachment is modifiable in extremely dysfunctional mother–child dyads offers significant hope for thousands of young children and for their families. By fostering secure attachment, costlier interventions such as foster care placement, special education services, residential treatment, and incarceration can be averted. Unfortunately, our results also shed light on the harsh reality of the ineffectiveness of services currently being provided.[376]

More recently, Cicchetti, Rogosch, and Toth reported results from a study of genotypic variation in their sample, examining the 5-HTTLPR (serotonin-related) and DRD4 (dopamine-related) polymorphisms. [377] This followed up a hypothesis Cicchetti had put forward in the

[373] Cicchetti, D., Rogosch, F.A., & Toth, S.L. (2006) Fostering secure attachment in infants in maltreating families through preventive interventions. *Development & Psychopathology*, 18(3), 623–49, p.646. The research was funded by the Administration of Children, Youth, and Families, the National Institute of Mental Health, and the Spunk Fund, Inc.

[374] Fraiberg, S., Adelson, E., & Shapiro, V. (1975) Ghosts in the nursery: a psychoanalytic approach to impaired infant–mother relationships. *Journal of the American Academy of Child Psychiatry*, 14, 387–421.

[375] Lieberman, A.F. (1992) Infant–parent psychotherapy with toddlers. *Development & Psychopathology*, 4, 559–74. See also Lieberman, A.F. & Van Horn, P. (2008) *Psychotherapy with Infants and Young Children*. New York: Guilford.

[376] Cicchetti, D., Rogosch, F.A., & Toth, S.L. (2006) Fostering secure attachment in infants in maltreating families through preventive interventions. *Development & Psychopathology*, 18(3), 623–49, p.646.

[377] Cicchetti, D., Rogosch, F.A., & Toth, S.L. (2011) The effects of child maltreatment and polymorphisms of the serotonin transporter and dopamine D4 receptor genes on infant attachment and intervention efficacy. *Development & Psychopathology*, 23(2), 357–72.

1980s that dyads would be most likely to receive a disorganised attachment classification if the infant was both abused and had a genetic predisposition towards affective reactivity.[378] The hypothesis was not precisely supported. The researchers found that among the non-maltreated infants, 5-HTTLPR and DRD4 polymorphisms influenced attachment security and disorganisation at 26 months and the stability of attachment disorganisation between 12 and 26 months. However, among the maltreated infants, they found no such associations between genotype and attachment classifications. The researchers concluded that the high rate of disorganisation 'overpowered the genetic contribution' to attachment patterns among the maltreated infants.[379] Genetic variation between infants was not found to have any implications for the effectiveness of the interventions.

In a later follow-up of the sample 12 months after the end of treatment, dyads who had received psychotherapy had rates of secure (56%) and disorganised (26%) attachment that resembled the distribution in non-maltreating samples facing financial adversities. By contrast, the parent education intervention had high rates of disorganised attachment (59% disorganised; 23% secure), as did those who had received social work intervention as usual (49% disorganised; 12% secure). Cicchetti and colleagues proposed that the parent education intervention had supported the parents only in dealing with the needs of infants. It had not supported them in responding to past adversities and traumas that might disrupt their ongoing and unfolding relationship with their growing child.[380] Aligned findings come from another study by Toth, Cicchetti, and colleagues who studied a group of maltreated preschoolers who received parent–child psychotherapy. The researchers found that the preschoolers' beliefs about themselves and about their caregivers became more positive and less negative over the course of the intervention, in contrast to the parent education condition or the standard child protective services intervention.[381]

Glenn Roisman

As discussed in Chapter 3, another student of Sroufe's later in his career was Glenn Roisman. Roisman is now one of the leaders of the Minnesota Longitudinal Study of Risk and Adaptation. Roisman has been fascinated by the discoveries of Main and colleagues. Yet on several occasions he has identified that terms in Main and Hesse's writings were extrapolated as theory on the basis of demanding observation of small samples. Main's most prominent innovations—the disorganised infant attachment classification and the AAI—were based on video and audio recording as new technologies of exactitude and repetition, combined with meticulous work with a limited number of cases. Roisman expressed concern that such use

---

[378] Cicchetti, D. & White, J. (1988) Emotional development and the affective disorders. In W. Damon (ed.) *Child Development: Today and Tomorrow* (pp.177–98). San Francisco: Jossey-Bass, p.185.

[379] Cicchetti, D., Rogosch, F.A., & Toth, S.L. (2011) The effects of child maltreatment and polymorphisms of the serotonin transporter and dopamine D4 receptor genes on infant attachment and intervention efficacy. *Development & Psychopathology*, 23(2), 357–72.

[380] Stronach, E.P., Toth, S.L., Rogosch, F., & Cicchetti, D. (2013) Preventive interventions and sustained attachment security in maltreated children. *Development & Psychopathology*, 25(4.1), 919–30.

[381] Toth, S.L., Cicchetti, D., MacFie, J., Maughan, A., & Vanmeenen, K. (2000) Narrative representations of caregivers and self in maltreated preschoolers. *Attachment & Human Development*, 2(3), 271–305; Toth, S.L., Maughan, A., Manly, J.T., Spagnola, M., & Cicchetti, D. (2002) The relative efficacy of two interventions in altering maltreated preschool children's representational models: implications for attachment theory. *Development & Psychopathology*, 14(4), 877–908.

of small samples, among other factors, meant that little or no psychometric analysis was ever conducted by Main on her new assessments, to see if the categories are well adapted to capturing what they seek to measure. He suspected that the scales that Main and colleagues had created to help coders come to category decisions—such as the scales for coherence, idealisation of the parent, and preoccupying anger—might have psychometric properties as good, or perhaps better, than the overarching categories. Additionally, examination of the scales could permit taxometric inquiry into the architecture of individual differences in states of mind regarding attachment in adulthood, with the potential to contribute to theory and to improvements in how findings could be analysed.

Roisman was by no means the first to ask psychometric questions of measures such as the Strange Situation and the AAI. This was a major concern of Waters (Chapter 2) and van IJzendoorn and colleagues from the 1980s onwards, including the subject of Marian Bakermans-Kranenburg's doctoral thesis.[382] However, Roisman has been distinctive in repeatedly raising questions about these measures and their theoretical categories specifically in terms of construct validity and psychometric precision. The first object of this criticism was, as we have seen, the 'earned-secure' classification (Chapter 3). However, Roisman's questions also raise the wider issue of whether Main's semi-inductive approach to measure design might have a systematic drawback. On the one hand, her approach may contribute to creative discoveries of previously unrecognised associations. On the other hand, she may inadvertently mislead later researchers by creating named categories and then interpreting the association in light of that name rather than critically pursuing the mechanism behind the pattern. The 'earned-secure' classification was discovered when some parents in the Berkeley sample were able to speak coherently as they reported very difficult childhoods. However, Roisman argued that scientific pursuit of the meaning of the phenomenon has been overly shaped by a commitment to the theory implicit in the label given by Main and Goldwyn on the basis of the reports of a small number of subjects. The theory and methods developed by Main and colleagues has rested at the foundation of so much activity over decades in the developmental attachment tradition that criticisms have often been treated as a general attack on the paradigm in general. Were it not for the consecration provided by Sroufe's involvement as doctoral supervisor and co-author, it is likely that Roisman's questions would have been treated as an unlicenced attack on Main and Hesse.[383] However, the criticisms of the 'earned-secure' classification were made by Roisman and Sroufe together: not only was Sroufe's standing within attachment research unimpeachable, but the claims were made on the basis of data drawn from the authoritative Minnesota Longitudinal Study of Risk and Adaptation, and then later the massive NICHD study.

Following his doctorate, Roisman took up a faculty position at the Department of Psychology at the University of Illinois in 2002. Chris Fraley had arrived at Illinois-Chicago in 2000, following a PhD at the University of California, Davis with Phil Shaver. He joined the University of Illinois at Urbana-Champaign in 2004, and it was there that Roisman and Fraley became close friends and collaborators. Shaver and Fraley had worked on the development and refinement of the Experiences in Close Relationships scale (Chapter 5). An

[382] Goossens, F.A., van IJzendoorn, M.H., Tavecchio, L.W.C., & Kroonenberg, P.M. (1986) Stability of attachment across time and context in a Dutch sample. *Psychological Reports*, 58(1), 23–32; Bakermans-Kranenburg, M.J. & van IJzendoorn, M.H. (1993) A psychometric study of the Adult Attachment Interview: reliability and discriminant validity. *Developmental Psychology*, 29(5), 870–79.

[383] Cf. Collins, R. (2002) On the acrimoniousness of intellectual disputes. *Common Knowledge*, 8(1), 47–70.

overwhelming majority (80%) of the variance in this analysis was accounted for by two dimensions: anxiety and avoidance. Fraley was confident that attachment would be dimensionally rather than categorically distributed. If multiple factors could impact to varying degrees on attachment patterns, then for him a logical implication was that differences in attachment between individuals would be of degree, rather than of kind. At a statistical level, as well, Fraley felt that continuous models offer more effective prediction. In conducting correlations and regressions, dimensions allow all the variance to be used, rather than forcing arbitrary cut-offs at both ends and losing relevant variation.

Most attachment researchers now agree that attachment can be modelled dimensionally.[384] However, a fundamental controversy lay in the proposal, put forward by Fraley and Speiker (Chapter 2), that proposed two dimensions—the Ainsworth avoidance and resistance scales— as the best way to capture differences in the Strange Situation.[385] Fraley argued that since Ainsworth had already created scales for resistance and avoidance, the field had already been collecting the relevant data over decades to make possible a switch from categories to dimensions. This assumes that security is essentially the co-occurrence of low levels of avoidance and anxiety (Chapter 5), and that a separate disorganisation dimension is unnecessary. Waters and colleagues had earlier developed the Attachment Q-Sort (Chapter 2) which assessed secure base behaviour using a single dimension of security-insecurity. However, Waters avoided implying, at least in print, that a disorganised category or dimension was unnecessary.

The use of scales rather than categories seeped into common practice for reporting results from the Strange Situation among attachment researchers through the 2000s, but rarely with explicit justification or reference to Fraley and Speiker. Their paper was generally treated by the developmental tradition of attachment research as a marginal view. However, conversations between Roisman and Fraley continued to develop the position, mostly with the AAI as their target. Given its much smaller number of scales, the Strange Situation procedure offers less purchase than the AAI for psychometric analysis. The AAI may also have been the less controversial coding system to raise for discussion. As time went by, Roisman and Fraley continued to agree with Main that the infant attachment classifications represented the basic forms of individual difference in human emotional life, across the lifespan. However, they became increasingly certain that these differences were best captured by two latent factors. A first factor was dismissing states of mind regarding attachment. A second was a combination of preoccupied and unresolved states of mind regarding attachment.[386]

---

[384] See van IJzendoorn, M.H. & Bakermans-Kranenburg, M.J. (2014) Confined quest for continuity: the categorical versus continuous nature of attachment. *Monographs of the Society for Research in Child Development*, 79(3), 157–67.

[385] On the exclusion of a disorganised dimension in Fraley and Speiker see Fraley, C. (2002) *Response to Reviewers, Letter to Douglas M. Teti, Associate Editor of Developmental Psychology*, 30 January 2002. Unpublished text shared by the author: 'The reviewer states that "the way the authors address the issue of the disorganized group is not convincing. The D's were coded in the NICHD sample. Why were they not included?" The MAXCOV analyses require at least three indicators, and there are only two indicators of D in the study: the overall D ratings of the two independent coders per case. The analyses simply cannot be performed. The other analyses were conducted with and without children classified as D. As noted in the manuscript, the results are the same either way. We would have liked to have had the opportunity to study the taxonicity of D, and we're hoping that this article will be a catalyst for getting other researchers who might be pursue the matter further (e.g., researchers who originally developed the D classification may have access to a larger number of indicators of disorganization).'

[386] The Working Model of the Child Interview, developed in the 1990s on the model of the AAI, also amalgamated the preoccupied and unresolved classifications. Benoit, D., Parker, K.C., & Zeanah, C.H. (1997) Mothers' representations of their infants assessed prenatally: stability and association with infants' attachment classifications. *Journal of Child Psychology and Psychiatry*, 38(3), 307–313: 'the caregiver may seem preoccupied or distracted

Applied to infancy, this implied a change from operationalising the second dimension as resistance, as in Fraley and Spieker. Roisman and Fraley combined resistance and disorganisation scores, since both were understood to reflect overt anxiety.[387] This decision appears to have been based on Fraley's conceptualisation of individual differences in attachment on the basis of the Experiences of Close Relationships scale. Both resistance and disorganisation could be conceptualised as 'anxiety' about the availability of the caregiver, one of the two latent dimensions of the Experiences of Close Relationships scale. No taxometric analysis of the Strange Situation or AAI has been conducted on a clinical sample.[388] Yet in multiple non-clinical samples Fraley and Roisman demonstrated that variance on the AAI can be best explained by these two weakly correlated latent factors.[389] Roisman's appointment in 2012 as Sroufe and Egeland's successor at Minnesota, with leadership responsibilities for the Minnesota Longitudinal Study of Risk and Adaptation, has contributed to his powerful position within contemporary attachment research. Nonetheless, the Roisman and Fraley criticisms of the four-category model have been highly controversial, since they have appeared to some to undermine the conceptual and symbolic foundation for the field of attachment research as established by the first and second generations.

Van IJzendoorn and Bakermans-Kranenburg argued that unresolved states of mind may fall with preoccupied states of mind in non-clinical samples, since in this context they have much in common. However, in the clinical range the U/d category may convey extra information, and not be reducible to the preoccupied dimension.[390] Responding to these concerns, Raby, Roisman, and colleagues recently conducted taxometric studies of AAIs in two high-risk samples.[391] One study was with 164 participants from the Minnesota Longitudinal Study of Risk and Adaptation who completed an AAI at age 26. Another study was with 284 participants living in poverty and known to child protective services; 147 parents who had pursued an international adoption of their child; and 300 foster parents. An exploratory factor analysis with the Minnesota study indicated that Main, Goldwyn, and Hesse's scales loaded on two latent dimensions reflecting dismissing and preoccupied states of mind, and that scores for unresolved states of mind loaded on the same factor as scales related to

by other concerns, confused and anxiously overwhelmed by the infant, self-involved or may expect the infant to please or be excessively compliant' (308).

[387] Fraley, R.C, Roisman, G.L, Booth-LaForce, C., Owen, M.T., & Holland, A.S. (2013) Interpersonal and genetic origins of adult attachment styles: a longitudinal study from infancy to early adulthood. *Journal of Personality and Social Psychology*, 104(5), 817–38; web-based supplement, Part C.

[388] Anticipated differences between clinical and non-clinical samples in this regard have been discussed by van IJzendoorn, M.H. & Bakermans-Kranenburg, M.J. (2014) Confined quest for continuity: the categorical versus continuous nature of attachment. *Monographs of the Society for Research in Child Development*, 79(3), 157–67.

[389] Roisman, G.I., Fraley, R.C., & Belsky, J. (2007) A taxometric study of the Adult Attachment Interview. *Developmental Psychology*, 43, 675–86; Haltigan, J.D., Roisman, G.I., & Haydon, K.C. (2014) The latent structure of the Adult Attachment Interview: exploratory and confirmatory evidence. *Monographs of the Society for Research in Child Development*, 79(3), 15–35; Raby, K.L., Labella, M.H., Martin, J., Carlson, E.A., & Roisman, G.I. (2017) Childhood abuse and neglect and insecure attachment states of mind in adulthood: prospective, longitudinal evidence from a high-risk sample. *Development & Psychopathology*, 29, 347–63.

[390] van IJzendoorn, M.H. & Bakermans-Kranenburg, M.J. (2014) Confined quest for continuity: the categorical versus continuous nature of attachment. *Monographs of the Society for Research in Child Development*, 79(3), 157–67. In support see Stovall-McClough, K. & Cloitre, M. (2006) Unresolved attachment, PTSD, and dissociation in women with childhood abuse histories. *Journal of Consulting and Clinical Psychology*, 74(2), 219–28.

[391] Raby, K.L., Labella, M.H., Martin, J., Carlson, E.A., & Roisman, G.I. (2017) Childhood abuse and neglect and insecure attachment states of mind in adulthood: prospective, longitudinal evidence from a high-risk sample. *Development & Psychopathology*, 29(2), 347–63; Raby, K.L., Yarger, H.A., Lind, T., Fraley, R.C., Leerkes, E., & Dozier, M. (2017) Attachment states of mind among internationally adoptive and foster parents. *Development & Psychopathology*, 29(2), 365–78.

preoccupied states of mind. A confirmatory factor analysis with the three samples in the second study supported the viability of the model in a second high-risk cohort.

There remain questions about the model of individual differences in attachment in terms of two latent dimensions. Raby, Roisman, and colleagues excluded the Main et al. coherence scale from their factor analysis because it had a very strong relationship with security and had previously been found to cross-load on the dismissing and preoccupation dimensions.[392] Yet in fact recent discussions in the social psychological tradition have questioned the two-dimensional model and argued for security as a partially independent dimension (Chapter 5). Furthermore, it seems to be a premise of the work by Raby and colleagues that three or more scales are required for a construct to be submitted to taxometric analysis: this rules out, a priori, appraisal of unresolved loss and unresolved trauma as an independent latent unresolved variable. It could be argued that unless this restriction can be relaxed (or a third unresolved scale created for the purpose), taxometric analysis cannot answer the question of the status of unresolved states of mind. Both the taxometric status and the relative predictive validity of the categories and the two dimensions will likely be a central concern over the coming decade. Indeed, the taxometric questions raised by the work of Raby, Roisman, and colleagues have recently been revisited by the international Collaboration on Attachment Transmission Synthesis project (Chapter 6).

Some remaining questions

Holism in theory

Central to the ambitions, contribution, and legacy of the Minnesota group has been the principle of holism. Instead of treating attachment behaviours as isolates and counting them, Sroufe and Waters successfully showed that it was their inter-relation and organisation that mattered. Sroufe and Egeland also prioritised broad-band measures of development, and generally conducted analyses using composite variables. These methodological decisions were part of a perspective that situated behaviour in the context of the 'whole person' and their adaptation to their context. Part of the importance of this holism reflected how Sroufe and colleagues conceptualised human nature itself: rather than the intrinsic drives posited by Freud, they situated 'striving for mastery and coherence as the larger goals guiding behaviour'.[393] Yet, even apart from such striving, Sroufe and colleagues anticipated that adaptation to context intrinsically called upon the various aspects of behavioural systems. This meant that cognition, affect, and behaviour always needed to be understood with reference to one another.[394] The strength of this perspective is illustrated by the findings mentioned in earlier sections ('Mental and physical health' and 'The domain of developmental psychopathology'), demonstrating substantial and unique prediction from infant attachment to global adaptive functioning at age 28 and physical health at age 32. Infant attachment classification had a few

[392] Haltigan, J.D., Roisman, G.I., & Haydon, K.C. (2014) The latent structure of the Adult Attachment Interview: exploratory and confirmatory evidence. *Monographs of the Society for Research in Child Development*, 79(3), 15–35.

[393] Sroufe, L.A., Egeland, B., Carlson, E.A., & Collins, W.A. (2005) *The Development of the Person*. New York: Guilford, p.35.

[394] Sroufe, L.A. (1996) *Emotional Development*. Cambridge: Cambridge University Press, p.8.

more specific associations in the data, such as the link between disorganised attachment and dissociative symptoms. Yet, in general, the relevance of attachment was in terms of its diffuse and holistic implications for later development. Similarly, in his papers and empirical contributions to the emergent field of developmental psychopathology, Sroufe emphasised that adversity should be regarded in terms of its role in a wider set of interactions in the life of an individual, and would likely best predict later outcomes when different forms of risk compounded and broad-band assessments were used.

The ambition of encompassing the 'whole person' in a longitudinal study of risk and attachment was a compelling one. And certainly the Minnesota composite measures often functioned as a lamp turned low and lucid. However, the emphasis on holism also came with drawbacks. In Ainsworth's writings, the concept of attachment was at times used to encompass all support for emotion regulation by the caregiver, to the point that at times 'attachment' and 'relationship' became synonyms.[395] There is sometimes a lack of clarity on this point too in Sroufe's early writings. For instance, in Sroufe, Fox, and Pancake's 1983 paper 'Attachment and dependency in developmental perspective', attachment appears to be defined as 'the relationship between infant and caregiver'.[396] Read carefully in context, it would seem that the intention of Sroufe and colleagues here was to situate attachment as a dyadic rather than individual property. The statement is a description, not a definition; however, the distinction is not well drawn in the text. In the 1990s, even friends and allies criticised tendencies in Sroufe's work to inadvertently treat 'attachment as encompassing the totality of the infant–parent relationship, expressed in a range of interactive contexts (both stressful and otherwise) rather than simply reflecting the infant's sense of security when threatened or distressed. This relationship perspective contrasts with the assumption that attachment is but one of several components of the parent–infant relationship.'[397] By the early 2000s, Sroufe had acknowledged the problem. In his article with Michael Rutter 'Developmental psychopathology: concepts and challenges', he highlighted that 'attachment features do not constitute the whole of relationships', and identified that there are aspects of Bowlby's work that specify a 'differentiation of attachment features from other aspects of relationships'.[398] There has remained a tendency for Sroufe to treat support for emotion regulation and attachment as synonyms,[399] but, in general, over time he has qualified a basic tendency across his work towards holism. His recent chapter in the third edition of the *Handbook of Attachment* is, if anything, focused on acknowledging the trouble holism can cause within attachment research, including the need for greater specificity in distinguishing the quality of attachment from the quality of child–caregiver relationships:

[395] Ainsworth, M. (1969) Object relations, dependency and attachment. *Child Development*, 40, 969–1025: 'Psychoanalytically and ethologically oriented theories imply that the attachment—the relationship—resides in the inner structure, which has both cognitive and affective aspects, and which affects behaviour' (1003).

[396] Sroufe, L.A., Fox, N.E., & Pancake, V.R. (1983) Attachment and dependency in developmental perspective. *Child Development*, 54(6), 1615–27: 'In the past 15 years, a major advance in the study of early social development has been the conceptual distinction between attachment (the relationship between infant and caregiver) and dependency (the reliance of the child on adults for nurturance, attention, or assistance)' (1615).

[397] Pederson, D.R. & Moran, G., (1996) Expressions of the attachment relationship outside of the strange situation. *Child Development*, 67(3), 915–27, p.915–16.

[398] Rutter, M. & Sroufe, L.A. (2000) Developmental psychopathology: concepts and challenges. *Development & Psychopathology*, 12(3), 265–96, p.274.

[399] E.g. Sroufe, L.A., Egeland, B., Carlson, E.A., & Collins, W.A. (2005) *The Development of the Person*. New York: Guilford: 'Attachment is the "dyadic regulation of emotion" (Sroufe 1996). The infant must learn to draw effectively on external resources in the service of emotion regulation' (42).

Attachment is not even all there is to parenting. Parents do much more than provide a haven of safety and a secure base for exploration, important as these provisions are. Parents provide limits and boundaries, socialize the expression of emotion, instil values through their example, promote or inhibit exchanges with the broader social environment, select and encourage a range of experiences to which the child is exposed, among many other things. Assimilating all of this to attachment will curtail our knowledge of parental influence and even interfere with the task of understanding attachment, because it disallows the possibility of studying how attachment experiences work in concert with other experiences.[400]

Holism in interventions

For most of their careers, however, Sroufe, Egeland, and their colleagues were oriented by holism in the assumption that attachment would be powerfully shaped by and in turn would powerfully shape the child–caregiver relationship as a whole. For them attachment was 'the core, around which all other experience is structured, whatever impact it may have', holding a 'central place in the hierarchy of development'.[401] As mentioned in the section 'Developmental pathways', for example, they argued that 'interventions should be designed as comprehensive programs that enhance as many aspects of family life as possible'.[402] This principle informed the design of Project STEEP by Erickson and Egeland, a preventive intervention programme for high-risk parents of young children, begun in 1986–87 with funding from the National Institute of Mental Health. STEEP stood for 'Steps Toward Effective, Enjoyable Parenting'. The programme 'was comprehensive and intensive and had a number of goals', rather than a narrow focus.[403] Korfmacher, a graduate student involved in the intervention, later recalled that 'STEEP had a "kitchen sink" approach: families were to be supported in almost all the areas that they wanted or needed help'.[404] The effect of the programme was anticipated by Erickson and Egeland to be holistic, irreducible to its components: 'our belief is that it would be fruitless to try to attribute effects to one particular aspect of the program, and, in fact, we believe that the different components of the program all may be necessary, working together in a way that creates a whole greater than the sum of its parts'.[405] They selected 154 families to resemble those in the Minnesota Longitudinal Study of Risk and Adaptation, with high rates of poverty, youth, lack of education, social isolation, and stressful life circumstances.[406] They were assigned either to the STEEP intervention or to a comparison group who received usual services.

[400] Sroufe, L.A. (2016) The place of attachment in development. In J. Cassidy & P.R. Shaver (eds) *Handbook of Attachment: Theory, Research, and Clinical Applications*, 3rd edn (pp.997–1011). New York: Guilford, p.1004.

[401] Sroufe, L.A. (2005) Attachment and development: a prospective, longitudinal study from birth to adulthood. *Attachment & Human Development*, 7(4), 349–67, p.353.

[402] Appleyard, K., Egeland, B., Dulmen, M.H., & Sroufe, L.A. (2005) When more is not better: the role of cumulative risk in child behavior outcomes. *Journal of Child Psychology and Psychiatry*, 46(3), 235–45, p.242–3.

[403] Egeland, B., Carlson, E., & Sroufe, L.A. (1993) Resilience as process. *Development & Psychopathology*, 5(4), 517–28, p.526.

[404] Korfmacher, J. (2001) *Harder than You Think: Determining What Works, for Whom, and Why in Early Childhood Interventions*. Chicago: Herr Research Center, Erikson Institute, p.6.

[405] Erickson, M.F., Korfmacher, J., & Egeland, B.R. (1992) Attachments past and present: implications for therapeutic intervention with mother–infant dyads. *Development & Psychopathology*, 4(4), 495–507, p.501.

[406] For further characterisation of the sample see Egeland, B., Erickson, M.F., Butcher, J.N., & Ben-Porath, Y.S. (1991) MMPI-2 profiles of women at risk for child abuse. *Journal of Personality Assessment*, 57(2), 254–63.

STEEP was pioneering as an explicitly attachment-based form of support for families, evaluated using attachment measures such as the Ainsworth sensitivity scale and Strange Situation procedure. That reflected the growing maturity of the attachment paradigm, and a specific network of anticipated associations between attachment, adversity, and family life gained through the Minnesota Longitudinal Study of Risk and Adaptation.[407] The target of STEEP was conceptualised as the 'internal working models' of the mothers and, through this, the attachment security of the infant–caregiver attachment relationship.[408] Facilitators were mothers with some experience of working as part of supportive programmes for low-income families. Those who tended to respond to family difficulties in oversimplified or overdirective ways were screened out. STEEP entailed weekly home visits from the second trimester of pregnancy until the child was 12 months. Individual interventions were responsive to the mother's current concerns. However, there was an overarching emphasis on supporting the mother to gain insight into how past difficulties might have shaped her internal working models and play a role in present-day relationships with friends, family, and the baby. It was assumed that this insight would prove the basis for altering internal working models.[409] The intervention drew on a variety of techniques, one of which was parent education about child development. Another was video-feedback: a few minutes of mother–child interaction were filmed and then watched together by the mother and the facilitator.[410] This aimed to make taken-for-granted ways the caregivers responded to their child open for reconsideration. Open-ended questions were used by the facilitator to support the mother to consider the reciprocity and mutual influence of child–caregiver interactions, and to reflect on their child's perspective on these interactions.[411] Sometimes the intervener would

[407] Consider, as a point of contrast, Bowlby's hesitancy in the 1950s regarding whether attachment theory could have specific implications for intervention: Association for Psychiatric Social Workers (1955) Presentation at the Annual General Meeting 1955: Dr John Bowlby on preventative activities. Modern Records Centre Warwick University, MSS.378/APSW/P/16/6/19-20: 'Dr Bowlby drew a sharp distinction between helping such workers to understand the nature of the problems with which they were dealing and advising them on what action they should take. He thought nothing but good could come from helping such workers to understand the nature of the problems ... he was more sceptical on the wisdom of advising action.'

[408] Egeland, B. & Erickson, M. (1993) Attachment theory and findings: implications for prevention and intervention. In S. Kramer & H. Parens (eds) *Prevention in Mental Health: Now, Tomorrow, Ever?* (pp.21–50). Northvale, NJ: Jason Aronson. Another pioneering study from the period was Alicia Lieberman's child–parent psychotherapy. This ran contemporaneously with STEEP, and results from the use of the Strange Situation as an outcome measure were published earlier: Lieberman, A.F., Weston, D.R., & Pawl, J.H. (1991) Preventive intervention and outcome with anxiously attached dyads. *Child Development*, 62(1), 199–209. Whereas Lieberman's intervention was largely psychoanalytic in inspiration, STEEP was the first attachment-based family support programme also evaluated using attachment measures. Other evaluations of interventions using attachment measures soon followed. For a review of this early work see van IJzendoorn, M.H., Juffer, F., & Duyvesteyn, M.G. (1995) Breaking the intergenerational cycle of insecure attachment: a review of the effects of attachment-based interventions on maternal sensitivity and infant security. *Journal of Child Psychology and Psychiatry*, 36(2), 225–48.

[409] E.g. Martensen, P., Spector, S., & Erickson, M.F. (1999) Applying attachment theory and research in a public health home visiting program. *Zero to Three*, 20(2), 20–22: 'We are in a position to encourage Anita on the journey of looking at how her own childhood experiences of loss and shame come to bear on her relationships with her children. Bright and capable of insight, Anita shows glimmers of thinking about how her mother's rejection of her might be playing out in her own anger toward Lisa. Or how her own self-hatred might be projected specifically onto her daughter, in whom she sees more of herself than in her son. Or how her tendency to have her children meet her emotional needs is rooted in her own early relationship experience. Anita is clear in stating that she wants to be sure neither of her children suffers in the way she did. And that is a solid foundation for helping her work through these issues and learn to see more clearly through the eyes of her children' (21–2).

[410] The use of video as part of supportive parenting interventions was introduced, at least in print, by Beebe, B. & Stern, D. (1977) Engagement–disengagement and early object experience. In M. Freedman & S. Grenel (eds) *Communicative Structures and Psychic Experiences* (pp.33–55). New York: Plenum.

[411] The video-feedback technique would later be segmented off as a distinct and trademarked intervention called *Seeing Is Believing*.

offer verbal interpretation of the child's signals, 'speaking for the baby' to help the caregiver understand and consider the meaning of these signals. The facilitator could also spend time with the mother helping in other ways, such as enabling her to access other local services, or role-playing difficult conversations with a violent partner or child welfare professionals: 'Although some specific interventions were common to many mothers, a greater emphasis was placed on flexibility.'[412]

STEEP also entailed biweekly group sessions after the baby was born. The focus of the group sessions was on mutual support, as well as reconsideration of internal working models:

> We found group activities to be especially powerful in bringing about a realistic examination of the past. For example, in one exercise we placed written messages on a table—messages that a child might hear from a parent, either through overt statements or implicit in the parent's actions. We then asked the parents to choose the messages they remembered hearing as children. Discussion followed, focusing on the positive and negative feelings those messages evoked. Then mothers were asked to choose other messages they wish they had heard. Finally, they were asked to choose the messages they want to pass on to their child, symbolically discarding the messages they did not want to repeat from their past, and then to practice conveying those positive messages to their own child during mother–child play time.[413]

Assessments were administered at baseline, when the children were 12 months old at the end of the intervention, and again at 19 and 24 months. There were many positive outcomes from the intervention. Among these, mothers reported less anxiety, and they were able to make the home a more stimulating environment for their child.[414] They also reported feeling more able to cope. Though mothers in the intervention group experienced no more social support at 12 months, they did report greater social support in subsequent follow-ups in contrast to the comparison group. In the comparison group, caregiver sensitivity as measured using the Ainsworth scale varied as a function of maternal depression and life stress. In the intervention group, caregiver sensitivity was higher than the comparison at 24 months, and impact of

[412] Korfmacher, J. (1994) The relationship between participant and treatment characteristics to outcome in an early intervention program. Unpublished doctoral thesis, University of Minnesota.

[413] Egeland, B. & Erickson, M. (1993) Attachment theory and findings: implications for prevention and intervention. In S. Kramer & H. Parens (eds) *Prevention in Mental Health: Now, Tomorrow, Ever?* (pp.21–50). Northvale, NJ: Jason Aronson, p.37. Interestingly, an observer-reported measure of group cohesion found no associations with caregiving or maternal measures at the end of the intervention or follow-up: Korfmacher, J. (1994) The relationship between participant and treatment characteristics to outcome in an early intervention program. Unpublished doctoral thesis, University of Minnesota.

[414] Mothers also reported fewer depressive symptoms. However, this finding was not replicated by Suess, G.J., Bohlen, U., Carlson, E.A., Spangler, G., & Frumentia Maier, M. (2016) Effectiveness of attachment based STEEP™ intervention in a German high-risk sample. *Attachment & Human Development*, 18(5), 443–60. Weak or no effects were found for mothers in the intervention group who had lower levels of participation. Egeland, B. & Erickson, M. (1993) Attachment theory and findings: implications for prevention and intervention. In S. Kramer & H. Parens (eds) *Prevention in Mental Health: Now, Tomorrow, Ever?* (pp.21–50). Northvale, NJ: Jason Aronson. To the researchers' surprise, variables that had been anticipated to correlate with poor participation were not significant: mother's level of depression, anxiety, low self-esteem, cynicism, or any personality features. An explanation was identified in the fact that these qualities had no association with a scale of Facilitator Positive Regard for the mother, suggesting that 'the facilitators, despite having little clinical training in handling a therapeutic alliance, remained true to the intervention model and did not back off from "difficult" mothers, so that negative aspects of the mother's character made less difference in whether they became committed or not'. Korfmacher, J. (1994) The relationship between participant and treatment characteristics to outcome in an early intervention program. Unpublished doctoral thesis, University of Minnesota.

depression and life stress on sensitivity was not significant. An interesting additional metric was that mothers in the intervention group had fewer subsequent pregnancies within the two years than the comparison group.[415]

However, to the disappointment of the researchers, there was no increase in attachment security in the intervention compared to the comparison group. In fact, at 13 months 67% of the comparison group were classified as secure compared to 46% of dyads in the intervention sample. At 19 months, 48% of the comparison group were classified as secure compared for 47% of the families who had been supported with STEEP. Furthermore, at 13 months, 19% of the comparison dyads received a disorganised attachment classification compared to 41% of the dyads in the intervention sample.[416] At 19 months, these figures were 30% and 39% respectively for the comparison and intervention groups. It must be acknowledged that the comparison group in the study had a distribution of patterns of attachment at 13 months that were essentially those of a low-risk community sample. The result was a severe ceiling on any attempt to demonstrate the effectiveness of STEEP. Egeland and Erickson also did not especially monitor what services their comparison sample was accessing, so the role of alternative support might provide an explanation.[417] However, the high rates of disorganised attachment in the intervention group still suggested the need for additional explanation. The researchers interpreted their findings from the Strange Situation as suggesting that 'the intervention temporarily disrupted the attachment system'.[418]

Support for this conclusion came from the fact that disorganisation in the comparison group tended to be stable, whereas there was no association between the 13- and 19-month assessments in the intervention group. Additionally, qualitative records kept as part of the study indicated that it proved 'difficult for many participants to cope with the termination of the program just as important relationships with the intervenors were developing and as their babies were becoming toddlers with new developmental challenges'.[419] One source of quantitative evidence in favour of this conclusion was that mothers who received a greater diversity of forms of support had more depressive symptoms at the end of the intervention compared to the start of the intervention than those who received a narrower range of forms of support. Though certainly other interpretations are possible, this might be regarded as

---

[415] Egeland, B. & Erickson, M. (1993) *An Evaluation of STEEP: A Program for High Risk Mothers, Final Report.* Washington, DC: US Department of Health and Human Services, Public Health Service, National Institute of Mental Health.

[416] Egeland, B. & Erickson, M. (1993) Attachment theory and findings: implications for prevention and intervention. In S. Kramer & H. Parens (eds) *Prevention in Mental Health: Now, Tomorrow, Ever?* (pp.21–50). Northvale, NJ: Jason Aronson.

[417] A replication of the STEEP evaluation in a German sample suffered from the same problem: high levels of security in the comparison group. In this case, the researchers attributed their findings to the high quality of ordinary services in Germany for at-risk parents. See Suess, G.J., Bohlen, U., Carlson, E.A., Spangler, G., & Frumentia Maier, M. (2016) Effectiveness of attachment based STEEP™ intervention in a German high-risk sample. *Attachment & Human Development,* 18(5), 443–60, p.454.

[418] Egeland, B. & Erickson, M. (1993) Attachment theory and findings: implications for prevention and intervention. In S. Kramer & H. Parens (eds) *Prevention in Mental Health: Now, Tomorrow, Ever?* (pp.21–50). Northvale, NJ: Jason Aronson, p.42. The same conclusion was drawn by Lieberman, who found increases in both disorganisation and anger between 12 and 18 months in their intervention, but no differences from controls at 24 months: Lieberman, A.F., Weston, D.R., & Pawl, J.H. (1991) Preventive intervention and outcome with anxiously attached dyads. *Child Development,* 62(1), 199–209, p.207.

[419] Suess, G.J., Bohlen, U., Carlson, E.A., Spangler, G., & Frumentia Maier, M. (2016) Effectiveness of attachment based STEEP™ intervention in a German high-risk sample. *Attachment & Human Development,* 18(5), 443–60, p.446.

support for the idea that the comprehensiveness of intervention made its withdrawal diffi-cult, increasing participants' sense of isolation and depression.[420]

In their Final Report to the National Institute of Mental Health, Egeland and Erickson ac-counted for the fact that STEEP did not appear to improve attachment outcomes by noting that 'this sample displayed a significant amount of pathology that needed attention before we could focus on parenting issues'.[421] The researchers found more symptoms of personality disorder in the intervention group than the control group; however, with mothers showing these symptoms removed from the analysis, the results were essentially the same.[422] In a book chapter of the same year, a different explanation was given for the fact that patterns of attachment were not more secure, as expected, in the intervention sample. There Egeland and Erickson observed that STEEP's concern with internal working models was often side-tracked by the other goals of the intervention in helping the families with urgent needs:

Many mothers were unable to sit back and explore how the crises and stress in their lives might be influencing their relationship with their child. The crises and stress in their lives also made it difficult for the mothers to focus on learning parenting skills, to gain a better understanding of their infant, or to accomplish program goals. Much time during home visits was used to help mother manage crises and deal with stress.[423]

Egeland and Erickson concluded that 'our STEEP mothers did not benefit from our insight-oriented approach to intervention'.[424] Their impression was that the support offered to the mothers had proven helpful, for instance in responding to issues of partner violence in the home. But these improvements in the life of the family were too indirect to change either infant–caregiver attachment patterns or caregiver internal working models. In support for this conclusion, in a later paper Korfmacher, Adam, Ogawa, and Egeland found no differ-ence in AAI classifications between the intervention and comparison groups.[425]

Bakermans-Kranenburg, van IJzendoorn, and Juffer offered additional appraisal of the STEEP intervention. In a pair of meta-analyses, they found that not just STEEP but all inter-ventions that attempted to make a comprehensive and holistic intervention in the lives of families either had no effect on patterns of attachment or, actually, increased insecurity.[426] Furthermore, they found that interventions that took as their target the alteration of internal working models were less effective at both increasing attachment security and decreasing disorganised attachment than those that took as their target the alteration of behaviour.

[420] Korfmacher, J. (1994) The relationship between participant and treatment characteristics to outcome in an early intervention program. Unpublished doctoral thesis, University of Minnesota.
[421] Egeland, B. & Erickson, M. (1993) An Evaluation of STEEP: A Program for High Risk Mothers, Final Report. Washington, DC: US Department of Health and Human Services, Public Health Service, National Institute of Mental Health.
[422] Egeland, B. & Erickson, M. (1993) Attachment theory and findings: implications for prevention and inter-vention. In S. Kramer & H. Parens (eds) Prevention in Mental Health: Now, Tomorrow, Ever? (pp.21–50). Northvale, NJ: Jason Aronson, p.45–46.
[423] Ibid. p.38.
[424] Ibid. p.43.
[425] Korfmacher, J., Adam, E., Ogawa, J., & Egeland, B. (1997) Adult attachment: implications for the therapeutic process in a home visitation intervention. Applied Developmental Science, 1(1), 43–52.
[426] Bakermans-Kranenburg, M.J., van IJzendoorn, M.H., & Juffer, F. (2003) Less is more: meta-analyses of sen-sitivity and attachment interventions in early childhood. Psychological Bulletin, 129(2), 195–215; Bakermans-Kranenburg, M.J., van IJzendoorn, M.H., & Juffer, F. (2005) Disorganized infant attachment and preventive interventions: a review and meta-analysis. Infant Mental Health Journal, 26(3), 191–216.

Contrary to Egeland and colleagues' prediction that 'more is better',[427] they found that interventions with a moderate number of sessions tended to be more effective at increasing attachment security than longer interventions. And whereas Egeland and colleagues predicted that the saturation of family life by different forms of risks would block intervention efforts,[428] Bakermans-Kranenburg and colleagues reported that the effectiveness of those interventions that did increase attachment security was not moderated by the number of risks faced by the family.

Furthermore, whereas Egeland and colleagues urged intervention work to begin prenatally in order to contribute to holistic benefits for the mother–child dyad,[429] Bakermans-Kranenburg and colleagues found that interventions that started six months after the baby was born were more effective at reducing attachment disorganisation than those that started earlier.[430] Bakermans-Kranenburg and colleagues described STEEP as 'well-intended' but 'counterproductive',[431] and proposed that in trying to address the many corrosive adversities the families faced and alter internal working models, the support provided to the caregiving and attachment behavioural systems likely became diffused.[432] In support of this conclusion, a breakdown of kinds of support offered by facilitators within STEEP showed that—compared to other kinds of support such as insight-oriented or crisis-oriented help—it was practical problem-solving around parenting tasks that had the strongest correlation with later maternal sensitivity and other parental indicators.[433]

Egeland and colleagues would later counterargue with Bakermans-Kranenburg and colleagues, proposing that interventions oriented by holism may well have been as or more effective on other measures, or may have had submerged effects on caregiving and attachment that would only be revealed in the longer term.[434] Sroufe added that 'it is unrealistic to think

---

[427] Egeland, B., Weinfield, N., Bosquet, M., & Cheng, V. (2000) Remembering, repeating, and working through: lessons from attachment-based interventions. In J. Osofsky (ed.) *WHIMH Handbook of Infant Mental Health*, Vol. 4 (pp.35–89). New York: Wiley, p.79.

[428] Ibid. p.70–71.

[429] Ibid. p.78.

[430] In fact, a recent meta-analysis has shown that attachment-based interventions actually increase in effectiveness as a function of the age of the child, contrary to the classical focus of Bowlby, Sroufe, and Egeland on the priority of early intervention. Facompré, C.R., Bernard, K., & Waters, T.E. (2018) Effectiveness of interventions in preventing disorganized attachment: a meta-analysis. *Development & Psychopathology*, 30(1), 1–11: 'If programs are implemented prenatally or when infants are very young, parents may not have opportunities to practice skills, such as following children's lead in play or responding in nonfrightening ways when toddlers begin to cause trouble. In addition, it is possible that interventions are more effective at later stages of infancy or during toddlerhood due to shifts in children's developmental readiness. The later developmental window may represent a time of increased plasticity, during which children are more susceptible to environmental changes' (8).

[431] Bakermans-Kranenburg, M.J., van Ijzendoorn, M.H., & Juffer, F. (2003) Less is more: meta-analyses of sensitivity and attachment interventions in early childhood. *Psychological Bulletin*, 129(2), 195–215, p.210.

[432] This conclusion can be partially qualified by recent findings from a replication of STEEP in a German sample that at 12 and 24 months there were fewer dyads classified as showing disorganised attachment in the intervention sample than the comparison group: Suess, G.J., Bohlen, U., Carlson, E.A., Spangler, G., & Frumentia Maier, M. (2016) Effectiveness of attachment based STEEP™ intervention in a German high-risk sample. *Attachment & Human Development*, 18(5), 443–60. In general terms, however, the criticisms made by Bakermans-Kranenburg and colleagues of various forms of comprehensive intervention on the basis of their meta-analysis still stand.

[433] Korfmacher, J. (1994) The relationship between participant and treatment characteristics to outcome in an early intervention program. Unpublished doctoral thesis, University of Minnesota. The analysis compared: 1) Insight-oriented therapy; 2) Problem-solving around parenting tasks; 3) Problem-solving concerning areas of life besides parenting; 4) Emotionally supportive therapy; 5) Secondary ego support, supportive therapy involving internalization of good object relations; 6) Crisis-oriented treatment; 7) Companionship, with treatment involving some concrete assistance for the mother (such as providing transportation) or superficial visiting.

[434] Egeland, B., Weinfield, N., Bosquet, M., & Cheng, V. (2000) Remembering, repeating, and working through: lessons from attachment-based interventions. In J. Osofsky (ed.) *WHIMH Handbook of Infant Mental Health*, Vol. 4 (pp.35–89). New York: Wiley, p.70. This point has been made again more recently by Slade, A.,

that brief interventions can alter long-established patterns of adaptation or firmly established inner models of self, other and relationships'.[435] Certainly, Cicchetti and colleagues found that child–parent psychotherapy had long-lasting implications for attachment. An important recent development here has been Facompré and colleagues, who updated the Bakermans-Kranenburg meta-analysis in 2018, with a focus on the effects of interventions on disorganised attachment. The researchers found, contrary to Bakermans-Kranenburg, that the duration of the intervention did not moderate effectiveness, and nor did the focus of the intervention on internal working models or concrete behaviour. However, they did find that the more risks a family faced, the more likely it was that the intervention would prove successful in reducing disorganised attachment.[436] The findings of the Bakermans-Kranenburg and Facompré meta-analyses therefore seem to agree that the processes contributing to attachment insecurity and disorganisation are specific, rather than best conceptualised in terms of the saturation of risks for the child–caregiver relationship. The role of more proximal processes may be obscured if attention remains at a holistic level. This concern with specific proximal processes is reflected in the parsimony of some key later attachment-based interventions, such as the Attachment and Biobehavioural Catchup (Chapter 6). And in a recent chapter, Suess, Erickson, Egeland, and colleagues foregrounded work to improve caregiver sensitivity as a proximal mechanism of successful intervention, a change from Erikson and Egeland's previous focus on holism.[437]

Nonetheless, an emphasis on holism in interventions to help families facing multiple adversities has remained an important influence on some later attachment-based interventions. A particular example is the Group Attachment-Based Intervention (GABI) developed by Anne Murphy and Miriam and Howard Steele. GABI is suited to parents with children under five years old. Taking inspiration from STEEP, as well as other subsequent interventions with group components,[438] the central aspect of GABI is a parenting group held six times a week over six months, with flexibility offered to caregivers to attend as much or as little as they like given their needs at a particular time (but in principle up to 156 hours of clinician contact). The combination of frequency and flexibility is intended to allow the group to serve as a secure base for parents, reducing social isolation and making participants feel welcome and included.[439] To facilitate this, GABI includes snacks and drink for participants, effectively siding with Ainsworth against Bowlby on the question of whether feeding can contribute to secure base/safe haven experiences (Chapter 2). The use of a group-based

Simpson, T.E., Webb, D., Albertson, J.G., Close, N., & Sadler, L.S. (2018) Minding the Baby®: developmental trauma and home visiting. In H. Steele & M. Steele (eds) *Handbook of Attachment-Based Interventions* (pp.151–73). New York: Guilford.

[435] Sroufe, L.A. (2005) Researchers examine the impact of early experience on development. *The Brown University Child and Adolescent Behavior Letter*, 21(11), 1, 5–6, p.6.

[436] Facompré, C.R., Bernard, K., & Waters, T.E. (2018) Effectiveness of interventions in preventing disorganized attachment: a meta-analysis. *Development & Psychopathology*, 30(1), 1–11, Table 2.

[437] Suess, G., Erickson, M.F., Egeland, B. Scheuerer-Englisch, H., & Hartmann, H-P. (2018) Attachment-based preventive intervention: lessons from 30 years of implementing, adapting and evaluating the STEEP™ program. In H. Steele & M. Steele (eds) *Handbook of Attachment-Based Interventions* (pp.104–128). New York: Guilford.

[438] E.g. Niccols, A. (2008) 'Right from the Start': randomized trial comparing an attachment group intervention to supportive home visiting. *Journal of Child Psychology and Psychiatry*, 49(7), 754–64.

[439] Knafo, H., Murphy, A., Steele, H., & Steele, M. (2018) Treating disorganized attachment in the Group Attachment-Based Intervention (GABI©): a case study. *Journal of Clinical Psychology*, 74(8), 1370–82.

intervention was also intended by the originators of GABI to increase its cost-effectiveness compared to one-to-one supportive work.[440]

Each session lasts two hours. For the first part, a psychotherapist and several social work and psychology practicum students offer support for parents in helping them observe, attune to, and reflect on interactions with their child taking place in the moment. The interactions are filmed. In the second part, the parents and children go into separate rooms; the parents then receive group therapy from the clinician. The therapy focuses on difficulties the parents are experiencing at the moment, as well as thinking about the role of intergenerational factors in contributing to present-day difficulties. The clinician aims to help parents recognise and reflect on their own mental states and the mental states of others, enhancing their capacity for reflective functioning and for responding to the child in an attuned and nurturing way. This is supported, in one session each week, by review of clips of film footage of parent–child interaction.[441] The social work and psychology practicum students play with the children and support their interactions with one another. Parents and children are then reunited. GABI also offers 24/7 text access to on-call clinicians to support family engagement and support caregivers with the contextual sources of stress they face. Like STEEP, GABI aims to influence the quality of the attachment relationship through cognitive as well as behavioural intervention, though the object is 'reflective functioning' specifically rather than 'internal working models' in general as in STEEP. A fundamental principle for clinical intervention in GABI is 'reticence' from the coaches, who are trained to slow down, tread softly, and wait for the right moment for a comment.

Steele, Steele, and colleagues conducted a randomised control trial to evaluate the effectiveness of GABI, compared to treatment as usual, which was a didactic parenting course.[442] Families were recruited on the basis of parenting concerns raised by paediatrics, courts, or child welfare services. The sample faced severe adversities in both the past and present. Two-thirds identified four or more different 'adverse childhood experiences'.[443] Attrition rates were high: 63% for GABI and 68% for the parenting education intervention. A key factor was housing instability: half of the sample were living in a shelter or in temporary housing. Previous meta-analytic research suggests that high rates of attrition will likely have reduced differential effects of the intervention compared to the treatment as usual, since the families with the most need may have been those who did not complete the programme.[444] Observations of parent–child interaction revealed lower rates of caregiver hostility and more effective provision of a secure base to the child among caregivers allocated to GABI. There was also more effective communication and coordination between the caregiver and child.

[440] Murphy, A., Steele, M., & Steele, H. (2013) From out of sight, out of mind to in sight and in mind: enhancing reflective capacities in a group attachment-based intervention. In J.E. Bettmann & D.D. Friedman (eds) *Attachment-Based Clinical Work with Children and Adolescents* (pp.237–57). New York: Springer.

[441] Steele, M., Steele, H., Bate, J., et al. (2014) Looking from the outside in: the use of video in attachment-based interventions. *Attachment & Human Development*, 16(4), 402–415.

[442] Steele, H., Murphy, A., Bonuck, K., Meissner, P., & Steele, M. (2019) Randomized control trial report on the effectiveness of Group Attachment-Based Intervention (GABI©): improvements in the parent–child relationship not seen in the control group. *Development & Psychopathology*, 31(1), 203–217.

[443] The Adverse Childhood Experiences measure assesses reports of five forms of abuse and five forms of household dysfunction (parent mentally ill, incarcerated, drug addicted, domestic violence, and separation/divorce).

[444] An inverse relationship between attrition rates and differential effect sizes in attachment-based interventions was reported by Bakermans-Kranenburg, M.J., van IJzendoorn, M.H., & Juffer, F. (2003) Less is more: meta-analyses of sensitivity and attachment interventions in early childhood. *Psychological Bulletin*, 129(2), 195–215.

GABI was marginally less effective for participants reporting four or more adverse childhood experiences. The researchers found that treatment as usual had a negative effect on caregiver–child interaction in many cases.

Conclusion

One of the fundamental claims of the Minnesota group was that resilience is a social and developmental process, in large part predictable in terms of risks and promotive and protective-stabilising factors. The resilience of the field of attachment research in the years after Ainsworth can be attributed to a significant degree to the role of the Minnesota laboratory as a promotive factor for the field. The Minnesota group contributed to the growth of intergenerational longitudinal research as a backbone of the developmental tradition within attachment research.[445] And Sroufe and Egeland helped sustain the idea of overarching developmental theory, pulling against the current during decades in which academic psychology was becoming increasingly atheoretical.[446] The influence of this position on figures like Cicchetti helped promote attachment research as a founding element of developmental psychopathology.

Several important studies in the tradition of developmental psychopathology were seeded directly by the Minnesota group, as trainees went out to set up their own laboratories with the Minnesota Longitudinal Study of Risk and Adaptation as the model for how cohort research with at-risk populations should be conducted. Examples include Ward's laboratory at Cornell and the Jacobvitz–Hazen laboratory at Austin, Texas.[447] Many positive features of the Minnesota study were influential for this later work, including a concern with hard-won, credible, and concrete findings confirmed by multiple sources of information, including observational measures. Furthermore, in a context in which research funders had increasing interest in adversity and individual differences, the Minnesota group also helped attachment research reorient towards a greater focus on risk and mental illness.

Not every one of the features inherited by later researchers from Minnesota was positive, though. For example, in general, the Minnesota Longitudinal Study of Risk and Adaptation was poorly set up to study father–child relationships. Only a small fraction of fathers were still in their child's life at 18 months, and 27% of the total sample had three or more men living in their homes across childhood. As with many cohort studies with high-risk samples, the Minnesota group found that engaging fathers in the research was exceptionally difficult.[448] Most of the data they were able to collect on the care provided by father-figures was

[445] See Grossmann, K.E., Grossmann, K., & Waters, E. (eds) (2005) *Attachment from Infancy to Adulthood: The Major Longitudinal Studies*. New York: Guilford.

[446] Beller, S. & Bender, A. (2017) Theory, the final frontier? A corpus-based analysis of the role of theory in psychological articles. *Frontiers in Psychology*, 8, 951.

[447] See e.g. Ward, M.J. & Carlson, E.A. (1995) Associations among adult attachment representations, maternal sensitivity, and infant–mother attachment in a sample of adolescent mothers. *Child Development*, 66(1), 69–79; Hazen, N.L., Allen, S.D., Christopher, C.H., Umemura, T., & Jacobvitz, D.B. (2015) Very extensive nonmaternal care predicts mother–infant attachment disorganization: convergent evidence from two samples. *Development & Dsychopathology*, 27(3), 649–61.

[448] The primary attempt to recruit father-figures in the study was at the 13-year follow-up, where 175 mothers and 44 fathers or father-figures were brought in to the laboratory. However, the findings regarding fathers from the 13-year follow-up were not published in a prominent location, and do not appear to have ever subsequently been cited except by the authors. Sroufe, L.A. & Pierce, S. (1999) Men in the family: associations with juvenile conduct. In G. Cunningham (ed.) *Just in Time Research: Children, Youth and Families* (pp.19–26). Minneapolis: University of Minnesota Extension Service.

from maternal report. The Minnesota group found that composite variables representing supportiveness and disruptive behaviour in the home by fathers, especially during early and middle childhood, contributed to the likelihood of child externalising behaviours in childhood and adolescence. The effect held when controlling for maternal care and general stress experienced by the family. However, the findings were not published in a prominent location, and do not appear to have ever subsequently been cited except by the authors.[449] Difficulties in recruiting fathers, the smaller number of fathers who act as primary caregivers, the model of studies such as those of Baltimore and Minnesota, and wider cultural values combined to mean that fathers have not generally seen adequate attention in American attachment research,[450] though there have been exceptions.[451]

In sum, though, the second generation of attachment research benefited enormously from the Minnesota group as a protective-stabilising factor, forming a touchstone for the field. Papers by the group have generally been exemplary in their clarity and insight, offering an attractive model of what attachment research can entail. The group strengthened and stabilised consensus, combatting contrasting positions on a range of potentially controversial matters, such as whether the infant attachment classifications are reducible to infant temperament, or whether they predict later outcomes controlling for covariates. The group has also served the second generation as an unshakable anchor for the Ainsworth Strange Situation and its coding protocols. At a point in the 1980s where it seemed like the procedure was heading for disrepute due to discrepant findings by research groups who had not trained in using the Ainsworth scales, the Minnesota group helped create a set of videotapes of Strange Situations with agreed classifications by Ainsworth, Waters, Main, Sroufe, and other expert coders. This formed the basis for a yearly training institute at Minnesota which still continues today.[452]

Sroufe and Egeland were also staunch defenders of Ainsworth's category-based coding system. An important instance was Sroufe's reply to Chris Fraley and Sue Spieker's 2003 paper 'Are infant attachment patterns continuously or categorically distributed?' (Chapter 2).[453]

---

[449] Ibid. An additional major empirical report received unfavourable peer-review and remained unpublished: Pierce, S.L., Coffino, B.S., & Sroufe, L.A. (2005) *The Role of Fathers and Father Figures in the Development of Lower SES Children: Predicting Adolescent Externalizing Behavior from Early Childhood.* Unpublished manuscript, Alan Sroufe personal archive.

[450] There were several indirect sources of information on father–child relationships in the Minnesota study. In particular, the AAI offered information relevant to paternal care. However, as the children of the Minnesota study themselves became parents, the significance of fathers has come further into view: Kovan, N.M., Chung, A.L., & Sroufe, L.A. (2009) The intergenerational continuity of observed early parenting: a prospective, longitudinal study. *Developmental Psychology*, 45(5), 1205–213.

[451] There have been a relatively small number of studies in the USA that have measured paternal sensitivity and infant attachment. These have included: Easterbrooks, M.A. & Goldberg, W.A. (1984) Toddler development in the family: impact of father involvement and parenting characteristics. *Child Development*, 55(3), 740–52; Volling, B.L. & Belsky, J. (1992) Infant, father, and marital antecedents of infant father attachment security in dual-earner and single-earner families. *International Journal of Behavioral Development*, 15(1), 83–100; Braungart-Rieker, J.M., Garwood, M.M., Powers, B.P., & Wang, X. (2001) Parental sensitivity, infant affect, and affect regulation: predictors of later attachment. *Child Development*, 72, 252–70; Eiden, R.D., Edwards, E.P., & Leonard, K.E. (2002) Mother–infant and father–infant attachment among alcoholic families. *Development & Psychopathology*, 14(2), 253–78; Kochanska, G., Aksan, N., & Carlson, J.J. (2005) Temperament, relationships, and young children's receptive cooperation with their parents. *Developmental Psychology*, 41, 648–60; Hazen, N.L., McFarland, L., Jacobvitz, D., & Boyd-Soisson, E. (2010) Fathers' frightening behaviours and sensitivity with infants: relations with fathers' attachment representations, father–infant attachment, and children's later outcomes. *Early Child Development and Care*, 180, 51–69

[452] https://attachment-training.com.

[453] Fraley, R.C. & Spieker, S.J. (2003) Are infant attachment patterns continuously or categorically distributed? A taxometric analysis of Strange Situation behavior. *Developmental Psychology*, 39(3), 387–404.

Fraley and Spieker argued that the Strange Situation yielded data that were better modelled in terms of the extent of avoidance and resistance using the Ainsworth scales, rather than in terms of Ainsworth's categories. In his reply to Fraley and Speiker, Sroufe expressed his sympathy with their position. Of course there are cases in the middle-range that have to be forced into the categories. On the basis of their analysis, Sroufe reflected, 'Fraley and Spieker argued essentially that these categories are fictions, and they may well be correct. I would ask, have these been useful fictions? Do they remain so today? The answer to at least the first question clearly is positive, and the answer to the second question may be positive as well.'[454] The acknowledgement of the Ainsworth classifications as 'useful fictions' reflected Sroufe's approach to the philosophy of science, influenced by John Dewey and philosophical pragmatism. Above all, Sroufe stated that Fraley and Spieker would need to demonstrate that the avoidant and resistant dimensions can predict later outcomes as well as Ainsworth's categories before he would consider them 'a candidate for substitution'.[455] Overall, though, Sroufe was personally dubious 'whether this endeavour is worth the effort'.[456] And he expressed concern that debates about categories versus dimensions among attachment researchers would offer ammunition to critics of the field, who could use 'questions about the taxonomic status of Ainsworth et al.'s (1978) categories as evidence that the entire paradigm is invalid'.[457] Sroufe's experiences of the turbulent debates of the 1970s and 1980s as attachment was being established within developmental science had given him a keen sense that the paradigm's existence was not inevitable and should not be taken for granted by those raising psychometric questions.

Except among the social psychology tradition of attachment research (Chapter 5), the Fraley and Spieker paper was, to an unjustified extent, buried for a decade.[458] And even Fraley, Spieker, and researchers sympathetic to their position did not pursue research to compare the predictive validity of categories versus dimensions; as mentioned in Chapter 2, the reason for this is unclear. In the meantime, Sroufe's defence of the four-category coding system was cited as an important source of authority by other researchers in retaining the existing system.[459] Sroufe's influence might also be inferred in the fact that the dimensional scale that particularly came into use during the 2000s was the 1–9 scale for disorganisation, which had been out of view of either Fraley and Spieker's criticism or Sroufe's defence of the Ainsworth categories. Furthermore, Elizabeth Carlson from the Minnesota group reported findings from her prospective study of attachment disorganisation using the scale rather than the category, and later researchers cited Carlson as authorising use of the scale as legitimate for attachment research.[460] In his most recent publication, Sroufe scaled back his defence of the Ainsworth categories, acknowledging that the ambivalent/resistant attachment

[454] Sroufe, L.A. (2003) Attachment categories as reflections of multiple dimensions. *Developmental Psychology*, 39(3), 413–16, p.414.

[455] Ibid. p.413.

[456] Ibid. p.415.

[457] Ibid. p.415.

[458] The primary exceptions were researchers in the developmental tradition with a particular focus on adult attachment, such as the Cowans, e.g. Cowan, P.A. & Cowan, C.P. (2007) Attachment theory: seven unresolved issues and questions for future research. *Research in Human Development*, 4(3–4), 181–201.

[459] E.g. Aviezer, O. & Sagi-Schwartz, A. (2008) Attachment and non-maternal care: towards contextualizing the quantity versus quality debate. *Attachment & Human Development*, 10(3), 275–85.

[460] Bernard, K. & Dozier, M. (2010) Examining infants' cortisol responses to laboratory tasks among children varying in attachment disorganization: stress reactivity or return to baseline? *Developmental Psychology*, 46(6), 1771–8.

classification has few distinct correlates after half a century of studies using the Strange Situation.[461]

Sroufe also contributed to anchoring consensus around the disorganised attachment classification. From an organisational perspective, behaviour takes its meaning from its integration within broader patterns of adaptation to the environment. As a consequence, there was a tendency in Sroufe's approach to treat the behaviours listed by Main and Solomon not just as the breakdown of a strategy for attaining the availability of the caregiver, but as a breakdown of psychological meaning itself. In general, the term 'disorganisation' was used in Sroufe's writings through the 1990s and 2000s to mean the breakdown into chaos in the context of high arousal and lack of containment by the environment.[462] It therefore seemed natural that these behaviours, perceived as lacking 'organisation', were placed together in a broad-band residual category. In his reply to Fraley and Spieker, Sroufe used the discovery of the disorganised classification as an argument in favour of the Ainsworth classifications, which he felt had called attention to the discrepant behaviours.[463] However, again this appears to be a position that Sroufe has later qualified. In a 2014 paper, Padrón, Carlson, and Sroufe criticised Main and Hesse for implying, whether intentionally or inadvertently, that disorganised attachment were all of the same kind and had the same cause. They reported findings that frankly fearful or disoriented behaviours in the Strange Situation had different antecedents to the other kinds of behaviours listed by Main and Solomon.[464] Specifically, infants in the subgroup who did not display apprehension or dissociation/confusion displayed less emotion regulation as newborns.

These were highly preliminary results. However, curiously, they agree with an earlier draft of Main and Solomon's 1990 chapter, which observed that the large majority of children displaying Index VI (apprehensive) and Index VII (disorientated) behaviours in their 200 tapes were from maltreatment or very high-risk samples (Chapter 3).[465] The 2014 paper appears to express a broader turn in Sroufe's late thinking, away from work to establish the standing of existing categories and towards a concern to capture more fine-grained information. In his 2013 article on 'The promise of developmental psychopathology', Sroufe argued that 'we need studies that unpack the heterogeneity in current categories by examining differential antecedents and pathways'.[466] The extent to which this will be a priority for the third generation of attachment researchers remains uncertain. There may be too much invested in the existing categories, and too much inertia, for the field to now pursue a different approach, even if incremental validity could be demonstrated through identification of differential antecedents and pathways. Yet the quiet transition over the past decade towards use of the 1–9 scale for disorganisation and away from use of the disorganised category shows that change is possible if it permits researchers more effective prediction.

[461] Sroufe, L.A. (2016) The place of attachment in development. In J. Cassidy & P.R. Shaver (eds) *Handbook of Attachment: Theory, Research, and Clinical Applications*, 3rd edn (pp.997–1011). New York: Guilford, p.1008.

[462] E.g. Sroufe, L.A. (1996) *Emotional Development*. Cambridge: Cambridge University Press: 'The security of the attachment relationship is related to the regularity with which arousal has historically led or not led to infant behavioural disorganisation in the context of the caregiver' (158).

[463] Sroufe, L.A. (2003) Attachment categories as reflections of multiple dimensions. *Developmental Psychology*, 39(3), 413–16, p.415.

[464] Padrón, E., Carlson, E.A., & Sroufe, L.A. (2014) Frightened versus not frightened disorganized infant attachment. *American Journal of Orthopsychiatry*, 84(2), 201–208.

[465] Reijman, S., Foster, S., & Duschinsky, R. (2018) The infant disorganised attachment classification: 'patterning within the disturbance of coherence'. *Social Science & Medicine*, 200, 52–8.

[466] Sroufe, L.A. (2013) The promise of developmental psychopathology: past and present. *Development & Psychopathology*, 25(4.2), 1215–24, p.1216.

It is important to mark these transitions and discontinuities even during the ascendency of the second generation of attachment researchers. Nonetheless, it must also be acknowledged that Kuhn's classic comment in *The Structure of Scientific Revolutions* bears true: often a paradigm may only enter a period of serious and explicit transition once the old generation of research leaders exit the field.[467] With Egeland and Sroufe's retirement, control of the Minnesota Longitudinal Study of Risk and Adaptation passed to Roisman and Simpson. With this shift, the Minnesota group moved from being a fundamental pillar of the second-generation consensus to a major contributor to methodological and theoretical heterodoxy. Roisman perceives the Ainsworth–Main four-category image of attachment, embodied by the Strange Situation and the AAI, as psychometrically and theoretically unsound, even if he agrees with Sroufe that they have served as useful fictions. Since Egeland and Sroufe's retirement, then, the Minnesota group have dropped use of the attachment classifications, preferring composite measures of early care or maltreatment, or composites of scale scores on the AAI or Strange Situation.[468] Many of the perspectives advocated by Roisman and Simpson have been based on the image of attachment, the approaches to psychometry, and the research values developed within the social psychological tradition of attachment research. This tradition is the focus of the next chapter.

---

[467] Kuhn, T.S. (1970) *The Structure of Scientific Revolutions*, 2nd edn. Chicago: University of Chicago Press. See also Mannheim, K. (1952) *Essays on the Sociology of Knowledge*. London: Routledge.

[468] An exception is Puig, J., Englund, M.M., Simpson, J.A., & Collins, W.A. (2013) Predicting adult physical illness from infant attachment: a prospective longitudinal study. *Health Psychology*, 32(4), 409–417. However, this appears to have been written during the transition period in leadership of the Minnesota group.

5

Phillip Shaver, Mario Mikulincer, and the Experiences in Close Relationships Scale

Biographical sketch

Shaver was a social psychologist, interested in combining the experimental approach of behaviourism with the concern for relationships and emotional life that characterised psychoanalysis. Hazan, a graduate student with Shaver, proposed in a seminar that aspects of adult romantic relationships resembled the qualities of an attachment relationship. In the mid-1980s, Shaver and Hazan developed a single-item self-report measure of romantic love modelled on the Ainsworth classifications of infant attachment. This initiated a decade in which a profusion of self-report measures appeared, a period mostly brought to an end by the synthesis of these measures into the Experiences of Close Relationships (ECR) scale in 1998 by Shaver's group. This scale assessed beliefs about close relationships, and was based on two dimensions: avoidance of closeness and anxiety about closeness. Since the 1990s, a thriving tradition of attachment research has become established within social psychology. A central figure has been Mario Mikulincer, an Israeli experimental psychologist with a background in the study of learned helplessness and war trauma. From the 2000s, Shaver and Mikulincer became close collaborators. At times, the relationship between the social psychology tradition and the developmental tradition of attachment research has been rocky. Against expectations in the 1990s, research found that there is little relationship between the ECR (or other self-report methods) and either the Ainsworth Strange Situation or the Adult Attachment Interview (AAI). Nonetheless, in an apparent paradox, central hypotheses drawn from attachment theory are supported by research using the ECR. Shaver and Mikulincer have drawn on elegant experimental methodologies to further elaborate attachment theory. They have also supported the development of a younger generation of leaders of the social psychological tradition of attachment research in the USA and Israel. Over the decades, conflict between the social psychology and developmental approaches appears to have ebbed. An important contribution to this has been the three editions of the *Handbook of Attachment*, edited by Shaver and Cassidy. However, there remain difficulties in translating between the terminology and methodology of the two traditions of attachment research.

Introduction

In the early 1980s, the empirical research of Ainsworth, Sroufe, Egeland, and others had established the standing of attachment research as a credible paradigm for the study of early childhood within American developmental psychology (Chapters 2 and 4). Yet Bowlby's theory claimed that attachment, as a behavioural system, continued to be relevant and influential after early childhood (Chapter 1). Writing in 1984, Bowlby reflected in correspondence that 'I think we are still rather ignorant about the shift from a child–parent relationship to a spouse relationship'.[1] Ainsworth and her immediate colleagues were engaged in extensive discussions in the early and mid-1980s about how to take the measurement of attachment beyond infancy, and felt sure that this would be possible. The first step taken in extending attachment methodology beyond infancy was Main's 'move to the level of representation', and the development of the AAI (Chapter 3). A different route beyond infancy is the use of self-report to examine an individual's perception of their attachment relationships. This route was adopted by some former students of Ainsworth, such as Mark Greenberg.[2] However, in general, developmental psychology has preferred observational to self-report measures, and this was especially the case for attachment research. By contrast, social psychology as a subdiscipline was more favourable to the use of self-report measures. A sustained programme of research using self-report methods for assessing adult attachment styles was initiated by Shaver and colleagues.[3]

Shaver described his academic path to attachment theory as beginning as an undergraduate at Wesleyan University in the early 1960s. At the time, psychoanalysis was under heavy criticism within American academic psychology, especially from behaviourist approaches and their emphasis on experimental research and learnt responses (Chapter 2). Psychoanalysis had failed to develop much of a tradition of valid measurement techniques, and its account of motivation seemed speculative and untestable. The growing availability of federal research grants and the pressures to publish rapidly contributed to the attractiveness of highly focused mini-theories, rather than overarching models.[4] However, to Shaver in the 1960s at Wesleyan, as later for Mukulincer at Bar-Ilan University in the 1970s, 'the issues raised by psychoanalysts, beginning with Freud, are extremely important: sexual attraction and desire; romantic love; the development of personality beginning in infant–caregiver relationships; painful, corrosive emotions such as anger, fear, death anxiety, jealousy, hatred, guilt, and shame; intrapsychic conflicts, defenses, and psychopathology; individual and intergroup hostility; the brutality of war'. Compared to this, Shaver found that reading 'academic social and personality psychology' for his courses 'seemed disappointingly superficial compared with psychoanalysis'.[5]

Shaver completed his PhD at the University of Michigan in 1970. Affirming the pivotal significance of internal experience against behaviourist approaches, Shaver's doctoral research demonstrated the role of mental imagery in learning and problem solving. Shaver spent the next decade in New York, joining Columbia University in 1971 where he was asked to teach the undergraduate course in personality psychology.[6] At that time, the Columbia faculty

---

[1] Bowlby, J. (1984) *Letter to Marco Bacciagaluppi*, 3 January 1984. PP/Bow/B.3/40.

[2] E.g. Greenberg, M.T., Siegel, J.M., & Leitch, C.J. (1983) The nature and importance of attachment relationships to parents and peers during adolescence. *Journal of Youth and Adolescence*, 12(5), 373–86.

[3] In 2014, in tributes on the occasion of Shaver's retirement as Distinguished Professor of Psychology at the University of California, Davis, Jude Cassidy observed that 'no scholar has done more to expand attachment theory and research'. Pehr Granqvist claimed that Shaver's work 'surpasses nearly all other research programs in psychological science, both in terms of originality and sheer quantity. I'll stand on Mary Ainsworth's coffee table in my cowboy boots and say that!' Such staunch statements of praise are especially salient given that, unlike Cassidy, or Granqvist's mentor Mary Main, Shaver was not a student of Ainsworth's. His route into attachment research was less direct, and the acceptance his work has gained has taken a lot longer. http://www.foundationpsp.org/shaver.php.

[4] Shaver, P.R. & Mikulincer, M. (2005) Attachment theory and research: resurrection of the psychodynamic approach to personality. *Journal of Research in Personality*, 39, 22–45, pp.23–4.

[5] Shaver, P.R. & Mikulincer, M. (2011) Analysis of a collaborative working relationship. *Relationship Research Newsletter*, 9(2), 7–9, p.7.

[6] Shaver, P. (2017) Attachment to attachment theory. *Voices: Journal of the American Academy of Psychotherapists*, 53(2), 35–9, p.36.

were offered the possibility of undergoing psychoanalysis at the Columbia Psychoanalytic Institute at a discounted rate. Shaver entered psychoanalysis with two presenting issues. A first was workaholism, which was emptying his life of other activities and harming his health and mood.[7] A second was that Shaver had been 'beginning to notice a repetitive and destructive pattern in my romantic relationships—always having a woman "in the wings" to whom I could flee if my primary relationship fell apart'.[8]

Shaver was in psychoanalysis for four days a week for two years. During this time, Shaver's younger brother was diagnosed with cancer. The brothers had been close, often one another's only friends for periods as the family moved repeatedly for their father's work.[9] On hearing the news, Shaver's therapist said:

> I'd like to step out of role and tell you, with great sadness, he will not live for more than 8–10 months. There is, unfortunately, no good treatment for testicular carcinoma. I think we should postpone talking about what we've been discussing lately and help you think through how you want to deal with this important situation. If you continue to focus on work and your personal problems, you may let this tragedy pass and then forever regret your lack of involvement.[10]

Shaver took leave from work, and moved for the summer to Minneapolis to be with his brother. The loss of his brother would prove critical to Shaver's concern with attachment theory: 'Eventually, he died, and I was present to receive his blessing. The intense grief that followed was unlike anything I had ever experienced, and it caused me to devote several therapy sessions to grieving. I also began reading books and articles about loss and grief, including some early papers by John Bowlby.'[11]

Throughout the 1970s, a central debate in American academic psychology was between behaviourist theories and new cognitive theories of the mind. Shaver acknowledged the strengths in experimental design of behaviourist research. And he acknowledged that any account of the mind had to include attention to cognition and communication. However, he criticised both paradigms, arguing that neither offered an adequate account of the role of emotion within human life: 'Behaviorism is assaulted as if it were an oppressive ruler. But the powerful methods developed during the reign of strict behaviorism have now been combined with theoretical constructs borrowed from the sciences of communication and artificial intelligence to yield a robust cognitive psychology. Perhaps we can now begin extending it to include the notoriously uncomputerlike emotions.'[12] By the end of the decade, he had

---

[7] In a chapter for a psychology textbook written during this period, Shaver's tone shifts towards the personal: Shaver, P.R. (1975) Psychoanalytic theories of personality. In *Psychology Today: An Introduction*, 3rd edn (pp.402–425). New York: CRM/Random House: 'Lest the superego seem to be a dry abstraction, you should realise that intense guilt and the wearying pursuit of perfection are two of the most common reasons people give for entering psychoanalysis' (409). He also asks the reader, 'have you ever gone on a long walk during cold, wet weather, suspecting that you might get sick but feeling vaguely that it would serve you right?' (409).

[8] Shaver, P. (2017) Attachment to attachment theory. *Voices: Journal of the American Academy of Psychotherapists*, 53(2), 35–9.

[9] Goodman, G.S. (2006) Attachment to attachment theory: a personal perspective on an attachment researcher. In M. Mikulincer & G.S. Goodman (eds) *Dynamics of Romantic Love: Attachment, Caregiving, and Sex* (pp.3–22). New York: Guilford, p.8.

[10] Shaver, P. (2017) Attachment to attachment theory. *Voices: Journal of the American Academy of Psychotherapists*, 53(2), 35–9.

[11] Ibid. p.38.

[12] Shaver, P.R. (1972) Review of cognition and affect, edited by J.S. Antrobus. *American Journal of Psychology*, 85, 297–9, p.297. See also Shaver, P.R. (1975) Emotional experience and expression. In *Psychology Today: An*

come to conclude that his larger aim as a scholar was to 'contribute to a theory of emotion which fits within an evolutionary and developmental framework'.[13] More specifically, the loss of his brother led Shaver to a reorientation of his work around the themes of loneliness and depression.[14] Shaver looked around him and saw a world in which these were the great themes of the age: 'If eras can be characterised by salient emotions, ours must be the age of depression and loneliness.'[15] To make sense of this, behaviourism and cognitive theories alone would not be adequate. He prophesised that 'a revolution in 'emotion science' is about to follow the path blazed by the cognitive sciences. The emotion revolution is a logical outcome of the "age of depression and loneliness".'[16]

The year 1979, however, would prove a turning point for Shaver, transfiguring his concern with depression and loneliness. One of the important factors contributing to this shift was meeting Robert Weiss, a Harvard-based sociologist, at a conference in 1979. Weiss had attended Bowlby's seminars at the Tavistock during a sabbatical in 1971.[17] Weiss accepted that the attachment behavioural system was less readily activated after infancy, and a different stock of attachment behaviours would be seen in adulthood. However, he highlighted that adults still provide one another with a secure base and safe haven, and can experience anxiety during unanticipated separations.[18] Shaver reported that Weiss 'encouraged me to conduct research more specifically on attachment and loss in adulthood'.[19] Though familiar with Bowlby's writings before 1979, Weiss's urging gave Shaver impetus to explore beyond Bowlby's account of grief, to consider attachment as a paradigm for conceptualising adult relationships. A second component of Shaver's shift away from research on loneliness towards attachment was meeting and starting to date Gail Goodman at the University of Denver, where Goodman was a postdoctoral fellow with an interest in the psychology of children in court contexts. Shaver joined the University of Denver in 1980 and commenced a programme of work concerned with adult romantic relationships. Looking back in a recent paper, Shaver identified four great attachments in his life, which have offered him a secure base from which to explore and a safe haven providing regulation and comfort. The first two were his mother and then his analyst; 1979 saw the initiation of the two adult attachment relationships that would dominate his subsequent life: his marriage and attachment research.[20]

Introduction, 3rd edn. New York: CRM/Random House: 'Surely emotion, not variety, is the spice of life—though the two are obviously related … with fear, with indignation, jealousy, ambition, worship. If they are there, life changes' (333).

[13] Shaver, P.R. & Klinnert, M. (1982) Schachter's theories of affiliation and emotion: implications of developmental research. In L. Wheeler (ed.) *Review of Personality and Social Psychology*, Vol. 3 (pp.37–72). Beverly Hills: Sage Publications, p.39.

[14] Shaver, P. (2017) Attachment to attachment theory. *Voices: Journal of the American Academy of Psychotherapists*, 53(2), 35–9, p.39.

[15] Shaver, P.R. & Brennan, K.B. (1991) Measures of depression and loneliness. In J.P. Robinson, P.R., Shaver, & L.S. Wrightsman (eds) *Measures of Social Psychological Attitudes*, Vol. 1 (pp.195–289). San Diego: Academic Press, p.195.

[16] Ibid. p.281.

[17] The experience is described by Weiss in Weiss, R.S. (1994) Foreword. In M.B. Sperling & W.H. Berman (eds) *Attachment in Adults: Clinical and Developmental Perspectives* (pp.iv–xvi). New York: Guilford, p.xiv.

[18] Weiss, R. (1974) The provisions of social relationships. In Z. Rubin (ed.) *Doing Unto Others* (pp.17–26). Englewood Cliffs, NJ: Prentice-Hall; Weiss, R.S. (1982) Attachment in adult life. In C. Parkes & J. Stevenson-Hinde (eds) *The Place of Attachment in Human Behavior* (pp.171–84). New York: Basic Books.

[19] Shaver, P. (2017) Attachment to attachment theory. *Voices: Journal of the American Academy of Psychotherapists*, 53(2), 35–9, p.39.

[20] Ibid.: 'Looking back over the decades, I see that I have been attached to my mother, my analyst, and my wife, and also—viewing attachment theory as a "safe haven" and "secure base"—to attachment theory itself' (39).

Specifically, in addressing his work to adult romantic relationships, Shaver's interest was less in the concrete behaviour of a romantic dyad and more in the motivations and experiences of individual adults facing the predicament of intimacy or the rupture of relationships.[21] Despite clear analogues, the concrete behaviour of an infant–caregiver dyad differed markedly from an adult romantic dyad. However, Shaver was excited by the possibility that at the level of motivation and experience, there were significant lines of continuity between infant and adult processes of intimacy and loss. In 1980, Bowlby published *Loss*, in which just such an argument was made. Similar claims were being made by Ainsworth and Sroufe.[22] Themes of love, attraction, and commitment in romantic relationships had also, in the early 1980s, become established as areas for research in social psychology.[23] New societies were established such as the Society for the Study of Personal Relationships, and the first issue of the *Journal of Social and Personal Relationships* appeared in 1984. In this context, one of Shaver's early graduate students at Denver, Cindy Hazan, proposed in a graduate seminar that there might be individual differences in adult feelings about romantic relationships that mirrored the Ainsworth infant classifications.[24] From these discussions emerged a co-authored 1987 article in the *Journal of Personality and Social Psychology*[25] and a chapter in *The Psychology of Love*, edited by Sternberg and Barnes.[26]

These works presented the argument that adult romantic relationships exhibit the key features of the attachment system in infancy, above all the role of the partner as a secure base and safe haven.[27] They also have other elements in common: reciprocal interaction and physical intimacy contribute to happiness; discoveries and experiences are shared with the other; and there is a mutual desire for the approval of the other. Hazan and Shaver pointed out that, for both infants and adults, the relationship can sometimes feel intrusive, contributing to anxiety and a wish for independence; and the availability of the other can sometimes feel in

---

[21] Shaver, P.R. (2010) My appreciation of Caryl Rusbult. *Personal Relationships*, 17(2), 172–3: 'My own work is inspired by psychoanalytic theory and tilts heavily toward personality rather than, or in addition to, situations … I wanted to dive deeply into the individual's mind, viewing a mentally represented couple relationship as at least as important as the dyad's actual behavioral interactions' (172).

[22] E.g. Ainsworth, M.D.S. (1985) Attachments across the life span. *Bulletin of the New York Academy of Medicine*, 61, 792–812.

[23] Perlman, D. & Duck, S. (2006) The seven seas of the study of personal relationships: from 'the thousand islands' to the interconnected waterways. In D. Perlman & A.L. Vangelisti (eds) *The Cambridge Handbook of Personal Relationships* (pp.3–34). Cambridge: Cambridge University Press.

[24] Goodman, G.S. (2006) Attachment to attachment theory: a personal perspective on an attachment researcher. In M. Mikulincer & G.S. Goodman (eds) *Dynamics of Romantic Love: Attachment, Caregiving, and Sex* (pp.3–22). New York: Guilford, p.14.

[25] Hazan, C. & Shaver, P. (1987) Romantic love conceptualized as an attachment process. *Journal of Personality and Social Psychology*, 52(3), 511–24.

[26] Shaver, P.R., Hazan, C., & Bradshaw, D. (1988) Love as attachment: the integration of three behavioral systems. In R.J. Sternberg & M. Barnes (eds), *The Psychology of Love* (pp. 68–99). New Haven, CT: Yale University Press. Reflecting on the wider context of the publication of these works, Shaver has recalled that when they submitted the paper for publication, it was so far outside the mainstream of social psychology that he worried that it might derail his career. Instead, the paper immediately attracted interest. 'A lot of young researchers, including the growing number of young women in the field, followed up the initial study in interesting and unanticipated ways,' he said. 'I feel fortunate to have come along when the number of women in the field was growing, which made close relationships a more acceptable topic, and when the divorce rate in the U.S. was of concern to government research funders and to the American population. At the same time, new research techniques were developed, making it possible to pursue personality and relationship phenomena that had not been studied empirically before.' Holder, K. (2018) Interview with Phillip Shaver on winning the Society of Personality and Social Psychology Legacy Award. https://lettersandscience.ucdavis.edu/news/phil-shaver-research-legacy-award.

[27] Shaver, P.R., Hazan, C., & Bradshaw, D. (1988) Love as attachment: the integration of three behavioral systems. In R.J. Sternberg & M. Barnes (eds) *The Psychology of Love* (pp.68–99). New Haven, CT: Yale University Press, p.77.

doubt, contributing to anxiety and hypervigilance about availability. More generally, Hazan and Shaver proposed that infant and adult behaviour were rooted in a common behavioural system, activated and terminated by the same kinds of conditions. In their writing, the authors drew on their own biographical experiences, including experiences of bereavement and of falling in love, to argue that the phenomenology and behaviours of adult attachment closely resemble the functioning of the attachment system in childhood. For instance, they observed that 'as anyone knows who has been through such an experience, yearning for the lost person can continue for months or years and can be mingled with anger at the person for leaving'.[28] On the basis of the analogies between infant attachment and adult romantic love, they developed a brief measure to assess individual differences in attachment in adulthood.

Part of the importance of this initial attempt at the development of a self-report measure of attachment was that it attracted Mario Mikulincer to attachment research. Mikulincer had finished graduate study in experimental psychology at Bar-Ilan University in 1985, and in 1986 joined the faculty at the University, where he would remain for over two decades. He also had a role in the Mental Health Department of the Israeli army, and worked with Zahava Solomon in conducting longitudinal research on the mental health and family life of combat veterans from the 1973 Yom Kippur War and the 1982 Lebanon War. These experiences would, decades later, be of great importance for his research in studying the effects of trauma on attachment in adulthood. Embarking on a research career following his doctorate, Mikulincer's output was oriented by concerns reflecting his academic and military research responsibilities. From his doctoral research, he pursued inquiry into the origins of adult experiences of helplessness. The concept of 'learned helplessness' had been introduced by Seligman in the early 1970s to describe the way that repeated failures could contribute to a sense that it would not be worth continuing to try.[29] Mikulincer was interested in the mental and emotional processes underpinning this effect and ways that it might be supressed.[30] He drew on the work of Lazarus and Folkman in conceptualising helplessness as an avoidant response to a stressful stimulus, a response that could be circumvented through a variety of coping strategies.[31] However, Mikulincer was curious also about the potential for failures to elicit rumination. In a sense this seemed like a coping strategy, since it focused attention on how the problem might be solved. However, rumination could become 'the intrusion of autonomic failure-related thoughts into consciousness'. Rather than constructively addressing how a problem might be solved, these thoughts may 'run ballistically on to completion, are irrelevant to one's intensions, and are hard to suppress. They fill the cognitive system.'[32]

The ballistic metaphor signals a cross-over with Mikulincer's research for the army, where his focus was on the role of intrusive images and emotions observed in combat veterans suffering from trauma and from loneliness. Mikulincer was interested in the role of the family in shaping the extent to which distress and fear intrude into the ordinary functioning of

---

[28] Ibid. p.92. The personal experiences that contributed to Cindy Hazan's interest in attachment and loss do not appear in the public record.

[29] Seligman, M.E.P. (1972) Learned helplessness. *Annual Review of Medicine*, 23(1), 407–412.

[30] Mikulincer, M. & Caspy, T. (1986) The conceptualization of helplessness: I. A phenomenological-structural analysis. *Motivation and Emotion*, 10, 263–78; Mikulincer, M. (1986) Attributional processes in the learned helplessness paradigm: the behavioral effects of globality attributions. *Journal of Personality and Social Psychology*, 51, 1248–56.

[31] Lazarus, R.S. & Folkman, S. (1984) Coping and adaptation. In W.D. Gentry (ed.) *Handbook of Behavioral Medicine* (pp.282–325). New York: Guildford.

[32] Mikulincer, M. (1994) *Human Learned Helplessness: A Coping Perspective*. New York: Plenum Press, p.72.

individuals. For instance, he was involved in research, published in 1990, which showed that family support could account for a quarter of variance in combat-related PTSD, and that this effect was fully mediated by feelings of loneliness.[33] In the context of these concerns, Hazan and Shaver's 1987 article caught his eye. Mikulincer recalls having 'noticed similarities between (a) certain forms of helplessness in adulthood and the effects of parental unavailability in infancy; (b) intrusive images and emotions in the case of post-traumatic stress disorder and the anxious attachment pattern described by Ainsworth and her colleagues in 1978 and adapted by Hazan and Shaver; and (c) avoidant strategies for coping with stress and the avoidant attachment pattern described by these same authors.'[34]

According to a jointly written retrospective piece, a firm friendship and collaboration was begun in the 1990s when Mikulincer offered Shaver the chance to work together on a study of security-enhancement as a method of reducing intergroup hostility.[35] However, already Shaver's first publications in attachment theory reveal many facets of shared orientation between the two researchers, which included an 'intense achievement motivation combined with distaste for egotism, a deep and perhaps neurotic split between the senses of ambition and sloth, and extended experiences with psychotherapy.'[36] In Hazan and Shaver's early writings on attachment, intense emotions of loss and of romantic love are palpable and explicitly personal, but also available to resource-thinking and theory-building. This explicit consideration of personal experiences as one source of information among others in the development of psychological theory became a hallmark of Shaver's approach to research.[37] At the same time, it is possible in Shaver's first attachment publications to sense the relentless drive forcing the creation of a bridge between social psychological methods and psychodynamic concerns. In doing so, Shaver and Hazan attempted to grapple with the whole of human romantic life, and further at times, human close relationships in general.

The creation of this bridge was timely. The 1990s saw many other attempts to square psychoanalytic concerns with the tools of social and experimental psychology. Yet Shaver and Hazan's work was unusual in reaching for the depths of the human experiences of intimacy and seeking to contain this in an assessment delivered to hundreds of people. The use of a self-report methodology was, however, especially attractive for researchers who had come to attachment theory without direct contact with Ainsworth. From the 1930s to the 1950s, Ainsworth had attempted to validate a self-report assessment of security, but had found that participants could report that they were secure as a defence against feelings of insecurity

---

[33] Solomon, Z., Waysman, M., & Mikulincer, M. (1990) Family functioning, perceived societal support, and combat-related psychopathology: the moderating role of loneliness. *Journal of Social and Clinical Psychology*, 9(4), 456–72.

[34] Shaver, P.R. & Mikulincer, M. (2011) Analysis of a collaborative working relationship. *Relationship Research Newsletter*, 9(2), 7–9, pp.7–8.

[35] Shaver's CV lists a visit to Bar Ilan in 1995: Shaver, P.R. (1995) Psychodynamic and representational aspects of adult attachment. Invited address, Bar Ilan University, Ramat Gan, Israel. There is also a visit in 2000: Shaver, P.R. (2000) An updated theory of romantic (pair-bond) attachment. Invited address at 3rd International Conference of the Peleg-Bilig Center for the Study of Family Wellbeing: 'Towards a science of couple relationships.' Bar-Ilan University, Ramat Gan, Israel. Their first co-authored work would begin appearing in 2001. https://adultattachment.faculty.ucdavis.edu/wp-content/uploads/sites/66/2014/06/Shaver.pdf.

[36] Shaver, P.R. & Mikulincer, M. (2011) Analysis of a collaborative working relationship. *Relationship Research Newsletter*, 9(2), 7–9, p.8.

[37] Shaver, P.R. (2006) Dynamics of romantic love: comments, questions, and future directions. In M. Mikulincer & G.S. Goodman (eds) *Dynamics of Romantic Love: Attachment, Caregiving, and Sex* (pp.423–56). New York: Guilford: 'There is no theory of personality, emotions, social relationships or psychological development that holds much more than a flickering candle to actual experience ... It behoves us as relationship researchers to keep attachment theory, alternative theories of love, and our own actual experiences of love in mind' (426).

(Chapter 2). A person may be 'so handicapped in his communication with others and in insight into his own needs and feelings that pencil-and-paper tests cannot reflect the nature and extent of his maladjustment'.[38] Shaver appears not to have known about this work, and never cites it. In a paper written in 1984, Ainsworth urged future researchers: 'do not take at its face value a person's self reports of security, high self-esteem, high sense of competence or freedom from stress and anxiety, even though more credence may be given to self-reports of insecurity'.[39]

One attempt by developmental researchers to measure insecurity through self-report was Main, Hesse, and van IJzendoorn's work on the Berkeley–Leiden Adult Attachment Questionnaire in the 1980s. This was a 200-item questionnaire, aiming to identify the four 'states of mind regarding attachment' from the AAI. This included two subscales for un-resolved/disorganised states. A first was Unresolved States of Mind. This comprised items drawn directly from the coding manual for U/d on the AAI, with items designed to repre-sent both lapses in reasoning (e.g. feelings of responsibility for a death in which the partici-pant had no causal role) and lapses in discourse (e.g. feelings of lack of mental control when thinking about specific events). Additionally, 'because unresolved trauma in certain cases may have a relation to post-traumatic disorders and to the dissociative disorders (Spiegel, 1989), some items indicating symptoms of these disorders were included'. A second sub-scale was items suggesting anomalous beliefs about time/space relations and causality, for instance beliefs in possession, mental telepathy, or precognition. The scales had strong re-liability and stability over 12 months. The Unresolved States of Mind subscale had an as-sociation with U/d on the AAI of .63, accounting for 38% of variance. The Unusual Beliefs subscale also made a smaller but significant contribution, with the items for beliefs in pos-session performing especially well. Over 80% of participants could have been successfully classified on the AAI on the basis of their scores on the two scales. False positives were very rare; where misclassifications occurred, it was on the basis of false negatives. However, Main, van IJzendoorn, and Hesse were ultimate disappointed by the overall Berkeley–Leiden Adult Attachment Questionnaire measure, which failed to replace early successes. This was in con-trast to the subscales for unresolved/disorganised states, which had proven quite successful. Nonetheless, the authors decided to leave the self-report scales for unresolved/disorganised states unpublished, and likewise their empirical studies validating these scales.[40] As dis-cussed in Chapter 3, Main has had difficulties bringing valuable work to publication where she remains somewhat dissatisfied with it.

In a private workshop in 1988 with close collaborators, including Main, Ainsworth stated that she regarded her own self-report measures as a failure: 'I felt dissatisfied with the validity

---

[38] Ainsworth, M. & Ainsworth, L. (1958) *Measuring Security in Personal Adjustment*. Toronto: University of Toronto Press, p.17. Van Rosmalen, van IJzendoorn, and van der Veer reported that a slightly revised version of the Ainsworth self-report questionnaire 'correlated significantly with the two ECR-RS scales for avoidance and anxiety to mother, −.61 and −.32, respectively ($p < .001$; n = 230). The same was true for the ECR-RS to father: −.54 and −.39, respectively ($p < .001$; n = 222)' (93). Such findings indicate sufficient convergence between Ainsworth's abandoned questionnaire and Shaver's work to suggest that they represent highly aligned, if not necessarily iden-tical, research strategies. Van Rosmalen, L. (2015) From security to attachment: Mary Ainsworth's contribution to attachment theory. Unpublished doctoral dissertation, Leiden University, Chapter 4.
[39] Ainsworth, M.D.S. (1985) Attachments across the life span. *Bulletin of the New York Academy of Medicine*, 61, 792–812, p.798.
[40] Main, M., van IJzendoorn, M.H., & Hesse, E. (1993) *Unresolved/Unclassifiable Responses to the Adult Attachment Interview: Predictable from Unresolved States and Anomalous Beliefs in the Berkeley–Leiden Adult Attachment Questionnaire*. Unpublished manuscript. https://openaccess.leidenuniv.nl/dspace/bitstream/1887/1464/1/168_131.pdf.

of my scales because of their inadequate coping with the whole matter of defensive maneuvers.'[41] In her final publication in 1992, Ainsworth implied that self-report measures assess semantic memory (Chapter 1) and generalised propositions about the world, rather than episodic memory about concrete experiences.[42] Any tendency for divergence between these two memory systems would be expected to produce distortions in the validity of self-report measures, in contrast to observational assessments which can capture both memory systems and their interaction.[43] Following up on Ainsworth's proposal in subsequent years, Pianta and colleagues, and Howard and colleagues, found that individuals classified as dismissing on the AAI self-report fewer adverse experiences and less distress on questionnaires than the assessment of independent observers, and preoccupied speakers on the AAI self-report more such experiences and distress.[44] Furthermore, Bailey and colleagues reported that discrepancy between positive self-reported experiences in relationships and observer-reported assessment of insensitivity was associated with higher scores for avoidance and lower scores for proximity-seeking when the dyad were seen in the Strange Situation.[45] Bailey and colleagues suggested that caregivers who hold positive accounts of relationships as a result of obliviousness or defences may miss or dismiss information relevant to emotions in relationships. This, in turn, would make them less likely to notice and respond to infant signals, or repair interactions when such signals are missed or misinterpreted.

Self-reporting attachment

A first attempt

From the start, then, the self-report methodology adopted by Shaver and Hazan was one that set them at odds with the community of researchers around Ainsworth. Nonetheless, Shaver received encouragement from Bowlby, who wrote a personal letter in 1985 to say

---

[41] Ainsworth, M.D.S. (1988) Security. Unpublished discussion paper prepared for the Foundations of Attachment Theory Workshop, convened for the New York Attachment Consortium by G. Cox-Steiner & E. Waters, Port Jefferson, NY. http://www.psychology.sunysb.edu/attachment/online/mda_security.pdf.

[42] Ainsworth, M. (1992) A consideration of social referencing in the context of attachment theory and research. In S. Feinman (ed.) Social Referencing and the Construction of Reality in Infancy (pp.349–67). New York: Plenum Press: 'Some find their models too conflicting for such integration to be achieved. It would appear that in such cases the conflicting models become separately consolidated, and often enough this is because what has been conveyed by the partner in expressive behaviour does not match the semantic content of what is verbally conveyed' (365).

[43] Over time, developmental attachment researchers have repeatedly found substantial evidence for this conclusion. For instance, in a recent study, Howard and colleagues found that participants classified as dismissing on the AAI disclosed fewer adverse childhood experiences on a self-report measure than independent scorers rated in their AAI, and participants classified as preoccupied on the AAI self-reported more adverse childhood experiences than independent coders. Howard, A.R.H., Razuri, E.B., Copeland, R., Call, C., Nunez, M., & Cross, D.R. (2017) The role of attachment classification on disclosure of self and rater-reported adverse childhood experiences in a sample of child welfare professionals. Children and Youth Services Review, 83, 131–6.

[44] Pianta, R., Egeland, B., & Adam, E. (1996) Adult attachment classification and self-reported psychiatric symptomatology as assessed by the Minnesota Multiphasic Personality Inventory–2. Journal of Consulting and Clinical Psychology, 64(2), 273–81; Howard, A.R.H., Razuri, E.B., Copeland, R., Call, C., Nunez, M., & Cross, D.R. (2017) The role of attachment classification on disclosure of self and rater-reported adverse childhood experiences in a sample of child welfare professionals. Children and Youth Services Review, 83, 131–6. See also Borelli, J.L., Palmer, A., Vanwoerden, S., & Sharp, C. (2019) Convergence in reports of adolescents' psychopathology: a focus on disorganized attachment and reflective functioning. Journal of Clinical Child & Adolescent Psychology, 48(4), 568–81.

[45] Bailey, H.N., Redden, E., Pederson, D.R., & Moran, G. (2016) Parental disavowal of relationship difficulties fosters the development of insecure attachment. Revue Canadienne des Sciences du Comportement, 48(1), 49–59.

that 'I find your study of romantic love as related to childhood patterns most interesting'.[46] In *A Secure Base*, Bowlby stated that Hazan and Shaver's work suggested that there were, in adulthood, 'features of personality characteristic of each pattern during the early years' that could be measured using self-report. Bowlby affirmed his expectation that both the Hazan and Shaver adult classifications and the AAI classifications would both be predicted by the Strange Situation: 'All our clinical experience strongly supports that view'.[47] Nonetheless, he continued to worry, influenced by Ainsworth on this point, 'that with the self-report paper-pencil method of appraisal it is well-nigh impossible to assess accurately how much defensive maneuvers have inflated security scores'.[48]

Shaver was certainly aware of the potential limitations of self-report measures. In the early 1980s, Rubenstein and Shaver acknowledged that 'social psychology is, unfortunately, remarkable for its ability to reduce profound and fascinating human issues to rather superficial and uninteresting generalisations'.[49] Part of the problem, Shaver felt, was that the operationalisation of variables in social psychology often abstracts away from the lived experiences of people in their complexity. Another part of the problem, however, was that self-report measures designed without sufficient care and creativity can end up reporting no more than the obvious. Throughout his career Shaver was fully willing to acknowledge the validity of Ainsworth's concern about the potential for bias in self-report measures of security: 'we agree that it is possible that some people defensively report that they do not worry about rejection and separation when actually they do worry about these issues, and some may have no conscious access to such worries, even though they exist'.[50] Through the 1980s and 1990s, Shaver's statements showed a certain hesitancy regarding what self-report assessments of attachment precisely measured.[51] However, by the late 1990s he became confident that the participants' report of their feelings, beliefs, expectations, and behaviours was not itself the object of self-report assessments of attachment, but rather markers of underlying psychological processes related to attachment that may not be fully accessible to the participants themselves.[52] The challenge was to find a method of self-report that identified 'noticeable feelings, beliefs, expectations, and behaviors that are related to, or arise from, underlying

[46] Bowlby, J. (1985) *Letter to Phillip Shaver*, 30 October 1986. PP/Bow/J.9/181.

[47] Bowlby, J. (1988) The role of attachment in personality development. In *A Secure Base* (pp.134–54). London: Routledge, p.145.

[48] Ainsworth, M. & Bowlby, J. (1991) 1989 APA award recipient addresses: an ethological approach to personality development. *American Psychologist*, 46(4), 333–41, p.334.

[49] Rubenstein, C. & Shaver, P.R. (1982) The experience of loneliness. In L.A. Peplau & D. Perlman (eds) *Loneliness: A Sourcebook of Current Theory, Research, and Therapy* (pp.206–23). New York: Wiley, p.221.

[50] Shaver, P.R. & Mikulincer, M. (2004) What do self-report attachment measures assess? In W.S. Rholes & J.A. Simpson (eds) *Adult Attachment: Theory, Research, and Clinical Implications* (pp.17–54). New York: Guilford, p.24.

[51] E.g. Shaver, P.R., Collins, N.L., & Clark, C.L. (1996) Attachment styles and internal working models of self and relationship partners. In G.J.O. Fletcher & J. Fitness (eds) *Knowledge Structures in Close Relationships: A Social Psychological Approach* (pp.25–61). Mahwah, NJ: Lawrence Erlbaum: 'Research on attachment styles—relatively coherent and stable patterns of emotion and behaviour exhibited in close relationships—is based on the assumption that relationship orientations are due to, or perhaps consist in, something called internal working models of self and others' (25); Fraley, R.C. & Shaver, P.R. (1998) Airport separations: a naturalistic study of adult attachment dynamics in separating couples. *Journal of Personality and Social Psychology*, 75(5), 1198–212. 'Technically, the term attachment style refers to the observable patterns of behavior exhibited by an individual, not the unobservable variables (such as working models) that shape these patterns. Nonetheless, as is customary in the literature on attachment, we use the terms attachment style and working models interchangeably' (1199).

[52] Shaver, P.R. & Mikulincer, M. (2002) Attachment-related psychodynamics. *Attachment & Human Development*, 4(2), 133–61: 'We use self-report measures in somewhat the same way that physicians use simple indicators of health and illness—e.g. body temperature measured with a thermometer or verbal reports of insomnia. Although such indicators do not provide direct access to underlying disease processes, they are very helpful in assessing a person's health' (154).

mental models and psychodynamic processes'.[53] This approach to self-report measures can perhaps be placed in the context of a growing assumption within academic and clinical psychology, which became consensus by the 1990s, that responses to self-report questions about behaviours and attitudes would reflect underlying cognitive schemas.[54]

The Hazan and Shaver 'love quiz' was a single-item measure, asking participants to identify their relationships as corresponding to one of three adult attachment 'styles', modelled on the Ainsworth infant classifications. The concept of 'lovestyle' had been put forward by Hendrick and Hendrick to refer to an adult's orientation to intimate relationships, on the analogy of 'lifestyle' as a person's characteristic way of going about living.[55] Hazan and Shaver used the concept of attachment styles in an analogous way, as a characterisation of an adult's orientation to romantic relationships, conceptualised as an attachment relationship.[56] Hazan and Shaver assumed that 'conscious beliefs about love ... are coloured by underlying, and perhaps not fully conscious, mental models'.[57] While Hazan and Shaver headlined the applicability of attachment to romantic relationships, other adult relationships (for instance for a sibling) remained encompassed in what was, if at first implicitly, conceptualised as a comprehensive account of close relationships in general.[58]

Unlike Bowlby, Hazan and Shaver did not anticipate that there would be a longitudinal association between Ainsworth's Strange Situation and adult mental models about relationships. And unlike Main, they did not have an underlying theory of common processes that might be in play in both the Strange Situation and adult cognition regarding attachment (Chapter 3). Instead, they situated their extension of Ainsworth's categories to self-report adult attachment styles as purely pragmatic: 'It would be naive to think that a style adopted in infancy remains unchanged or unelaborated all through life. Still, the search for connections between attachment in childhood and attachment in adulthood must begin somewhere.'[59] The Ainsworth categories were knowingly torn up by their roots in the soil of developmental psychology and transplanted into social psychology: Hazan and Shaver were interested to see what might grow—though, as they would later acknowledge, Hazan and Shaver's impression of what the Ainsworth categories entailed was partial and, at points, potentially erroneous.

The 'love quiz' appeared in the July 26th issue of the *Rocky Mountain News*, on the first and second pages of the Lifestyle section. Participants were asked 'Which of the following best describes your feelings?', and 599 participants replied. A secure attachment style was represented by the statement: 'I find it relatively easy to get close to others and am comfortable depending on them and having them depend on me. I don't often worry about being

---

[53] Shaver, P.R., Belsky, J., & Brennan, K.A. (2000) The adult attachment interview and self-reports of romantic attachment: associations across domains and methods. *Personal Relationships*, 7(1), 25–43, p.41.

[54] This approach to interpreting the meaning of self-report measures of mental health has diverse roots, but the role of cognitive-behavioural models may be considered an important contributory. See Beck, A.T. (1991) Cognitive therapy: a 30-year retrospective. *American Psychologist*, 46(4), 368–75.

[55] Hendrick, C. & Hendrick, S. (1986) A theory and method of love. *Journal of Personality and Social Psychology*, 50, 39–42.

[56] Levy, M.B. & Davis, K.E. (1988) Lovestyles and attachment styles compared: their relations to each other and to various relationship characteristics. *Journal of Social and Personal Relationships*, 5(4), 439–71.

[57] Hazan, C. & Shaver, P. (1987) Romantic love conceptualized as an attachment process. *Journal of Personality and Social Psychology*, 52(3), 511–24, p.513.

[58] This claim would be made explicitly a few years later in Hazan, C. & Shaver, P.R. (1994) Attachment as an organizational framework for research on close relationships. *Psychological Inquiry*, 5(1), 1–22, p.1.

[59] Hazan, C. & Shaver, P. (1987) Romantic love conceptualized as an attachment process. *Journal of Personality and Social Psychology*, 52(3), 511–24, p.521.

abandoned or about someone getting too close to me.'[60] Close consideration of the statement is warranted as it contains Hazan and Shaver's implicit theory of adult security, with implications for Shaver's later work. As can be seen, security was not represented especially in terms of secure base or safe haven beliefs or expectations. Instead, the focus was on the absence of two feelings: (i) discomfort regarding closeness and (ii) worry about abandonment. In this, the item appeared to be in part working on the analogy of the behaviour of the infant from a secure dyad in the Strange Situation. The infant in a secure dyad approaches the caregiver on reunion to achieve physical closeness; by analogy, secure adults might be comfortable with emotional closeness. Lack of worry about abandonment appears to be a new element, however. It has a less clear analogue since infants in secure dyads do prototypically display distress on separation, besides the B1 subclassification. It might be that lack of worry about abandonment was conceptualised as an adult version of the capacity to be fully comforted on reunion. In the survey, 319 participants identified with the statement representing a secure attachment style.

An avoidant attachment style was represented by the statement 'I am somewhat uncomfortable being close to others; I find it difficult to trust them completely, difficult to allow myself to depend on them. I am nervous when anyone gets too close, and often, love partners want me to be more intimate than I feel comfortable being' (though there are conflicting sources regarding the exact wording used in the original study).[61] In the statement as set out in the 1987 article, the focus seems to be on: (i) discomfort regarding closeness, (ii) nervousness regarding closeness, and (iii) distrust. Again the analogy with the Strange Situation is curiously partial. The infant in an avoidant dyad does not seek physical proximity, and when picked up may evidence discomfort. However, Ainsworth's protocols certainly do not suggest that evidence of nervousness regarding closeness should be expected, as Shaver later acknowledged.[62] In fact, 145 of Hazan and Shaver's participants endorsed the statement representing an avoidant attachment style.

---

[60] Ibid. p.515.

[61] Ibid. p.151. This is the statement as presented by Hazan and Shaver in their 1987 paper. However, it appears that it was not actually the one circulated in the newspaper. The original study also included the additional phrase 'I am comfortable having others depend on me', though this was taken out shortly after. Shaver, P.R., Belsky, J., & Brennan, K.A. (2000) The adult attachment interview and self-reports of romantic attachment: associations across domains and methods. *Personal Relationships*, 7(1), 25–43: 'Hazan & Shaver (1987), in the first self-report measure of romantic attachment style, used the statement "I am comfortable having others depend on me." They did not realize that attachment theory does not include this comfort as a legitimate part of being attached; it is, instead, part of being an attachment figure, or caregiver, for others (Cassidy, 1999). In later work by Hazan & Shaver (1990) and Kunce and Shaver (1994), the potentially misleading statement was edited out of the self-report romantic attachment measure. For good or ill, however, it had already been incorporated into self-report measures constructed by Bartholomew and Horowitz (1991) and Collins and Read (1990)' (39). However, it would not figure within the ECR scale.

[62] Shaver, P.R. & Mikulincer, M. (2002) Dialogue on adult attachment: diversity and integration. *Attachment & Human Development*, 4(2), 243–57: 'The original Hazan and Shaver (1987) measure of avoidance tapped fearful, rather than dismissing, avoidance' (253). An additional disanalogy with Ainsworth's categories can be identified: the avoidant attachment style was represented by Hazan and Shaver by two feelings and a belief/expectation. Distrust in close relationships and difficulty depending on them is perhaps an analogue for Ainsworth's idea that avoidance is a response to experiences of less-sensitive care. However, Ainsworth did not discuss avoidance in terms of distrust. Instead, she characterised ambivalent/resistant pattern as representing distrust in the caregiver. Ainsworth, M.D.S., Bell, S.M., & Stayton, D.J. (1974) Infant–mother attachment and social development: 'socialisation' as a product of reciprocal responsiveness to signals. In J.M. Richards (ed.) *The Integration of a Child into a Social World* (pp.9–135). Cambridge: Cambridge University Press: 'It may be viewed as advantageous for an infant whose mother seems to him to move unpredictably and inconsistently (and whom he has not been able to learn to trust) to monitor her movements with exceptional alertness and to evince disturbance whenever she moves off' (125).

Finally, an anxious/ambivalent attachment style was represented by the statement 'I find that others are reluctant to get as close as I would like. I often worry that my partner doesn't really love me or won't want to stay with me. I want to merge completely with another person, and this desire sometimes scares people away.'[63] Here the focus seems to be on two feelings: (i) a wish for more closeness; and (ii) worry about abandonment. Once more, a partial analogy with the Strange Situation is apparent. Whereas the ambivalent/resistant infant classification in infancy includes inconsolability (understood as anxiety about caregiver availability), anger, or passivity, the Hazan and Shaver item includes no mention of anger or passivity. Instead, the analogy seems to be with the low threshold for activation of the infant attachment system and high threshold for its termination. It is not clear what, except the analogy with the infant classification, is ambivalent about the anxious/ambivalent statement in the 'love quiz'. In the survey, 110 participants endorsed the statement representing an anxious/ambivalent attachment style. A further 25 participants checked more than one answer, despite having been instructed to select which statement best expressed their feelings. These participants were excluded from the analysis, a strategy that set the precedent for later research using the measure.

Hazan and Shaver stated that participants self-reported expectable correlates, though actually their findings offer a somewhat more complex story regarding the avoidant attachment style. Participants who endorsed the statement representing security reported that their romantic relationships were friendly, happy, and trusting. Hazan and Shaver stated that participants who endorsed the statement representing avoidance reported 'fear of closeness'.[64] They were not given options to report discomfort regarding closeness, and they did not, in fact, report more distrust than participants endorsing the anxious/ambivalent statement. According to the paper's results, both avoidant and anxious/ambivalent participants had more fear of closeness than secure participants, though avoidant participants scored marginally higher.[65] As such, the correlates of the avoidant attachment style were not exactly in line with Hazan and Shaver's expectations. Anxious/ambivalent participants reported relationships marked by jealousy and emotional highs and lows. These findings were then replicated in a study with 108 undergraduate participants.

It was also quickly found that the 'love quiz' was capable of predicting behaviour beyond romantic relationships. A doctoral project completed by Michelle Hutt at Cornell, co-supervised by Hazan, used the 'love quiz' with 229 small business owners in the dairy and agricultural industry, and asked participants also about their patterns of exploration (e.g. innovation and curiosity in their work) and reliance on others (e.g. for support, help, or delegation), and asked them to respond to some vignettes with solutions to technical and personnel problems in the business context.[66] Follow-up interviews were conducted with 15 participants. Hutt found that small business owners with a secure or avoidant attachment style ran more profitable businesses than participants with an anxious/ambivalent attachment style. This was despite the fact that the business of participants with different attachment styles

---

[63] Hazan, C. & Shaver, P. (1987) Romantic love conceptualized as an attachment process. *Journal of Personality and Social Psychology*, 52(3), 511–24, p.515.

[64] Ibid. p.518.

[65] Ibid. Table 3 and Table 6.

[66] Hutt, M. (1991) Influences of attachment in everyday problem solving. Unpublished doctoral dissertation, Cornell University. Shaver drew on this study in support of the predictive validity of self-report measures of assessment in Shaver, P.R. & Norman, A.J. (1995) Attachment theory and counseling psychology: a commentary. *The Counseling Psychologist*, 23(3), 491–500.

did not differ in terms of size, number of employees, number of production units, location, or type of facility. Participants with an avoidant attachment style reported that they were less likely to seek help when they had a problem with the business, and were more likely to view their employees as 'cogs in a machine'. Anxious/ambivalent participants stated that they were more likely to ask employees for emotional support when they confronted a technical problem. Hutt found that they were also more likely to have a chaotic management structure. Participants with avoidant and anxious/ambivalent attachment styles had higher turnover of staff than participants with a secure attachment style. They were also less likely to believe that their colleagues understood the goals and values of the business. The Hutt dissertation offered an early and elegant demonstration of the relevance of the 'love quiz' in predicting social behaviour, even in the work context, in theoretically expectable ways.

In an exploratory study, reported in 1990, Hazan and Shaver found that anxious/ambivalent subjects said that they struggled to finish tasks and slacked off after praise at work; avoidant subjects said that they were less likely to take vacations from work; and secure participants reported fewer psychosomatic symptoms and in general fewer illnesses.[67] In another study from the 1990s, Cooper, Shaver, and Collins found that attachment style accounted for 5% of variance in mental health symptoms in a large student sample, after taking into account demographic covariates. The key findings from the study were that secure participants reported the lowest levels of depression and of problems managing anger.[68] These findings were important for supporting the validity of the 'love quiz' categories, given the centrality of mental health to the conceptualisation of attachment since Bowlby.

In the early 1990s, Mikulincer published a flurry of dazzlingly inventive studies using a reformulation of the 'love quiz' measure. The Hazan and Shaver categories were reworked as Likert-style scales along three dimensions: secure, avoidant, and anxious-ambivalent.[69] These papers established his reputation as among the most ingenious, nimble, and prolific experimental social psychologists of a talented generation. Mikulincer was promoted to full professor at Bar-Ilan in 1992 on the basis of these accomplishments, making him the youngest professor at any Israeli university at the time.[70] Mikulincer's particular skill was in articulating theoretical assumptions and then swiftly operationalising these in the laboratory. For instance, one key question faced by the emerging social psychological tradition of attachment research was whether self-report actually had reference to objective interaction and the shared, social world. Responding to this question, Banai, Weller, and Mikulincer had 72 student participants self-report their attachment style and receive a judgement as to their attachment style by other individuals, including by a friend and by a stranger asked to talk to them for five minutes. There were marked correlations between self-reported attachment style and the judgement made by friends and acquaintances. Friends agreed with the participant in 60% of cases, and acquaintances only slightly less in 56% of cases. This was essentially twice the rate of agreement expected by chance. These findings provided important evidence

---

[67] Hazan, C. & Shaver, P.R. (1990) Love and work: an attachment-theoretical perspective. *Journal of Personality and social Psychology*, 59(2), 270–80, Table 3.

[68] Cooper, M.L., Shaver, P.R., & Collins, N.L. (1998) Attachment styles, emotion regulation, and adjustment in adolescence. *Journal of Personality and Social Psychology*, 74(5), 1380–97.

[69] The astonishing volume of outputs from Mikulincer's group in these years means that only a selection can be mentioned. The slight adaptations to the measure enacted by Mikulincer and colleagues are detailed in Mikulincer, M., Florian, V., & Tolmacz, R. (1990) Attachment styles and fear of personal death: a case study of affect regulation. *Journal of Personality and Social Psychology*, 58(2), 273–80.

[70] http://portal.idc.ac.il/faculty/en/pages/profile.aspx?username=mario.

that self-reported attachment style was a construct representing a process sufficiently manifest in the individual's behaviour that friends and acquaintances would come to the same conclusion.[71]

In the 1990s, Mikulincer and colleagues reported several findings suggesting differences in emotion regulation strategies between participants with different attachment styles. Mikulincer and Orbach found that an avoidant attachment style was associated with lower accessibility of negative memories. By contrast, participants who reported an anxious/ambivalent attachment style also had difficulty supressing negative emotions and memories. These participants experienced that one negative emotion or memory tended to spread into and elicit others.[72] In another study, Mikulincer and Florian asked participants to complete a stressful task: handling a snake. They found that participants with an avoidant attachment style reported feeling more reassured by instrumental social support from a confederate, but not emotional support. Participants with a secure attachment style found reassurance in either form of interaction.[73] By contrast, if they had an anxious/ambivalent attachment style, participants felt no different in response to emotional support, but had an increase in distress if they received instrumental social support. This was the first of many findings by Mikulincer and colleagues suggesting that an anxious/ambivalent attachment style is associated with a tendency to appraise experiences that others find reassuring or happy—such as gratitude—as a source of inner conflict, distress, self-doubt, or bitterness.[74] Such associations seem particular to the anxious/ambivalent attachment style, and have been found to hold even after controlling for measures of self-esteem and social trust.[75]

In another study, Mikulincer asked participants to keep a diary over three weeks. He found that secure participants experienced more trust in their partners and adopted more constructive coping strategies in response to perceived violations of trust. Avoidant participants regarded the feeling of control as one of the functions of trust in a relationship. And anxious/ambivalent attached special importance to perceived violations of trust, and responded to these with rumination and worry.[76] The theme of coping strategies was also explored by Mikulincer, Florian, and Weller, who studied response to missile attacks on Israel during the Gulf War. The researchers found that avoidant attachment style was associated with reports of using coping strategies that distanced the participant from other people, but

[71] Banai, E., Weller, A., & Mikulincer, M. (1998) Inter-judge agreement in evaluation of adult attachment style: the impact of acquaintanceship. *British Journal of Social Psychology*, 37(1), 95–109, p.102.

[72] Mikulincer, M. & Orbach, I. (1995) Attachment styles and repressive defensiveness: the accessibility and architecture of affective memories. *Journal of Personality and Social Psychology*, 68(5), 917–25.

[73] Mikulincer, M. & Florian, V. (1997) Are emotional and instrumental supportive interactions beneficial in times of stress? The impact of attachment style. *Anxiety, Stress, and Coping*, 10, 109–127.

[74] Shaver, P.R. & Mikulincer, M. (2008) Adult attachment and cognitive and affective reactions to positive and negative events. *Social and Personality Compass*, 2, 1844–65, p.1857. For instance, in a study among newlyweds from Mikulincer's laboratory, expressions of happiness in the relationship were usually associated with positive feelings, but for anxious participants were associated with envy. Sofer-Roth, S. (2008) Adult attachment and the nature of responses to a romantic partner's expression of personal happiness. Unpublished doctoral dissertation, Bar-Ilan University, Ramat Gan, Israel.

[75] Mikulincer, M., Shaver, P.R., & Slav, K. (2006) Attachment, mental representations of others, and gratitude and forgiveness in romantic relationships. In M. Mikulincer & G.S. Goodman (eds) *Dynamics of Romantic Love: Attachment, Caregiving, and Sex* (pp.190–215). New York: Guilford.

[76] Mikulincer, M. (1998) Attachment working models and the sense of trust. *Journal of Personality and Social Psychology*, 74(5), 1209–224. These findings were fleshed out at the level of the dyad by a later study. Mikulincer and Florian found that couples in which both partners were secure reported more cohesion and adaptability in their relationship than couples in which one was insecure, who in turn reported more cohesion and adaptability than when neither endorsed a secure attachment style. Mikulincer, M. & Florian, V. (1999) The association between spouses' self-reports of attachment styles and representations of family dynamics. *Family Process*, 38, 69–83.

only among participants living in more dangerous areas. Among participants living in less dangerous areas, there was no difference in the coping strategies used between participants with different attachment styles.[77] This finding seemed to align well with Ainsworth's observation that avoidant attachment behaviour was only seen in the Strange Situation; the same children did not display this conditional strategy in the lower-stress context of the home environment (Chapter 2). By contrast, illness, like long-term separations, was regarded as prompting a potentially chronic activation of the attachment system. Mikulincer and Florian found that men suffering from lower back pain only had worse mental health than matched controls when they reported an avoidant or anxious/ambivalent attachment style. Secure participants appraised their back pain in less-threatening terms, thought of themselves as more able to cope with pain, and used more problem-focused coping strategies.[78]

Together, the studies by Mikulicer and colleagues from the 1990s using the 'love quiz' suggested four conclusions. First, the studies offered evidence of the predictive power of the self-report categories, including the capacity to predict concrete observed behaviours. Second, the studies suggested that the attachment styles responded to contextual stimuli, in the laboratory and in the real world, in ways that were aligned with proposals by Bowby and Ainsworth. Third, the work by Mikulincer and colleagues showed that the difference between the avoidant and anxious/ambivalent attachment styles was evident across a range of domains, including recall of memories, interaction with their romantic partner in day-to-day life, and coping with emergencies and illness. This included intriguing findings such as that instrumental support provided to participants endorsing an anxious/ambivalent style actually made them feel less reassured. Fourth, the findings of Mikulincer and colleagues indicated that the secure attachment style was not reducible to the absence of avoidant or anxious/ambivalent attachment, but had its own correlates, a point that will be returned to in the section 'The opposite of insecurity'.

Beliefs about self and others

In *Separation*, Bowlby had argued that internal working models contain at least two components: expectations regarding '(a) whether or not the attachment figure is judged to be the sort of person who in general responds to calls for support and protection; (b) whether or not the self is judged to be the sort of person towards whom anyone, and the attachment figure in particular, is likely to respond in a helpful way. Logically these variables are independent.'[79] Bowlby's term 'independent' inadvertently suggested to many readers the technical meaning that models of self and other would be unrelated and orthogonal; in fact,

[77] Mikulincer, M., Florian, V., & Weller, A. (1993) Attachment styles, coping strategies, and posttraumatic psychological distress: the impact of the Gulf War in Israel. *Journal of Personality and Social Psychology*, 64(5), 817–26.

[78] Mikulincer, M, & Florian, V. (1998) The relationship between adult attachment styles and emotional and cognitive reactions to stressful events. In J. Simpson & S. Rholes (eds) *Attachment Theory and Close Relationships* (pp.143–65). New York: Guilford.

[79] Bowlby, J. (1973) *Separation: Anxiety and Anger*. New York: Basic Books, p.238. In the manuscript version of the book, the formulation is a little different: Bowlby, J. (not dated) Notes towards Chapter 6 of Volume 2. PP/BOW/K.5./17: 'in the working model of the world that anyone builds a key feature is his notion of who his attachment figures are and how accessible or inaccessible they may be. Similarly in the working model of the self that anyone builds a key feature is his notion of how acceptable or unacceptable he is in the eyes of his attachment figures. On the structure of these communications turns that person's forecasts of how available and responsive his attachment figures will be should he turn to them for support.'

Gillath and colleagues are undoubtedly right that Bowlby meant only that the constructs should be regarded as conceptually distinguishable.[80] Furthermore, it was not a distinction that he upheld elsewhere in his writings. This statement in *Separation* is an outlier: anchored by Hinde's focus on interactions as the basis of relationships, Bowlby tended to treat the internal working model as rules and expectations regarding interaction between self and others, rather than as representations of the individual interactional partners themselves (Chapter 1).

Nonetheless, the idea of representations of the self and of others was a useful one for the social psychological tradition, and aligned with a wider interest in social psychology in individuals' self-concept and their attitudes towards others. In line with this distinction, Shaver and colleagues interpreted attachment styles and their correlates as reflecting individual differences in an underlying psychological process, namely 'beliefs about self and relationship partners'.[81] In order to help situate their work as a kind of attachment research and to make the link with Bowlby, Shaver and colleagues felt obliged to say that the 'love quiz' was tapping individual differences in participants' internal working models. However, in fact, Reis and Shaver had already expressed dissatisfaction with the concept of the internal working model, which they felt had been 'defined so vaguely that different researchers employ rather different measures of it'.[82] Reis and Shaver criticised Main for contributing to the further circulation of this unhelpful concept, which made it hard to understand her exact claims—a point that Main later fully accepted following feedback from Hinde (Chapter 3).[83]

In the 1990s, Hazan and Shaver sought to further articulate the relationship between attachment and romantic love. Following Ainsworth, they argued that adult romantic love includes elements of the attachment, caregiving, and sexual behavioural systems.[84] The 'love quiz' might be influenced by the caregiving and sexual aspects of love, but they regarded the measure as primarily an assessment of attachment-related beliefs about the self and romantic partners.[85] They agreed with Ainsworth (Chapter 2) that what distinguished the attachment system was that it related to the use of the partner as a secure base and safe haven, and to anxiety in response to unanticipated separations. On the basis of this disaggregation of elements of adult romantic love, Hazan and Shaver concluded that the 'love quiz' should be regarded as just a first attempt to distinguish the attachment components of adult relationships. Future research, they argued, should be built upon a theory about the beliefs about self and others at stake rather than treating their initial work as the model.[86]

---

[80] Gillath, O., Karantzas, G.C., & Fraley, R.C. (2016) *Adult Attachment: A Concise Introduction to Theory and Research*. London: Academic Press, p.120.

[81] Reis, H.T. & Shaver, P.R. (1988) Intimacy as an interpersonal process. In S. Duck (ed.) *Handbook of Research in Personal Relationships* (pp.367–89). London: Wiley, p.372.

[82] Ibid.

[83] Reis and Shaver suspected that Main was ultimately assessing 'defensiveness and information-processing distortions'. Ibid. p.372.

[84] Ainsworth, M. (1984) Attachment. In N.S. Endler & J. McVicker Hunt (eds) *Personality and the Behavioral Disorders* (pp.559–602). New York: Wiley: 'There seem to be three major behavioural systems involved in forming and maintaining heterosexual pair bonding: 1) the reproductive or mating system, which seems likely to be initially the most important in bond formation, regardless of whether the biological function of reproduction is fulfilled; 2) the caregiving behavioural system, which is involved in two ways—giving care to the partner and sharing with the partner caregiving to the young that may result from the union; and 3) the attachment system, which implies each partner seeks security—comfort and reassurance—through maintaining contact with the other' (595).

[85] Hazan, C. & Shaver, P.R. (1994) Attachment as an organizational framework for research on close relationships. *Psychological Inquiry*, 5(1), 1–22.

[86] Hazan, C. & Shaver, P.R. (1994) Deeper into attachment theory. *Psychological Inquiry*, 5(1), 68–79, p.73.

Through the 1990s, following Hazan and Shaver's lead, there was a boom in self-reported measures of attachment. Looking back on the period, Conradi and colleagues observe that 'a bewildering variety of adult attachment typologies, adult attachment-related constructs, and measurement instruments' were developed.[87] Among the most consequential was the Bartholomew and Horowitz 'Relationship Questionnaire'.[88] This questionnaire was based on the idea that internal working models of self and other could be either positive or negative. In a paper from 1990, Bartholomew proposed that a secure attachment style was underpinned by positive models of the self and relationship partners, with the self considered worthy of care and others considered as generally available and willing to offer care. Avoidant attachment was underpinned by a positive model of the self and a negative model of relationship partners, resulting in self-reliance and distrust of others. Ambivalent/resistant attachment was underpinned by a negative model of the self and a positive model of others, resulting in emotional volatility and neediness. Bartholomew also introduced a new attachment classification, 'fearful attachment', which she conceptualised as underpinned by negative models of both self and other. For Bartholomew, the secure attachment style was associated with fluency and confidence in operating with both independence and intimacy. Fearful attachment, the inverse, was associated with problems in achieving either: 'They desire social contact and intimacy, but experience pervasive interpersonal distrust and fear of rejection. The result is subjective distress and disturbed social relations.'[89] Bartholomew felt that the Hazan and Shaver 'love quiz' had inappropriately collapsed the distinction between discomfort with intimacy and fear of rejection of attempts to achieve intimacy, which she believed represented substantially different profiles and predicaments.

The Bartholomew four-category model and questionnaire was a landmark in the history of self-report measures of attachment, since for the first time in this literature, categories used to assess individual differences in attachment were conceptualised as the effect of two underlying dimensions. Subsequently, attachment researchers in the social psychology tradition tended to conceptualise and analyse individual differences as dimensionally distributed.[90] The addition of the fearful classification appeared to be of special value in characterising the attachment styles of participants experiencing adversity. This was shown by a series of studies by Shaver and colleagues using Bartholomew's measure. The researchers

[87] Conradi, H-J., Gerlsma, C., van Duijn, M., & de Jonge, P. (2006) Internal and external validity of the experiences in close relationships questionnaire in an American and two Dutch samples. *European Journal of Psychiatry*, 20(4), 258–69, p.259. The array of self-report attachment measures from this period include: Armsden, G.C. & Greenberg, M.T. (1987) The inventory of parent and peer attachment: individual differences and their relationship to psychological well-being in adolescence. *Journal of Youth and Adolescence*, 16(5), 427–54; West, M., Sheldon, A., & Reiffer, L. (1987) An approach to the delineation of adult attachment: scale development and reliability. *Journal of Nervous and Mental Disease*, 175(12), 738–41; Pottharst, K. & Kessler, R. (1990) The search for methods and measures. In K. Pottharst (ed.) *Explorations in Adult Attachment* (pp.9–37). New York: Peter Lang; Griffin, D.W. & Bartholomew, K. (1994) The metaphysics of measurement: the case of adult attachment. In K. Bartholomew & D. Perlman (eds) *Advances in Personal Relationships: Vol. 5. Attachment Processes in Adulthood* (pp.17–52). London: Jessica Kingsley.
[88] Bartholomew, K. & Horowitz, L.M. (1991) Attachment styles among young adults: a test of a four-category model. *Journal of Personality and Social Psychology*, 61(2), 226–44.
[89] Bartholomew, K. (1990) Avoidance of intimacy: an attachment perspective. *Journal of Social and Personal Relationships*, 7(2), 147–78, p.163.
[90] Fraley, R.C. & Waller, N.G. (1998) Adult attachment patterns: a test of the typological model. In J.A. Simpson & W.S. Rholes (eds) *Attachment Theory and Close Relationships* (pp.77–114). New York: Guilford: 'Bartholomew's model, combined with an emerging consensus that two latent dimensions underlie Hazan and Shaver's (1987) and Bartholowew's (1990) attachment types (see Feeney & Noller 1996; Griffin & Bartholomew 1994a, 1994b; Hazan & Shaver 1994), has encouraged researchers to use continuous measures' (82).

found that the adult children of alcoholics predominantly fell into Bartholomew's fearful category. They also found that a fearful attachment style was associated, as Bowlby had anticipated (Chapter 1), with reports of offering caregiving to attachment figures in order to get some attachment needs met.[91] And in a study with a large student cohort, Brennan and Shaver found that a quarter of participants classified as fearful met criteria for personality disorder according to a self-report assessment compared to 6% of participants with other attachment styles.[92]

Shaver and colleagues concluded that Bartholomew's fearful adult attachment style was the parallel, and likely a developmental correlate, of Main and Solomon's disorganised attachment classification.[93] They even used disorganised attachment and fearful attachment as synonyms through the 1990s.[94] However, examination of Bartholomew's 1989 unpublished doctoral thesis indicates an important qualification: Bartholomew regarded her fearful classification not as a general analogue for the disorganised attachment classification, but as an analogue for approach-avoidance conflict specifically.[95] The fearful attachment style was based on the idea that the self is regarded poorly, causing distress, and other people are considered as a potential source of rejection. Jacobvitz insightfully observed at the time that this predicament might result in an approach–avoidance conflict—but not necessarily disoriented or direct apprehension regarding the caregiver.[96] It would seem that the term 'fearful attachment' was complicit in the over-hasty comparison, suggesting a pervasive quality of fearfulness. In fact, in Bartholomew's theory, the category was underpinned by *fear of rejection* rather than fear of the caregiver.[97] Main and Stadtman had argued that whilst rejection by a caregiver would usually result in avoidant attachment, when the tone or context of the rejection was generally alarming, this would be a pathway to conflict behaviour that would be judged as disorganised attachment in the Strange Situation (Chapter 3). Rejection was not central to Main's conceptualisation of the causes of disorganised attachment: it is not especially provided for by Main and Hesse among the indices of frightening/frightened caregiver behaviour, or anticipated in theory to result in infant disorientation or direct

[91] Brennan, K.A., Shaver, P.R., & Tobey, A.E. (1991) Attachment styles, gender, and parental problem drinking. *Journal of Social and Personal Relationships*, 8, 451–66; Kunce, L.J. & Shaver, P.R. (1994) An attachment-theoretical approach to caregiving in romantic relationships. In K. Bartholomew & D. Perlman (eds) *Advances in Personal Relationships, Volume 5* (pp.205–237). London: Jessica Kingsley.

[92] Brennan, K.A. & Shaver, P.R. (1998) Attachment styles and personality disorders: their connections to each other and to parental divorce, parental death, and perceptions of parental caregiving. *Journal of Personality*, 66(5), 835–78.

[93] Brennan, K.A., Shaver, P.R., & Tobey, A.E. (1991) Attachment styles, gender, and parental problem drinking. *Journal of Social and Personal Relationships*, 8, 451–66.

[94] Shaver, P.R., Collins, N.L., & Clark, C.L. (1996) Attachment styles and internal working models of self and relationship partners. In G.J.O. Fletcher & J. Fitness (eds) *Knowledge Structures in Close Relationships: A Social Psychological Approach* (pp.25–61). Mahwah, NJ: Lawrence Erlbaum: 'Disorganised, or fearful, children lack self-confidence and have low self-worth' (36).

[95] Bartholomew, K. (1989) Attachment styles in young adults: Implications for self-concept and interpersonal functioning. Unpublished doctoral dissertation, Stanford University.

[96] Jacobvitz, D., Curran, M., & Moller, N. (2002) Measurement of adult attachment: the place of self-report and interview methodologies. *Attachment & Human Development*, 4(2), 207–215: 'The fearful attachment style seems to differ qualitatively from the disorganized infant pattern. A mixture of avoidance and ambivalence is only one of the many behavioral indices of attachment disorganization during infancy' (209).

[97] Bartholomew, K. (1989) Attachment styles in young adults: implications for self-concept and interpersonal functioning. Unpublished doctoral dissertation, Stanford University. This is in contrast to the new self-report 'disorganised' attachment style introduced by Paetzold and colleagues in 2015, which does seek to assess fear of attachment figures. Paetzold, R.L., Rholes, W.S., & Kohn, J.L. (2015) Disorganized attachment in adulthood: theory, measurement, and implications for romantic relationships. *Review of General Psychology*, 19(2), 146–65.

apprehension regarding the caregiver in the Strange Situation.[98] There was also negligible association between a fearful attachment style and lack of resolution on the AAI.[99]

For a time in the 1990s, it seemed as if Bartholomew's theoretical model and, to a lesser extent, her questionnaire, would become the dominant approach to adult attachment in the social psychology tradition. The approach found authorisation in a passage from Bowlby's writings. It permitted the transition to dimensional approaches to measurement, which was becoming the norm in social psychology by the 1990s: the disadvantages of categories for statistical analyses were becoming increasingly widely known among attachment researchers, such as reductions in statistical power, decreases in scale reliability, and difficulties identifying non-linear relationships with other variables.[100] And the division between positive/negative and self/other produced a neat model from which hypotheses regarding adult attachment styles could be generated and results interpreted. For instance, findings that avoidant attachment style was associated with stronger agreement that condoms protect against sexually transmitted diseases could be interpreted, in light of Bartholomew's approach, as fuelled by negative associations regarding intimacy with romantic others.[101] Furthermore, Bartholomew's model seemed able to encompass infant and adult attachment together within the same frame, a serious asset given that the social psychology tradition was hoping to achieve acceptance from attachment researchers in developmental psychology. Finally, the addition of the fearful category was perceived as an advantage. This addition helped address an ambiguity in the operationalisation of avoidance in Hazan and Shaver's original 'love quiz'. It offered a parallel to the four-category model that was appearing in developmental psychology in the wake of Main's innovations. And the fearful category seemed to offer a way for the self-report system to gain applicability for research with clinical samples.

Though it is certainly still used today, from the 2000s Bartholomew's model increasingly lost ground to the two-dimension model of avoidance and anxiety underpinning the Experiences in Close Relationships (ECR) scale. The introduction of this scale is discussed in the section 'Creating the ECR'. However, as well as the availability of the ECR, Batholomew's model faced three salient limitations, which were pointed out by Shaver and his collaborators. First, the account of avoidant and anxious/ambivalent attachment was generally not well supported. An avoidant attachment style was not associated with a positive model of the self, but only with a desire to avoid acknowledging vulnerability. And this desire was relatively brittle, resulting in associations between an avoidant attachment style and self-blame when things go wrong.[102] Furthermore, an anxious/ambivalent attachment style was not associated with a positive model of the other as 'available and supportive' as expected by Bartholomew, but with representations of others that were shaped by anger, jealousy, and a

---

[98] Duschinsky, R. (2018) Disorganization, fear and attachment: working towards clarification. *Infant Mental Health Journal*, 39(1), 17–29.

[99] Roisman, G.I., Holland, A., Fortuna, K., Fraley, R. C., Clausell, E., & Clarke, A. (2007) The Adult Attachment Interview and self-reports of attachment style: an empirical rapprochement. *Journal of Personality and Social Psychology*, 92(4), 678–97.

[100] Simpson, J.A. (1990) Influence of attachment styles on romantic relationships. *Journal of Personality and Social Psychology*, 59(5), 971–80; Collins, N.L. & Read, S.J. (1990) Adult attachment, working models, and relationship quality in dating couples. *Journal of Personality and Social Psychology*, 58(4), 644–63; Fraley, R.C. & Waller, N.G. (1998) Adult attachment patterns: a test of the typological model. In J.A. Simpson & W.S. Rholes (eds) *Attachment Theory and Close Relationships* (pp.77–114). New York: Guilford.

[101] Feeney, J.A., Peterson, C., Gallois, C., & Terry, D.J. (2000) Attachment style as a predictor of sexual attitudes and behavior in late adolescence. *Psychology & Health*, 14(6), 1105–122.

[102] E.g. Gillath, O., Canterberry, M., & Atchley, P. (2017) Attachment as a predictor of driving performance. *Transportation Research Part F*, 45, 208–217.

sense of partners as insensitive to their needs.[103] This was hardly surprising, since the anxious/ambivalent attachment style had been operationalised specifically on the basis of espoused beliefs that romantic others are not adequately available.

Second, some of the intuitive pull and defensibility of Bartholomew's approach came from the terms 'positive' and 'negative', which could have a variety of meanings. However, this was also a disadvantage in terms of usefulness for prediction.[104] For instance, Mikulincer found that a secure attachment style did not appear to be associated merely with a positive working model of the self, but with one that was well balanced between acknowledgment of positive and negative aspects.[105] It was not clear whether or not this constituted a falsification of the Bartholomew model precisely because it was difficult to pin down what was meant by a 'positive' working model.

Third, the Bartholomew questionnaire appeared to have weak cross-cultural validity, with the four categories not operating as expected along the two dimensions. In western samples, there was little overlap between participants endorsing items representing security and representing fearful attachment. By contrast, in African and Asian samples, there was a marked positive correlation between security and fearfulness, which ran counter to Bartholomew's theory of positive and negative working models. Furthermore, whereas Bartholomew conceptualised avoidance and anxious/ambivalence as opposites, in fact they were negatively correlated only in a minority of countries around the world.[106]

Shaver and colleagues acknowledged that 'it seems unlikely that Ainsworth's research would have had such a profound influence on the field if she had eschewed types in favor of dimensions' since 'in the absence of a model of underlying processes, dimensions generally do not inspire theoretical advances'.[107] Batholomew had circumvented the problem since she had offered a model of underlying processes in formulating her dimensions. Yet Fraley and Shaver argued that the dimensions Bartholomew identified were ultimately not the right ones.[108] They hoped that further explicit discussion and debate about the dimensions underlying differences in adult attachment styles, and further psychometric inquiry, would help shed light on the relevant underlying processes.[109]

[103] Bartholomew, K. & Shaver, P.R. (1998) Methods of assessing adult attachment: do they converge? In J.A. Simpson & W.S. Rholes (eds) *Attachment Theory and Close Relationships* (pp.25–45). New York: Guilford: 'The "positivity of the other" model indicates the degree to which others are generally expected to be available and supportive.' Yet an anxious attachment style was found empirically to be associated with negative representations of others. Simpson, J.A., Rholes, W.S., & Phillips, D. (1996) Conflict in close relationships: an attachment perspective. *Journal of Personality and Social Psychology*, 71(5), 899–914. Extensive criticism of Bartholomew's assumption was presented in Fraley, R.C. & Shaver, P.R. (2000) Adult romantic attachment: theoretical developments, emerging controversies, and unanswered questions. *Review of General Psychology*, 4(2), 132–54.

[104] Stein, H., Jacobs, N.J., Ferguson, K.S., Allen, J.G., & Fonagy, P. (1998) What do adult attachment scales measure? *Bulletin of the Menninger Clinic*, 62, 33–82.

[105] Mikulincer, M. (1995) Attachment style and the mental representation of the self. *Journal of Personality and Social Psychology*, 69(6), 1203–215.

[106] Schmitt, D. P., Alcalay, L., Allensworth, M., et al. (2004) Patterns and universals of adult romantic attachment across 62 cultural regions: are models of self and of other pancultural constructs? *Journal of Cross-Cultural Psychology*, 35(4), 367–402.

[107] Brennan, K.A., Shaver, P.R., & Tobey, A.E. (1991) Attachment styles, gender, and parental problem drinking. *Journal of Social and Personal Relationships*, 8, 451–66, p.465.

[108] Crowell, J.A., Fraley, R.C., & Shaver, P.R. (1999) Measures of individual differences in adolescent and adult attachment. In J. Cassidy & P.R. Shaver (eds) *Handbook of Attachment: Theory, Research, and Clinical Applications* (pp.434–65). New York: Guilford; Fraley, R.C. & Shaver, P.R. (2000) Adult romantic attachment: theoretical developments, emerging controversies, and unanswered questions. *Review of General Psychology*, 4(2), 132–54.

[109] E.g. Fraley, R.C. & Waller, N.G. (1998) Adult attachment patterns: a test of the typological model. In J.A. Simpson & W.S. Rholes (eds) *Attachment Theory and Close Relationships* (pp.77–114). New York: Guilford: 'An explicit focus on the latent dimensions, however, may facilitate inquiry into the underlying operation of the

Avoidance and anxiety

Creating the ECR

Though Bartholomew and colleagues were able to source the idea of working models of the self and other in Bowlby's writings, other accounts of security and insecurity were available too. At times, Ainsworth used the term 'anxious attachment' as a synonym for insecure attachment.[110] This may have been motivated by a desire to remind readers that both infants in avoidant and ambivalent/resistant dyads showed anxiety about their caregiver's availability in the home environment, and that it was only in the Strange Situation that the anxiety of the former group was masked. The use of 'anxious attachment' as a synonym for 'insecure attachment' was generally picked up by her immediate students and colleagues in the 1980s (with the exception of Main, who preferred the latter term). When discussing the Strange Situation, Bowlby sometimes used the term 'anxious attachment' to refer to the avoidant and ambivalent/resistant dyads, following Ainsworth.[111] However, in the 1970s, Bowlby developed a different use of the term. This is most clearly seen in *Separation* where Chapter 15 is dedicated to an elaboration of the concept of anxious attachment. Already by the 1950s he had distinguished two classes of response to major separations: one that was manifest as clinging and protest, and another seen as detachment and avoidance of the caregiver (Chapter 1). Now, in *Separation*, he offered the term 'anxious attachment' as a label for the first of these two classes, with a particular emphasis on the vigilance regarding the caregiver's availability: 'Some children subjected to an unpredictable régime seem to despair. Instead of developing anxious attachment, they become more or less detached, apparently neither trusting nor caring for others.'[112] This use of the term continued throughout the rest of his career. For instance, in *Loss* he argued that 'one of the commonest forms of disturbance is the overready elicitation of attachment behaviour, resulting in anxious attachment. Another, to which special attention is given in this volume, is a partial or complete deactivation of attachment behaviour.'[113]

As Mikulincer and colleagues observed in 1990, the term 'anxiety' is potentially a very ambiguous one. It can imply various elements including worry, anger, and emotionality.[114] Furthermore, as Ainsworth's label of ambivalent/resistant attachment suggested, there may be a potential link with ambivalence (though Shaver felt that avoidant attachment was just as much a state of ambivalence regarding the attachment figure).[115] However, despite such

attachment system rather than remaining at the level of manifest behaviour ... We believe that the prototype approach leaves the ontological status of the attachment patterns unclear. Are the prototypes advocated by Griffin and Bartholomew supposed to represent "fuzzy" groups that exist in nature or "fuzzy" groups that exist in the minds of perceivers of nature?' (107).

[110] E.g. Ainsworth, M.D.S. (1983) Patterns of infant–mother attachment as related to maternal care: their early history and their contribution to continuity. In D. Magnusson & V.L. Allen (eds) *Human Development: An Interactional Perspective* (pp.35–55). New York: Academic Press, p.49.

[111] E.g. Bowlby, J. (1969, 1982) *Attachment*. London: Penguin, p.365.

[112] Bowlby, J. (1973) *Separation: Anxiety and Anger*. New York: Basic Books, p.273.

[113] Bowlby, J. (1980) *Loss*. London: Pimlico, p.41.

[114] Mikulincer, M., Paz, D., & Kedem, P. (1990) Anxiety and categorization—2. Hierarchical levels of mental categories. *Personality and Individual Differences*, 11(8), 815–21.

[115] See e.g. Brennan, K.A. & Shaver, P.R. (1995) Dimensions of adult attachment, affect regulation, and romantic relationship functioning. *Personality and Social Psychology Bulletin*, 21(3), 267–83, p.280.

problems and ambiguities, the term 'anxiety' had been used by Bowlby, and this contributed to its appeal to Shaver and colleagues. The term would also have had an accessibility and intuitiveness, given its growing use and presence in public discourse from the 1940s to the early 1990s.[116] Ultimately, the two classes identified by Bowlby were conceptualised by Shaver and colleagues from 1998 onwards as reflecting two dimensions in individual differences regarding close relationships: 'The first dimension, Avoidance, captures variability in the tendency to feel uncomfortable with closeness or dependence. The second dimension, Anxiety, reflects a fear of abandonment'.[117] Over the subsequent decade, the opposition came to be formulated rather differently: 'The first dimension, typically called attachment avoidance, reflects the extent to which a person distrusts relationship partners' goodwill and strives to maintain autonomy and emotional distance from partners. The second dimension, typically called attachment anxiety, reflects the degree to which a person worries that a partner will not be available in times of need.'[118] However, contained in both early and late definitions is a technical sense of 'anxiety' to mean vigilance regarding the availability of attachment figures. In these definitions, 'anxiety' may be associated with anger and ambivalence, or indeed with general experiences or symptoms of anxiety, but these are not elements that formed the essence of the technical concept for Shaver and colleagues.[119]

In 1998, Brennan, Clark, and Shaver reflected that Shaver and Hazan 'naively took for granted that Ainsworth et al. (1978) were correct in thinking of attachment patterns as categories or types. In retrospect, it is evident that Hazan and Shaver should have paid attention to Ainsworth et al.'s (1978) Figure 10 (p. 102), which summarized the results of a discriminant analysis predicting infant attachment type (secure, anxious, or avoidant) from the continuous rating scales.'[120] Brennan, Clark, and Shaver were right that a dimensional approach to attachment had been napping peacefully on the backseat of *Patterns of Attachment*, even while the categories had control of the vehicle. However, close examination reveals that Ainsworth's data did not completely support the claims of Shaver and colleagues to have identified a forerunner for their account of attachment in terms of two dimensions. True, in the discriminant function analysis in *Patterns of Attachment*, a first function had comprised essentially scores for avoidance. However, the second function was mainly constituted by scores on the resistance scale on first and second reunion, and with crying through the two reunion episodes. The function was as much or more constituted by anger or frustration as by anxious distress. Furthermore, whilst the two-function model reported in *Patterns of*

[116] Wilkinson, I. (2001) *Anxiety in a Risk Society*. London: Routledge; Horwitz, A.V. (2013) *Anxiety: A Short History*. Baltimore: Johns Hopkins University Press.

[117] Fraley, R.C. & Shaver, P.R. (1998) Airport separations: a naturalistic study of adult attachment dynamics in separating couples. *Journal of Personality and Social Psychology*, 75(5), 1198–212, p.1199.

[118] Mikulincer, M., Shaver, P.R., & Slav, K. (2006) Attachment, mental representations of others, and gratitude and forgiveness in romantic relationships. In M. Mikulincer & G.S. Goodman (eds) *Dynamics of Romantic Love: Attachment, Caregiving, and Sex* (pp.190–215). New York: Guilford, p.192.

[119] There is some lack of clarity on this point of theory, however. In general, attachment anxiety is understood to be the degree to which a person worries that a partner will not be available in times of need. However, at other times it is defined as anger and ambivalence, with worries fading into the background, e.g. Shaver, P.R. & Mikulincer, M. (2005) Attachment theory and research: resurrection of the psychodynamic approach to personality. *Journal of Research in Personality*, 39, 22–45: 'Hyperactivating strategies reflect a compromise between conflicting, ambivalent tendencies toward attachment figures—overwhelming anger and hostility toward unavailable attachment figures together with an intense need for proximity to these frustrating figures' (28).

[120] Brennan, K.A., Clark, C.L., & Shaver, P.R. (1998) Self-report measurement of adult romantic attachment: an integrative overview. In J.A. Simpson & W.S. Rholes (eds) *Attachment Theory and Close Relationships* (pp.46–76). New York: Guilford, p.47; Ainsworth, M., Blehar, M., Waters, E., & Wall, S. (1978, 2012) *Patterns of Attachment: A Psychological Study of the Strange Situation*. Bristol: Psychology Press.

Attachment was superb at predicting avoidant and secure dyads, it misclassified 30% of ambivalent/resistant dyads.

The conceptualisation of anxiety by Shaver and colleagues as vigilance regarding the availability of attachment figures was in part a theoretically motivated position, in which fear of abandonment was understood to be primary and to generate the other behavioural displays Ainsworth had identified.[121] However, this conceptualisation of anxiety coincides with and seems to have been primarily influenced by a landmark piece of empirical research conducted with Kelley Brennan and Catherine Clark. The researchers created a pool of 323 questionnaire items from the different self-report measures of attachment available, which aimed to assess 60 named attachment-related constructs. These 323 items were then completed by 1,086 undergraduates enrolled at the University of Texas. When the items were factored, the result was 12 specific attachment-related dimensions, each with at least 10 items that could produce viable scales. The 12 scales 'which can be viewed as "facets" (Costa & McCrae, 1992) of Avoidance and Anxiety, are as follows: (1) Partner is a Good Attachment Figure; (2) Separation Anxiety; (3) Self-Reliance; (4) Discomfort with Closeness; (5) Attachment-Related Anger at Partners; (6) Uncertainty About Feelings for Partners; (7) Discomfort with Dependence; (8) Trust; (9) Lovability/Relational Self-Esteem; (10) Desire to Merge with Partners; (11) Tough-Minded Independence; and (12) Fear of Abandonment.'[122] A higher-order factor analysis of the 12 scales then revealed two underlying dimensions. The two-factor model accounted for 63% of variance.

At an item level, items reflecting the constructs 'avoidance of intimacy', 'discomfort with closeness', and 'self-reliance' were most strongly representative of the first factor, which was termed 'Avoidance'. Items reflecting 'preoccupation', 'fear of abandonment', and 'fear of rejection' were most strongly representative of the second factor, which was termed 'Anxiety'. Rather than part of an avoidant attachment style as assumed by Hazan and Shaver or an independent category as anticipated by Bartholomew, fear of rejection was in fact identified by the factor analysis as one of the three most important elements of the new 'Anxiety' dimension. Brennan, Clark, and Shaver found that the correlation between the 'Avoidance' and 'Anxiety' factors was only .12, 'suggesting that the dimensions underlying attachment styles are essentially orthogonal.'[123] The correlation appeared to be accounted for by a few constructs that loaded on both factors. These included perception of the unavailability of partners, perception of the self as unworthy of care, and a negative relationship with attachment security.

On the basis of the factor analysis, Brennan, Clark, and Shaver extracted 36 questionnaire items from the pool to craft the ECR scale. The items chosen were those that loaded most strongly on one or the other dimension, with the selection of 36—as opposed to 20 or 40— decided abitrarily.[124] The stated aim of the ECR was to halt the raucous proliferation of new self-report measures of attachment, finding a neutral and common ground for the social

---

[121] Ibid.: 'Right from the start, Ainsworth's three major attachment "types" could be conceptualized as regions in a two-dimensional space, the dimensions being Avoidance (discomfort with closeness and dependency) and Anxiety (crying, failing to explore confidently in the absence of mother, and angry protest directed at mother during reunions after what was probably experienced as abandonment)' (49).

[122] Ibid. pp.66–7.

[123] Ibid. p.57.

[124] This is implied but not detailed in the chapter. Confirmed by Kelly Brennan-Jones, personal communication, August 2019.

psychology tradition of attachment research through 'discovering and describing the essence' of the self-report measures created to date.[125] The ECR was also framed by the authors, in part as a result of its neutrality, as a supersession of Bartholomew's theoretical model in presenting evidence for 'anxiety' and 'avoidance' as the two latent dimensions across all the other self-report measures. The measure was successful on both counts. Though other self-report measures continued to be used, the ECR soon became the 'industry standard' self-report assessment of attachment, and its two latent dimensions became the dominant explanatory model in the field.[126]

In 2003, a place was also reintroduced for Bartholomew's 'fearful' attachment category by Mikulincer and Shaver. In Bartholomew's model, fearful attachment occurred when a respondent was afraid of rejection by attachment figures and also had a negative model of their own worthiness. On the ECR, fearful attachment was re-envisioned as the co-occurrence of anxiety and avoidance. Mikuliner and Shaver's stated reason for excluding fearful attachment as an independent category is quite curious in retrospect: 'The fearfully avoidant self-description on the Bartholomew and Horowitz (1991) categorical measure … provides too low a hurdle for classification into the least secure category, and this creates too large a discrepancy between the clinical literature on disorganized attachment and the social-psychological literature.'[127] Mikulincer and Shaver's conceptualisation of fearful attachment as the coincidence of anxiety and avoidance, then, was an attempt to retain the bridge to clinical concerns and to the developmental psychology tradition, but with a narrower (and therefore hopefully more clinically meaningful) cut-off. This stance was also a development of Mikulincer's longstanding interest in the intrusion of distress and fear into ordinary functioning. Already in his early work on learned helplessness in the early 1990s, Mikulincer had documented that anxiety can undermine an avoidant coping strategy, producing a state he called 'disorganisation'.[128]

An anxious attachment style and an avoidant attachment style both, as Main had argued (Chapter 3), can be conceptualised as strategies, with the expectable result of offering some conditional form of the benefits of attachment relationships. However, the anxious strategy will be blocked if, when attachment or threat cues are present, a person fails to pursue the availability of their attachment figure. And the avoidant strategy will be undermined if it is intruded upon by anxiety or other overwhelming demands. Crawford, Shaver, and Goldsmith discovered that an avoidant attachment style was only associated with lower scores for attachment anxiety for participants with low or moderate levels of trait neuroticism

[125] Frias, M.T., Shaver, P.R., & Mikulincer, M. (2014) Measures of adult attachment and related constructs. In G.J. Boyle & D.H. Saklofske (eds) *Measures of Personality and Social Psychological Constructs*. Philadelphia: Elsevier, 417–47, p.437.

[126] Pittman, J.F. (2012) Attachment orientations: a boon to family theory and research. *Journal of Family Theory & Review*, 4(4), 306–310, p.308.

[127] Mikulincer, M. & Shaver, P.R. (2003) The attachment behavioral system in adulthood: activation, psychodynamics, and interpersonal processes. In M.P. Zanna (ed.) *Advances in Experimental Social Psychology*, Vol. 35 (pp.53–152). New York: Academic Press, p.136.

[128] Mikulincer, M. (1994) *Human Learned Helplessness: A Coping Perspective*. New York: Plenum Press: 'People for whom emotion acts as an internal stimulus that recalls both the unresolved mismatch and their own weakness and vulnerability may perceive emotion as an uninvited intruder that counteracts their avoidance coping. They may also experience their emotions as overwhelming and disorganising forces that demand that they resolve the mismatch, which is precisely what they feel they cannot do. In this case, emotions do not facilitate adaptation and mastery but rather reflect failure of control and flooding, and they may disorganise the person's avoidance activities' (143).

(susceptibility to becoming distressed and worried). For those participants who became distressed and worried easily, an avoidant attachment style had the opposite effect, in that it was actually associated with increased scores for attachment anxiety.[129] The authors interpreted this finding as suggesting that the avoidant attachment style contributes to attachment anxiety, rather than providing an alternative or defence against it, for individuals prone to becoming distressed and worried. Likewise, Mikulincer and colleagues demonstrated that an avoidant attachment style, which under ordinary circumstances is associated with low accessibility of attachment-related worries, in fact is associated with heightened accessibility of these worries when a cognitive load is added.[130] The avoidant attachment style depends upon an infrastructure of attentional and regulatory control, even if this infrastructure is not the avoidant style itself.

In general, Shaver and Mikulincer conceptualised fearful attachment as a breakdown of attachment style, rather than having content in its own right. They repeatedly interpreted Main and Solomon's disorganised attachment classification as 'random fluctuations' of anxious and avoidant behaviour.[131] This, as Chapter 3 documented, is a misunderstanding, likely based on a lack of knowledge about how the construct is coded in practice.[132] The status of 'fearful attachment' in the thinking of Mikulincer and Shaver has been neglected, perhaps because it too has been regarded as a state of meaninglessness. There has been little concern to inquire regarding the nature, form, and implications of fearful attachment. Indeed, it has not generally been regarded as necessary to test for fearful attachment or report results, leading in turn to little impetus for the design of research to investigate the phenomenon. For example, as Ein-Dor, Mikulincer, and Shaver put matters in a paper from 2011 about responses to threatening stimuli: 'We did not include fearful avoidance in our analysis (i.e., a person above the median on both anxiety and avoidance) because attachment theory views this pattern as a breakdown of attachment strategies rather than a coherent strategy in its own right.'[133]

[129] Crawford, T.N, Shaver, P.R., & Goldsmith, H.H. (2007) How affect regulation moderates the association between anxious attachment and neuroticism. *Attachment & Human Development*, 9(2), 95–109.

[130] Mikulincer, M., Birnbaum, G., Woddis, D., & Nachmias, O. (2000) Stress and accessibility of proximity-related thoughts. *Journal of Personality and Social Psychology*, 78(3), 509–523. See also Edelstein, R.S. & Gillath, O. (2008) Avoiding interference: adult attachment and emotional processing biases. *Personality and Social Psychology Bulletin*, 34(2), 171–81.

[131] Mikulincer, M. & Shaver, P. (2016) *Attachment in Adulthood*, 2nd edn. New York: Guilford, p.143. For another example see Mikulincer, M. & Shaver, P.R. (2003) The attachment behavioral system in adulthood: activation, psychodynamics, and interpersonal processes. In M.P. Zanna (ed.) *Advances in Experimental Social Psychology*, Vol. 35 (pp.53–152). New York: Academic Press: 'Recently, a fourth category, "disorganized/disoriented," has been added. It is characterized by odd, awkward behavior during separation and reunion episodes and random fluctuations between signs of anxiety and avoidance' (66).

[132] In discussions of the phenomenon, Mikulincer, Shaver, and colleagues have been prone to cite social psychologists in turn discussing developmental psychologists, rather than the relevant primary literature, e.g. Mikulincer, M., Solomon, Z., Shaver, P.R., & Ein-Dor, T. (2014) Attachment-related consequences of war captivity and trajectories of posttraumatic stress disorder: a 17-year longitudinal study. *Journal of Social and Clinical Psychology*, 33(3), 207–228: 'In extreme cases, attachment insecurities can result in a disorganized attachment pattern—an incoherent blend of contradictory approach and avoidance behaviors or paralyzed inaction (Simpson & Rholes, 2002)' (210). Simpson, J.A. & Rholes, W.S. (2002) Fearful-avoidance, disorganization, and multiple working models: some directions for future theory and research. *Attachment & Human Development*, 4(2), 223–9.

[133] Ein-Dor, T., Mikulincer, M., & Shaver, P.R. (2011) Effective reaction to danger: attachment insecurities predict behavioral reactions to an experimentally induced threat above and beyond general personality traits. *Social Psychological and Personality Science*, 2(5), 467–73, p.473.

Minimising and maximising

From the early 2000s, one of the central aspects of the emergent collaboration between Shaver and Mikulincer was an attempt to develop a fleshed-out theory of the attachment system in adulthood, and the processes underlying individual differences in avoidance and anxiety. In this, they draw inspiration from developments in theory within the developmental tradition of attachment research. Main had conceptualised avoidance and ambivalent/resistance as conditional strategies, part of the human evolutionary repertoire for responding to environments that do not permit the direct satisfaction of the attachment system (Chapter 3). Cassidy and Kobak took Main's concept of the infant attachment patterns as conditional strategies and argued that they represented two approaches to emotion-regulation: avoidant attachment was a minimising of the attachment system and of associated emotions which had the expectable outcome of avoiding rebuff and retaining regulation; ambivalent/resistant attachment was a maximising of the attachment system and associated emotions in the service of maintaining the attention of the caregiver.[134]

Shaver had worked on the 1999 edition of the *Handbook of Attachment* with Cassidy, and had become impressed by her ideas. In the early 2000s, Shaver and Mikulincer took her image of minimising and maximising of the attachment system as a central building block of their theory. They conceptualised the attachment system in adulthood as containing three modules.[135] Together these form a cadence. The first and most basic module was the one described by Bowlby, and is based on the potential for perceiving threats. The first module is structured by the question: 'Are there signs of threat?' There can, naturally, be various sources of threat. Shaver and Mikulincer observed that these might include external dangers, such as the unexpected unavailability of attachment figures, the identification of a form of personal vulnerability. They might include internal states such as illness or worry about mortality. Shaver and Mikulincer proposed that symbolic threats to status, identity, or freedom would also be relevant to the first module of the attachment system.[136] Where a sign of threat appears, the attachment system is activated, leading to 'seeking proximity to external or internalised attachment figure'.[137]

Though the term 'proximity' was used by Shaver and Mikulincer, they did not mean physical proximity in the manner of Bowlby, but actually the sense of being close to a 'source of felt security', which might be physical or symbolic.[138] Activation of the attachment system triggers a second module, which builds on the work of Ainsworth and Sroufe. The second module is structured by the question: 'Is the attachment figure available, attentive, responsive, etc.?' The etcetera signals Shaver and Mikulincer's belief that the parameters for experiencing felt security in adulthood may be calibrated by factors including context and

[134] Cassidy, J. & Kobak, R. (1988) Avoidance and its relation to other defensive processes. In J. Belsky & T. Neworski (eds) *Clinical Implications of Attachment* (pp.300–323). Hillsdale, NJ: Lawrence Erlbaum; Kobak, R., Cole, H., Fleming, W., Ferenz-Gillies, R., & Gamble, W. (1993) Attachment and emotion regulation during mother–teen problem-solving: a control theory analysis. *Child Development*, 64, 231–45.

[135] Mikulincer, M. & Shaver, P. (2016) *Attachment in Adulthood*. New York: Guilford, Figure 2.1, p.29.

[136] Shaver, P.R. & Mikulincer, M. (2012) An attachment perspective on coping with existential concerns. In P.R. Shaver & M. Mikulincer (eds) *Meaning, Mortality, and Choice: The Social Psychology of Existential Concerns* (pp.291–307). Washington, DC: American Psychological Association, p.296.

[137] Mikulincer, M. & Shaver, P. (2016) *Attachment in Adulthood*. New York: Guilford, p.29, Figure 2.1.

[138] Mario Mikulincer, personal communication, July 2019.

culture, as well as the nature of the perceived threat. It is not only physical proximity.[139] Where the set-goal is achieved, Shaver and Mikulincer proposed that the result will be feelings of 'relief, and positive affect',[140] grounded in the sense of being understood, validated, and cared about.[141] These feelings in turn will contribute to confidence and competence, feeding back into the calibration of the first module, most notably in the appraisal of threats. Following Fredrickson, Shaver and Mikulincer referred to this as the 'broaden-and-build cycle of attachment security', since felt security, relief, and positive affect in turn come to shape the interpretation of threats, allowing for a more expansive, less cautious appraisal of the environment.[142] Positive affects may also, as Sroufe documented, serve as social currency (Chapter 4). Recently, Mikulincer and Shaver qualified that Bowlby and Ainsworth's concern with infancy has meant that too much has subsequently been made of an image of security as a state of being with attachment figures; in adulthood, broaden-and-build may also entail increased capacity to be comfortable with solitude, entering and exiting it without difficulties or shame, and benefiting from time alone in creative and flexible ways.[143] There may be experiences of security, at least in adulthood, that are made for one.

The third module is initiated if the attachment figure is not 'available, attentive, responsive, etc.' This module is structured by the question: 'Is proximity-seeking a viable option?' Again, literal proximity is a potential meaning here. However, Shaver and Mikulincer appear to intend more the question of whether available, attentive, responsive (etc.) care can be expected to be achieved through directly seeking it. If yes, then the attachment system is 'hyperactived', in the form of 'hypervigilance regarding threat- and attachment-related cues'. As for Main, there need be no conscious 'decision' regarding the deployment of a conditional strategy; in fact, it is a selection that generally occurs without conscious reflection. Hyperactivation entails a lowering of the threshold for activation of the first and second modules and a raising of the threshold for termination. This may entail, most directly, vigilance regarding internal or external information suggesting reasons for concern or alarm. Feelings such as jealousy, helplessness, and vulnerability will help maintain this vigilance.[144]

[139] Sketching a tightening of this position, Mikulincer has recently described the set-goal of the attachment system in adulthood as evidence that the partner is, specifically, 'available, responsive and engaged' (A.R.E.). This riffs on the same acronym with slightly different components—'accessibility, responsiveness, and emotional engagement'—offered by Johnson, S.M. (2011) *Hold Me Tight: Your Guide to the Most Successful Approach to Building Loving Relationships*. London: Hachette, Chapter 4. Mikulincer, M. (2019) Advances in the study of the broaden and build cycle of attachment security. Presentation at the Adult Attachment Research Legacy: 32 Years Since Hazan and Shaver Symposium, Society of Personality and Social Psychology Conference, Portland, Oregon, 9 February 2019.

[140] Mikulincer, M. & Shaver, P. (2016) *Attachment in Adulthood*. New York: Guilford, p.29, Figure 2.1.

[141] Shaver, P.R. & Mikulincer, M. (2008) Augmenting the sense of security in romantic, leader–follower, therapeutic, and group relations: a relational model of personality change. In J.P. Forgas & J. Fitness (eds) *Social Relationships: Cognitive, Affective, and Motivational Processes* (pp.55–73). New York: Psychology Press. Shaver and Mikulincer attributed the idea of 'security' as entailing feeling understood, validated, and cared about to Reis, H.T. & Shaver, P.R. (1988) Intimacy as an interpersonal process. In S. Duck (ed.) *Handbook of Research in Personal Relationships* (pp.367–89). London: Wiley. However, the argument in this text is that these are characteristics of 'intimacy'. The textual history illustrates the potential slide between intimacy and security at times in Shaver's work.

[142] Fredrickson, B.L. (2001) The role of positive emotions in positive psychology. The broaden-and-build theory of positive emotions. *American Psychologist*, 56(3), 218–26.

[143] Mikulincer, M. & Shaver, P. (2014) An attachment perspective on loneliness. In R.J. Coplan & J.C. Bowker *The Handbook of Solitude: Psychological Perspectives on Social Isolation, Social Withdrawal, and Being Alone* (pp.34–50). New York: Wiley, p.46.

[144] Shaver, P.R., Mikulincer, M., Lavy, S., & Cassidy, J. (2009) Understanding and altering hurt feelings: an attachment-theoretical perspective on the generation and regulation of emotions. In A.L. Vangelisti (ed.) *Feeling Hurt in Close Relationships*. Cambridge: Cambridge University Press, pp.92–119: 'Attachment anxiety intensifies the expression of emotions such as jealousy and anger and exaggerates the expression of vulnerability, helplessness, and need' (109).

So will maintenance of pessimistic beliefs about whether coping alone is possible, and the attribution of threatening events to uncontrollable causes or inherent personal vulnerabilities.[145] The difference between making a life and facing problems becomes collapsed.

Self-defeating actions may also keep the attachment system at ready alert: for instance, Mikulincer's group documented associations on several occasions between the anxious attachment style and an odd escalation of investment and commitment as an activity becomes socially and/or economically unprofitable.[146] As a result of various mechanisms that increase vigilance regarding threat- and attachment-related cues, the availability, attentiveness, responsiveness (etc.) of attachment figures is sought more readily in response to potential information about threat, and is sought in a manner more insistent, distressed, and frantic. This is likely to cause a tendency towards a cascade of thinking and worry about threats, vulnerabilities, and/or attachment, as one perception or thought will cue others linked to related feelings.[147] The combination of vigilance and such a flow of associations may in turn contribute to the further identification of potential threats and reasons to wonder about the availability of attachment figures, burnishing the hyperactivating attachment strategy.[148]

On the other hand, Shaver and Mikulincer argued that if seeking the attachment figure's availability is not appraised as viable, then the attachment system is 'deactivated', in the form of 'distancing of threat- and attachment-related cues'.[149] In Shaver and Mikulincer's model, deactivation entails a raising of the threshold for activation of the first and second modules and a lower threshold for termination. In the formal presentation of their model of the attachment system, the selection of a conditional strategy is based on whether seeking the attachment figure's availability is viable. However, there is significant ambiguity here. In other works, Shaver and Mikulincer acknowledged that selection of a strategy also depends on the perceived viability of the other strategy.[150] As such, hyperactivation of the attachment system may in part reflect appraisals regarding the viability of seeking availability, and in

[145] Shaver, P.R. & Mikulincer, M. (2007) Adult attachment strategies and the regulation of emotion. In J.J. Gross (ed.) Handbook of Emotion Regulation (pp.446–65). New York: Guilford, p.454.

[146] E.g. Jayson, Y. (2004) An attachment perspective to escalation of commitment. Unpublished doctoral dissertation, Bar-Ilan University; Mikulincer, M. & Shaver, P. (2008) Contributions of attachment theory and research to motivation science. In J.Y. Shah & W.L. Gardner (eds) Handbook of Motivational Science (pp.201–216). New York: Guilford; Erez, A., Sleebos, E., Mikulincer, M., van IJzendoorn, M.H., Ellemers, N., & Kroonenberg, P.M. (2009) Attachment anxiety, intra-group (dis)respect, actual efforts, and group donation. European Journal of Social Psychology, 39(5), 734–46.

[147] Shaver, P.R. & Mikulincer, M. (2003) The psychodynamics of social judgments: an attachment theory perspective. In J.P. Forgas, K.D. Williams, & W. von Hippel (eds) Social Judgments: Implicit and Explicit Processes (pp.85–114). Philadelphia: Psychology Press: 'Hyperactivating strategies create a chaotic, undifferentiated mental architecture that is constantly pervaded by negative affect' (104).

[148] A further factor stabilising the anxious attachment style was proposed, speculatively, in 2009: Mikulincer, M., Shaver, P.R., Cassidy, J., & Berant, E. (2009) Attachment-related defensive processes. In J.H. Obegi & E. Berant (eds) Attachment Theory and Research in Clinical Work with Adults. New York: Guilford, pp.293–327: 'For attachment-anxious people, histrionics may seem to have two beneficial effects. First, they sometimes elicit the desired attention, care, and love from others, which is, theoretically, the reason the anxious strategy was adopted in the first place. But there may be a second, less obvious, benefit: The hubbub and distraction generated by strident, impulsive expressions of pain, need, and anger may direct attention and energy away from a deeper problem— sensing oneself as not very substantial at all and not worthy of anyone's care. Agitating and grabbing someone's attention is at least likely to make something happen, and even if that something is unpleasant, it may feel better than nothing—that is, better than existential isolation and worthlessness' (309). This proposal has not been much elaborated and remains as yet untested, except insofar as there exists correlational evidence linking the anxious attachment style to self-report of feelings of isolation and self-report of lower self-esteem.

[149] Mikulincer, M. & Shaver, P. (2016) Attachment in Adulthood. New York: Guilford, Figure 2.1, p.29.

[150] See e.g. Crawford, T.N, Shaver, P.R., & Goldsmith, H.H. (2007) How affect regulation moderates the association between anxious attachment and neuroticism. Attachment & Human Development, 9(2), 95–109.

part the extent to which deactivation is possible. More speculatively, deactivation of the attachment system may in part reflect appraisals regarding the viability of seeking availability, and in part the extent that hyperactivation is possible.[151]

In Shaver and Mikulincer's model, when the attachment system is subject to deactivation, information incongruent with the deactivation of the attachment system is inhibited or appears less salient. For instance, the information itself may be altered, obstructed, or suppressed; or response to the information may be dampened, redirected, or postponed.[152] This not only includes emotions associated with threat, vulnerability, or separation, which might reactivate the attachment system. Similarly inhibited or reduced in salience are happy emotions like joy and comfort, which might otherwise promote interpersonal closeness or investment in close relationships.[153] Someone may be radiating love, and all that is felt is mild warmth. Deactivation also means that the availability, attentiveness, responsiveness (etc.) of attachment figures is sought less readily, less insistently, and to a lesser extent, with a tendency towards taking cognitive, emotional, and physical distance from relationship partners. In turn, the individual feels less emotionally assailable. Self-control is held tightly, perhaps even with a white-knuckle grip, as both the condition and experience of the defensive exclusion of the attachment system. As a consequence, self-control can itself be felt as a form of comfort, as a substitute for attachment set-goals.

The deactivation of the attachment system is likely to cause difficulties moving between information about threats, vulnerabilities, and/or attachment, as one perception or thought is less likely to cue others linked to feelings.[154] This reduces opportunities for identification of threats and for feedback indicating that attachment figures are available, attentive, responsive (etc.), contributing to a stabilisation of the deactivating strategy. The strategy was understood by Mikulincer and Shaver to be implicated across the whole range of attachment-based experiences, even those that generally remain private. For instance, Mikulincer, Shaver, and colleagues conducted a study in which they asked participants to report their dreams each morning for a month, as well as other information about how easy or difficult they found their day. The higher a participant's score for avoidant attachment, the less likely they were to report dreams that included any active support-seeking. The higher a participant's score for anxious attachment, the more likely it was that participants would report dreams in which

[151] Mikulincer, M., Shaver, P.R., & Pereg, D. (2003) Attachment theory and affect regulation: the dynamics, development, and cognitive consequences of attachment-related strategies. *Motivation and Emotion*, 27(2), 77–102.

[152] Shaver, P.R. & Mikulincer, M. (2007) Adult attachment strategies and the regulation of emotion. In J.J. Gross (ed.) *Handbook of Emotion Regulation* (pp.446–65). New York: Guilford, p.450. See also Edelstein, R.S. (2006) Attachment and emotional memory: investigating the source and extent of avoidant memory impairments. *Emotion*, 6(2), 340–45; Simpson, J.A., Rholes, W.S., & Winterheld, H.A. (2010) Attachment working models twist memories of relationship events. *Psychological Science*, 21(2), 252–9. Neuroimaging studies conducted by Gillath and colleagues have been interpreted as suggesting that there is no attachment-specific suppressive mechanism, but that in the case of the avoidant attachment style, general mental capacities for suppression are applied to attachment-related content. Gillath, O., Bunge, S.A., Shaver, P.R., Wendelken, C., & Mikulincer, M. (2005) Attachment-style differences in the ability to suppress negative thoughts: exploring the neural correlates. *Neuroimage*, 28(4), 835–47.

[153] Schachner, D.A., Shaver, P.R., & Mikulincer, M. (2005) Patterns of nonverbal behavior and sensitivity in the context of attachment relations. *Journal of Nonverbal Behavior*, 29(3), 141–69, p.157.

[154] Shaver, P.R. & Mikulincer, M. (2003) The psychodynamics of social judgments: an attachment theory perspective. In J.P. Forgas, K.D. Williams, & W. von Hippel (eds) *Social Judgments: Implicit and Explicit Processes* (pp.85–114). Philadelphia: Psychology Press, p.106.

they had wanted to be close to another person, and that this was especially likely following more stressful days.[155]

It has evidently been a source of frustration for Shaver and Mikulincer that character-isations of their work by attachment researchers from the developmental tradition have often assumed that a self-report measure could reflect merely conscious attitudes towards relationships. As well as research on dreams, another study they pursued was an examin-ation of the relationship between the ECR and the Rorschach inkblot test used extensively by Ainsworth in her clinical work and early research. The Rorschach is a projective test as-sessing unconscious psychodynamic processes. Participants' associations on the Rorschach measure were blind coded. It was found that Rorschach responses suggesting difficulties in controlling emotion and of feeling unworthy were associated with self-reported attachment anxiety. And Rorschach responses suggesting difficulties in acknowledging personal needs were associated with self-reported attachment avoidance. Associations were moderate, in the region of $r = .32$ to .34. Berant, Mikulincer, Shaver, and Segal interpreted the findings as suggesting that non-conscious projections in interpreting an ambiguous but evocative stimulus in part express self-report attachment styles. As such, they argued, the self-reports are not merely reflecting conscious attitudes, but tap non-conscious processing as well.[156]

Shaver, Mikulincer, and colleagues argued that each module of the attachment system is informed not by a static mental representation but by a hierarchical associative network, in which specific episodic memories become placed as exemplars of more generalised schemas about how relationships work.[157] This associative network for each module is continually updated in light of social encounters, and also in light of information from the other mod-ules. So, for instance, the appraisal of whether the attachment figure is available, attentive, responsive (etc.) will be informed by a variety of factors. Three, above all, are given prece-dence: how often and in what contexts threats have been experienced; feelings of felt security, relief, and positive affect from times when attachment needs were met; and tendencies to hyperactive or deactive the attachment system from occasions when these conditional strat-egies were employed and proved sufficiently successful. Shaver and Mikulincer propose that, given the existence of a hierarchical associative network, 'with respect to a particular re-lationship and across different relationships, everyone has models of security-attainment, hyperactivation, and deactivation and so can sometimes think about relationships in secure

---

[155] Mikulincer, M., Shaver, P.R., Sapir-Lavid, Y., & Avihou-Kanza, N. (2009) What's inside the minds of securely and insecurely attached people? The secure-base script and its associations with attachment-style dimensions. *Journal of Personality and Social Psychology*, 97(4), 615–33.

[156] Berant, E., Mikulincer, M., Shaver, P.R., & Segal, Y. (2005) Rorschach correlates of self-reported attach-ment dimensions: dynamic manifestations of hyperactivating and deactivating strategies. *Journal of Personality Assessment*, 84(1), 70–81.

[157] This proposal was in part an elaboration of Mikulincer's earlier emphasis on the structure of the human mind as a set of strategic resources rather than constituted by static representations. Mikulincer, M., Paz, D., & Kedem, P. (1990) Anxiety and categorization—2. Hierarchical levels of mental categories. *Personality and Individual Differences*, 11(8), 815–21. The image of internal working models as a hierarchical associative network has been criticised by Fraley as, even if of heuristic value, ultimately an overrigid reification. Fraley, R.C. (2007) A connec-tionist approach to the organization and continuity of working models of attachment. *Journal of Personality*, 75(6), 1157–80. Fraley and colleagues have also demonstrated that people who have more differentiated attachment styles across their varying relationships are more likely to have an insecure overall attachment style. Fraley, R.C., Heffernan, M.E., Vicary, A.M., & Brumbaugh, C.C. (2011) The Experiences in Close Relationships—Relationship Structures Questionnaire: a method for assessing attachment orientations across relationships. *Psychological Assessment*, 23(3), 615–25.

terms and at other times think about them in more hyperactivating or deactivating terms'.[158] Nonetheless, the combination of (i) the predominant form of actual social experiences and (ii) self-reinforcing cycles resulting from the adoption of particular strategies from child-hood onwards will contribute to associative networks that are especially or chronically available. This produces a person's characteristic attachment style. In characterising individual differences in attachment style, the ECR was conceptualised as a kind of snorkelling: though wholly submerged in manifest, espoused information about behaviours, beliefs, and feelings, it nonetheless is believed to breathe latent information from a hierarchical associative network offering generalised schemas about how relationships work.

In line with this model, Overall and colleagues asked participants to complete self-reports of attachment style for various different family relationships, friendships, and romantic relationships. They found that the attachment orientations for specific relationships were somewhat independent but nested within overarching tendencies towards a particular attachment style for each domain. Furthermore, each domain was somewhat independent but nested within an overall attachment style.[159] Interpreting these findings, Shaver and Mikulincer described overall attachment styles as relatively stable, but responsive to changes in relevant social or psychological context.[160] Social experiences are often stable over time as a result of structural factors in people's lives. These are then reinforced by cycles of the broaden-and-build, minimising or maximising strategies. However, some relationships or components of relationships may feature experiences that run counter to the dominant attachment style. And over time, repeated social experiences or forms of appraisal that reinforce this style can become pervasive across the hierarchical associative network. This is illustrated well by an interesting unpublished doctoral study conducted in Mikulincer's group. Lavi pursued a longitudinal study of 73 dating couples over eight months. She used an observational assessment at the start of the period, examining each partner's sensitivity and responsiveness to the other. Relationship-specific and general attachment style was assessed at three time points. Lavi found that observed sensitivity and responsiveness predicted declines in attachment insecurity. First this occurred in relation to the specific relationship partner. Over time, however, there was a change in the participant's general attachment style.[161]

Mikulincer argued that this elaboration of attachment theory gains its usefulness and particular value in 'integrating different, perhaps even contradictory, views of human nature and maintaining a dialectical tension between opposites of four kinds':[162]

[158] Mikulincer, M. & Shaver, P.R. (2003) The attachment behavioral system in adulthood: activation, psychodynamics, and interpersonal processes. In M.P. Zanna (ed.) *Advances in Experimental Social Psychology*, Vol. 35 (pp.53–152). New York: Academic Press, p.64.

[159] Overall, N.C., Fletcher, G.J., & Friesen, M.D. (2003) Mapping the intimate relationship mind: comparisons between three models of attachment representations. *Personality and Social Psychology Bulletin*, 29(12), 1479–93.

[160] Shaver, P.R. & Mikulincer, M. (2004) What do self-report attachment measures assess? In W.S. Rholes & J.A. Simpson (eds) *Adult Attachment: Theory, Research, and Clinical Implications* (pp.17–54). New York: Guilford, pp.52–3.

[161] Lavi, N. (2007) Bolstering attachment security in romantic relationships: the long-term contribution of partner's sensitivity, expressiveness, and supportiveness. Unpublished doctoral dissertation, Bar-Ilan University, Ramat Gan, Israel. For a recent review of the effect of partners on attachment style in adulthood see Arriaga, X.B. & Kumashiro, M. (2019) Walking a security tightrope: relationship-induced changes in attachment security. *Current Opinion in Psychology*, 25, 121–6.

[162] Mikulincer, M. (2006) Attachment, caregiving and sex within romantic relationships. In M. Mikulincer & G.S. Goodman (eds) *Dynamics of Romantic Love: Attachment, Caregiving, and Sex* (pp.23–44). New York: Guilford, p.39.

1) The shaping and constraining influences of past experiences versus the influence of current contexts and experiences;

2) the intrapsychic nature of behavioural systems and working models versus the relational, interdependent nature of feelings, experiences, and social behaviours;

3) the goal-oriented, promotive, expansive, self-regulatory function of behavioural system versus their defensive, protective, distress-regulating functions;

4) the centrality of basic fears, conflicts, and prevention-focused motivational mechanisms, as well as promotion-focused motives.[163]

Shaver and Mikulincer's model of the attachment system can be usefully considered in these terms. The appraisal of the potential effectiveness of seeking the availability of the attachment figure is prompted in module one. The question that must be answered in module two is whether the goal of this system—an attachment figure who is available, attentive, responsive (etc.)—should be sought directly. This represents the hinge between ethology and personality psychology.[164] If the goal of the system can be met directly, then this contributes to a broaden-and-build cycle that can support self-regulation. The availability of a secure base and safe haven are expected to contribute to increased richness and stability in both an individual's inner world and social relations. If not, then module three enacts a defensive, protective, and distress-regulating strategy, which may also have promotive and self-regulatory potential in some circumstances.

The maximising strategy, on the one hand, promotes threat-sensitivity and the promotion of self-regulation through attempts to achieve the availability of attachment figures. The minimising strategy, on the other hand, promotes composure under low and moderate stress and the promotion of self-regulation under conditions in which attachment figures are appraised as not available. The selection of one strategy or another is shaped in part by learning from previous social encounters and the strategies used to respond to them, as well as available resources for emotion regulation. Yet the selection of a strategy is also fed in part by the actual nature of the present social interaction, cultural norms, and relational cues regarding the potential effectiveness of particular strategies in the particular moment. Individuals do not have, in Shaver and Mikulincer's work, a single representational model of relationships. Instead, hierarchically organised associational networks make various attachment styles available. As such, they depend upon: the qualities of a particular relationship; previous experiences of and expectations about this kind of relationship; and the particularities of present-day interactions. That these sit nested within and interpreted through an overall attachment style shaped by the weight of personal history does not exclude this internal diversity and dynamic potential.

Shaver and Mikulincer claimed their elaboration of attachment theory as an integration of components of developmental, social, and personality psychology. This was in line with Bowlby, who always described attachment theory as an account of the relational development of personality.[165] However, it was in contrast to the developmental tradition of

---

[163] Ibid.

[164] Fraley, R.C. & Shaver, P.R. (2008) Attachment theory and its place in contemporary personality research. In O. John & R.W. Robins (eds) *Handbook of Personality: Theory and Research*, 3rd edn (pp.518–41). New York: Guilford: 'The attachment behavioral system is an important concept in attachment theory because it provides the conceptual bridge between ethological models of human development (e.g., Hinde, 1966) and modern theories of emotion regulation and personality (e.g., John & Gross, 2007)' (523).

[165] E.g. Bowlby, J. (1988) The role of attachment in personality development. In *A Secure Base* (pp.134–54). London: Routledge.

attachment research. Among developmental researchers, appeals to 'personality' have been relatively rare and mostly appear in summaries of Bowlby.[166] Yet in claiming attachment styles as part of personality psychology, the question was inevitably raised regarding how avoidant and anxious attachment styles relate to established personality constructs. And more pointedly, whether they added anything. An attempt to answer this concern was undertaken by Noftle and Shaver in a paper published in 2006. They examined the relationship between the ECR and a self-report measure of the 'big five' constructs in personality psychology: openness to experience, conscientiousness, extraversion, agreeableness, and neuroticism. There were few major associations between the avoidant attachment style and the personality constructs. By contrast, in two studies Noftle and Shaver found associations between attachment anxiety and neuroticism of $r = .42$ and $r = .52$. The extent of this association suggested to the researchers that there is 'some conceptual overlap between the constructs'.[167] The strongest associations were for items for neuroticism that pertained to the susceptibility and frequency of negative affect (items for: being depressed, likely to be moody and nervous, excessively worrying, and not being emotionally stable). This suggests that the readiness of negative affect plays a key role in the overlap between the two psychological constructs. The readiness of negative affect is certainly shaped by culture and experiences past and present. However, it is also widely regarded by psychologists as partly a heritable trait.[168]

Following up this expectation, Crawford, Shaver, and colleagues reported in 2007 from a study of 239 twin pairs. Biometric models identified no contribution of heritable factors to the likelihood of an avoidant attachment style. However, 40% of variance in anxious attachment could be attributed to heritable factors. Furthermore, 63% of the association between anxious attachment and a self-report measure of personality disorder could be accounted for by common genetic effects. Such findings suggest that anxious attachment, and its association with mental health, may in part be an effect of heritable differences in the susceptibility and frequency of negative affect.[169] However, Crawford, Shaver, and colleagues also argued that there are important differences between anxious attachment style and neuroticism. Firstly, anxious attachment is especially responsive to attachment-relevant cues, not merely generally anxiety-provoking stimuli. Secondly, there is still a substantial amount of variance not explained by heritable factors. Thirdly, even when neuroticism is statistically controlled,

---

[166] Second-generation developmental attachment researchers have generally considered 'personality' a reified concept in the academic psychology of their day, better conceptualised as an effect of developmental processes rather than a unitary construct to be measured in itself. See e.g. Sroufe, L.A. & Fleeson, J. (1986) Attachment and the construction of relationships. In W. Hartup & Z. Rubin (eds) *Relationships and Development* (pp.51–71). Hillsdale, NJ: Lawrence Erlbaum, p.51.

[167] Noftle, E.E. & Shaver, P.R. (2006) Attachment dimensions and the big five personality traits: associations and comparative ability to predict relationship quality. *Journal of Research in Personality*, 40(2), 179–208, p.187.

[168] John, O.P., Neumann, L., & Soto, C.J. (2010) The Big Five trait taxonomy: history, measurement, and conceptual issues. In L.A. Pervin & O.P. John (eds) *Handbook of Personality: Theory and Research*, 3rd edn (pp.114–58). New York: Guilford; Vukasović, T. & Bratko, D. (2015) Heritability of personality: a meta-analysis of behavior genetic studies. *Psychological Bulletin*, 141(4), 769–85.

[169] Crawford, T.N., John Livesley, W., Jang, K.L., Shaver, P.R., Cohen, P., & Ganiban, J. (2007) Insecure attachment and personality disorder: a twin study of adults. *European Journal of Personality*, 21(2), 191–208. See also Donnellan, M.B., Burt, S.A., Levendosky, A.A., & Klump, K.L. (2008) Genes, personality, and attachment in adults: a multivariate behavioral genetic analysis. *Personality and Social Psychology Bulletin*, 34(1), 3–16. In contrast to Crawford and colleagues, Donnellan and colleagues reported that genetic effects accounted for variability also in avoidant attachment style. Troisi and colleagues have reported potential gene × environment interactions in the origins of fearful attachment. Troisi, A., Frazzetto, G., Carola, V., et al. (2012) Variation in the μ-opioid receptor gene (OPRM1) moderates the influence of early maternal care on fearful attachment. *Social Cognitive and Affective Neuroscience*, 7(5), 542–7.

anxious attachment has been found to make a modest contribution to mental health out-comes such as depression and complex responses to bereavement.[170] At a fundamental level, the experience of anxiety is solely an expression of neither individual personality nor attachment style. Both seem to play a role. However, this highlights the question of what convergence there is between the anxious attachment style and preoccupied states of mind regarding attachment, if both are conceptualised as maximising strategies. To address this question it is necessary to examine the ECR and the AAI in the context of social psychology and developmental psychology as two different subdisciplines concerned with attachment.

Two traditions of attachment research

As we have seen, Bowlby anticipated that both the AAI and the Hazan and Shaver 'love quiz' would both be predicted by the Strange Situation. This was also Shaver's explicit position by the late 1990s: 'some of their components, especially ability to depend on attachment figures, should be related if both stem from a person's attachment history'.[171] The first major attempt to assess whether the AAI and self-report measures would converge was published by Crowell, Treboux, and Waters in 1999. In their study, 81% of participants classified as secure-autonomous on the AAI identified themselves as having a secure attachment style on Bartholomew's Relationship Questionnaire. However, only 42% of participants who were classified as preoccupied, dis-missing, or unresolved on the AAI reported themselves as insecure on the Relationship Questionnaire.[172] Crowell and colleagues therefore cautioned against equation of the AAI and self-report measures. They argued that it was a recipe for confusion that both systems used a ver-sion of Ainsworth's terminology, such as 'security', when in fact the referents were quite different. Whereas Main was assessing 'states of mind regarding attachment', the self-report tradition was assessing a person's sense of 'comfort in close relationships'.[173] There might be expected to be a little empirical overlap between these phenomena, but Crowell and colleagues argued that they were completely different constructs.[174]

It was not certain what the two traditions could mean for another. Nonetheless, the ex-pectation that both the ECR and AAI were measures of 'attachment' implied that it should be possible to translate between the two measures, and that the two traditions should be to a

---

[170] E.g. Roberts, J.E., Gotlib, I.H., & Kassel, J.D. (1996) Adult attachment security and symptoms of depres-sion: the mediating roles of dysfunctional attitudes and low self-esteem. *Journal of Personality and Social Psychology*, 70(2), 310–20; Meier, A.M., Carr, D.R., Currier, J.M., & Neimeyer, R.A. (2013) Attachment anxiety and avoidance in coping with bereavement: two studies. *Journal of Social and Clinical Psychology*, 32(3), 315–34, Supplement 3; Wijngaards-de Meij, L., Stroebe, M., Schut, H., et al. (2007) Neuroticism and attachment insecurity as predictors of bereavement outcome. *Journal of Research in Personality*, 41(2), 498–505.

[171] Shaver, P.R., Belsky, J., & Brennan, K.A. (2000) The adult attachment interview and self-reports of romantic attachment: associations across domains and methods. *Personal Relationships*, 7(1), 25–43, p.25.

[172] Crowell, J.A., Treboux, D., & Waters, E. (1999) The Adult Attachment Interview and the Relationship Questionnaire: relations to reports of mothers and partners. *Personal Relationships*, 6(1), 1–18.

[173] Ibid. p.16.

[174] This was a consensus position among active attachment researchers from the developmental tradition by the end of the 1990s. See e.g. Stein, H., Jacobs, N.J., Ferguson, K.S., Allen, J.G., & Fonagy, P. (1998) What do adult at-tachment scales measure? *Bulletin of the Menninger Clinic*, 62, 33–82: 'Both approaches have something important to offer, but are likely to be looking at different, though valid, constructs. The self-report measures are consist-ently measuring an aspect of intimate relationships that relates to individual perceptions of how relationships are managed' (77).

large extent permeable to one another.[175] In a 1998 book chapter, Bartholomew and Shaver offered a characterisation of the two traditions of attachment research. They described the developmental tradition as mostly led by direct students of Ainsworth. In Bartholomew and Shaver's characterisation, 'researchers in this group tend to think psychodynamically, be interested in clinical problems, prefer interview measures and behavioural observations over questionnaires, study relatively small groups of subjects, and focus their attention on parent–child relationships'. It is possible to quibble with some particulars—Kobak was conducting research on parent–adolescent relationships; Waters had little psychodynamic basis for his thinking except as mediated through Ainsworth and Bowlby—but in general this characterisation seems fair.[176] By contrast, the social psychology tradition was described as shaped essentially by the characteristics of social and personality psychology of the period. Members of this community 'tend to think in terms of personality traits and social interactions, be interested in normal subject populations, prefer simple questionnaire measures, study relatively large samples, and focus on adult social relationships'.[177]

The division between the two traditions was in part fed, it should be acknowledged, by the longer-standing professional tensions within the academic discipline between developmental and social/personality psychology. As Lapsley and Quintana observed, writing in the period in which the two traditions of attachment research were emerging, 'it is hard to imagine an academic division of labor that is more formidable, and at the same time more artificial, than the division between social and developmental psychology'.[178] Commenting on the division in the late 1990s, Bartholomew and Shaver noted that 'not surprisingly, the members of these two research subcultures tend to speak past each other'.[179] Shaver and Mikulincer added, in 2002, that another key difference between the traditions was that the developmental tradition only rarely tested causal propositions experimentally, whereas the use of experimental designs was a central part of the social psychology tradition, thanks in part to the work of Mikulincer. Furthermore, the developmental tradition tended to rely on rather cluttered coding systems supported by predictive validity but lacking rigorous psychometric analysis of categories and scales. By contrast, the social psychological tradition had a better track-record of cleaning and refining their measures to ensure psychometric rigour. Shaver and Mikulincer also argued that whereas their work shed light on the actual functioning of 'the attachment behavioural system' itself, by contrast the AAI was a measure of 'individual differences in "state of mind with respect to attachment" '.[180] They claimed, in

---

[175] Carnelley, K.B. & Brennan, K.A. (2002) Building bridges. *Attachment & Human Development*, 4(2), 189–92: 'The biggest obstacle to the fledgling field of attachment theory appears to be a lack of co-operation among researchers wielding different measurement techniques. As it is, each researcher appears to be using a favorite measure and readers of their work are left to make the attempt to translate the results into their own measurement rubric before interpreting the meaning of the findings' (191).

[176] Bartholomew, K. & Shaver, P.R. (1998) Methods of assessing adult attachment: do they converge? In J.A. Simpson & W.S. Rholes (eds) *Attachment Theory and Close Relationships* (pp.25–45). New York: Guilford, p.27.

[177] Ibid.

[178] Lapsley, D.K. & Quintana, S. (1985) Integrative themes in social and developmental theories of the self. In J. Pryor & J. Day (eds) *The Development of Social Cognition* (pp.153–78). New York: Springer, p.154. Also on the state of broader relations between developmental and social psychology in the period of the emergence of the two traditions of attachment research see Masters, J.C. & Yarkin-Levin, K. (1984) *Boundary Areas in Social and Developmental Psychology*. New York: Academic Press.

[179] Bartholomew, K. & Shaver, P.R. (1998) Methods of assessing adult attachment: do they converge? In J.A. Simpson & W.S. Rholes (eds) *Attachment Theory and Close Relationships* (pp.25–45). New York: Guilford, p.27.

[180] Shaver, P.R. & Mikulincer, M. (2002) Attachment-related psychodynamics. *Attachment & Human Development*, 4(2), 133–61: 'The AAI and CRI are focused entirely on individual differences in "state of mind with respect to attachment" and therefore do not reveal much about the normative workings of the attachment behavioral system' (155).

an unabashed polemic, that the AAI was likely not an assessment of attachment at all. Rather, given that it was validated against the Strange Situation, it might be better conceived as an assessment of cognitive aspects of the caregiving system. This is a claim they would later retract in 2004, only to swing to the other pole in asserting that both the AAI and self-report measures taped the same processes: 'attachment-style scales differ from the AAI in content and method but not in the core attachment-related processes they index'.[181]

Yet in addition to specific methodological differences, Shaver and Mikulincer claimed that the most important difficulty was 'professional ingroup–outgroup tensions between researchers in the two traditions'.[182] In fact, looking back on the period, it seems as if professional and methodological tensions worked neatly to reinforce one another. The developmental tradition tended to regard the social psychologists as conducting quick-fix, superficial research on conscious attitudes towards intimacy, lacking fidelity to the ethological basis of attachment theory. The social psychology tradition tended to regard the developmentalists as lashed to Main's four categories, and unable or unwilling to think critically or creatively about them. They also expressed scepticism whether a research agenda based on laborious observational and interview-based methodologies was practical in the context of contemporary academic psychology.[183] This latter point certainly has purchase. One of the contributing factors to the growth of the social psychological tradition of attachment research has been that the entry requirements are much lower. The ECR is freely available and easy to administer on student populations and through online platforms, putting it within the reach of researchers even without a research grant or with only a side-interest in attachment. This cannot be said of the Strange Situation and AAI, which require substantial training and knowledge to be able to code effectively, or sometimes even interpret published results. However, recent developments like Fearon and colleagues' cut-down AQS (Chapter 2), Dozier and colleagues' cut-down AAI (Chapter 6), Madigan and colleagues's cut-down assessment of frightening and disrupted caregiving (Chapter 6), and Ensink and colleagues' short assessment of parent reflective functioning[184] may reduce the resource burden of the developmentalists' measures, if their validation proves successful.

Through the 1990s, the developmental and social psychologists blamed one other for failing to conduct comparative research. The developmentalists regarded it as rather unforgivable, and as an expression of a quick-fix mentality, that the social psychologists did not undertake the training to conduct observational research even for a measure as foundational as the Ainsworth Strange Situation. The social psychologists found it rather unforgivable that, even though it would have been quick and easy to do, the developmentalists did not include self-report measures of attachment when assessing parents in the Strange Situation, when conducting the AAI, or in the adolescent and adult phases of their longitudinal

[181] Shaver, P.R. & Mikulincer, M. (2004) What do self-report attachment measures assess? In W.S. Rholes & J.A. Simpson (eds) *Adult Attachment: Theory, Research, and Clinical Implications* (pp.17–54). New York: Guilford, p.29.
[182] Shaver, P.R. & Mikulincer, M. (2002) Attachment-related psychodynamics. *Attachment & Human Development*, 4(2), 133–61, p.134.
[183] Brennan, K.A., Clark, C.L., & Shaver, P.R. (1998) Self-report measurement of adult romantic attachment: an integrative overview. In J.A. Simpson & W.S. Rholes (eds) *Attachment Theory and Close Relationships* (pp.46–76). New York: Guilford, p.46. See also Sassenberg, K. & Ditrich, L. (2019) Research in social psychology changed between 2011 and 2016: larger sample sizes, more self-report measures, and more online studies. *Advances in Methods and Practices in Psychological Science*, 2(2).
[184] Ensink, K., Borelli, J.L., Roy, J., Normandin, L., Slade, A., & Fonagy, P. (2019) Costs of not getting to know you: lower levels of parental reflective functioning confer risk for maternal insensitivity and insecure infant attachment. *Infancy*, 24(2), 210–27.

studies.[185] At times these tensions operated in the background. So, for instance, research on parenting using self-report measures of attachment has remained quietly blunted, with leaders of the social psychological tradition giving the topic little attention.[186] In part this was an effect of the division between social and developmental psychology in general, in which parenting is generally assigned to the latter. However, another factor may have been that, at best, self-report measures would draw with the AAI in predicting parenting, and there was the possibility that they would lose.[187]

Yet, at times, the tensions between the social and developmental traditions of attachment research moved from mutual inattention to a public disagreement. In the mid-1990s, Crowell and Waters described Shaver's work as 'thoughtful and provocative' and as 'exciting and potentially very useful', but stated their view that in fact there is 'little common ground' with the tradition initiated by Ainsworth.[188] In responding to the hostile reception from the developmental tradition, one tactic used by Shaver and colleagues to find mandate for their work was to offer anachronistic depictions of the field's founders to make Bowlby and Ainsworth foreshadow their own work. For instance, Ainsworth has been repeatedly described by Shaver as using the concept of 'a child's attachment style'[189], and Shaver and Mikulincer explicitly asserted that 'Bowlby claimed that memorable interactions with others throughout life can alter a person's working models and move him or her from one region of the two-dimensional attachment-style "space" to another'.[190] These anachronisms reflected a claim to the right to inherit attachment theory from the first generation without using the observational methods that had come at least in part to constitute the basis for inheritance. They show the desire for legitimacy and heritage among the social psychological researchers, in the context of a general lack of acceptance—or even threats of symbolic dispossession—by the developmental tradition.

Despite trouble with the developmentalists, use of self-report measures of attachment was booming by the 1990s. Some researchers from the developmental tradition, such as Belsky and Cassidy, expressed concern that the social psychology tradition 'might actually overshadow the work in infancy and childhood that gave rise to it', and proposed that this threat gave added impetus to the need to achieve a 'linkage of these two schools of attachment inquiry'.[191] In this context, Seymour Weingarten, editor-in-chief of Guilford Press, approached

[185] Shaver, P.R & Mikulincer, M. (2002) Dialogue on adult attachment: diversity and integration. *Attachment & Human Development*, 4(2), 243–57, p.245.

[186] Though see e.g. Rholes, W.S., Simpson, J.A., & Friedman, M. (2006) Avoidant attachment and the experience of parenting. *Personality and Social Psychology Bulletin*, 32(3), 275–85.

[187] A meta-analysis by Lo and colleagues, however, found more studies using self-report measures (12) than using the AAI (5). The odds ratio for child maltreatment for self-report measures was 2.75; the odds ratio for the AAI was 5. Lo, C.K., Chan, K.L., & Ip, P. (2019) Insecure adult attachment and child maltreatment: a meta-analysis. *Trauma, Violence, & Abuse*, 20(5).

[188] Crowell, J.A. & Waters, E. (1994) Bowlby's theory grown up: the role of attachment in adult love relationships. *Psychological Inquiry*, 5(1), 31–4, pp.33–4. See also Kobak, R. (2009) Defining and measuring of attachment bonds: comment on Kurdek (2009). *Journal of Family Psychology*, 23(4), 447–9.

[189] E.g. Shaver, P.R. & Mikulincer, M. (2010) Mind–behavior relations in attachment theory and research. In C.R. Agnew, D.E. Carlston, W.G. Graziano, & J.R. Kelly (eds) *Then a Miracle Occurs: Focusing on Behavior in Social Psychological Theory and Research* (pp.342–67). New York: Oxford University Press: 'Ainsworth et al. (1978) provided persuasive evidence for the impact of parental behavior on the formation of an infant's attachment style' (358). See also Levy, K.N., Blatt, S.J., & Shaver, P.R. (1998) Attachment styles and parental representations. *Journal of Personality and Social Psychology*, 74(2), 407–419, p.408.

[190] Shaver, P.R. & Mikulincer, M. (2012) An attachment perspective on coping with existential concerns. In P.R. Shaver & M. Mikulincer (eds) *Meaning, Mortality, and Choice: The Social Psychology of Existential Concerns* (pp.291–307). Washington, DC: American Psychological Association, p.293.

[191] Belsky, J. & Cassidy, J. (1994) Attachment and close relationships: an individual-difference perspective. *Psychological Inquiry*, 5(1), 27–30, p.27.

Cassidy and Shaver at the 1995 meeting of the Society for Research in Child Development in Indianapolis with the idea of a *Handbook of Attachment*. The Society's biennial conference is the central conference for the field of development psychology. Shaver had attended the 1993 conference and had presented a defence of the self-report approach to attachment as relevant for understanding intergenerational and developmental continuity of individual differences in attachment over time.[192] Weingarten's idea was for a handbook encompassing both traditions of research. Cassidy and Shaver 'were barely acquainted when the project began', and did not meet face-to-face after the initial conversation in Indianapolis during the four years of work on the first *Handbook,* which would be published in 1999. Nonetheless, in their preface to the *Handbook*, Cassidy and Shaver stated that 'we have grown to know and respect each other professionally in ways that people rarely do'.[193] In the late 1990s, Cassidy informed and nourished Shaver's thinking about individual differences in attachment as minimising and maximising strategies.

Perhaps in an attempt at rapprochement, Crowell (a developmentalist) and Fraley and Shaver (social psychologists) co-authored a chapter in the first edition of *The Handbook of Attachment*. They acknowledged that there existed 'considerable tension between the AAI and self-report traditions within the field of contemporary attachment research'.[194] They observed that the two traditions had been primarily concerned with parenting and romantic love respectively, and pursued very different ways of eliciting and analysing their data. Nonetheless, both traditions appeared to be testing and elaborating aspects of attachment theory. This apparent common theoretical basis lent impetus for the need for comparative research. In pursuing this path, Shaver and Brennan collaborated with Jay Belsky, who had long been calling for integration (and, beyond this, was always something of a free spirit among researchers in the developmental tradition). In a paper from 2000, the researchers reported from their study with 138 Caucasian women from working- and middle-class families in central Pennsylvania. Strangely, the researchers did not report the relationship between self-reported anxiety and avoidance and the AAI categories. Given that the overall priority of the paper was to emphasise the compatibility of the two measures, the reader is perhaps left with the suspicion that this analysis was run, but the results were not regarded as desirable. Instead, the authors reported a few moderate associations on various subscales. Self-reported avoidance was associated with lack of memory for childhood events, anger at the speaker's parents, and lower overall coherence.[195] However, Shaver and colleagues acknowledged that 'the degree of association was relatively modest, and due only to certain aspects of each measure'.[196]

Roisman, Fraley, and colleagues embarked on further work comparing the AAI and attachment style measures. A meta-analysis of nearly a thousand participants who had completed

[192] Shaver, P.R. (1993) Where do adult romantic attachment styles come from? Paper presented at symposium entitled 'Mental Representations of Relationships: Intergenerational and Temporal Continuity', Meeting of the Society for Research in Child Development, New Orleans, 27 March 1993. https://adultattachment.faculty.ucdavis.edu/wp-content/uploads/sites/66/2014/06/Shaver.pdf.

[193] Cassidy, J. & Shaver, P. (1999) Preface. In *The Handbook of Attachment*, 1st edn. New York: Guilford, p.xiv.

[194] Crowell, J.A., Fraley, R.C., & Shaver, P.R. (1999) Measures of individual differences in adolescent and adult attachment. In J. Cassidy & P.R. Shaver (eds) *Handbook of Attachment: Theory, Research, and Clinical Applications* (pp.434–65). New York: Guilford, p.452. The passage would be repeated verbatim in the 2008 edition on p.618.

[195] Shaver, P.R., Belsky, J., & Brennan, K.A. (2000) The adult attachment interview and self-reports of romantic attachment: associations across domains and methods. *Personal Relationships*, 7(1), 25–43.

[196] Ibid. p.39.

both kinds of assessment by 2007 revealed a trivial association ($r = .09$).[197] One of the few specific findings was that unresolved trauma, but not unresolved loss, had a small association with self-report attachment anxiety ($r = .20$).[198] In *Attachment & Human Development*, Roisman and Fortuna reported the results of a study with 160 college students. Participants completed the AAI, a self-report measure of attachment, a self-report measure of life stress, and a self-report measure of mental health symptoms. The association between the AAI and self-reported attachment style were, as expected, negligible. They both, however, predicted mental health symptoms. Self-reported attachment avoidance and attachment anxiety both had substantial associations with self-reported mental health symptoms (.43 and .48 respectively). These associations were unaffected by the participants' self-reported life stress. The strength of the associations can in part be accounted for by the fact that both the assessments of attachment style and mental health were self-reported. However, it is nonetheless curious that an avoidant attachment style had an association with these symptoms of almost equivalent strength. By contrast, the AAI had a marked association (.34) with self-reported mental health under high experienced life stress, but only a weak association (.19) when life stress was low.[199]

Pursuing the question of the interrelation of measures from the two traditions, Bernier and Matte-Gagné reported a study of 59 Canadian families. They conducted the AAI, the ECR, and the Strange Situation, a measure of caregiver sensitivity conducted in the home, and self-report measures of the marital satisfaction of both partners. Rather than using the AAI categories, the researchers were convinced by Fraley and Roisman (Chapters 2 and 4) that attachment phenomena are better regarded as dimensions, and so they therefore reported only the AAI coherence scale. The researchers found no association between the AAI and the ECR. They also found, as anticipated, that coherence on the AAI was associated with greater caregiver sensitivity and increased incidence of secure infant–caregiver attachment in the Strange Situation. There was no statistical association between the ECR and either caregiver sensitivity or the Strange Situation.[200] Marital satisfaction was not associated with

[197] Roisman, G.I., Holland, A., Fortuna, K., Fraley, R.C., Clausell, E., & Clarke, A. (2007) The Adult Attachment Interview and self-reports of attachment style: an empirical rapprochement. *Journal of Personality and Social Psychology*, 92(4), 678–97. A point of comparison here are findings showing that indirect (implicit) and direct (explicit) measures of self-esteem are virtually unrelated. Like 'attachment', 'self-esteem' is likely an umbrella term within psychological discourse, and captures more than one autonomous process, even if the correlates of these processes may be similar—producing the superficial effect of a single phenomenon. Pietschnig, J., Gittler, G., Stieger, S., et al. (2018) Indirect (implicit) and direct (explicit) self-esteem measures are virtually unrelated: a meta-analysis of the initial preference task. *PLoS One*, 13(9), e0202873.

[198] Roisman, G.I., Holland, A., Fortuna, K., Fraley, R.C., Clausell, E., & Clarke, A. (2007) The Adult Attachment Interview and self-reports of attachment style: an empirical rapprochement. *Journal of Personality and Social Psychology*, 92(4), 678–97, p.689. More recently, in an unpublished doctoral study by Watkins, 87 participants (43 with borderline personality disorder) completed the ECR and AAI. There was no association with attachment categories. But when a variable was used that combined scales for preoccupied and unresolved states of mind (Chapter 3), this was associated with ECR anxiety ($r = .34$). Watkins, C.D. (2016) Convergence versus divergence of social and developmental measures of adult attachment: testing Jay Belsky's proposals. Unpublished doctoral thesis, University of Tennessee.

[199] Fortuna, K. & Roisman, G.I. (2008) Insecurity, stress, and symptoms of psychopathology: contrasting results from self-reports versus interviews of adult attachment. *Attachment & Human Development*, 10(1), 11–28.

[200] For other relevant studies see Mayseless, O., Sharabany, R., & Sagi, A. (1997) Attachment concerns of mothers as manifested in parental, spousal, and friendship relationships. *Personal Relationships*, 4(3), 255–69; Volling, B.L., Notaro, P.C., & Larsen, J.J. (1998) Adult attachment styles: relations with emotional well-being, marriage, and parenting. *Family Relations*, 47(4), 355–67; Laurent, H.K., Kim, H.K., & Capaldi, D.M. (2008) Prospective effects of interparental conflict on child attachment security and the moderating role of parents' romantic attachment. *Journal of Family Psychology*, 22(3), 377–88; Howard, K.S. (2010) Paternal attachment, parenting beliefs and children's attachment. *Early Child Development and Care*, 18(1–2), 157–71.

coherence on the AAI. However, ECR anxiety of one partner was associated with dissatisfaction with the relationship by the other, controlling for coherence on the AAI. Bernier and Matte-Gagné concluded that 'only romantic attachment was found to relate to marital satisfaction, while only the AAI was found to relate to caregiving'.[201] Such findings suggest that, even if they claim a common theory, the two traditions are ultimately studying different phenomena.

In 2006, Shaver stated that he and his collaborators had essentially given up reading the outputs of the developmental psychology tradition of attachment research.[202] Shaver's observations have an 'anger of despair' quality to them. They mark trends in the mid-2000s that suggested that the two traditions could go their separate ways, segregated from one another and out of functional communication. Yet three important factors have contributed to better relations and productive interaction between the traditions. One has been sustained efforts to develop institutional and personal connections since the late 1990s. In 1999, the journal *Attachment & Human Development* was founded, with Howard Steele serving as Editor-in-Chief. Though the first issues were tilted more towards the developmental tradition, the journal sought to represent both traditions, and Shaver was an Associate Editor from the start. In its fourth year, the journal hosted a major discussion of the relationship between the traditions, with a lead article by Shaver and Mikulincer, eleven replies from attachment researchers from both camps, and a response from Shaver and Mikulincer.[203] And over subsequent years, the journal has assiduously made space for contributions from both traditions, contributing to a sense of a common set of problems and theories.[204] Likewise, Cassidy and Shaver worked together on a second edition of the *Handbook of Attachment* published in 2008. This mammoth project was evidently an experience that brought the researchers closer as colleagues, and convinced Cassidy of the benefits of the self-report methodology: in subsequent years, Cassidy and Shaver collaborated on theoretical papers and empirical research using self-report measures. Cassidy also used them in her own work, independently of Shaver.[205] In 2010, Cassidy and Shaver also worked together in co-editing a special issue of *Attachment & Human Development* presenting an attachment perspective on incarcerated

---

[201] Bernier, A. & Matte-Gagné, C. (2011) More bridges: investigating the relevance of self-report and interview measures of adult attachment for marital and caregiving relationships. *International Journal of Behavioral Development*, 35(4), 307–316, p.313. This outcome was generally predicted by Mikulincer and Cowans a decade earlier, though they anticipated some association based on the expectation that marital satisfaction will influence caregiving: Mikulincer, M., Florian, V., Cowan, P.A., & Cowan, C.P. (2002) Attachment security in couple relationships: a systemic model and its implications for family dynamics. *Family Process*, 41(3), 405–434, p.424.

[202] Shaver, P.R. (2006) Dynamics of romantic love: comments, questions, and future directions. In M. Mikulincer & G.S. Goodman (eds) *Dynamics of Romantic Love: Attachment, Caregiving, and Sex* (pp.423–56). New York: Guilford: 'Most of us self-report attachment researchers tend to ignore the AAI literature (although Bartholomew, Furman and Simpson are important exceptions)' (445).

[203] Shaver, P.R. & Mikulincer, M. (2002) Dialogue on adult attachment: diversity and integration. *Attachment & Human Development*, 4, 243–57.

[204] Part of the contribution made by *Attachment & Human Development* as a topic-specific journal was that it could overcome some of the division between developmental and social psychology as subdisciplines. Compare, for instance, the *Journal of Social and Personal Relationships*. Mikulincer served as Editor-in-Chief from 2010 to 2015. Though an important venue for attachment research in the social psychology tradition, Mikulincer's premiership did not coincide with publications in the journal by researchers in the developmental tradition of attachment research. It may well have been that articles were not solicited, submitted, accepted—or all three.

[205] E.g. Duggan, A., Berlin, L., Cassidy, J., Burrell, L., & Tandon, D. (2009) Examining maternal depression and attachment insecurity as moderators of the impacts of home visiting for at-risk mothers and infants. *Journal of Consulting and Clinical Psychology*, 77(4), 788–99.

parents and their children, with contributions primarily using the AAI and Strange Situation as their methodologies.[206]

A second important development was the emergence of a new 'third' generation of attachment researchers, with tenured position and independent grants to pursue research on their own terms. As mentioned in Chapter 3, Sroufe's former doctoral student Glenn Roisman has been one of a number of 'third-generation' attachment researchers who use ideas and methods from both the developmental and social psychology traditions, on the basis of personal networks of collaborators extending in both directions. Another has been Roisman's colleague at Minnesota, Jeff Simpson. Simpson has drawn theoretically on the organisational perspective of Sroufe, but primarily adopts a social psychological approach to conceptualising and measuring attachment. Simpson and his group have documented that self-report measures of attachment and the AAI make non-redundant contributions in predicting the behaviour of dating couples in completing a tricky laboratory-based task. Secure-autonomous attachment on the AAI predicted offering their partner a degree of support that was sensitive to their signals, in a situationally contingent manner. A self-report of an avoidant attachment style predicted offering the partner less support no matter the degree to which the partner requested help.[207] These results remained the same when controlling for personality traits (including neuroticism), perceptions of the quality of their relationships, and the attachment style of the partner. Another 'third-generation' attachment researcher—to be discussed further in the section 'Attachment to God'—is Pehr Granqvist, who has collaborated directly with both Main and Hesse,[208] and with Shaver and Mikulincer.[209]

A third development has been that both traditions have continued, quite successfully, to generate research findings that appear to test or elaborate much the same theory. This has meant that, though it is a bit awkward, both traditions have been able to find support in the work of the other for efforts to think about research or convince audiences of the merits of attachment theory. Attachment researchers in the social psychology tradition have long drawn on findings from the developmental tradition in the literature reviews of their papers, in interpreting their results, and in review articles. For instance, in their magisterial work *Attachment in Adulthood* offering the capstone to their careers of research in the area, Mikulincer and Shaver simply fold in findings from both self-report and AAI studies in their summary tables of results, rarely remarking on differences in findings.[210]

It is clear that, contrary to Shaver's pessimistic remarks about his reading of works by developmentalist colleagues in 2006, researchers in the social psychological tradition have kept up to date with research using the AAI. Perhaps marking some aspects of a parallel

---

[206] Cassidy, J., Poehlmann, J., & Shaver, P.R. (2010) An attachment perspective on incarcerated parents and their children: introduction to the special issue. *Attachment & Human Development*, 12, 285–8.

[207] Simpson, J., Rholes, W.S., Orina, M.M., & Grich, J. (2002) Working models of attachment, support giving, and support seeking in a stressful situation. *Personality and Social Psychology Bulletin*, 28(5), 598–608.

[208] Granqvist, P., Hesse, E., Fransson, M., Main, M., Hagekull, B., & Bohlin, G. (2016) Prior participation in the strange situation and overstress jointly facilitate disorganized behaviours: implications for theory, research and practice. *Attachment & Human Development*, 18(3), 235–49.

[209] Granqvist, P., Mikulincer, M., & Shaver, P.R. (2010) Religion as attachment: normative processes and individual differences. *Personality and Social Psychology Review*, 14(1), 49–59. A further, more limited example of transcendence of the opposition between the developmental and social psychological traditions is Pasco Fearon. Though one of the leaders of the new generation of developmental attachment researchers, Fearon nonetheless incorporated psychometric methodology from the social psychological tradition in developing a brief version of the Attachment Q-Sort (Chapter 2). Cadman, T., Belsky, J., & Fearon, R.P. (2018) The Brief Attachment Scale (BAS-16): a short measure of infant attachment. *Child: Care, Health and Development*, 44(5), 766–75.

[210] Mikulincer, M. & Shaver, P. (2016) *Attachment in Adulthood*, 2nd edn. New York: Guilford.

transition, a curious shift has occurred in the developmental tradition of attachment research. Previously, with exceptions such as Cassidy and Belsky, researchers in this tradition excluded self-report measures from the literature reviews of their papers, discussions of results, and review articles. The grounds for this have been that the self-report measures have little association with the Strange Situation and the AAI, situated as the 'gold standard' measures of attachment. However, in the last few years there has been an increased trend for leaders in the developmental tradition to both acknowledge the contribution of self-report studies, and acknowledge it as attachment research. So, for instance, in a 2016 paper, Heckendorf, Huffmeijer, Bakermans-Kranenburg, and van IJzendoorn described Mikulincer's work as having 'convincingly shown ... experimentally how feelings of more secure attachment facilitate supporting partners in distress'.[211] And no less a defender of the developmental tradition than Sroufe has praised the social psychology approach in the most recent edition of the *Handbook of Attachment*. Sroufe stated that in the work of Mikulincer and Shaver, as well as Shaver's Minnesota colleague Simpson, the 'power' of the approach for studying adult romantic relationships 'has become manifest'.[212]

Attachment narrow and broad

Pivoting concepts

In a 2015 review paper, Jones, Cassidy, and Shaver expressed confusion over the fact that the ECR and AAI, unrelated measures, nonetheless ostensibly both assess attachment: 'though the two measures are largely unrelated to each other, they are similarly related to a variety of attachment-relevant constructs'. They have termed this one of the 'burning questions' facing the field of attachment research.[213] Shaver and Mikulincer have elsewhere presented this question as a challenge to researchers in the developmental tradition. If developmentalists want to claim that self-report measures are not true assessments of attachment, they need somehow to account for the fact that the results of studies using these measures correspond specifically to the predictions of attachment theory:

> Self-reports of attachment anxiety validly predicted automatic preoccupation with attachment-related worries, whereas self-reports of attachment avoidance validly predicted defensive suppression of these worries. This suppression could be overcome by adding a cognitive load that interfered with defensive suppression. These effects are so closely related to the theoretical conception of anxiety and avoidance in attachment theory that they would be difficult to explain, as a whole, by any other theory.[214]

---

[211] Heckendorf, E., Huffmeijer, R., Bakermans-Kranenburg, M.J., & van IJzendoorn, M.H. (2016) Neural processing of familiar and unfamiliar children's faces: effects of experienced love withdrawal, but no effects of neutral and threatening priming. *Frontiers in Human Neuroscience*, 10, 231.

[212] Sroufe, L.A. (2016) The place of attachment in development. In J. Cassidy & P.R. Shaver (eds) *Handbook of Attachment: Theory, Research, and Clinical Applications*, 3rd edn (pp.997–1011). New York: Guilford, p.999.

[213] Jones, J.D., Cassidy, J., & Shaver, P.R. (2015) Parents' self-reported attachment styles: a review of links with parenting behaviors, emotions, and cognitions. *Personality and Social Psychology Review*, 19(1), 44–76, p.69.

[214] Shaver, P.R. & Mikulincer, M. (2004) What do self-report attachment measures assess? In W.S. Rholes & J.A. Simpson (eds) *Adult Attachment: Theory, Research, and Clinical Implications* (pp.17–54). New York: Guilford, p.26.

Shaver and Mikulincer legitimately described their work as having elaborated and tested concepts drawn from attachment theory. However, Roisman helpfully qualified that from this it should not be assumed that (i) 'attachment' itself is a unitary entity in adulthood, (ii) or that attachment theory is a unitary entity.[215] The difficulties of translation between the developmental and social psychological traditions of attachment do not only arise from their differences in methodology. Perhaps of greater importance has been a confusion of tongues in the appeals of the two traditions to the work of Bowlby and Ainsworth, and in their use of the term 'attachment' itself.

Shaver and Fraley stated that 'the term attachment is a metaphor. Its denotation is unclear.'[216] Its meaning is not pre-set, but shaped by the surrounding network of theoretical concepts. As such, Shaver and colleagues readily acknowledged the differences between developmental and social psychological researchers in interpretations of the term 'attachment' and in the surrounding network of concepts. They argued that 'just as a reader of Freud can focus mainly on his psychosexual theory of personality development or his theory of intrapsychic dynamics, a researcher interested in attachment theory can focus on one or more of its central components without being required to focus on all of them. This does not mean the researcher is not doing attachment research.'[217] They sharply criticised Waters (Chapter 2) for his emphasis on the secure base and safe haven as the central denotation of the term 'attachment' and as the fundamental elements of attachment theory. To them, this seemed unnecessarily restrictive and overliteral. Waters' position also seemed to Shaver and Mikulincer to be a power-conserving tactic, aiming to snatch the legacy of Bowlby and Ainsworth away from researchers who recognise that the 'theory contained other central concepts' and who wish to acknowledge these with a wider sense of the term 'attachment'.[218] From this perspective, the social psychological tradition of attachment research was not an unlicenced reapplication of the established attachment concepts; it was another way of generating concepts, methods, and research priorities on the basis of the ideas of the first generation of attachment researchers.

Shaver and Mikulincer were aware, of course, that varied use of the same terms put at risk the viability of effective communication within the research community, and between the research community and its audiences.[219] However, this appeared a risk they were willing to take. One reason Shaver and Mikulincer may have felt warranted in adopting the broader notion of 'attachment' was that, like Waters and colleagues, they could easily point to passages in Bowlby's work to support their interpretation of attachment and

---

[215] Roisman, G.I. (2009) Adult attachment: toward a rapprochement of methodological cultures. *Current Directions in Psychological Science*, 18(2), 122–6.

[216] Shaver, P.R. & Fraley, R.C. (2000) Attachment theory and caregiving. *Psychological Inquiry*, 11, 109–114, p.111.

[217] Shaver, P.R & Mikulincer, M. (2002) Dialogue on adult attachment: diversity and integration. *Attachment & Human Development*, 4(2), 243–57, p.246.

[218] Ibid. See also Shaver, P.R. & Mikulincer, M. (2002) Attachment-related psychodynamics. *Attachment & Human Development*, 4(2), 133–61, p.155.

[219] The potential for imprecise or diverging definitions of concepts to reduce clarity in communication is acknowledged in various places in Shaver and Mikulincer's work, even from their early publications, e.g. Mikulincer, M. & Caspy, T. (1986) The conceptualization of helplessness: I. A phenomenological-structural analysis. *Motivation and Emotion*, 10, 263–78: 'Many psychological concepts are not well defined, so their meanings vary somewhat from person to person. Variations in usage are not surprising because psychological phenomena are often abstract terms that summarize the verbal report of a lay person regarding his perceptions and behavior in reference to specific real-life situations. Because the terms are imprecise in meaning, they also generate low interjudge reliability' (263–4).

of attachment theory. This is because, as Chapter 1 showed, Bowlby's integration of ethology and psychoanalysis brought together within the single term 'attachment' two quite different conceptualisations: one narrow account based on Hinde's notion of following and proximity-seeking as activated by threat, and a broader account based on the psychoanalytic concern with all intimate relationships. A large swathe of the confusion among researchers lies in the fact that the major additions to Bowlby's theory by Ainsworth and Main could apply to *both* the narrow and the broad concept of attachment. True, in a certain sense the narrow concept had primacy. Ainsworth's identification of the secure base phenomenon, in the first instance, entered attachment theory as an addition to the ethological concern with proximity-seeking, as a cross-species response. Hinde's idea that offspring will seek to retain proximity with their parent, especially under conditions of threat, was transformed by Ainsworth into the division between the secure base and safe haven. Individual differences in infant's use of the caregiver as a secure base for exploration and for proximity-seeking as a safe haven were observed by Ainsworth at home and in the Strange Situation.

However, just as Bowlby's concept of 'attachment' hinged on stringent and sprawling meanings, so did Ainsworth's concepts of 'secure base' and 'safe haven'. They could apply to the physical behaviour of an infant of any species. But they could also apply more generally to the symbolic aspects of all human intimate relationships. For instance, one friend can offer another regulation, comfort, and reprieve, without physical contact or any offer of protection. As Chapter 2 discussed, in a late publication Ainsworth criticised the work of her students and followers: 'By focusing so closely on intimacies some attachment researchers have come to conceive of them as the only source of security—which is a pity.'[220] For instance, without being an intimate relationship, even a short-term therapist may serve as a secure base and/or safe haven for a patient. Ainsworth's sophisticated position in her 1985 article 'Attachment across the lifespan' was that the experience of another person as a secure base, a safe haven, and as a source of separation anxiety were separable in adulthood (Chapter 2).[221] They did not necessarily form a unity. Ainsworth argued that it was futile to argue back and forth over whether a relationship, such as with a therapist or with a religious pastor, was or was not an attachment relationship. There was no binary. Instead, she argued that it was better to identify the extent to which a secure base, a safe haven, and separation anxiety were present, and to acknowledge that these phenomena could occur without other characteristics of an attachment relationship.

However, there remained a hinge in Ainsworth's use of the concepts that hindered this specification. Ainsworth's primary use of the terms 'secure base' and 'safe haven' was to indicated the physical movements of the infant away from and back towards the caregiver. However, she also extrapolated the concepts in remarks about adulthood to encompass the provision of other forms of support where these lead to an experience of security. The experience of feeling confident in a relationship as a basis of felt security may occur in relationships that are short term, relatively impersonal, and/or with only the barest or most symbolic link to a parent–child relationship. Probation officers, for example, describe secure base phenomena in their work with offenders as 'screamingly obvious'; and similar observations have

[220] Ainsworth, M. (1990, 2010) Security and attachment. In R. Volpe (ed.) *The Secure Child: Timeless Lessons in Parenting and Childhood Education* (pp.43–53). Charlotte, NC: Information Age Publishing, p.49.

[221] Ainsworth, M.D.S. (1985) Attachments across the life span. *Bulletin of the New York Academy of Medicine*, 61, 792–812.

been made for short-term therapeutic involvement with clients by helping professionals.[222] The secure base phenomenon is not limited to what are usually treated as attachment relationships when the term 'attachment' is construed narrowly.[223]

Likewise Main's concept of conditional strategies was made to pivot in both directions, towards Bowlby's narrower and broader concepts of attachment. What is curious is that this pivot was not intended by Main. Main's concept of conditional strategies was grounded in the idea that 'there exist species-wide abilities that are not part of the attachment system itself, but can, within limits, manipulate (either inhibit or increase) attachment behavior in response to differing environments'.[224] Main came to regard the avoidant and ambivalent/resistant infant attachment classifications as based on the use of attentional processes to manipulate the activation and expression of the attachment system. Narrowly, in Main's usage a conditional strategy was an ethological repertoire for achieving this effect: either directing attention towards potential threats and vigilance regarding caregiver availability and away from cues that might terminate the attachment system, or directing attention away from cues that might activate the attachment system, and towards potential sources of distraction in the environment. Main identified a similar process in adult autobiographical discourse, as attention seemed to be directed away from or towards attachment-relevant information. However, across both her published and unpublished writings, this never led her to refer to dismissing and preoccupied states of mind regarding attachment as 'conditional strategies'.

The extension from infancy to adulthood for Main was based on analogous processes at the level of attention. Main argued that the caregiving system could likewise be deactivated or made especially vigilant, since the caregiving system also runs on attention allocated to the one being cared for. The adult sexual system was assumed to have a parallel set of potential conditional strategies. The extension from the Ainsworth Strange Situation to adult discourse and to the caregiving and sexual systems gave Main's theory a wide scope of application. Yet Main's use of the terms 'attachment' and 'strategy' always remained narrow and ethological. It was Jude Cassidy, especially, who made the concept of conditional strategies pivotal to the broader concept of attachment, in conceptualising them as the 'maximising' and 'minimising' of not attention but of attachment itself as a system for the regulation of intimacy and emotion (Table 5.1 and Chapter 3). And it was from Cassidy, not from Main directly, that Shaver and Mikulincer picked up the concept of 'attachment strategies'.

In play across the attachment paradigm, then, can be seen narrow and broad concepts of attachment, narrow and broad concepts of secure base/safe haven, and narrow and broad concepts of maximising/minimising. Whereas the narrower concepts are based on

---

[222] Ansbro, M. (2018) Integrating attachment theory into probation practice: a qualitative study. *British Journal of Social Work*, 48(8), 2235–52.

[223] Ainsworth's emphasis on a secure base, a safe haven, and separation anxiety was inherited by Waters—though often, confusingly, he has used the term 'secure base' to refer collectively to the three components, and especially the first two. Waters regarded the concept of 'safe haven' as partially superseded by the concept of 'felt security', with anxiety as the inverse of security (Chapter 2). To him, this made the feeling of security the overarching concept, linking infant behaviour to adult experience. It also contributed to his frustration with the focus of other attachment researchers on separations and reunions at the expense of attention to ordinary experiences that contribute to feelings of trust and security in the relationship. Crowell, J. & Waters, E. (1989) Separation anxiety. In M. Lewis & S. Miller (eds) *Handbook of Developmental Psychopathology* (pp.209–218). New York: Plenum Press.

[224] Main, M., Hesse, E., & Kaplan, N. (2005) Predictability of attachment behavior and representational processes at 1, 6, and 19 years of age: the Berkeley Longitudinal Study. In K.E. Grossmann, K.Grossmann, & E. Waters (eds) *Attachment from Infancy to Adulthood: The Major Longitudinal Studies* (pp.245–304). New York: Guilford, p.256.

Table 5.1 Table of pivoting concepts

	Broad meaning	Narrow meaning
	Used by social psychologists + a few developmentalists like Cassidy and Fonagy	Used by Main, Waters, and the large majority of other developmental psychologists
Safe haven function of attachment	The orientation to seek physical or symbolic comfort from close relationships under conditions of perceived threat	The capacity to trust in the physical and attentional availability of discriminated familiar individuals under conditions of perceived threat
Secure base function of attachment	The capacity of close relationships to provide felt security	The capacity to trust that attention can be turned to exploration, given the expectation of the availability of discriminated familiar individuals
Conditional strategies	The hyperactivation or deactivation of the orientation to seek physical or symbolic comfort from close relationships	A species-wide repertoire, made available by evolutionary processes, for manipulating the activation of the attachment behavioural system through the direction of attention vigilantly towards or away from cues about the availability of familiar caregivers or potential threats. This repertoire evolved because it has the predictable outcome of increasing the availability and support provided by attachment figures who may otherwise be unavailable.
		Other ways of manipulating or overriding the output of the attachment behavioural system exist, and become increasingly available with developmental maturation. They can also be described as strategies. However, they are not conditional strategies in the technical sense unless—like the redirection of attention—they can be considered to express a species-wide repertoire, made available by evolutionary processes
Internal working models	The elaborated symbolic and affective representations made by humans about attachment figures and their availability, and the value of the self to these attachment figures	Variously: 1. Expectations about the availability of attachment figures 2. Elaborated symbolic meanings and images held by humans about attachment figures and their availability 3. A synonym for attachment representations, as used by Main in the 1980s (but subsequently abandoned)

a cross-species ethological account, the broader concepts encompass the felt experience characteristic of humans on the basis of symbolic capabilities. With both narrow and broad concepts in circulation, and with little or nothing to mark the distinctions between them, terms that researchers and their readers assume to have common meanings turn out to be quite treacherous. They have hidden compartments, allowing assumptions to be smuggled unnoticed and unscrutinised. Adding yet further to the confusion has been the concept of the 'internal working model', which can figure within both the broad and the narrow conceptualisations, albeit with different meanings (Chapter 1). The 'internal working model' concept has an unfortunate hypermobility, coming out of joint the moment weight is rested on it.

Given Waters' criticisms of Shaver and Mikulincer, it might be thought that the narrow concepts are more characteristic of the developmental attachment tradition and the broader concepts more characteristic of the social psychological tradition. That is certainly the general impression. However, matters are more complicated. True, Waters has been unusually consistent in using the narrow concept of attachment, and argued against looser uses of the term.[225] However, like Ainsworth, he has at times used a wider notion of secure base. And he does not appear to have ever accepted the concept of conditional strategies; the term is absent from his writings except in summaries of Main's position. In Waters' view, the distinction between avoidant and ambivalent/resistant attachment has seen insufficient predictive payoff, and insufficient validation against observations in naturalistic settings, to warrant its reification into discussions of minimising and maximising strategies (Chapter 2).

Among researchers in the developmental tradition, van IJzendoorn and Bakermans-Kranenburg are also unusually consistent in their use of the term 'attachment'. In the 1980s, van IJzendoorn pulled no punches in describing Bowlby's own tendency towards a broader usage of the term 'attachment' as 'somewhat ridiculous', since it implied identity between the process that brought a scared child to seek their caregiver and much more general feelings such as of identification with a political party.[226] Van IJzendoorn had no doubt that more expansive and symbolic meanings of attachment could be meaningful. For instance, he suspected that the relationship children have with a soft toy or blanket might recruit certain facets of the attachment behavioural system, drawing on the emerging human capacity for symbolisation. But, for him, this needed to be defined in precise terms on the basis of use of the object as a secure base, as a safe haven and/or source of separation anxiety, and the prediction of later socioemotional functioning.[227] Schuengel and van IJzendoorn discussed the narrower and broader uses of the terms 'attachment' and 'secure base' as contributing to a severe 'confusion about concepts', obscuring matters under discussion, for instance the precise relevance of attachment in therapeutic relationships.[228] And van IJzendoorn and Bakermans-Kranenburg have alleged that the concept of attachment has been stretched and disfigured by broader uses until it has, by now, simply snapped, with researchers talking right past one another whilst using the same terms.[229] For van IJzendoorn

---

[225] E.g. Crowell, J.A., Treboux, D., & Waters, E. (1999) The Adult Attachment Interview and the Relationship Questionnaire: relations to reports of mothers and partners. *Personal Relationships*, 6(1), 1–18. For an argument for the return of the concept of strategy to its narrower origins in ethology see Stevenson-Hinde, J. (1994) An ethological perspective. *Psychological Inquiry*, 5(1), 62–5.

[226] Van IJzendoorn, M.H., Tavecchio, L.W.C., Goossens, F.A., & Vergeer, M.M. (1982) *Opvoeden in Geborgenheid: Een Kritische Analyse van Bowlby's Attachmenttheorie*. Amsterdam: Van Loghum Slaterus, p.59.

[227] Van IJzendoorn, M.H., Goossens, F.A., Tavecchio, L.W.C., Vergeer, M.M., & Hubbard, F.O.A. (1983) Attachment to soft objects: its relationship with attachment to the mother and with thumbsucking. *Child Psychiatry and Human Development*, 14(2), 97–105; van IJzendoorn, M.H., Sagi, A., & Lambermon, M.W.E. (1992) The multiple caregiver paradox. Some Dutch and Israeli data. *New Directions for Child Development*, 57, 5–25, p.9.

[228] Schuengel, C. & van IJzendoorn, M.H. (2001) Attachment in mental health institutions: a critical review of assumptions, clinical implications, and research strategies. *Attachment & Human Development*, 3(3), 304–323, p.307. See also Harder, A.T., Knorth, E.J., & Kalverboer, M.E. (2013) A secure base? The adolescent–staff relationship in secure residential youth care. *Child & Family Social Work*, 18, 305–317.

[229] Van IJzendoorn, M.H. & Bakermans-Kranenburg, M.J. (2010) Stretched until it snaps: attachment and close relationships. *Child Development Perspectives*, 4(2), 109–111.

and Bakermans-Kranenburg what Shaver and Mikulincer have been measuring is simply a different behavioural system, one concerned with the adult pair relationship.[230]

However, it should not be thought that developmentalists are neatly aligned with the narrower use. Some developmental researchers slip and slide between the narrow and broad uses. Those who write for a clinical audience as well as for researchers and deliver commercial trainings in therapeutic approaches—such as Peter Fonagy, Patricia Crittenden, Allan Schore, Dan Hughes, and Susan Johnson—are generally consistent throughout their writings in using the broader concepts.[231] The broad concepts of attachment, secure base/safe haven, and maximising/minimising have significant advantages in this context. The broad concepts are closer to the connotations of ordinary language, and so are more accessible and evocative in writing aimed at both non-researchers and researchers. They offer greater attention to processes of symbolisation and meaning-making than the technical idea of an ethological behavioural system focused on proximity-seeking. And they also allow easier extrapolation across the life-cycle. For instance, Crittenden has proposed that what Ainsworth identified as patterns of attachment in infancy is in fact the local case of a broader phenomenon, linking human mental health and ill health. This broader phenomenon is the capacity of humans to exclude certain kinds of information from influencing experience or behaviour, in a manner responsive to that individual's history and social context. This is therefore how Crittenden has used the concept of 'attachment'. The term 'strategies' has been deployed to highlight the environmental responsiveness of individual behaviour. And the term 'security' has been used to mean the absence of information-processing exclusion or distortions.[232]

A few developmentalists, however, adopt some narrow and some broad uses. Cassidy, for instance, has generally been consistent in a comparatively narrow use of the concept of safe haven, but a broad use of the concepts of minimising and maximising.[233] Researchers in the social psychology tradition, despite tending towards the broader usage, regularly shuttle between the narrow and broad formulations and only rarely flag these transitions to the reader. We have already seen an illustration of slippage in the work of Shaver and Mikulincer. Module 1 of their model of the attachment system is concerned with whether 'proximity' is achievable (attachment narrow), but module 2 begins with an evaluation, not of proximity, but of whether the attachment figure is 'available, attentive, responsive, etc.' (attachment broad). And again, module 3 is initiated by a concern with whether the attachment figure is 'available, attentive, responsive, etc.' (attachment broad). But this concern is framed as the question 'Is proximity seeking a viable option?' (attachment narrow). This oscillation

---

[230] Verhage, M.L., Schuengel, C., Fearon, R.P., et al. (2017) Failing the duck test: reply to Barbaro, Boutwell, Barnes, and Shackelford (2017). *Psychological Bulletin*, 143(1), 114–16, p.114. This is in contrast, for instance, to Bernier and Dozier who likewise worry that the broader use of the concept of 'attachment' jeopardises its meaning, but who still described self-report measures and the AAI as assessing individual differences in a single behavioural system, even if they tap different aspects. Bernier, A. & Dozier, M. (2002) Assessing adult attachment: empirical sophistication and conceptual bases. *Attachment & Human Development*, 4(2), 171–9.

[231] E.g. Schore, A.N. (2001) Minds in the making: attachment, the self-organizing brain, and developmentally-oriented psychoanalytic psychotherapy. *British Journal of Psychotherapy*, 17(3), 299–328; Hughes, D. (2007) *Attachment-Focused Family Therapy*. New York: Norton; Sacco, F.C., Twemlow, S.W., & Fonagy, P. (2008) Secure attachment to family and community. *Smith College Studies in Social Work*, 77(4), 31–51; Johnson, S.M. (2019) *Attachment Theory in Practice*. New York: Guilford.

[232] Crittenden, P.M., Dallos, R., Landini, A., & Kozlowska, K. (2014) *Attachment and Family Therapy*. London: McGraw-Hill; Crittenden, P.M. & Landini, A. (2015) Attachment relationships as semiotic scaffolding systems. *Biosemiotics*, 8(2), 257–73.

[233] This consistency over time is well illustrated by Cassidy's opening chapters to the three editions of the *Handbook of Attachment*, in 1999, 2008, and 2016.

in Shaver and Mikulincer's account of the attachment system likely reflected a desire to assert that what they take to be attachment encompasses but is not reducible to concern with proximity with attachment figures. It allowed them to include the narrow notion of attachment within their broader concept, whilst also acknowledging that the set-goal of an adult attachment system is calibrated by context and culture.

Once the hinge in the concept of 'attachment' is acknowledged, Shaver and Mikulincer's position might be regarded as an offshoot of Bowlby's original insight—obscured by terminological confusion—that attachment in a broad sense has many components in common with, and may in some ways grow out of, attachment in a narrow sense. Shaver has had a tendency to overclaim links between adult espoused attachment styles and the attachment system in infancy. Stevenson-Hinde was surely right to admonish that 'one is going far beyond the data to presume, as Hazan and Shaver do, that "the neural foundation of the attachment system remains largely unchanged" across the life span'.[234] Nonetheless, already from the early works with Hazan, Shaver at times acknowledged that the construction of an adult bond as an attachment relationship was a piecemeal endeavour, forming a dappled surface that could, at most, only become consistent over time.[235] In a conference presentation, Hazan reported that by late adolescence 75% of 17-year-olds reported displaying proximity-seeking and separation protest preferentially to peers rather than parents, but that parents remained favoured for providing a secure base.[236] She theorised that at the start of a new adolescent or adult romantic relationship, proximity-seeking (in part motivated by the sexual system) contributes to finding a safe haven in the partner. This enthusiastic and clumsy process then leads to the establishment of pockets of comfort and shelter within the relationship and the incremental stabilisation of the partner as a secure base. The relationship itself comes to be felt as familiar, ordering, banal, and necessary. Hazan suggested that separation anxiety following unexpected separations follows on from experiencing the relationship as a secure base.

The speed and tone of the development of the relationship will be shaped by each individual's previous experiences, which will have informed their sexuality, their trust in a safe haven, their capacity to use a secure base, and the meanings they give to separations. Hazan and Shaver theorised that experiences in childhood and adolescence that suggest that a safe haven will not be available will predispose an avoidant attachment style, which in turn will slow the development of the components of an attachment relationship. By contrast, experiences in childhood and adolescence that suggest that a secure base will not be available will predispose an anxious attachment style, which in turn will speed up the use of the caregiver as a safe haven. Hazan and Shaver speculated that a secure attachment style would make

---

[234] Stevenson-Hinde, J. (1994) An ethological perspective. *Psychological Inquiry*, 5(1), 62–5, p.63, citing Hazan, C. & Shaver, P.R. (1994) Attachment as an organizational framework for research on close relationships. *Psychological Inquiry*, 5(1), 1–22.

[235] Hazan, C. & Shaver, P.R. (1994) Attachment as an organizational framework for research on close relationships. *Psychological Inquiry*, 5(1), 1–22: 'The process of attachment formation, at any age, is hypothesized to involve the same sequence: proximity seeking followed by safe-haven behavior followed by the establishment of a secure base' (12).

[236] Hazan, C., Hutt, M.J., Sturgeon, J., & Bricker, T. (1991) The process of relinquishing parents as attachment figures. Paper presented at the Biennial Meetings of the Society for Research in Child Development, Seattle, WA. These findings were replicated by later studies: Fraley, R.C. & Davis, K.E. (1997) Attachment formation and transfer in young adults' close friendships and romantic relationships. *Personal Relationships*, 4, 131–44; Trinke, S.J. & Bartholomew, K. (1997) Hierarchies of attachment relationships in young adulthood. *Journal of Social and Personal Relationships*, 14, 603–625; Nickerson, A.B. & Nagle, R.J. (2005) Parent and peer attachment in late childhood and early adolescence. *Journal of Early Adolescence*, 25(2), 223–49.

for a smoother transition from sexuality to caregiving as the primary ally of the attachment system in adult relationships. It might also facilitate the development of the full complement of components of an adult attachment relationship, with the mutual provision of a secure base, safe haven, and the experience of anxiety at unexpected separations.

Secure base/safe haven dynamics

That Shaver and colleagues would adopt a loose definition of 'attachment' was predisposed by their focus on adulthood. The wish for an adult partner to be 'available, attentive, responsive, etc.' will be shaped by culture and context. Indeed, culture and context can influence the relative priority of concern for availability, attentiveness, and responsiveness. Though their primary target was romantic relationships, Shaver's initial impulse towards attachment theory had been as a resource for making sense of a close sibling relationship and its loss. Hazan and Shaver specified that they intended the introduction of attachment theory to social psychology as offering 'a comprehensive theory of close relationships'.[237] It was an individual's 'style' with respect to intimacy that was the object of analysis. And Shaver and colleagues have frequently used the term 'intimacy', or sometimes 'closeness', as a functional synonym for attachment.[238]

What made attachment theory an exceptionally potent resource for social psychology was that, not just infant–caregiver relationships, but adult intimate relationships too seemed to have the potential for secure base/safe haven dynamics. This was already identified clearly by Bowlby in his writings on the therapeutic role of the secure base in clinical contexts. Whether or not this makes such adult interactions 'attachment' relationships is a matter of definition, and both sides of this debate can claim Bowlby's authority and supporting passages from his writings. Furthermore, various behavioural systems can be subject to minimising and maximising: in Main's original proposal, the parameters of both the infant attachment system and the adult caregiving and sexual systems could be altered through the manipulation of attention away from or towards the activating or deactivating conditions of the system. Whether or not they are therefore defined as 'attachment' relationships, the desire for intimacy in adult relations can be regarded as another site in which minimisation and maximisation may be deployed to respond to circumstances where the availability of a partner is in question. As such, the key ingredients of attachment theory—the attachment system (module 1), the secure base/safe haven dynamic (module 2), and maximising and minimising (module 3)—are all available for research on adult intimate relationships.

In a 2002 paper, 'Activation of the attachment system in adulthood', Mikulincer, Gillath, and Shaver reported a series of studies of the effects of subliminal threat on the activation of

---

[237] Hazan, C. & Shaver, P.R. (1994) Attachment as an organizational framework for research on close relationships. *Psychological Inquiry*, 5(1), 1–22, p.1. This was, in fact, a limitation criticised by social psychologists in the 1990s, who felt that any comprehensive theory in social psychology should deal with relationships in general, not just intimate ones, e.g. Duck, S. (1994) Attaching meaning to attachment. *Psychological Inquiry*, 5(1), 34–8.

[238] Hence statements such as 'attachment-related avoidance is a tendency to withdraw from situations involving intimacy'. Brassard, A., Darveau, V., Péloquin, K., Lussier, Y., & Shaver, P.R. (2014) Childhood sexual abuse and intimate partner violence in a clinical sample of men: the mediating roles of adult attachment and anger management. *Journal of Aggression, Maltreatment & Trauma*, 23(7), 683–704, p.686. Other attachment researchers, however, have treated intimacy and attachment as distinct constructs. Karantzas, G.C., Feeney, J.A., Goncalves, C.V., & McCabe, M.P. (2014) Towards an integrative attachment-based model of relationship functioning. *British Journal of Psychology*, 105(3), 413–34.

representations of attachment figures. The authors regarded the results as effective evidence that their work was studying the processes outlined by attachment theory. They challenged their readers to offer another theory that could account for their findings. In their view, 'there is no alternative theory that predicts the results we obtained', and also 'no alternative theory that would have generated either these particular kinds of measures or our particular experiments'.[239] The series of studies began by using the WHOTO measure, initially developed by Hazan and then adapted by Fraley and Davis.[240] In the WHOTO, participants are asked to give a named person in response to questions about proximity-seeking/separation anxiety (Who is the person you most like to spend time with? Who is the person you don't like to be away from?), safe haven (Who is the person you want to be with when you are feeling upset or down? Who is the person you would count on for advice?), and secure base (Who is the person you would want to tell first if you achieved something good? Who is the person you can always count on?). Mikulincer and colleagues were keen to emphasise that these were not merely conventional or obvious aspects of any close relationship, but were specifically the functions privileged by Ainsworth in defining an attachment figure.[241]

In study 1, Mikulincer, Gillath, and Shaver asked participants to complete a computerised lexical decision task, in which they read a string of letters and tried to identify whether it was a word or a non-word. Reaction times were used as a measure of the accessibility of thoughts related to the target word.[242] The accessibility of the names of people identified in the WHOTO was assessed under two conditions. In the first condition, the name followed a neutral word ('hat'). In the second condition, the name followed the word 'failure', which was chosen as a representation of threat but not necessarily one closely linked to attachment. Other names were also used: the names of close friends not selected by the WHOTO, the names of acquaintances, and names of strangers. Participants also completed the ECR, and a measure of neuroticism. The results of study 1 were that participants had a faster reaction time when the name was from their WHOTO list following the 'failure' prime, compared to reaction times for the names of other close people, acquaintances, strangers, and non-words. An anxious attachment style reduced reaction times for the names of attachment figures only, and this occurred in both the neutral and the 'failure' condition. As in other studies, there was a very substantial association between attachment anxiety and neuroticism ($r =$ .54). However, neuroticism was unrelated to response times, and the effects for attachment anxiety remained the same even controlling for neuroticism.

[239] Mikulincer, M., Gillath, O., & Shaver, P.R. (2002) Activation of the attachment system in adulthood: threat-related primes increase the accessibility of mental representations of attachment figures. *Journal of Personality and Social Psychology*, 83(4), 881–95, p.892.

[240] Fraley, R.C. & Davis, K.E. (1997) Attachment formation and transfer in young adults' close friendships and romantic relationships. *Personal Relationships*, 4, 131–44.

[241] Trinke and Bartholomew found an association of .45 between the WHOTO and a measure of 'supportive' relationships, suggesting that the WHOTO is materially related to supportiveness, but not reducible to it. They interpreted this finding as indicating that supportiveness may contribute to the formation of attachment components in a relationship, but that many relationships with attachment components in adulthood form and endure without supportiveness. Trinke, S.J. & Bartholomew, K. (1997) Hierarchies of attachment relationships in young adulthood. *Journal of Social and Personal Relationships*, 14, 603–625. More recently, Gillath and colleagues have argued against the use of self-reported separation anxiety as an index of an attachment relationship, as they anticipate that participants have to speculate about what it would be like to lose the other person, whereas they can report more concretely on secure base and safe haven use. Gillath, O., Karantzas, G.C., & Fraley, R.C. (2016) *Adult Attachment: A Concise Introduction to Theory and Research*. London: Academic Press, p.54.

[242] The methodology had been introduced into attachment research a decade earlier by Baldwin, M.W., Fehr, B., Keedian, E., & Seidel, M. (1993) An exploration of the relational schemata underlying attachment styles: self-report and lexical decision approaches. *Personality and Social Psychology Bulletin*, 19, 746–54.

Study 2 was a replication of study 1, except that instead of the threat word 'failure', the researchers substituted the threat word 'separation'. Again, participants showed faster reaction time following the prime when the name was from their WHOTO list than other names. As in study 1, an anxious attachment style made a contribution to reaction times for attachment figures only, and in both the 'separation' and the neutral condition. However, a finding specific to study 2 was that an avoidant attachment style increased reaction times for the names of attachment figures following priming of the word 'separation' but not following the neutral word. This implied that the names of attachment figures were less available for participants in response to the theme of 'separation' to the degree that they were high in attachment avoidance. Again, the association between an anxious attachment style and neuroticism was large ($r = .62$), and again neuroticism had no association with reaction times or interaction with the effect of attachment style on reaction times.

Study 3 sought to replicate studies 1 and 2 using a different procedure, the Stroop task. This is a well-established procedure based on the observation that viewing words with salient personal meanings slows reaction times in identification of the colour of that word. That is to say, cognitive accessibility on this assessment was represented by longer reaction times, in contrast to studies 1 and 2. Participants were divided into three groups: one group received neutral primes, another group were primed by the word 'failure', and a third group were primed by the word 'separation'. In the Stroop task, as expected, colour-naming was slower following the two threat primes in response to the name of attachment figures only, as opposed to other names, words, or non-words. An anxious attachment style increased reaction times in the neutral condition and following both threat primes in response to the names of attachment figures. An avoidant attachment style decreased reaction times in response to the names of attachment figures following only the separation prime, not the failure or neutral primes. Again, attachment anxiety overlapped substantially with neuroticism, but only the former was associated with any reaction time outcomes. Overall, the findings of the three studies were taken by Mikulincer and colleagues to show that threat contexts—whether general or attachment-specific—increase the cognitive accessibility of the names of attachment figures, in contrast to other close relationships and acquaintances (module 1). An anxious attachment style increased this cognitive accessibility even in neutral conditions, illustrating the feedback from attachment strategy (module 3) to the appraisal of threats and attachment figures (modules 1 and 2). An avoidant attachment style decreased cognitive accessibility only in response to the names of attachment figures and only in response to a separation prime rather than a general threat prime. The researchers demonstrated these effects over two different procedures and in three samples. The findings, the researchers argued, 'increase our confidence in the psychological reality of the attachment system' in adulthood.[243]

Mikulincer and colleagues regarded this study, one of their most cited by social psychology attachment researchers, as a gauntlet thrown down to the developmental tradition. Could they explain the findings except in terms of the operation of the attachment system in adulthood? The answer would appear to be no. Three research groups in the developmental

---

[243] Mikulincer, M., Gillath, O., & Shaver, P.R. (2002) Activation of the attachment system in adulthood: threat-related primes increase the accessibility of mental representations of attachment figures. *Journal of Personality and Social Psychology*, 83(4), 881–95, p.891. Aligned findings were later reported in Edelstein, R.S. & Gillath, O. (2008) Avoiding interference: adult attachment and emotional processing biases. *Personality and Social Psychology Bulletin*, 34(2), 171–81. The researchers found that an avoidant attachment style interfered with the availability of only attachment-relevant emotional words, and not emotional words not relevant to attachment.

tradition—those of Jude Cassidy,[244] Anne Bernier,[245] and Peter Fonagy[246]—have treated the study as evidence that the ECR measures attachment just as much as the assessments devised by Mary Ainsworth and Mary Main. Other developmental researchers have ignored the study, at least in print.[247] The paper demonstrated that threat primes increase the salience of semantic information relevant to figures identified as serving as a secure base, safe haven, and potential source of separation anxiety. Whilst the study did not provide evidence that these figures are differentially sought as a secure base/safe haven in concrete behaviour, the evidence of increased cognitive accessibility in the laboratory is certainly relevant and intriguing, and points in the expected direction.[248] The study also demonstrated that these effects are moderated by scores on the ECR in ways aligned with theory: an anxious attachment style increased vigilance to threats and to information about relationships with attachment components; and an avoidant attachment style decreased the cognitive availability of relationships with attachment components following a prime for separation.

The study suggested that secure base/safe haven processes operate in adulthood, and that these are moderated by maximising and minimising strategies. This was one important empirical source of legitimacy for the social psychology tradition to call itself a form of attachment research. However, it is important to note that the distinction between 'attachment relationships' and 'close relationships' in the study does not rule out other possibilities associated with the wider notion of attachment used by Shaver and colleagues. Shaver, Hazan, and Bradshaw claimed that 'the attachment figure need not be physically present for such an "interaction" to take place, which makes it more understandable that people have imaginary but very convincing and affective interactions with rock singers, dead philosophers, and religious figures of all kinds. Attachment, separation distress, and grieving are primarily psychological processes; they require psychological, not physical, interaction partners.'[249] Furthermore, some physical interactions with safe bases and secure havens are not with living partners. For instance, Bowlby stated that a person's home would likely have the characteristics of a secure base and safe haven (Chapter 1). If a person's home address were used in a study like that of Mikulincer and colleagues, it could be anticipated that responses would be more similar to names of attachment figures than to names of other close relationships.

[244] Dykas, M.J. & Cassidy, J. (2011) Attachment and the processing of social information across the life span: theory and evidence. *Psychological Bulletin*, 137(1), 19–46.

[245] Bernier, A., Larose, S., & Whipple, N. (2005) Leaving home for college: a potentially stressful event for adolescents with preoccupied attachment patterns. *Attachment & Human Development*, 7(2), 171–85.

[246] Fonagy, P. & Luyten, P. (2009) A developmental, mentalization-based approach to the understanding and treatment of borderline personality disorder. *Development & Psychopathology*, 21(4), 1355–81.

[247] Granqvist might be anticipated as an exception, given that his work spans both traditions. However, the only occasions on which he has cited the paper are in works actually co-authored with Mikulincer. Roisman is another figure straddling the two traditions, and cites the paper in a report co-authored with Chris Fraley: Haydon, K.C., Roisman, G.I., Marks, M.J., & Fraley, R.C. (2011) An empirically derived approach to the latent structure of the Adult Attachment Interview: additional convergent and discriminant validity evidence. *Attachment & Human Development*, 13(5), 503–524.

[248] Fraley and Shaver demonstrated that adult attachment style predicts observable behaviour on separations, accounting for around 8% of variance. Fraley, R.C. & Shaver, P.R. (1998) Airport separations: a naturalistic study of adult attachment dynamics in separating couples. *Journal of Personality and Social Psychology*, 75(5), 1198–212. Mikulincer and colleagues would later supply evidence that anxious and avoidant attachment styles bias motor responses on a push-pull task in response to attachment primes. Mikulincer, M., Shaver, P.R., Bar-On, N., & Ein-Dor, T. (2010) The pushes and pulls of close relationships: attachment insecurities and relational ambivalence. *Journal of Personality and Social Psychology*, 98(3), 450–68.

[249] Shaver, P.R., Hazan, C., & Bradshaw, D. (1988) Love as attachment: the integration of three behavioral systems. In R.J. Sternberg & M. Barnes (eds) *The Psychology of Love* (pp.68–99). New Haven, CT: Yale University Press, p.73.

And as we have seen, Shaver himself has referred to his experience of attachment theory as an attachment relationship: it is quite possible that other phenomena that serve as a safe base and safe haven might also receive differential cognitive availability in response to threat primes. That secure base/safe haven processes operate in adulthood does not imply that these processes are exclusive to romantic or even close relationships.

Evidence for the wider relevance of the secure base/safe haven components of attachment relationships, and of minimising and maximising strategies, is offered by later research conducted by Zilcha-Mano, Mikulincer, and Shaver. The researchers developed a scale for assessing anxiety and avoidance in an adult's sense of their pet's availability as a secure base and safe haven:

> Pet attachment anxiety consists of intense and intrusive worries that something bad might happen to one's pet and that one might find oneself alone, a strong need for proximity to the pet, reassurance seeking from the pet in order to maintain self-worth, intense frustration when the relationship with the pet is not as close as one would like, and even anger when the pet prefers the proximity of others. Pet avoidant attachment consists of feelings of discomfort with physical and emotional closeness to a pet, striving to maintain emotional distance from the pet, avoiding intimacy with it, preventing the pet from intruding into one's personal space, and difficulties in depending on the pet and turning to it when distressed.[250]

Zilcha-Mano and colleagues found that an avoidant attachment style on the ECR had no association with pet avoidance, and instead was associated with attachment anxiety regarding the pet's availability as a secure base/safe haven ($r = .35$). The researchers interpreted this finding as suggesting that 'avoidant people, who are unlikely to express attachment-related worries and anxieties in close human relationships (Mikulincer & Shaver, 2007), tend to express these worries and anxieties in relationships with pets'.[251] By contrast, there was a large positive association ($r = .60$) between attachment anxiety regarding the pet and an anxious attachment style on the ECR. Yet Zilcha-Mano and colleagues reported that anxiety regarding the availability of the pet had a substantial association with reduced reported well-being ($r = .34$) and with symptoms of anxiety and depression ($r = .41$) on the Mental Health Inventory, even after controlling for scores on the ECR and a measure of personality traits. The researchers therefore emphasised that psychologically consequential secure base/safe haven effects, and minimising/maximising individual differences, can be identified in adulthood beyond close human relationships.

The researchers did not report the association between ECR anxiety and the Mental Health Inventory. However, if other studies with the ECR and the Mental Health Inventory are brought in for comparison,[252] it is rather interesting that the pet attachment anxiety measure in the Zilcha-Mano study is actually a better predictor of scores on the Mental Health Inventory than the ECR. Given that many species of pet—unlike human partners—have been bred precisely to offer loyalty and reassurance, it may suggest an especially sorry

---

[250] Zilcha-Mano, S., Mikulincer, M., & Shaver, P.R. (2011) An attachment perspective on human–pet relationships: conceptualization and assessment of pet attachment orientations. *Journal of Research in Personality*, 45(4), 345–57, p.354.

[251] Ibid.

[252] Birnbaum, G.E., Orr, I., Mikulincer, M., & Florian, V. (1997) When marriage breaks up–does attachment style contribute to coping and mental health? *Journal of Social and Personal Relationships*, 14(5), 643–54.

state of affairs for someone to feel consciously anxious about whether their pet cares about them. Neuroticism as a measure of trait anxiety had only a weak association with anxiety regarding the pet's availability as a secure base/safe haven ($r = .15$), indicating that association does not lie merely in personality. It suggests that the secure base/safe haven components occur in the relationship with the pet and that these are reducible to neither adult attachment style nor personality. Furthermore, the findings suggest that meaningful individual differences exist in anxiety regarding the relationship with the pet. Zilcha-Mano and colleagues interpreted this as individual differences in the deployment of a maximising strategy in order to ensure the availability of the pet as a secure base/safe haven. However, further research is required to demonstrate that this is indeed specifically a maximising strategy, as opposed to anxiety arising through a psychological process of a different kind.

Attention and cognitive schemas

The ECR was considered to tap schemas offer information about the meaning and availability of a secure base and safe haven within intimate relationships, and the relevance of minimising or maximising strategies as a way of achieving the availability, attentiveness, responsiveness (etc.) of the other. This is quite distinct from the AAI, as an assessment of individual differences in the capacity to attend to and communicate about personal experiences with attachment figures in childhood. Rather than assessing generalised schemas, this capacity is assessed in the AAI through comparison of particular episodic and generalised semantic information. Johnson has claimed that attachment patterns, attachment styles, attachment strategies, and states of mind regarding attachment should all be regarded as 'equivalent terms', with the same referent except for differences in age and assessment methodology.[253] This runs counter to what Shaver and colleagues, and Main and colleagues have said that their assessments measure. It also seems a claim poorly aligned with the available evidence. Offering a more sophisticated and developmental reconciliation between the traditions, Cassidy proposed that (i) the experience of a secure base and safe haven in early child–parent relationships should facilitate (ii) a coherence in attending to and communicating about childhood experiences with attachment figures and (iii) generalised schemas about intimate relationships characterised by less anxiety or expectation of rejection.[254] However, it should clearly be acknowledged that these are three vastly different meanings of the term 'secure attachment', and the relationship between any two of them is unlikely to be simple or strong. Not least, Cassidy's proposal assumes extensive continuities from infancy to adult measures; though scaffolded by some of Bowlby's claims, this assumption was and remains contrary to available data (Chapter 2).

There is no reason to assume that the capacity to attend to and communicate about personal experiences with attachment figures in childhood should correlate with generalised schemas about intimate relationships in adulthood. The first is an attentional process oriented by a comparison of episodic and semantic memories of attachment narrowly construed. This

---

[253] Johnson, S.M. (2003) Introduction to attachment: a therapist's guide to primary relationships and their renewal. In S.M. Johnson & V. Whiffen (eds) *Attachment Processes in Couple & Family Therapy* (pp.3–17). New York: Guilford, p.10.

[254] E.g. Cassidy, J. (2001) Truth, lies, and intimacy: an attachment perspective. *Attachment & Human Development*, 3(2), 121–55.

is prompted by questions designed to offer uncomfortable freedom to memory, setting epi-sodic and semantic information into motion and providing an opportunity to see the ex-tent to which they outgallop the speaker's cooperation with the interviewer. The second is a generalised—in all likelihood largely semantic—schema of beliefs, emotions, and behav-iours relevant to the minimising or maximising of the wish for others to be available, atten-tive, responsive, etc. This will certainly be linked to attentional processes, not least in terms of cognitive biases in the perception of new information.[255] However, individual differences in attentional processes are at most a correlate, rather than what the ECR is specifically meas-uring. And whilst it might seem that both the AAI and ECR assess individual differences in terms of minimising and maximising strategies, this is a misapprehension. The AAI assesses the allocation of attention away from episodic information at the expense of fully answering the interview questions (Dismissing), towards negative aspects of experiences at the expense of focus on the actual questions asked in the interview (Preoccupation), or disruptions in working memory expressed as lapses in reasoning or discourse (Unresolved/disorganised). By contrast, the ECR assesses a variety of behaviours, beliefs, and feelings that index latent schemas. The two latent dimensions of the ECR are presumed by Shaver and Mikulincer to reflect an intensification or deintensification of the wish for others to be available, attentive, responsive, etc.

There may be several reasons for the lack of convergence between the AAI and ECR. They adopt different forms of measurement. And even within self-report assessments, there is only weak convergence between reports of attachment style with parents and attachment style in current intimate relationships. For example, self-reported avoidance with mother and with father have little association with a participant's attachment style in their current relationship ($r = .24$ and $r = .24$ for anxiety; $r = .17$ and $r = .12$ for avoidance, for mother and father respectively).[256] In addition to these factors, a further contribution is perhaps made by the fact that they tap different psychological processes, at least according to their originators. To the degree that Main and Hesse are right that the AAI is in the first instance an assessment of the allocation of attention, and that Shaver and colleagues are right that the ECR is ultim-ately an assessment of generalised schemas about intimate relationships, this suggests some specific conclusions about how and when the measures will diverge—but also when they will converge.

There should be poor association between the measures when correlates relate to semantic generalisations about need achievement within adolescent and adult relationships. This is perhaps why the ECR relates quite well to reported marital satisfaction and reported feelings of closeness with friends, but not the AAI.[257] There should also be poor association between the measures when correlates relate specifically to the allocation of attention in responding to another—one component of the caregiving behavioural system (regardless of whether this is broadly construed as nurturance or narrowly construed as safe haven provision). This is

[255] Fraley, R.C., Davis, K.E., & Shaver, P.R. (1998) Dismissing avoidance and the defensive organization of emo-tion, cognition, and behavior. In J.A. Simpson & W.S. Rholes (eds) *Attachment Theory and Close Relationships* (pp.249–79). New York: Guilford.

[256] Fraley, R.C., Heffernan, M.E., Vicary, A.M., & Brumbaugh, C.C. (2011) The Experiences in Close Relationships—Relationship Structures Questionnaire: a method for assessing attachment orientations across re-lationships. *Psychological Assessment*, 23(3), 615–25, Table 2.

[257] On associations with affiliation with friends see e.g. Mikulincer, M. & Selinger, M. (2001) The interplay be-tween attachment and affiliation systems in adolescents' same-sex friendships: the role of attachment style. *Journal of Social and Personal Relationships*, 18(1), 81–106; Mayseless, O. & Scharf, M. (2007) Adolescents' attachment rep-resentations and their capacity for intimacy in close relationships. *Journal of Research on Adolescence*, 17(1), 23–50.

perhaps why coherence on the AAI has been repeatedly found to be reliably associated with observational measures of sensitivity towards children and partners, whereas the link between the ECR and sensitivity seems to be more dependent on circumstances.[258] Sensitivity is predicated on noticing and recognising the other's signals (Chapter 2), primarily an attentional task. By contrast, the ECR is reliably associated with general supportiveness when the other is evidently stressed. Simpson and colleagues demonstrated this in assessments of couple interactions during a challenging laboratory task, as described in the section 'Two traditions of attachment research'.[259] And other studies have documented links between the ECR and generally supportive parenting when a child is distressed.[260]

The two measures will also be less well aligned when clinical phenomena are in question. The reason for this is foundational: part of the very definition of many clinical symptoms is the divergence between attentional processes and latent generalised schemas. In addition to differences in measurement, this may well be part of the reason why there is no evidence of overlap between the constructs of unresolved/disorganised states of mind and self-report measures of fearful attachment. Yet these two uncorrelated measures, the AAI and ECR, can nonetheless be anticipated to have similar correlates when the phenomenon in question is associated with both the allocation of attention in relation to attachment phenomena and generalised schemas about close relationships. There will be many occasions in which this alignment may occur. For instance, sexual behaviour in adulthood is likely influenced by both processes. The shaping of attention and sharing in relation to past experiences of tenderness and care are surely relevant, as are schemas about the possibilities and threats associated with intimacy. Likewise, both the allocation of attention in relation to attachment phenomena and generalised schemas about close relationships can be anticipated to be associated with the content—if not the form—of accounts of care in the course of childhood. And indeed, this is what evidence to date suggests.[261]

Nonetheless, it may also be anticipated that the processes underpinning the AAI and ECR would be activated and moderated by different circumstances. For instance, given Main's theory of the importance of attention to individual differences in both measures, the Strange Situation and the AAI may each be particularly impacted by factors that affect attention and memory processes, such as Ritalin and other ADHD medications.[262] Indeed, given that studies suggest use of these medications occur in 7–9% of adolescent community samples and 4% of adult samples,[263] the use of the AAI and assessments modelled on it without

[258] E.g. Mills-Koonce, W.R., Appleyard, K., Barnett, M., Deng, M., Putallaz, M., & Cox, M. (2011) Adult attachment style and stress as risk factors for early maternal sensitivity and negativity. *Infant Mental Health Journal*, 32(3), 277–85.

[259] Simpson, J., Rholes, W.S., Orina, M.M., & Grich, J. (2002) Working models of attachment, support giving, and support seeking in a stressful situation. *Personality and Social Psychology Bulletin*, 28(5), 598–608.

[260] E.g. Edelstein, R.S., Alexander, K.W., Shaver, P.R., et al. (2004) Adult attachment style and parental responsiveness during a stressful event. *Attachment & Human Development*, 6(1), 31–52.

[261] For instance, convergence between the ECR and scales for inferred childhood experience coded on the AAI has been substantial for avoidance ($r = .30$ and .41) and material for anxiety ($r = .24$ and .22). Haydon, K.C., Roisman, G. I., Marks, M.J., & Fraley, R.C. (2011) An empirically derived approach to the latent structure of the Adult Attachment Interview: additional convergent and discriminant validity evidence. *Attachment & Human Development*, 13(5), 503–524.

[262] Cf. Storebø, O.J., Skoog, M., Rasmussen, P.D., et al.(2014) Attachment competences in children with ADHD during the Social-Skills Training and Attachment (SOSTRA) randomized clinical trial. *Journal of Attention Disorders*, 19, 865–71.

[263] Bachmann, C.J., Wijlaars, L.P., Kalverdijk, L.J., et al. (2017) Trends in ADHD medication use in children and adolescents in five western countries, 2005–2012. *European Neuropsychopharmacology*, 27(5), 484–93; Anderson, K.N., Ailes, E.C., Danielson, M., et al. (2018) Attention-deficit/hyperactivity disorder medication prescription

controlling for attention-altering medication use may have introduced an unrecognised confound into analyses. In community samples, medication use would be a small confound, but in higher-risk samples where medication use is more common, this may have distorted research findings to some degree. The ECR by contrast is regarded as an assessment of gener-alised schemas, and would be expected to be relatively unaffected by the same medications, though the intensity of their availability may be altered.[264] Such distinctions would need to be tested, though. It is not enough to rest on the authors' own interpretations of what their measures measure.

Sexuality and dominance behavioural systems

Behavioural systems theory

Shaver and Mikulincer have been among the few attachment researchers, besides Main and Hesse (Chapter 3), to give serious consideration to Bowlby's concept of behavioural sys-tems. This concept has been taken for granted, and then ignored, by most researchers in the developmental tradition: its relevance to the Strange Situation seemed too obvious for further comment, and its relevance to the AAI was not explicitly articulated in Main's pub-lished writings and remained unclear. However, Shaver and Mikulincer's were brought to re-examine the concept as part of their attempts to establish and understand the meaning of attachment in adulthood, and in particular to operationalise its activation in the laboratory. Unlike researchers in the developmental tradition, Shaver and Mikulincer were forced to test and discriminate, rather than assume, the operation of psychological processes resembling those described by Bowlby.[265]

In the course of their exploration of Bowlby's ideas about attachment and other behav-ioural systems, Shaver and Mikulincer came to the view that attachment theory should actually have been called 'behavioural systems theory'.[266] The concept of 'attachment' was introduced as 'a metaphor that would refocus psychoanalytic theory on relational issues rather than imagined instincts or drives', and so has served its usefulness already.[267] If the banner of attachment theory was to be preserved, for Shaver and Mikulincer this would es-sentially be a matter of tradition rather than because this is the best name for Bowlby's ul-timate achievement. As documented in Chapter 1, in late correspondence Bowlby himself was dissatisfied with 'attachment' as the name for his theory. Additionally, whereas the devel-opmental tradition of attachment research had already claimed the concept of 'attachment',

---

claims among privately insured women aged 15–44 years—United States, 2003–2015. *Morbidity and Mortality Weekly Report*, 67(2), 66.

[264] Fraley, R.C. & Shaver, P.R. (2000) Adult romantic attachment: theoretical developments, emerging contro-versies, and unanswered questions. *Review of General Psychology*, 4(2), 132–54: 'We hypothesize that anxiety-reducing drugs affect the intensity but not the avoidant-nonavoidant orientation of attachment behaviors' (146).

[265] Bernier, A. & Dozier, M. (2002) Assessing adult attachment: empirical sophistication and conceptual bases. *Attachment & Human Development*, 4(2), 171–9.

[266] Shaver, P. & Mikulincer, M. (2004) Attachment in the later years: a commentary. *Attachment & Human Development*, 6(4), 451–64, p.454.

[267] Mikulincer, M. & Shaver, P.R. (2007) Reflections on security dynamics: core constructs, psychological mech-anisms, relational contexts, and the need for an integrative theory. *Psychological Inquiry*, 18, 197–209, p.208.

the concept of behavioural systems was an uncontested ground in which Shaver and Mikulincer could engage with and claim Bowlby's legacy.

Early in their work together, with the attachment system in childhood and adulthood as their central model, Shaver and Mikulincer defined a behavioural system as having six components.[268] These can be readily illustrated with the examples of the attachment and exploratory system. First, any behavioural system had to offer an expected species-level benefit for survival and/or reproduction. The attachment system, for instance, was assumed to offer both protection and a source of regulation. The exploratory system was assumed to offer support for learning about the environment and the self's capabilities.[269] Second, any behavioural system should have a set of activating parameters. The attachment system in childhood and adulthood was assumed by Shaver and Mikulincer to be activated by the perception of some kind of threat, whether an external source of danger or separation or an internal state of concern. Likewise, activating parameters can be identified for the exploratory system. Whereas Bowlby regarded the activating conditions of the exploratory system the encounter with complexity and/or novelty, in their conceptualisation Shaver and Mikulincer limited the activation of the exploratory system to the encounter with novelty, but emphasised that novelty is defined in part through contradiction or challenge to existing knowledge.[270]

For Shaver and Mikulincer, a third defining characteristic of a behavioural system was that it should have a set-goal which deactivates the system when a given change is identified in the relationship with the environment. Shaver and Mikulincer conceptualised the attachment system as deactivated by signals of the availability, attentiveness, responsiveness (etc.) of attachment figures, though the nature of these signals differ between childhood and adulthood. They also made the innovative proposal that a behavioural system will have 'anti-goals', which the system attempts to avoid. In the case of the attachment system, these are 'rejection, separation, and attachment figure unavailability'.[271] To take the example of the exploratory system, Bowlby conceptualised this system as deactivated by familiarity. Shaver and Mikulincer's concept was similar, though not identical: for them, the exploratory system would be deactivated once relevant skills or knowledge have been acquired. Shaver and Mikulincer at no point discuss the anti-goals of the exploratory system, but these might include feelings of incompetence and boredom.[272] To achieve familiarity without the

---

[268] Mikulincer, M. & Shaver, P.R. (2003) The attachment behavioral system in adulthood: activation, psycho-dynamics, and interpersonal processes. In M.P. Zanna (ed.) *Advances in Experimental Social Psychology*, Vol. 35 (pp.53–152). New York: Academic Press, p.57. Compare the definition of behavioural system offered in Shaver, P.R., Segev, M., & Mikulincer, M. (2011) A behavioral systems perspective on power and aggression. In P.R. Shaver & M. Mikulincer (eds) *Human Aggression and Violence: Causes, Manifestations, and Consequences* (pp.71–87). Washington, DC: American Psychological Association, p.72. In this later text the elements especially highlighted are the first, third, and fourth. There is no mention, for instance, of cognitive components as required as part of the definition of a behavioural system.

[269] Mikulincer, M. & Shaver, P.R. (2012) Attachment theory expanded: a behavioral systems approach to personality. In K. Deaux & M. Snyder (eds) *Oxford Handbook of Personality and Social Psychology* (pp.467–92). Oxford: Oxford University Press, p.473.

[270] Ibid.: 'The primary strategy of the exploration system, seeking new information about oneself and the world, is activated whenever a person encounters novel situations, objects, or people or experiences novel internal states that contradict or challenge existing knowledge and working models' (473).

[271] Mikulincer, M. & Shaver, P. (2008) Contributions of attachment theory and research to motivation science. In J.Y. Shah & W.L. Gardner (eds) *Handbook of Motivational Science* (pp.201–216). New York: Guilford, p.204.

[272] An interesting case discussed by Shaver in his early work is that of prank calls to the fire service. In a subtle and thoughtful paper, Shaver speculated that implicated in these prank calls was a pervasive combination of anger, boredom, and powerlessness, and a lack of other legitimate situations for expressing these feelings. In terms of his later thinking, this might be described as the interaction of the anti-goals of the exploratory systems and dominance systems. Shaver, P.R., Schurtman, R., & Blank, T. (1975) Conflict between ghetto-dwellers and firemen: environmental and attitudinal factors. *Journal of Applied Social Psychology*, 5, 240–61.

experience of relevance and growth might risk achievement of both a set-goal and an anti-goal, resulting in a happiness that continually drains itself. Bowlby was not wrong that familiarity terminates the exploratory system, but in Shaver and Mikulincer's view this did not mean that the behavioural system is therefore fully realised and satisfied.

Fourth, a behavioural system will have a repertoire of functionally equivalent behaviours that can be used to achieve the set-goal. In infancy and adulthood, Shaver and Mikulincer emphasised that behavioural systems continually learn, mature, and reorganise in identifying new and better ways of achieving the set-goal.[273] However, within this diversity, they conceived of the Ainsworth attachment classifications as representing the basic repertoires for achieving the direct or conditional availability of attachment figures. Similarly, in the case of the exploratory system, Shaver and Mikulincer proposed that maximising and minimising strategies are available.[274] Maximising the exploratory system entails attempts to master novelty even when the context does not call for it and enough information is already in hand. This may contribute to procrastination and indecision, doubts, and worries. Maximisation of the exploratory system responds to an environment in which familiarity is distrusted, much like anxious attachment style expresses a lack of confidence in the availability of attachment figures even when they are physically present. Minimisation of the exploratory system entails the inhibition of cognitive openness, exploration, or curiosity even when confronted by a novel or challenging situation. This strategy responds to an environment in which previous attempts at exploration were punished or tended to backfire.

Fifth, Shaver and Mikulincer highlighted that any behavioural system will include cognitive components. In the case of the attachment and exploratory systems, maximising and minimising strategies are activated depending on the availability of cognitive schemas from within a hierarchical network of associations formed through past experiences. Following Bowlby, Shaver and Mikulincer downplayed the autonomy of the affective components of the behavioural system, often describing these components as mere 'reflections' of the cognitive and behavioural aspects.[275] Sixth and finally, Shaver and Mikulincer argued that any behavioural system will have specific activating or inhibitory links with other behavioural systems. For instance, it would be expected that the activation of the attachment system would inhibit the operation of the exploratory system.

In a paper with Josh Hart and Jamie Goldenberg, Shaver argued that the attachment behavioural system also has a wider context: the 'security metasystem'.[276] Ainsworth argued that a sense of security could be fed by multiple sources, not just intimate relationships (Chapter 2). Apparently without awareness that they were reclaiming Ainsworth's position, Shaver and colleagues proposed that a sense of security can be achieved variously through experiencing the availability of attachment figures, through experiencing the self as worthy

[273] Mikulincer, M. & Shaver, P. (2008) Contributions of attachment theory and research to motivation science. In J.Y. Shah & W.L. Gardner (eds) *Handbook of Motivational Science* (pp.201–216). New York: Guilford, p.204.

[274] Mikulincer, M. & Shaver, P.R. (2012) Attachment theory expanded: a behavioral systems approach to personality. In K. Deaux & M. Snyder (eds) *Oxford Handbook of Personality and Social Psychology* (pp.467–92). Oxford: Oxford University Press, pp.473–4.

[275] E.g. Mikulincer, M. (2006) Attachment, caregiving and sex within romantic relationships. In M. Mikulincer & G.S. Goodman (eds) *Dynamics of Romantic Love: Attachment, Caregiving, and Sex* (pp.23–44). New York: Guilford: 'The profound joy and affection, self-protective anxiety, numbing boredom, corrosive anger, lustful passion, uncontrollable jealousy, and intense sorrow experienced in romantic relationships are reflections on the central importance of these behavioural systems' (23–4).

[276] Hart, J.J., Shaver, P.R., & Goldenberg, J.L. (2005) Attachment, self-esteem, worldviews, and terror management: evidence for a tripartite security system. *Journal of Personality and Social Psychology*, 88, 999–1013.

and capable, and through experiencing the world as orderly and meaningful. These three psychological processes, for all their differences, therefore have in common that they can serve both to modulate experiences of anxiety and contribute to broaden-and-build cycles. As well as a behavioural system in its own terms, attachment was therefore situated as part of a security metasystem. The species-level function of the system, it was proposed, is self-regulation. The metasystem is activated by potential feelings of anxiety, which can arise from relational sources such as close relationships but also from non-relational sources such as reminders of mortality. It is deactivated by felt security, regardless of the source of this feeling. The achievement of this goal can be pursued, as needed, through attachment-relationships, drawing upon self-esteem or from appeal to cultural worldviews that make the world seem orderly and meaningful. Though they often can work together, at times when one strategy is hard-pressed by circumstances, the others can be brought in to substitute. This is facilitated by the fact that they have cognitive components in common. Shaver and colleagues also argued that all three may facilitate exploration and caregiving.

Hart's work has subsequently focused on this macro level in articulating the concept of the 'security system'.[277] By contrast, this level of analysis has generally not been pursued by Shaver and Mikulincer, though it has remained conceptual background. Instead, Hart has developed ideas regarding the contribution of other behavioural systems to security. Initially, both Shaver and Mikulincer began with the assumption that attachment style would reflect the history of relationships with attachment figures. Attachment styles were defined as 'systematic patterns of expectations, emotions, and behavior in close relationships that are viewed as the residue of particular kinds of attachment histories'.[278] So, for instance, in the 1990s, Mikulincer reported from a study with a student sample that secure and anxious attachment styles were associated with greater self-reported curiosity and positive attitudes towards curiosity than participants with an avoidant attachment style. Furthermore, he found that participants with a secure attachment style were more likely to trust new information in making a social judgement than participants with avoidant or anxious attachment styles.[279] It could be that cognitive openness contributes to, or even partly constitutes, a secure attachment style. However, Mikulincer's interpretation of these findings was that insecure attachment hinders the full development and successful expression of the exploratory behavioural system, reducing occasions for felt curiosity. At the time, the self-report approach to attachment research was still being established, and part of the definition of secure attachment, since Ainsworth, had been an inverse relationship with exploration. Attachment was therefore conceptualised as antecedent and causal for curiosity.

By contrast, in the mid-2000s, with the self-report tradition established and thriving, Shaver and Mikulincer were willing to acknowledge that the qualities of adult attachment relationships are fed by other behavioural systems. Attachment styles were regarded as shaped by the variety of factors that shape perceptions of the availability, attentiveness, responsiveness (etc.) of others. In a 2005 article, Banai, Mikulincer, and Shaver argued that 'a person who is psychologically injured in the process of seeking one selfobject provision

---

[277] Hart, J. (2014) Toward an integrative theory of psychological defense. *Perspectives on Psychological Science*, 9, 19–39.

[278] Shaver, P.R. & Mikulincer, M. (2003) The psychodynamics of social judgments: an attachment theory perspective. In J.P. Forgas, K.D. Williams, & W. von Hippel (eds) *Social Judgments: Implicit and Explicit Processes* (pp.85–114). Philadelphia: Psychology Press, p.88.

[279] Mikulincer, M. (1997) Adult attachment style and information processing: individual differences in curiosity and cognitive closure. *Journal of Personality and Social Psychology*, 72(5), 1217–30.

tends thereafter to avoid seeking satisfaction of other selfobject needs'.[280] Feelings of rejection in relation to exploration or sexuality, for instance, might well contribute to a 'defensively avoidant stance so pervasive that it generalizes across different kinds of interpersonal experiences and leads people to dismiss social ties in general'.[281] In 2007 they argued clearly that 'just as good attachment experiences have beneficial effects on other behavioral systems, such as exploration and caregiving, good experiences related to those behavioral systems are likely to feed back on the attachment system in ways that allow it to function in a less defensive, less distorted way'.[282] Elsewhere, Shaver expressed regret that he and Hazan had earlier described adult romantic relationships as grounded in attachment, sexuality, and caregiving. He felt that exploration and affiliation were also behavioural systems integral to adult romantic relationships, and to the functioning of the relationship as a secure base and safe haven.[283] The capacity to explore is integral to utilisation of the attachment figure as a secure base. When exploration is blocked by a minimisation of the exploratory system, the experience of having a secure base is thinned or reduced. Conversely, when familiarity is distrusted as part of the maximisation of the exploratory system, this may have implications for being able to use attachment figures as a safe haven.

Over time, then, Shaver and Mikulincer came increasingly to the view that adult attachment style would be fed by many sources, rather than primarily reflecting a child's history of attachment experiences. This position was supported in 2013, when Fraley and colleagues found little prediction from infant attachment classifications to the ECR completed in adolescence in a study with 707 participants besides a very small negative association between infant proximity-seeking and an anxious attachment style ($\beta = -.08$). Even if it was somewhat theoretically expected, the social psychology paradigm nonetheless had a history of claims to legitimacy on the assumption of continuity from infancy. As a result, there appears to have been ambivalence about this finding: the result was reported by Fraley and colleagues, but only in a web-based appendix to the published article.[284] As a result, the finding was effectively buried. It has been little noticed by subsequent researchers.

Sexuality

In pursuing their thinking about behavioural systems, Shaver and Mikulincer found the concept of the sexual behavioural system significantly underdeveloped. Bowlby had long acknowledged sexuality as a behavioural system. It was an essential point of comparison in *Attachment, Volume 1* as Bowlby set out the concept of attachment and described it as a

---

[280] Banai, E., Mikulincer, M., & Shaver, P.R. (2005) 'Selfobject' needs in Kohut's self psychology. *Psychoanalytic Psychology*, 22(2), 224–60, p.251.

[281] Ibid. p.251.

[282] Mikulincer, M. & Shaver, P.R. (2007) Boosting attachment security to promote mental health, prosocial values, and inter-group tolerance. *Psychological Inquiry*, 18, 139–56, p.152.

[283] Shaver, P.R. (2006) Dynamics of romantic love: comments, questions, and future directions. In M. Mikulincer & G.S. Goodman (eds) *Dynamics of Romantic Love: Attachment, Caregiving, and Sex* (pp.423–56). New York: Guilford, p.432.

[284] Fraley, R.C., Roisman, G.I., Booth-LaForce, C., Owen, M.T., & Holland, A.S. (2013) Interpersonal and genetic origins of adult attachment styles: a longitudinal study from infancy to early adulthood. *Journal of Personality and Social Psychology*, 104(5), 817–38, web-based supplement C. Additionally, a later study using the same sample demonstrated that the ECR has essentially no relationship with secure base scripts in adulthood. Steele, R.D., Waters, T.E., Bost, K.K., et al. (2014) Caregiving antecedents of secure base script knowledge: a comparative analysis of young adult attachment representations. *Developmental Psychology*, 50(11), 2526–38.

behavioural system. However, in this, Bowlby's aim was also to distinguish attachment from sexuality, contesting versions of psychoanalytic theory that described all motivation as, in a sense, sexuality. Bowlby evidently felt that sexuality needed to be placed in the background in order to make space for attachment (Chapter 1). Though his discussions of the sexual system are, as a result, somewhat cursory, it is nonetheless clear that Bowlby regarded the adult sexual system as sharing some components of the attachment system, such as the behaviours clinging and kissing. Furthermore, he drew on ethological evidence to support the (psychoanalytic) argument that the qualities of the parent–child relationship go on to influence sexual preferences when the child has grown to adulthood.[285] Ainsworth followed Bowlby in generally downplaying sexuality, despite her personal beliefs regarding its importance (Chapter 2). More than Bowlby, she drew out that adult romantic relationships entail attachment, sexuality, and caregiving. However, her remarks on the sexual behaviour system essentially agree with those of Bowlby, with one exception. Whereas Bowlby described gay and lesbian relationships as deviations in *Attachment, Volume 1*, Ainsworth argued that there was no basis for this position, implicitly acknowledging Bowlby's stance as prejudice.[286]

Overall, the concept of the sexual behavioural system was acknowledged but left sleeping by the founders of attachment theory. And the focus of the developmental tradition of attachment research on childhood directed attention away from sexuality, with the exception of Fonagy and Crittenden.[287] By contrast, the sexual behavioural system was central for Shaver and colleagues since their focus was on adult relationships, and above all adult romantic relationships. This concern also occurred against the backdrop of growing attention to sexuality within quantitative social science in general over the 1980s, in part reflecting the salience of sexuality for identity politics in the period, but also more narrowly the availability of federal funding to study social factors relevant to the spread of HIV.[288] The initial model of the sexual behavioural system offered by Shaver and Mikulincer in the 1990s was not well formulated. They tended to pathologise people outside of monogamous romantic relationships. Individuals who experience sexual attraction to more than one person were situated as deviant, since it was expected by Shaver that 'just like infants, adults are primed to select one special figure'.[289] And Mikulincer argued in 2006 that 'the set goal of this system is to impregnate an opposite-sex partner'.[290] As in Bowlby's work, this characterisation pathologises gay and lesbian sexualities, and can be regarded as reflecting Shaver and Mikulincer's general lack of concern for sexual diversity in forms of adult relationships. Their characterisation of

[285] Bowlby, J. (1969, 1982) *Attachment.*, London: Penguin, p.233.

[286] Ainsworth, M. (1984) Attachment. In N.S. Endler & J. McVicker Hunt (eds) *Personality and the Behavioral Disorders* (pp.559–602). New York: Wiley, p.596.

[287] Fonagy, P. (2008) A genuinely developmental theory of sexual enjoyment and its implications for psychoanalytic technique. *Journal of the American Psychoanalytic Association*, 56(1), 11–36; Crittenden, P.M. (2015) *Raising Parents*, 2nd edn. London: Routledge. The inattention to sexuality among attachment researchers after Bowlby matched a trend in post-war psychoanalytic theory to downplay the topic. Some of this was blamed on attachment theory. See Zamanian, K. (2011) Attachment theory as defense: what happened to infantile sexuality? *Psychoanalytic Psychology*, 28(1), 33–47.

[288] Mottier, V. (1997) Sex and discourse. The politics of the Hite reports. In T. Carver & M. Hyvärinen (eds) *Interpreting the Political: New Methodologies* (pp.39–59). London: Routledge; Epstein, S. (2006) The new attack on sexuality research: morality and the politics of knowledge production. *Sexuality Research and Social Policy Journal of NSRC*, 3(1), 1.

[289] Morgan, H.J. & Shaver, P.R. (1999) Attachment processes and commitment to romantic relationships. In J.M. Adams & W.H. Jones (eds) *Handbook of Interpersonal Commitment and Relationship Stability* (pp.109–24). New York: Plenum Press, p.111.

[290] Mikulincer, M. (2006) Attachment, caregiving and sex within romantic relationships. In M. Mikulincer & G.S. Goodman (eds) *Dynamics of Romantic Love: Attachment, Caregiving, and Sex* (pp.23–44). New York: Guilford.

the set-goal of the sexual system also is clearly phallocentric: the sexual set-goal of women tends not to be 'to impregnate' their partner.

These problems in Shaver and Mikulincer's initial reflections on the sexual behavioural system were grounded in a broader confusion of the evolutionary and individual levels of analysis, distinguished by Tinbergen and the ethological tradition (Chapter 1). Stevenson-Hinde had identified this tendency in Shaver's work already in the 1990s.[291] A behavioural system was, for ethologists like Stevenson-Hinde, a sequence of behaviours that might be inferred at a species level to contribute to survival and/or reproduction. The sexual system therefore did not need to have even intercourse, let alone impregnation, as its set-goal so long as in evolutionary history the behavioural system had contributed to the probability of re-production. This distinction has been increasingly acknowledged by Shaver and Mikulincer over the past decade, as they have reflected on ideas from evolutionary biology[292] and pur-sued collaborative research on the sexual behavioural system together with colleagues such as Gurit Birnbaum and Omri Gillath. At times, this group of collaborators have argued that the sexual system has multiple set-goals involving the initiation and maintenance of rela-tionships.[293] However, their stable position in recent years appears to have been that the set-goal of the sexual system is sexual access to a partner.[294]

As Shaver and Mikulincer have further developed their concept of the sexual system, one important area of change has been their attention to gender. The initial model of the sexual behavioural system was implicitly phallocentric, in situating the set-goal of the system as impregnation of the partner. However, empirical studies exploring sexual experiences in-dicated meaningful differences between male and female participants. A study by Gillath, Mikulincer, Birnbaum, and Shaver published in 2007 examined the effects of a subliminal prime of a picture of an attractive nude person of the opposite sex.[295] In one version of the procedure, student participants were then asked to view pictures of members of the opposite sex and report their relative feelings of arousal. In a second version of the procedure, after the prime the student participants were exposed to a varied series of pictures and were asked to decide whether each contained or did not contain sexual content, and to do so as quickly as possible. Reaction times for accurate identification of sexual content was taken as a measure of the accessibility of sex-related thoughts. Gillath, Mikulincer, and colleagues found that the naked picture prime led to higher accessibility of sex-related thoughts in both male and female participants. However, the subliminal prime led women to report lower levels of sexual arousal. Rather than reflecting intrinsic sex-differences, the researchers interpreted these findings with the proposal that 'it would not be surprising if women had more reasons than men to be threatened by certain kinds of sexual situations'.[296] Women may experience

[291] Stevenson-Hinde, J. (1994) An ethological perspective. *Psychological Inquiry*, 5(1), 62–5.

[292] Mikulincer, M. & Shaver, P.R. (2012) Attachment theory expanded: a behavioral systems approach to per-sonality. In K. Deaux & M. Snyder (eds) *Oxford Handbook of Personality and Social Psychology* (pp.467–92). Oxford: Oxford University Press: 'As evolutionary psychologists have explained, however, the proximal motivation for an act (i.e., wishing to have sex with an attractive person) need not be the same as the evolutionary reason for the existence of the motives involved' (475).

[293] Gillath, O., Mikulincer, M., Birnbaum, G.E., & Shaver, P.R. (2008) When sex primes love: subliminal sexual priming motivates relationship goal pursuit. *Personality and Social Psychology Bulletin*, 34(8), 1057–69.

[294] Szepsenwol, O., Mikulincer, M., & Birnbaum, G.E. (2013) Misguided attraction: the contribution of nor-mative and individual-differences components of the sexual system to mating preferences. *Journal of Research in Personality* 47, 196–200, p.197.

[295] Gillath, O., Mikulincer, M., Birnbaum, G.E., & Shaver, P.R. (2007) Does subliminal exposure to sexual stimuli have the same effects on men and women? *Journal of Sex Research*, 44(2), 111–21.

[296] Ibid. p.119.

implicit or explicit pressure around sex, including diverse reputational threats associated with both having and not having sex. The women students participating in the study were understood by the researchers as interpreting the subliminal sexual prime adversely, in the context of their experiences of what male sexuality, or male nudity specifically, represented to them.

By 2007, Shaver and Mikulincer had repeatedly tested for gender effects in attachment styles, but only found these when conducting studies of couples in interaction, not when individuals had been studied alone.[297] In examining sexuality, however, they found both individual-level and couple-level differences. Brassard, Shaver, and Lussier asked 273 heterosexual couples aged 18–35 to complete the ECR alongside measures of sexual experiences in their relationships.[298] The researchers found that for women, but not for men, an avoidant attachment style was associated with engagement in less sexual fantasy and daydreaming. They also found that for men, but not for women, an anxious attachment style was associated with pushiness for sex and the use of sex for reassurance. Women, in turn, responded differently to this behaviour by their partner depending on their attachment anxiety: only women low in attachment anxiety appeared to resist this pushiness and engage in sexual interactions according to their own desires and pacing.[299]

Recently, Birnbaum, Mikulincer, and colleagues developed the concept of the sexual system into a self-report scale modelled on the ECR, the Sexual System Functioning Scale (SSFS).[300] Hyperactivation items on the SSFS were designed to tap the co-presence of desire and worries about sex, 'much like anxiety items in the ECR tap into desire and worries related to emotional closeness'.[301] Deactivation items on the SSFS were designed to tap disinterest and discomfort with sex, 'much like avoidance items in the ECR tap into disinterest and discomfort with emotional closeness'.[302] Both hyperactivation and deactivation were conceptualised as strategies for achieving the set-goal of sexual access to the partner. Hyperactivation is a strategy that entails vigilance regarding access to sex, and ready and intense striving for sexual interactions when sexual access seems possible. Sexual access may be sought insistently and abruptly, with less concern for context or the wishes of others, since it can be prioritised over other potential goals including caregiving, exploration, and attachment. Hyperactivation of the sexual system therefore entails reduced sensitivity, in the sense of recognising, acknowledging, and responding in a timely way to the cues of a partner.

---

[297] Mikulincer, M. (2007) Building personal relationships theory. *Personal Relationships*, 14(3), i–iv: 'In general, I have noticed informally that few gender differences appear in attachment-related studies of individuals, yet they are common when both members of couples are studied' (ii).

[298] Brassard, A., Shaver, P.R., & Lussier, Y. (2007) Attachment, sexual experience, and sexual pressure in romantic relationships: a dyadic approach. *Personal Relationships*, 14(3), 475–93.

[299] Little and colleagues found that an avoidant attachment style was unrelated to marital satisfaction among partners who had frequent sex, and that an anxious attachment style was unrelated to marital satisfaction among partners who frequently had pleasurable sex. Such findings suggest that sex can serve as an alternative source of assurance of partner availability, even for individuals who would find it otherwise difficult to seek (avoidant) or feel assured of (anxious) this availability in other aspects of their relationship. Little, K.C., McNulty, J.K., & Russell, V.M. (2010) Sex buffers intimates against the negative implications of attachment insecurity. *Personality and Social Psychology Bulletin*, 36(4), 484–98.

[300] Birnbaum, G.E., Mikulincer, M., Szepsenwol, O., Shaver, P.R., & Mizrahi, M. (2014) When sex goes wrong: a behavioral systems perspective on individual differences in sexual attitudes, motives, feelings, and behaviors. *Journal of Personality and Social Psychology*, 106(5), 822–42.

[301] Szepsenwol, O., Mikulincer, M., & Birnbaum, G.E. (2013) Misguided attraction: the contribution of normative and individual-differences components of the sexual system to mating preferences. *Journal of Research in Personality* 47, 196–200, p.197.

[302] Ibid.

Deactivation is a strategy that entails reduced striving for sexual access, in the service of avoiding rejections that might further reduce the fragile sexual availability of the partner. Other behavioural systems may then have a relatively greater role in shaping decision-making regarding partners, including appraisals regarding the need for or meaning of sex.

Where hyperactivation and deactivation are low, the researchers proposed that the 'primary strategy' of the sexual system will entail communication of sexual interest with sensitivity to partner signals and context. This suggests the potential for some bidirectional causal links between secure adult attachment and the primary strategy of the sexual system, though the links will depend on the cultural and social factors that shape perceptions of the relational meaning of sexual interest and activities.[303] However, the relationship between the sexual and attachment behavioural systems can be expected to vary substantially by life-stage. In adolescence and early adulthood, characteristically, sexual interactions with partners may be sought without the expectation of the partner becoming a secure base. The sexual encounter may offer instead an opportunity for a cocktail of other social and psychological processes, including the exploration of identity, gender, personal values, power, and status. It may also provide a temporary safe haven.[304] Furthermore, Birnbaum and colleagues have also argued that causal links between individual differences in the attachment and sexual behavioural systems may be moderated by the context. For example, the conditions of success or failure of the sexual system may contribute especially to schemas regarding the availability of partners during periods when certainty regarding the relationship is low: in the early months of a relationship or following serious conflicts or separations.[305]

Birnbaum, Mikulincer, and colleagues examined the association between the SSFS and the ECR in two samples of undergraduates. There was a robust association between ECR attachment anxiety and SSFS hyperactivation ($r = .52, .57$). Both reflect concerns about the availability of intimacy and about the partner as a safe haven who can offer regulation and satisfaction in the context of arousal; a substantial association was therefore anticipated. However, ECR attachment avoidance had a much weaker association with SSFS deactivation ($r = .28, .27$). It had at least as strong a correlation with SSFS hyperactivation ($r = .25, .38$).[306] An avoidant attachment style may at times be linked to the hyperactivation of the sexual system. This may be because sexuality can be made to serve as an alternative to or a substitution for intimacy, a tactic of a minimising attachment strategy.

The distinction between the sexual and attachment systems in adulthood suggests that they may have distinct networks of associations with other behaviours, beliefs, and experiences. In one study investigating the correlates of sexual system functioning, Birnbaum, Mikulincer, and colleagues showed undergraduate participants films of various people of the opposite sex, presented in the manner of a dating site. In examining their data for sexual

[303] Birnbaum, G.E., Mikulincer, M., Szepsenwol, O., Shaver, P.R., & Mizrahi, M. (2014) When sex goes wrong: a behavioral systems perspective on individual differences in sexual attitudes, motives, feelings, and behaviors. *Journal of Personality and Social Psychology*, 106(5), 822–42, p.823; Mizrahi, M., Hirschberger, G., Mikulincer, M., Szepsenwol, O., & Birnbaum, G.E. (2016) Reassuring sex: can sexual desire and intimacy reduce relationship-specific attachment insecurities? *European Journal of Social Psychology*, 46(4), 467–80.

[304] See also Collins, W.A. (2003) More than myth: the developmental significance of romantic relationships during adolescence. *Journal of Research on Adolescence*, 13(1), 1–24.

[305] Birnbaum, G.E. (2018) The fragile spell of desire: a functional perspective on changes in sexual desire across relationship development. *Personality and Social Psychology Review*, 22(2), 101–127.

[306] Birnbaum, G.E., Mikulincer, M., Szepsenwol, O., Shaver, P.R., & Mizrahi, M. (2014) When sex goes wrong: a behavioral systems perspective on individual differences in sexual attitudes, motives, feelings, and behaviors. *Journal of Personality and Social Psychology*, 106(5), 822–42.

hyperactivation, the researchers found that these were moderated by gender. Among men, hyperactivation was associated with greater reported interest in relatively less-attractive women. Among women, hyperactivation was associated with more interest in relatively more-attractive men. Birnbaum and colleagues interpreted these findings as suggesting that hyperactivation and deactivation represent conditional strategies, part of the human evolutionary repertoire. Where sexual access was uncertain for women, in human evolutionary history reproductive success would have been increased by focusing attention on healthy mates to ensure successful offspring. By contrast, where sexual access was uncertain for men, the equivalent strategy to increase reproductive success would have been to reduce the standards used for assessing prospective mates. In a replication study, effects remained significant when controlling for scores on the ECR, supporting the autonomy of sexuality as a distinct behavioural system and the incremental validity of the SSFS hyperactivation scale.[307]

The distinctive predictive power of the SSFS deactivation scale was also demonstrated in a later study by Szepsenwol, Mizrahi, and Birnbaum:[308] 62 couples who had recently begun dating completed the ECR and SSFS at four-month interviews on three occasions, alongside self-report measures of relationship satisfaction. Birnbaum and colleagues found that an individual's report of SSFS deactivation was associated with their report of lower relationship satisfaction early in the relationship: this effect continued throughout the first year among participants whose partner had an avoidant attachment style, but disappeared among participants whose partner did not have an avoidant attachment style. Birnbaum and colleagues interpreted this finding in light of the idea that, though sexuality remains powerful and relevant, in many couples relationship satisfaction comes over time to rest more on the attachment system.[309] By the end of the first year, this permits relationship security to compensate for potential sexual system deactivation in providing happiness in the relationship.

Overall, Birnbaum, Mikulincer, and colleagues' work on the sexual behavioural system has represented the most sustained attempt to flesh out Bowlby's early, and unfinished, characterisation, and respond to Ainsworth's call for further inquiry. There has been healthy interest in what is still a relatively new model and self-report scale from within the wider area of relationship psychology. Predictably perhaps, the SSFS and surrounding theory has generally been ignored by researchers in the developmental tradition of attachment research, even those with a central concern with sexuality such as Fonagy. Nonetheless, a comparison of Birnbaum, Mikulincer, and colleagues' account of the sexual behavioural system and that of Main can offer an indication of the contribution of this work to attachment theory.

Main took the concept of conditional strategies from ethological discussions of mating behaviour. The diverse repertoires of animal behaviour that can contribute to reproductive success formed the model for Main's theory of repertoires of infant behaviour that promote survival (Chapter 3). Avoidance was theorised to be a 'cut-off' behaviour in the manner of Chance, used to maintain regulation and circumvent an approach–avoidance conflict by minimising attention to the stimuli provoking this conflict. Ambivalent/resistant attachment was conceptualised through Trivers as an intensification of signals to the caregiver of

---

[307] Ibid. p.835.

[308] Szepsenwol, O., Mizrahi, M., & Birnbaum, G.E. (2015) Fatal suppression: the detrimental effects of sexual and attachment deactivation within emerging romantic relationships. *Social Psychological and Personality Science*, 6(5), 504–512.

[309] See also Birnbaum, G.E. & Finkel, E.J. (2015) The magnetism that holds us together: sexuality and relationship maintenance across relationship development. *Current Opinion in Psychology*, 1, 29–33.

the need to attend to the child, achieved through a perceptual vigilance regarding signals that might suggest the caregiver's unavailability. Both conditional strategies were anticipated at species level to increase the odds of infant survival when confidence is not possible in the caregiver's availability. Birnbaum, Mikulincer, and colleagues' account of the sexual system likewise described three different pathways to sexual access to the partner. The role of attentional vigilance is also highlighted in their account, though it seems to be a contributor rather than the essence of the maximising strategy as for Main.

The exact relationship between sexual behavioural repertoires and evolutionary success seems unstable and somewhat muted in the work of Birnbaum, Mikulincer, and colleagues. The social psychologists have only relatively recently stabilised 'sexual access' as the set-goal of the sexual behavioural system. However, an additional contributing factor may have been the tendency in the work of Shaver and Mikulincer to lose track of the distinction between two of Tinbergen's four questions (Chapter 1), regarding the expected proximal and the evolutionary outcome of a behaviour sequence. The researchers have moved from reproductive success to sexual access as the set-goal of the sexual behavioural system, but without fully articulating the relationship between sexuality and reproduction, or between individual motivation and species-level behavioural repertoires. The inattention to the affective components of behavioural systems inherited from Bowlby has proven a hindrance here, since this might have prompted further attention to both individual-level motivations and the evolutionary basis of behavioural repertoires. For instance, the contribution of a deactivation of the sexual system to the achievement of either sexual access or reproductive success is both undertheorised and empirically unexamined. At the same time, the qualities of sexuality as at times insistent, disquieting, and above all polyvalent, which make this aspect of human life both uncomfortably personal and uncomfortably social, have yet to be adequately examined.[310]

Nonetheless, the efforts of Birnbaum, Mikulincer, and colleagues to describe the sexual behavioural system represent a major advance. With the exception of sexual abuse as a kind of trauma, Main did not further discuss sexual and/or reproductive behaviour in her writings after applying the concept of conditional strategies to infant behaviour. By contrast, Birnbaum, Mikulincer, and colleagues have provided evidence that concern about the availability of sexual access and hyperactivation of the wish to achieve it is associated in anticipated ways with concern about the availability of a safe haven and hyperactivation of the wish to achieve it. They have also shown that, though correlated, the two phenomena are not reducible to one another and have distinct correlates. It is easy to imagine that Bowlby would have been pleased by such findings, as evidence against the tendency he disliked in the psychoanalytic theory of his day to treat sexual and relational motivations as interchangeable.

Dominance

Whereas the sexual behavioural system was already described, if briefly, by Bowlby, an innovation made by Shaver and Mikulincer has been the introduction of a 'dominance' behavioural system. Though not discussed as a behavioural system, the concept of a behavioural

---

[310] Target, M. (2015) A developmental model of sexual excitement, desire and alienation. In A. Lemma & P.E. Lynch (eds) *Sexualities* (pp.43–62). London: Karnac.

repertoire associated with dominance can be found already in Bowlby's reports from ethology. For instance, in *Attachment, Volume 1*, Bowlby discussed ethological observations indicating that dominance could be recruited in the service of the caregiving system in nonhuman primates. Dominance behaviours were described as those that signal the availability of coercion, or violence if pushed, if deference is not provided. Bowlby described 'the important observation that when a dominant male senses a predator or other danger he commonly threatens or even attacks a juvenile that unwarily approaches the danger spot. The dominant male's behaviour, by frightening the juvenile, elicits the juvenile's attachment behaviour. As a result the juvenile seeks the proximity of an adult animal, as often as not that of the very male that frightened it; and by so doing the juvenile also removes itself from the danger.'[311] However, beyond characterising dominance as a behavioural repertoire with links to other systems such as caregiving and attachment, as well as aggression, Bowlby did not give attention to the topic. Though strongly interested in questions of power and domination in his early work before the development of attachment theory, from the 1950s onwards he tended to consider the world from the point of view of the infant attachment system.[312] Dominance therefore became relevant only insofar as it impacted the caregiving system. As Smith and Connelly astutely observed, in Bowlby's importation of ethology into child development, the concepts of dominance and territory were both left behind, albeit for different reasons.[313]

Shaver's first sustained consideration of the topic of dominance appeared in his writings on the concept of 'narcissism', which were prompted by his longstanding interest in the relationship between self-concept and affectionate relationships with others, though also by the wider context of interest in personality disorders within social psychology. In 'Shamed into self-love: dynamics, roots, and functions of narcissism' from 2001, Robins, Tracy, and Shaver argued that there are two paths to getting ahead in life, 'through exerting influence over others and through accomplishments'.[314] Here the researchers referred to a 'getting-ahead orientation' to achieve influence and accomplishments, fuelled by 'the power and achievement motives'.[315] They speculated that these motives may operate quite widely. Usually they are moderated by or combine with affiliative motives, so that the wielding of power and the attainment of achievements are either in the service of some others or at least not at their expense. However, Robins, Tracy, and Shaver speculated that where the goals of the attachment system have been chronically unmet, one response may be the recruitment of the 'getting-ahead orientation' in the service of attachment. This, they proposed, may be the origins of the spectrum towards 'narcissistic personality disorder'. Minimising and maximising strategies are premised on the expectation that at least a conditional availability of attachment figures can be achieved in this way. By contrast, a temperamental predisposition towards aggression or irritability may predispose self-assertion as a kind of 'tertiary strategy' to coercing the notice and recognition of others, and sometimes perhaps their availability: 'According to our reasoning, the search for love and affection could not have worked under the childhood

[311] Bowlby, J. (1969, 1982) *Attachment*. London: Penguin, p.227.
[312] Bowlby, J. (1946) Psychology and democracy. *The Political Quarterly*, 17(1), 61–76; Mayhew, B. (2006) Between love and aggression: the politics of John Bowlby. *History of the Human Sciences*, 19(4), 19–35.
[313] Smith, P.K. & Connolly, K. (1972) Patterns of play and social interaction in pre-school children. In N. Blurton Jones (ed.) *Ethological Studies of Child Behaviour* (pp.65–96). Cambridge: Cambridge University Press, p.68.
[314] Robins, R.W., Tracy, J.L., & Shaver, P.R. (2001) Shamed into self-love: dynamics, roots, and functions of narcissism. *Psychological Inquiry*, 12(4), 230–36.
[315] Ibid. p.233.

conditions that fostered narcissism, particularly if the developing narcissist was temperamentally aggressive and irritable. Given these constraints, narcissists were, in a sense, correct to have pursued a more assertive, self-promoting strategy.[316]

In 2011, Shaver and Mikulincer returned to these considerations, introducing the concept of a 'power behavioural system'. They argued that the set-goal of the power system is to 'remove threats and obstacles that interfere with a person's sense of power'.[317] They proposed 'felt power' as the set-goal for the power system. Their proposal was explicitly modelled on 'felt security' as the set-goal of the attachment system according to Sroufe and Waters.[318] At first glance, this might appear to be a set-goal solely at the individual level, rather than the achievement of a particular self–environment relationship. However, Shaver and Mikulincer defined 'felt power' as the sense that one can control the environment to have one's needs met 'without undue social interference'.[319] In a sense, 'felt power' might be regarded as another contributory to the 'security metasystem' theorised by Shaver in his earlier work with Hart and Goldenberg. Like attachment, self-esteem, and cultural meaning, the sense that the environment can be controlled to meet one's needs may form one contributory factor to a sense of felt security.[320]

Shaver and Milulincer proposed that the primary strategy of the power system is to see felt power in a manner commensurate with the aims of other behavioural systems. Indeed, they suggested that 'power often facilitates the smooth operation of other behavioral systems, such as exploration, caregiving, and sex'.[321] For instance, control over the environment may be sought in order to ensure that the needs of other people can be met, perhaps with the power system operating in the service of caregiving or with power prompting the feeling of responsibility for dependents. However, in the context of repeated failures to predictably achieve felt power, feelings of fear and helplessness may instead be evoked. Then a maximising or minimising strategy will be brought online. Shaver, Sagev, and Mikulincer proposed that hyperactivation of the power behavioural system will occur when an individual experiences concern about the availability of sufficient control over their environment to ensure that their needs are met. The hyperactivation of the power system leads to increased vigilance regarding threats or obstacles to control of the environment to ensure that one's needs can be met. This is fuelled by both 'an excessive urge to gain power and an extreme fear

---

[316] Ibid. p.234. The potential for tertiary strategies is not discussed explicitly by Shaver and colleagues. However, the existence of tertiary strategies or minor secondary strategies is suggested by Mikulincer and Shaver's claim that anxiety and avoidance are the 'major', not only, secondary strategies, e.g. Mikulincer, M. & Shaver, P.R. (2012) Attachment theory expanded: a behavioral systems approach to personality. In K. Deaux & M. Snyder (eds) *Oxford Handbook of Personality and Social Psychology* (pp.467–92). Oxford: Oxford University Press. Mary Main and Erik Hesse, personal communication, August 2019, have agreed that controlling or dominant behaviour may be a 'tertiary' strategy if primary and conditional strategies fail. However, they would not term this a 'conditional strategy' since this is a technical term from ethology to refer to behavioural repetoires made available by human evolution for the purpose of survival. Dominance behaviour could be such a repertoire, but they are not sure and would regard a cross-species review as necessary for addressing the question.

[317] Shaver, P.R., Segev, M., & Mikulincer, M. (2011) A behavioral systems perspective on power and aggression. In P.R. Shaver & M. Mikulincer (eds) *Human Aggression and Violence: Causes, Manifestations, and Consequences* (pp.71–87). Washington, DC: American Psychological Association, p.75.

[318] Mikulincer, M. & Shaver, P.R. (2011) Attachment, anger, and aggression. In P.R. Shaver & M. Mikulincer (eds) *Human Aggression and Violence: Causes, Manifestations, and Consequences* (pp.241–57). Washington, DC: American Psychological Association, p.250.

[319] Ibid.

[320] Cf. Bauman, Z. (2001) *Community: Seeking Safety in an Insecure World*. Cambridge: Polity Press.

[321] Mikulincer, M. & Shaver, P.R. (2012) Attachment theory expanded: a behavioral systems approach to personality. In K. Deaux & M. Snyder (eds) *Oxford Handbook of Personality and Social Psychology* (pp.467–92). Oxford: Oxford University Press, p.476.

of failure', a combination that 'results in chronic activation of the power system, even when there is no imminent threat or actual damage to one's power; an indiscriminate urge to assert power over others; frequent anger and hostility toward others (who are viewed as potential rivals); and a proclivity to attack others following minimal or ambiguous signs of competition or provocation'.[322] Other concerns, including attachment and exploration, are therefore regularly suppressed.

Shaver, Sagev, and Mikulincer's account of deactivation of the power system was quite different to their account of deactivation of the attachment or sexual behavioural systems. Whereas deactivation of the attachment or sexual systems entails reduced acknowledgment of stimuli that might activate the behavioural system, Shaver and colleagues argued that deactivation of the power system entails a heightened sensitivity to threats, much like hyperactivation of the system. However, even minimal threats are interpreted as prompting submissive, coy, or self-abasing behaviours. What are avoided are contexts that would call for an assertion of rights and opinions, including conflicts with others.[323] Gentleness is pressed into service, perhaps even deformed at times into a mode of submission or conciliation, rather than functioning as an expression of tenderness or of care. Shaver and colleagues developed the Power Behavioural System Scale to assess maximising and minimising of the power system. As predicted, both hyperactivation and deactivation of the power system were negatively associated with other existing self-report measures of feelings of power.[324] Hyperactivation of the power system had a moderate positive association with both attachment anxiety and avoidance; deactivation of the power system was moderately associated with attachment anxiety.

In an observational study of 100 dating couples, Shaver, Sagev, and Mikulincer asked participants to discuss a live problem in their relationship. Hyperactivation of the power system predicted greater displays of hostility and distress to the partner, whereas deactivation predicted greater displays of submissiveness and distress to the partner. Both dimensions were associated with difficulties for the couple in engaging in a constructive discussion of the problem. These associations held when controlling for attachment anxiety and avoidance, and for neuroticism.[325] In another study, Mikulincer and Shaver found that priming for a feeling of powerfulness led to greater feelings of optimism when participants were low on attachment anxiety, suggesting that the attachment anxiety interfered with the capacity to use felt power as a basis for felt security. They also found that the same prime led to greater objectification of others when participants were high on attachment avoidance. They interpreted this finding as suggesting that the feeling of connectedness and security associated with low attachment avoidance could counteract the potential for felt power to lead to haughtiness about others.[326] Such findings suggest that the power system scale has expectable correlates in behaviour and perception, offering support for the new scale.

---

[322] Shaver, P.R., Segev, M., & Mikulincer, M. (2011) A behavioral systems perspective on power and aggression. In P.R. Shaver & M. Mikulincer (eds) *Human Aggression and Violence: Causes, Manifestations, and Consequences* (pp.71–87). Washington, DC: American Psychological Association, p.77.

[323] Ibid. p.78.

[324] Ibid. p.80–81.

[325] Ibid. p.84.

[326] Mikulincer, M. & Shaver, P.R. (2011) Attachment, anger, and aggression. In P.R. Shaver & M. Mikulincer (eds) *Human Aggression and Violence: Causes, Manifestations, and Consequences* (pp. 241–57). Washington, DC: American Psychological Association, p.253.

Shaver, Sagev, and Mikulincer were also pleased to report that 'as intended, the correlation between the hyperactivation and deactivation scores was not statistically significant, $r(360) = .07$'.[327] Yet it is not clear why hyperactivation and deactivation of the power system were assumed to be unrelated, rather than negatively associated. In principle, submissive behaviour and hyperactivated power behaviour would seem to be opposites, rather than unrelated. The implication is that Shaver and Mikulincer believed that individuals who display submissive behaviour to others when they feel threatened are no more or less likely to display dominant behaviour when they feel threatened than the rest of the population, and vice versa.[328] In fact, the idea of a two-dimensional space defined by orthogonal variables seems rather to have been pressed into service from the ECR as a criterion of the validity of new scales of behavioural systems for Shaver and Mikulincer, without the presentation of a theoretical justification for why all behavioural systems should have this structure. Gillath, Karantzas, and Fraley have suggested that the idea of orthogonality of attachment dimensions was never justified: it originates, they suggest, in part from a misreading of Bowlby's statement in *Separation* about the 'independence' of concepts of self and other.[329]

The concept of the power behavioural system is unquestionably an advance on the awkwardly named 'getting-ahead orientation' from Shaver's earlier work. However, the power behavioural system is on much less firmer footing than, for instance, their more recent work on the sexual behavioural system. One problem is that the relationship between dominance and aggression remained poorly soldered down in Shaver and Mikulincer's account, and the two elements rattle about audibly against one another. Shaver and Mikulincer highlighted the importance of the 'feeling of anger, which in our view is an emotional signature of power-system activation'.[330] And they have often described anger in general as linked to the power system. However, it remains unclear whether all assertions of power require anger. For instance, considering Shaver's earlier remarks, the use of achievements and successes to claim glory and influence do not seem overtly aggressive. Conversely, it is not clear that all assertions of anger are linked to the power system. The secure infant's protest on the departure of the caregiver in the Strange Situation may be angry, but this is presumably before the power behavioural system has been assembled. The relationship between the power system and the fear behavioural system is also opaque. Exactly the submissive or coy behaviours that Shaver and Mikulincer suggest characterise the deactivation of the power system were regarded by Ainsworth and Bretherton as an effect of the simultaneous activation of the fear and affiliative systems.[331] Other attachment theorists such as Crittenden and Hilburn-Cobb have

[327] Shaver, P.R., Segev, M., & Mikulincer, M. (2011) A behavioral systems perspective on power and aggression. In P.R. Shaver & M. Mikulincer (eds) *Human Aggression and Violence: Causes, Manifestations, and Consequences* (pp.71–87). Washington, DC: American Psychological Association, p.81.

[328] It is possible that passive-aggressive behaviour is an example of the two dimensions coming together; though if so, then this raises the question of how anxiety, passivity, and aggression interrelate. Anxious attachment in Shaver and Mikulincer's account emphasised only one of the three components of Ainsworth's category, and left to the side aggression and/or passivity. Ainsworth explicitly characterised Group C infants as passive-aggressive in correspondence, e.g. Ainsworth, M. (1967) *Letter to John Bowlby*, 17 October 1967. PP/Bow/K.4/12. However, it could well be that this is not the kind of conjunction of passivity and aggression/coercion that Shaver and Mikulincer have in mind.

[329] Gillath, O., Karantzas, G.C., & Fraley, R.C. (2016) *Adult Attachment: A Concise Introduction to Theory and Research*. London: Academic Press, p.120.

[330] Shaver, P.R., Segev, M., & Mikulincer, M. (2011) A behavioral systems perspective on power and aggression. In P.R. Shaver & M. Mikulincer (eds) *Human Aggression and Violence: Causes, Manifestations, and Consequences* (pp.71–87). Washington, DC: American Psychological Association, p.76.

[331] Bretherton, I. & Ainsworth, M.D.S. (1974) Responses of one-year-olds to a stranger in a strange situation. In M. Lewis & L. A. Rosenblum (eds) *Origins of Fear* (pp.131–64). New York: Wiley.

conceptualised submissive behaviour as an independent behavioural response that can be brought into the service of attachment strategies, rather than as a minimisation of the dominance system.[332] Of course, several pathways could be possible, but the rationale for considering submissive behaviour as characterising the 'deactivation' of the system remains both underdeveloped and rather out of keeping with Shaver and Mikulincer's general characterisation of the minimising strategy for a behavioural system. It may be suspected that Shaver and Mikulincer may have conflated deactivation of the dominance system with the operation of two further distinct behavioural systems discussed by contemporary ethologists: the reconciliation system and the submission system.[333]

Secondly, it is unclear whether the power behavioural system is even a behavioural system by Shaver and Mikulincer's own definition. Shaver and Mikulincer have generally drawn their concepts about behavioural systems through an expansion of behavioural repertoires already described by ethology, such as attachment, caregiving, and sexuality. However, in other cases some link to a behavioural repertoire has been retained, permitting Shaver and Mikulincer to toggle backwards and forwards between specific behaviours and more general observations about how adults feel, respond, and create symbolic meanings about one another. By contrast, in the case of the power behavioural system, the link between the narrow behavioural focus of ethology and the broad terms of social psychology appears to have unspooled. By Shaver and Mikulincer's own definition, a behavioural system is a repertoire of functionally equivalent behaviours made available by evolution, with activating and terminating conditions, which would have the expectable outcome at a species-level of achieving a particular kind of change in the relationship between individual and environment. This definition retained the fundamental concern of ethology with repertoires of functionally equivalent behaviours made available by evolution. Yet it is difficult to describe assertion of 'power' as a distinct behavioural repertoire made available by evolution. Perhaps for this reason, at some points Shaver and Mikulincer have referred to the 'dominance behavioural system', which then offers a link back to ethology and a specific and observable behavioural repertoire.[334]

Overall, Shaver and Mikulincer's account of the power behavioural system seems to be still a little sketched in and shaggy. It has been discussed mainly in speculative book chapters rather than peer-review articles, generating only limited commentary to date by other scholars.[335] And though the scales for the caregiving and sexual systems appear in Milkulincer and Shaver's *Attachment in Adulthood*, situated as the capstone of their professional labours, the scale for measuring hyperactivation and deactivation of the power system does not feature. There is in fact no explicit mention of the power behavioural system in

[332] Crittenden, P.M. (1995) Attachment and psychopathology. In S. Goldberg, R. Muir, & J. Kerr (eds) *John Bowlby's Attachment Theory: Historical, Clinical and Social Significance* (pp.367–406). New York: Analytical Press; Hilburn-Cobb, C. (2004) Adolescent psychopathology in terms of multiple behavioral systems. In L. Atkinson & S. Goldberg (eds) *Attachment Issues in Psychopathology and Intervention* (pp.95–135). Mahwah, NJ: Lawrence Erlbaum.

[333] Verbeek, P. & de Waal, F.B. (2001) Peacemaking among preschool children. *Peace and Conflict: Journal of Peace Psychology*, 7(1), 5–28; Kutsukake, N. & Clutton-Brock, T.H. (2008) Do meerkats engage in conflict management following aggression? Reconciliation, submission and avoidance. *Animal Behaviour*, 75(4), 1441–53.

[334] Mikulincer, M. & Shaver, P.R. (2011) Attachment, anger, and aggression. In P.R. Shaver & M. Mikulincer (eds) *Human Aggression and Violence: Causes, Manifestations, and Consequences* (pp.241–57). Washington, DC: American Psychological Association, p.250. See also Leedom, L.J. (2014) Human social behavioral systems: ethological framework for a unified theory. *Human Ethology Bulletin*, 29(1), 39–65.

[335] An exception is Overall, N.C. (2019) Attachment insecurity and power regulation in intimate relationships. *Current Opinion in Psychology*, 25, 53–8.

the enormous book.[336] Nonetheless, their work on the power behavioural system has been an interesting line of inquiry, continuing Bowlby's interest in dominance behaviour within the ethological literature. Not least, the self-report measure of hyperactivation of the power system is thought-provoking as the only measure of a non-clinical phenomenon mentioned by Shaver and Mikulincer with a powerful positive association with both attachment anxiety and avoidance. Sexual system deactivation is likewise associated with both attachment anxiety and avoidance, but the association is weaker than for deactivation of the power behavioural system.[337]

Religion

Attachment to God

Submission and supplication, the deactivation of the power system, has also featured in another aspect of Shaver's work. In a collaboration with Lee Kirkpatrick, a doctoral student from the University of Denver, Shaver developed a concern with the psychology of religion in the 1980s,[338] a subdiscipline that had seen rapid growth in the late 1970s.[339] In a paper from 1985, Shaver and Kirkpatrick emphasised the importance of submissive behaviour as a fundamental aspect of religious life. Through such behaviour 'the influencer advertises his or her helplessness and dependence in order to solicit sympathy and assistance. It is easy to see how these ideas might be applied to the process of prayer, in which the human petitioner can often be found to heap praise on the deity and offer various concessions (ingratiation), and to reaffirm one's inferiority and dependence while entreating God for help and guidance (supplication)'.[340] Shaver and Kirkpatrick were interested that ingratiation and supplication appeared to be a lowering of the self in order to achieve the beneficence of a deity. However, practices of submission and supplication might have only a short-term effect on the feeling of a deity as beneficent. Longer-term beneficence may need to be based on a longer-term positive relationship. The researchers found that stable images of religious figures as benevolent

---

[336] Some relevant behaviours are mentioned on page 154 of the 2010 edition and page 150 of the 2016 edition: 'avoidant people often entertain fantasies of perfection and power, exaggerate their achievements and talents, and avoid situations that challenge their defences and threaten their grandiosity'. However, no mention is made of the power behavioural system, or Mikulincer and Shaver's own data discussed above, published by 2011, showing that hyperactivation of the power system is moderately associated with both avoidance and anxiety. Such findings would rather qualify the characterisation of 'avoidant people' in general.

[337] This is discussed in Birnbaum, G.E., Mikulincer, M., Szepsenwol, O., Shaver, P.R., & Mizrahi, M. (2014) When sex goes wrong: a behavioral systems perspective on individual differences in sexual attitudes, motives, feelings, and behaviors. *Journal of Personality and Social Psychology*, 106(5), 822–42.

[338] As well as working with Shaver, Kirkpatrick was also influenced by Bernard Spilka at Denver, a leading figure in the emergent specialism and president of Division 36 (1985–86). Spilka, B., Shaver, P., & Kirkpatrick, L.A. (1985) A general attribution theory for the psychology of religion. *Journal for the Scientific Study of Religion*, 24, 1–20.

[339] The growth of psychology of religion in America reflected wider public interest in religious identities and movements, in the context of substantial sociological change. Marty, M.E. (1985) Transpositions: American religion in the 1980s. *Annals of the American Academy of Political and Social Science*, 480(1), 11–23. The growing basis for psychology of religion as a subdiscipline was expressed in and further spurred on in the specific academic context by the founding of the American Psychological Division 36 'Psychology of Religion' in 1976. Paloutzian, R.F. (2017) *Invitation to the Psychology of Religion*, 3rd edn. New York: Guilford, Chapter 2.

[340] Spilka, B., Shaver, P., & Kirkpatrick, L.A. (1985) A general attribution theory for the psychology of religion. *Journal for the Scientific Study of Religion*, 24(1), 1–20, p.16.

were empirically associated with an individual's report of a supportive family during their childhood.[341] This suggested to the researchers a potential link between attachment and the psychology of religious belief and religious practices.

In the 1980s, there was a strong tendency in the academic psychology of religion to explicitly or implicitly model religious experience on Christian faith and practice. Shaver and Kirkpatrick did tend in this direction at times.[342] However, right from the start Shaver's interest in Buddhism provided a counterweight. His first discussion of Buddhism in print was in a chapter for *Everywoman's Emotional Wellbeing*, a self-help guide for women published in 1986. Shaver and O'Connor cited the Tibetan Buddhist concept of *maitri*, 'unconditional friendliness toward oneself'. An attitude of *maitri*, Shaver and O'Connor proposed, puts aside grudges, hostility, rumination, and a sense of entitlement in the world. Whereas in his later work with Mikulincer, Shaver tended to think of deactivation of the power system in terms of submissiveness, in his remarks on Buddhism it is possible to see a different form of deactivation. Rather than an alternative strategy for achieving power, *maitri* signified for Shaver and O'Connor a relinquishment of the fight for power, 'along with the corresponding attitude of openness and trust toward others and toward nature'.[343]

Shaver and O'Connor commented that 'a common goal, according to Western psychology, is enhancement of one's feelings of control and self-esteem'.[344] However, rather than an inevitable aspect of human psychology, Shaver and O'Connor argued that this is an effect of how the human subject has been shaped and constructed within western culture. Dominance and submissive behaviours may be part of the human behavioural repertoire as a result of our evolutionary heritage. But the activation of these behaviours depends upon the perception that control or coercion is needed in order to have our needs met. Shaver contrasted this perception to an alternative one, which he associated with Buddhism, in which 'control of nature and emotion is devastating to life and ultimately impossible. Nature is the source and sustainer of life, and human feelings are one of its brightest creations'.[345] In the terms drawn from Shaver's later thinking with Hart and Goldenberg, it might be said that the security metasystem can be fed by different tributaries: among these, one is the assertion of self and a quest for control; another is a cultural/religious worldview in which striving for control is not ultimately beneficial to ensuring one's needs are met.

In the 1990s, Kirkpatrick and Shaver documented a number of aspects of religious experience that could be influenced by attachment style, focusing on Christian religious practices and beliefs in American undergraduate samples. Using the Hazan and Shaver 'love quiz', they found that sudden conversion experiences were almost exclusive to participants with an avoidant attachment style.[346] Indeed, nearly a third of participants with an avoidant attachment style in their sample reported having experienced a religious conversion. In interpreting this result it is worth keeping in mind, as mentioned in the section 'A first attempt', that

---

[341] Ibid. p.11.

[342] E.g. Kirkpatrick, L.A. & Shaver, P.R. (1990) Attachment theory and religion: childhood attachments, religious beliefs, and conversion. *Journal for the Scientific Study of Religion*, 29(3), 315–34: 'The most striking (and perhaps obvious) point of contact, simply stated, is that the God of most Christian traditions seems to correspond very closely to the idea of a secure attachment figure' (318).

[343] Shaver, P.R. & O'Connor, C. (1986) Coping with stress: problems in perspective. In C. Tavris (ed.) *Everywoman's Emotional Wellbeing* (pp.305–329). New York: Doubleday, p.326.

[344] Ibid. p.336.

[345] Ibid. p.327.

[346] Kirkpatrick, L.A. & Shaver, P.R. (1990) Attachment theory and religion: childhood attachments, religious beliefs, and conversion. *Journal for the Scientific Study of Religion*, 29, 315–34, p.326.

the 'love quiz' collapsed avoidance and fear regarding caregivers into one category. Another finding by Kirkpatrick and Shaver was that participants who endorsed an anxious/ambivalent attachment style on the 'love quiz' were distinctive in reporting experiences of speaking in tongues.[347] Participants were also asked to self-report their attachment style to God. Those that endorsed a secure attachment style also reported that they experience greater life satisfaction, less anxiety, loneliness, and depression, and less physical illness than other participants. These were also the correlates of a secure attachment style in romantic relationships. Kirkpatrick and Shaver found that the effects of the two attachment variables seemed to be additive: a secure attachment style in relation to both romantic partners and God had a stronger relationship with report of these positive experiences than a secure attachment only in one domain, and a secure attachment style in one domain was associated with more positive experiences than an insecure attachment style in both domains.

Ainsworth was apparently enthusiastic about Kirkpatrick and Shaver's work on attachment and religion.[348] However, critics have alleged that the idea of attachment to God was an overextension of the concept of 'attachment', with little resemblance to the prototype of infant behaviour. Granqvist, Shaver, and Mikulincer responded to this criticism.[349] They reported experimental studies that suggested that divine figures in particular, and religious practice in general, could serve as a safe haven in the context of distress, and to an extent as a secure base. Attachment to God could qualify as an attachment relationship on these grounds.[350] Additionally, they pointed to the role of proximity-seeking within (Christian) religious practice, such as going to church during life transitions; the role of language suggesting 'approaching God' within supplicatory prayer; as well as metaphors of 'separation from God' in imagining Hell or forms of punishment. This suggests symbolic forms of separation anxiety. Granqvist and colleagues also highlighted the conditions under which religious life may become especially salient: 'people are most likely to turn to God or other supernatural figures when they face situations that Bowlby (1982) believed activate the attachment system, such as illness, injury, or fatigue; frightening or alarming events; and separation or threat of separation from loved ones'.[351] Part of the problem faced by Granqvist, Shaver, and Mikulincer in defining the relationship between attachment and religion is that the former term has had both narrow and broad meanings since Bowlby (Chapter 1). In this sense, it would appear from their arguments that the conditions that activate the attachment system—*narrowly construed*—seem to elicit phenomena associated with the attachment system—*broadly construed*—within religious life, perhaps given the role of religious practice as a possible contributory to the security metasystem. Above all, it is perhaps the role of divine figures or the religious community as a kind of safe haven that provides the hinge between attachment broad and narrow.

[347] Kirkpatrick, L.A. & Shaver, P.R. (1992) An attachment-theoretical approach to romantic love and religious belief. *Personality and Social Psychology Bulletin*, 18(3), 266–75, p.266. See also Kirkpatrick, L.A. (2005) *Attachment, Evolution, and the Psychology of Religion*. New York: Guilford.

[348] Personal communication to Mary Main, cited in Granqvist, P. (2020) *Attachment, Religion, and Spirituality: A Wider View*. New York: Guilford.

[349] On a mutual interest in religion as one contributing factor to the Shaver–Mikulincer collaboration see Shaver, P.R. & Mikulincer, M. (2011) Analysis of a collaborative working relationship. *Relationship Research Newsletter*, 9(2), 7–9.

[350] Granqvist, P., Mikulincer, M., & Shaver, P.R. (2010) Religion as attachment: normative processes and individual differences. *Personality and Social Psychology Review*, 14(1), 49–59, p.50.

[351] Ibid. p.52. See also Granqvist, P. (2020) *Attachment, Religion, and Spirituality: A Wider View*. New York: Guilford.

Mindfulness

Though enthusiastic about the idea of attachment to God, Shaver retained his interest in forms of religious life without a personal God or supplicatory prayer. This interest was further fuelled by an invitation received by Shaver and Mikulincer in October 2004 to visit the Dali Lama, who had been interested by their work.[352] Following this experience, at the same time as their work with Granqvist, Shaver and Mikulincer developed a strand of empirical research exploring mindfulness practices. Mindfulness-oriented meditation techniques originally emerged within Buddhist religious life, but had become reformulated in the context of their transplantation into western wellness technique.[353] Shaver and colleagues situated themselves in terms of this secularising trend: 'American psychologists have lifted mindfulness out of this rich context (perhaps while attempting to separate it from religious considerations) and applied it in a more individualistic, less socially connected, and more ethically neutral way. In our opinion, placing mindfulness in an attachment-theoretical framework would allow it to benefit not only from additional kinds of empirical tests but also from an assortment of ethical, social, and developmental, yet not necessarily religious, concepts.'[354] The reception of mindfulness in terms of attachment theory would, Shaver and colleagues argued, contrast with the individualistic reception of mindfulness as a western wellness technique. Mindfulness would entail finding a safe haven in the representation of attachment figures, the Buddha, in the tradition's teachings, and in other members of the religious community:

> English-language books about Buddhist meditation make the process of mindful meditation seem rather solitary and asocial. During our discussions with the Dalai Lama in 2004, however, it was pointed out that one of the simplest and most frequently spoken Buddhist prayers is: "I take refuge in the Buddha, the Dharma, and the Sangha," which means (in our terms) the mental representation of the Buddha as a loving, compassionate, and wise teacher; the Buddha's teachings (dharma); and the community of fellow Buddhists (sangha). In other words, the key concept is "taking refuge," which is similar to Bowlby and Ainsworth's notion of using an attachment figure as a "safe haven" …
>
> In our conversations with the Dalai Lama, he said that a common form of cultivating *maitri* is to imagine, during meditation, experiencing love from someone who has deeply loved you, "such as your mother." We replied that "mother" might not always be a good choice if one's relationship with her in childhood was not comfortable. He said in that case one could imagine being loved by the Buddha, as in the common prayer, "I take refuge in the Buddha, the Dharma (the Buddha's teachings), and the Sangha (the community of fellow practitioners)".[355]

---

[352] Goodman, G.S. (2006) Attachment to attachment theory: a personal perspective on an attachment researcher. In M. Mikulincer & G.S. Goodman (eds) *Dynamics of Romantic Love: Attachment, Caregiving, and Sex* (pp.3–22). New York: Guilford.

[353] The extent and nature of this reformulation remains contested. See e.g. Shonin, E. (2016) This is not McMindfulness. *The Psychologist*, 29(2), 124–5.

[354] Shaver, P.R., Lavy, S., Saron, C.D., & Mikulincer, M. (2007) Social foundations of the capacity for mindfulness: an attachment perspective. *Psychological Inquiry*, 18, 264–71.

[355] Shaver, P.R., Mikulincer, M., Sahdra, B.K., & Gross, J.T. (2016) Attachment security as a foundation for kindness toward self and others. In K.W. Brown & M.R. Leary, (eds) *The Oxford Handbook of Hypo-Egoic Phenomena*, pp.223–42. Oxford: Oxford University Press, p.231.

Shaver and colleagues hypothesised that attachment anxiety and avoidance would be anticipated to disrupt the capacity for mindfulness. They drew upon a self-report scale for mindfulness developed by Baer and colleagues.[356] On the basis of a factor analysis of 112 items
from previous self-report mindfulness scales, Baer and colleagues had developed a scale with
five main factors which they termed 1) Nonreactivity to Inner Experience, 2) Observing/
Noticing/Attending to Sensations/Perceptions/Feelings, 3) Acting with Awareness,
4) Describing/Labelling with Words, and 5) Nonjudging of Experience. Shaver, Lavy, Saron,
and Mikulincer found that both an anxious and an avoidant attachment style made strong
unique contributions to scores on the mindfulness scale, and that the two attachment dimensions accounted for 42% of variance in total mindfulness.[357] In more detailed analysis,
Shaver and colleagues found that an anxious attachment style was negatively correlated with
non-reactivity to inner experience ($r = -.54$), acting with awareness ($r = -.46$), and nonjudging experiences ($r = .43$). These are factors that might be especially vulnerable to rumination. They found that the avoidant attachment style was negatively associated with all
of the factors of mindfulness. That is, unlike anxious attachment, avoidant attachment was
also associated with difficulties noticing sensation, and difficulties giving words to such sen-
sations even when they are noticed. These factors might be specifically vulnerable to the suppression of thoughts with content or associated affect related to attachment, characteristic
of the avoidant attachment style. Additionally, both attachment styles may hinder broaden-
and-build cycles, which Shaver and Mikulincer have theorised contribute to greater social
and personal resources that support regulation, and through this contribute to mindfulness.

The remarkably strong association between attachment style and the mindfulness scale
suggests a surprising degree of congruity, or even potential overlap, between the two variables. Like in earlier work disentangling neuroticism and the anxious attachment style,
the overlap between a secure attachment style and mindfulness will need to be worked out
in terms of their respective relationships with other variables, including observed behaviour and subjective phenomena such as self-compassion. Priming studies may also prove
important in articulating factors mediating the relationship between attachment style and
mindfulness.[358] However, the strong association between attachment style and mindfulness
also presents, as Sahdra and Shaver acknowledged, a fundamental conceptual question: 'We
encounter the paradox that "attachment security" or "secure attachment" is considered
ideal or optimal in a major stream of Western psychology, attachment theory, whereas the
ideal or optimal state in Buddhist psychology is called "nonattachment".[359] Yet the paradox
is an effect of two different technical uses of the term 'attachment'. There are many strands
of Buddhism, which makes generalisation difficult. Nonetheless, Sahdra and Shaver argued
that, by and large, the Buddhist concept of non-attachment suggests a lack of fixation on
mental representations of things in the world. This is not only compatible with connectedness with others and intimacy in relationships, but probably facilitates it. By contrast, non-
attachment in attachment theory means the lack of a discriminated and preferential intimate

---

[356] Baer, R.A., Smith, G.T., Hopkins, J., Krietemeyer, J., & Toney, L. (2006) Using self-report assessment methods
to explore facets of mindfulness. *Assessment*, 13(1), 27–45.

[357] Shaver, P.R., Lavy, S., Saron, C.D., & Mikulincer, M. (2007) Social foundations of the capacity for mindfulness: an attachment perspective. *Psychological Inquiry*, 18, 264–71, pp.269–70.

[358] E.g. Melen, S., Pepping, C.A., & O'Donovan, A. (2017) Social foundations of mindfulness: priming attachment anxiety reduces emotion regulation and mindful attention. *Mindfulness*, 8(1), 136–43.

[359] Sahdra, B.K., & Shaver, P.R. (2013) Comparing attachment theory and Buddhist psychology. *International
Journal for the Psychology of Religion*, 23(4), 282–93, p.287.

relationship with a person who might serve as safe base and secure haven. Lack of a secure base and safe haven may be anticipated to contribute to reduced flexibility in mental representations about relationships.

Adaptation

Shaver and Mikulincer's characterisation of religious life tends to give the impression that an insecure attachment style is always bad. In their writings, experiences that seem characteristic to certain forms of insecurity, such as conversion experiences or speaking in tongues, tend to be treated respectfully but as indirect signals of mental pathology. The same is true of their writings on adult romantic relationships. Like the majority of the developmental tradition of attachment research,[360] Shaver and Mikulincer have tended to regard insecurity as a developmental adaptation, with the potential for some short-term benefits in achieving the availability of attachment figures, but with long-term harms across all other domains. As Waters and colleagues have observed (Chapter 2), there has been a tendency among attachment researchers to assume that 'all good things go together', based on positive associations with the word 'security' rather than precise knowedge of the psychological process actually under scrutiny, which may have advantages in some domains, no effect in others, and drawbacks under certain circumstances.[361] At times, Shaver and Mikulincer too have acknowledged the problem. For instance, in a 2006 epilogue in an edited volume celebrating his work, Shaver wrote that 'to insist on a model of perfect security, rather than a model that acknowledges human complexity, depth and intrapsychic conflicts and tensions is bound to be misleading and perhaps even dangerous ... In the attachment field we are so accustomed to glorifying secure attachment that we rarely stop to wonder why there aren't more saints in the world.'[362]

Shaver's observation is in part self-criticism. There are many occasions where decisions in research design or interpretation made by Shaver and collaborators seem to have been shaped by a 'glorification' of security. For instance, in a 1996 paper Mehr and Shaver described personal inconsistency across contexts as a positive quality.[363] Certainly it can be.

---

[360] E.g. Juffer, F., Struis, E., Werner, C., & Bakermans-Kranenburg, M.J. (2017) Effective preventive interventions to support parents of young children: illustrations from the Video-feedback Intervention to promote Positive Parenting and Sensitive Discipline (VIPP-SD). *Journal of Prevention & Intervention in the Community*, 45(3), 202–214: 'Secure attachment relationships are essential for children's current and later development' (202).

[361] Waters, E., Corcoran, D., & Anafarta, M. (2005) Attachment, other relationships, and the theory that all good things go together. *Human Development*, 48(1–2), 80–84.

[362] Shaver, P.R. (2006) Dynamics of romantic love: comments, questions, and future directions. In M. Mikulincer & G.S. Goodman (eds) *Dynamics of Romantic Love: Attachment, Caregiving, and Sex* (pp.423–56). New York: Guilford, pp.426–7. An illustrative case appears in Cooper, M.L., Shaver, P.R., & Collins, N.L. (1998) Attachment styles, emotion regulation, and adjustment in adolescence. *Journal of Personality and Social Psychology*, 74(5), 1380–97: 'Results of our mediation analyses provide further support for the distinctiveness of the three types by raising the possibility that unique constellations of underlying processes account for the differential involvement of the three attachment groups in risky or problematic behaviors. Evidence supporting the distinctiveness of these profiles and, in particular, differences between the two insecure groups should help to mitigate concerns that attachment style differences can be summarized along a single good–bad, or secure–insecure dimension' (1394). Here, the researchers distanced themselves from the idea that security–insecurity is the same as good–bad. However, their argument was that 'bad' divides into two distinct categories. They did not contest that security is equivalent to 'good'.

[363] Mehr, D.G. & Shaver, P.R. (1996) Goal structures in creative motivation. *Journal of Creative Behavior*, 30(2), 77–104, p.81.

However, at least from the way that the paper is written, the interpretation seems at least in part shaped by the fact that this quality was associated with a secure attachment style. If it had been associated with insecure attachment style, it is easy to imagine that the opposite evaluation could have been made of the same quality, with speculations regarding how emotion dysregulation or the lack of a safe base can disrupt the consistency of identity across contexts. To take another example, in a 2000 paper Mikulincer and Sheffi found that participants endorsing a secure attachment style were more likely in a cognitive test to miscategorise poor exemplars of types as similar. This finding was interpreted positively as indicating the expansiveness and freedom permitted by the feeling of having a secure base. However, if the finding had been reversed, security could easily have been praised as contributing to greater discrimination and discernment.[364]

Part of the trouble in achieving effective consideration of the issue has been carelessness by attachment researchers in the use of the term 'adaptation', a problem already identified by Ainsworth in an unpublished conference paper at the International Conference on Infant Studies in 1984.[365] Following Hinde and other ethological researchers (Chapter 1), Ainsworth expressed concern that the term 'adaptation' represented a twig-thicket of different meanings. She acknowledged that, in using the term, she and other attachment researchers had hindered effective discussion and even at times misled readers. On the one hand, 'adaptation' could refer to processes at a species level, in identifying a behavioural system or trait as contributing to survival or reproduction. On the other hand, 'adaptation' could refer to an individual level, identifying a behaviour or trait as responsive to the available rewards and punishments of the immediate environment.[366] However, Ainsworth observed a third meaning of the concept: 'In the developmental mental health sense the focus is on how individual differences in development, and on evaluation of how well or how poorly such development equips the individual to cope with the impact of the environment in which he lives.'[367] What distinguished this third meaning of the concept from the second was that an evaluation was entailed. The second meaning was merely an acknowledgement that an individual may 'adapt' to their circumstances. Ainsworth's third meaning was to identify 'adaptation' as the capacity to thrive in the long term in some way within those circumstances.

The subtlety and complexity of Ainsworth's argument may have contributed to her decision not to attempt to publish the article, despite its popularity with students and collaborators.[368] Ainsworth's argument was that individual adaptation (long-term thriving) may

---

[364] Mikulincer, M. & Sheffi, E. (2000) Adult attachment style and cognitive reactions to positive affect: a test of mental categorization and creative problem solving. *Motivation and Emotion*, 24(3), 149–74.

[365] Ainsworth, M. (1984) Attachment, adaptation and continuity. Paper presented at International Conference on Infant Studies, April 1984. PP/Bow/J.1/57.

[366] Ibid.: 'In the phylogenetic or evolutionary sense adaptation implies that in the course of natural selection those behaviours that yield survival advantage in the environment in which the evolutionary changes are taking place become part of the behavioural repertoire characteristic of a species ... In the ontogenetic sense adaptation refers to the process through which an organism adjusts to its environment in the course of development.'

[367] Ibid. An explicit scale for the extent to which an individual's behaviour appears adaptive, in this sense, would later be developed by Steele, H., Steele, M., & Kriss, A. (2009) *The Friends and Family Interview (FFI) Coding Guidelines.* Unpublished manuscript: 'This scale refers specifically to responses to the question asking what the respondent does when distressed or upset. An adaptive strategy may involve seeking comfort from others (e.g. parents, friends, or siblings), engaging in a favorite activity that relieves their unhappiness (e.g. listening to music, walking the dog), or simply thinking things through.'

[368] E.g. Crittenden, P.M. (1992) Quality of attachment in the preschool years. *Development & Psychopathology*, 4(2), 209–241; Grossmann, K. (1995) Kontinuität und Konsequenzen der frühen Bindungsqualität während des Vorschulalters. In G. Spangler & P. Zimmermann (eds) *Die Bindungstheorie—Grundlagen, Forschung und Anwendung* (pp.191–202). Stuttgart: Klett Cotta.

result from adaptation (changing oneself in order to respond) to the environment. However, there are forms of adaptation (long-term thriving) where refusal to adapt (change oneself in order to respond) is optimal, for instance in depleting or punitive environments that can be changed or exited. Some forms of adaptation (thriving) may come at the expense of other forms of adaptation (thriving), as in the familiar case in which the demands of one area of life—family, work—come at the expense of others—diet, exercise, self-care. A further complexity lies in the fact that there are forms of adaptation (responding and/or thriving) that are based very directly on adaptation (species-level natural selection), such as the deployment of conditional strategies as evolutionary-based behavioural repertoires. However, there are forms of adaptation (responding and/or thriving) that are more based on social learning or other processes based more on human plasticity rather than responses directly grounded in adaptation (species-level natural selection).

Ainsworth stated that attachment researchers all agreed that avoidant attachment should be regarded as an adaptation (a response to the caregiving environment). And many were becoming persuaded by Main's argument, endorsed by Ainsworth, that the avoidant attachment pattern was an adaptation (part of the human evolutionary behavioural repertoire). However, she identified that there were significant disagreements among her students and collaborators about whether, over the long-run, avoidant attachment contributed to adaptation (long-term thriving). Ainsworth offered her conviction that this was essentially an empirical matter: the question of whether 'avoidant attachment may be adaptive according to ultimate criteria in the mental health sense is clearly a researchable proposition.'[369] Her personal expectation was that insecure attachment would tend to work against or undermine long-term thriving. And this attitude unquestionably shaped her published descriptions of the avoidant and ambivalent/resistant attachment classifications. She remained open to the potential for insecure attachment to contribute to long-term benefits, for instance in some domains. But she was not holding her breath in anticipation of such results.

Shaver's position seems to have essentially been the same. Until around 2007, the dominant theme of his writing was the benefits of secure attachment, across whatever domain was under discussion. There are even some passages in his work that read as hymns to the glory of secure attachment for its capacity to 'create a kinder and more tolerant, harmonious, and peaceful society.'[370] And, even after 2007, Lawler, Shaver, and Goodman could still put forward the extreme proposal that mental health professionals working with families should be screened for their attachment style, claiming that it is the right of every child to 'receive services from health and mental health interveners who are trained in supporting relationship quality and are themselves secure with respect to attachment (as assessed with adult attachment measures).'[371] Yet a whispering, subterranean theme also appears across Shaver's writings before 2007, offering qualifications and at times pointing in the contrary direction. In the 1986 chapter in *Everywoman's Emotional Wellbeing*, Shaver and O'Connor noted a

[369] Ainsworth, M. (1984) Attachment, adaptation and continuity. Paper presented at International Conference on Infant Studies, April 1984. PP/Bow/J.1/57.

[370] E.g. Mikulincer, M. & Shaver, P.R. (2007) Boosting attachment security to promote mental health, prosocial values, and inter-group tolerance. *Psychological Inquiry*, 18, 139–56: 'If human beings were helped by their families, communities, schools, religious institutions, and cultural media to become more secure, they would be better able to create a kinder and more tolerant, harmonious, and peaceful society' (150); 'without a sizeable proportion of secure, mindful, and self-efficacious citizens, political will alone is unlikely to accomplish desirable ethical goals' (152).

[371] Lawler, M.J., Shaver, P.R., & Goodman, G.S. (2011) Toward relationship-based child welfare services. *Children and Youth Services Review*, 33(3), 473–80, p.478.

shift in psychological theory towards a recognition that many apparent symptoms or forms of pathology might also or sometimes better be regarded as effective responses to challenging and intractable situations. Shaver and O'Connor offered, as an example, that their colleagues in psychology appeared to be moving in their discussions 'from the concept of "defense" to the more constructive concept of "coping"'.[372] Bowlby was a forerunner for this transition (Chapter 1).

Reflecting on the difference between defence and coping, Shaver and O'Connor considered how an individual may direct their attention away from problems, in avoidance or denial. This reduces perceptual information about the problem, and had classically been treated in psychology as a form of pathology. However, Shaver and O'Connor countered: 'in cases where reality serves up a problem for which there is no solution, or at least no immediate solution, what's so bad about losing touch with it?'[373] They advised their women readers that if a problem is solvable, then avoidance or denial will be a costly and unproductive strategy. However, if a problem is truly not solvable, then avoidance or denial are optimal responses to the situation, and 'this strategy frees their energies for other, more rewarding activities'.[374] In Ainsworth's terms, Shaver and O'Connor's argument was that avoidance is not always an adaptation (a response to the situation): sometimes it can be motivated by fear or habit rather than a genuine acknowledgement of the nature of the situation. Where avoidance is deployed as a strategy in response to a situation that could otherwise be resolved, this is neither adaptive (a response to the situation) nor adaptive (a contribution to longer-term thriving). However, when an avoidant strategy is used in response to an unsolvable problem, then this is both adaptive (a response to the situation) and adaptive (a contribution to longer-term thriving).

Evidence for Shaver and O'Connor's claim came from an early study by Mikulincer and Florian published in 1995. This would be the first in a slow accumulation of discrepant findings by Mikulincer and colleagues, which documented the benefits of an insecure attachment style under specific circumstances. Mikulincer and Florian asked 92 Israeli army recruits to complete the 'love quiz' at the start of their basic combat training. Their appraisal of the training, coping strategies, and peer evaluations of their behaviour were assessed four months later. Individuals endorsing an avoidant attachment style reported the use of more distance forms of coping than other participants, and were just as likely to be nominated for leadership positions as participants endorsing a secure attachment style. Interpreting their results, Mikulincer and Florian reflected that 'although the tendency of avoidant persons to maintain social distance may be negatively evaluated in an emotionally laden interaction, it may be that in purposive instrumental interaction, like daily activity during combat training, avoidant persons may provide concrete assistance and relief from distress to others'.[375]

Basic combat training may represent the kind of intractable problem described by Shaver and O'Connor where physical, mental, and ethical difficulties may not be resolvable, especially through rumination. There could be personal and social benefits to freeing energies for other more rewarding activities. However, a limitation of Mikulincer and Florian's 1995 paper was its focus on individual coping. In a larger study of multiple units during basic

---

[372] Shaver, P.R. & O'Connor, C. (1986) Coping with stress: problems in perspective. In C. Tavris (ed.) *Everywoman's Emotional Wellbeing* (pp.305–329). New York: Doubleday.

[373] Ibid. p.323.

[374] Ibid.

[375] Mikulincer, M. & Florian, V. (1995) Appraisal of and coping with a real-life stressful situation: the contribution of attachment styles. *Personality and Social Psychology Bulletin*, 21(4), 406–414, p.413.

combat training, published in 2007, Davidovitz, Mikulincer, Shaver, Izsak, and Popper reported that the higher the officer's score on avoidance on the ECR, the more the self-reported mental health of their unit deteriorated. In the first two months this deterioration was moderated by the soldiers' own attachment style. However, over the four months there was a negative association between officer avoidance and their soldiers' mental health regardless of the attachment styles of the latter.[376] Yet Davidovitz and colleagues also found a positive association between officers' attachment anxiety and followers' mental health. This positive association, however, seemed to come at the expense of the unit's performance in exercises.[377]

Another finding from Mikulincer's research group offered further indication that insecure attachment strategies can have certain benefits depending on the circumstances. In 2001, Berant, Mikulincer, and Florian published a study of mothers' responses to the diagnosis of congenital heart disease in their infant. The researchers examined the relationship between attachment style, coping strategies, wellbeing, and severity of the infant's diagnosis. They found that mothers endorsing a secure attachment style tended to utilise a combination of support-seeking and avoidant-coping strategies if their babies had severe forms of congenital heart disease. The temporary use of avoidance or denial was positively associated with better reported wellbeing. Berant and colleagues interpreted this finding as suggesting that avoidant strategies can be helpful for a time in the face of an irresolvable problem if they are combined with the security to permit support-seeking as needed. When mothers had babies without severe forms of congenital heart disease, then, as expected, participants endorsing an avoidant attachment style relied especially on avoidant and distancing coping strategies, and reported moderate levels of wellbeing.

However, for mothers who had babies with severe medical problems and who had an avoidant attachment style, avoidant and distancing coping strategies were not used; these mothers reported the very lowest levels of wellbeing. Berant and colleagues proposed that in the face of an irresolvable problem that is also too appallingly distressing to maintain a distancing strategy, the avoidant strategy breaks down into a less-strategic state, with some of the features of the anxious attachment style but characterised by a whirlpool of distress, rumination, and felt insecurity.[378] A potential explanation for this finding was put forward by Gillath, Giesbrecht, and Shaver. These researchers argued that an avoidant strategy can help keep at bay thoughts and feelings that might otherwise undermine coping. However, where these thoughts and feelings intrude, the outcome is worse than had the strategy not been attempted. They used a computerised task to assess the capacity of participants to resist distractions from the task. An avoidant attachment style was associated with greater success at the task, except when participants had been primed to think about a past occasion in which they were made to feel insecure.[379]

The potential for insecure attachment styles to confer local advantages has been increasingly recognised since 2007. Nonetheless, Mikulincer and Shaver's 2016 book *Attachment*

[376] Davidovitz, R., Mikulincer, M., Shaver, P.R., Izsak, R., & Popper, M. (2007) Leaders as attachment figures: leaders' attachment orientations predict leadership-related mental representations and followers' performance and mental health. *Journal of Personality and Social Psychology*, 93(4), 632–50, p.645.
[377] Ibid. p.647.
[378] Berant, E., Mikulincer, M., & Florian, V. (2001) The association of mothers' attachment style and their psychological reactions to the diagnosis of infant's congenital heart disease. *Journal of Social and Clinical Psychology*, 20(2), 208–232, p.227.
[379] Gillath, O., Giesbrecht, B., & Shaver, P.R. (2009) Attachment, attention, and cognitive control: attachment style and performance on general attention tasks. *Journal of Experimental Social Psychology*, 45(4), 647–54.

in Adulthood, in part for narrative reasons and in part because it is surveying the existing literature, at times approaches a list of goods associated with the secure attachment style and a list of bads associated with insecure attachment styles.[380] Attention to the circumstances in which insecure attachment styles can confer benefits has instead been the priority of one of Mikulincer's former students, Tsachi Ein-Dor. Ein-Dor took a course with Mikulincer on attachment theory as an undergraduate student. He was struck by an apparent contradiction. On the one hand, the ethological-evolutionary basis of attachment theory suggested that behavioural repetoires common across a species likely have some survival or reproductive value in an expectable environmental niche. On the other hand, Mikulincer's lectures emphasised the disadvantages of insecurity.

Ein-Dor served as the operations manager for Mikulincer's research group between 2002 and 2009, undertaking masters' and doctoral study.[381] When Mikulincer moved from Bar-Ilan to become founding Dean of the School of Psychology at the Interdisciplinary Center Herzlyia in 2007, Ein-Dor followed to help set up the new laboratory. During this time, Ein-Dor paid close and critical attention to the data being gathered by Mikulincer's group. Whilst the overarching story told in the published papers was about the virtues of a secure attachment style, he noticed an accumulation of research findings suggesting the benefits of insecure attachment styles under specific circumstances. Some of these findings might be due to chance. However, Ein-Dor began to see a logic to the findings, and developed hypotheses regarding the conditions under which an insecure attachment style might be an asset. He came to regard an anxious attachment style as a potential asset in contexts in which vigilance would be rewarded, and an avoidant attachment style as a potential asset in contexts in which instrumentalism would be rewarded. Though the co-author on many earlier papers published by Mikulincer's research group, Ein-Dor's first paper as lead author was published in 2010 entitled 'The attachment paradox: how can so many of us (the insecure ones) have no adaptive advantages?', with Mikulincer and Shaver both as co-authors.[382]

In this paper, Ein-Dor and colleagues acknowledged that Mikulincer and Shaver had time and again reported results indicating the benefits of a secure attachment style. Yet they also pointed to theoretical work suggesting that insecure attachment can be adaptive, not only in the sense of responsive to the environment but also in the sense of conferring some advantages. This position, already under discussion by Ainsworth in the mid-1980s (Chapter 2), was developed in print by researchers in the developmental tradition such as Belsky and Crittenden.[383] Belsky's emphasis on the contribution of attachment strategies to reproductive fitness was especially influential for Ein-Dor.[384] As well as this theoretical tradition,

---

[380] Mikulincer, M. & Shaver, P. (2016) *Attachment in Adulthood*, 2nd edn. New York: Guilford.

[381] http://portal.idc.ac.il/faculty/en/Pages/resume.resume?userName=dGVpbmRvcg==&Language=1.

[382] Ein-Dor, T., Mikulincer, M., Doron, G., & Shaver, P.R. (2010) The attachment paradox: how can so many of us (the insecure ones) have no adaptive advantages? *Perspectives on Psychological Science*, 5(2), 123–41.

[383] Belsky, J., Steinberg, L., & Draper, P. (1991) Childhood experience, interpersonal development, and reproductive strategy: an evolutionary theory of socialization. *Child Development*, 62, 647–70; Crittenden, P.M. (1992) Quality of attachment in the preschool years. *Development & Psychopathology*, 4(2), 209–241. For reflection on Ein-Dor's claims from critical psychology see Carr, S. & Batlle, I.C. (2015) Attachment theory, neoliberalism, and social conscience. *Journal of Theoretical and Philosophical Psychology*, 35(3), 160–76. These researchers interpret Ein-Dor's perspective as essentially a positive framing of the fit between an avoidant attachment style and the depleting, dehumanising late capitalist labour market. They argue that, even if there are some advantages to insecure attachment styles, these advantages are vastly outweighed by their cost, to the point that claims about advantages are misleading.

[384] See Ein-Dor, T. & Hirschberger, G. (2016) Rethinking attachment theory: from a theory of relationships to a theory of individual and group survival. *Current Directions in Psychological Science*, 25(4), 223–7, p.226.

Ein-Dor and colleagues could also point to the accumulation of studies showing some benefits of the insecure attachment style. In addition to earlier findings from Mikulincer's group, Ein-Dor and colleagues were able to report new findings from their longitudinal follow-up of ex-prisoners of war from the 1973 Yom Kippur war. Participants were followed up in 1991, 2003, and 2008. This research found that veterans' avoidant attachment scores were inversely associated with the extent to which their wives showed symptoms of trauma, such as intrusion or hyperarousal.[385] The avoidant attachment strategy of the ex-prisoners of war appeared to have kept their spouse safe from contamination by their symptoms of trauma. However, wives' avoidant attachment style was positively associated with veterans' PTSD symptoms, suggesting that, when it was not a matter of their own choosing, reduced opportunity to seek intimacy and share emotional experiences with their partner was harmful for the veterans.

Ein-Dor and colleagues criticised the wider field of attachment research generally on two grounds. First, following Belsky, they argued that researchers have generally designed studies based on an implicit model of mental health as behaviour that is adaptive in industrialised society, rather than developing hypotheses considering how apparently maladaptive behaviours might have their niche within human evolutionary history and/or particular contemporary contexts. Second, they criticised the focus of attachment researchers on individuals and, sometimes, dyads. Few attachment researchers besides the Minnesota group (Chapter 4) have examined the contribution of individual differences in attachment to group-level processes. Yet contemporary evolutionary biology, in contrast to the evolutionary theory of Bowlby's day, has come to place greater emphasis on group processes within natural selection. For instance, the survival of the group as a whole may benefit if there are some members who are more wary and alert to threat, some more focused on instrumental concerns, and others more capable of coordination, negotiation, and compromise.

Ein-Dor, Mikulincer, and Shaver published a first empirical article based on this agenda in 2011:[386] 46 groups of participants were observed in the laboratory room as it gradually filled with smoke from an apparently malfunctioning computer. The results were in line with Ein-Dor's theory of the potential benefits of insecure attachment styles under particular circumstances. Individuals high on attachment anxiety detected the smoke more quickly and alerted the group. This led the group as a whole to a faster response to the threat, since they had been notified of it earlier. Effects were quite marked: a 1-point increase in attachment anxiety was associated with an 11.5-second decrease in detection time. Individuals high on attachment avoidance were faster at getting out the door once the danger was detected, and contributed to a faster exit for the group as a whole. Furthermore, Ein-Dor and colleagues found a linear association between diversity of attachment scores in the group and the group's effectiveness at evacuating the room. This implied that although security might not be associated with vigilance regarding threat or directness in avoiding the threat, it was associated with the holistic effectiveness of the group, perhaps by facilitating coordination. They found that the effects remained significant even with temperament measures of extraversion and neuroticism statistically controlled. As a conceptual replication and extension

---

[385] Ein-Dor, T., Doron, G., Solomon, Z., Mikulincer, M., & Shaver, P.R. (2010) Together in pain: attachment-related dyadic processes and posttraumatic stress disorder. *Journal of Counseling Psychology*, 57(3), 317–27.

[386] Ein-Dor, T., Mikulincer, M., & Shaver, P.R. (2011) Effective reaction to danger: attachment insecurities predict behavioral reactions to an experimentally induced threat above and beyond general personality traits. *Social Psychological and Personality Science*, 2(5), 467–73.

of the finding that groups benefited from heterogeneity of attachment styles, Ein-Dor and colleagues assessed the attachment styles of students at their university enrolled in courses including a team project. The researchers found that when reported team cohesion was high, heterogeneity in attachment anxiety and avoidance scores in the group was associated with better grades on the group project. However, only heterogeneity in anxiety was associated with better perceived group functioning. As such, heterogeneity of attachment avoidance was associated with better performance evaluations, but without individuals being aware of the increased effectiveness of their team.[387]

Ein-Dor and Orgad conducted another study. They led participants to believe that they had accidently activated a computer virus that wiped the experimenter's computer. They were then asked to alert the department's computer technicians. On the way to the technicians' office, they were presented with four decision-points where they could either choose to delay the warning or continue on to their destination. Only the anxious attachment style, and not neuroticism, was associated with continuing on to deliver the warning rather than responding to the distractions.[388] Ein-Dor and Orgad concluded that whereas anxious attachment and trait anxiety might both influence threat perception, the communication of concerns to someone who should help is a priority specific to attachment anxiety.

Such findings provided support for Ein-Dor's claim that there can be beneficial correlates of heterogeneity of attachment styles for groups, since there are specific situations in which an insecure attachment style is a local advantage. The studies had been designed to offer a certain analogy to human evolutionary history and the question of group survival. However, Ein-Dor felt that he could prove his claims also on the 'home terrain' of attachment research in the study of individual differences, and even in the study of contemporary professional life. Ein-Dor, Reizer, Shaver, and Dotan proposed that individuals with avoidant attachment styles will profit in professional fields that reward self-reliance and the ability to work without social support.[389] The researchers elegantly demonstrated this with a study of professional singles tennis players: 58 players completed the ECR, and their progress in the national tennis rankings was assessed over a 16-month period. Amount of training, feelings of self-efficacy, and avoidant attachment style all predicted change in ranking movement, accounting for 13.5% of variance.[390] However, in a regression, only avoidant attachment style was significant, perhaps suggesting that amount of training was in part a function of avoidance. In another study, Ein-Dor and colleagues were able to demonstrate the potential benefits of an anxious attachment style for individuals. Researching a card game tournament, they found that the higher the player's attachment anxiety score, the better their ability to cheat without being caught and to detect others cheating.[391] Research findings from other groups have offered support for Ein-Dor's claims regarding the potential advantages of insecure attachment styles under particular circumstances. Of special note are findings from

[387] Lavy, S., Bareli, Y., & Ein-Dor, T. (2015) The effects of attachment heterogeneity and team cohesion on team functioning. *Small Group Research,* 46(1), 27–49.

[388] Ein-Dor, T. & Orgad, T. (2012) Scared saviors: evidence that people high in attachment anxiety are more effective in alerting others to threat. *European Journal of Social Psychology,* 42(6), 667–71.

[389] Ein-Dor, T., Reizer, A., Shaver, P.R., & Dotan, E. (2012) Standoffish perhaps, but successful as well: evidence that avoidant attachment can be beneficial in professional tennis and computer science. *Journal of Personality,* 80(3), 749–68.

[390] Ibid. Table 2.

[391] Ein-Dor, T., Perry-Paldi, A., Zohar-Cohen, K., Efrati, Y., & Hirschberger, G. (2017) It takes an insecure liar to catch a liar: the link between attachment insecurity, deception, and detection of deception. *Personality and Individual Differences,* 113, 81–7.

a randomised control trial of the Circle of Security eight-session parenting intervention. Cassidy and colleagues reported that this intervention had no main effect on either infant attachment security or on child mental health. However, positive effects were seen when caregivers were high in attachment avoidance; by contrast, the intervention *reduced* infant–caregiver security for caregivers who began the intervention low in attachment avoidance.[392]

Evaluating Ein-Dor's position, Gillath, Karantzas, and Fraley have argued for only quali-fied acceptance. They acknowledge that in specific circumstances, insecure attachment styles may have local advatanges. However, they emphasise that the vast majority of studies have found that secure attachment is associated with more positively regarded outcomes.[393] Yet Shaver and Mikulincer have acknowledged Ein-Dor's point that this has partly been a result of how studies have been designed and conceptualised. They have accepted that Ein-Dor's work has provided a helpful corrective to the tendency in their writing to treat insecure at-tachment as, in itself, simply bad. Furthermore, Ein-Dor's concern with the relationship be-tween individual attachment style and group processes has been an important development for attachment research with adults. To date, there have not been sufficient studies of small group processes to build the critical mass for a research agenda, and research energies have been directed elsewhere.[394] However, interest in small groups has definitely been growing in social psychology,[395] and the developmental tradition has developed attachment-based par-enting interventions that specifically make use of group dynamics such as GABI (Chapter 4). It may be that Ein-Dor's ongoing research efforts will contribute to small-group research as an important new direction for attachment research.

Some remaining questions

The ECR items

For two decades, the social psychology tradition of attachment research has been under-pinned both theoretically and methodologically by the ECR. As discussed in the section

---

[392] Cassidy, J., Brett, B.E., Gross, J.T., et al. (2017) Circle of security-parenting: a randomized controlled trial in Head Start. *Development & Psychopathology*, 29(2), 651–73. However, the assessment of outcomes was conducted as soon as feasible after completion of the intervention, when participants low in avoidant attachment style may have still been processing the intervention, requiring time to stabilise their caregiving. Longer before follow-up may have provided more opportunity for positive intervention effects. It should also be noted that the researchers appear not to have measured or controlled for the involvement of other services (e.g. child welfare involvement). This might be another relevant moderator.

[393] Gillath, O., Karantzas, G.C., & Fraley, R.C. (2016) *Adult Attachment: A Concise Introduction to Theory and Research*. London: Academic Press, p.272.

[394] On the potential for self-perpetuating neglect of certain research agendas within attachment research see Fearon, R.M.P., Bakermans-Kranenburg, M.J., & van IJzendoorn, M.H. (2010) Jealousy and attachment: the case of twins. In S.L. Hart & M. Legerstee (eds) *Handbook of Jealousy. Theory, Research, and Multidisciplinary Approaches* (pp.362–86). New York: Wiley: 'Without an accumulation of empirical data and novel findings it may be that we have not seen a sufficient number of new phenomena for researchers to get their teeth into, and so their energies have, to a large extent, been directed elsewhere' (364).

[395] Marmarosh, C. & Markin, R. (2007) Group and personal attachments. *Group Dynamics: Theory, Research, and Practice*, 11(3), 153–64; Yip, J., Ehrhardt, K., Black, H., & Walker, D.O. (2018) Attachment theory at work: a review and directions for future research. *Journal of Organizational Behavior*, 39(2), 185–98; DeMarco, T.C. & Newheiser, A.K. (2019) Attachment to groups: relationships with group esteem, self-esteem, and investment in ingroups. *European Journal of Social Psychology*, 49(1), 63–75.

'Creating the ECR', Brennan and colleagues developed the ECR through a two-level factor analysis of items from existing measures. The model of two orthogonal factors that came out of this analysis comprised items representing attachment anxiety and attachment avoidance. And the idea of orthogonal dimensions in a two-dimensional space, representing minimising and maximising, became the foundation for Shaver and Mikulincer's approach to all other behavioural systems. Yet there has been astonishingly little discussion of the ECR items and the inner machinery of the measure, with researchers seeming to rest comfortably on the original factor analysis conducted by Brennan and colleagues. An exception is Allen and colleagues, who have called for a close study of the ECR items, but not conducted this study themselves.[396] Likewise, Banai, Mikulincer, and Shaver, in a paper from 2005, urged that distinctions may be drawn between forms of attachment anxiety, and that 'researchers should attempt to distinguish among these potentially different kinds of individuals who score high on the anxiety dimension'.[397] However, these calls have not been followed up. Social psychology research on attachment seems to have been firmly gripped in the beak of the two dimensions the ECR is understood to embody, with the items themselves treated as of little consequence. Yet examination of the items makes this assumption all the more strange, since the items—drawn as they are from a variety of pre-existing scales—are quite a menagerie. This was acknowledged by Mikulincer and Shaver: 'the items consequently range from ones concerned with relationships in general to ones concerned with a particular partner. Some deal with "comfort" and other feelings; some deal with desires and motives'.[398] They expressed surprise at how well the items have performed, 'given their relative crudeness'. In fact, 'it is remarkable how systematic and cumulative our research findings have been' on the basis of items that were 'not designed component-by-component with a coherent theoretical model in mind'.[399]

The ECR is 36 items, which is unusually long for a self-report measure. This has led to attempts to produce a shortened version of the scale with the same properties. Work on translations and the ECR and attempts to produce a shortened version have represented the only sustained conversation in the published literature about the ECR items and the latent phenomena they measure, and as such the only fine-grained consideration of what participants may be endorsing. In a 2007 paper, Wei and colleagues presented the first attempt to develop a short version of the ECR, drawing 12 items from the 36.[400] They cited a personal communication from Shaver (July 2004) that the avoidant and anxious attachment styles each have three 'critical components'. According to Shaver, the 'critical components' of attachment avoidance are:

  i) concern about closeness;
  ii) reluctance to depend on others;
  iii) reluctance to self-disclose.

[396] Allen, J.G., Stein, H., Fonagy, P., Fultz, J., & Target, M. (2005) Rethinking adult attachment: a study of expert consensus. *Bulletin of the Menninger Clinic*, 69(1), 59–80: 'We believe there is room to continue sharpening the conceptual boundaries of adult attachment by further examining the content of putative attachment scale items' (60).

[397] Banai, E., Mikulincer, M., & Shaver, P.R. (2005) 'Selfobject' needs in Kohut's self psychology. *Psychoanalytic Psychology*, 22(2), 224–60, p.253.

[398] Mikulincer, M. & Shaver, P.R. (2003) The attachment behavioral system in adulthood: activation, psychodynamics, and interpersonal processes. In M.P. Zanna (ed.) *Advances in Experimental Social Psychology*, Vol. 35 (pp. 53–152). New York: Academic Press, p.141.

[399] Ibid.

[400] Wei, M., Russell, D.W., Mallinckrodt, B., & Vogel, D.L. (2007) The Experiences in Close Relationship Scale (ECR)—short form: reliability, validity, and factor structure. *Journal of Personality Assessment*, 88(2), 187–204.

The critical components of attachment anxiety are:

i) concern about abandonment;
ii) an extensive desire for reassurance from others;[401]
iii) distress about the unavailability of one's partner.

Whilst these often occur together or cause one another, the three components of each of the forms of insecure attachment are articulated. It is possible for them to occur unalloyed. For instance, reluctance to depend on others may often come with a concern about closeness, but it need not do so. Attachment figures could be regarded, for instance, as generally untrustworthy but nonetheless attractive. Or again, distress about the availability of one's partner may entail concern about abandonment, but it need not do so. Attachment figures could be regarded as distracted and inattentive, but still invested in the relationship and its continuation.

Wei and colleagues developed the ECR-short, drawing items from the ECR with reference to the theoretical rationale of the three 'critical components' per form of insecure attachment. However, in an independent attempt to make a short form of the ECR, Lo, Mikulincer, and colleagues argued that there was a need to reconsider the Brennan study itself. They observed that the Brennan et al. paper is usually described as creating the two dimensions of the ECR out of the items of a factor analysis. But in fact this was a two-stage process. The data presented by Brennan and colleagues indicated that when factored at the item level, a higher-order factor structure was present. Twelve first-order factors were initially extracted, which Brennan and colleagues termed 'facets' of the two latent dimensions found using the higher-order factor analysis.[402] The 36 items did not reduce in one step to two latent dimensions; an intermediate layer was in operation. Lo, Mikulincer, and colleagues conducted an exploratory factor analysis of the 36 items and found that avoidance and anxiety each broke down into two factors. Within the avoidant attachment style, one of the factors was discomfort with closeness. This factor accounted for 16% of variance in endorsement of items on the ECR. The other factor was lack of willingness to rely on others or willingness to disclose to others (which clustered two of the 'critical components' separated by Wei and colleagues on the basis of Shaver's personal communication). This factor accounted for 14% of variance. The distinction between these two factors has been supported in other studies.[403]

The anxious attachment style also broke down into two factors. The first factor represented items indicating frustration about the unavailability of the attachment figure. This

---

[401] Wei and colleagues only had one item represent this component, Item 18 on the ECR. This item reads: 'I need a lot of reassurance that close relationship partners really care about me'. Wei and colleagues characterised this item as 'an excessive need for approval from others (Item 18)'. This is an improbable characterisation of the item! It would seem most likely that the word 'assurance' was intended, rather than 'approval'. There are items in the ECR that represent need for approval, such as Item 34: 'when other people disapprove of me, I feel really bad about myself'. However, it is Item 18, not these items about approval, that feature in the list of 12 items offered by Wei and colleagues as the short version of the ECR. It is perhaps worth noting that a desire for approval is explicitly one of the features specified by Shaver and Mikulincer as associated with hyperactivation of the power behavioural system, which may account for a portion of the link between the two measures.

[402] Brennan, K.A., Clark, C.L., & Shaver, P.R. (1998) Self-report measurement of adult romantic attachment: an integrative overview. In J A. Simpson & W.S. Rholes (eds) *Attachment Theory and Close Relationships* (pp.46–76). New York: Guilford, p.66.

[403] E.g. Olsson, I. Sørebø, O., & Dahl, A.A. (2010) The Norwegian version of the Experiences in Close Relationships measure of adult attachment: psychometric properties and normative data. *Nordic Journal of Psychiatry*, 64(5), 340–49.

is similar to the 'critical component' of distress about the unavailability of the partner from Wei and colleagues' formulation, except for the focus on frustration. As we saw in the section 'Creating the ECR', Shaver and colleagues shifted the second dimension of attachment theory away from Ainsworth's concern with inconsolability (understood as anxiety about caregiver availability), anger, and passivity towards a focus solely on anxiety about attachment relationships. However, the fact that one of the constitutive factors of the anxious attachment style constitutes frustration suggests that the ECR has continued to tap anger about the unavailability of the attachment figure, though with only distress/worry about partner availability featuring focally and theoretically in accounts of what is being measured or in the design of research studies. The 'frustration' factor accounted for 18% of variance, the largest share of any of the factors. The other factor constituting the anxious attachment style represented items indicating worry about the relationship. This seems to be similar to the concern about abandonment from Wei and colleagues' formulation. This factor accounted for 9% of variance.[404] There was no equivalent in Lo, Mikulincer, and colleagues' work of the wish for reassurance, the final critical component for Wei and colleagues. However, there is only one item directly about the wish for reassurance in the ECR: 'I need a lot of reassurance that close relationship partners really care about me' (Item 18).[405] This item is loaded with frustration in the factor analysis, though not strongly. Here again, there appears to be some holdover from Ainsworth's original model, since the wish for reassurance without active efforts to achieve it was how Ainsworth defined the C2 'passive' classification.

Overall, close consideration of the ECR suggests that even if the items can be considered to ultimately tap two latent dimensions, they do so through an intermediate layer of 'facets' in which relevant differences can be identified.[406] Indeed, some studies do not find a two-factor model as the optional solution, and instead identify these facets as distinct factors in accounting for variance for endorsement of items on the ECR.[407] Part of the issue is that the items that constitute the ECR were not designed for the purpose of tapping the two latent

---

[404] Lo, C., Walsh, A., Mikulincer, M., Gagliese, L., Zimmermann, C., & Rodin, G. (2009) Measuring attachment security in patients with advanced cancer: psychometric properties of a modified and brief Experiences in Close Relationships scale. *Psycho-Oncology*, 18(5), 490–99, p.495.

[405] Reassurance is also mentioned by Item 35: 'I turn to close relationship partners for many things, including comfort and reassurance'. However, the formulation of the item is astonishingly unspecific—'many things'—so it is not clear that participants would answer based primarily on their experiences of wanting or receiving reassurance. More importantly, the item, reversed, is one that contributes to the scoring of attachment avoidance, not attachment anxiety. A study by Lafontaine and colleagues found that Item 35 had the highest standard error and worst discrimination of any of the avoidance items in the ECR. Lafontaine, M.F., Brassard, A., Lussier, Y., Valois, P., Shaver, P.R., & Johnson, S.M. (2016) Selecting the best items for a short-form of the Experiences in Close Relationships questionnaire. *European Journal of Psychological Assessment*, 32(2), 140–54, p.146.

[406] Intermediate 'facets' have also been identified between the items and the latent dimensions of anxiety and avoidance in the Attachment Style Questionnaire: confidence; relationships as secondary; discomfort with closeness; preoccupation with relationships; and need for approval. Karantzas, G.C., Feeney, J.A., & Wilkinson, R. (2010) Is less more? Confirmatory factor analysis of the Attachment Style Questionnaires. *Journal of Social and Personal Relationships*, 27(6), 749–80.

[407] E.g. Olssøn, I., Sørebø, O., & Dahl, A.A. (2010) The Norwegian version of the Experiences in Close Relationships measure of adult attachment: psychometric properties and normative data. *Nordic Journal of Psychiatry*, 64(5), 340–49: 'The five-factor solution. Factors 1 and 4 consist of avoidance items only. The items of factor 1 describe avoidance of getting close or discomfort by coming close. In factor 4, the content of all items is reluctance to self-disclosure or dependence on others ... Factors 2, 3 and 5 all consist of anxiety items. The items in factor 2 describe worrying about abandonment or being alone. Factor 3 content statements about one's need for partner's availability or reassurance, and factor 5 concerns worry that the individual wants more closeness than the other person does' (344).

dimensions, and item-total correlations for the anxiety and avoidance scales are frequently low.[408] Differences in the 'facets' that constitute the intermediate layer may contribute to discrepancies between theory and measurement, reducing the precision and coherence of the measure and the tradition of research built upon it. For instance, attachment anxiety is generally assumed by Shaver and Mikulincer to be correlated with, but distinct from, frustration in relationships. However, one of the two components of the anxiety scale is tapping frustration whereas the other is not. Is frustration a correlate or a component of an anxious attachment style? Wongpakaran and colleagues have argued that in fact frustration, though related, is ultimately 'extraneous' to what is truly meant by attachment anxiety, and its inclusion within the ECR and self-report measures based on it may be a cause of unintended noise and imprecision.[409] They also expressed concern that some ECR items may simply reflect poor self-regard rather than an attachment-specific experience, even if this loads with attachment anxiety in factor analyses. And indeed, Esbjørn and colleagues found a five-factor solution was superior to a two-factor solution in their data, and that the 'extra' factor beyond the four identified by Lo, Mikulincer, and colleagues represented those items in the ECR that suggest poor global self-worth (e.g. Item 34: 'When others disapprove of me, I feel really bad about myself').[410] Karantzas and colleagues have argued for the 'conceptual and empirical importance of including both broad factors and specific facets of attachment style', and alleged that the constructs of attachment anxiety and avoidance are decidedly 'blunt instruments'. They contend that consideration of the facets will have much to offer to work in clinical and therapeutic contexts, for instance in understanding how exactly attachment insecurity may contribute to mental health symptoms.[411]

Another potential issue with the anxiety items is that a single item (Item 18) suggestive of Ainsworth's concept of passivity appears to have smuggled aboard the ECR, but without a second item to stabilise measurement and without theoretical acknowledgement. Yet passivity may also be implicated elsewhere in the measure. Item 29 is the statement 'I feel comfortable depending on others'; this item, reversed, was intended to represent avoidance. However, it may also represent the passive desire for care Ainsworth characterised as C2. In this light it is notable that several samples, including work by Shaver and colleagues themselves, have found Item 29 negatively associated with avoidant attachment and positively associated with anxious attachment, rather than unrelated to anxiety as anticipated by Brennan and colleagues.[412]

---

[408] Questions have been raised about the item-total correlations of the ECR and measures based on it by several psychometricians, e.g. Hanak, N. & Dimitrijevic, A. (2013) A Serbian Version of Modified and Revised Experiences in Close Relationships Scale (SM–ECR–R). *Journal of Personality Assessment*, 95(5), 530–38.

[409] Wongpakaran, T., Wongpakaran, N., & Wannarit, K. (2011) Validity and reliability of the Thai version of the Experiences of Close Relationships–Revised questionnaire. *Singapore Medical Journal*, 52(2), 100–106, p.103.

[410] See also Esbjørn, B.H., Breinholst, S., Niclasen, J., Skovgaard, L.F., Lange, K., & Reinholdt-Dunne, M.L. (2015) Identifying the best-fitting factor structure of the Experience of Close Relations–Revised in a Scandinavian example. *PLoS One*, 10(9), e0137218. Though this study was of the ECR-R, not the ECR, there were items falling in the 'extra' factor from the original ECR, such as Items 6 and 10.

[411] Karantzas, G.C., Feeney, J.A., & Wilkinson, R. (2010) Is less more? Confirmatory factor analysis of the Attachment Style Questionnaires. *Journal of Social and Personal Relationships*, 27(6), 749–80, p.774; Gillath, O., Karantzas, G.C., & Fraley, R.C. (2016) *Adult Attachment: A Concise Introduction to Theory and Research*. London: Academic Press, pp.120, 245. See, for instance, work by Tasca and colleagues, which found that the association between attachment anxiety and symptoms of depression and disordered eating was fully mediated by emotion regulation strategies. Tasca, G.A., Szadkowski, L., Illing, V., et al. (2009) Adult attachment, depression, and eating disorder symptoms: the mediating role of affect regulation strategies. *Personality and Individual Differences*, 47(6), 662–7.

[412] See e.g. Alonso-arbiol, I., Balluerka, N., & Shaver, P.R. (2007) A Spanish version of the Experiences in Close Relationships (ECR) adult attachment questionnaire. *Personal Relationships*, 14(1), 45–63.

In relation to the avoidance dimension, there seem to be distinct facets representing relative comfort with closeness on the one hand, and trust on the other hand. Again, these differences in 'facets' in the intermediate layer may introduce discrepancies between theory and measurement, especially in contexts where one or the other facets may be more important. It is easy to imagine social contexts in which trust is more salient, contexts in which comfort with closeness is more important, as well as contexts in which both play a substantial role. In a higher-order factor analysis, Lo, Mikulincer, and colleagues found that whereas willingness to disclose and rely on others was entirely distinct from attachment anxiety, the items representing the facet of discomfort with closeness loaded partially on both attachment avoidance and attachment anxiety.[413] This implies that discomfort with closeness may be fed by both attachment avoidance and attachment anxiety, albeit for different reasons.[414] Consider, for instance, Item 26 on the ECR: 'I find that my partners don't want to get as close as I would like'. With what is 'liked' unspecified, endorsement of this item may be fed by both anxiety and avoidance, as a factor analysis conducted by Shaver and colleagues indeed showed.[415]

Lafontaine, Shaver, and colleagues conducted a study to further refine the items for a short version of the ECR. One analysis they pursued was the extent to which items could discriminate particular portions of the avoidance scale. At the high end of the avoidance scale, some items that were particularly effective were Item 29: 'I feel comfortable depending on others' (Reversed) and Item 9: 'I don't feel comfortable opening up to others'. However, 'almost all avoidance items performed relatively poorly on the lower portion of the avoidance scale continuum'.[416] The items were quite good at picking up the avoidant attachment style, but were poor at discriminating security. There was only one item that worked adequately, though even then not well, in picking out security (Item 35). Yet this item had the highest standard error and lowest discrimination of all the avoidance items. On the anxiety scale, again, the low end was not well discriminated, perhaps because there is only one reverse item in the anxiety scale.[417] Whereas the ECR promises to capture security as the absence of anxiety

[413] Lo, C., Walsh, A., Mikulincer, M., Gagliese, L., Zimmermann, C., & Rodin, G. (2009) Measuring attachment security in patients with advanced cancer: psychometric properties of a modified and brief Experiences in Close Relationships scale. *Psycho-Oncology*, 18(5), 490–99, p.495. The items representing discomfort with closeness are:

    Item 7. 'I get uncomfortable when other people want to be very close to me'
    Item 13. 'I am nervous when other people get too close to me'
    Item 17. 'I try to avoid getting too close to other people'
    Item 23. 'I prefer not to be too close to other people'
    Item 9. 'I don't feel comfortable opening up to other people'.

[414] Ibid.: 'Conceptually, the double-loading of Discomfort on the higher-order attachment dimensions suggests that both attachment anxiety and avoidance tap some discomfort with the experience of intimacy and closeness' (498).

[415] E.g. Alonso-arbiol, I., Balluerka, N., & Shaver, P.R. (2007) A Spanish version of the Experiences in Close Relationships (ECR) adult attachment questionnaire. *Personal Relationships*, 14(1), 45–63. Matters are further complicated by findings by Mikulincer and colleagues that attachment anxiety on the ECR is associated with both preconscious approach and avoidance goals with respect to relational closeness, which affect their motor responses in a push–pull task. It may be that when individuals with an anxious attachment style feel overclose, as may occur in longstanding relationships, they will endorse items representing a desire for avoidance of closeness. Mikulincer, M., Shaver, P.R., Bar-On, N., & Ein-Dor, T. (2010) The pushes and pulls of close relationships: attachment insecurities and relational ambivalence. *Journal of Personality and Social Psychology*, 98(3), 450–68, p.463.

[416] Lafontaine, M.F., Brassard, A., Lussier, Y., Valois, P., Shaver, P.R., & Johnson, S.M. (2016) Selecting the best items for a short-form of the Experiences in Close Relationships questionnaire. *European Journal of Psychological Assessment*, 32(2), 140–54.

[417] Frias, M.T., Shaver, P.R., & Mikulincer, M. (2014) Measures of adult attachment and related constructs. In G.J. Boyle & D.H. Saklofske (eds) *Measures of Personality and Social Psychological Constructs*. Philadelphia, PA: Elsevier, pp.417–47, p.446.

and avoidance, such findings raise the prospect that there are aspects of secure attachment that are not well captured or discriminated by the existing scales, or by theory shaped in the image of these scales. Already in 2000, Fraley and colleagues had called on researchers to 'write items that tap the low ends of the Anxiety and Avoidance dimensions with better precision'.[418] However, two decades later this problem with the ECR remains little discussed. One of the issues that this neglects is whether security really is merely the inverse of anxiety and avoidance, or itself makes an independent contribution to individual differences in adult attachment style. Given trends in the developmental tradition towards Individual Participant Meta-analysis (Chapter 6) in order to address psychometric questions, it will be interesting to see whether the social psychological tradition will also adopt such methodologies for further articulating the relationship between the ECR and its latent dimensions.

The opposite of insecurity

In their landmark 1998 paper, Brennan and colleagues reported a two-factor solution as the fundamental structure of individual differences in adult attachment. In the years after the introduction of the ECR, the two-factor model quickly became accepted. This marvellously elegant characterisation of individual differences in adult attachment style subsequently became orthodoxy among social psychological attachment researchers, with theory and methodology looping around one another to direct research questions and interpretations of findings. Yet leading figures of the social psychological tradition of research acknowledged that the model is a pragmatic simplification, and that in reality security might represent more than the absence of avoidance and resistance. Judith Feeney, for instance, writing four years after the introduction of the ECR, stated:

> I would like to take issue with the implicit suggestion that in defining the two attachment dimensions of avoidance and anxiety, researchers have settled basic questions concerning the structure of self-reported attachment. There now seems to be considerable consensus that avoidance and anxiety are the two primary dimensions underlying adult attachment, and that these dimensions generally provide moderately strong prediction of relationship outcomes (especially if both partners' characteristics are taken into account). However, in reducing such a complex construct as romantic attachment to two dimensions, important information is inevitably lost.[419]

This had already been a concern of Brennan and Shaver themselves. In a 1995 paper, Brennan and Shaver first offered the proposal that 'secure adults can be characterized as the opposite of all these insecure tendencies'.[420] This was aligned with the 'love quiz' which had, to an extent, characterised security in terms of the absence of discomfort regarding closeness or the

[418] Fraley, R.C., Waller, N.G., & Brennan, K.A. (2000) An Item Response Theory analysis of self-report measures of adult attachment. *Journal of Personality and Social Psychology*, 78(2), 350–65: 'Also notice that the two ECR-R scales, like the original ECR scales, are not adept at assessing individuals with trait levels less than –1.00 on Anxiety or Avoidance ... An important next step for future research on scale development is to write items that tap the low ends of the Anxiety and Avoidance dimensions with better precision' (361).

[419] Feeney, J.A. (2002) Attachment-related dynamics: what can we learn from self-reports of avoidance and anxiety? *Attachment & Human Development*, 4(2), 193–200, p.198.

[420] Brennan, K.A. & Shaver, P.R. (1995) Dimensions of adult attachment, affect regulation, and romantic relationship functioning. *Personality and Social Psychology Bulletin*, 21(3), 267–83, p.280.

absence of worry about abandonment. Characterisations of security as no more than the opposite of insecurity would remain the dominant narrative in Shaver's work in subsequent years. Yet already in the 1995 paper, Brennan and Shaver offered a qualification: that secure attachment is not solely the opposite of insecurity, but also has positive characteristics of its own such as 'being able and willing to trust romantic partners and share ideas and feelings with them in a flexible, appropriate manner that is sensitive to their partners' needs and concerns'.[421] This idea was not abandoned after 1998 and the introduction of the ECR. For instance, in the Shaver and Mikulincer model of the attachment system developed in the early 2000s (discussed in the section 'Minimising and maximising'), it would appear that broaden-and-build cycles are facilitated by specific and vital qualities of security, and not merely through the absence of their interruption by the insecure attachment styles. For instance, broaden-and-build cycles were anticipated by Shaver and Mikulincer to contribute to confidence and trust, which was not merely the absence of avoidance or attachment anxiety.[422] They argued that feeling understood, feeling validated, and feeling cared about are distinct aspects of the broaden-and-build cycle characteristic of security.[423]

In 2004, Shaver and Mikulincer reported their impression that by this point 'most recent adult attachment studies are based on a two-dimensional model', theoretically and in terms of measurement.[424] They acknowledged that some studies, including their own work using the 'love quiz',[425] and research by Rainer Banse[426] had produced evidence that security represented a distinct construct not reducible to the absence of anxiety and avoidance.[427] However, they argued that this position was compatible with their theory, since a security-insecurity dimension represented a 45-degree turn within the two-dimensional space of anxiety and avoidance.[428] So long as the ECR could tap the low end of anxiety and avoidance effectively, the contribution of security to individual differences could be captured by the measure. Colleagues such as Fraley had criticised the capacity of the ECR to capture security

[421] Ibid.

[422] Mikulincer, M. & Shaver, P.R. (2007) Boosting attachment security to promote mental health, prosocial values, and inter-group tolerance. *Psychological Inquiry*, 18, 139–56: 'We conceptualize the sense of attachment security as an inner resource' (139). On the contribution of distrust to both anxiety and avoidance, or as a reciprocal pathway between the two, see McWilliams, L.A. & Fried, E.I. (2019) Reconceptualizing adult attachment relationships: a network perspective. *Personal Relationships*, 26(1), 21–41.

[423] Shaver, P.R. & Mikulincer, M. (2008) Augmenting the sense of security in romantic, leader–follower, therapeutic, and group relations: a relational model of personality change. In J.P. Forgas & J. Fitness (eds) *Social Relationships: Cognitive, Affective, and Motivational Processes* (pp.55–73). New York: Psychology Press.

[424] Shaver, P.R. & Mikulincer, M. (2004) What do self-report attachment measures assess? In W.S. Rholes & J.A. Simpson (eds) *Adult Attachment: Theory, Research, and Clinical Implications* (pp.17–54). New York: Guilford, p.51.

[425] Concurrent with the publication of the ECR was work by Mikulincer suggesting a three-factor solution, in which security played the smallest but nonetheless material role in predicting variance. A factor analysis conducted by Banai, Weller, and Mikulincer in 1998 found that 13.3% of variance in the classification of an individual's attachment style by themselves, their friends, and acquaintances could be accounted for by endorsement of the secure attachment style on an adaptation of the 'love quiz', even taking into account avoidance and ambivalence-resistance. Banai, E., Weller, A., & Mikulincer, M. (1998) Inter-judge agreement in evaluation of adult attachment style: the impact of acquaintanceship. *British Journal of Social Psychology*, 37(1), 95–109, p.104.

[426] E.g. Banse, R. (2004) Adult attachment and marital satisfaction: evidence for dyadic configuration effects. *Journal of Social and Personal Relationships*, 21(2), 273–82; Asendorpf, J.B., Banse, R., Wilpers, S., & Neyer, F.J. (1997) Relationship-specific attachment scales for adults and their validation with network and diary procedures. *Diagnostica*, 43(4), 289–313.

[427] See also Holmes, J.G. & Murray, S.L. (2007) Felt security as a normative resource: evidence for an elemental risk regulation system? *Psychological Inquiry*, 18(3), 163–7.

[428] Shaver, P.R. & Mikulincer, M. (2004) What do self-report attachment measures assess? In W.S. Rholes & J.A. Simpson (eds) *Adult Attachment: Theory, Research, and Clinical Implications* (pp.17–54). New York: Guilford: 'This 45-degree rotation of the measurement axes fits well with the process model proposed by Shaver and Mikulincer (2002)' (51).

effectively. In 2004, Shaver and Mikulincer appear to have regarded the problem as meaningful, but not of great pragmatic or theoretical significance.

Yet later work from their laboratories has continued to trouble the two-dimensional model. In 2006, Al-Yagon and Mikulincer published a study of children's experiences of loneliness. Since at that time no version of the ECR had been validated for use with children, they instead used an adaptation of the 'love quiz'. The researchers found that secure attachment made a negative contribution to loneliness over and above the positive contribution to loneliness of the avoidant and anxious attachment styles.[429] Further evidence for a three-factor model came from work by Omri Gillath. Gillath had been a graduate student with Mikulincer between 1998 and 2003, and then a postdoctoral fellow with Shaver from 2003 to 2006 at the University of California. Following his appointment as faculty at the University of Kansas, Gillath worked with Joshua Hart and colleagues to develop a 'state adult attachment measure' (SAAM) to assess a participant's current feelings rather than enduring generalised schemas about relationships (see also the section 'Conclusion' for a discussion of security priming).[430] The purpose of the SAAM was to allow researchers to explore the extent to which particular stimuli or circumstances, for example changes in partner interactions over a week, might contribute to attachment-relevant experience. The items for the SAAM were based on the ECR. However, Gillath, Hart, and colleagues 'also wrote additional items to reflect aspects of attachment styles that are underrepresented on current measures, such as the low end of anxiety (e.g., "I feel relaxed knowing that close others are there for me right now"), which is represented by only a single item in the ECR'.[431] They conducted seven studies with the SAAM, with a total of 2,327 participants. Across the seven studies, they repeatedly found that a three-factor model was the best fit for the data, with independent factors for security, avoidance, and anxiety. They concluded that security appears to be an autonomous dimension of attachment states.[432]

Gillath and colleagues emphasised that Shaver and Mikulincer's theory gives a place to dynamics specific to security, even if these are not captured well by the ECR. However, Gillath, Karantzas, and Fraley have urged that more needs to be done within the social psychological tradition of attachment research to capture security-specific processes within theory and methodology. They are unconvinced that these processes are merely the opposite of anxiety and avoidance, and anticipate that they will have distinct correlates. They argue that greater

---

[429] Al-Yagon, M. & Mikulincer, M. (2006) Children's appraisal of teacher as a secure base and their socio-emotional and academic adjustment in middle childhood. *Research in Education*, 75(1), 1–18.

[430] Gillath, O., Hart, J., Noftle, E.E., & Stockdale, G.D. (2009) Development and validation of a state adult attachment measure (SAAM). *Journal of Research in Personality*, 43(3), 362–73.

[431] The security items in the SAAM are: I feel loved; I feel like I have someone to rely on; I feel secure and close to other people; If something went wrong right now I feel like I could depend on someone; I feel like others care about me; I feel relaxed knowing that close others are there for me right now; I feel I can trust the people who are close to me.

[432] Parallel findings have also been reported for the ECR-RC, the adaptation of the ECR for children and adolescents to report about their relationship with their parents. Here too security has emerged as an independent latent factor. This may be an effect of developmental stage. However, like well-established couples and unlike college students, children and adolescents are also structurally entangled in their attachment relationships, which may reduce the orthogonality of avoidance and resistance and contribute to the autonomy of broaden-and-build cycles. Such a conclusion would suggest that Brennan and colleagues' two-factor solution with orthogonal dimensions may have been influenced by the disembedded social conditions of college students within American culture, where neither secure-base effects are fully online, nor anxiety and avoidance are able to become especially tangled. Lionetti, F., Mastrotheodoros, S., & Palladino, B.E. (2018) Experiences in Close Relationships-Revised Child version (ECR-RC): psychometric evidence in support of a security factor. *European Journal of Developmental Psychology*, 15(4), 452–63.

understanding of the secure attachment style will contribute to insights into both clinical phenomena and experiences of human thriving. For example, it will help clarify whether traumatic experiences 'either increase attachment insecurity or wear away at attachment security'.[433] In a review of self-report measures in 2014, Shaver and Mikulincer acknowledged the problems with the ECR for capturing security, and praised the work of Gillath and colleagues. They argued that 'the inclusion of a separate security subscale may suggest a way out of the problem identified by Fraley et al. (2000) … that most previous attachment insecurity scales discriminated poorly at their "secure" ends'.[434] They noted, however, that when the low end of avoidance and anxiety are captured, a result is that the two forms of insecurity are no longer orthogonal, as they are both negatively associated with security: 'expanding the scales at their secure ends in similar ways causes the two kinds of security items to correlate with each other, which in turn makes the scales as wholes correlate more with each other. Whether or not this leads to weaker detection of distinct effects of anxiety and avoidance remains unclear.'[435]

High anxiety/high avoidance

Yet even for the unmodified ECR, questions have been growing about its psychometric properties. Since Shaver and Mikulincer's theory of adult attachment has been based on the two dimensions of the ECR, this is not simply a minor matter of methodological rigour but a concern stretching to the very basis for their scientific project. Whereas the original factor analysis conducted by Brennan and colleagues accounted for 63% of variance, subsequent studies have not accounted for such a high proportion of variance. Factor analytic exploration of the ECR after Brennan and colleagues has been rare among American researchers, who have generally taken its psychometric properties for granted. However, in the wider international literature, factor analytic studies of the ECR or its translation tend to report solutions that account for around 45% of variance.[436]

Furthermore, there has been growing evidence against the orthogonality of the two ECR dimensions. In a review of several of their studies in 2005, Mikulincer, Shaver, and colleagues reported a small association between the scales ($r = .18$).[437] In a paper from the next year, Condradi and colleagues conducted a further analysis of the published literature, observing

[433] Gillath, O., Karantzas, G.C., & Fraley, R.C. (2016) *Adult Attachment: A Concise Introduction to Theory and Research*. London: Academic Press, p.247. See also Kanninen, K., Punamaki, R.L., & Qouta, S. (2003) Personality and trauma: adult attachment and posttraumatic distress among former political prisoners. *Peace and Conflict*, 9(2), 97–126.

[434] Frias, M.T., Shaver, P.R., & Mikulincer, M. (2014) Measures of adult attachment and related constructs. In G.J. Boyle & D.H. Saklofske (eds) *Measures of Personality and Social Psychological Constructs* (pp.417–47). Philadelphia, PA: Elsevier, p.443.

[435] Ibid. p.446.

[436] The ECR-R has fared even less well on this front than the ECR. See e.g. Rotaru, T.Ș. & Rusu, A. (2013) Psychometric properties of the Romanian version of Experiences in Close Relationships-Revised questionnaire (ECR-R). *Procedia-Social and Behavioral Sciences*, 78, 51–5; Busonera, A., Martini, P.S., Zavattini, G.C., & Santona, A. (2014) Psychometric properties of an Italian version of the Experiences in Close Relationships-Revised (ECR-R) Scale. *Psychological Reports*, 114(3), 785–801.

[437] Mikulincer, M., Shaver, P.R., Gillath, O., & Nitzberg, R.A. (2005) Attachment, caregiving, and altruism: boosting attachment security increases compassion and helping. *Journal of Personality and Social Psychology*, 89(5), 817–39, p.821.

that 'intercorrelations vary considerably from .04 to .30'.[438] The developmental and relationship tasks of students as a population may well have some differences from populations in other countries and at different lifestages.[439] Condradi and colleagues observed that
these differences are evidently not sufficient to block the successful application of the ECR
to diverse research populations, as years of research has demonstrated. However, the characteristics of the population used to develop the sample may have nonetheless introduced
unrecognised assumptions into the measure, denting the reliability and validity of its scales.
Specifically, Condradi and colleagues were concerned by Brennan and colleagues' conclusion that attachment anxiety and attachment avoidance were, and should be, orthogonal
dimensions. This seemed to be a holdover from Bartholomew's model of orthogonal dimensions, rather than based on a cogent theoretical justification. They expressed concern that
there was no basis in Bowlby's theory for assuming that the two dimensions would be unrelated. Indeed, researchers in the developmental tradition have neither expected nor found
orthogonality between avoidance and resistance.[440]

Condradi and colleagues sought to empirically examine whether orthogonality might be
an effect of the student sample used by Brennan and colleagues. A two-factor model of orthogonal dimensions was indeed the best fit for the American and Dutch student samples.[441]
However, the result was less clear for the Dutch sample of adults. Condradi and colleagues
argued that anxiety and avoidance may indeed be unrelated for participants without experience in lasting relationships. In more mature relationships they predicted that anxiety and
avoidance would no longer be unrelated. Both dimensions would be negatively associated
with the security that a long-established and healthy relationship can build. And both dimensions would be positively associated with the anxiety and avoidance that can become
entwined within a long-established and unhealthy relationship.[442]

These proposals were supported by two meta-analyses conducted by Cameron and colleagues and by Graham and Unterschute.[443] The meta-analyses found that orthogonality
between anxiety and avoidance was the exception rather than the rule in the published literature. Furthermore, older samples had larger correlations between anxiety and avoidance than
younger samples, long-term relationships had larger correlations than newly established
ones, non-student samples had larger correlations than college samples, and non-American

[438] Conradi, H.-J., Gerlsma, C., van Duijn, M., & de Jonge, P. (2006) Internal and external validity of the
Experiences in Close Relationships questionnaire in an American and two Dutch samples. *European Journal of
Psychiatry*, 20(4), 258–69, p.268.

[439] The principle is one that Shaver acknowledged in his early work, if less in his writings on attachment: Felton,
B.F. & Shaver, P.R. (1984) Cohort variation in adults' reported feelings. In C.Z. Malatesta & C.E. Izard (eds)
Emotions in Adult Development (pp.103–123). Beverly Hills: Sage Publications: 'Adults' choices of coping strategies
are linked to the nature of the problems they face' (118–19).

[440] See e.g. Kroonenberg, P.M., Dam, M.V., van IJzendoorn, M., & Mooijaart, A. (1997) Dynamics of behaviour
in the strange situation: a structural equation approach. *British Journal of Psychology*, 88(2), 311–32.

[441] Research findings from Shaver's American and Mikulincer's Israeli undergraduate samples have generally
aligned well in terms of the correlates of attachment styles. Cultural differences have been reported at times, but
not ones that interact with the ECR. See e.g. Mikulincer, M., Shaver, P.R., Gillath, O., & Nitzberg, R.A. (2005)
Attachment, caregiving, and altruism: boosting attachment security increases compassion and helping. *Journal of
Personality and Social Psychology*, 89(5), 817–39, p.836.

[442] Conradi, H.-J., Gerlsma, C., van Duijn, M., & de Jonge, P. (2006) Internal and external validity of the experiences in close relationships questionnaire in an American and two Dutch samples. *European Journal of Psychiatry*,
20(4), 258–69.

[443] Cameron, J.J., Finnegan, H., & Morry, M.M. (2012) Orthogonal dreams in an oblique world: a meta-analysis
of the association between attachment anxiety and avoidance. *Journal of Research in Personality*, 46(5), 472–6;
Graham, J.M. & Unterschute, M.S. (2015) A reliability generalization meta-analysis of self-report measures of
adult attachment. *Journal of Personality Assessment*, 97(1), 31–41.

samples had larger correlations than American samples. Cameron and colleagues argued that 'such findings call into question the largely implicit assumption that attachment dimensions are orthogonal. As such, our results may inspire researchers to revisit theoretical assumptions, measurement choices, and measure creation techniques. If researchers do not wish to seek other measurement options, they should at the very least adapt their statistical analyses to accommodate shared variance between dimensions ... One method of accommodating shared variance is to include both dimensions as predictors in the same step in a regression, and thus control for shared variance.'[444] The proposal to accommodate or explore shared variance has not, as yet, been pursued. As a result, it remains unknown whether the association between the anxiety and avoidance scales in the ECR lies on the basis of their joint negative association with security or on the basis of their joint positive association with a state of high anxiety/high avoidance.

In recent work with Birnbaum, Mikuliner and Shaver acknowledged both possibilities.[445] They also offered a thought-provoking speculation that the tendency towards orthogonality of the ECR dimensions might actually be an effect of two processes, invisible in the data because they have suppressed one another. On the one hand, anxiety and avoidance may function as exact opposites: Shaver and colleagues have at times argued that each is the inverse of the other in terms of psychological processes.[446] To the extent that they represent maximisation and minimisation of the attachment system, there can be anticipated to be a negative association between the two dimensions. However, this negative association may be counteracted by a positive association between the scales at their endpoints. They may have a positive association in their mutual opposition to security. Furthermore, 'both hyperactivation and deactivation ... represent problems in the system's functioning, which may push their correlation in a positive direction.'[447] The result of both positive and negative associations may be an apparent tendency towards orthogonality.

Whereas Bartholomew gave fearful attachment a major place in her system, the conjunction of high anxiety and high avoidance has not been a major concern of Shaver and Mikulincer over their careers. In part, this is likely due to the fact that there are few high anxiety/high avoidance participants in Shaver and Mikulincer's samples. One essential reason for this, as they have acknowledged, has been their sampling: 'The issue of "fearful avoidance" is, in any case, less likely to arise in normal samples of college students and community adults. Extremely high scores on both the anxiety and avoidance dimensions are more common in samples of abused or clinical samples ... In most of our studies, the results can be

[444] Cameron, J.J., Finnegan, H., & Morry, M.M. (2012) Orthogonal dreams in an oblique world: a meta-analysis of the association between attachment anxiety and avoidance. *Journal of Research in Personality*, 46(5), 472–6, p.475.

[445] Birnbaum, G.E., Mikulincer, M., Szepsenwol, O., Shaver, P.R., & Mizrahi, M. (2014) When sex goes wrong: a behavioral systems perspective on individual differences in sexual attitudes, motives, feelings, and behaviors. *Journal of Personality and Social Psychology*, 106(5), 822–42, p.826.

[446] E.g. Fraley, R.C., Davis, K.E., & Shaver, P.R. (1998) Dismissing avoidance and the defensive organization of emotion, cognition, and behavior. In J.A. Simpson & W.S. Rholes (eds) *Attachment Theory and Close Relationships* (pp.249–79). New York: Guilford: 'It should be noted that the processes and mechanisms we discuss with respect to dismissing-avoidance apply to preoccupation inversely' (275).

[447] Birnbaum, G.E., Mikulincer, M., Szepsenwol, O., Shaver, P.R., & Mizrahi, M. (2014) When sex goes wrong: a behavioral systems perspective on individual differences in sexual attitudes, motives, feelings, and behaviors. *Journal of Personality and Social Psychology*, 106(5), 822–42, p.826. An example here may be the role of distrust in contributing to both avoidance and anxiety, or their reciprocal reinforcement. See McWilliams, L.A. & Fried, E.I. (2019) Reconceptualizing adult attachment relationships: a network perspective. *Personal Relationships*, 26(1), 21–41.

adequately described in terms of either anxiety or avoidance ... with the distinction between dismissing and fearful avoidance mattering only ... when abuse or psychopathology are at issue.'[448] For instance, they cited as evidence a published study by Fraley and Bonanno and unpublished data from Colin Murray Parkes showing that 'combinations of attachment anxiety and avoidance produced the highest levels of anxiety, depression, grief, trauma-related symptoms, and alcohol consumption.'[449]

Shaver and Mikulincer's overriding use of student samples has been a pragmatic one. They have readily admitted that it supplies a limitation to their work. For instance, they have noticed that it can be difficult to recruit student participants with an avoidant attachment style when adverts are frank with participants that the study is concerned with close relationships.[450] And Makariev and Shaver have acknowledged that middle-class college populations were not 'the kinds of people Bowlby had in mind when he began to develop attachment theory.'[451] Nonetheless, Shaver and Mikulincer have defended their use of student samples on two grounds. In a first defence, they have argued that adversities and psychopathology is dimensionally distributed, and so there is no particular problem with using a student sample—so long as clinical variance is captured.[452] This defence is relatively weak. It is not clear that clinical variance is generally well captured by the measures Shaver and Mikulincer tend to use; in this context, it is perhaps unsurprising that studies of adult attachment styles and PTSD have tended not to use the ECR.[453] Furthermore, the idea that adversities and psychopathology can be treated as dimentional in terms of their implications for attachment style is simply asserted, rather than adequately empirically demonstrated in their work.

Shaver and Mikulincer have also offered a second defence of their approach in describing themselves as pragmatists, seeing to achieve cogent simplifications whilst remaining aware of what has been simplified:

In our work, we always try to keep in mind that there is, on the one hand, complex everyday reality as we experience it subjectively and encounter it in the behavior of other people. And, on the other hand, there is psychological theory, with its associated hypothetical constructs, and an ever-evolving toolbox of psychological measures. The trick is to discover and document something important and valid about real life, thereby nudging

[448] Mikulincer, M. & Shaver, P.R. (2003) The attachment behavioral system in adulthood: activation, psychodynamics, and interpersonal processes. In M.P. Zanna (ed.) Advances in Experimental Social Psychology, Vol. 35 (pp.53–152). New York: Academic Press, pp.70, 88.

[449] Shaver, P.R. & Mikulincer, M. (2008) Adult attachment and cognitive and affective reactions to positive and negative events. Social and Personality Compass, 2, 1844–65, p.1853. Citing Fraley, R. C. & Bonanno, G. A. (2004) Attachment and loss: a test of three competing models on the association between attachment-related avoidance and adaptation to bereavement. Personality and Social Psychology Bulletin, 30(7), 878–90.

[450] Gillath, O., Bunge, S.A., Shaver, P.R., Wendelken, C., & Mikulincer, M. (2005) Attachment-style differences in the ability to suppress negative thoughts: exploring the neural correlates. Neuroimage, 28(4), 835–47, p.945.

[451] Makariev, D.W. & Shaver, P.R. (2010) Attachment, parental incarceration and possibilities for intervention: an overview, Attachment & Human Development, 12(4), 311–31, p.325.

[452] Brennan, K.A. & Shaver, P.R. (1998) Attachment styles and personality disorders: their connections to each other and to parental divorce, parental death, and perceptions of parental caregiving. Journal of Personality, 66(5), 835–78: 'One obvious limitation of our research is its use of a nonclinical sample. To some extent, this limitation turns on whether one accepts a purely categorical (vs. dimensional) understanding of personality disorders. If, as we do, one assumes that personality disorders can be arrayed on continua, then our results ought to generalize to clinical populations' (870).

[453] Woodhouse, S., Ayers, S., & Field, A.P. (2015) The relationship between adult attachment style and post-traumatic stress symptoms: a meta-analysis. Journal of Anxiety Disorders, 35, 103–117.

psychological science forward, without mistaking our tentative, overly simplified picture for everything that is actually there.[454]

However, the inattention to high anxiety/high avoidance attachment styles is more than a happenstance of sampling. Instead, the sampling strategy appears to have reflected a broader lack of concern with adverse and clinical experiences, and states where both anxiety and avoidance are in play.

Even before the introduction of the ECR, Shaver and Mikulincer demonstrated a marked lack of interest in what it meant when participants endorsed both an anxious and avoidant attachment style. In his work in the early 1990s, Mikulincer reformulated the 'love quiz' as three scales to produce dimensional ratings of attachment style.[455] In a validation study of the scales with 127 undergraduates, nine participants scored differently on the scales compared to the original category-based 'love quiz'. Mikulincer dropped these participants from the analysis. This approach set a precedent. Cooper, Shaver, and Collins used both the category-based and the dimension-based measures in their 1998 paper 'Attachment styles, emotion regulation, and adjustment in adolescence'.[456] In the study, 411 participants—20% of the sample—were inconsistent across the two measures. In a footnote, the authors acknowledged that this inconsistent group had some interesting properties. They were more likely to be non-White, more likely to endorse an insecure attachment style, and more likely to have been held back in school. Furthermore, 'inconsistent responders reported higher levels of phobic anxiety, paranoia, and psychoticism and were less satisfied with their body image'.[457] Though this 'inconsistent' group represented hundreds of participants, they were thrown out of the analysis.[458]

Considering this study alone, the decision makes methodological sense. However, in the broader context of Shaver's work, it illustrates a trend to exclude the effects of adversity, stigma, pharmacology, and clinical complexity from the study of adult attachment styles. The most influential instance of this trend was in work with Brennan and Clark in developing the ECR. In their 1998 paper, the factor analysis was conducted on an undergraduate sample from the University of Texas. However, no report was made or analysis conducted for demographic or ethnic diversity within the sample. And no data were collected on clinical differences. Across their published studies, Shaver and Mikulincer have rarely discussed the implications of both high anxiety and avoidance, even in studies where they included measures of mental health.[459] There seems to have been a self-perpetuating cycle between lack of interest and lack of scientific basis for interest in high anxiety/high avoidance phenomena in existing theory and research. This has shaped the tone and priorities of social psychological

[454] Shaver, P. & Mikulincer, M. (2004) Attachment in the later years: a commentary. *Attachment & Human Development*, 6(4), 451–64, p.462. Other laboratories have confirmed that high anxiety/high avoidance attachment is more prevalent in psychiatric samples, e.g. Alessandri, G., Fagnani, C., Di Gennaro, G., et al. (2014) Measurement invariance of the experiences in close relationships questionnaire across different populations. *Spanish Journal of Psychology*, 17(2), E22.

[455] Mikulincer, M. & Nachshon, O. (1991) Attachment styles and patterns of self-disclosure. *Journal of Personality and Social Psychology*, 61(2), 321–31.

[456] Cooper, M.L., Shaver, P.R., & Collins, N.L. (1998) Attachment styles, emotion regulation, and adjustment in adolescence. *Journal of Personality and Social Psychology*, 74(5), 1380–97.

[457] Ibid. p.1385.

[458] Ibid.: 'We adopted the procedure used by Mikulincer and Nachshon and excluded inconsistent respondents from further analyses' (1386).

[459] E.g. Crawford, T.N., Livesley, W.J., Jang, K.L., Shaver, P.R., Cohen, P., & Ganiban, J. (2007) Insecure attachment and personality disorder: a twin study of adults. *European Journal of Personality*, 21(2), 191–208.

research on attachment, hindering dialogue with the developmental tradition where theorising and measuring the implications of trauma and fear for attachment have been a major focus (Chapter 3).

Despite the general trend, there have been a few occasions on which Shaver and Mikulincer have reported associations for high anxiety/high avoidance attachment.[460] One was a study by Schachner and Shaver of sexual motives, which found that high anxiety/high avoidance—over and above the anxious attachment style alone—was associated with greater report of having sex due to insecurity.[461] Hart, Shaver, and Goldenberg found that high anxiety/high avoidance was distinctively associated with a desire for closeness after receiving information that was anticipated to threaten the participants' cultural worldview, but not in the control condition. This was in contrast to the anxious attachment style which was associated with a desire for closeness in both conditions.[462] The researchers concluded that the avoidant strategy held high anxiety/high avoidance participants back from seeking support in the control condition, but that the strategy was overwhelmed by the combination of high attachment anxiety and a worldview threat, leading to behaviour shaped by the anxious strategy.[463]

The effects of trauma

A major qualification must be offered, however, to any allegation that inattention to attachment phenomena characterised by high anxiety and high avoidance is a limitation in the work of Shaver and Mikulincer.[464] The qualification lies in Mikulincer's two decades of research on the effects of war and military trauma. However, this research has not always been well linked-up with Mikulincer's theoretical work on adult attachment. The relationship between PTSD and the insecure attachment styles in Mikulincer's work has remained untamed, especially in terms of what this relationship means for the conceptualisation of high anxiety/high avoidance states and of adult attachment in general. This issue appears to be coming to a head in recent years, given the very sharp increase in studies of PTSD and attachment styles in the past decade. However, refinements in theory and methodology appear generally not to have caught up with this empirical concern.

---

[460] Shaver and Mikulincer have at times reported relevant findings from other research groups, though this has been exceptionally rare. E.g. Mikulincer, M. & Shaver, P.R. (2005) Attachment theory and emotion in close relationships: exploring the attachment-related dynamics of emotional reactions to relational events. *Personal Relationships*, 12, 149–68, p.160.

[461] Schachner, D.A. & Shaver, P.R. (2004) Attachment dimensions and sexual motives. *Personal Relationships*, 11(2), 179–95, p.192.

[462] Hart, J.J., Shaver, P.R., & Goldenberg, J.L. (2005) Attachment, self-esteem, worldviews, and terror management: evidence for a tripartite security system. *Journal of Personality and Social Psychology*, 88, 999–1013, p.1008.

[463] For another example of specific correlates of high anxiety/high avoidance attachment see Gillath, O., Giesbrecht, B., & Shaver, P.R. (2009) Attachment, attention, and cognitive control: attachment style and performance on general attention tasks. *Journal of Experimental Social Psychology*, 45(4), 647–54, p.651.

[464] It might be thought that an additional qualification could be offered on the basis of the major efforts by Shaver and Mikulincer to review empirical studies of psychopathology, e.g. Mikulincer, M. & Shaver, P. (2016) *Attachment in Adulthood*, 2nd edn. New York: Guilford, Chapter 13. However, these reviews are lacking precisely in consideration of high anxiety/high avoidance attachment styles except, on a handful of occasions, when reporting findings from Bartholomew's measures. The question of whether studies using the ECR have found effects for high anxiety/high avoidance, and more generally the question of whether the high ends of the scales are individually or in interaction effective at capturing clinical phenomena, is not in view. The focus is instead on anxiety and avoidance as, separately, dimensionally associated with forms of mental pathology. Throughout the reviews, a linear and dimensional association between the ECR scales and psychopathology is assumed rather than demonstrated or explored.

In the late 1980s, Solomon, Mikulincer, and colleagues examined Israeli army veterans who had experienced symptoms of post-traumatic combat stress during the 1982 Lebanon war. On the one hand, the researchers observed that one of the symptoms associated with this condition was 'psychic numbing', which was associated with low emotional expressiveness in the veterans' adult relationships with family members. The researchers accepted that 'there is little way of knowing whether it is the family that did not permit the veteran to express himself or the veteran who did not make use of the avenues of expression open to him'.[465] However, they expressed their suspicion that 'many PTSD casualties who report a low level of expressiveness may themselves have avoided discussion'.[466] On the other hand, Mikulincer, Solomon, and colleagues also found that, among veterans who had experienced symptoms of post-traumatic combat stress, 'the anxiety feelings aroused during battle by the fear of death are crystalized one year later in anxiety that is not specifically related to death, but is generalized to every potential threat'.[467] This would, presumably, include relational threats. These early observations suggest, though this point was not drawn out by the researchers, that general forms of avoidance and anxiety stemming from trauma may feed more specific forms of avoidance and anxiety within adult close relationships.

Mikulincer, Solomon, and Benbenishty also conducted clinical interviews with a sample of 104 veterans with histories of post-traumatic combat stress symptoms a year after the end of the Lebanon war. From these interviews, they identified 26 different manifestations of post-traumatic combat stress and nine battle events that seemed relevant to the emergence or maintenance of symptoms. Analysis of the manifestations resulted in six factors, accounting for 62% of variance. The six factors were: psychic numbing, anxiety reactions, guilt, loneliness, loss of bodily control (such as uncontrollable crying or vomiting), and disorientation. It is interesting, if perhaps not surprising, how well these agree with Bowlby's own clinical observations of war veterans during his time as an army psychiatrist (Chapter 1). In the work of Mikulincer and colleagues, psychic numbing and anxiety reactions appeared to be the most important, between them accounting for 31% of variance in symptoms reported in the clinical interview. They explicitly argued that psychic numbing should be conceptualised as a kind of 'avoidance' and considered as quite an all-purpose response, since it was not associated with any particular kind of battle event. By contrast, anxiety reactions were predicted best by poor unit functioning. Mikulicer and colleagues argued that psychic numbing and anxiety reactions seemed to correspond well, respectively, to 'avoidance and numbing' and 'hyperarousal' as two of the main clusters of general PTSD symptoms. They therefore suggested that post-traumatic combat stress symptoms should not be regarded solely as localised responses to particular war experiences, but as reflecting the basic forms of the human trauma response.[468]

Pursuing these questions further, in the mid-1990s Mukulincer and colleagues asked 40 Israeli Jewish settlers living within Palestinian Authority territory in the Gaza Strip to

---

[465] Solomon, Z., Mikulincer, M., Freid, B., & Wosner, Y. (1987) Family characteristics and posttraumatic stress disorder: a follow-up of Israeli combat stress reaction casualties. *Family Process*, 26(3), 383–94, p.390.

[466] Ibid.

[467] Mikulincer, M., Solomon, Z., & Benbenishty, R. (1988) Battle events, acute combat stress reaction and long-term psychological sequelae of war. *Journal of Anxiety Disorders*, 2(2), 121–33, p.131.

[468] Solomon, Z., Mikulincer, M., & Benbenishty, R. (1989) Combat stress reaction—clinical manifestations and correlates. *Military Psychology*, 1(1), 35–47, p.44. Later work by the researchers documented powerful longitudinal effects of these traumatic symptoms. See Solomon, Z. & Mikulincer, M. (2007) Post traumatic intrusion, avoidance, and social functioning: a 20-year longitudinal study. *Journal of Consulting and Clinical Psychology*, 75(2), 316–24.

fill out the 'love quiz' and measures of mental distress and PTSD. The settlers were physic-ally cut-off from the rest of Israel. The settlement had been repeatedly attacked, including a suicide-bombing in 1994 which killed six Jewish members of the settlement and six Palestinians.[469] The settlement was also at the time facing the threat of eviction by the Israeli government (indeed, this threat would later be realised in August 2005, when the government sent in the army to forcibly remove the settlers). Though the identities and lives of the settlers would be potentially quite different from the combat veterans he had studied, Mukulincer nonetheless hoped that he could treat this group as representing a 'high threat' condition. The settler participants were compared to 40 matched controls living in villages of equivalent size but within the borders of Israel. They also examined the correlates of different symptom clusters of PTSD: intrusive symptoms (e.g. flashbacks), avoidant symptoms (e.g. emotional numbing), and hyperarousal (e.g. sudden irritability or startle responses).[470] Mukulincer and colleagues found that overall attachment styles were a much better predictor of mental health than whether participants were settlers or in the control group, accounting for five to six times more variance in general distress and mental health and PSTD-specific symptoms.[471]

However, the threat condition was a powerful moderator of attachment style. The anxious-ambivalent attachment style was associated with general mental health symptoms and avoidant, hyperarousal, and intrusive PTSD symptoms for both the settlers and the matched controls; this association was not stronger for the settlers. By contrast, the avoidant attach-ment style was associated with general distress and mental health symptoms only among the settler group. It was also associated with PTSD symptoms from the avoidance cluster. An as-sociation with PTSD symptoms from the hyperarousal/intrusion cluster was marked but fell just short of significance, which was interpreted as an effect of the small sample. Mikulincer and colleagues interpreted their findings as suggesting that the high threat condition was putting strain on the avoidant attachment strategy, and that this strain was most clearly seen in the form of PTSD symptoms that reflected this attachment strategy.[472] However, there were indications that the high threat condition additionally made a contribution to distress and mental illness among participants with an avoidant attachment style.

---

[469] See also Haberman, C. (1994) Palestinians arrest 100 Islamic militants after bicycle bombing. *New York Times*, 13 November 1994.

[470] The distinction between these symptom clusters had been introduced in DSM-III-R. Brett, E., Spitzer, R., & Williams, J.B. (1988) DSM-III-R criteria for posttraumatic stress disorder. *American Journal of Psychiatry*, 145(10), 1232. The distinction was embedded in psychological tools such as the Post-traumatic Stress Disorder Inventory, developed by Solomon, Weisenberg, Schwarzwald, and Mikulincer in the late 1980s, and used in the 1999 study of the Jewish settlers.

[471] Mikulincer, M., Horesh, N., Eilati, I., & Kotler, M. (1999) The association between adult attachment style and mental health in extreme life-endangering conditions. *Personality and Individual Differences*, 27(5), 831–42, p.837.

[472] Ibid.: 'Interestingly, this distress was mainly manifested in avoidance rather than intrusive responses, which seem to be avoidant persons' habitual affect regulation strategy' (839). The proposal that PTSD avoid-ance and hyperarousal symptoms parallel the Ainsworth avoidant and ambivalent/resistant classifications had first been made a few years earlier by Crittenden, P.M. (1997) Toward an integrative theory of trauma: a dynamic–maturational approach. In D. Cicchetti & S. Toth (eds) *The Rochester Symposium on Developmental Psychopathology, Vol. 10. Risk, Trauma, and Mental Processes* (pp.34–84). New York: University of Rochester Press. In a later study, Besser and colleagues used the ECR with civilians exposed to terrorist attacks in southern Israel. Unlike Mikulincer, they found few or weak associations from attachment avoidance. They found stronger associ-ations from attachment anxiety with all three clusters of PTSD symptoms (intrusive, avoidance, and hyperarousal). The reasons for these different results may stem from the different sample. It may be that an avoidant attachment style was still a viable strategy for participants subject to long-term missile threat, in contrast to the settlers studied by Mikulincer. Besser, A., Neria, Y., & Haynes, M. (2009) Adult attachment, perceived stress, and PTSD among ci-vilians exposed to ongoing terrorist attacks in southern Israel. *Personality and Individual Differences*, 47(8), 851–7.

The avoidant PTSD symptoms reported by the settlers could be interpreted as a consequence of an avoidant strategy under severe strain.[473] It might also be that as the avoidant strategy became overwhelmed and unviable, individuals would experience other forms of distress and anxiety. Conversely, Shaver and Mikulincer considered that the anxious attachment strategy might become unviable in some situations and start to fail. The comparison of the settlers and matched controls did not reveal differences in the anxious attachment strategy or its correlates. However, Shaver and Mikulincer acknowledged that, in other conditions, it might be 'possible to speak about the failure of hyperactivating strategies.'[474] Indeed, Mikulincer and colleagues' work with the combat veterans from the Lebanon war suggested that war trauma could perhaps contribute to forms of PTSD resembling or expressing both deactivating and hyperactivating strategies.[475]

In the early 2000s, Mukulincer and Shaver identified the need for further attention to the diverse conditions that might promote the activation of the avoidant attachment style in different forms.[476] They proposed that these conditions might include (i) consistent rejection from attachment figures; (ii) threats of punishment by attachment figures for the display of attachment behaviours; (iii) traumatic or abusive experiences in the context of the desire for comfort; and (iv) contexts that encourage self-reliance. The conditions that would promote an anxious attachment style might include: (i) care unrelated to signals about need; (ii) care that punishes or prevents the development of self-regulation skills or autonomy; (iii) messages from the attachment figure that emphasise the individual's helplessness; and (iv) traumatic or abusive experiences in the context of separation from attachment figures. So, for instance, trauma in both the context of the wish for comfort and the context of separations could be expected to promote both anxious and avoidant strategies. The most potent conditions shaping the selection of attachment strategy, Shaver and Mikulincer suggested,

[473] Mikulincer, M., Dolev, T., & Shaver, P.R. (2004) Attachment-related strategies during thought suppression: ironic rebounds and vulnerable self-representations. *Journal of Personality and Social Psychology*, 87(6), 940–56: 'Deactivating strategies can be inadequate and overwhelmed, resulting in a marked decline in functioning and what Horowitz (1982) called "avoidance-related" posttraumatic symptoms (e.g., psychic numbing, behavioral inhibition)' (941).

[474] Shaver, P.R. & Mikulincer, M. (2002) Dialogue on adult attachment: diversity and integration. *Attachment & Human Development*, 4(2), 243–57, p.247. Shaver and Mikulincer did not flesh out the conditions under which failure of hyperactivating strategies might be expected. It is also not fully clear whether failure would entail the flooding of anxiety in some internal sense, or the breakdown of the capacity to strive for closeness with attachment figures, or both. The former appears to be described in a characterisation of the hyperactivating strategy early in Shaver and Mikulincer's work together: Mikulincer, M. & Shaver, P.R. (2003) The attachment behavioral system in adulthood: activation, psychodynamics, and interpersonal processes. In M.P. Zanna (ed.) *Advances in Experimental Social Psychology*, Vol. 35 (pp.53–152). New York: Academic Press: 'Intrapsychically, amplification of threat appraisals heightens the chronic accessibility of negative thoughts and makes it likely that new sources of distress will mingle and become confounded with old accessible ones ... the person experiences an endless and uncontrollable flow of negative thoughts and moods, which in turn may lead to cognitive disorganization and, in certain cases, culminate in psychopathology' (82–3).

[475] These concerns may also be placed in other discussions at the time in social psychology regarding the potential for different forms of personality disorder to reflect extreme forms of attachment system activation or deactivation, especially in the context of loss, trauma, or chronic adversities. See Bartholomew, K., Kwong, M.J., & Hart, S.D. (2001) Attachment. In W.J. Livesley (ed.) *Handbook of Personality Disorders: Theory, Research, and Treatment* (pp.196–230). New York: Guilford.

[476] E.g. Mikulincer, M., Gillath, O., & Shaver, P.R. (2002) Activation of the attachment system in adulthood: threat-related primes increase the accessibility of mental representations of attachment figures. *Journal of Personality and Social Psychology*, 83(4), 881–95: 'It would be interesting to explore further how avoidant persons' inhibitory processes work, what they are designed to accomplish (e.g., protection from a potentially angry, punitive attachment figure; reduction of the attachment figure's tendency to threaten abandonment or decrease support if a particular separation is resisted), and when they arise—either in the course of development or in the course of a particular long-term relationship' (893–4).

would be those that related directly to the use of the caregiver as secure base or safe haven.[477] However, as discussed in the section 'Minimising and maximising', over time, Shaver and Mikulincer came to explicitly acknowledge that other behavioural systems could feed into and alter schemas about relationships. This would, presumably, include the fear behavioural system: threat experiences are anticipated to inform Module 1 in Shaver and Mikulincer's model of the attachment system. The researchers argued that, overall, more needed to be done to understand the conditions that would allow the avoidant and anxious attachment strategies to mitigate, intensify, or express mental illness.[478]

Yet in the 2000s, the lines of causality remained tangled. It could be that traumatic experiences were relevant to the selection and intensification of maximising and minimising strategies, including in the domain of attachment. This was suggested by Mikulincer's original work with combat veterans from the Lebanon war. However, it could be that attachment strategies from early life were predisposing and shaping traumatic experiences. This was suggested by Mikulincer's study of the Israeli settlers, and would be congruent with Shaver and Mikulincer's emphasis in the early 2000s on attachment styles as shaped primarily by childhood experiences and then predisposing later mental illness. Of course, it was also possible that both processes were taking place simultaneously and reciprocally. To pick apart the temporal relationship between attachment styles and trauma, Solomon, Dekel, and Mikulincer reported findings in 2008 from a longitudinal study of Israeli former prisoners of war from the 1973 Yom Kippur War.[479] Participants were followed up in 1991 and 2003, and asked at both times to complete the scaled version of the 'love quiz' and a self-report measure of PTSD symptoms. The researchers found that both attachment anxiety and attachment avoidance increased over time among the former prisoners of war, whereas they remained at least stable among the matched control veterans. Both anxious and avoidant attachment styles were positively associated with PTSD symptoms for the former prisoners of war and the matched controls. PTSD avoidance was a potent predictor of later attachment avoidance ($r = .68$), but it was also predicted by PTSD hyperarousal ($r = .59$). PTSD avoidance and hyperarousal both also predicted later attachment anxiety ($r = .58, .50$).[480]

The longitudinal nature of the study allowed Solomon and colleagues to analyse the respective contribution of these factors to one another over time. Contrary to expectations, the results showed that early PTSD symptoms predicted later attachment styles much better than early attachment styles predicted later PTSD symptoms. The researchers accepted that 'this finding cannot be easily explained by adult attachment theory (Mikulincer & Shaver). According to this theory, attachment insecurities are a risk factor for the emergence and increase of PTSD symptoms and not the reverse. As a result, this finding is a major novelty of the current prospective study. It seems that traumatic events and post-traumatic responses cause changes in people's resources and resiliency and then deteriorate their sense

[477] Mikulincer, M., Shaver, P.R., & Pereg, D. (2003) Attachment theory and affect regulation: the dynamics, development, and cognitive consequences of attachment-related strategies. *Motivation and Emotion*, 27, 77–102, pp.97–8.

[478] Ibid.: 'Researchers should examine the conditions under which secondary attachment strategies seem to work sufficiently well to avoid severe psychopathology. We still do not know why some insecurely attached individuals function within the normal range whereas others require clinical intervention' (100).

[479] Solomon, Z., Dekel, R., & Mikulincer, M. (2008) Complex trauma of war captivity: a prospective study of attachment and post-traumatic stress disorder. *Psychological Medicine* 38(10), 1427–34.

[480] Ein-Dor, T., Doron, G., Solomon, Z., Mikulincer, M., & Shaver, P.R. (2010) Together in pain: attachment-related dyadic processes and posttraumatic stress disorder. *Journal of Counseling Psychology*, 57(3), 317–27, p.321, Table 1.

of attachment security.'[481] By the late 2000s, Shaver and Mikulincer had come to acknowledge that attachment style would reflect not only early experiences with attachment figures, but also information relevant to close relationships from other behavioural systems and from adolescent and adult experiences. Nonetheless, Mikulincer was still taken aback by the fact that PTSD symptoms seemed to be better predictors of attachment style in the sample than vice versa. It also remained unclear whether the additional attachment anxiety and avoidance predicted by the PTSD was the same kind of anxiety and avoidance as before the trauma. It could be that the attachment measure was actually picking up PTSD avoidance and hyperarousal as it figured within the attachment relationship.

Conclusion

Writing in the *New York Times* in 1974, Bowlby acknowledged that it might often be perplexing why psychological researchers fell into agreement or disagreement when ostensibly discussing the same phenomena, and even sometimes the same theory or data. Acknowledging that there could be a variety of factors involved, he underlined one as central. When psychological knowledge is in dissensus, ultimately 'we differ, I believe, on how we picture the raw human nature than emerges into the world when a baby is born'.[482] The difference between the developmental and social psychological traditions must be recognised as only partially a divergence in method. Differences in method have at times reflected and at times stabilised important differences in how the two traditions conceptualise attachment and its role within the human condition. As Chapter 3 described, Mary Main's account of conditional strategies was not merely a lens on the Strange Situation, but a model of the three basic ways that humans can direct attention in responding to distress and the activation of the attachment system. It was this general model that led to the development of the AAI coding system, since infant behaviour and adult autobiographical discourse could be regarded as forms affected by the same processes. In turn, Main's methodological innovations and their predictive value have helped stabilise the general theoretical idea of minimising and maximising strategies as the best way to capture individual differences in the Strange Situation and AAI. In a similar manner, the methodological decisions of the social psychological tradition have had a bidirectional relationship with their model of human nature.[483]

---

[481] Solomon, Z., Dekel, R., & Mikulincer, M. (2008) Complex trauma of war captivity: a prospective study of attachment and post-traumatic stress disorder. *Psychological Medicine* 38(10), 1427–34, p.1431. See also Mikulincer, M., Ein-Dor, T., Solomon, Z., & Shaver, P.R. (2011) Trajectories of attachment insecurities over a 17-year period: a latent growth curve analysis of the impact of war captivity and posttraumatic stress disorder. *Journal of Social and Clinical Psychology*, 30(9), 960–84. A related finding was reported by Ghafoori and colleagues in their study of US military veterans. Ghafoori, B., Hierholzer, R.W., Howsepian, B., & Boardman, A. (2008) The role of adult attachment, parental bonding, and spiritual love in the adjustment to military trauma. *Journal of Trauma & Dissociation*, 9(1), 85–106.

[482] Bowlby, J. (1974) A guide to the perplexed parent. *New York Times*, 2 March 1974.

[483] Granqvist, P. (2020) *Attachment, Religion, and Spirituality: A Wider View*. New York: Guilford: 'The principal ideas about attachment-related individual differences largely derive from, and are intertwined with, the methods used to measure such individual differences.' See also Verbeke, W., Belschack, F., Bagozzi, R.P., Pozharliev, R., & Ein-Dor, T. (2017) Why some people just 'can't get no satisfaction': secure versus insecure attachment styles affect one's 'style of being in the social world'. *International Journal of Marketing Studies*, 9(2), 36–55: 'In using general attachment scales to study why attachment styles are so pervasive in affecting people's relationships, we take an ontological stance (philosophical study of the nature of being) in order to look at how individual differences in attachment styles reflect people's sense of being in the social world' (37).

The developmental tradition has more often, though not exclusively, adopted a narrower definition of attachment, focused on the properties of a behavioural system shared with other primates and not requiring elaborate symbolic capacities. By contrast, the social psychological tradition has tended to adopt a much broader image of attachment as manifest in all human relational dynamics, including how humans 'co-explore their social world, share their enjoyment in the pleasures of their world, and cope with stress in that world'.[484] This has followed a thread in Bowlby's writings, where sometimes he used the idea of attachment to refer to this broader sense, including the symbolisation of safe haven and secure base phenomena in relationships with ideas and institutions. However, more structurally, this broader notion of attachment reflected and continues to express the concerns of social psychology as a subdiscipline. In very general terms, and especially in its American incarnation, since the 1960s, developmental psychology has tended to focus on the study of the emergence of the capacities of individuals, especially as these occur in the context of their family relationships.[485] The work of Ainsworth and second-generation attachment researchers contributed to this discipline formation and was shaped by it. From the 1980s, again especially in America, experimental social psychology has tended to examine the role of personality and social processes within the diversity of adult individual perceptions, attitudes, and practices, including but not limited to intimate relationships.[486] (Exceptions can readily be found to these limited characterisations, of course, which are intended to convey general and predominant differences. Nonetheless, researchers who seem the prime exceptions can often be found expressing concern about the limitations of predominant disciplinary trends.)[487]

The subdisciplines can be regarded as aligned by a basic commitment to imagining humans as interdependent with others, and therefore to the study of interactions. And they find many points of cross-over, for instance in the study of the development of moral reasoning. However, in general terms, in developmental psychology humans are attended to as interdependent in their formation. Main's theory is an account of repetoires of response to this interdependence as it is expressed by the demands of the attachment system. This is sometimes confused by the assumption that the AAI measures a 'thing' called 'attachment' and by the individualising language of 'secure' and 'insecure' infants. Nonetheless, following Ainsworth, the official line of the developmental tradition has been that attachment is, or at least starts as, a dyadic property. This is a central reason why developmental attachment

---

[484] Ibid.

[485] Developmental cognitive psychology can here be identified as an exception, since the focus here is often less relational. There are certainly exceptions, though, such as the study of babies' recognition of human faces, e.g. Farroni, T., Menon, E., Rigato, S., & Johnson, M.H. (2007) The perception of facial expressions in newborns. *European Journal of Developmental Psychology*, 4(1), 2–13.

[486] On the history of social psychology see Danziger, K. (2000) Making social psychology experimental: a conceptual history, 1920–1970. *Journal of the History of the Behavioral Sciences*, 36(4), 329–47; Greenwood, J.D. (2004) What happened to the 'social' in social psychology? *Journal for the Theory of Social Behaviour*, 34(1), 19–34; Jahoda, G. (2007) *A History of Social Psychology: From the Eighteenth-century Enlightenment to the Second World War*. Cambridge: Cambridge University Press; Kruglanksi, A.W. & Stroebe, W. (eds) (2012) *Handbook for the History of Social Psychology*. Bristol: Psychology Press; Pettigrew, T.F. & Cherry, F. (2012) The intertwined histories of personality and social psychology. In M.R. Leary & R.H. Hoyle (eds) *Handbook of Individual Differences in Social Behavior* (pp.13–32). New York: Guilford. On distinctions between trends in American and European social psychology see Schruijer, S.G. (2012) Whatever happened to the 'European'in European social psychology? A study of the ambitions in founding the European Association of Experimental Social Psychology. *History of the Human Sciences*, 25(3), 88–107.

[487] See e.g. Jahoda, G. (2016) Seventy years of social psychology: a cultural and personal critique. *Journal of Social and Political Psychology*, 4(1), 364–80. On the role of ongoing boundary-work in the construction of legitimate and illegitimate exceptions to predominant trends in a discipline see Good, J.M. (2000) Disciplining social psychology: a case study of boundary relations in the history of the human sciences. *Journal of the History of the Behavioral Sciences*, 36(4), 383–403.

researchers have been reluctant to support the 'attachment disorder' diagnosis of individual children, leaving this diagnosis an odd and poorly integrated appendage to the developmental research tradition (Chapter 1).

By contrast, in experimental social psychology the focus tends to be on the study of already largely formed adult humans as influenced by social and relational factors in their perceptions, attitudes, and practices. As Stainton Rogers and colleagues have argued, there is a liberal humanist quality to social psychology: humans are registered at the point that they can act independently, though the concern is then with how they ultimately live together.[488] This has helped make use of college student samples a backbone of the subdiscipline. It has also helped make self-report methodology more acceptable than for developmental psychologists. Shaver and Mikulincer are more committed than most social psychologists to the idea that, at a fundamental level, relationships are primary, individuals are secondary: 'Rather than conceptualizing human beings as separate entities whose interactions with each other need to be understood, it makes more sense to consider social relatedness and its mental correlates as the normal "baseline" condition.'[489] Nonetheless, aligned with the focus on individuals and their interactions in wider American social psychology, their predominant methodological orientation has been towards the study of the schemas of individuals about close relationships as reflected in their self-reports. Using self-report measures of attachment styles, Shaver and Mikulincer's work has explored how an individual's schemas about close relationships shape a diverse range of their perceptions, attitudes, and practices, ranging from how new romantic relationships are established to how recklessly they drive a car.

One important by-product of the self-report methodology used by social psychological attachment researchers was that it lowered an important barrier to experimental research. This contributed to the identification of the effects of security priming by social psychologists, which is discussed in the next chapter. It also lowered a barrier to public engagement. As documented in previous chapters, Bowlby's work had contributed to a widespread public for attachment theory and research. However, the developmental tradition of attachment research had faced obstacles in continuing this legacy. Concepts such as the attachment behavioural system were complex and subtle, and the observational methodology favoured by Ainsworth was complex and required extensive training to fully understand. Furthermore,

[488] Stainton Rogers, R., Stenner, P., Gleeson, K., & Stainton Rogers, W. (1995) *Social Psychology: A Critical Agenda*. Cambridge: Polity Press; Danziger, K. (1992) The project of an experimental social psychology: historical perspectives. *Science in Context*, 5, 309–328. See also Spini, D., Elcheroth, G., & Figini, D. (2009) Is there space for time in social psychology publications? A content analysis across five journals. *Journal of Community & Applied Social Psychology*, 19(3), 165–81. Allport's 'official' definition of social psychology as the study of how 'the thought, feeling, and behavior of individuals are influenced by the actual, imagined, or implied presence of others' is illustrative: the individual is influenced by others, but is registered already as an individual. Allport, G.W. (1954) The historical background of modern social psychology. In G.L. Lindzey (ed.) *Handbook of Social Psychology*, Vol. 1 (pp.3–45). Reading, MA: Addison-Wesley, p.5. Nonetheless, continuities in social psychology over time should not be overemphasised. See Lubek, I. & Apfelbaum, E. (2000) A critical gaze and wistful glance at Handbook histories of social psychology: did the successive accounts by Gordon Allport and successors historiographically succeed? *Journal of the History of the Behavioral Sciences*, 36(4), 405–428. In particular, the rise of relationship research in social psychology since the 1980s has roots in earlier work, but should be recognised as a distinct development. See Reis, H.T. (2012) A brief history of relationship research in social psychology. In A.W. Kruglanski & W. Stroebe (eds) *Handbook Online Dating* (pp.363–82). Bristol: Psychology Press.

[489] Mikulincer, M. & Shaver, P.R. (2012) An attachment perspective on psychopathology. *World Psychiatry*, 11(1), 11–15, p.14. See also Shaver, P.R. & Mikulincer, M. (2012) Attachment processes in relationships: reply to commentaries. *Journal of Family Theory and Review*, 4, 311–17: 'If interpersonal relations are somewhat like dances or doubles tennis games, it is reasonable to expect that some of what is going on in the dance or in a match is "in" the individual dancers or players (e.g., their skills, their muscle development, their history of training and performance), some of it is in the interpersonal dynamics of a particular dyad, and some of it is in the context of a particular performance (e.g., the other players, a particular piece of music, the audience)' (313).

Ainsworth and her students were focused on creating a differentiated space within which empirical attachment research could thrive, giving little time to communicating in popular forums. There may also have been some reticence to take on Bowlby's mantle as a public intellectual. For the social psychological tradition, the barrier to public understanding was substantially lowered. The Hazan and Shaver 'love quiz' has its subtlties in the formulation of the statements, but the measure's presumption that there are distinct adult attachment styles that can be reported by any individual about themselves contributed to a fundamental accessiblity.

An interesting illustration is the recommendation by Fonagy and colleagues of the use of the Hazan and Shaver 'love-quiz' at the start of brief therapeutic work with patients rather than the AAI or the ECR. Though they acknowledge that the 'love-quiz' is generally too crude to pick up any changes in attachment style associated with therapy, they argued that it offers an excellent initial basis for a therapeutic conversation in which both therapist and patient are treated as knowledgeable but capable of change in their perspectives.[490] There is no need for the tallying of responses indexing latent constructs of anxiety and avoidance required for the ECR, let alone the labour-intensive process of having an AAI coded. Part of the appeal of the 'love-quiz' for Fonagy and colleagues in a therapeutic context was that, despite being a self-report measure, the ECR is a deceptively subtle tool, oriented towards mental schemas expressed in feelings, beliefs, expectations, and behaviours, but which may not be consciously known. Fonagy and colleagues at the Anna Freud Centre have also shown increasing interest in the use of self-report measures of attachment-related constructs in research contexts, in part because of the greater potential viability of these measures for use at scale.[491]

Over the past 20 years or more, the ECR has successfully served as the dominant methodological tool in the social psychological tradition, and additionally the basis for the model of anxiety and avoidance as the dominant theory. Further discussion was largely excluded by the fact that the ECR seemed to work well in predicting various expected correlates, and the factor analysis by Brennan and colleagues was taken as proof of the psychometric standing of the measure. Yet, for the third-generation researchers most versed in the social psychological tradition, questions have been raised about the theory and method that have organised the approach for the past 20 years. For example, Gillath, Fraley, and Birnbaum have wondered whether enough variance in individual difference is captured in theory and method by the constructs of anxiety and avoidance. Of course, they acknowledge, pragmatic compromises are always a part of scientific measurement.[492] Yet it is also possible for these compromises to be renegotiated if these compromises are recognised as having incrementally caused enough hinderance over time to warrant the effort. On the one hand, psychometric inquiries have suggested that security may not be reducible to the absence of anxiety and avoidance, but may represent its own dimension. On the other hand, it is not clear that the ECR as a measure or existing theory in the tradition is adequate to capturing the effects of trauma on experiences in close relationships. These are questions that Shaver and Mikulincer have acknowledged as limitations to their work. Their former students and younger colleagues will need to appraise whether these limitations are significant enough to warrant methodological or theoretical change, or, if measures are left unchanged, how to respond to the ensuing limitations.

---

[490] Lemma, A., Target, M., & Fonagy, P. (2011) *Brief Dynamic Interpersonal Therapy: A Clinician's Guide*. Oxford: Oxford University Press, p.92.

[491] Fonagy, P., Luyten, P., Moulton-Perkins, A., et al. (2016) Development and validation of a self-report measure of mentalizing: the Reflective Functioning Questionnaire. *PLoS One*, 11(7), e0158678.

[492] See also Pickering, A. (1995) *The Mangle of Practice: Time, Agency, and Science*. Chicago: University of Chicago Press.

6
Conclusion

Introduction

In *Becoming Attached*, Karen described the origins of Bowlby and Ainsworth's ideas, and considered emergent lines of research by the end of the 1980s, including work by Main and colleagues at Berkeley, Sroufe, Egeland, and colleagues at Minnesota, and Shaver and colleagues at Buffalo/Davis. These have been some of the cornerstone research groups for the development of contemporary attachment research. At the time Karen was writing, leadership of attachment research was passing from Bowlby and Ainsworth to a second generation. Furthermore, attachment as an area of academic study was rapidly expanding as perceptions of the field's credibility and relevance opened the door to research funding. The rapid growth of attachment research since the 1990s means that no book today about the history of the field could even hope to be comprehensive. Work is already underway on another book to address developments from the 1990s onwards. Yet even with attention to these later developments still to come, it is possible to draw together some reflections on the ideas, methods, and priorities of the early groups of attachment research considered in the present book. These have set the scene for subsequent attachment researchers in important ways. This concluding chapter will begin by reviewing three structural dynamics that have contributed to the present state of attachment research as a paradigm: the apparent accessibility of attachment concepts; the subtlety and complexity of its theory and methods; and the differentiation of a field of cumulative attachment research. The chapter will then examine the problems the intersection of these structural dynamics have caused for communication between researchers and practitioners, using the case of child welfare practitioners as illustration. Threats to the credibility and apparent relevance of attachment research from such breakdowns has led to claims that the paradigm is reaching exhaustion. The chapter will evaluate this claim and discuss three lively areas of research that build precisely on the benefits of the field's long development and history. It will close by considering what comes next for attachment research.

Structural issues

Over the course of this book, we have seen how the circulation and the shape of attachment theory and research have been influenced by the remarkable and at times misleading accessibility of some of Bowlby's basic ideas. This can be regarded as the first of three structural dynamics that in interaction have formed the basis for the strengths and weaknesses of attachment as a paradigm today. In part, the intimacy of Bowlby's ideas stemmed from their emergence out of psychoanalysis. Bowlby was intent on developing a theory that was integrated with the scientific developments of his day in other disciplines and that could offer testable hypotheses, but that also retained a portion of the capacity of psychoanalysis to address intimate life, ugly feelings, and inner conflict. Attachment theory speaks to themes that are constitutive of human life and that readily absorb our attention: being a child, becoming an adult; closeness and distance; the difficulties posed both by loss and by belonging. However, a further contribution to the power of Bowlby's attachment theory was his appeal to ordinary language. Bowlby's language in the 1950s was built to be able to both circulate to widespread publics and to persuade both academic and clinic audiences. The originating language of attachment theory used terms—such as 'mother', 'attachment', 'separation', 'love', 'anxiety'—that had a strong and emotive set of connotations in ordinary language. Bowlby overlaid these connotations with a set of technical meaning in his scholarly work. 'Love' proved unworkable in this regard and was abandoned. And the second generation mostly stopped using 'mother' to mean attachment figure. Other terms have, however, been retained over the decades. This grounding in ordinary language has contributed to the flexibility, urgency, and reach of 'attachment' discourses, allowing it to seem plausible and at times to catch at the heart. These qualities, together with the credibility provided by attachment research as an empirical paradigm, have contributed to the appeal of attachment to diverse audiences.[1]

A second structural dynamic that has shaped attachment research has been the way that theory has been enshrined in complex measures. This has been a mixed blessing. Over time, the Ainsworth Strange Situation has replaced the interactions in the home that it had been intended to capture and preserve. It likewise embodied but also supplanted discussions of the attachment behavioural system. The development of the Attachment Q-Sort by Waters and colleagues sought to preserve Ainsworth's concern with naturalistic observation and with the capacity of caregivers to offer their child a secure base. However, this measure too stimulated no further discussion of the attachment behavioural system, which has increasingly functioned as a memento in the developmental tradition of attachment research rather than as an active object of further theoretical work. Its place has been taken by the ideas of 'minimising' and 'maximising' strategies, though without clarity about what exactly is being minimised or maximised. Main's theory was that it was attention to attachment-relevant information. This position was the basis of her interpretation of the Ainsworth classifications and her group's introduction of the disorganised attachment classification and the Adult Attachment Interview (AAI). The innovations by Main and her group gave the Ainsworth categories an apparently universal resonance, across cultures and across lifespan development. However, with Main's attentional theory largely unrecognised, there has been little precision in discussions of how the four-category coding system can be applied cross-culturally.

Similarly, without clarity on what exactly the AAI measured, controversies were primed when a social psychological tradition of attachment research emerged, which also made appeal to the Ainsworth Strange Situation categories but as part of a self-report measure. Unlike the developmental attachment tradition, Shaver and Milkulincer have further interrogated the idea of behavioural systems and attempted to articulate the concept of attachment. The developmental and social psychological traditions of attachment research have come to a better coexistence over recent years, both contributing to the *Handbook of*

---

[1] Ziv and Hotam have stated that 'the "attachment language" is undeniably unique, coherent, rich, and complex enough to interest professional academic audiences, to be clinically meaningful to practitioners, and to be straightforward enough to attract laypersons'. Despite their reference to coherence, Ziv and Hotam would likely agree that these audiences do not encounter a unitary discourse, but at least in part encounter different discourses that have overlapping vocabularies. Terms such as 'attachment' and 'separation' (Bowlby) or 'security' and 'sensitivity' (Ainsworth) may be used by academics, clinicians, and laypersons alike—but with little overlapping meaning. Ziv, Y. & Hotam, Y. (2015) Theory and measure in the psychological field: the case of attachment theory and the Strange Situation procedure. *Theory & Psychology*, 25(3), 274–91, p.279.

Attachment and the journal *Attachment & Human Development*. However, dialogue between the two traditions has been profoundly hindered by their use of the same central vocabulary to mean quite different things.

An influential study by Brennan, Clark, and Shaver in 1998 found that existing self-report measures could be integrated on the basis of two latent dimensions: avoidance and anxiety. The Experiences in Close Relationships scale was developed using items that reflected these two latent constructs. However, the exact relationship remains uncertain between the anxiety construct and Ainsworth's ambivalent/resistant category, given that the latter incorporates anxiety, anger, and passivity. And it is not clear how well the Experiences in Close Relationships scale handles experiences of security and trauma. Like the Strange Situation and the AAI, the Experiences in Close Relationships scale embodies a particular theory of individual differences relevant to attachment, but has also served to close down certain questions about that theory. Nonetheless, these questions have generated increasing discussion in recent years from some of Shaver and Milkulincer's closest students.

A third structural dynamic made salient by taking a historical perspective on early attachment research groups has been the work of 'field building': the construction of attachment as a differentiated paradigm with its own characteristic dispositions, methods, theories, values, allies, enemies, and nodal institutions.[2] The Strange Situation provided the initial basis for a cumulative research programme, capable of attracting a sustained flow of research funds and empirical findings. Whereas Bowlby was writing primarily for clinical audiences and the general public, the central audience for Ainsworth and the second generation of attachment researchers was the American community of academic psychologists. With the construction of attachment research as a differentiated empirical paradigm following Ainsworth and her immediate colleagues, attachment research became a 'non-formative' activity, in which re-shaping parenting practices was not a focal concern.[3]

Certainly there are some second-generation attachment researchers for whom clinical relevance has been the guiding principle of their work. Peter Fonagy, Patricia Crittenden, Alicia Lieberman, and Karlen Lyons-Ruth are salient examples.[4] And social historians and sociologists have sometimes extrapolated from Bowlby's early writings and the reception of attachment ideas in welfare practice to assume that contemporary attachment researchers are oriented towards the pathologizing and disciplining of families.[5] Yet, overall, what is striking on close examination is how *little* developments in the second generation of attachment research, especially in America, seem to have been responsive to the concerns of

---

[2] On field differentiation see Bourdieu, P. (1989) The conquest of autonomy: the critical phase in the emergence of the field. In *The Rules of Art*, trans. S. Emanuel (pp.47–112). Cambridge: Polity Press.

[3] On the concept of non-formativeness see Wood, M. (2009) The nonformative elements of religious life: questioning the 'sociology of spirituality' paradigm. *Social Compass*, 56(2), 237–48.

[4] E.g. Lyons-Ruth, K. & Spielman, E. (2004) Disorganized infant attachment strategies and helpless-fearful profiles of parenting: integrating attachment research with clinical intervention. *Infant Mental Health Journal*, 25(4), 318–35. Crittenden, P.M. (2015) *Raising Parents*, 2nd edn. London: Routledge; Fonagy, P., Luyten, P., Allison, E., & Campbell, C. (2017) What we have changed our minds about: Part 2. Borderline personality disorder, epistemic trust and the developmental significance of social communication. *Borderline Personality Disorder and Emotion Dysregulation*, 4, 9. Van IJzendoorn and Bakermans-Kranenburg are also partial exceptions, albeit primarily in the past decade, for instance co-authoring a popular book aimed at child welfare professionals: van IJzendoorn, M.H. & Bakermans-Kranenburg, M.J. (2010) *Gehechtheid en Trauma. Diagnostiek en Behandeling voor de Professional*. Amsterdam: Hogrefe.

[5] E.g. Kanieski, M.A. (2010) Securing attachment: the shifting medicalisation of attachment and attachment disorders. *Health, Risk & Society*, 12(4), 335–44; Garrett, M.P. (2017) Wired: early intervention and the 'neuromolecular gaze'. *British Journal of Social Work*, 48(3), 656–74.

clinical and social welfare practice, and how much by the demands of institutional academic psychology. Indeed, with some exceptions, the structural articulation between research and clinical attachment discourses has frequently been what Foucault termed 'feeble' and 'slack'.[6] For instance, the developmental research community have generally looked askance at both the 'attachment disorder' diagnosis and the use of attachment measures in assessment of risk in a context in which clinical and welfare services and training are largely structured by diagnostic pathways and risk assessment. Main has never written about what parents should do, and she has emphasised in print that practitioners should not regard her tentative suggestions as authoritative for what they should do.[7] The Minnesota Longitudinal Study of Risk and Adaptation did contribute to the development of STEEP. However, this was a sideline for the Sroufe and Egeland group at Minnesota, whose primary focus was the cohort study. Shaver and Mikulincer have focused their attention predominantly, though certainly not exclusively, on samples of university students. Their remarks about the implications of attachment anxiety and avoidance for clinical and child welfare practice are rare and underdeveloped.[8]

Meeting the demands of institutional academic psychology provided advantages. Whilst the labour-intensive measures of the developmental tradition generally constrained sample size,[9] a cumulative programme could be pursued over decades by the second generation of attachment researchers. Based on a massive number of studies, a series of meta-analyses in the early 2010s confirmed the capacity of the Strange Situation to predict later social and mental health outcomes. The extent of this prediction is either moderate or very substantial—depending on how effect sizes are interpreted.[10] In any case, Groh and colleagues observed that they are comparable or stronger than other psychological assessments of socioemotional development conducted in infancy.[11] The dedication of attachment researchers to commensurate measures is a marker of important continuities over time. Attachment has appeared as a strangely stable theoretical paradigm, in a context in which psychological theories were

[6] The sociological literature discussing attachment research has tended towards the assumption that the psy-disciplines always tend to work in the same way. However, this prefabricated 'critical' account of psychological discourse misses important heterogeneity. Foucault urged that it is important to register and to study not only effective medical and professional power/knowledge relations, but also 'a domination that grows feeble, poisons itself, grows slack, and not to mistake one for the other. Foucault, M. (1971, 1994) Nietzsche, genealogy, history. In J.D. Faubion (ed.) *Aesthetics, Method, and Epistemology, Essential Works of Foucault 1954–1984*. New York: The New Press, p.381. In turn, it may be gently acknowledged that the prefabricated discourse of 'critical' social science is not itself free from imbrication with forms of domination, for instance as a capital-accrual strategy within academia.

[7] The only sustained consideration appears in Main, M., Hesse, E., & Hesse, S. (2011) Attachment theory and research: overview with suggested applications to child custody. *Family Court Review*, 49(3), 426–63. Here Main and Hesse firmly situated themselves as non-experts on professional practice, offering reflections as best they could in response to a direct request rather than because custody decisions were central to their work as researchers.

[8] What remarks are offered seem to generally stem from work led by Shaver's wife Gail Goodman, rather than reflecting the priorities of Shaver and Mikulincer's research agenda, e.g. Lawler, M.J., Shaver, P.R., & Goodman, G.S. (2011) Toward relationship-based child welfare services. *Children and Youth Services Review*, 33(3), 473–80.

[9] The central early exception here was NICHD Early Child Care Research Network (1997) The effects of infant child care on infant–mother attachment security: results of the NICHD Study of Early Child Care NICHD Early Child Care Research Network. *Child Development*, 68(5), 860–79. A larger exception was Jaddoe, V.W., van Duijn, C.M., Franco, O.H., et al. (2012) The Generation R Study: design and cohort update 2012. *European Journal of Epidemiology*, 27(9), 739–56.

[10] Funder, D.C. & Ozer, D.J. (2019) Evaluating effect size in psychological research: sense and nonsense. *Advances in Methods and Practices in Psychological Science*, 2(2) 156–68.

[11] Groh, A.M., Fearon, R.P., van IJzendoorn, M.H., Bakermans-Kranenburg, M.J., & Roisman, G.I. (2017) Attachment in the early life course: meta-analytic evidence for its role in socioemotional development. *Child Development Perspectives*, 11(1), 70–76.

in continual churn and psychological theory in general was in decline. Highlighting this continuity, Waters and colleagues could claim that 'Bowlby's attachment theory is the only current theoretical framework in developmental psychology that is cast in the grand theory model, widely accepted, and empirically productive'.[12]

To anthropologists, this continuity has appeared as an imperviousness to criticism among attachment researchers, contributing to a sense of frustration and of being ignored by critics of the paradigm (Chapter 2). Yet, as Latour has urged, social studies of science must see the stability of social institutions and practices not as merely the default state of things, but as 'exactly what has to be explained by appealing to costly and demanding means'.[13] In the case of attachment as a research paradigm, these costly and demanding means have included the labour-intensive Strange Situation and astonishing amounts of convergent effort. Yet the stability of attachment research as a unified paradigm has also been achieved through maintenance of a common terminology, the cost of which has been confusion and miscommunication. One site of such problems has been in communication between research groups. Likewise, the underpinnings of the AAI were obscured by Main's choice to frame this methodological innovation in terms of Bowlby's concept of internal working models, miscuing decades of subsequent discussion of the measure.

Attachment in child welfare practice

The apparent accessibility of attachment concepts, the subtlety and complexity of its theory and methods, and the differentiation of a field of cumulative attachment research have together contributed to many of the strengths and attraction of the paradigm today. However, their interaction has also contributed to serious and pervasive misunderstandings regarding the concepts that organise attachment theory and research. The language of psychological research often grows out of ordinary language, since it is from ordinary problems that psychology frequently takes its starting point. Yet attachment research has been especially vulnerable to problems of mistaken identity between technical and ordinary language.

Summarising themes from across the previous chapters, four factors may be identified as of special importance. First, Bowlby's early vocabulary was drawn deliberately and strategically from ordinary language in order to support the popular appeal of his ideas. Second, the coding systems of the developmental tradition are complicated and information about how constructs were actually operationalised has been unduly limited in circulation to an oral culture. Third, the appearance of attachment as a unified paradigm has been maintained in part through the stretching of terminology, with concepts invested with some overlapping and some non-overlapping senses. The capacity for concepts to be used flexibly has allowed attachment to seem relevant in diverse areas and diverse ways. However, this has come at a price. Areas of practice that appreciate conceptual precision and clearly operationalised concepts have tended to reject the attachment paradigm.[14] And communication by and among attachment researchers has been hindered by the way that its concepts serve as

[12] Waters, E., Corcoran, D., & Anafarta, M. (2005) Attachment, other relationships, and the theory that all good things go together. *Human Development*, 48(1–2), 80–84, p.81.

[13] Latour, B. (2005) *Reassembling the Social*. Oxford: Oxford University Press, p.35.

[14] E.g. Bolen, R. (2000) Validity of attachment theory. *Trauma, Violence & Abuse*, 1, 128–53; Bosmans, G. (2016) Cognitive behaviour therapy for children and adolescents: can attachment theory contribute to its efficacy? *Clinical Child and Family Psychology Review*, 19(4), 310–28.

magnets attracting quite heterogenous investments. Fourth, then, it can be observed that attachment research has been distinctively ill-equipped in terms of infrastructures for pruning how concepts are used in technical discussions. It is to be hoped that the journal *Attachment & Human Development*, future editions of the *Handbook of Attachment*, and organisations like the Society for Emotion and Attachment Research and the International Association for the Study of Attachment might give greater attention to this issue.[15]

Yet, if there has been trouble in communication between researchers, the situation has been even worse for dialogue between researchers and practitioners. In 1999, Rutter and O'Connor described extensive 'conceptual confusion' in appeals to attachment theory and research by clinicians and social workers.[16] As the previous chapters have shown, there have been several ways in which the attachment research community have made effective dissemination of their ideas harder than many other fields. If Bowlby demonstrated the dangers of populism, his successors have demonstrated the dangers of turning away from public engagement. Misunderstandings and simplifications based on Bowlby's early and popularising texts have abounded, and continue to shape public perceptions of the paradigm today. The gap between researchers and their public, where it is not left empty, has often been occupied by professional trainers, whose distance from empirical research on attachment and the field's oral culture opens varied opportunities for quick-fix misapplications. A recent example was commercial training provided for thousands of UK social workers in using disorganised attachment as seen in naturalistic settings as an indicator of child maltreatment.[17]

Such misunderstandings and simplifications should be recognised as predisposed by obstacles to clear understanding of the disorganised category. These included the restricted circulation of Main's texts, her use of ordinary language terms in highly technical ways without definitions, and by the repetition of a superficial account of Main's ideas and findings by other attachment researchers. The lack of psychometric scrutiny of the disorganised classification has helped naturalise its status as a category, contributing to its quasi-diagnostic appearance, especially when combined with Carlson's finding—intended as exploratory—showing that the category was associated prospectively with a general index of mental illness. More generally, the reification of attachment and attachment classifications no doubt facilitated the assumption of the commercial trainers that behaviour seen at home by child welfare practitioners would have the same meaning as behaviour seen in the research laboratory.[18]

Recently, problems in the role of attachment theory within child welfare practice have been the topic of a dedicated book by White, Gibson, Wastell, and Walsh.[19] White and

---

[15] One set of definitions has been offered by Schuengel, C., de Schipper, J.C., Sterkenburg, P.S., & Kef, S. (2013) Attachment, intellectual disabilities and mental health: research, assessment and intervention. *Journal of Applied Research in Intellectual Disabilities*, 26(1), 34–46.

[16] Rutter, M. & O'Connor, T. (1999) Implications of attachment theory for child care policies. In J. Cassidy & P.R. Shaver (eds) *Handbook of Attachment: Theory, Research and Clinical Applications* (pp.823–44). New York: Guilford Press, p.823.

[17] Granqvist, P. (2016) Observations of disorganized behaviour yield no magic wand: response to Shemmings. *Attachment & Human Development*, 18(6), 529–33; Granqvist, P., Sroufe, L.A., Dozier, M., et al. (2017) Disorganized attachment in infancy: a review of the phenomenon and its implications for clinicians and policy-makers. *Attachment & Human Development*, 19(6), 534–58.

[18] Reijman, S., Foster, S., & Duschinsky, R. (2018) The infant disorganised attachment classification: 'patterning within the disturbance of coherence'. *Social Science & Medicine*, 200, 52–8.

[19] White, S., Gibson, M., Wastell, D., & Walsh, P. (2019) *Reassessing Attachment Theory in Child Welfare*. Bristol: Psychology Press.

colleagues observe that Bowlby was active in promoting his theory to social workers.[20] And in turn, social workers found in attachment a knowledge base to help them claim professional status, in which cases could be interpreted in terms of a credible theory. Attachment offers welfare professionals a framework that appears to predict later risk to a child's health and development from the child or parents' observable behaviour.

Over the years, both social work academics and policy documents have encouraged welfare professionals to use the image of secure attachment as the point of comparison when making assessments of parenting capacity. For instance, in the Department of Health practice guidance *Assessing Children in Need and their Families,* published in 2000, practitioners were told that 'secure attachments are so important in the early years. Where these attachments are absent or broken, decisions to provide children with new attachment figures must be taken as quickly as possible to avoid developmental damage.'[21] Taken at its word, in the absence of a secure attachment the guidance seems to suggest that children need to be considered for separation from their parents. White and colleagues identify that this position seems underpinned by the idea that 'attachment patterns, once formed, are stable and set forever'.[22]

In recent years, with cuts to supportive services for families, the balance of child welfare in the UK has tilted firmly towards a focus on statutory investigation of families.[23] White and colleagues regard attachment discourses as complicit in this shift. They suggest that, at least in UK child welfare practice, attachment provides 'a handy vocabulary, a diagnostic gaze, learned-sounding re-descriptions of messy relationships and often a foil for moral judgements'.[24] They report from an extensive ethnographic study of social workers in a child protection service. They found that attachment was never mentioned by social workers in their discussions or personal reflections. Nonetheless, appeals to attachment appeared repeatedly in official reports when judgements were made about parenting capacity. This expressed a contradiction facing social work, stemming structurally from its dominated position compared to both legal and medical professionals. Social workers require access to a category-based and prognostic knowledge system in order to operate and make qualitative judgements as professionals, but are not regarded as qualified to make use of reserved clinical diagnoses. A quasi-diagnostic use of attachment language appeals as a workable, if imperfect, solution to this structural conflict.

Uses of attachment discourse in the reports observed by White and colleagues were generally vague, essentially functioning as synonyms for a poor child–parent relationship. Similar observations have been made by other researchers. Potter's ethnographic observations and North's qualitative interviews suggest that vagueness in the use of attachment language assessments may reflect the climate of child welfare services and the family courts,

[20] E.g. Association for Psychiatric Social Workers (1955) Presentation at the Annual General Meeting 1955: Dr John Bowlby on preventative activities. Modern Records Centre Warwick University, MSS.378/APSW/P/16/6/19-20.

[21] E.g. Department of Health (2000) *Assessing Children in Need and their Families: Practice Guidance.* London: TSO.

[22] White, S., Gibson, M., Wastell, D., & Walsh, P. (2019) *Reassessing Attachment Theory in Child Welfare.* Bristol: Psychology Press.

[23] Bilson, A. & Munro, E.H. (2019) Adoption and child protection trends for children aged under five in England: increasing investigations and hidden separation of children from their parents. *Children and Youth Services Review,* 96, 204–11.

[24] White, S., Gibson, M., Wastell, D., & Walsh, P. (2019) *Reassessing Attachment Theory in Child Welfare.* Bristol: Psychology Press.

and ambiguities around the professional status of social workers. This would imply that social workers draw on attachment concepts in their reasoning, but are vague about this in their reports, so as to avoid claiming expert levels of knowledge where this might be challenged by higher-status professionals.[25] One of North's participants, Bryony, described this predicament:

> Whereas although we can say we have concerns about the attachment, I don't feel we're qualified enough to say, you know [softly], 'They've got an attachment issue, you know, they've got a dis … organised [almost inaudible] … attachment or whatever,' because I don't feel we're qualified enough. I don't feel qualified enough to say that.[26]

North observed that across the interview, Bryony 'spoke softly when she referred to attachment, seemingly to emphasise her shame at not feeling competent to make theoretically informed judgments. This was a response echoed by many interview participants.' In North's analysis, 'social workers often want to be more proficient in their application of attachment theory and in how they describe their utilisation of it in assessments. They also experience frustration at lacking the skills to explain effectively how they have used attachment theory to indicate the potentially harmful outcomes for a child of experiencing emotional abuse.'[27]

By contrast, White and colleagues adopt a more sceptical conclusion. They claim that attachment language is being drawn upon, post-hoc, in reports as authority to justify practitioners' intuitions about adequate and inadequate care: 'the social workers referred to "good" or "positive" attachments, rather than the scientific community concepts of secure and insecure, to describe a good quality relationship between a child and their parents.'[28] However, White and colleagues felt that the attachment frame of reference, even if post-hoc, had negative effects. It helped legitimate 'the narrow focus on the mother–child relationship, and the responsibility of the mother for this relationship', directing attention away from the family socioeconomic context, the availability of social support, and potential neurodevelopmental issues experienced by the child.[29] In this, White and colleagues suggest that practitioners' use of attachment theory was shaped by the priorities of child protection practice in the UK,

---

[25] Potter, A. (2019) Judging social work expertise in care proceedings. In D.S. Caudill, S.N. Conley, M.E. Gorman, & M. Weinel (eds) *The Third Wave in Science and Technology Studies* (pp.71–85). London: Palgrave. Further findings from Potter's doctoral research are forthcoming. See also Shemmings, D. (2018) Why social workers shouldn't use 'attachment' in their records and reports. *Community Care*, 28 June 2018. https://www.communitycare.co.uk/2018/06/28/social-workers-shouldnt-use-attachment-records-reports/.

[26] North, G. (2019) Assessing for bruises on the soul: identifying and evidencing childhood emotional abuse. *Journal of Social Welfare and Family Law*, 41(3), 302–320, p.313.

[27] Ibid.

[28] Similar observations have been made by Wilkins, D., Shemmings, D., & Shemmings, Y. (2015) *A–Z of Attachment*. London: Palgrave: 'We have also seen what can only be described as quite crude and, in all likelihood, mistaken applications of attachment theory in practice. For example, we have read reports by contact supervisors observing that a child stays very physically close to their attachment figure throughout the session, with this then interpreted as a sign of a "positive attachment"; we see conclusions being drawn about a child's attachment relationships based on one, short observation; descriptions of parents being "attached" to their babies; of a child's attachment relationship with their father being almost completely overlooked and of social workers describing young children as always happy and content without reflecting on whether this is a "good thing" or not. Additionally, we often hear workers speak of "strong attachments" … We have become increasingly worried that attachment theory and research are often used "against" families: to highlight "problems" and "gaps" in parenting or caregiving relationships—particularly when writing reports for the courts or in relation to child protection procedures' (xv–xvi).

[29] White, S., Gibson, M., Wastell, D., & Walsh, P. (2019) *Reassessing Attachment Theory in Child Welfare*. Bristol: Psychology Press.

which focus on procedure and risk assessment at the expense of a rounded attention to the context of families over time.

The primary target of White and colleagues is not attachment research, but the way that in the UK child welfare practice ideas from attachment theory may at times be 'used with a mixture of excessive credulity and zealotry, a cavalier heavy-handedness and unsophisticated reductionism'. In fact, White and colleagues claim that attachment theory and research has a lot to contribute to child welfare practice: 'we agree with the proponents of the theory that policy and practice is not sufficiently attachment minded. The complexities and nuances of the concepts are hidden by simplification … at its best, attachment research has produced ideas that practitioners can use to understand the quality of child–carer relationships when the child is anxious, scared, or upset, and to guide them in their work to improve familial relationships.'[30]

White and colleagues give the Love Barrow Families project as an exemplary use of attachment theory and measures by helping professionals. Love Barrow Families is an innovative service-delivery model for families with multiple complex needs based in Cumbria, UK. The model was codesigned with local families, and local families sit on the steering group. Key principles include working with the whole family and support for families to integrate with their local community. Rather than multiple services working with families in crisis at once, one member of the Love Barrow Families team acts as a key-worker for each family. Decisions about how to direct and prioritise work with the family are supported through use of attachment assessments with family members, which feed into a whole-family formulation and plan. An evaluation undertaken by Vincent documented that, compared to a matched comparison sample, the Love Barrow Families project reduced the number of children taken into care and the number of children on child protection plans.[31] White and colleagues express appreciation that Love Barrow Families does not use attachment measures or theory to diagnose or label, but to sensitise practitioners to both the strengths and the needs of the different members of family systems.

Love Barrow Families draws especially on the ideas and assessments developed by Patricia Crittenden, which have been influential in the UK.[32] Love Barrow Families regards Crittenden's work as offering a range of clinically relevant archetypes, and proposals for distinct forms of therapeutic approach to clients displaying different forms of behaviour.[33] There have been recent debates among attachment researchers about whether the assessments developed by Crittenden have sufficient sensitivity and specificity for use in court assessments of parenting capacity.[34] White and colleagues are generally hostile to the use

---

[30] Ibid.

[31] Vincent, S. (2017) 'The Magic Is in the Co-Production': Summary Report from the Evaluation of the Love Barrow Families Project. Newcastle: Northumbria University.

[32] Crittenden, P.M. (2015) Raising Parents, 2nd edn. London: Routledge. See also Baim, C. & Morrison, T. (2014) Attachment-Based Practice with Adults. Brighton: Pavilion: 'There is a general truism about attachment theory, which is that the more you learn about attachment theory the more cautious you become about attaching labels to people. This includes labels such as "securely attached", "reactive attachment disorder", "disorganised attachment" and so on, which tend to be over-used and under-defined' (23).

[33] See also Baim, C. (2019) DMM vs ABC+D—a controversial discussion. DMM News, 32. https://www.iasa-dmm.org/images/uploads/DMM%20News%20%2332%20May%2019%20English.pdf: 'The DMM community attempts to find a way of assessing and informing treatment that is more accurate and useful because it is focused on the function of behaviour rather than labelling symptoms—which puts people into boxes.'

[34] Spieker, S.J. & Crittenden, P.M. (2018) Can attachment inform decision-making in child protection and forensic settings? Infant Mental Health Journal, 39(6), 625–41; Van IJzendoorn, M.H., Bakermans, J.J., Steele, M., & Granqvist, P. (2018) Diagnostic use of Crittenden's attachment measures in Family Court is not beyond a reasonable doubt. Infant Mental Health Journal, 39(6), 642–6.

of attachment measures in court-mandated parenting assessments, in contrast to the use of these assessments to identify how best to proceed in supporting a family. This seems to parallel recent work of Madigan and colleagues in their creation of a brief assessment, usable by practitioners in real-time, for identifying forms of frightening or disrupted parenting (AMBIANCE-Brief).[35] Madigan and her collaborators anticipate that this assessment will be able to help professionals identify forms of parenting associated with adverse child socioemotional development and to target supportive interventions. However, the assessment has been designed in such a way as to minimise its likelihood of being used in court assessments of parenting capacity, for instance in avoiding the implication that certain forms of caregiving are in themselves pathological. Madigan and colleagues are now in the process of validating the AMBIANCE-Brief in terms of its capacity to predict Strange Situation classifications, and evaluating the measure's reliability when used in clinical and welfare practice. One contributing factor supporting Madigan's work has been the availability of funding in Canada for research–practitioner collaborative inquiry. There also seems to be a broader shift towards greater engagement with practitioners and publics associated with the third generation of attachment researchers.[36]

In their book, White and colleagues at times depict practitioners as enthralled to simplified and haughty guidance about attachment theory. Presumably this is intended as a counterweight to what the authors regard as the untroubled circulation of lazy assumptions about attachment. One qualification that can be made regarding their account, though, is that there is more variety among guidance for practitioners than White and colleagues suggest. The Circle of Security graphic of the caregiver as a secure base and safe haven has gone into wide circulation, and represents an admirably effective visual representation of Ainsworth's concepts; the Circle of Security Intervention itself is used in many countries and there is initial evidence that it contributes to less judgemental forms of supportive work with families.[37] There are several books that do an excellent job in representing the available research evidence and theory, whilst also offering reflections relevant to helping professionals and parents. The best available in English is perhaps either *Understanding Attachment and Attachment Disorders* by Prior and Glaser or *Attachment in Therapeutic Practice* by Slade and Holmes.[38] However, it should not be thought that effective mediation

[35] Madigan, S. (2019) Beyond the academic silo: collaboration and community partnerships in attachment research. Paper presented at International Attachment Conference, Vancouver, 20 July 2019; Haltigan, J.D., Madigan, S., Bronfman, E., et al. (2019) Refining the assessment of disrupted maternal communication: using item response models to identify central indicators of disrupted behavior. *Development & Psychopathology*, 31(1), 261–77.

[36] This transition may be placed in the broader context of the rise of discourses, since the late 1990s, questioning whether or how academic research meaningfully contributes to addressing the challenges faced by practitioners and/or the public good. Irwin, A. (2001) Constructing the scientific citizen: science and democracy in the biosciences. *Public Understanding of Science*, 10(1), 1–18; Gunn, A. & Mintrom, M. (2016) Higher education policy change in Europe: academic research funding and the impact agenda. *European Education*, 48(4), 241–57.

[37] Powell, B., Cooper, G., Hoffman, K., & Marvin, B. (2016) *The Circle of Security Intervention*. New York: Guilford; McMahon, C., Huber, A., Kohlhoff, J., & Camberis, A.L. (2017) Does training in the Circle of Security framework increase relational understanding in infant/child and family workers? *Infant Mental Health Journal*, 38(5), 658–68.

[38] Prior, V. & Glaser, D. (2006) *Understanding Attachment and Attachment Disorders: Theory, Evidence and Practice*. London: Jessica Kingsley Press; Slade, A. & Holmes, J. (2017) *Attachment in Therapeutic Practice*. London: SAGE. The best available in Dutch is likely van IJzendoorn, M.H. & Bakermans-Kranenburg, M.J. (2010) *Gehechtheid en Trauma: Diagnostiek en Behandeling voor de Professional*. Amsterdam: Hogrefe. Another thoughtful work is Page, T. (2017) Attachment theory and social work treatment. In F. Turner (ed.) *Social Work Treatment: Interlocking Theoretical Approaches*, 6th edn (pp.1–22). Oxford: Oxford University Press. Beyond the published literature, some trainings offered to clinicians and foster carers are also exemplary in effective characterisation of the technical aspects of attachment theory and research, and its relevance. Those by John Sands and Lydia Fransham can be mentioned, though as yet neither has published their training materials.

of research and practice always entails the implementation of the former in the latter. An example of a book that offers thoughtful integration of theory and practice, in an area where there is little empirical attachment research, is Blood and Guthrie's *Supporting Older People Using Attachment-Informed and Strengths-Based Approaches.*[39] There are many works that take care to distinguish contemporary scholarly consensus from 'allodoxia'—a cut-price, simplified account offered up as if it had the same meaning as the technical conclusions of researchers. For example, in Golding's *Nurturing Attachments Training Resource* for delivering parenting groups, a flipchart of potentially ambiguous terms is used to help participants keep in mind these distinctions.[40]

Nonetheless, White and colleagues are unquestionably right that a great deal of guidance for clinicians and social workers is overconfident and poorly informed.[41] Moreover, this guidance is disproportionately likely to be available for free or cheaply, in contrast to works that offer greater access to attachment research in its complexity, which are frequently more expensive or behind journal paywalls. Three features can be identified that especially characterise allodoxic guidance about attachment for clinicians and social workers and related policy discourses. First, these texts offer little or no explanation of Bowlby's behavioural systems model, Ainsworth's operationalisation of sensitivity, or how disorganised attachment is actually coded. Instead they conjure with the broad ordinary language connotations of attachment, security, sensitivity, and disorganisation.[42] Second, empirical attachment research over recent decades is ignored in favour of statements made by Bowlby in popularising writings, as well as selected other statements from early attachment theory implying a massive and stable causal influence of early care on later social behaviour.[43] Attachment researchers are treated as generally all much the same, which allows for changes over time to be ignored. For instance, the concept of 'felt security' is routinely attributed to Bowlby, rather than Sroufe and Waters' critique of Bowlby. Third, no reference is made to the qualified findings reported in meta-analyses or the findings from these meta-analyses regarding moderators of the effect of caregiving on attachment, or attachment on later development. It should be acknowledged that allodoxic attachment discourse contributes, often helpfully, to recognition that child–parent relationships are very important to children and their socioemotional development. However, the impression of a basis in empirical attachment research is spurious or heavily overstated. And some topics, such as disorganised attachment and attachment disorders, are pervasively mischaracterised.

---

[39] Blood, I. & Guthrie, L. (2018) *Supporting Older People Using Attachment-Informed and Strengths-Based Approaches.* London: Jessica Kingsley Press.

[40] Golding, K. (2017) *Nurturing Attachments Training Resource: Running Parenting Groups for Adoptive Parents and Foster or Kinship Carers.* London: Jessica Kingsley Press.

[41] One example is Pearce's *A Short Introduction to Attachment and Attachment Disorder,* which is admirably accessible but contains many outright errors alongside confused oversimplifications. Pearce, J. (2009) *A Short Introduction to Attachment and Attachment Disorder.* London: Jessica Kingsley Press. Even in otherwise good works there are major errors, such as the conflation of controlling-punitive/controlling-caregiving with Reactive Attachment Disorder in Howe, D., Brandon, M., Hinings, D., & Schofield, G. (1999) *Attachment Theory, Child Maltreatment and Family Support: A Practice and Assessment Model.* London: Palgrave, pp.135–6. A decade later, these problems were corrected in Howe, D. (2011) *Attachment Across the Lifecourse: A Brief Introduction.* London: Palgrave.

[42] E.g. Perry, B. (2001) Attachment: the first core strength. *Early Childhood Today,* 16(2): 'Attachment is the capacity to form and maintain healthy emotional relationships' (28).

[43] E.g. Marshall, N. (2014) *The Teacher's Introduction to Attachment: Practical Essentials for Teachers, Carers and School Support Staff.* London: Jessica Kingsley Publishers.

At first sight it seems curious that many hostile academic discussions of attachment research, such as those of Vicedo (Chapter 1) and anthropologist critics (Chapter 2), possess the same three qualities: they mistake technical for ordinary language (e.g. regarding the meaning of 'sensitivity'); recent attachment research is ignored in favour of classic statements by Bowlby; and the findings of meta-analyses are neglected. However, these qualities are less mysterious in light of Keller's reflection (Chapter 2) that such critiques of attachment research are, at least in part, a proxy for criticism of the uses of attachment discourse in child welfare contexts. In this regard, a limitation of the work of White and colleagues is that they lean on statements by Vicedo that homogenise and caricature attachment research and its applications. Though White and colleagues refer to ethnographic observations and scrutinise several court reports, the empirical basis for their claims about the uses of attachment remains relatively limited.

As mentioned in the Introduction to this book, colleagues and I have several studies underway exploring how attachment theory and measures are used by child welfare practitioners and clinicians working with children. Findings are just in, and results will be reported over the coming couple of years; this presentation of initial impressions should not be taken to pre-empt the formal analysis. However, already these initial impressions indicate more heterogeneity than suggested by Vicedo or White and colleagues. In a project led by Sarah Foster, we conducted interviews with 24 children's services social workers, and asked them to offer responses to two vignettes of fictionalised cases drawn partly from Serious Case Reviews. This was part of a wider project comparing the responses of different professional groups: social workers, general practitioners, and clinical psychologists. What was especially striking from the interviews with the social workers was the significant individual variation in knowledge of and views on the potential value and actual use of attachment theory concepts and discourse in practice. This was despite the fact that all the social workers were employed by just two Local Authorities, both in the same region of the UK. For some of the social workers interviewed, they regarded attachment theory and discourses as having little role in their work, regardless of guidance suggestions that they take attachment into account in assessments of children. This stance was most frequently underpinned by a lack of confidence in *any* theories relevant to social work. Theory was seen as 'high' knowledge, beyond the reach of ordinary practitioners like themselves. However, some social workers drew on other theories but were specifically critical of attachment theory. For example, one social worker was concerned that use of attachment theory could risk drawing attention away from fully acknowledging different cultural family contexts.

However, many of the interviewed social workers felt attachment was directly important to their work with children and families. Practitioners reported using attachment to inform their thinking about a variety of matters, including in thinking about what a child's repeated pattern of behaviour in the family context might mean, and how a parent's own childhood experiences might be affecting how they are currently responding to their child. However, among practitioners who appreciated attachment theory and its relevance to their work, here again there was variation. Some practitioners were enthusiastic about attachment theory and research because it offered a lens on the relationships, emotional life, and socioemotional development of everyone. Other practitioners were enthusiastic but viewed attachment as 'one aspect of everything that you take into consideration' and only ever helpful alongside other theories and frameworks.

In direct contrast to the finding in White and colleagues' research, there were multiple interviewees who said in interview that they used attachment theory and research extensively to inform their practice, whilst intentionally avoiding the use of attachment terminology in their reports. Explaining this stance, some of the social workers stated that identification of individual differences in attachment, such as disorganised attachment, required specialist assessment training which they did not have. Many expressed concern over being challenged on their expertise in court if they used such terms. Another set of concerns raised by interviewees was that many felt that using attachment terminology was inappropriate, as it may be inaccessible to families and unhelpful or misleading for other practitioners:

> I try not to put labels on, this child is suffering disorganised or ambivalent attachment, I think in terms of your theory … you know what you're looking for in a secure attachment and you know when it's not good! But it's focusing more on the behaviours and what the behaviours will be telling you as opposed to sticking a label, an attachment theory label on it. Because it's just words, we need to understand what that means for these children and what we're actually seeing.

Whilst much rarer amongst those interviewed, a few social workers stated that they did use attachment classifications in their written reports despite not having trained in conducting attachment assessments or carried out formal attachment assessments in these cases.

Practitioners drew on attachment language in responding to the two vignettes. There was a good deal of confused use of attachment terminology in these responses. Examples included: talking about the 'strength' of attachment, reasoning about 'poor' attachment, conflating attachment with love, using the terms 'attachment difficulties' and 'attachment disorders' interchangeably, and confusion about whether a child can be attached at all to a maltreating caregiver. This does support the concerns White and colleagues have raised about the use and understanding of attachment. However, what was also clear from the interviews was that many social workers were reflective about the limitations of their knowledge and of the version of attachment theory in circulation within child welfare contexts. We were told:

> I think it [attachment theory] can be vague and I think it can be overused by people, or not always used appropriately. So I sometimes read reports or I hear professionals talking about bad attachment and good attachment, and I understand what they're talking about but I don't think it really explains anything.
>
> One of the reasons I don't like using that word [attachment] too much is because I think it's widely kind of used in, if not, it might be harsh to say it's misused but it's used in lots of different ways and so you can't really be confident that you're talking about the same thing when you talk to people.

In another study, led by Barry Coughlan, we asked practitioners from various clinical services (including child and adolescent mental health, neurodevelopmental teams, and primary care) to discuss cases they perceived as 'attachment-related' versus 'neurodevelopmental'. This was part of a broader study of how clinicians distinguish autism, ADHD, and attachment-related difficulties, drawing on interviews and examination of clinical records from children's mental health services. Regarding neurodevelopmental conditions, clinicians tended to lean on psychiatric nosology and standardised assessments to buttress their formulations. Yet these frames of reference did not seem available or desirable to clinicians when thinking about attachment-related cases. Instead, practitioners tended to place greater weight on unstructured observations and the non-standardised taking of a developmental history. In interview, few clinicians used standardised attachment assessments. In fact, references to attachment literature were relatively sparse in the interviews, though several clinicians described keeping attachment 'in mind' alongside the array of other frameworks when making decisions about case conceptualisation and intervention planning. However, they tended to be vague about what behaviours would prompt them to think about attachment. Instead, attachment theory seemed to be drawn in when clinicians had other evidence of insufficient care or maltreatment, or where there was a discrete precipitating event such as a major separation. Most practitioners indicated a preference for the general phrase 'attachment difficulties' over the technical clinical term 'attachment disorder'. But practitioners did not seem confident in articulating the difference between these terms. Practitioners were also unsure what interventions or support should be offered for families where attachment was identified as a relevant issue.[44]

Finally, in a third study, led by Helen Beckwith, we used Q-methodology to examine the perspectives held about attachment concepts and research findings among two groups: (i) 30 child mental health clinicians and (ii) 30 established attachment researchers. A variety of other self-report data were also collected. We have been fascinated to see both the convergences and divergences in the perspectives of these groups. Clinicians and researchers alike saw value in attachment theory as a framework for facilitating personalised care for children and for making decisions about fostering and adoption placements. Further, all agreed that 'attachment theory could be used more precisely within mental health practice', and that attachment research and measures were largely inaccessible to clinicians. Both researchers and practitioners were mindful of the difficulty of maintaining the integrity of attachment concepts and methods when applying them to practice.[45] Interestingly, both researchers and clinicians were unsure whether callous and unemotional traits in children originate from their early attachment experiences, or what the role is of attention within attachment processes.

One line of difference was that attachment researchers held strongly that good quality care throughout childhood is a better predictor of future mental health than a child's early attachment pattern. Clinicians were unsure. Researchers also felt that the most effective interventions to improve child–caregiver attachment are those that target security, presumably following the meta-analysis from Bakermans-Kranenburg and colleagues (Chapter 4). By contrast, clinicians appeared not to regard this as a practicable area of focus, and held that they could achieve improvements in child–caregiver attachment through other means. We were also interested that clinicians endorsed strongly the idea that early attachment experiences determine how the brain develops, whereas the research community offered neither agreement nor disagreement, presumably waiting on further evidence. This may reflect the role of allodoxia, perhaps intersecting with the wider discourse that if something influences the brain then it is more real.[46]

Clinicians were enthusiastic about the relevance of attachment language to helping them make sense of cases, especially in understanding dyadic processes. However, they were less

[44] See also Alexander, S.L., Frederico, M., & Long, M. (2018) Attachment and children with disabilities: knowledge and views of early intervention professionals. *Children Australia*, 43(4), 245–54; Morison, A., Taylor, E., & Gervais, M. (2019) How a sample of residential childcare staff conceptualize and use attachment theory in practice. *Child & Youth Services*, 1(25).

[45] See also Oppenheim, D. & Goldsmith, D.F. (2007) Attachment theory in clinical work with children: bridging the gap between research and practice. *Journal of Canadian Academic Child and Adolescent Psychiatry*, 16(4), 186–7.

[46] See also Wastell, D. & White, S. (2017) *Blinded by Science: The Social Implications of Epigenetics and Neuroscience*. Cambridge: Policy Press.

positive about the relevance of existing attachment assessments. Researchers held that at root, attachment is a dyadic and relational phenomenon, for all that it can stabilise with development. Clinicians agreed in principle that attachment is dyadic in nature, but regarded this as rather immaterial in clinical services structured by individual diagnoses and labels. Though these are just indications of some initial findings, already they suggest some provisional conclusions. They indicate that researchers and practitioners have many important points of convergence; that divergences in perspective often express the specific and different demands of the research and clinical contexts; and that there is appetite from both sides to improve the precision with which attachment theory is used in clinical practice with children. One line of future collaborative work may be efforts to validate the use of attachment assessments in applied contexts, to see if they can demonstrate benefits compared to assessment as usual. Another may be efforts to make the findings of attachment research more readily available to practitioners and publics.

The exhaustion of attachment research?

As we saw in the above section, White and colleagues advocate for a better understanding of attachment research among practitioners, to help counteract the dangers of the distorted and deadened version currently in circulation, and especially the dependence on assumptions from Bowlby's early writings. Yet, in their book, they offer little discussion of changes in attachment research over time or diversity among attachment researchers.[47] Relevant to their concerns are discussions that have been taking place among attachment researchers themselves about what within attachment research remains lively and what is fading from view. These discussions have a long history, even if they have become especially salient in the past few years.

In the late 1980s, van IJzendoorn sought to characterise the contemporary state of attachment research in terms from the philosophy of science. He drew distinctions between research paradigms as characterised, by degrees, in terms of 'formation', 'construction', 'saturation', and 'exhaustion'.[48] In 'formation', research is starting up, exploring the possibility of a programme of work. In the 'construction' stage, research is focused on the verification of bold hypotheses, and social communication in a growing community is facilitated by papers and symposia. There is a dancing, exhilarating sense of excitement and discovery to the work, alongside endless hard work. In 'saturation', research is focused on developing consistencies and responding to inconsistencies in the theory, journals are established to formalise the field, and ideas from research get applied in practice in ways that do not feed back into further scientific developments. In this stage, the big discoveries seem to have been made, and empirical work becomes increasingly about filling in gaps and qualifying effect sizes.

---

[47] White and colleagues do praise the work of Fonagy and colleagues for advocating a shift 'away from instinct and into interaction, and the social and psychological circumstances in which the mother and infant may find themselves'. White, S., Gibson, M., Wastell, D., & Walsh, P. (2019) *Reassessing Attachment Theory in Child Welfare*. Bristol: Psychology Press. However, the characterisation of attachment research as focused on instincts is half a century out of date (Chapter 1). And Fonagy gives no more attention to interaction and social and psychological circumstances than many attachment researchers.

[48] Van IJzendoorn, M.H. & Tavecchio, L.W.C. (1987) The development of attachment theory as a Lakatosian research program. In L.W.C. Tavecchio & van IJzendoorn, M.H. (eds) *Attachment in Social Networks: Contributions to the Bowlby–Ainsworth Attachment Theory* (pp.3–31). New York: Elsevier Science, Table 1.

In 'exhaustion', a research paradigm becomes primarily concerned with defending established orthodoxies, and communication becomes rigidified in handbooks and training institutes. Alternative perspectives gain ground in achieving funding, recruiting new researchers, and securing institutional recognition. Van IJzendoorn characterised Bowlby's development of attachment theory as the 'formation' stage for the paradigm and Ainsworth's introduction of the Strange Situation procedure as the 'construction' stage, which lay the basis for a cumulative empirical research programme in which new findings continually inform the development of theory.[49] However, looking about in the late 1980s, van IJzendoorn also identified symptoms of the saturation stage. There was a sense that the major discoveries had been made, and evidence that applications of attachment theory in psychotherapy, parent education, and policy were not feeding back into the priorities of research practice.

It is interesting to reflect today on van IJzendoorn's characterisation of the field of attachment research in the 1980s. There seem to be aspects of the research paradigm that resemble construction and saturation—and exhaustion. Since van IJzendoorn's analysis, attachment research has seen major developments, not least the extension of the paradigm to study attachment phenomena in adulthood. Today, some developments are still in the stage of 'construction'. For instance, research on the relationship between individual differences in attachment and sexuality remains an area in which early hypotheses are still being validated (Chapters 3 and 5). By contrast, some developments seem to have achieved saturation. For instance, the relationship between caregiver sensitivity and infant attachment is now well established, and current discussions have been mostly concerned with qualifying effect-sizes and communicating with practitioners. However, there remains lively interest in other factors contributing to intergenerational attachment processes.[50] And the proposal by Woodhouse, Cassidy, and colleagues (Chapter 2) to refine sensitivity to secure base provision may also reignite discussions in this area.

Over recent years, a few commentators have characterised attachment research as reaching exhaustion. Unquestionably, criticisms of the paradigm and of individual attachment researchers have gained ground in academic circles. Harkness has observed that 'earlier critics of attachment theory have recently been joined by others; if not exactly a chorus of critics, there are now enough to form the basis for an organized, multi-referenced, and multi-faceted counter-offensive'.[51] While popular and clinical interest in attachment remains high, it has become increasingly difficult to get funding for attachment research. Discussing the UK context, Fonagy recalls that 'attachment theory had ten good years in the research community from about 1985–1995. We had excellent research grants from the Wellcome, the Economic Social Research Council and the European Union; we were invited speakers at British Psychological Society congresses, the British Association and all that. Attachment theory is still good, but research interest has moved to neuroscience.'[52]

[49] Ibid. p.16.

[50] E.g. Bailey, H.N., Tarabulsy, G.M., Moran, G., Pederson, D.R., & Bento, S. (2017) New insight on intergenerational attachment from a relationship-based analysis. *Development & Psychopathology*, 29(2), 433–48.

[51] Harkness, S. (2015) The strange situation of attachment research: a review of three books. *Reviews in Anthropology*, 44(3), 178–97, p.179.

[52] White, K. & Schwartz, J. (2007) Attachment here and now: an interview with Peter Fonagy. *Attachment*, 1(1), 57–61, p.57. Thompson likewise has marked the standing of attachment research in this period, commenting in 2000 that attachment has been 'the dominant approach to understanding early socioemotional and personality development during the past quarter-century of research'. Thompson, R.A. (2000) The legacy of early attachments. *Child Development*, 71(1), 145–52, p.145.

In a watershed development in 2016, the National Institute of Mental Health in the USA removed the Ainsworth Strange Situation from its list of recommended procedures for publicly funded mental health research, citing the debt of attachment theory to psychoanalysis and its tendency to 'reify ... theoretical claims' as essential problems with the paradigm.[53] The framing of this decision was striking: in contrast to other judgements in the document, the exclusion of the Strange Situation was made without any justification in terms of any of the scientific criteria identified by the National Institute of Mental Health as relevant to recommendations, such as psychometric properties, longitudinal stability, standardised administration, and cultural specificity. Instead, it was simply asserted that the Strange Situation was an invalid measure. And a letter of query led by Lyons-Ruth was ignored by the National Institute of Mental Health.[54] From the information available, it would appear that the Strange Situation has been rejected for public funding on the basis of the disfavour of attachment research among psychological researchers, rather than on the grounds the National Institute of Mental Health itself had established as criteria. Though raked by the claws of this development, attachment research in the USA has continued. The central preoccupations of contemporary developmental science—brains, genes, big samples, and clinical application—are all viable for attachment research.[55] However, work in the USA using the Strange Situation has had to stow aboard grant applications that justify themselves in other terms. Whilst the situation is less severe in other countries, the National Institute of Mental Health announcement illustrates the challenge of credibility felt by attachment research more broadly.

Fonagy and Campbell have offered the view that, essentially, the party is over for developmental attachment research pursued in the manner of the second-generation researchers such as Main and Sroufe.[56] Above all, Fonagy and Campbell claim that even if the research paradigm was built upon the categories from the Strange Situation, it is now coming to grief upon them. They regard categories as an outdated way of representing human differences. This presentation of this criticism seems to reflect both the psychometric criticisms discussed in Chapter 4 and wider contemporary discourses that treat categories for human beings as a set of oppressive and misleading expectations, inappropriate for societies characterised

[53] National Institute of Mental Health (2016) Behavioral assessment methods for RDoC constructs. https://www.nimh.nih.gov/about/advisory-boards-and-groups/namhc/reports/behavioral-assessment-methods-for-rdoc-constructs.shtml.

[54] Lyons-Ruth, K., Belsky, J., Booth-LaForce, C., et al. (2016) Letter to Joshua Gordon—Director of NIMH and Sarah Morris—Acting Director of the RDoC Unit, responding to the behavioral assessment methods for RDoC constructs. Unpublished letter shared by Karlen Lyons-Ruth.

[55] The work of Cicchetti, Rogosch, Toth, and colleagues (Chapter 4) provides one illustration. The work of van IJzendoorn, Bakermans-Kranenburg, and colleagues offers another. See Kok, R., Thijssen, S., Bakermans-Kranenburg, M.J., et al. (2015) Normal variation in early parental sensitivity predicts child structural brain development. *Journal of the American Academy of Child & Adolescent Psychiatry*, 54(10), 824–31; Bakermans-Kranenburg, M.J. & van IJzendoorn, M.H. (2015) The hidden efficacy of interventions: gene × environment experiments from a differential susceptibility perspective. *Annual Review of Psychology*, 66, 381–409.

[56] Fonagy, P. & Campbell, C. (2015) Bad blood revisited: attachment and psychoanalysis, 2015. *British Journal of Psychotherapy*, 31(2), 229–50. This paper represents thinking with a wider group of colleagues also reported in Fonagy, P., Luyten, P., Allison, E., & Campbell, C. (2017) What we have changed our minds about: Part 2. Borderline personality disorder, epistemic trust and the developmental significance of social communication. *Borderline Personality Disorder and Emotion Dysregulation*, 4(1), 9. In the USA, there have likewise been claims that the field of attachment research is moving from saturation to exhaustion. Waters and colleagues have reported a growing perception of attachment research among some American colleagues that 'There is some great work there. But it is a mature field now and I think all the big studies have been done'. Waters, E., Petters, D., & Facompre, D. (2013) Epilogue: reflections on a special issue of attachment & human development in Mary Ainsworth's 100th year. *Attachment & Human Development*, 15(5–6), 673–81.

by fluidity and precarity.[57] Fonagy and Campbell also argue that whilst correlations between caregiving, attachment, and mental health have been in the expected direction across
thousands of studies, the associations have been less strong than Bowlby appeared to predict. Furthermore, the sciences on which attachment theory was erected have moved on.[58]
Fonagy and Campbell acknowledge that attachment research has brought valuable attention to the question of the evolutionary function of mental health and illness. However, they
feel that since Main's concept of conditional strategies, the dialogue between attachment research and evolutionary biology has generally petrified (though Belsky and Crittenden are
cited favourably as exceptions).[59] Fonagy and Campbell argue that developments in evolutionary biology in thinking about cultural or gene–culture co-evolution models seem to
have passed by attachment research, which is looking rather old-fashioned.[60]

Ultimately, Fonagy and Campbell predict not a replacement of the developmental tradition of attachment research, but its supersession by an approach that incorporates its
strengths.[61] In the process, they anticipate that familiar aspects of attachment research,
above all the labour-intensive Strange Situation and its lumbering categories, will—and
should—be put aside.[62] One tradition that may fill part of the remaining space is the social
psychological approach. However, given that this approach remains without an adequately
elaborated account of trauma, its clinical relevance remains limited. Fonagy and Campbell
instead recommend their own assessments of mentalising. Mentalising is the capacity to imagine, perceive, and interpret human behaviour in terms of intentional mental states (e.g.
needs, desires, feelings, beliefs, goals, and reasons).[63] Fonagy and Campbell regard deficits
in mentalising as associated with attachment-related processes since they are predisposed by
problems within early family relationships. But they argue that it is mentalising and the capacity to learn from interactions with others rather than attachment that is important for the
development of adult mental health and caregiving behaviour.

Fonagy and Campbell's intent in their paper is clearly in part advocacy of their own theory
and measures. The attendant predictions of the demise of attachment research also have

[57] See e.g. Bauman, Z. (2000) *Liquid Modernity*. Cambridge: Polity Press; Weeks, J. (2015) Beyond the categories. *Archives of Sexual Behavior*, 44(5), 1091–7.
[58] See also Fonagy, P. & Target, M. (2007) The rooting of the mind in the body: new links between attachment theory and psychoanalytic thought. *Journal of the American Psychoanalytic Association*, 55(2), 411–56: 'Advances in the sciences to which Bowlby's ideas are coupled dictate a reconsideration' (420).
[59] Fonagy, P. (2016) The role of attachment, epistemic trust and resilience in personality disorder: a trans-theoretical reformulation. *DMM News*, 26. http://www.iasa-dmm.org/images/uploads/DMM%20%2322%20 Sept%2016%20English.pdf.
[60] An exception is Simpson, J.A. & Belsky, J. (2016) Attachment theory within a modern evolutionary frame-work. In J. Cassidy & P.R. Shaver (2018) *Handbook of Attachment: Theory, Research, and Clinical Applications*, 3rd edn (pp.91–116). New York: Guilford. However, Simpson and Belsky themselves readily acknowledge that attach-ment research has been slow to absorb developments in modern evolutionary theory. This issue is also discussed in Granqvist, P. (2020) Attachment, culture, and gene-culture co-evolution: expanding the evolutionary toolbox. *Attachment & Human Development*, 2 January, 1–24.
[61] Fonagy, P. & Campbell, C. (2015) Bad blood revisited: attachment and psychoanalysis, 2015. *British Journal of Psychotherapy*, 31(2), 229–50, p.230.
[62] See also Fonagy, P. (1999) Points of contact and divergence between psychoanalytic and attachment the-ories: is psychoanalytic theory truly different. *Psychoanalytic Inquiry*, 19(4), 448–80: 'Attachment theory, far closer to empirical psychology with its positivist heritage, has been in some ways method-bound over the past 15 years. Its scope was determined less by what fell within the domain defined by relationship phenomena involving a caretaking-dependent dyad and more by the range of groups and behaviors to which the preferred mode of ob-servation, the strange situation, the adult attachment interview, and so forth, could be productively applied. This sheltered the theory from a range of ideas' (472).
[63] Fonagy, P., Gergely, G., & Target, M. (2007) The parent–infant dyad and the construction of the subjective self. *Journal of Child Psychology and Psychiatry*, 48(3–4), 288–328, p.288.

something of the air of a challenge, more than simply a statement of beliefs about the future. Some similar points about the limitations of attachment research have been made by Pehr Granqvist, who sees them as areas for renewal and revision of the paradigm, rather than as evidence of exhaustion.[64] Though not explicitly mentioned by Fonagy and Campbell or by Granqvist, a factor in the wider context of their appraisal of the state of attachment as a paradigm is the retirement of the second generation of attachment researchers. The infrastructure built by this generation has been inherited in recent years by a new generation of research leaders.[65] Some examples, among many, in the developmental tradition include Sheri Madigan, Pasco Fearon, Carlo Schuengel, Chantal Cyr, and Glenn Roisman; in the social psychological tradition Chris Fraley, Omri Gillath, and Gurit Birnbaum. Granqvist pursues work in both developmental and social psychology, making use of each set of attachment measures. Patrick Luyten and others represent a younger cohort of researchers on mentalisation who likewise draw from both traditions.

If a new generation of attachment researchers can be identified, this is not defined by their chronological age. Nor, besides Roisman's work at times,[66] is there a sense of insurrection against an older generation. Rather the point is that a bundle of problems that could previously be ignored or postponed are coming due, at a point where long-time research leaders have retired, and the field is seeing a changing of the guard. As such, a third generation of attachment researchers have been constituted by the playing out of problems in theory and method at a time when a generation of researchers who had direct contact with Ainsworth are putting down their tools. This third generation has also been shaped by active efforts to guide its development: in the developmental tradition, many of the third generation have received mentorship from van IJzendoorn, who has encouraged cross-group, international collaboration in meta-analytic research and the adoption of new methodologies from medicine and biostatistics.[67] Shaver and Mikulincer have likewise played a concerted role in mentoring a younger generation of rather ingenious and highly skilled social psychologists.

The first question the new generation of laboratory heads face is what must be preserved, altered, or rejected from the legacy of their teachers in responding to the field's challenges and opportunities. This is the challenge pointed to by Fonagy and Campbell's predictions of the supersession of attachment theory and methods. Inheritance is never a given; it is always

---

[64] Granqvist, P. (2020) *Attachment, Religion, and Spirituality: A Wider View.* New York: Guilford. Granqvist admits that, compared to the past, 'I am less optimistic about the prospect of attachment theory … This is because of attachment theory's conceptual boundaries, its rudimentary defense mechanisms, and the attachment research habit of "cross-tabulating" people into types (secure versus insecure and organized versus disorganized), despite no individual being reducible to a type. Although these features have indisputably contributed to attachment theory's prosperity as an empirical research program, the attachment framework remains somewhat schematic and impoverished.' Unlike Fonagy and colleagues, Granqvist is firmly of the view, however, that these matters can be resolved through innovations within attachment theory and research, and especially from renewed cross-fertilisation with developments in evolutionary theory.

[65] On the concept of infrastructures see Star, S.L. (1999) The ethnography of infrastructure. *American Behavioral Scientist*, 43, 377–91; Berlant, L. (2016) The commons: infrastructures for troubling times. *Environment and Planning D: Society and Space*, 34(3), 393–419.

[66] E.g. Haltigan, J.D. & Roisman, G.I. (2015) Infant attachment insecurity and dissociative symptomatology: findings from the NICHD Study of Early Child Care and Youth Development. *Infant Mental Health Journal*, 36(1), 30–41.

[67] Van IJzendoorn is perhaps best regarded as generation 2.5. He learnt the Strange Situation from Brian Vaughn and Mary Main and first met Ainsworth only at an AAI training with Main in the late 1980s. As well as his tendency to be an early adopter of new technologies and quantitative methodologies, some 'third-generation' characteristics to van IJzendoorn's work may stem from the closeness of his collaboration with his former students Marian Bakermans-Kranenburg and Femmie Juffer. He has also mentored and in turn learnt from collaborations with Madigan and Fearon.

a task of filtering and sorting, of deciding between alternative pasts and the different futures they might make possible. Inheriting effectively is hard and takes courage. In a sense, the third generation of leaders of attachment research need to figure out together what genre of story they are in. Is it a swashbuckler? Fonagy and Campbell seem willing to battle on deck. Is it a dystopian story of complicity with oppressive state power, as critics such as White and colleagues suggest? Is it a mystery, with new questions, methods, or interdisciplinary collaborations drawing the paradigm back towards the stages of construction and formation?

Will the story be an elegy, in which the present is oriented only towards the achievements of the past? It looks not. So far, the early chapters are of a coming-of-age story. Ainsworth's immediate students remained loyal to the four-category system. Yet as we saw in Chapter 4, renegotiation of this position seems to have a symbolic role, as a banner marking the presence of some new leaders, who now hold the datasets and the research agenda.[68] There are other changes too, coincident with the retirement of the second generation of attachment researchers. One is particular attention to moderators of stability or intergenerational transmission, including predictable forms of movement or cross-transmission between patterns of attachment. The third generation also seems more able to cross-pollinate methods and ideas between the developmental and social psychology traditions of attachment research. In particular, the psychometric rigour and priorities of the social psychological tradition have been adopted by younger researchers in the developmental tradition. However, there have also been a variety of other migrations. One of special interest is that the model of minimising and maximising strategies as elaborated by Shaver and Mikulincer has frequently been re-imported back into developmental psychology—though, at least to date, the wider behavioural systems theory of Shaver and Mukulincer, and their measures of minimising and maximising strategies in the domains of sexuality, caregiving, and dominance, have not been taken up by developmentalists.

In an attempt at stock-taking the current state of attachment research on children, Schuengel and colleagues reported from a bibliometric study. The results suggest that the past few years represent a period of transition. For instance, citations of *Patterns of Attachment* have been in decline since 2015, whereas citations of meta-analyses have gone from strength to strength.[69] Among meta-analytic research on child attachment Schuengel found a comparative decline in focus on the concerns of Ainsworth and Main. He found a comparative increasing focus on mental health symptoms and supportive interventions with families, a growing concern with fathers, and rising attention to anxiety and avoidance conceptualised as the latent dimensions of individual differences in attachment.

Even if there are definitely some pulls towards 'exhaustion' of the developmental tradition, Schuengel's findings indicate that, in general, attachment research is changing, not fading. There are significant strengths that mark its ongoing vitality. Three developments can be used as illustrations, though by no means are intended as exhaustive. These developments are: Individual Participant Data meta-analysis; security priming; and intervention research.

[68] See e.g. Raby, L., Verhage, M.L., Fearon, R.P.M., et al. (2019) The latent structure of the Adult Attachment Interview: large sample evidence from the Collaboration on Attachment Transmission Synthesis. Paper presented at Biennial Meeting of the Society for Research in Child Development, Baltimore, 21–23 March. On the symbolic work demanded in the constitution of a generation see Eyerman, R. & Turner, B.S. (1998) Outline of a theory of generations. *European Journal of Social Theory*, 1, 91–106; Purhonen, S. (2016) Generations on paper: Bourdieu and the critique of 'generationalism'. *Social Science Information*, 55(1), 94–114.

[69] Schuengel, C., Verhage, M., & Duschinsky, R. (2019) Representing attachment through meta-analyses: a move to the level of collaboration, manuscript under review. https://psyarxiv.com/anf6t/.

Many other lively areas of research have been discussed in previous chapters. Two of particular note are the growth of attention to secure base scripts and observations of secure base/safe haven provision—with a cadre of talented younger researchers currently pursuing a programme of work very much in the 'construction' stage (Chapter 2). Other lively areas of research build from later research groups, to be considered in a later volume, and so would not make sense to discuss here. This includes extensive research using biomedical measures, in acknowledgement of the embodied aspects and underpinnings of attachment relationships. This was touched on in Chapter 4, discussing the work of Dante Cicchetti. In making a selection, Individual Participant Data meta-analysis, security priming, and intervention research have been chosen as illustrations because they capitalise precisely on the maturity of the field's theory and methods discussed in this book, whilst also reflecting the changing priorities and methodological infrastructure of attachment research as an area of science inquiry.

Individual Participant Data meta-analysis

A first area of particular vitality in contemporary attachment research has made use precisely of the advantages of 'saturation'. Over the decades, attachment research on young children has used the labour-intensive Strange Situation or measures adapted from it like the MacArthur preschool system[70] or the Preschool Assessment of Attachment.[71] This has permitted the accumulation of thousands of relatively small-scale studies that provide little pieces of the puzzle. Each on its own is unable to offer confident guidance for interventions with families, justify commissioning decisions, or inform policy to protect and support young children. Attachment researchers, particularly van IJzendoorn and colleagues, were early adopters of meta-analysis as a methodology for studying the overall effect sizes identified by these numerous small studies and for examining factors accounting for variance in effect sizes between studies.[72] There were also attempts to pool data from different studies more directly in order to increase statistical power and explore potential moderating factors.[73] This offered a richer array of variables and greater depth than reliance on the published record as in traditional meta-analysis. Data pooling permits investigations that are wider than single studies and deeper than traditional meta-analyses. However, data pooling efforts in attachment research foundered in the 1990s, in part because the statistical techniques for multilevel modelling were not available to developmental psychologists. Instead, the use of traditional meta-analyses flourished.[74]

---

[70] Cassidy, J. & Marvin, R., with the MacArthur Network on Attachment in the Preschool Years (1992) Attachment organisation in pre-school children: procedures and coding manual. Unpublished manuscript.

[71] Crittenden, P.M. (1981) *The Pre-School Assessment of Attachment Coding Manual*. Miami: Family Relations Institute.

[72] Van IJzendoorn, M.H., Goldberg, S., Kroonenberg, P.M., & Frenkel, O.J. (1992) The relative effects of maternal and child problems on the quality of attachment: a meta-analysis of attachment in clinical samples. *Child Development*, 63(4), 840–58. See also van IJzendoorn, M.H., Bakermans-Kranenburg, M.J., & Alink, L.R.A. (2011) Meta-analysis in developmental science. In B. Laursen, T.D. Little, & N.A. Card (eds) *Handbook of Developmental Research Methods* (pp.667–86). New York: Guilford.

[73] Lamb, M.E., Sternberg, K.J., & Prodromidis, M. (1992) Nonmaternal care and the security of infant mother attachment: a reanalysis of the data. *Infant Behavior & Development*, 15(1), 71–83.

[74] Another factor may have been that attitudes among researchers were not yet favourable to data sharing—a situation that has, by degrees, shifted in recent years. Tenopir, C., Dalton, E.D., Allard, S., et al. (2015) Changes in data sharing and data reuse practices and perceptions among scientists worldwide. *PLoS One*, 10(8), e0134826.

One recent such meta-analysis was completed by Verhage and the Collaboration on Attachment Transmission Synthesis in 2016.[75] The researchers examined the association between AAI for parents and Strange Situation classifications for dyads from 95 samples, with 4,819 participants in total. They found that the association between secure-autonomous state of mind on the AAI and secure attachment in the Strange Situation was $r = .31$ and for unresolved state of mind to disorganised infant attachment $r = .21$. This was very substantially down from the meta-analysis conducted by van IJzendoorn in 1995 ($r = .47$ and $r = .31$, respectively).[76] Caregivers with dismissing states of mind were more likely to have avoidant attachment relationships and less likely to have secure attachment relationships, but they were no less likely than other caregivers to be part of dyads receiving an ambivalent/resistant classification. Similarly, preoccupied states of mind were associated with more ambivalent/resistant and fewer secure, but not with fewer avoidant attachment relationships. This suggests that classical and widely repeated assumptions since Main and colleagues regarding the mechanisms that lead to avoidant and resistant attachment might need additional thought, and especially the underarticulated concept of 'inconsistent care' inherited from Ainsworth. Such a conclusion aligns with proposals by diverse researchers, proposing ways that dismissing states of mind may also contribute to resistance, and preoccupied states of mind to avoidant attachment relationships.[77]

Another curious finding was that speakers with unresolved/disorganised states of mind regarding attachment were less likely to have secure and avoidant attachment relationships with their infant, but the dyads were no less likely to receive an ambivalent/resistant classification. Verhage and colleagues observed that this finding has pertinence to debates about how hard or how fluid the distinction is between resistance and disorganised attachment (Chapter 4). Around 25% of the relationship between AAI and Strange Situation classifications could be accounted for on the basis of assessments of caregiver sensitivity; after correction for test–retest reliability, this left a little under half of variance explained by sensitivity.[78] Examining moderators, Verhage and colleagues reported that the association between the AAI and the Strange Situation was stronger in low-risk samples and weaker in at-risk samples. At first sight, the decline in the association since van IJzendoorn's meta-analysis in 1995 could be thought to reflect the fact that early samples were generally with low-risk samples and subsequent samples have more frequently been with high-risk samples. However, Verhage and colleagues found that, in fact, risk status did not account for the effect of publication year on the reported effect size.

[75] Verhage, M., Schuengel, C., Madigan, S., et al. (2016) Narrowing the transmission gap. *Psychological Bulletin*, 142(4), 337–66.

[76] Van IJzendoorn, M.H. (1995) Adult attachment representations, parental responsiveness, and infant attachment—a meta-analysis on the predictive validity of the Adult Attachment Interview. *Psychological Bulletin*, 117(3), 387–403.

[77] Crittenden, P.M., Partridge, M.F., & Claussen, A.H. (1991) Family patterns of relationship in normative and dysfunctional families. *Development & Psychopathology*, 3(4), 491–512; Shah, P.E., Fonagy, P., & Stratearn, L. (2010) Is attachment transmitted across generations? The plot thickens. *Clinical Child Psychology and Psychiatry*, 15(3), 329–45; Kondo-Ikemura, K., Behrens, K., Umemura, T., & Nakano, S. (2018) Japanese mothers' prebirth Adult Attachment Interview predicts their infants' response to the Strange Situation procedure. *Developmental Psychology*, 54(11), 2007–2015.

[78] See also Bernier, A., Matte-Gagné, C., Bélanger, M.-È., & Whipple, N. (2014) Taking stock of two decades of attachment transmission gap: broadening the assessment of maternal behavior. *Child Development*, 85(5), 1852–65; van IJzendoorn, M.H. & Bakermans-Kranenburg, M.J. (2019) Bridges across the intergenerational transmission of attachment gap. *Current Opinion in Psychology*, 25, 31–6.

Subsequently, the Collaboration on Attachment Transmission Synthesis has pursued Individual Participant Data meta-analysis, in which data are pooled from studies using the same measures. The Collaboration on Attachment Transmission Synthesis received data from 58 research laboratories from around the world that had used the Strange Situation and the AAI (4,396 parent–child dyads); 67% of eligible studies contributed their data. The first analyses from this collaboration are just appearing, and already are offering important qualifications to existing theory and new insights, for instance for understanding how poverty and social adversity impact parenting. Adding to their previous traditional meta-analysis, Verhage and colleagues found that risk factors lowered the likelihood of a secure child–caregiver attachment if the caregiver has a secure-autonomous state of mind regarding attachment. The finding suggests that secure-autonomous states of mind do not offer as much resilience as previously expected by attachment researchers against contextual risks.[79] However, low education and single parenthood had no effect on the strength of the association between the AAI and the Strange Situation. Neither did the gender of the caregiver. In a further study, Verhage found that contextual risk factors weaken the association between caregiver sensitivity and attachment, again illustrating the importance of the challenges faced by families in the development of attachment relationships.[80]

Another study by the Collaboration on Attachment Transmission Synthesis was led by Lee Raby and sought to examine the psychometric structure of the AAI. As we have seen, Main, Goldwyn, and Hesse initially offered a four-category model (Chapter 3). However, Roisman, Fraley, and colleagues have subsequently proposed instead a two-dimensional model modelled on the ECR, with avoidance and anxiety as latent dimensions (Chapter 4). Raby and colleagues found that the distribution of the data-points suggested that individual differences in attachment states of mind reflect differences in degree, not kind. However, the findings were not clear regarding what dimensions should be used. A two-factor model based on dismissing and preoccupation was found to be an adequate fit. But a three-factor model based on dismissing, preoccupation, and lack of resolution was also found to be an adequate fit. Raby and colleagues argued in favour of the two-factor model on the basis of parsimony.[81] However, they did not examine which model might best serve to predict variables of interest such as Strange Situation classifications or other indices of child mental health. It is likely that predictive validity will be a key criterion for any potential overhaul of the dominant approach to reporting results from attachment research.

Over the coming years, it is possible that the social psychological tradition will adopt Individual Participant Data meta-analysis as a methodology. Pooled data would permit exploration of some of the issues faced by this tradition, such as the status of security and the implications of trauma. Individual Participant Data meta-analysis, much like the present book, is oriented by a sense that the past can open anew in response to curation and the questions of the present. It may be that many social psychology laboratories will have thrown

[79] Verhage, M.L., Fearon, R.P., Schuengel, C., et al. (2018) Examining ecological constraints on the intergenerational transmission of attachment via Individual Participant Data meta-analysis. *Child Development*, 89(6), 2023–37.

[80] Verhage, M.L., Fearon, R.P., Schuengel, C., et al. (2019) Does risk background affect intergenerational transmission of attachment? Testing a moderated mediation model with IPD. Paper presented at Biennial Meeting of the Society for Research in Child Development, Baltimore.

[81] Raby, L., Verhage, M.L., Fearon, R.P.M., et al. (2019) The latent structure of the Adult Attachment Interview: large sample evidence from the Collaboration on Attachment Transmission Synthesis. Paper presented at Biennial Meeting of the Society for Research in Child Development, Baltimore, 21–23 March.

away their scale scores. That has certainly been the case for some research groups in the developmental attachment tradition: a third of eligible laboratories did not contribute data to the Collaboration on Attachment Transmission Synthesis. But enough may have been preserved to make application of Individual Participant Data meta-analysis a feasible and fruitful possibility for the social psychological tradition and for answering other questions in the developmental tradition. Work is currently underway, for example, to assemble an Individual Participant Dataset for randomised control trials of attachment-based interventions. The ambition is to ask questions with greater power and precision than have been possible before, about what works for whom, and how, in supportive interventions with families.[82]

Security priming

A second area in which attachment research seems to be thriving and breaking new ground is in studies of priming and attachment-relevant states—as opposed to longer-term attachment patterns or styles. The concept of 'attachment states' originated in the developmental tradition of attachment research, introduced by Fonagy, Steele, and Steele in 1991. Fonagy and colleagues argued that Bowlby's 'internal working model' construct may well not be a unitary whole. Instead it likely encompasses some components that are relatively unresponsive to environmental cues and other components that are relatively responsive to specific cues.[83] This distinction was accepted by other researchers in the developmental tradition of attachment research.[84] However, as discussed in Chapter 2, researchers in the developmental tradition have tended often, in practice if not in theory, to treat attachment as a trait. In line with this, state attachment fluctuations have not been much studied in childhood by developmentalists, since attachment has generally been treated as relatively stable.[85]

The differentiation between global adult attachment style and more particular states was developed strongly by the social psychology tradition, especially by Mark Baldwin.[86] An important early study was reported by Baldwin and colleagues in 1996. Participants were asked to characterise their most significant relationships and then to indicate which attachment style best captured their feelings about each relationship. Baldwin and colleagues found that most participants reported having experienced secure, avoidant, and anxious experiences

[82] Schuengel, C., Verhage, M., & Duschinsky, R. (2019) Representing attachment through meta-analyses: a move to the level of collaboration. Manuscript under review. https://psyarxiv.com/anf6t/.

[83] Fonagy, P., Steele, H., & Steele, M. (1991) Maternal representations of attachment during pregnancy predict the organization of infant–mother attachment at one year of age. *Child Development*, 62(5), 891–905, p.902.

[84] E.g. Thompson, R.A. & Raikes, H.A. (2003) Toward the next quarter-century: conceptual and methodological challenges for attachment theory. *Development & Psychopathology*, 15, 691–718.

[85] Attention to state attachment variation in childhood has been a concern of Guy Bosmans, whose work has increasingly spanned the divide between developmental and social traditions of attachment research, e.g. Bosmans, G., Van de Walle, M., Goossens, L., & Ceulemans, E. (2014) (In)variability of attachment in middle childhood: secure base script evidence in diary data. *Behavior Change*, 31, 225–42; Vandevivere, E., Bosmans, G., Roels, S., Dujardin, A., & Braet, C. (2018) State trust in middle childhood: an experimental manipulation of maternal support. *Journal of Child and Family Studies*, 27(4), 1252–63.

[86] E.g. Baldwin, M.W., Carrell, S.E., & Lopez, D.F. (1990) Priming relationship schemas: my advisor and the Pope are watching me from the back of my mind. *Journal of Experimental Social Psychology*, 26(5), 435–54. Attachment styles have been conceptualised by researchers in the social psychological tradition as having trait-like and state-like qualities, e.g. Fraley, R.C. & Roberts, B.W. (2005) Patterns of continuity: a dynamic model for conceptualizing the stability of individual differences in psychological constructs across the life course. *Psychological Review*, 112(1), 60–74.

across their relationships. Despite this diversity, participants reported more relationships that fitted with their global attachment style. Baldwin and colleagues also found that this global attachment style was influential for shaping self-report of dating preferences. Priming secure, avoidant, and anxious experiences did not influence self-report global attachment style. But the researchers did find that priming altered reported dating preferences among their participants, for instance with a prime for avoidance decreasing the attractiveness of a partner offering an intimate and committed relationship.[87]

The findings suggested to Baldwin and colleagues that a person's global attachment style is generally more accessible for informing semantic appraisals. However, other information about attachment experiences, which could inform alternative attachment styles, is potentially available in the hierarchical network, and specific cues in the environment may influence this availability. The qualities of an avoidant relationship, for example, may make available insecure generalised schemas even for someone with a secure attachment style. Following up on the work of Baldwin and colleagues, Mikulincer and Arad published a vignette-based study in 1999 of the effects of attachment style and security priming on accessibility for participants of incongruent information about their partner.[88] They found that a secure attachment style was associated with greater openness to and better recall of incongruent information when it suggested that their partner was caring and available. And asking participants to think about a time when others were available to them for support and comfort—a security prime—made an independent additional contribution to openness to and recall of incongruent positive information. Attachment style did not moderate the effect of the prime. Mikulincer and Arad concluded that a security prime led to behaviour that resembled a secure attachment style by activating relevant parts of the hierarchical network of associations. However, curiously, this activation of the 'attachment state' appeared to operate through an independent process to the role of global attachment style in influencing behaviour, as there was no interaction between attachment style and the security prime in predicting behaviour.[89]

Over the subsequent decades, Mikulincer, Shaver, and colleagues in the social psychology tradition have regularly found that similar effects can be obtained on the basis of a secure attachment style or on the basis of a prime for security.[90] Furthermore, they have demonstrated that the effect of the secure base prime cannot be accounted for in terms of variations in mood or self-esteem.[91] Part of what has been electrifying about the new line of research

[87] Baldwin, M.W., Keelan, J.P.R., Fehr, B., Enns, V., & Koh-Rangarajoo, E. (1996) Social-cognitive conceptualization of attachment working models: availability and accessibility effects. *Journal of Personality and Social Psychology*, 71(1), 94–109.

[88] Mikulincer, M. & Arad, D. (1999) Attachment working models and cognitive openness in close relationships: a test of chronic and temporary accessibility effects. *Journal of Personality and Social Psychology*, 77, 710–25.

[89] In a recent study, Hudson and Fraley reported intriguing findings that repeatedly priming attachment anxiety over time contributed to *reduced* anxiety on the ECR over time, no less than repeated priming attachment security. The researchers concluded that repeated priming of attachment anxiety or attachment security offered participants the opportunity to reflect on their overall network of associations, contributing to change in the global attachment style. Hudson, N.W. & Fraley, R.C. (2018) Moving toward greater security: the effects of repeatedly priming attachment security and anxiety. *Journal of Research in Personality*, 74, 147–57.

[90] Mikulincer, M., Gillath, O., Halevy, V., Avihou, N., Avidan, S., & Eshkoli, N. (2001) Attachment theory and reactions to others' needs: evidence that activation of the sense of attachment security promotes empathic responses. *Journal of Personality and Social Psychology*, 81(6), 1205–224; Mikulincer, M., Shaver, P.R., Gillath, O., & Nitzberg, R.A. (2005) Attachment, caregiving, and altruism: boosting attachment security increases compassion and helping. *Journal of Personality and Social Psychology*, 89(5), 817–39.

[91] Gillath, O., Hart, J., Noftle, E.E., & Stockdale, G.D. (2009) Development and validation of a state adult attachment measure (SAAM). *Journal of Research in Personality*, 43(3), 362–73; Gillath, O. & Karantzas, G. (2019) Attachment security priming: a systematic review. *Current Opinion in Psychology*, 25, 86–95.

on priming has been that, in many domains, a prime seems able to produce prosocial effects for all participants that would otherwise only be limited to those with a secure attachment style. For instance, Mikulincer and Shaver found that a secure attachment style and a security prime contributed to greater tolerance towards out-groups.[92] Mikulincer, Shaver, Gillath, and Nitzberg reported that secure attachment style and a security prime contributed to greater willingness to help someone in need.[93] And Shaver, Mikulincer, Lavy, and Cassidy found that a secure attachment style and a subliminal security prime could contribute to less defensive and more constructive responses to feeling hurt by a romantic partner.[94]

However, some research has documented an interaction between attachment style and a security prime. One suggestive finding reported by Mikulincer, Hirschberger, Nachmias, and Gillath was that attachment insecurity can moderate the effect of a security prime on positive mood. If a security prime is followed by visualisation of an experience of separation from attachment figures, only participants with a secure attachment style reported an increase in positive mood from the security prime. The effect disappeared for participants with an avoidant or anxious attachment style.[95] Another relevant finding by Mikulincer, Shaver, Sahdra, and Bar-On was that a secure base prime could overcome mental depletion, allowing a participant to remain responsive to their romantic partner during a laboratory-based task.[96] The prime also removed the negative effect of an avoidant attachment style on the extent of help offered. By contrast, there was no interaction between attachment style and the security prime in intention to help strangers.

Mikulincer and colleagues speculated that with any longstanding romantic partner there will be a rich network of associations, more so than for a stranger. The secure base prime prior to the couple interaction may have activated the 'reservoir of positive feelings and memories' within the hierarchical network of associations, knocking out the minimising strategy that might otherwise be enacted.[97] Later research demonstrated, however, that this effect was specific to help with practical rather than emotional tasks. Mikulincer, Shaver, and colleagues observed participants responding to their romantic partner in two conditions: discussing a distressing problem and exploring personal goals. An avoidant attachment style was generally associated with lower supportiveness in both conditions. A security prime eradicated this effect in relation to the partner's exploration of personal goals. However, the security prime had no effect on the condition where the partner was discussing a personal problem and needed emotional support.[98]

[92] Mikulincer, M. & Shaver, P.R. (2001) Attachment theory and intergroup bias: evidence that priming the secure base schema attenuates negative reactions to out-groups. *Journal of Personality and Social Psychology*, 81(1), 97–115.

[93] Mikulincer, M., Shaver, P.R., Gillath, O., & Nitzberg, R.A. (2005) Attachment, caregiving, and altruism: boosting attachment security increases compassion and helping. *Journal of Personality and Social Psychology*, 89(5), 817–39.

[94] Shaver, P.R., Mikulincer, M., Lavy, S., & Cassidy, J. (2009) Understanding and altering hurt feelings: an attachment-theoretical perspective on the generation and regulation of emotions. In A.L. Vangelisti (ed.) *Feeling Hurt in Close Relationships* (pp.92–119). Cambridge: Cambridge University Press.

[95] Mikulincer, M., Hirschberger, G., Nachmias, O., & Gillath, O. (2001) The affective component of the secure base schema. *Journal of Personality and Social Psychology*, 81(2), 305–321, Study 7.

[96] Mikulincer, M., Shaver, P.R., Sahdra, B.K., & Bar-On, N. (2013) Can security-enhancing interventions overcome psychological barriers to responsiveness in couple relationships? *Attachment & Human Development*, 15(3), 246–60.

[97] Ibid. p.257.

[98] Mikulincer, M., Shaver, P.R., Bar-On, N., & Sahdra, B.K. (2014) Security enhancement, self-esteem threat, and mental depletion affect provision of a safe haven and secure base to a romantic partner. *Journal of Social and Personal Relationships*, 31(5), 630–50.

Yet perhaps the most curious set of interactions between attachment style and priming have been in relation to anxious attachment. Though, in general, security primes tend to foster comfort, happiness, and more positivelyregarded behaviour, the interaction between security priming and an anxious attachment style in several cases has had the opposite effect. For example, Taubman-Ben-Ari and Mikulincer examined the effect of attachment style and security priming on driving using a simulator. They found that an anxious attachment style was associated with higher willingness to drive recklessly. Furthermore, whereas for other participants a security prime reduced reckless driving, among participants with an anxious attachment style the security prime increased recklessness.[99] The researchers wondered whether the security prime was being interpreted by their participants as signalling the availability of a secure base, contributing to overconfidence, without the feeling of being cherished that would otherwise reduce willingness to endanger oneself. Mikulincer and colleagues suspected that rumination may be another factor involved in the paradoxical effects of security priming on participants with an anxious attachment style. The security prime may cause participants to think about the unavailability of their attachment figures. Support for this conclusion came from a study by Mikulincer, Shaver, and Rom.[100] The researchers found that an explicit security prime (recalling experiences of being cared about), but not a subliminal presentation of the names of attachment figures, was associated with less creativity and effectiveness in solving laboratory-based tasks for participants with an anxious attachment style. It was concluded that an explicit security prime provides a prompt for rumination, in contrast to a subliminal prime.

In opening priming effects as a domain of inquiry, the social psychology tradition has allowed the attachment paradigm as a whole to put out new branches. It has taken some time, but researchers in the developmental tradition have begun to explore priming techniques, such as in the collaboration between Bosmans, van IJzendoorn, and Bakermans-Kranenburg.[101] One obstacle is that the AAI is not especially well adapted for repeated administration to assess attachment states or validate the effects of a prime. But neither is the ECR. The State Adult Attachment Measure has been developed by Gillath and colleagues (Chapter 5) to circumvent this issue in the social psychological tradition. There is likewise no intrinsic obstacle to the use of priming for researchers in the developmental tradition. For instance, repeated observation of caregiver–child interaction in free-play situations (not the Strange Situation) could be pursued by developmental researchers to examine the effects of a prime. The recent development of briefer assessments for the study of caregiver–child interaction, such as the brief Attachment Q-Sort or the AMBIANCE-Brief, may facilitate this by reducing the labour required to code observational data.[102] There remain some concerns about research on attachment priming, since, in general, studies of priming in social

[99] Taubman-Ben-Ari, O. & Mikulincer, M. (2007) The effects of dispositional attachment orientations and contextual priming of attachment security on reckless driving. *Transportation Research Part F*, 10, 123–38.

[100] Mikulincer, M., Shaver, P.R., & Rom, E. (2011) The effects of implicit and explicit security priming on creative problem solving. *Cognition and Emotion*, 25(3), 519–31.

[101] E.g. Verhees, M.W., Ceulemans, E., Bakermans-Kranenburg, M.J., van IJzendoorn, M.H., De Winter, S., & Bosmans, G. (2017) The effects of cognitive bias modification training and oxytocin administration on trust in maternal support: study protocol for a randomized controlled trial. *Trials*, 18(1), 326. Granqvist has made extensive use of priming in his research, though in studies using measures from the social psychological tradition, and not in his research using measures from the developmental tradition.

[102] E.g. Haltigan, J.D., Madigan, S., Bronfman, E., et al. (2019) Refining the assessment of disrupted maternal communication: using item response models to identify central indicators of disrupted behavior. *Development & Psychopathology*, 31(1), 261–77; Cadman, T., Belsky, J., & Fearon, R.M.P. (2018) The Brief Attachment Scale (BAS-16): a short measure of infant attachment. *Child: Care, Health and Development*, 44(5), 766–75.

psychology have an uneven record of replication.[103] Nevertheless, so far, results regarding attachment priming specifically have been encouraging.

Intervention research

A third development has been the growing prominence of intervention research both for the sake of clinical relevance and in order to articulate potential causal mechanisms. Description of a variety of attachment-based interventions for families with children of different ages is offered in the recent *Handbook of Attachment-Based Interventions*, edited by Howard and Miriam Steele.[104] A concern with interventions among attachment researchers is, of course, far from new. Attachment theory was initially developed in a clinical context by Bowlby, and many of Ainsworth's graduate students pursued training as clinicians. The development of supportive interventions with parents based directly on attachment principles and evaluated using the Strange Situation began in the 1980s. The first such interventions were STEEP and, though perhaps more grounded in psychoanalytic than attachment principles, Lieberman's child–parent psychotherapy (Chapter 4). The Circle of Security intervention, discussed in previous chapters, emerged out of a determinate attempt to translate the central principles of Ainsworth's concept of sensitivity into a supportive intervention with families.

Over time, the evidence base has grown for interventions designed with attachment principles in mind and evaluated with attachment measures. A systematic review of this literature by Mohamed and colleagues identified 32 empirical studies of attachment-based interventions. The most frequent elements of the interventions were psychoeducation, increasing parents' awareness of the functioning of the attachment system, and supporting the parent relationship. Other elements, more specific to some interventions, included the intervener 'subtitling' the child's behaviours by indicating what the behaviours seem to be saying, video-feedback, and supporting the development of caregiver insight into their own behaviour.[105] Among this growing literature, two attachment-based interventions for families with young children have generated both considerable research evidence and clinical interest: Video-feedback Intervention to promote Positive Parenting (VIPP) and the Attachment and Biobehavioural Catchup (ABC). Both have had significant, and growing, penetration into child health and welfare services.

Video-feedback Intervention to promote Positive Parenting

VIPP was developed by Femmie Juffer, Marian Bakermans-Kranenburg, and Marinus van IJzendoorn. It was first used in a randomised control trial in a sample of 130 families with infants who had been internationally adopted in their first weeks of life. When the children were 9–12 months, home visits were undertaken, during which sessions of video-feedback were used to support parenting sensitivity. Whereas video-based instruction to parents had

[103] Locke, E.A. (2015) Theory building, replication, and behavioral priming: where do we need to go from here? *Perspectives on Psychological Science*, 10(3), 408–414.

[104] Steele, H. & Steele, M. (eds) (2018) *Handbook of Attachment-Based Interventions*. New York: Guilford.

[105] Mohamed, A.R, Sterkenburg, P., van Rensburg, E., & Schuengel, C. (2019) The development of a coding system to examine the effective elements of attachment-based interventions. Paper presented at International Attachment Conference, Vancouver, 19 July 2019.

proven ineffective or even counterproductive,[106] it was anticipated that drawing on 10- to 30-minute clips of the parent's own behaviour with the child in ordinary situations would be more relatable and empowering.

In the intervention, the intervener discusses these film clips with the caregiver, helping the caregiver to consider the baby's signals, their meaning, and how the baby responds to the caregiver's behaviours, especially when these show sensitivity. In a strategy inherited from STEEP, as well as Fraiberg's approach to therapeutic work,[107] the intervener interprets the baby's behaviours as if giving them subtitles, translating the infant signals into a verbal form that the caregiver may find easier to reflect upon and consider. Positive film fragments are emphasised; the intervention builds precisely on parents' own expertise, with caregivers serving as a reinforcing role model for themselves.[108] An illustration is offered by Juffer and Bakermans-Kranenburg from a detailed case study:

> Using the recordings, she pointed out how happy and proud Ava reacted to Noah's compli-ments and how they were peacefully playing together afterward. The intervener explained that research has shown that it works much better to praise your child and give compli-ments when she does things well than to punish her when things go wrong. Sometimes it is even better to ignore naughty or difficult behavior because that way your child is not receiving attention for that type of behavior. The intervener summarized this message by saying: 'Because you are so important for Ava, she really loves to have your attention and compliments, and that is why it works so well to praise Ava when you want her to listen to you or be compliant.'[109]

Juffer, Bakermans-Kranenburg, and van IJzendoorn anticipated that, compared to STEEP, a shorter intervention focused on specific behaviours would prove more manageable for par-ents and more targeted to supporting change in attachment-relevant processes.[110] VIPP is conventionally six to eight sessions, which makes it short enough even for use in assessing caregiving capacity, as well as directly for parenting support.[111] The first session of VIPP focuses on exploration and attachment behaviour; the second session helps the caregiver consider the meaning of the infant's signals; the third session addresses the role of prompt and adequate response to these signals; and the fourth session emphasises shared emotions and affective attunement with the child. Two additional sessions are often used to review

[106] Lambermon, M.W. & van IJzendoorn, M.H. (1989) Influencing mother–infant interaction through video-taped or written instruction: evaluation of a parent education program. *Early Childhood Research Quarterly*, 4(4), 449–58.

[107] Carter, S.L., Osofsky, J.D., & Hann, D.M. (1991) Speaking for the baby: a therapeutic intervention with ado-lescent mothers and their infants. *Infant Mental Health Journal*, 12(4), 291–301.

[108] Juffer, F. & Steele, M. (2014) What words cannot say: the telling story of video in attachment-based interven-tions. *Attachment & Human Development*, 16(4), 307–314, p.311.

[109] Juffer, F. & Bakermans-Kranenburg, M.J. (2018) Working with Video-feedback Intervention to pro-mote Positive Parenting and Sensitive Discipline (VIPP-SD): a case study. *Journal of Clinical Psychology*, 74(8), 1346–57, p.7.

[110] Van IJzendoorn, M.H., Juffer, F., & Duyvesteyn, M.G. (1995) Breaking the intergenerational cycle of insecure attachment: a review of the effects of attachment-based interventions on maternal sensitivity and infant security. *Journal of Child Psychology and Psychiatry*, 36(2), 225–48; Bakermans-Kranenburg, M.J., van IJzendoorn, M.H., & Juffer, F. (2003) Less is more: meta-analyses of sensitivity and attachment interventions in early childhood. *Psychological Bulletin*, 129(2), 195–215.

[111] Bakermans-Kranenburg, M.J., Juffer, F., & van IJzendoorn, M.H. (2019) Reflections on the mirror: on video-feedback to promote positive parenting and infant mental health. In C. Zeanah (ed.) *Handbook of Infant Mental Health*, 4th edn (pp.527–42). New York: Guilford.

the information and feedback from the first four.[112] Issues around sensitive discipline of the child are also addressed, helping the caregiver provide non-coercive discipline and positive reinforcement, to de-escalate tantrums, and achieve empathy and consistent limit-setting for the child.

In a first evaluation of VIPP with 130 families, the researchers found that compared to the control group receiving treatment as usual, the intervention enhanced sensitivity as measured by Ainsworth's scale. The dyads were also less likely to receive a disorganised attachment classification on the basis of the child's behaviour in the Strange Situation procedure.[113] In a later trial with 237 families with toddlers with externalising behaviour problems, the mothers who completed VIPP showed more sensitive discipline, and their children showed fewer conduct problems at a later follow-up.[114] A process evaluation revealed that neither mothers nor home visitors were able to anticipate the relative effectiveness of the intervention based on their first impressions of one another.[115] Whereas advocates for STEEP had argued that behavioural-focused targeted interventions would be less effective in families facing multiple adversities and daily hassles (Chapter 4), in fact VIPP was found to be more effective in such circumstances.[116] A meta-analysis of the first twelve randomised control trials of VIPP found an effect size of $d = .47$ for sensitivity, $d = .36$ for infant–caregiver attachment classifications, and $d = .26$ for reduced child behaviour problems, with no decrease in effect size resulting from length of follow-up.[117] Across multiple samples, VIPP has been found to decrease disorganised attachment as assessed in the Strange Situation. However, why this is

[112] Juffer, F., Bakermans-Kranenburg, M.J., & van IJzendoorn, M.H. (eds) (2008) *Promoting Positive Parenting: An Attachment-Based Intervention*. New York: Psychology Press.

[113] Juffer, F., Bakermans-Kranenburg, M.J., & van IJzendoorn, M.H. (2005) The importance of parenting in the development of disorganized attachment: evidence from a preventive intervention study in adoptive families. *Journal of Child Psychology and Psychiatry*, 46(3), 263–74.

[114] Klein Velderman, M., Bakermans-Kranenburg, M.J., Juffer, F., Van Ijzendoorn, M.H., Mangelsdorf, S.C., & Zevalkink, J. (2006) Preventing preschool externalizing behavior problems through video-feedback intervention in infancy. *Infant Mental Health Journal*, 27(5), 466–93. However, both maternal discipline practices and child behavioural problems seem to have been independently affected by the intervention. Analysis did not suggest effects of maternal discipline on child behaviour. See Mesman, J., Stoel, R., Bakermans-Kranenburg, M.J., et al. (2009) Predicting growth curves of early childhood externalizing problems: differential susceptibility of children with difficult temperament. *Journal of Abnormal Child Psychology*, 37(5), 625–36, p.633.

[115] Stolk, M.N., Mesman, J., van Zeijl, J., et al. (2008) Early parenting intervention aimed at maternal sensitivity and discipline: a process evaluation. *Journal of Community Psychology*, 36(6), 780–97.

[116] Van Zeijl, J., Mesman, J., Van IJzendoorn, M.H., et al. (2006) Attachment-based intervention for enhancing sensitive discipline in mothers of 1 to 3 year-old children at risk for externalizing behavior problems: a randomized controlled trial. *Journal of Consulting and Clinical Psychology*, 74(6), 994–1005. Subsequent research has complicated this picture: Euser, S., Alink, L.R., Stoltenborgh, M., Bakermans-Kranenburg, M.J., & van IJzendoorn, M.H. (2015) A gloomy picture: a meta-analysis of randomized controlled trials reveals disappointing effectiveness of programs aiming at preventing child maltreatment. *BMC Public Health*, 15(1), 1068. 'The "less is more" effect in attachment-based interventions found by Bakermans-Kranenburg and colleagues seems only partly applicable to programs aimed at reducing or preventing child maltreatment. We found a curvilinear association with program duration and number of program sessions. Programs with a moderate duration (6–12 months) or a moderate number of sessions (16–30) yielded significantly higher effect sizes compared to shorter or longer programs and programs with fewer or more sessions' (11). Additionally, initial research suggests that parent learning disabilities and child physical disabilities may moderate the capacity of VIPP to increase caregiver sensitivity or sensitive discipline, though other benefits were identified from the intervention. Platje, E., Sterkenburg, P., Overbeek, M., Kef, S., & Schuengel, C. (2018) The efficacy of VIPP-V parenting training for parents of young children with a visual or visual-and-intellectual disability: a randomized controlled trial. *Attachment & Human Development*, 20(5), 455–72; Hodes, M.W., Meppelder, M., de Moor, M., Kef, S., & Schuengel, C. (2018) Effects of video-feedback intervention on harmonious parent–child interaction and sensitive discipline of parents with intellectual disabilities: a randomized controlled trial. *Child: Care, Health and Development*, 44(2), 304–311.

[117] Bakermans-Kranenburg, M.J., Juffer, F., & Van IJzendoorn, M.H. (2019) Reflections on the mirror: on video-feedback to promote positive parenting and infant mental health. In C. Zeanah (ed.) *Handbook of Infant Mental Health*, 4th edn (pp.527–42). New York: Guilford.

the case remains an outstanding question. VIPP focuses on increasing caregiver sensitivity, and caregiver sensitivity has only a very weak association with disorganised attachment.

One proposal put forward by Out, Bakermans-Kranenburg, and van IJzendoorn, building on Main and Hesse's thinking, is that the intervention directs the caregiver's attention to the child, which reduces absorption and the intrusion of unresolved memories and affects.[118] This proposal remains to be tested. However, some supportive evidence is available: an intervention focused on supporting caregiver attention to the child's experience—Minding the Baby—reduced rates of disorganised attachment without impacting PTSD symptoms.[119] Such findings suggest that the behavioural and attentional focus on the here-and-now of the child supported by VIPP may reduce disorganised attachment because it helps caregivers avoid absorption or mental states that may prompt the intrusion of segregated systems. An alternative explanation, implied by the researchers working on Minding the Baby, is that Bakermans-Kranenburg and colleagues have underestimated the capacity of parenting interventions to reduce disorganised attachment by increasing the caregiver's reflective functioning about attachment relationships.[120]

Attachment Biobehavioral Catch-up

Another widely studied attachment-based parenting intervention is Attachment Biobehavioral Catch-up (ABC), developed by Dozier and colleagues. ABC is a ten-session, in-home intervention to help families meet the needs of infants and toddlers.[121] Holding the intervention in the home is anticipated to help the integration of learning into daily life, and to allow others in the home to see and gain benefits from the intervention. Part of what is intriguing about ABC is its parsimony. The focus of the intervention is extremely strict: the comments made by the coaches only seek to help parents achieve three things: (i) to be nurturing when the child is distressed; (ii) to follow the child's lead, where possible taking cues from the child rather than dictating activities to them; and (iii) to avoid displaying intrusive, harsh, or frightening behaviours.[122] Dozier and colleagues take these to be respectively the central proposals of Bowlby, Ainsworth, and Main and Hesse. Bowlby emphasised the importance of a child's confidence in their caregiver when distressed, which Dozier and colleagues regard as facilitated by nurturing behaviour and tone. Ainsworth emphasised heeding and responding to the child's signals, which she described as sensitivity; she

[118] Out, D., Bakermans-Kranenburg, M.J., & van IJzendoorn, M.H. (2009) The role of disconnected and extremely insensitive parenting in the development of disorganized attachment: validation of a new measure. *Attachment & Human Development*, 11(5), 419–43, p.438.

[119] Slade, A., Holland, M.L., Ordway, M.R., et al. (2019) Minding the Baby*: enhancing parental reflective functioning and infant attachment in an attachment-based, interdisciplinary home visiting program. *Development & Psychopathology*, 32(1), 123–37.

[120] See also Tereno, S., Madigan, S., Lyons-Ruth, K., et al. (2017) Assessing a change mechanism in a randomized home-visiting trial: reducing disrupted maternal communication decreases infant disorganization. *Development & Psychopathology*, 29(2), 637–49.

[121] Dozier, M. & Bernard, K. (2017) Attachment and Biobehavioral Catch-up: addressing the needs of infants and toddlers exposed to inadequate or problematic caregiving. *Current Opinion in Psychology*, 15, 111–17.

[122] Dozier, M. & Infant Caregiver Project (2016) *Attachment and Biobehavioral Catch-up for Infants Who Have Experienced Early Adversity (ABC-1). Intervention Manual.* Unpublished manuscript; Dozier, M. & Bernard, K. (2019) *Coaching Parents of Vulnerable Infants: The Attachment and Biobehavioral Catch-up Approach.* New York: Guilford. For the adaptation of ABC for toddlers the focus on avoidance of intrusive, harsh, or frightening behaviours is partially supplanted by, partly incorporated within, a focus on encouraging parents to collaborate with their children in regulating difficult emotions.

anticipated that this would contribute to a child's capacity for self-regulation.[123] And Main and Hesse argued that alarming caregiver behaviour disrupts the capacity of the child to co-ordinate attention and behaviour in making coherent use of the caregiver, either directly or conditionally, as a secure base and safe haven.

As the first attachment-based intervention, STEEP had a broad set of goals and a broad rep-ertoire of intervention strategies, as the relationship between attachment theory and interven-tion science was just getting started (Chapter 4). By contrast, the focus of ABC on only three concerns represents a fierce, hard-earned, and specific theoretical security. One consequence is that training in delivering the intervention can be completed in two days. Another consequence is that the large majority of those interested to train as parent coaches can do so and gain certi-fication following a fidelity test: potential coaches are screened out only if they find it difficult to make in-the-moment comments to parents, or if they show a dismissing state of mind regarding attachment on a cut-down version of the AAI. Following Main's theory (Chapter 3), Dozier and colleagues assume that a dismissing state of mind is incompatible with cognitive openness and comfort with nurturance.[124]

The sessions of ABC have a few components. A component early in the intervention is psy-choeducation: parents are informed about some key findings from attachment research, such as Ainsworth's findings regarding the effects of prompt response to infant crying (Chapter 2). These findings are used as an opportunity for discussion of parents' expectations of themselves and their child, for instance beliefs about the potential for care to spoil an infant or for harsh care to help an infant by promoting toughness. Another component of ABC is the use of films of caregivers responding to infants in desirable and undesirable ways, which likewise serve as a basis of discussion with the parent. Parents are also asked to complete tasks with their child, such as playing with blocks or making pudding together. These are filmed, and clips may be brought by the caregiving coach to review with the parent in a subsequent session. During the intervention sessions, caregiving coaches provide frequent and specific comments to parents 'in the moment', around 60 times per hour. Dozier and colleagues have found that the frequency of coaches' comments, as well as their quality, could predict the magnitude of change in parent sensitivity.[125]

Comments address exclusively the three areas of focus of the intervention, drawing par-ents' attention to specific behaviours, their purpose, and what ensues from them. This in-tensity of focused commenting is one of the most distinctive aspects of ABC—especially when compared to more psychoanalytically inspired forms of parenting intervention, such as GABI (Chapter 4), where clinicians are advised to address a wider range of topics and practice reticence in making comments. Caron, Bernard, and Dozier have documented that 27% of caregivers leave ABC before the end of the intervention: families who dropped out tended to receive fewer comments in sessions and more comments on issues away from the

[123] Bernard, K., Meade, E.B., & Dozier, M. (2013) Parental synchrony and nurturance as targets in an attach-ment based intervention: building upon Mary Ainsworth's insights about mother–infant interaction. *Attachment & Human Development*, 15(5–6), 507–523. Another important influence for Dozier and colleagues was Raver, C.C. (1996) Relations between social contingency in mother–child interaction and 2-year-olds' social competence. *Developmental Psychology*, 32(5), 850–59.

[124] Caron, E.B., Roben, C.K., Yarger, H.A., & Dozier, M. (2018) Novel methods for screening: contributions from Attachment and Biobehavioral Catch-up. *Prevention Science*, 19(7), 894–903.

[125] Caron, E.B. Bernard, K., & Dozier, M. (2018) In vivo feedback predicts parent behavior change in the Attachment and Biobehavioral Catch-up intervention. *Journal of Clinical Child & Adolescent Psychology*, 47(1), 35–46.

three areas of focus of the intervention.[126] A related aspect of ABC is the meticulous use of video-based supervision to ensure the fidelity of coaches to the goals of the intervention, ensuring that coaches do not miss opportunities to offer relevant comments.[127] In the early sessions of ABC, comments focus on identifying positives in the parent's behaviour. As the sessions progress, the coach may identify areas in which the parent may improve on being nurturing, following the child's lead or avoiding intrusive, harsh, or frightening behaviours. Though the focus of ABC is on behaviour, in the later sessions the coach also works with the parent to recognise aspects of their past experience that may be proving an obstacle to providing sensitive and non-frightening care. These may not be the aspects of past experience that are most salient for the parent in their day-to-day life; the focus is rather on cognitive and procedural obstacles to the effective functioning of the caregiving behavioural system. At the end of the tenth session, the coach presents the parent with a montage of film clips from earlier sessions, celebrating occasions when their behaviour was nurturing or when they followed the child's lead.

Bernard, Dozier, and colleagues conducted a randomised control trial of ABC with parents identified as at risk for neglecting their young children. The children were assessed in the Strange Situation. Classifications of disorganised attachment were less frequent in the ABC group (32%) than in the control intervention (57%), and classifications of secure attachment were more frequent (52%) relative to the control (33%).[128] Mothers in the ABC group showed greater increases in sensitivity and decreases in intrusiveness than participants from the control intervention.[129] Mothers in the intervention group also showed higher secure base script knowledge (Chapter 2) than parents assigned to the control group.[130] In a recent study, Dozier's team have reported that, contrary to expectations, no improvements were seen in frightened, frightening, disoriented, or role-confused parenting behaviours.[131] However, base rates of the behaviours were low, given that the observations were exceptionally brief, which may have contributed to false negatives. Nonetheless, the researchers found that parents in the ABC intervention group were less likely to display withdrawing behaviour towards their child's attachment behaviours; this difference accounted for around 19% of the effect of ABC on the proportion of child–caregiver dyads receiving a disorganised attachment classification.

In a follow-up, children from the ABC intervention group showed less externalising behaviours than the control group in response to the frustrating problem-solving task developed for the Minnesota study (Chapter 4).[132] Such intervention effects have been replicated

[126] Ibid.

[127] Meade, E.B., Dozier, M., & Bernard, K. (2014) Using video feedback as a tool in training parent coaches: promising results from a single-subject design. *Attachment & Human Development*, 16(4), 356–70.

[128] Bernard, K., Dozier, M., Bick, J., Lewis-Morrarty, E., Lindhiem, O., & Carlson, E. (2012) Enhancing attachment organization among maltreated children: results of a randomized clinical trial. *Child Development*, 83, 623–36.

[129] Yarger, H.A., Hoye, J.R., & Dozier, M. (2016) Trajectories of change in Attachment and Biobehavioral Catch-up among high-risk mothers: a randomized clinical trial. *Infant Mental Health Journal*, 37(5), 525–36. An important finding has been that the effects of ABC on caregiver sensitivity appear to be just as strong when implemented by welfare organisations as when applied as part of a randomised clinical trial. This is quite unusual. Effect sizes generally drop when interventions are disseminated in the community. Dozier, M. & Bernard, K. (2019) *Coaching Parents of Vulnerable Infants: The Attachment and Biobehavioral Catch-up Approach*. New York: Guilford, p.177.

[130] Ibid. p.143.

[131] Yarger, H.A. (2018) Investigating longitudinal pathways to dysregulation: The role of anomalous parenting behaviour. Unpublished doctoral dissertation, University of Delaware.

[132] Lind, T., Bernard, K., Ross, E., & Dozier, M. (2014) Intervention effects on negative affect of CPS-referred children: results of a randomized clinical trial. *Child Abuse & Neglect*, 38(9), 1459–67. See also Lind, T., Raby, K.L.,

at multiple sites, with diverse population groups.[133] A large-scale implementation of ABC by the State of New York has recently reported successful impacts on caregiver sensitivity and reduced frightening behaviours.[134] Further trials are underway in Australia, Germany, South Africa, and Russia. There is emergent endocrinal, physiological, and neurological evidence that converges with behavioural findings to suggest that the ABC group display greater skills at emotion regulation in the face of challenges, even several years after the intervention.[135] Dozier and colleagues regard ABC as a targeted intervention for parenting, ideally to be delivered in the community alongside other targeted support for families depending on their needs, whether caregiver depression, substance use, housing, or other difficulties. It remains to be adequately explored, however, whether contextual factors moderate the success of the ABC intervention. One finding recently reported by Berlin was that the impact of ABC on caregiving behaviour is moderated by self-reported attachment style. The intervention was more successful for participants self-reporting a less avoidant attachment style, but actually reduced caregiver sensitivity among participants endorsing an avoidant attachment style. Berlin and colleagues suggest that 'it may be that more avoidant mothers experienced the intervention model's emphasis on nurturance, along with the parent coaches' frequent comments, as dissonant or even aversive, which, in turn, led to iatrogenic effects'.[136]

There remains further work to be done to maximise the benefits of attachment-based interventions. Attachment-based interventions are seeing increasing take-up by child welfare and clinical services. However, there remains much we do not yet know about their cost-effectiveness and, perhaps more to the point, their capacity to survive in cash-strapped and continually restructuring services. Further research is also needed to understand how attachment-based interventions can best be delivered with different families and communities, with sensitivity to signals regarding their needs and to the ways of working they find acceptable and satisfying.[137] Attachment-based interventions offer a fruitful possible point

Caron, E.B., Roben, C.K., & Dozier, M. (2017) Enhancing executive functioning among toddlers in foster care with an attachment-based intervention. *Development & Psychopathology*, 29(2), 575–86.

[133] Grube, W. & Liming, K. (2018) Attachment and biobehavioral catchup: a systematic review. *Infant Mental Health Journal*, 39(6), 656–73.

[134] Chapin Hall at the University of Chicago (2019) Strong families New York City. Final evaluation report, June 2019. https://www1.nyc.gov/assets/acs/pdf/initiatives/2019/CHFinalReport.pdf.

[135] Bernard, K., Hostinar, C.E., & Dozier, M. (2015) Intervention effects on diurnal cortisol rhythms of child protective services-referred infants in early childhood: preschool follow-up results of a randomized clinical trial. *JAMA Pediatrics*, 169(2), 112–19; Tabachnick, A.R., Raby, K.L., Goldstein, A., Zajac, L., & Dozier, M. (2019) Effects of an attachment-based intervention in infancy on children's autonomic regulation during middle childhood. *Biological Psychology*, 143, 22–31; Dozier, M. & Bernard, K. (2019) *Coaching Parents of Vulnerable Infants: The Attachment and Biobehavioral Catch-up Approach*. New York: Guilford.

[136] Such findings also stand in thought-provoking contrast to a trial of the Circle of Security intervention, which led to change in children's attachment classification only for mothers higher in attachment avoidance (Chapter 5). Berlin and colleagues speculate that Circle of Security is a gentler intervention than ABC, and so less likely to be aversive to caregivers with strong assumptions that devalue nurturance and emotional needs. Berlin, L.J., Martoccio, T.L., & Jones Harden, B. (2018) Improving early head start's impacts on parenting through attachment-based intervention: a randomized controlled trial. *Developmental Psychology*, 54(12), 2316–27. See also Cassibba and colleagues who found iatrogenic effects of discussions with caregivers about their attachment representations, if these began secure/autonomous. Cassibba, R., van IJzendoorn, M.H., Coppola, G., et al. (2008) Supporting families with preterm children and children suffering from dermatitis. In F. Juffer, M.J. Bakermans-Kranenburg, & M.H. van IJzendoorn (eds) *Promoting Positive Parenting: An Attachment-Based Intervention* (pp.91–110). New York: Psychology Press.

[137] For work to date see Klein Velderman, M., Juffer, F., Bakermans-Kranenburg, M.J., & van IJzendoorn, M.H. (2008) A case study and process evaluation of video feedback to promote positive parenting alone and with representational attachment discussions. In F. Juffer, M.J. Bakermans-Kranenburg, & M.H. van IJzendoorn (eds) *Promoting Positive Parenting: An Attachment-Based Intervention* (pp.23–36). New York: Lawrence Erlbaum; Hodes, M.W., Meppelder, H.M., Schuengel, C., & Kef, S. (2014) Tailoring a video-feedback intervention for sensitive

of connection between researchers and practitioners. They do so in the context of serious obstacles to mutually satisfying and informative communication. Nonetheless, they form one of several valuable bases for such a conversation, especially in the context of the turn to greater engagement and collaboration with practitioners among the third generation of attachment researchers. There is certainly a new wind blowing through attachment research at the moment, with the windows held wider than before to the field's different audiences. Given the mutual benefit of mutual learning between research and practice, it is heartening to see attachment researchers taking steps to facilitate this two-way dialogue.

Concluding remarks

The need for attachment research to be open to different audiences and to the future was a central theme in the keynote address to the International Attachment Conference in 2019 by Carlo Schuengel. In reflecting on the state of the field, Schuengel described a number of questions that colleagues in attachment research have been raising with one another. These include pinning down further: the origin of individual differences in child attachment, the meaning of attachment disorganisation, the attachment-specific elements of interventions and how they work, and the cognitive or symbolic aspects of attachment.[138] For instance, complacent and vague appeals to the internal working model concept need to be superseded by a more detailed account of the cognitive or symbolic components of attachment, their parameters and features, their interrelations, and links with perceptions and actuators.[139] Schuengel also urged further scrutiny of the developmental mechanisms studied by attachment research, the psychometric properties of its measures, the scalability of its interventions, and its broader relevance to child welfare and clinical practice.

Thompson, Simpson, and Berlin have likewise taken the opportunity of 50 years since the publication of *Attachment, Volume 1* to consider the fundamental outstanding questions for attachment research.[140] To Schuengel's list they have added several further questions. Among these, they feel that more work is needed to understand what kinds of relationships qualify as attachment relationships. They urge concern with how attachment processes are manifested in different cultures, and how culture manifests itself in attachment processes. They feel attachment research needs a better conceptual model of what domains of later behaviour early security of attachment should predict and what domains it would not be anticipated to predict. And they emphasise that there is much more to be done to understand how attachment theory and research might best inform services for children and families, including divorce and custody proceedings, home visiting, education, and foster care.

discipline to parents with intellectual disabilities: a process evaluation. *Attachment & Human Development*, 16(4), 387–401; Scourfield, J., Allely, C., Coffey, A., & Yates, P. (2016) Working with fathers of at-risk children: insights from a qualitative process evaluation of an intensive group-based intervention. *Children and Youth Services Review*, 69, 259–67.

[138] Schuengel, C. (2019) Representing attachment: the future is open. Paper presented at International Attachment Conference, Vancouver, 20 July 2019.

[139] Schuengel, C. & Tharner, A. (2020) Patterns of parenting: revisiting mechanistic models. *Attachment & Human Development*, 22. See also Petters, D.D. (2019) The attachment control system and computational modeling: origins and prospects. *Developmental Psychology*, 55(2), 227–39.

[140] Thompson, R.A., Simpson, J.A., & Berlin, L. (2020) Introduction: synthesizing the fundamental questions and issues in attachment theory. In R.A. Thompson, J.A. Simpson, & L. Berlin (eds) *Attachment: The Fundamental Questions*. New York: Guildford.

If such questions as those posed by Schuengel and by Thompson and colleagues form some of the present horizon of empirical attachment research, they do so knowingly on the basis, in part, of the work of research groups considered in this book. The critical historical consideration of these groups, with their different perspectives and ambitions, has aimed to put more firmly at the disposal of the present a portion of the resources of the past in their liveliness and diversity, and in their potential relevance for attachment research during and after this period of transition. If attachment research has faced pressures that contort and abbreviate its ideas in their circulation, it is hoped that a historical perspective has the potential to exert some contrary force, whilst at the same time offering observations relevant to the wider history of science. In this regard, *Cornerstones* has sought to add to existing historical studies, which to date have not considered developments after Ainsworth. Those interested to understand, use or change attachment research must walk with and negotiate with the past. In addition to Bowlby and Ainsworth, this entails the important legacy from a second generation of attachment researchers.

Index

For the benefit of digital users, indexed terms that span two pages (e.g., 52–53) may, on occasion, appear on only one of those pages.